Body MRI

Evan S. Siegelman, MD

Associate Professor of Radiology
Chief, MRI Section
Department of Radiology
Hospital of the University of Pennsylvania
Philadelphia, PA

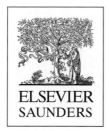

ELSEVIER
SAUNDERS

ELSEVIER
SAUNDERS

The Curtis Center
170 S Independence Mall W 300E
Philadelphia, Pennsylvania 19106

Body MRI   ISBN 0-7216-3740-X
Copyright © 2005, Elsevier Inc. All rights reserved.

No part of this publication may be reproduced or transmitted in any form or by any means, electronic or mechanical, including photocopying, recording, or any information storage and retrieval system, without permission in writing from the publisher.
Permissions may be sought directly from Elsevier's Health Sciences Rights Department in Philadelphia, PA, USA: phone: (+1) 215 238 7869, fax: (+1) 215 238 2239, e-mail: healthpermissions@elsevier.com. You may also complete your request on-line via the Elsevier homepage (http://www.elsevier.com), by selecting 'Customer Support' and then 'Obtaining Permissions.'

NOTICE

Radiology is an ever-changing field. Standard safety precautions must be followed, but as new research and clinical experience broaden our knowledge, changes in treatment and drug therapy may become necessary or appropriate. Readers are advised to check the most current product information provided by the manufacturer of each drug to be administered to verify the recommended dose, the method and duration of administration, and contraindications. It is the responsibility of the licensed health care provider, relying on experience and knowledge of the patient, to determine dosages and the best treatment for each individual patient. Neither the publisher nor the author assumes any liability for any injury and/or damage to persons or property arising from this publication.

Library of Congress Cataloging-in-Publication Data
Siegelman, Evan S.
    Body MRI / Evan S. Siegelman. — 1st ed.
        p. ; cm.
    Includes bibliographical references.
    ISBN 0-7216-3740-X
    1. Magnetic resonance imaging. 2. Body cavities–Imaging. I. Title.
    [DNLM: 1. Magnetic Resonance Imaging. WN 185 S571b 2005]
    RC78.7.N83S55 2005
    616.07'548—dc22
                                                        2004051092

Acquisitions Editor: Allan Ross
Project Manager: Mary Stermel

Printed in the United States of America

Last digit is the print number: 9 8 7 6 5 4 3 2 1

I dedicate this book to my father, Stanley S. Siegelman, MD, and to the memory of my mother, Doris F. Siegelman.

Contributors

Saroja Adusumilli, MD
*Assistant Professor of Radiology,
Department of Radiology, University of
Michigan Health System, Ann Arbor, MI*

Laura Carucci, MD
*Assistant Professor, Director of MR
Imaging, Director of Abdominal MR,
Department of Radiology, Virginia
Commonwealth University Medical Center,
Richmond, VA*

Adam Fisher, MD
*Staff Radiologist, Department of
Radiology, Crozer Chester Medical Center,
Upland, PA*

Anne M. Hubbard, MD
*Associate Professor of Radiology,
University of Pennsylvania Medical School;
Staff Radiologist, Department of
Radiology, Children's Hospital of
Philadelphia, Philadelphia, PA*

E. Scott Pretorius, MD
*Wallace T. Miller Sr. Chair of Radiologic
Education, Residency Program Training
Director, Department of Radiology,
Hospital of the University of Pennsylvania,
Philadelphia, PA*

David Roberts, MD, PhD
*Director of CT/MRI, Department of
Radiology, Kennedy Health System,
Voorhees, NJ*

Mark A. Rosen, MD, PhD
*Assistant Professor of Radiology,
Department of Radiology, Hospital of the
University of Pennsylvania,
Philadelphia, PA*

Evan S. Siegelman, MD
*Associate Professor of Radiology, Chief,
MRI Section, Department of Radiology,
Hospital of the University of Pennsylvania,
Philadelphia, PA*

Drew A. Torigian, MD, MA
*Assistant Professor of Radiology,
Department of Radiology, Hospital of the
University of Pennsylvania,
Philadelphia, PA*

Preface

MR is a powerful imaging tool in the evaluation of disease processes of the thorax, abdomen, and pelvis, but some radiologists are uncomfortable performing and interpreting body MR examinations. This book is an attempt to familiarize the target audience (radiology residents, fellows, and practicing radiologists trained before the maturation of body MR) with the MR findings of normal anatomy and common entities encountered in clinical practice. It is my hope that the reader will use this text to assist him or her in establishing specific MR tissue diagnoses (the "elusive tissue signature"[1]) and to accurately diagnose and stage neoplasms.

I have modeled the format of this textbook on the highly successful *Musculoskeletal MRI.*[2] Specific MR techniques and physical principles are addressed in individual chapters where appropriate. Some topics, such as MR techniques and physics, are not covered in this textbook. For those who desire supplementary material, dedicated textbooks and reviews are available.[3-5] Reviews of MR imaging of the small and large bowel are also available elsewhere.[6-8] MR techniques used to evaluate cardiac structure and function, myocardial viability and perfusion,[9-13] and the coronary arteries[14,15] are still evolving.[16] Those interested in additional reading can consult available texts[17,18] or a recent issue of the *MR Clinics of North America* devoted to this "hot topic."[19] Body applications of functional MR techniques have not been widely incorporated into clinical practice. I anticipate that we shall adopt functional techniques to evaluate tumor viability and to differentiate between reactive and malignant lymph nodes.[20,21]

I thank my friends-colleagues at the University of Pennsylvania Health System for their efforts in the preparation of this text. I would also like to acknowledge the patience and support of my wife, Debby Michelman, and our three sons, Daniel, Matthew, and Dylan.

Respectfully,

Evan S. Siegelman, MD

REFERENCES

1. Rogers LF. Imaging: a Sisyphean search for the elusive tissue signature. AJR Am J Roentgenol 2002;179(3):557.
2. Kaplan P, A., Helms CA, Dussault R, Anderson MW, Major NM, editors. Musculoskeletal MRI, 1st ed. Philadelphia, W. B. Saunders, 2001.
3. Horowitz AL. MR physics for radiologists: A visual approach. 3rd ed. New York, Springer, 1994.
4. Mitchell DG, Cohen. MS. MRI Principles. 2nd ed. Philadelphia, W. B. Saunders 2004.
5. Constable RT. MR physics of body MR imaging. Radiol Clin North Am 2003;41(1):1-15, v.
6. Lomas DJ. Techniques for magnetic resonance imaging of the bowel. Top Magn Reson Imaging 2002;13(6):379-387.
7. Umschaden HW, Gasser J. MR enteroclysis. Radiol Clin North Am 2003;41(2):231-248.
8. Lauenstein TC. Magnetic resonance imaging in bowel imaging. Top Magn Reson Imaging 2002;13(6):377.
9. Kim RJ, Wu E, Rafael A, Chen EL, Parker MA, Simonetti O, et al. The use of contrast-enhanced magnetic resonance imaging to identify reversible myocardial dysfunction. N Engl J Med 2000;343(20):1445-1453.
10. Earls JP, Ho VB, Foo TK, Castillo E, Flamm SD. Cardiac MRI: Recent progress and continued challenges. J Magn Reson Imaging 2002;16(2):111-127.
11. Duerinckx AJ. Myocardial viability using MR imaging: is it ready for clinical use? AJR Am J Roentgenol 2000;174(6):1741-1743.
12. Wagner A, Mahrholdt H, Holly TA, et al. Contrast-enhanced MRI and routine single photon emission computed tomography (SPECT) perfusion imaging for detection of subendocardial myocardial infarcts: an imaging study. Lancet 2003;361(9355):374-379.
13. Castillo E, Bluemke DA. Cardiac MR imaging. Radiol Clin North Am 2003;41(1):17-28.
14. Kim WY, Danias PG, Stuber M, Flamm SD, Plein S, Nagel E, et al. Coronary magnetic resonance angiography for the detection of coronary stenoses. N Engl J Med 2001;345(26):1863-1869.
15. Achenbach S, Daniel WG. Noninvasive coronary angiography—an acceptable alternative? N Engl J Med 2001;345(26):1909-1910.
16. Polak JF. MR coronary angiography: are we there yet? Radiology 2000;214(3):649-650.
17. Duerinckx AJ, editor. Coronary Magnetic Resonance Angiography. New York, Springer-Verlag, 2002.
18. Manning WJ, Pennell DJ. Cardiovascular Magnetic Resonance. Philadelphia, Churchill Livingstone, 2002.
19. Woodward P. Cardiac MR imaging. MR Clinics of North America 2003;11(1):1-191.
20. Choyke PL, Dwyer AJ, Knopp MV. Functional tumor imaging with dynamic contrast-enhanced magnetic resonance imaging. J Magn Reson Imaging 2003;17(5):509-520.
21. Koh DM, Cook GJ, Husband JE. New horizons in oncologic imaging. N Engl J Med 2003;348(25):2487-2488.

Contents

Protons dance and sing
Reveal our inner secrets
To the naked eye

Body MR Techniques and MR of the Liver

Adam Fisher, MD

Evan S. Siegelman, MD

Magnetic resonance (MR) imaging provides comprehensive evaluation of the liver including the parenchyma, biliary system, and vasculature. While computed tomography and sonography are often the initial studies used in evaluating the liver, MR is increasingly relied upon as a primary imaging modality in addition to its problem-solving capacity. MR provides soft tissue characterization unachievable with other imaging modalities. Lack of ionizing radiation and relative lack of operator dependence are additional advantages over computed tomography and ultrasound, respectively. Rapid breath-hold pulse sequences have largely supplanted older, slower pulse sequences, resulting in shortened examination times. After a brief review of current techniques, this chapter will focus on MR imaging manifestations of liver diseases, with an emphasis on pathologic correlation.

FIELD STRENGTH AND SURFACE COILS

Ideally, MR imaging of the liver is performed on high-field systems greater than 1.0 tesla (T), with open, low-field systems reserved for claustrophobic or obese patients. Phased-array surface coils provide improved signal-to-noise and contrast-to noise ratios, and better lesion detection and conspicuity in comparison with the conventional body coil surrounding the bore of the scanner.[1] Proximity of anterior abdominal wall subcutaneous fat to the surface coil can result in respiratory motion artifact "ghosts" projecting over the image. This artifact can be eliminated or minimized with breath-holding sequences or fat suppression.[1]

MR PULSE SEQUENCES

T1-Weighted Imaging (T1-WI)

The liver has a T1-relaxation time shorter than that of other abdominal tissues except for fat and pancreas. This short T1-relaxation time of liver has been attributed to abundant rough endoplasmic reticulum and high rate of protein synthetic activity (Box 1-1).[2] Hepatic lesions that are isointense or hyperintense to liver parenchyma on T1-weighted images (T1-WIs)

1-1 Causes of High Signal Intensity (SI) on Unenhanced T1-WI

- Protein (common; cause of normal high SI of hepatocytes)
- Lipid (common)
- Hemorrhage
- Paramagnetic substances (e.g., melanin, gadolinium)
- Blood flow

1-3 Signal Loss in Liver on Chemical Shift Imaging

Hepatocellular (Common)

Diffuse steatosis
Focal steatosis
Lipid containing hepatocellular neoplasms
    Common: hepatic adenoma
    Uncommon: well-differentiated hepatocellular
      carcinoma
    Rare: follicular nodular hyperplasia

Nonhepatocellular (Rare)

Hepatic angiomyolipoma
Metastatic germ cell tumor
Hepatic lipoma

---

are usually of hepatocellular origin (Box 1-2). Lesions of other cellular origin such as cysts, hemangiomas, and metastases typically have a longer T1-relaxation time than does liver and will appear hypointense to liver parenchyma on T1-WIs.

Breath-hold gradient-echo (GRE) pulse sequences can replace spin-echo (SE) images for T1-WI of the liver. T1-W GRE sequences can be performed with multishot or single-shot techniques.[3] The term shot refers to the number of excitation pulses used in a pulse sequence. Multishot spoiled GRE T1-W sequences utilize a short repetition time (TR), short echo time (TE), and a high flip angle of 70° to 90°.[3] The lack of 180° refocusing pulses in GRE sequences allow water and lipid protons to precess in and out of phase with varying echo times. At 1.5 T, water and lipid are in phase at a TE range of 4.2 to 4.6 ms and out of phase at a TE range of 2.1 to 2.3 ms. Dual GRE T1-W sequences enable simultaneous acquisition of in-phase and opposed-phase images with two echo times per excitation. On in-phase images, signal from water and lipid within the same voxel are additive, whereas on opposed phase images, destructive interference of water and lipid protons results in loss of signal intensity (SI).

The combination of in-phase and opposed-phase images, referred to as chemical shift imaging, allows detection of hepatic steatosis as well as intralesional lipid in hepatocellular neoplasms such as hepatic adenoma and well-differentiated hepatocellular

carcinoma (Box 1-3). Chemical shift refers to the difference in resonant frequency between two types of protons, with the resonant frequency of a proton dependent on its local molecular environment. Chemical shift imaging is optimal for detection of microscopic lipid, whereas chemically selective fat-suppression techniques are best for the macroscopic lipid present in subcutaneous and intraabdominal fat or macroscopic fat containing tumors such as adrenal myelolipoma (see Chapter 3), renal angiomyolipoma (see Chapter 4), and ovarian dermoid cysts (see Chapter 7).

In patients with limited breath-holding capacity, rapid T1-WIs can be obtained with magnetization-prepared GRE pulse sequences.[3] A single section can be obtained in less than 1.5 sec with negligible effects from respiratory motion. This sequence incorporates a section-selective 180° inversion pulse and produces T1-WIs with high SI blood vessels; most lesions will appear hypointense on this sequence. The inversion pulse and inversion time can also be manipulated to produce T1-WIs with low SI blood vessels, a feature that minimizes pulsation artifacts.

T2-Weighted Imaging (WI)

The T2-relaxation time of liver is shorter than for most other abdominal tissues, including spleen.[3] Nonsolid liver lesions have long T2-relaxation times and are easily detected on T2-WIs. Solid masses such as hepatocellular carcinoma and hepatic metastases have shorter T2-relaxation times compared with nonsolid lesions and may be relatively inconspicuous on T2-WIs.

Multishot or single-shot echo-train pulse sequences have replaced conventional spin-echo techniques for T2-WI of the liver (as well as for evaluation of other organs in the abdomen and pelvis). These pulse sequences utilize one or more excitation pulses followed by two or more 180° refocusing pulses, the echo train. Each of the multiple spin echoes within an echo-train sequence is acquired with a different amplitude phase-encoding gradient, and

---

1-2 Isointense-hyperintense Liver Lesions on Unenhanced T1-WI

Hepatocellular (Common)

Focal nodular hyperplasia
Hepatic adenoma
Focal hepatic steatosis (in-phase imaging)
Focal sparing of steatosis (opposed-phase imaging)
Regenerative nodule
Hepatocellular carcinoma

Nonhepatocellular (Uncommon)

Hematoma (methemoglobin within rim)
Hemorrhagic metastases (e.g., melanoma, choriocarcinoma)
Treated metastatic disease (e.g., radiofrequency ablation)

therefore the resulting image contains data with different TE values. The effective TE refers to the TE at which the lowest amplitude phase-encoding gradients are applied. Low amplitude phase-encoding gradients provide the high-contrast, low-resolution data of central k-space, whereas high amplitude phase-encoding gradients provide the high-resolution, low-contrast data of peripheral k-space.

Echo-train T2-W pulse sequences can be performed without or with breath-holding techniques. Non–breath hold echo-train T2-W pulse sequences benefit from use of fat suppression and respiratory triggering.[4,5] Respiratory triggering requires a pneumatic bellows that is wrapped around the patient's torso. As only a portion of the respiratory cycle is used for data acquisition, respiratory triggering necessitates a long TR and is therefore easily adapted to multishot echo-train T2-W pulse sequences. Single-shot echo-train T2-weighted pulse sequences incorporate half-Fourier reconstruction (interpolation of k-space data) to reduce acquisition time. The subsecond acquisition time of single-shot T2-W sequences is useful with patients unable to comply with breath holding or for whom rapid scanning is required.[3] In comparison with multishot echo-train T2-W sequences, single-shot techniques produce images with decreased signal-to-noise ratios and increased blurring and consequently are less sensitive in the detection of smaller or low-contrast lesions.[3] T2-W sequences utilizing a TE of at least 160 ms allow improved discrimination between non-solid hepatic lesions, such as cysts and hemangiomas, and solid lesions.[6,7] A T2-W sequence with an even longer TE (e.g., 600-700 ms) can discriminate between a hepatic cyst and hemangioma based on the higher persistent SI of the former.[8] Heavily T2-W sequences are also used for magnetic resonance cholangiopancreatography (MRCP; see Chapter 2).

Short Tau Inversion Recovery Imaging

Short tau inversion recovery (STIR) pulse sequences provide fat-suppressed images with additive T1-weighted and T2-weighted contrast. STIR pulse sequences incorporate a preparatory 180° inversion pulse prior to the excitation pulse. The interval between the inversion pulse and excitation pulse is referred to as the inversion time (TI). At a TI of 150 to 170 ms at 1.5 T, the SI of fat is null. Similar to T2-WIs, fluid and most pathologic tissues will appear hyperintense on STIR images. The echo-train technique can be incorporated into the STIR pulse sequence to shorten the acquisition time.

T2 Star (T2*)-Weighted Imaging

GRE T2*-weighted pulse sequences are used for optimal detection of hepatic iron deposition. GRE sequences lack the 180° refocusing pulses of SE or echo-train sequences and therefore do not correct for phase shifts incurred by magnetic field inhomogeneity or static tissue susceptibility gradients. T2*-contrast reflects the effective spin-spin relaxation time resulting from true T2-decay and inhomogeneity effects. The susceptibility effect of iron results in signal loss that is most conspicuous on T2*-WIs. T2*-W GRE sequences are used after the administration of iron-containing reticuloendothelial system contrast agents. These contrast agents are cleared from plasma by the Kupffer cells present in normal hepatic parenchyma and some hepatocellular lesions. The susceptibility effect induced by the iron-containing contrast results in signal loss in the normal hepatic parenchyma and renders nonhepatocellular lesions, such as metastases, hyperintense. While MR angiography is currently performed with gadolinium-enhanced techniques, T2*-W sequences can be useful for depicting the direction of flow when specific saturation pulses are applied. This information may be useful in evaluating the portal venous system or portosystemic collateral vessels/varices.[3]

Contrast-enhanced Imaging

Four major classes of intravenously administered contrast agents are used for hepatic and abdominal MR imaging: nonspecific extracellular, hepatocyte-specific, reticuloendothelial system-specific, and blood pool-specific.[9] The nonspecific extracellular agents are chelates of gadolinium, a paramagnetic metal that shortens the T1-relaxation time of surrounding molecules. Chelation is required because of the toxicity, biodistribution, and efficacy of the free gadolinium ion.[10] The nonspecific extracellular gadolinium chelates diffuse rapidly from the intravascular space into the extracellular space, similarly to the iodinated contrast agents used in CT. While iodinated contrast agents are directly imaged by radiographic techniques, it is the paramagnetic effect of gadolinium on surrounding protons that is detected by MR.[11] Nonspecific extracellular gadolinium chelates are excreted via glomerular filtration.

Hepatocyte-specific agents are chelates of gadolinium or manganese that show variable excretion through the hepatobiliary system. Increasing the lipophilicity of the gadolinium chelate allows hepatocyte uptake. Manganese-based compounds partially dissociate in the circulation; the manganese ions are excreted by the hepatobiliary system, kidneys, pancreas, and gastric mucosa.[9] Reticuloendothelial system–specific agents are superparamagnetic iron oxide formulations cleared from the plasma by the reticuloendothelial system of the liver (80%) and spleen (12%) and subsequently eliminated in the lymph nodes and bone marrow.[9] Blood pool–specific agents include ultrasmall iron oxide particles and proteinaceous or polymeric complexes of gadolinium that remain in the bloodstream for an extended period of time.

The nonspecific extracellular gadolinium chelates are the most widely used of the MR imaging contrast agents. For optimal detection and characterization of hepatic lesions with this class of agents, dynamic imaging is often needed. Prior to administration of gadolinium chelates, precontrast imaging is acquired to assess anatomic coverage and the patient's breath-hold capacity.[12] In addition, unenhanced images serve as a baseline for comparison to the enhanced images and can also be subtracted from contrast-enhanced images. Subtraction imaging can improve MR angiographic reconstructions and detection of enhancement in masses that are hyperintense on unenhanced T1-WIs.[12,13]

Postcontrast imaging is classified into three phases: hepatic arterial dominant, portal venous, and hepatic venous or interstitial.[9,14] The hepatic arterial-dominant phase occurs 15 to 30 seconds after rapid bolus injection of contrast agent. Images obtained during this phase show enhancement of the hepatic arteries and possibly the main portal veins. However, there is no enhancement of the hepatic veins and minimal hepatic parenchymal enhancement. The hepatic arterial-dominant phase is important in the detection of hypervascular lesions and the evaluation of the hepatic arterial system. The portal venous phase occurs 45 to 75 seconds after contrast agent administration. During this phase, the portal veins, hepatic veins and hepatic parenchyma are maximally enhanced. This phase is optimal for detection of hypovascular lesions. The hepatic venous, or interstitial, phase spans from 90 seconds to 5 minutes after injection of contrast agent. This phase is useful for characterizing lesions that show continued enhancement, such as hemangiomas, or lesions with a large extracellular space, such as intrahepatic cholangiocarcinoma.

The variable circulatory status of patients requires a reliable and reproducible method for coordinating imaging, particularly acquisition of central k-space data, with the hepatic arterial-dominant phase. Commercially available methods include timing-runs, automated bolus detection and triggering, and real-time or "fluoroscopic" bolus detection with operator triggering.[15] (See Chapter 11.) The use of a power injector standardizes injection rates,[16]

optimizes MR angiography, and has proven superior to manual injection.[17,18]

Dynamic gadolinium-enhanced imaging is performed with pulse sequences that enable coverage of the entire liver within a reasonable breath-hold (less than 25 s). Three-dimensional, or volumetric, GRE T1-W sequences confer several advantages over two-dimensional pulse sequences.[12] Three-dimensional GRE T1-W sequences enable acquisition of thinner sections without intersection gaps, fat suppression, higher signal-to-noise ratios, and similar image contrast within the same breath-hold duration as two-dimensional sequences. Volumetric acquisitions provide isotropic data sets that optimize postprocessing techniques, such as multiplanar reconstructions or volume rendering.

PRIMARY HEPATIC MASSES

Benign Hepatocellular Neoplasms: Adenoma and Focal Nodular Hyperplasia

HEPATOCELLULAR ADENOMA (BOX 1-4)

Hepatic adenoma is a benign hepatic neoplasm occurring most commonly in women taking oral contraceptive medications. The incidence of hepatic adenomas increases with the duration of oral contraceptive medication use and the dosage of estrogen.[19,20] Anabolic-androgenic steroids used for medical indications or abused by athletes are associated with a number of hepatic diseases including hepatic adenomas.[21] Hepatic adenomas, often multiple, develop with increased incidence in patients with glycogen storage diseases types I and III.[22] Hepatic adenoma may be incidentally detected at cross-sectional studies performed for unrelated reasons, or the patient may have acute or chronic pain, a palpable mass, or abnormal liver function tests.[23,24]

Hepatic adenoma is composed of benign hepatocytes arranged in large plates or cords without an

---

1-4   Hepatic Adenoma

Clinical

Benign hepatocellular neoplasm
Potential for hemorrhage (common) and malignant transformation (rare)
Risk factors: oral contraceptives (most common), anabolic-androgenic steroids, and glycogen storage diseases

Pathology

Mean diameter of 5 cm, multiple in 30%
Hepatocytes, Kupffer cells (usually nonfunctioning), no bile ducts, pseudocapsule of compressed parenchyma and/or fibrosis

MRI

T1-WI: SI varies with presence of lipid, hemorrhage, and necrosis; portions of tumor isointense to hyperintense to liver
Intratumoral lipid common, confirmed by chemical shift imaging
T2-WI: SI variable but usually hyperintense to liver
Hypervascular on dynamic CE imaging, but not as vascular as FNH
No central scar

acinar architecture.[25-27] The plates of hepatocytes are separated by dilated sinusoids, which in addition to feeding arteries produce the hypervascularity of adenomas.[26,27] Adenoma cells contain glycogen and lipid.[25,27] Kupffer cells may be present in adenomas but usually are nonfunctioning, and bile ducts are absent.[25,27] A fibrous capsule or pseudocapsule composed of compressed parenchyma and/or fibrosis is usually present.[26,28]

Complications of hepatic adenomas include hemorrhage with possible rupture of the liver[27,29-31] and rare malignant transformation to hepatocellular carcinoma.[30,32,33] Hemorrhage within an adenoma is thought to be related to infarction as the tumor outgrows its blood supply.[27] A hemorrhagic adenoma may rupture through the liver, resulting in hemoperitoneum with possible shock.[34] Rupture of a hemorrhagic adenoma is related to its proximity to the liver surface and the thickness of the fibrous tumor capsule, if present.[31] The true risk of malignant transformation is uncertain but was present in 5 of 39 patients in one series.[30] Although adenomas have been shown to resolve completely after the cessation of oral contraceptive medications,[35,36] this resolution does not preclude the subsequent development of hepatocellular carcinoma.[20] Liver cell dysplasia may develop within an adenoma and is an irreversible premalignant change.[20]

Hepatic adenomas range in size from 1 to 19 cm, with a mean diameter of 3 to 5 cm.[24,37,38] The heterogeneous MR appearance of hepatic adenoma reflects the variable presence of intralesional steatosis, hemorrhage, peliosis hepatis, necrosis, fibrous encapsulation, rare central scars, and large tumoral vessels.[24,27,28,37] On T1-WIs, adenomas reveal variable SI but often have components that are hyperintense to surrounding liver parenchyma.[24,28,37] Hyperintense T1 foci can be from intracellular lipid or hemorrhage (Figs. 1-1 and 1-2).[24] Chemical shift imaging can confirm the presence of intralesional steatosis (see Fig. 1-1). On T2-WIs adenomas have variable SI but usually have some hyperintense components.[24,28,37] Hemorrhage and necrosis result in the heterogeneous T2 SI.[37] Most adenomas show hypervascularity on the arterial phase of dynamic contrast-enhanced (CE) T1-WIs.[28,37]

A pseudocapsule of compressed hepatic parenchyma or fibrosis may be identified at MR.[24,28,37] On T1-WIs, this pseudocapsule is typically hypointense to adjacent liver parenchyma.[28] The T2-W appearance of this pseudocapsule is more variable, with an approximately equal number being hyperintense, isointense, or hypointense to adjacent liver parenchyma.[28]

The main differential diagnosis for hepatic adenoma includes two other hypervascular hepatocellular lesions: focal nodular hyperplasia and hepatocellular carcinoma. Except for the central scar, focal nodular hyperplasia is typically homogeneously isointense or nearly isointense to liver parenchyma on both T1- and T2-WIs, whereas adenoma is usually of heterogeneous SI. In addition, FNH usually contains a central scar, a rare finding in hepatic adenoma.[37]

Hepatic adenomas can be indistinguishable hepatocellular carcinoma based only on the MR imaging features of the lesion, although vascular invasion does not occur in hepatic adenomas. Hepatocellular carcinoma typically develops in patients with cirrhosis whereas hepatic adenomas occur in young women who have taken oral contraceptive medications. Serum α-fetoprotein is usually elevated with hepatocellular carcinoma but not with hepatic adenomas.

The management of hepatic adenomas is somewhat controversial. Surgical resection has been advocated to eliminate the known risks of life-threatening hemorrhage and malignant transformation.[31] A more selective approach to management has also been proposed.[38] In patients with lesions less than 5 cm and normal α-fetoprotein levels, cessation of oral contraceptives, counseling regarding pregnancy, and serial imaging could be considered as an alternative to surgery.[38] Hepatic arterial embolization is preferred over surgery for the acute management of hemorrhage.[38]

LIVER ADENOMATOSIS

Hepatic adenomatosis was initially described as 10 or more hepatic adenomas occurring in an otherwise normal liver (absence of glycogen storage disease), unrelated to the use of oral contraceptive medications or anabolic-androgenic steroids, with associated abnormalities in liver function tests (serum alkaline phosphatase and gamma-glutamyl transpeptidase) occurring in either women or men.[39] Recently, liver adenomatosis was defined as greater than three adenomas.[40] The majority of lesions in hepatic adenomatosis are not estrogen dependent.[41] Two forms of liver adenomatosis have been described: multifocal and massive.[42] Management of the multifocal form can be surgical resection of the larger or more complicated lesions. Liver transplantation is reserved for the more aggressive form of the disease.[42] One group advocates close surveillance for asymptomatic patients with small lesions (≤3 cm) because of the presumed lower risk of intraperitoneal hemorrhage.[40] The MR imaging characteristics of individual adenomas in liver adenomatosis (see Fig. 1-1) are similar to the more common solitary lesions that develop in women taking oral contraceptive medications.[41]

FOCAL NODULAR HYPERPLASIA (BOX 1-5)

Focal nodular hyperplasia (FNH) is a benign tumor thought to represent a hyperplastic response of the hepatic parenchyma to a preexisting arterial malformation.[43] FNH is the second most common benign liver tumor after hemangioma.[44] FNH is most commonly detected in women of reproductive age but can rarely occur in men and children.[43,45] Most cases of FNH are incidentally discovered at autopsy, surgery, or imaging studies and are asymptomatic. Large lesions may be symptomatic because of distention of the liver capsule or mass effect on adjacent organs.[43] Oral contraceptive medications do not initiate development of FNH; however, the relationship

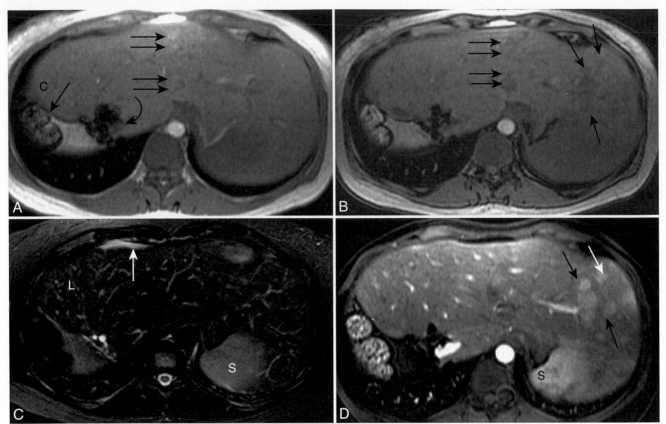

Figure 1-1 ▪ **MR illustration of multiple lipid-containing liver adenomas in a woman with a history of oral contraceptive medication use; prior right lobectomy established the diagnosis of adenomatosis. A** and **B,** T1-WIs show hypertrophy of the patient's remaining left lobe. No liver lesions are revealed on the in-phase image (**A**), but multiple hypointense liver lesions *(arrows)* are present on the opposed-phase image (**B**). Isointensity to liver on in-phase imaging and the presence of intracellular lipid (established by loss of SI on opposed-phase imaging) both indicate that the lesions are of hepatocellular origin. There is loss of SI on the in-phase image (with a longer TE) within right colon *(arrow* C) and adjacent to surgical clips *(curved arrow).* Round "pseudolesions" *(double black arrows)* of variable SI are located anterior to the hyperintense aorta. The high SI within the aorta and the pseudolesions are secondary to flow-related enhancement and pulsation artifact, respectively. Applying a superior saturation band to eliminate signal from arterial blood entering the top of the imaging volume could have minimized both. **C,** Fat suppressed T2-WI does not depict the liver lesions. Note the normal difference in T2 SI between the hypointense liver (L) and hyperintense spleen (S). The high SI anterior to the liver represents unsuppressed fat *(arrow)* and should not be mischaracterized as loculated fluid. Superiorly located perihepatic fat is not suppressed secondary to localized magnetic field inhomogeneity from adjacent lung parenchyma.[491] **D,** Arterial phase CE T1-WI shows multiple hypervascular masses *(arrows).* The heterogeneous enhancement of the spleen (S) is normal during this phase of enhancement.

between oral contraceptive medication use and growth of FNH is less clear. One study showed no relationship between oral contraceptive use and the number or size of FNH lesions,[46] whereas others showed lesion regression after discontinuation of oral contraceptive medications.[47]

FNH is solitary in 80% to 95% of patients.[43] The mass is composed of nodules of hyperplastic hepatocytes and small bile ductules surrounding a central fibrous scar.[26] The central scar contains dense connective tissue and blood vessels that may have thick, myxomatous walls.[26] Unlike neoplasms, growth of FNH is proportional to its vascular supply. Hemorrhage and necrosis are unusual, and rupture of FNH is extremely rare.[43] The mean diameter of

FNH is 5 cm.[45] Malignant transformation has not been reported.

MR has greater sensitivity and specificity in the diagnosis of FNH compared with either CT or sonography.[44] FNH is typically isointense or slightly hypointense to liver parenchyma on T1-WI (Fig. 1-3; see Fig. 3-4).[43,48-50] The rare presence of lipid within FNH is usually associated with diffuse hepatic steatosis.[51] FNH is isointense to slightly hyperintense on T2-WI. A central scar can be revealed at MR in 75% to 80% of FNH lesions.[44,48,52] The central scar is characteristically hypointense to the surrounding lesion on T1-WIs and hyperintense on T2-WIs (see Figs. 1-3 and 3-4).[43,48-50] Scar hyperintensity on T2-WIs is related to the presence of blood

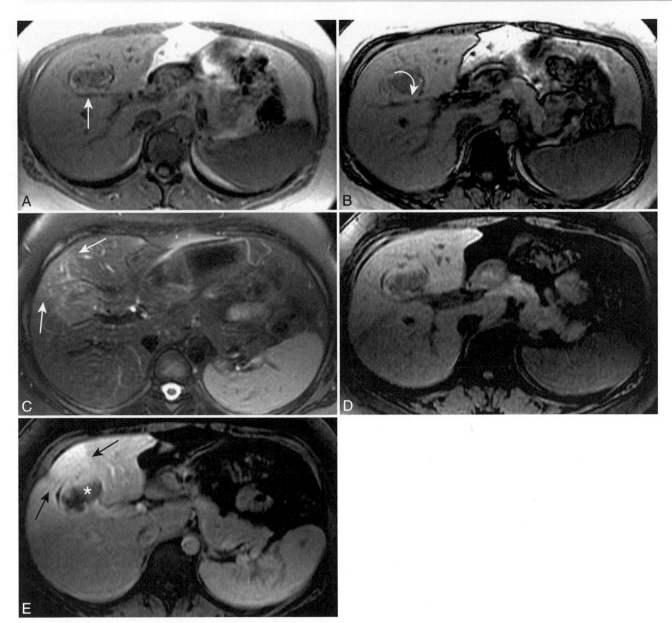

Figure 1-2 ■ Hemorrhagic hepatic adenoma revealed on MR in a 32-year-old woman. A, In-phase T1-WI (TE = 4.2) shows a mass with a hyperintense peripheral rim *(arrow)* relative to the surrounding liver. The central portion of the mass is hypointense to liver parenchyma. **B**, Opposed-phase image (TE = 2.5) shows that the rim remains hyperintense consistent with protein or blood rather than lipid. Dependent debris is present *(curved arrow)*. **C**, Fat-suppressed T2-WI shows the mass is slightly hyperintense to liver. A wedge-shaped area of increased SI *(arrows)* peripheral to the mass likely represents edema from venous outflow obstruction. **D** and **E**, Fat suppressed T1-WIs obtained before (**D**) and after (**E**) the arterial-phase of CE show that the hemorrhagic central portion (∗) of the mass does not enhance. A peripheral wedge-shaped area of increased enhancement *(arrows)* represents a transient-hepatic intensity difference, likely due to portal vein compression and compensatory increased hepatic arterial flow. It may be difficult to detect viable, enhancing portions of an adenoma that has bled. Subtraction imaging can reveal subtle enhancement within a hemorrhagic neoplasm.

vessels, bile ductules, and edema within myxomatous tissue.[43,44]

The three typical unenhanced MR imaging features of FNH—homogeneous T1 isointensity to hypointensity, homogeneous slight T2 hyperintensity, and T2 hyperintense central scar—are all present in approximately one third of lesions.[43] Atypical MR imaging findings of FNH include absence of the central scar, hypointensity of the scar on T2-WIs, non-enhancement of the scar, presence of a pseudocapsule, marked T1 or T2 lesion hyperintensity of the lesion, and heterogeneous SI.[49] Some of these atypical MR features are often present in the uncommon telangiectatic subtype of FNH.[44,53]

1-5 Focal Nodular Hyperplasia

Clinical

Benign, asymptomatic mass thought to represent hyperplastic response to preexisting arterial malformation
Most common in women of reproductive age
If a diagnosis can be established by MR, surgery can be avoided

Pathology

Hyperplastic hepatocytes, small bile ductules surrounding central fibrovascular scar, Kupffer cells present
Median diameter of 3 cm, mean diameter of 4 cm, multiple in approximately 20%

MRI

Mass

T1-WI: isointense to slightly hypointense to liver
T2-WI: isointense to slightly hyperintense to liver
Markedly hypervascular on dynamic CE imaging, isointense on portal venous phase, and slightly hyperintense on delayed phase

Central Scar

T1-WI: hypointense to surrounding mass
T2-WI: hyperintense to surrounding mass
CE imaging: hypovascular to mass on arterial phase with increased enhancement on delayed phase

On dynamic CE T1-WI, FNH shows marked arterial phase enhancement (see Fig. 1-3).[43,48,50,54] FNH becomes isointense to adjacent liver parenchyma on portal venous phase images and is slightly hyperintense on delayed images.[43,50,54] The central scar shows decreased enhancement relative to the surrounding lesion on arterial phase images[48] and almost always is hyperintense on delayed phase images (see Figs. 1-3 and 3-4).[43,48,50,52,54]

The management of asymptomatic FNH with typical MR imaging features is nonsurgical.[55,56] In contrast to hepatic adenoma, the negligible risk of hemorrhage and lack of malignant potential allow safe observation of FNH. If clinical, laboratory, or imaging data are inconsistent with a diagnosis of FNH, surgical biopsy is recommended.[56] In cases of indeterminate characterization after a gadolinium-enhanced MR examination, one could consider performing MR with a hepatocellular-specific contrast agent to confirm the hepatocellular origin of the lesion or the presence of a central scar.[44,57] Clinical history of chronic liver disease, malignancy, abnormal liver function tests, elevated serum α-fetoprotein, atypical imaging features, or increasing size should lead to biopsy for histologic confirmation. The risk of indeterminate or incorrect results with percutaneous biopsies has resulted in the use of large surgical biopsy specimens to establish a diagnosis of FNH and exclude hepatic adenoma.[55,56]

Fibrolamellar Hepatocellular Carcinoma (Box 1-6)

Fibrolamellar hepatocellular carcinoma (FL-HCC) is a rare subtype of hepatocellular carcinoma (HCC) with distinct clinical, pathologic, and imaging features. FL-HCC occurs in young patients, typically during the second or third decades, with an equal distribution between women and men.[58] As opposed to HCC, most patients who develop FL-HCC do not have a history of cirrhosis or other liver disease.[58] Clinically, patients may present with pain, hepatomegaly, palpable mass, and cachexia.[58] More than 85% of patients with FL-HCC have normal serum α-fetoprotein levels.[58]

1-6 Fibrolamellar Hepatocellular Carcinoma

Clinical

Rare; incidence of 1/million/year
M = F, present in second to third decades
Presentation may include pain, hepatomegaly, palpable mass, and cachexia
Serum α-fetoprotein usually normal (>85% of patients)

Pathology

Malignant hepatocytes separated by fibrous sheets (lamellae)
Central fibrous scar is common
Large and infiltrative, mean diameter of 13 cm

MRI

Mass

T1-WI: homogeneously hypointense to liver
T2-WI: heterogeneously hyperintense to liver
Dynamic gadolinium-enhanced: heterogeneous enhancement on arterial and portal venous phases
Aggressive lesions: possible portal vein invasion and/or extrahepatic extension

Central Scar

T1-WI: hypointense to mass and liver
T2-WI: hypointense to mass and liver
Scar usually does not enhance

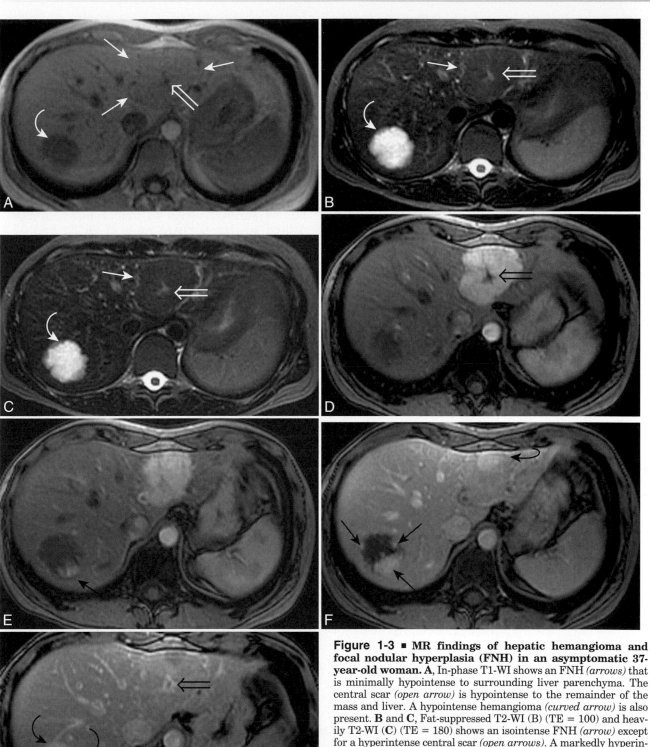

Figure 1-3 ■ MR findings of hepatic hemangioma and focal nodular hyperplasia (FNH) in an asymptomatic 37-year-old woman. A, In-phase T1-WI shows an FNH *(arrows)* that is minimally hypointense to surrounding liver parenchyma. The central scar *(open arrow)* is hypointense to the remainder of the mass and liver. A hypointense hemangioma *(curved arrow)* is also present. **B** and **C**, Fat-suppressed T2-WI (B) (TE = 100) and heavily T2-WI (**C**) (TE = 180) shows an isointense FNH *(arrow)* except for a hyperintense central scar *(open arrows)*. A markedly hyperintense hemangioma *(curved arrow)* is present. **D** and **E**, Arterial-phase CE T1-WIs show marked FNH enhancement and a nonenhancing central scar *(open arrow)* in **D** and peripheral nodular enhancement within the hemangioma in **E** *(black arrow)*. Portal (**F**) and delayed (**G**) CE T1-WI shows that the FNH becomes isointense to liver except for the hyperintense central scar *(open arrow)* that enhanced late. The hemangioma shows progressive centripetal enhancement *(black arrows)* and ultimately uniform hyperintensity *(curved arrows)*. Homogenous delayed enhancement is typical of hemangioma. The circular focus of high SI in **F** *(curved arrow)* represents phase encoding artifact from the aorta. This could have been minimized or eliminated by utilizing a superior saturation pulse.

FL-HCC is composed of sheets, cords, or trabeculae of malignant hepatocytes separated by fibrous sheets (lamellae).[25,26,58,59] The presence of intracellular glycogen or lipid has not been reported in FL-HCC.[58] Encapsulation is rare in FL-HCC but common in HCC.[58] Hemorrhage and necrosis are seen in approximately one third of cases microscopically but only 10% at gross pathology. FL-HCC is usually large, with a mean diameter of 13 cm.[60,61] A central fibrous scar is common.[58] Satellite nodules are often present.[25,26]

On T1-WI, FL-HCC is usually homogeneously hypointense to liver parenchyma, except for the central scar.[58,59] On T2-WIs, FL-HCC is usually heterogeneously hyperintense to liver parenchyma; isointensity is unusual.[58,59] The central fibrous scar is typically hypointense on both T1- and T2-WIs (Fig. 1-4).[58,59] The central scar and radiating fibrous septa are more often detected with MR imaging than with computed tomography.[59]

FL-HCC shows marked heterogeneous enhancement on arterial phase and portal venous phase gadolinium-enhanced images and becomes more homogeneous over time.[58] The central scar typically does not enhance and is most conspicuous on delayed images as the surrounding tumor becomes more homogeneous.[58,59] Hepatic vascular involvement and lymphadenopathy are frequent findings.[61]

FL-HCC is managed surgically when possible, either with partial hepatectomy or liver transplantation.[60,62] Involvement of the main portal vein or hepatic artery precludes surgical management.[60] Regional lymphadenopathy may be resected at the time of initial surgery.[60] Long-term survival has been achieved with aggressive surgical management; the largest surgical series to date reports cumulative 5- and 10-year survival rates of 66.2% and 47.4%, respectively.[60] In this series, patient survival was significantly associated with TNM staging. Vascular invasion and lymph node involvement were factors most associated with decreased survival. The prognosis for FL-HCC is considered to be better than for HCC.[58,60,61]

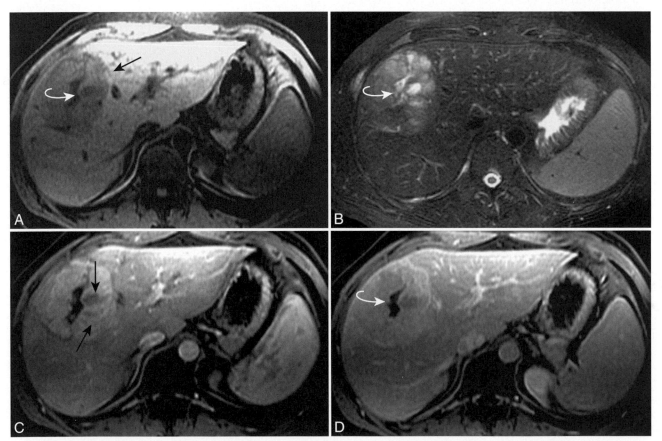

Figure 1-4 ■ **MR demonstration of a fibrolamellar hepatocellular carcinoma in a 28-year-old man. A**, Fat-suppressed T1-WI shows a slightly hypointense mass *(arrow)* compared with surrounding liver parenchyma with an even lower SI central scar *(curved arrow)*. **B**, Fat-suppressed T2-WI shows a lobular heterogeneous hyperintense mass. The central scar has both low and high SI components *(curved arrow)*. Scars within fibrolamellar hepatoma are usually fibrous and of relative low T2 SI. **C**, Arterial phase CE T1-WI shows hypointense radiating fibrous septa *(arrows)* and enhancing tumor. **D**, Delayed CE T1-WI shows that contrast has washed out of the tumor that is now isointense to liver. The nonenhancing scar remains of low SI *(curved arrow)*. The scar of FNH should have enhanced during the delayed phase of contrast enhancement.

Intrahepatic Peripheral Cholangiocarcinoma (Box 1-7)

Cholangiocarcinoma (CCA) is an adenocarcinoma that can develop from any segment of the biliary tract from the terminal ductules to the ampulla of Vater, and therefore may be intrahepatic or extrahepatic.[63] The four macroscopic growth patterns of CCA include exophytic (mass-forming), infiltrative (periductal), polypoid (intraductal), and combined.[63,64] Intrahepatic peripheral cholangiocarcinoma (IPC) accounts for approximately 10% of all cholangiocarcinomas, while lesions arising at the hilum or from the extrahepatic ducts account for 90%.[65] IPC is discussed here and the infiltrative and polypoid forms of CCA in Chapter 2. CCA is the second most common primary hepatic malignancy after HCC. Risk factors for the development of CCA include biliary lithiasis, primary sclerosing cholangitis, clonorchiasis, recurrent pyogenic cholangitis, Caroli's disease, and Thorotrast (thorium dioxide) exposure.[63,65-67] Most patients with CCA are in the fifth or sixth decade of life, and there is an approximately equal sex distribution.[25,26] Patients may present with abdominal pain, palpable mass, weight loss, or jaundice.[65]

IPC is thought to arise from the bile ducts distal to the second-order branches.[63,68] Histologically, the most common pattern of IPC is the small glandular adenocarcinoma with abundant sclerosis.[26] Adenosquamous, squamous, mucinous, or anaplastic carcinomas are uncommon variants.[69] IPC may spread through the liver via the sinusoids, vascular channels, lymphatic channels, perineural space, bile ducts, and periportal connective tissue.[69] Fibrosis, coagulative necrosis, hyalinization, and mucin are present in variable amounts within IPCs.[65,67,69-71]

IPC is usually hypointense to surrounding liver parenchyma on T1-WIs.[66-68,70-75] On T2-WIs, IPC is hyperintense to surrounding liver parenchyma. The majority of IPCs show heterogeneous T2 SI with central areas of either hypointensity or hyperintensity.[70] Foci of low T2 SI are secondary to fibrosis and/or coagulative necrosis. The rare variant of mucinous IPC is markedly hyperintense on T2-WIs.[70,76] Dynamic gadolinium-enhanced MR shows mild to moderate rim enhancement with heterogeneous centripetal progression.[66-68,70-75] Fibrosis accounts for the regions of delayed enhancement (Fig. 1-5).[70,71,77] Intratumoral foci of coagulative necrosis are not enhanced on delayed images.[70,71,77]

Intrahepatic biliary dilation peripheral to an IPC is shown in more than 50% of patients and is suggestive of an obstructive lesion of biliary ductal origin.[70,78] Vascular invasion is also a frequent finding with IPC.[67,68,70,72,78,79] Capsular retraction, a nonspecific sign suggestive of a desmoplastic reaction may be present with IPC[67,68,78] but can also be present in some liver metastases and hemangiomas.[80,81] Liver atrophy peripheral to IPC appears similar to capsular retraction and is likely due to portal venous invasion.[67,82]

The differential diagnosis for IPC includes colorectal metastases and hepatocellular carcinoma variants with intratumoral fibrosis (sclerosing hepatocellular carcinoma and fibrolamellar hepatocellular carcinoma).[63] Biliary dilation peripheral to hepatic colorectal metastases is rarely detected by imaging studies but is common with IPC.[70,83] Exclusion of a primary colorectal malignancy is necessary because of the pathologic similarity of IPC and hepatic colorectal metastases, especially in patients with ulcerative colitis who are at risk for both cancers. Sclerosing and fibrolamellar hepatocellular carcinomas can be distinguished from IPC with clinicopathologic features.[63] Management of IPC is surgical, and the prognosis usually is poor, because lymph node metastasis rarely is limited to regional nodes at the time of diagnosis.[84]

Biliary Cystadenoma and Cystadenocarcinoma (Box 1-8)

Biliary cystadenoma (BC) and biliary cystadenocarcinoma (BCCA) are rare cystic neoplasms of the liver

---

1-7 Intrahepatic Peripheral Cholangiocarcinoma

Clinical

Second most common primary hepatic malignancy after hepatocellular carcinoma
Risk factors: primary sclerosing cholangitis, biliary lithiasis, recurrent pyogenic cholangitis, clonorchiasis, Caroli's disease
M = F, presents in fifth to sixth decades
Signs and symptoms: abdominal pain, palpable mass, weight loss or jaundice

Pathology

Adenocarcinoma arising from bile ducts distal to second-order branches
Variable fibrosis, coagulative necrosis, hyalinization, and mucin

MRI

T1-WI: hypointense to liver
T2-weighted: hyperintense to liver, often with central areas of focally increased or decreased SI relative to hyperintense periphery; biliary dilation peripheral to mass present in >50%
Dynamic CE imaging: rim enhancement with heterogeneous centripetal progression with intratumoral fibrosis showing delayed enhancement

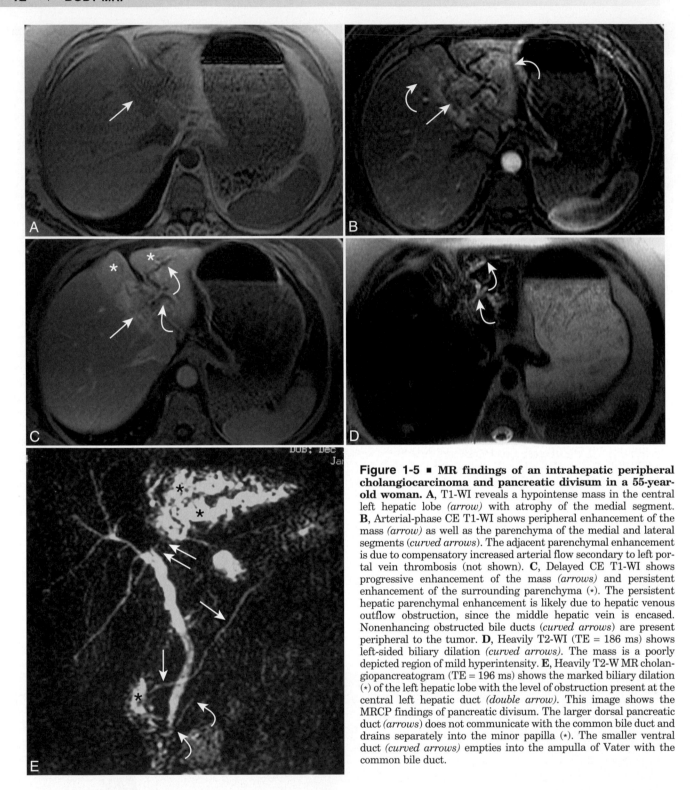

Figure 1-5 ■ MR findings of an intrahepatic peripheral cholangiocarcinoma and pancreatic divisum in a 55-year-old woman. A, T1-WI reveals a hypointense mass in the central left hepatic lobe *(arrow)* with atrophy of the medial segment. **B**, Arterial-phase CE T1-WI shows peripheral enhancement of the mass *(arrow)* as well as the parenchyma of the medial and lateral segments *(curved arrows)*. The adjacent parenchymal enhancement is due to compensatory increased arterial flow secondary to left portal vein thrombosis (not shown). **C**, Delayed CE T1-WI shows progressive enhancement of the mass *(arrows)* and persistent enhancement of the surrounding parenchyma (*). The persistent hepatic parenchymal enhancement is likely due to hepatic venous outflow obstruction, since the middle hepatic vein is encased. Nonenhancing obstructed bile ducts *(curved arrows)* are present peripheral to the tumor. **D**, Heavily T2-WI (TE = 186 ms) shows left-sided biliary dilation *(curved arrows)*. The mass is a poorly depicted region of mild hyperintensity. **E**, Heavily T2-W MR cholangiopancreatogram (TE = 196 ms) shows the marked biliary dilation (*) of the left hepatic lobe with the level of obstruction present at the central left hepatic duct *(double arrow)*. This image shows the MRCP findings of pancreatic divisum. The larger dorsal pancreatic duct *(arrows)* does not communicate with the common bile duct and drains separately into the minor papilla (*). The smaller ventral duct *(curved arrows)* empties into the ampulla of Vater with the common bile duct.

and represent less than 5% of intrahepatic cysts of biliary origin.[85] Most cases occur in middle-aged women.[85,86] Patients with BC are usually younger than those with BCCA.[86] While these lesions may be asymptomatic, clinical presentations may include abdominal pain, palpable mass, elevated liver function tests, jaundice, fever, and weight loss.[85-87]

Most instances of BC/BCCA arise from the intrahepatic bile ducts and occasionally from the extrahepatic bile ducts or gallbladder.[85,86,88] These masses are large,

1-8   Biliary Cystadenoma/Cystadenocarcinoma

Clinical

Rare cystic neoplasms of liver

Presents in middle-aged women with abdominal pain, palpable mass, elevated, liver function tests, jaundice, fever, possible weight loss

Pathology

Cystic lesion lined by cuboidal or columnar epithelium similarly to mucinous cystic neoplasms of the pancreas and ovary

Intratumoral ovarian (mesenchymal) stroma present only in women and associated with improved prognosis compared with lesions without ovarian stroma that can occur in both men and women

Internal septations and nodularity are frequent

Fluid may be hemorrhagic, bilious, clear, mucinous, or mixed

Biliary cystadenoma precursor lesion to cystadenocarcinoma

MRI

Multilocular cystic mass with internal septations/nodularity

T1 and T2 SI vary with type of fluid contents; proteinaceous/mucinous or hemorrhagic fluid is T1 hyperintense and T2 hypointense as compared with simple/bilious fluid

Cystadenoma not reliably distinguished from cystadenocarcinoma by MRI

---

ranging in size from 3 to 40 cm, with a mean diameter of 12 cm.[86] Histologically, BC/BCCA are similar to mucinous cystic neoplasms of the pancreas and ovary.[86] The presence or absence of ovarian (mesenchymal) stroma below the lining cuboidal or columnar epithelium classifies BC/BCCA into two subtypes.[86,88,89] The embryologic migration of primordial germ cells through the yolk stalk, a structure from which the hepatobiliary system and pancreas develop, accounts for the presence of ovarian stroma in BC/BCCA.[86] Lesions containing ovarian stroma occur only in women and have a better prognosis than those lesions without ovarian stroma that occur in women or men.[86,88] The fluid obtained from the loculi may be hemorrhagic, bilious, clear, mucinous, or mixed.[86] BC/BCCA may communicate with the biliary system and if mucin-secreting result in biliary obstruction.[90-92] In the absence of metastatic disease, neither gross lesions nor imaging studies can reliably distinguish between BC and BCCA. Only histopathologic studies can determine the presence of malignancy or differentiate lesions based on the presence or absence of ovarian stroma.[86]

MR imaging of BC/BCCA shows a multilocular cystic mass (Fig. 1-6). The SI of the cystic fluid varies with its components. Simple or bilious fluid is T1 hypointense and T2 hyperintense, whereas proteinaceous/mucinous or hemorrhagic fluid shows higher T1 and lower T2 SI. Fluid-fluid levels can be present in hemorrhagic lesions.[93,94] Internal septa and nodular projections are present in both BC and DCCA.[86] Internal septa without nodularity suggest a diagnosis of BC, whereas septations with nodularity are suggestive but not diagnostic of BCCA.[86]

The differential diagnosis for BC/BCCA includes other multiloculated cystic lesions of the liver, particularly liver abscess and hydatid disease.[86,95,96] Both hepatic abscess and hydatid disease of the liver

should be distinguishable from BC/BCCA by clinical and laboratory data.[86] Hepatic abscesses are often multifocal and show perilesional edema and a thick enhancing rim.[97] The presence of round or oval daughter cysts, thick walls, and detached germinative membrane may help differentiate hydatid cyst from BC/BCCA on imaging studies.[86,98,99]

BC is considered a precursor to BCCA because foci of benign epithelium are present in malignant lesions.[85,88,89] Malignant transformation of BC into BCCA, has been reported with serially observed lesions[100] and after surgical excision.[101] Complete excision is the treatment of choice for BC (as well as BCCA) to prevent recurrence and potential malignant transformation.[87,102] Drainage, marsupialization, or

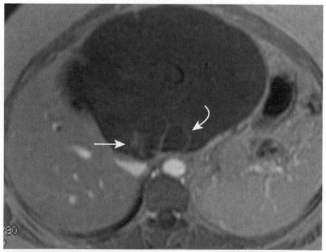

Figure 1-6 ▪ MR illustration of a biliary cystadenoma containing ovarian type stroma in a 33-year-old woman. CE T1-WI shows a multilocular cystic mass with enhancement of a small nodular component *(arrow)* and the loculus walls *(curved arrow)*.

sclerosis is not recommended.[87,102] Percutaneous or intraoperative aspiration/biopsy are not done because of the potential risk of peritoneal carcinomatosis.[103-105]

CYSTIC LESIONS ASSOCIATED WITH THE DUCTAL PLATE MALFORMATION

A unifying hypothesis for congenital diseases of the intrahepatic bile ducts centers on the embryologic ductal plate malformation (DPM).[106,107] The ductal plate is a layer of liver progenitor cells that forms a sleeve around the mesenchyme of the portal vein and develops into the intrahepatic bile ducts[106,107] DPM may involve any portion of the intrahepatic biliary tree and results in a spectrum of fibropolycystic disorders characterized by segmental dilation of the intrahepatic bile ducts and variable degrees of fibrosis.[106,107] These disorders include autosomal recessive and autosomal dominant polycystic kidney diseases, congenital hepatic fibrosis, Caroli's disease, von Meyenburg complexes (biliary hamartomas), and mesenchymal hamartomas.[106,107] Biliary hamartomas and the liver cysts associated with autosomal dominant polycystic kidney disease are discussed here and Caroli's disease in Chapter 2.

Biliary Hamartomas

A Meyenburg complex, or biliary hamartoma, is a small lesion composed of dilated bile ducts and interspersed fibrous or hyalinized stroma.[106,107] Biliary hamartoma is thought to represent a DPM of the smaller, more peripheral interlobular bile ducts[106,107] and can be identified macroscopically in 0.7% of autopsies.[108] Biliary hamartomas are usually less than 15 mm in size and asymptomatic. The importance of biliary hamartomas is their potential similarity to hepatic metastases on imaging studies.[109]

Biliary hamartomas are hypointense to liver parenchyma on T1-WIs and markedly hyperintense on T2-WIs.[110-117] Near isointensity to simple fluid on heavily T2-WIs has been reported.[111,112,117,118] Some lesions are hypointense to simple fluid on T2-WI.[110,115] No characteristic enhancement pattern has been identified. Solid, absent, and rim enhancement have been reported.[118] Thin rim enhancement has been attributed to surrounding compressed liver parenchyma or perilesional inflammatory cell infiltrate.[114]

The differential diagnosis for biliary hamartomas includes metastases, microabscesses, saccular dilation of the biliary system (Caroli's disease), and polycystic disease of the liver.[118] Features that suggest biliary hamartomas over metastases include small size (most hamartomas are less than 1 cm), thin rim enhancement with no centripetal progression, and high fluid content. Cystic or poorly vascularized hepatic metastases from ovarian carcinoma, sarcoma, gastrinoma, or chemotherapy-treated malignant lesions may appear similar to biliary hamartomas. The clinical setting should allow discrimination

between biliary hamartomas and microabscesses. MRCP has been useful in evaluation of biliary hamartomas, showing multiple cystic hyperintense lesions without communication with the bile ducts, allowing discrimination from Caroli's disease.

Autosomal-dominant Polycystic Kidney Disease

Hepatobiliary cysts are found in most patients with autosomal-dominant polycystic kidney disease (ADPCKD).[107,119,120] The incidence of hepatobiliary cysts in ADPCKD increases with patient age, increased severity of renal cystic disease and decreased creatinine clearance.[121] Women develop more and larger cysts than men.[121] Hepatobiliary cysts are usually asymptomatic but rarely produce symptoms related to hemorrhage, infection, or mass effect.[122-124] Infection of hepatic cysts in ADPCKD occurs more commonly after the development of end-stage renal disease (up to 3%).[125] Mass effect from cysts may cause inferior vena caval compression resulting in lower extremity edema or biliary compression with obstructive jaundice. Severe liver involvement may be complicated by liver failure or Budd-Chiari syndrome.[122]

Both intrahepatic and peribiliary cysts may be present in ADPCKD.[120,126] Intrahepatic cysts in ADPCKD have been attributed to cystic dilation of the Meyenburg complexes.[126] The peribiliary cysts are thought to arise from cystic dilation of the peribiliary glands of intrahepatic bile ducts.[126,127] Cystic dilation of these intrahepatic peribiliary glands occurs most commonly in ADPCKD and less often in patients with other hepatobiliary diseases. With severe liver disease, impaired intrahepatic hemodynamics may result in cystic dilation of the peribiliary glands, whereas in ascending cholangitis or septicemia, inflammatory destruction is the likely cause.[127] Hepatobiliary cysts are lined with cuboidal or columnar epithelium, contain serous fluid, and may be surrounded by a fibrous capsule.[107,122]

Hepatobiliary cyst size in ADPCKD may vary from less than 1 mm to greater than 10 cm.[120] Peribiliary cysts are defined as less than or equal to 10 mm.[120] On cross-sectional imaging, intrahepatic cysts of ADPCKD usually are round but may be polygonal or irregular when large cysts are densely distributed.[120] Peribiliary cysts are round, but multiple contiguous peribiliary cysts may appear as a tubular structure if the individual cyst walls are below the resolution of imaging and may mimic biliary dilation.[128,129] Peribiliary cysts are located along both sides of the portal triad, whereas dilated bile ducts are present on only one side.[130,131] Peribiliary cysts are present adjacent to the larger portal triads (up to third order), while intrahepatic cysts are located in the liver parenchyma and are not in contact with the larger portal triads.[120]

Uncomplicated hepatic cysts of ADPCKD have low T1 and high T2 SI and reveal no gadolinium

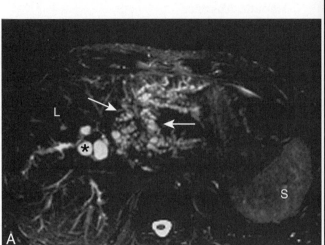
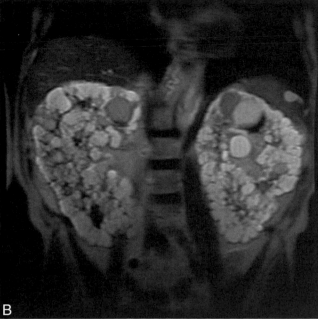

Figure 1-7 ■ MR demonstration of renal and peribiliary cysts in a man with autosomal-dominant polycystic kidney disease. A, Fat-suppressed heavily T2-WI shows larger cysts (*) and numerous smaller variably sized cysts *(arrows)* in a periportal distribution. **B**, Coronal T2-WI shows enlarged kidneys that contain numerous cysts, some of which contain hypointense hemorrhagic or proteinaceous fluid.

enhancement (Fig. 1-7).[122] Intracystic hemorrhage may result in cysts of varying SI including T1 hyperintensity, fluid-fluid levels, or thickened walls.[132] Asymptomatic hepatobiliary cysts of ADPCKD do not require treatment. Infected cysts require treatment that includes antibiotic therapy with or without percutaneous drainage.[125] Dominant cysts producing pain[133] or other complications due to mass effect may be treated with percutaneous drainage and sclerosis.[134,135]

Hepatic Cyst

Liver cysts are also thought to arise from cystic dilation of Meyenburg complexes.[126] Simple liver cysts are lined by cuboidal epithelium, surrounded by a thin fibrous stroma, and contain serous fluid.[26,122] Simple liver cysts have been detected sonographically in 2.5% of the population, are more common in women, and increase in incidence with age.[136] Simple liver cysts are more often multiple than solitary, measure between 1 and 5 cm, and are typically asymptomatic.[122,136] On MR uncomplicated hepatic cysts are homogeneously T1 hypointense and T2 hyperintense (see Figs. 1-7, 3-4, and 5-8). While cysts and hemangiomas may have similar SI on T2-WI with effective TEs of 160-180 ms, more heavily T2-WI with TEs in the range of 600-700 ms can effectively distinguish between the two; cysts show persistent marked hyperintensity, whereas hemangiomas do not.[8] Hepatic cysts do not enhance.[122] Cysts complicated by hemorrhage or infection may have variable T1 and T2 SIs and thickened walls.

INFLAMMATORY AND INFECTIOUS LIVER DISEASE

Inflammatory Myofibroblastic Tumor (Inflammatory Pseudotumor)

Inflammatory pseudotumor (IP)/inflammatory myofibroblastic tumor (IMT) is an uncommon mass composed of proliferating myofibroblasts and a lymphoplasmacytic infiltrate.[137] This lesion most commonly occurs in the lung but has been reported in virtually every organ of the body, including the liver.[138,139] The classification of this lesion continues to evolve. A subset of these lesions may represent, at least initially, a reactive pseudotumoral process to an infectious viral or bacterial agent.[137,138,140] Another distinct subset represents a true mesenchymal neoplasm of the myofibroblast, the inflammatory myofibroblastic tumor, and is considered synonymous with inflammatory fibrosarcoma.[137,138,141] Most cases of IMT occur in childhood and early adulthood.[138,139] Constitutional symptoms, present in 15% to 30% of cases, include fever and weight loss.[138] Hepatobiliary IMTs may present with abdominal pain or biliary obstruction. Laboratory abnormalities include anemia, thrombocytosis, leukocytosis, polyclonal hyperglobulinemia, and elevated erythrocyte sedimentation rate.[138]

Owing to the rarity of hepatic IMT, there are few reports of the MR imaging appearance, which is nonspecific.[142] IMT is hypointense to surrounding liver parenchyma on T1-WI and isointense to slightly hyperintense on T2-WI (Fig. 1-8).[143-149]

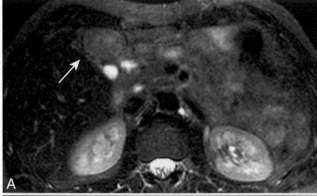
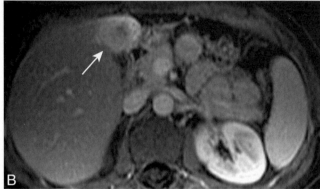
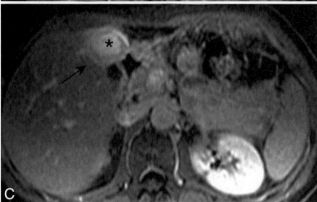

Figure 1-8 ■ MR findings of an inflammatory pseudo-tumor in a 50-year-old woman. A, Fat-suppressed T2-WI shows a hyperintense left lobe mass *(arrow)* with a small central area of higher SI. **B**, Portal venous phase CE T1-WI shows a peripheral rim of increased enhancement *(arrow)* and a central decreased enhancement. **C**, Delayed CE T1-WI shows peripheral washout of contrast *(arrow)* and increased central enhancement (∗). The progressive delayed enhancement reflects the fibrous content of the neoplasm. No other specific MR features are present, and surgery was required to establish the diagnosis.

The gadolinium-enhancement pattern is nonspecific, with peripheral, homogeneous, and heterogeneous patterns described.[144-146,148-150] If IMT is located in the hepatic hilum, biliary obstruction may occur and the clinical presentation and imaging studies may be similar to those of cholangiocarcinoma.[139,142,151-154] Although the prognosis generally is good and spontaneous resolution has been reported,[151,155] the neoplastic classification and potential malignant features of at least some of these lesions suggest that surgical resection is the treatment of choice when feasible.[138] IP of the spleen and IP of the bladder are discussed in Chapters 5 and 9, respectively.

Hepatic Abscess

Hepatic abscess, a collection of purulent material with associated destruction of hepatic parenchyma and stroma, may be bacterial, fungal, or amebic in etiology.[156-158] In developed countries, pyogenic abscesses are most common, but worldwide, amebic abscesses are most common.[157,158] Hepatic infection may occur through four pathways: portal veins, biliary ducts, hepatic arteries, or direct extension. Hepatic abscesses progress through three phases.[156] The acute phase occurs during approximately the first 10 days, with necrosis and small areas of lique-faction. From days 10 through 15, the subacute phase, there is progressive liquefaction with resorption of cellular debris. The chronic phase begins after day 15, when a thick, fibrous, peripheral wall envelops the central cavity containing a small amount of necrotic material.

PYOGENIC ABSCESS (BOX 1-9)

Currently, biliary tract infection is the most common cause of hepatic pyogenic abscesses.[97] Before the introduction of antibiotics, pylephlebitis complicating appendicitis or diverticulitis was the most common cause.[97,158] Approximately half of pyogenic abscesses are polymicrobial.[158,159] *Escherichia coli* is the most frequently isolated organism in adults.[97,157-159] *Bacteroides, Clostridium, Streptococcus faecalis, Klebsiella,* and *Staphylococcus aureus* may also be encountered.[97,157-159]

Pyogenic abscesses may be single but usually are multiple. Multiple pyogenic abscesses are more likely biliary in origin and single abscesses more likely cryptogenic in origin.[160] Single abscesses are larger than multiple abscesses.[160] Diabetes mellitus is present in up to half of patients with pyogenic abscess.[160] Clinical manifestations of pyogenic abscess include fever and chills, abdominal pain, abdominal tenderness, jaundice, and septic shock.[97,160] Pyogenic abscess may also present more insidiously with chronic abdominal pain and weight loss.[158,159] Laboratory abnormalities include leukocytosis, hypoalbuminemia, hyperbilirubinemia, elevated alkaline phosphatase and aspartase, and decreased hemoglobin.[97,160,161]

Pyogenic abscesses may be unilocular or multiseptate. The abscess cavity is typically hypointense to liver parenchyma on T1-WIs and hyperintense on T2-WIs (Fig. 1-9).[97,162,163] Small abscesses (less than 1.5 cm in diameter) are more conspicuous on T2- than T1-WIs.[163] The cluster sign refers to the grouping of multiple abscesses that may then coalesce into a single larger abscess.[164] This sign is considered suggestive of pyogenic abscesses, particularly those of biliary origin.[163,164] Perilesional edema, which may be circumferential or wedge-shaped, is

1-9   Pyogenic Hepatic Abscess

Clinical

Pathways of infection include biliary ducts (most common), portal veins, hepatic arteries, and direct extension
Presents with fever and chills, abdominal pain, jaundice, possible septic shock
Diabetes mellitus frequent comorbidity

Pathology

50% are polymicrobial; *E. coli* most frequently isolated organism in adults
Usually multiple abscesses
Three phases
Acute (first 10 days): necrosis, small areas of liquefaction
Subacute (days 10 to 15): progressive liquefaction and resorption of cellular debris
Chronic (after day 15): Thick fibrous wall envelops central necrotic cavity

MRI

T1-WI: hypointense to liver
T2-WI: hyperintense to liver and spleen and can have components that follow fluid
Cluster sign: coalescing of multiple small abscesses into single larger abscess
Perilesional edema: mildly T1 hypointense T1 and T2 hyperintense relative to liver
Dynamic CE imaging: abscess wall and septations show marked arterial phase enhancement that persists into
   the delayed phase

---

mildly hypointense to liver T1-WIs and mildly hyperintense on T2-WIs.[162,163] Perilesional edema is thought to reflect sinusoidal congestion due to the adjacent inflammation.[162]

After administration of gadolinium, the abscess wall shows marked arterial phase enhancement that persists on delayed imaging.[162,163] Septations will show a similar enhancement pattern.[97,162,163] Gadolinium increases the conspicuity of small abscesses.[162,163] Perilesional edema enhances on both arterial and delayed phase imaging.[162,163] Enhancement of the perilesional edema may be greater than that of the adjacent liver parenchyma but less than that of the abscess wall.[163] Wedge-shaped areas of arterial phase enhancement without concomitant abnormalities on unenhanced images have been attributed to inflammatory stenosis or occlusion of portal venules with compensatory increased hepatic arterial flow.[97,162,165,166]

Clinical and laboratory features help differentiate hepatic abscess from neoplastic lesions. Percutaneous drainage, along with antibiotics, has become a mainstay in the treatment of pyogenic hepatic abscesses with surgery reserved for treatment failure.[160,167,168] Multiple hepatic abscesses have a higher treatment failure rate than single hepatic abscesses with percutaneous aspiration and drainage.[160]

FUNGAL ABSCESSES (BOX 1-10)

Hepatic fungal abscesses develop most commonly in patients with neutropenia due to hematopoietic malignancies or intensive chemotherapy with or without bone marrow transplantation.[97,169-173] Hepatic fungal abscesses become clinically apparent as the neutrophil count recovers and an immune response is mounted.[172] The spleen is often concomitantly involved. Persistent fever after neutrophil recovery, despite coverage with broad spectrum antibiotics, may be the only clinical sign of hepatic abscesses, although abdominal pain, elevated liver function tests, and rebound leukocytosis may also be present.[172,174] *Candida albicans* is the most common fungal species causing hepatic abscesses.[170,172] Hematogenous dissemination of fungus may occur through bowel mucosa damaged by chemotherapy.[175]

1-10   Hepatosplenic Fungal Disease

Clinical

Develops in neutropenic patients (hematopoietic
   malignancies, intensive chemotherapy, bone marrow
   transplantation)
Manifests as neutrophil count recovers and immune
   response is mounted
Persistent fever despite broad-spectrum antibiotic
   coverage

Pathology

C. albicans most common fungal species
Route of infection: hematogenous dissemination
   of fungus through bowel damaged by chemotherapy

MRI

Multiple small (<1 cm) hepatic and splenic lesions
T1-WI: slightly hypointense to liver
T2-WI: markedly hyperintense to liver and mildly
   hyperintense to spleen (transfusional iron
   deposition, if present, increases abscess conspicuity)
CE: acute abscesses slightly hypointense and show
   perilesional enhancement

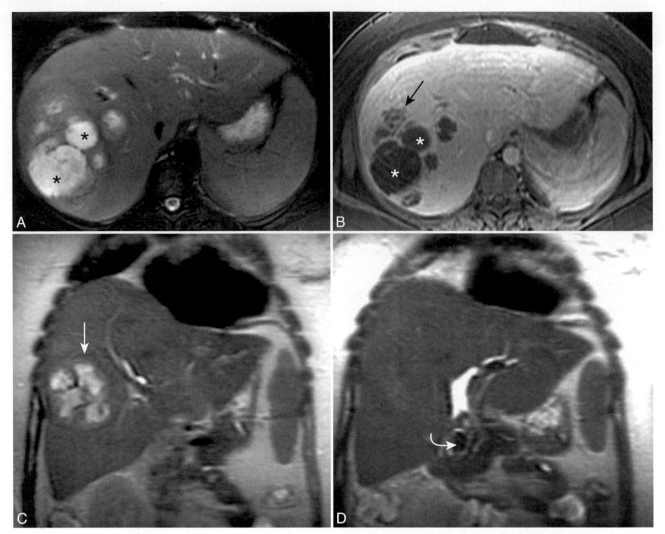

Figure 1-9 ■ **Multiple hepatic abscesses secondary to choledocholithiasis revealed by MRI and MRCP in a 37-year-old woman. A**, Fat-suppressed T2-WI shows multiple hyperintense hepatic masses (*). **B**, Delayed CE T1-WI shows rim enhancement of the multiple fluid-containing abscesses (*). The "cluster sign" of multiple coalescing small abscesses *(arrow)* is present adjacent to some of the larger lesions. **C** and **D**, Breath-hold coronal T2-WIs reveal a multi-locular hepatic abscess (**C**, *arrow*) and the contributory obstructing common bile duct calculus (**D**, *curved arrow*).

MR imaging has proved more sensitive than computed tomography or sonography for the detection of fungal hepatosplenic abscesses.[175,176] Fungal hepatosplenic abscesses are usually small (<1 cm) and diffusely distributed throughout the liver.[97,169] Fungal abscesses are slightly hypointense to liver on T1-WIs and markedly hyperintense on T2-WIs[169] (Fig. 1-10). Transfusional iron overload within the liver and spleen, common in the patient population susceptible to hepatosplenic fungal disease, increases the conspicuity of fungal abscesses on T2-WIs (see Fig. 1-10). On CE T1-WIs, acute fungal abscesses are slightly hypointense and usually do not show perilesional enhancement.[169]

A distinctive appearance of necrotizing fungal granulomas has been reported in leukemic patients with transfusional iron deposition during treatment with antimycotic medications.[177] Relative to liver, the lesions show mild central hyperintensity and a peripheral hypointense rim on T1-, T2-, and CE T1-WIs. Hemosiderin-laden macrophages in the periphery of the granulomas account for the hypointense ring.

MR imaging has shown very high sensitivity and specificity for the detection of acute hepatosplenic fungal disease and assumes an important role in the diagnosis.[169] Peripheral blood cultures are positive in only 50% of cases.[97] Absence of fungal organisms on liver biopsy and negative cultures of biopsy material do not exclude hepatic fungal abscesses.[97,172,178] Fever during neutrophil recovery is not specific for hepatosplenic fungal disease because extrahepatic infections and drug reactions may be responsible.[170]

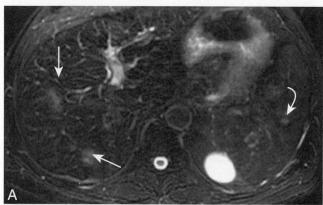

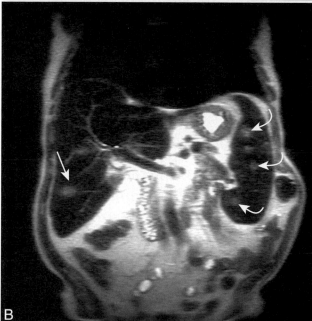

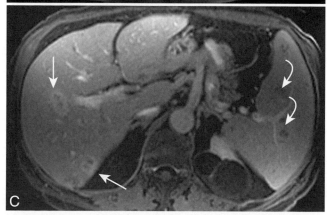

Figure 1-10 ▪ MR illustration of liver and splenic iron and multiple fungal abscesses in an immunosuppressed man with treated acute myelogenous leukemia. A and **B,** Axial fat-suppressed (**A**) and coronal (**B**) T2-WIs show multiple hyperintense lesions in the liver *(arrows)* and spleen *(curved arrows).* The liver and spleen are hypointense secondary to prior transfusions. **C,** Delayed CE T1-WI shows rim enhancement of some of the hepatic abscesses *(arrows)* and splenic *(curved arrows)* abscesses.

The MR differential diagnosis for hepatic fungal abscesses includes pyogenic abscesses, tuberculous abscesses, and metastases.[169,179] Hepatosplenic fungal disease is treated with antimycotic medical therapy.

AMEBIC ABSCESS

Amebic hepatic abscess is caused by the protozoan *Entamoeba histolytica.* This parasite colonizes the large bowel in approximately 12% of the world population.[180] Colonization occurs through ingestion of the infectious form of the parasite through contaminated water or food.[180] Only a small percentage of those colonized develop invasive amebiasis that presents clinically with intestinal or extraintestinal disease.[180]

Approximately one third of patients with amebic colitis will develop hepatic abscess that is the most common extraintestinal manifestation of amebiasis.[180,181] Amebic liver abscess is 10 times more common in men than in women.[182] The organisms infect the liver through the mesenteric and portal venous system.[180] Patients with amebic hepatic abscesses often present acutely with fever, right upper quadrant pain, leukocytosis, and elevated liver function tests.[180,183,184] Laboratory diagnosis can be established by light microscopy of stool or endoscopic biopsy specimens and serologic tests that identify amoeba-specific antigens or antibodies.[180,182]

On MR imaging, most amebic abscesses are well-circumscribed round or oval lesions. Amebic abscess is T1-hypointense and T2-hyperintense compared with surrounding liver.[185,186] The MR enhancement pattern of amebic hepatic abscesses is not well documented but has been reported to be similar to that of pyogenic abscesses.[97] MR imaging has been used to monitor the response to therapy.[185] Patients with hepatic amebic abscesses frequently have extrahepatic abnormalities such as right pleural effusion, perihepatic fluid collection, gastric or colonic involvement, and retroperitoneal extension.[187] Hepatic amebic abscesses are treated with amebicidal medications. Indications for percutaneous drainage include pyogenic superinfection and large, juxtacardiac abscesses that could potentially rupture into the pericardial space.[188]

HEPATIC TUBERCULOSIS

Tuberculosis is endemic in developing countries. An increase in tuberculosis in the West is largely related to the increased number of immunocompromised patients, predominantly due to AIDS.[97,189,190] *Mycobacterium tuberculosis* and *mycobacterium avium-intracellulare* are the two most commonly responsible organisms.[190] Mycobacteremia with granulomatous hepatitis has been reported after intravesical instillation of bacillus Calmette-Guérin for treatment of bladder carcinoma.[191]

The tubercle bacilli gain access to the liver through the hepatic artery, portal vein, or lymphatic system.[189] Hepatic tuberculosis has been classified into three forms.[189] The miliary form occurs during the course of generalized miliary tuberculosis typically without signs or symptoms referable to the liver. Tuberculous (granulomatous) hepatitis may result in unexplained fever, jaundice, and hepatomegaly. Localized hepatic tuberculosis, with signs and symptoms referable to the liver, may occur with or without biliary involvement. Hepatic parenchymal manifestations include solitary or multiple nodules, tuberculoma, or tuberculous hepatic abscess. Obstructive jaundice may result from compressive lymphadenopathy or inflammatory strictures due to tuberculous involvement of the biliary ductal epithelium.

The presence of caseating granulomas on liver biopsy is usually diagnostic for tuberculosis but is not invariably present.[189] If noncaseating granulomas are found, a positive acid-fast bacillus test or culture is necessary for confirmation but frequently these tests are negative.[189] The polymerase chain reaction (PCR) assay for detection of *M. tuberculosis* in liver biopsy specimens has increased the diagnostic yield over AFB and cultures.[192]

There are few reports describing the MR imaging appearance of hepatic tuberculomas, and the results are nonspecific.[193] With granulomatous hepatitis due to tuberculosis, numerous small lesions may be seen and are of low SI on T1-WIs and intermediate SI on T2-WIs and typically lack enhancement.[194] The differential diagnosis for the solitary macronodular tuberculoma or tuberculous abscess includes pyogenic or amebic abscess, necrotic tumors such as metastases or hepatocellular carcinoma, and lymphoma.[158,195,196] The differential diagnosis of miliary tuberculosis/granulomatous hepatitis includes metastases, fungal or bacterial microabscesses, sarcoidosis, and lymphoma.[197,198] Hepatic tuberculosis is treated medically, although tuberculous abscesses may be percutaneously drained.

HYDATID DISEASE

Hydatid disease is caused by infection with the larval form of *Echinococcus* tapeworms with *E. granulosus* being the most common and *E. multilocularis* much less common.[97,158,199,200] *E. granulosus*, which causes the unilocular form of hydatid disease, is endemic in sheep grazing regions of Mediterranean countries, Africa, South America, the Middle East, Australia, and New Zealand.[97,158,199,200] The definitive host of *E. granulosus* is the dog, and the intermediate host is most commonly sheep.[158,199,200] The human is an accidental intermediate host, becoming infected through contact with dogs or ingestion of contaminated water or food.[97,199,200] Infected patients are typically asymptomatic for years until the lesions produce mass effect, rupture, or become superinfected.[97,158,199,200] Rupture communicating with the vascular system may result in anaphylaxis.[199,200]

E. granulosus may infect any organ in the human body, but the liver is the most commonly involved site as the ingested embryos pass through the intestinal wall and travel to the liver via the portal venous system.[97,158,199,200] The hydatid cyst is composed of three layers. The inner germinal layer, or endocyst, produces the scolices (larval parasite) and daughter cysts as well as the surrounding laminated membrane.[97,158,199,200] The middle layer, the acellular laminated membrane, or ectocyst, allows passage of nutrients into the endocyst.[97,158,199,200] The outer layer, or pericyst, is produced by modified host cells that form a dense, fibrous protective zone.[97,158,199,200]

The MR imaging appearance of hydatid cysts is variable depending on the stage of the lesion and the presence of complications. The cyst wall and cyst contents of simple viable hydatid cysts are hypointense to liver on T1-WI.[98,158,200-202] On T2-WIs, the cyst fluid is hyperintense and the rim is hypointense to liver.[98,158,200-202] Daughter cysts are additional cysts attached to the germinal layer of the mother cyst and indicate early degeneration.[200] CE T1-WIs may or may not show enhancement of the cyst wall.[98] Liver abscesses secondary to *E. multilocularis* ("alveolar echinococcosis") shows multiple liver cysts with small amounts of associated enhancing solid components.[203]

The differential diagnosis of cystic echinococcosis includes other cystic lesions such as simple liver cyst, biliary cystadenoma/cystadenocarcinoma, pyogenic abscess, and cystic metastases. Traditionally, surgical resection has been the first line of treatment for hydatid disease. More recently, percutaneous techniques, combined with medication, have been used successfully in selected cases.[200,204,205]

Hepatic Sarcoidosis

Sarcoidosis is a systemic granulomatous disease of unknown etiology. After lymph nodes and lung, the liver is the most commonly involved organ.[206] Most patients with hepatic sarcoidosis show minimal clinical or laboratory findings of liver disease but rarely will develop cirrhosis, portal hypertension, or cholestasis.[206-208] The noncaseating granulomas are diffusely scattered throughout the liver parenchyma but may become confluent and result in scarring.[206,209] The granulomas are often more numerous in the periportal regions or portal tracts.[206,209] Granulomatous phlebitis of the portal veins and hepatic veins may lead to ischemia with resultant parenchymal fibrosis, cirrhosis, and portal hypertension.[206,207,209] Chronic cholestasis with progression to biliary cirrhosis may be the result of fibrosis-related ductopenia.[206] Biliary obstruction may also result from compressive hilar lymphadenopathy.

In nearly one third of patients with abdominal sarcoidosis, lymphadenopathy is present, with the porta hepatis, para-aortic, and celiac regions most often involved.[210] Hepatomegaly is present in one third of affected patients.[208] On MR imaging, hepatic nodules are typically small (2 to 15 mm) and revealed in approximately 5% to 15% of patients.[208,211,212] The nodules are isointense or slightly hypointense to liver on T1-WI and hypointense on T2-WI and show hypoenhancement on CE T1-WIs.[194,211,212] Splenic involvement by sarcoidosis is discussed in Chapter 5.

Radiation-induced Liver Disease

Radiation-induced hepatic injury may be due to inclusion of the liver in the treatment portal for extrahepatic malignancy, directed therapy for hepato-biliary malignancy, or total body irradiation in preparation for bone marrow transplantation. Histologically, radiation-induced hepatic injury is a veno-occlusive process of the centrilobular and lobular veins.[213,214] Dose-volume effects and the con-comitant use of chemotherapy are the two factors that are thought to affect the development of radiation-induced liver disease in patients with normal baseline liver function.[214]

Patients with partial liver irradiation may be asymptomatic.[213] Clinical manifestations of radiation-induced liver disease will typically become evident between 2 weeks and 4 months after completion of treatment and may include fatigue, right upper quadrant pain, ascites, hepatomegaly, and elevated alkaline phosphatase.[214] On MR imaging, areas of acute irradiation-induced injury will usually be hypointense to nonirradiated liver on T1-WIs and hyperintense on T2-WIs, reflecting edema.[215-217] Partial radiation-induced liver injury will show a sharp demarcation corresponding to the treatment portal.[217] Acute and chronic radiation injury may manifest as an area of fat sparing in an otherwise steatotic liver (Fig. 1-11).[218,219] Delayed enhancement of irradiated liver greater than that of nonirradiated liver has been attributed to decreased clearance of blood from occluded central veins in the irradiated area (see Fig. 1-11).[215]

Primary Sclerosing Cholangitis

Primary sclerosing cholangitis (PSC) is a chronic cholestatic liver disease of unknown etiology.[220] PSC is characterized by progressive inflammation, destruction and fibrosis of intrahepatic and extra-hepatic bile ducts resulting in secondary biliary cirrhosis, portal hypertension, and liver failure.[220] Diagnosis of PSC is based on clinical history, labora-tory and histologic data, and cholangiography. The biliary manifestations of PSC are fully discussed in Chapter 2. The hepatic parenchymal MR findings of PSC are reviewed here.

Approximately 75% of patients with PSC have inflammatory bowel disease, and of these patients, 80% to 90% have ulcerative colitis and 10% to 20% have Crohn's disease.[220] PSC is often asymptomatic in the early stages. Symptoms of pruritus, fatigue, jaundice, and weight loss indicate advanced disease.[220] Laboratory abnormalities may include early elevation of alkaline phosphatase and γ-glutamyltransferase and later increase in the bilirubin and/or decrease in serum albumin.[220] The characteristic pathologic find-ing in PSC, the "onionskin" pattern of periductal fibrosis around medium or large bile ducts, often cannot be identified on peripheral percutaneous biopsies that may show nonspecific portal tract inflammation and fibrosis.[220-221] The cholangio-graphic findings of multiple strictures, mural

irregularities, and diverticula of the intrahepatic and extrahepatic bile ducts are critical in establish-ing the diagnosis of PSC. Approximately 9% to 15% of patients with PSC develop cholangiocarcinoma.[220]

Several hepatic parenchymal abnormalities have been reported on MR in patients with PSC. Parenchymal changes are thought to be due to extension of the biliary inflammation into the parenchyma, retention of bile salts, and accumulation of copper in liver cells.[222] Peripherally distributed wedge-shaped areas of T2 hyperintensity may be present.[222] The periductal inflammation that obstructs the segmental bile ducts also involves the associated portal venules and lymphatics and is thought to result in the above-mentioned wedge-shaped edema with eventual segmental atrophy and scarring.[222] Periportal edema manifested as high T2 SI along the porta hepatis is a common but nonspecific finding in patients with PSC.[222,223] Less commonly present in PSC are areas of hyperintensity on T1-WI.[223] Biliary ductal dilation may be present in these areas, and the increased T1-weighted SI has been attributed to cholestasis and lipofuscin deposits in atrophic hepatocytes.[223-225]

Patchy, peripheral, or segmental areas of increased enhancement relative to adjacent liver parenchyma are seen on both arterial and delayed-phase images in approximately half of PSC patients.[223] The increased arterial phase enhancement may be due to the inflammation or a compensatory response to decreased portal venous flow.[223] The increased delayed-phase enhancement has been attributed to the hepatic fibrosis and atrophy.[223]

Hepatic morphologic changes in PSC-induced end-stage cirrhosis may be different from those seen in cirrhosis due to other etiologies.[226] The liver shows a lobular contour and is markedly deformed.[226] Caudate lobe hypertrophy is present in almost all cir-rhotic patients with PSC but in only 30% to 40% of patients with cirrhosis of other etiologies (Fig. 1-12).[226] The right main and left hepatic ducts are usually the most severely involved in PSC. The caudate ducts that drain just proximal to the ductal confluence may be relatively unobstructed, thus encouraging compensatory hypertrophy of the caudate lobe.[226] The lateral segment (frequently hypertrophied in cirrhosis due to other causes) and the posterior seg-ment are often atrophied.[223,226] Biliary dilation, biliary calculi, and regenerative nodules greater than 3 cm are also more common in PSC-induced cirrho-sis than in cirrhosis of other causes.[227]

HEPATIC HEMANGIOMA (BOX 1-11)

Cavernous hemangioma is the most common benign hepatic tumor. The reported incidence varies from 0.4% to 20% depending on the method of detection.[26] Most hemangiomas are small, asymptomatic, and incidentally detected at imaging or autopsy.[228-230] Most symptomatic hemangiomas are large lesions that may result in pain.[229,231] Rare rupture of

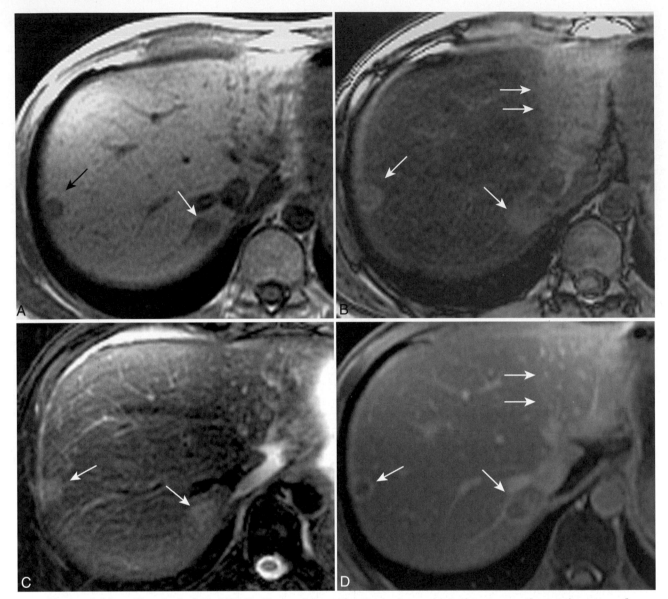

Figure 1-11 ■ **Chemical shift MR findings of hepatic steatosis, metastatic pancreatic carcinoma and radiation-induced liver disease. A,** In-phase T1-WI shows two hypointense metastases *(arrows)*. **B,** Opposed-phase T1-WI shows decreased SI of the right lobe representing hepatic steatosis. There is sparing of steatosis of the left lobe delimited by a straight edge *(double arrows)* that conforms to the radiation portal. The metastases are now hyperintense *(arrows)* relative to the hypointense steatotic liver. **C,** Fat-suppressed T2-WI shows hyperintense metastases *(arrows)* relative to liver. **D,** Delayed fat suppressed CE T1-WI shows rim-enhancing metastases *(arrows)*. The increased enhancement in the irradiated hepatic parenchyma is due to fibrosis and venous out-flow obstruction.

larger hemangiomas may occur spontaneously or following percutaneous biopsy or blunt abdominal trauma.[232]

Histologically, cavernous hemangioma is a well-circumscribed mass of blood-filled spaces lined by endothelium on thin, fibrous stroma.[25,26] Arterial branches and small bile ducts may be present in larger septa.[26] Arterial-portal shunts may occur.[26] Thrombi, calcification, fibrosis, and scarring are variably present.[25,26] Most hemangiomas are solitary and peripherally located.[26] Size range varies from a

few millimeters to greater than 20 cm,[26] with most measuring less than 5 cm.[25] Most hemangiomas remain stable in size, but interval growth of a minority of hemangiomas has been documented on serial imaging.[233]

On MR hemangiomas are well-circumscribed round or lobular lesions.[234,235] Hemangiomas are homogeneously hypointense to liver on T1-WIs and homogeneously hyperintense to liver parenchyma on T2-WIs (Figs. 1-13 and 1-14; see Fig. 1-3).[234-236] This hyperintensity persists on more heavily T2-WIs

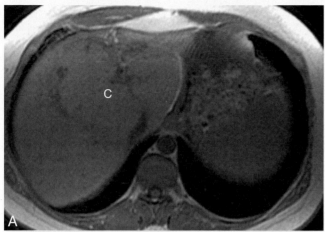

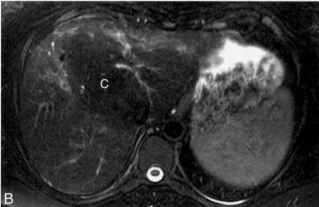

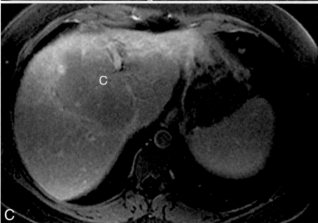

Figure 1-12 ■ MR depiction of cirrhosis with caudate lobe hypertrophy due to primary sclerosing cholangitis. **A** and **B**, In-phase T1 (**A**) and fat-suppressed T2-WI (**B**) show marked hypertrophy of the caudate lobe (C) that has relative T2 hypointensity compared with the remainder of the liver. **C**, Delayed CE T1-WI shows hyperintense peripheral liver parenchyma compared to more normal central SI within the caudate lobe (C) secondary to "hepatic atelectasis." The delayed enhancement can be secondary to either fibrosis or venous outflow obstruction. Caudate lobe hypertrophy is present more commonly in end-stage liver disease due to primary sclerosing cholangitis and Budd-Chiari syndrome compared with other etiologies.

1-11 Hemangioma

Clinical
Most common benign hepatic tumor
Almost always asymptomatic and incidentally detected

Pathology
Blood-filled spaces lined by endothelium on thin
    fibrous stroma
Size varies from a few millimeters to >20 cm;
    most <5 cm

MRI
T1-WI: hypointense to liver
T2-WI: markedly hyperintense to liver, hyperintense
    to spleen
Heavily T2-WI: hyperintense to liver and spleen,
    hypointense to CSF
Dynamic CE imaging: three patterns
    Immediate uniform hyperenhancement (typically
        smaller lesions)
    Peripheral nodular with centripetal progression to
        uniform enhancement (most common pattern)
    Peripheral nodular with centripetal progression but
        persistent central hypointensity (larger
        hemangiomas with nonenhancing central scar)

obtained with long echo times (>160 ms).[7,237] The long T2-relaxation time of hemangiomas allows differentiation from metastases in most cases.[7,237] The T2-relaxation time of hemangiomas is inversely proportional to the number of endothelial cells within the mass and proportional to the collective size of the vascular spaces that contain slowly flowing blood.[235]

Giant hemangiomas, defined as lesions greater than 6 cm in at least one dimension, show heterogeneous SI on T1- and T2-WI with internal cleft such as areas and septa (see Fig. 1-14).[231] The heterogeneous SI of these lesions has been attributed to the presence of hemorrhage, thrombosis, hyalinization, liquefaction, and myxoid degeneration.[231,238,239] The cleft-like areas are thought to represent cystic degeneration or myxoid change.[231,238] Round/oval, linear, or irregularly shaped internal cleft-like areas are hypointense to the main tumor on T1-WIs.[231] On T2-WIs, the main part of the tumor is hyperintense to liver parenchyma.[231] Internal septa appear as low SI on T2-WIs.[231] Hepatic capsular retraction adjacent to giant or large hemangiomas is related to intratumoral fibrosis.[240-242]

On dynamic gadolinium-enhanced MR imaging, three enhancement patterns have been described: immediate uniform enhancement (pattern 1), peripheral enhancement with centripetal progression to uniform enhancement (pattern 2; see Figs. 1-3 and 1-13), and peripheral nodular enhancement

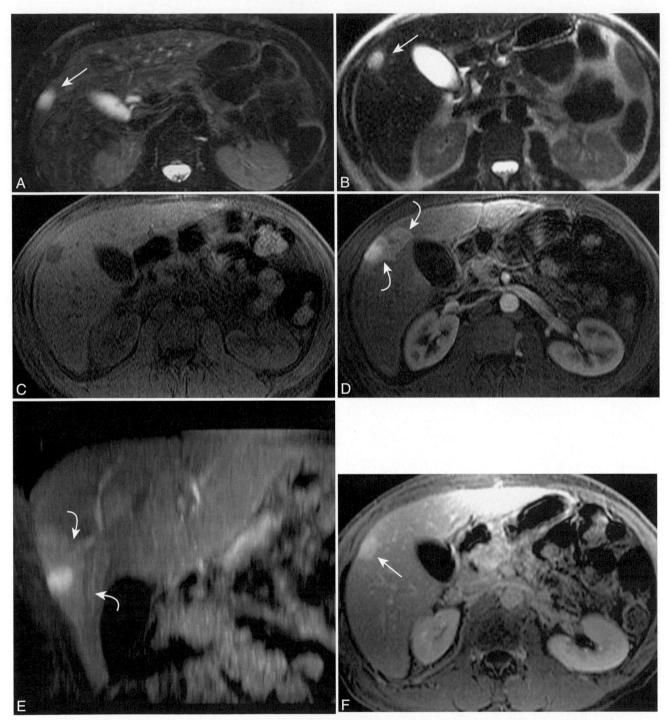

Figure 1-13 ▪ MR illustration of hepatic hemangioma with temporal peritumoral enhancement. A and **B,** Fat-suppressed T2 (**A**) and heavily T2-WIs (**B**) show a subcapsular liver mass *(arrow)* that is markedly hyperintense to liver parenchyma and almost isointense to bile within the gallbladder and cerebrospinal fluid. **C** and **D,** Fat-suppressed T1-WIs obtained before (**C**) and after (**D**) dynamic CE show marked hypervascularity of the hemangioma with a geographic region of increased enhancement in the surrounding liver *(curved arrows)*. **E,** Coronal reformatted arterial phase CE T1-WI reveals the wedge shape of the peritumoral enhancement *(curved arrows)*. **F,** Delayed CE T1-WI shows persistent enhancement of the hemangioma *(arrow)*. The peritumoral region of arterial enhancement is now isointense with liver.

and isointense to subcutaneous or retroperitoneal fat on T1-WIs and lose SI on fat-suppressed images.[266-271] Regions or lesions with minimal or no fat will be hypointense to liver on T1-WIs.[267,268,272] Intratumoral foci that contain both adipocytes and nonfatty tissue are better characterized with chemical shift (in-phase and opposed-phase) imaging. AMLs composed predominantly of fat will appear similar to lipomas at MR imaging and even at pathology, requiring careful search for smooth muscle cells.[273] AMLs can also be completely devoid of fat on MR imaging and histopathologic studies.[271] AMLs appear heterogeneous and are hyperintense to liver on T2-WIs.[263,266,267,269-272,274,275] Hepatic AML shows variable enhancement that correlates with tumor vascularity.[266,272,274,275] The MR imaging differential diagnosis of hepatic AML includes other fat containing hepatic masses: lipomas, focal steatosis, hepatocellular adenoma, hepatocellular carcinoma, metastases from fat-containing neoplasms such as liposarcoma or teratocarcinoma, and pseudomasses such as omental fat-packing, pseudolipoma of Glisson's capsule, and diaphragmatic indentation.[267,276] AMLs with minimal fat content may mimic hepatocellular carcinoma on MR imaging, and biopsy would be necessary to avoid surgical resection.[274] Larger lesions, such as those occurring in the kidney, may hemorrhage.

HEPATIC LIPOMA AND PSEUDOLIPOMA

True hepatic lipomas are rare nonencapsulated masses, composed entirely of mature adipose tissue (lipocytes), and are to be differentiated from focal hepatic steatosis and pseudolipoma of Glisson's capsule as well as other fat-containing lesions.[277,278] On MR imaging, lipomas follow the SI of fat on all pulse sequences and should not enhance.[278] Pseudolipoma of Glisson's capsule represents an entrapped and detached epiploic appendage in the hepatodiaphragmatic space.[279,280] As opposed to a true lipoma that is surrounded by hepatic parenchyma and located deep within the liver parenchyma, pseudolipoma of Glisson's capsule lies on the surface of the liver.[280]

HEPATIC LYMPHOMA

Lymphoma may involve the liver secondarily in patients with Hodgkin's disease or non-Hodgkin's lymphoma. Primary lymphoma of the liver is exceedingly rare. It has been reported in association with AIDS, chronic hepatitis C infection, primary biliary cirrhosis, and other immune system disorders.[281-285]

The liver also may be a primary or secondary site of post-transplant lymphoproliferative disorder. Identifying secondary hepatic lymphomatous involvement is important for staging and treatment.[286] In a series evaluating laparoscopic liver biopsy during the initial staging of lymphoma, hepatic involvement was identified in 8% of patients with Hodgkin's disease and 25% of those with non-Hodgkin's lymphoma.[286] At autopsy approximately half of patients with either type of lymphoma have liver disease.[206]

Hepatic involvement by Hodgkin's disease may result in fever, hepatomegaly, jaundice.[206] Identification of Reed-Sternberg cells is required for definitive histologic diagnosis. Hepatic infiltration by Hodgkin's disease almost always involves the portal tracts.[206] Diffusely distributed, uniformly small nodules, larger masses, or a combination of the two may be identified pathologically.[206]

In non-Hodgkin's lymphoma the liver is the most common site after lymph nodes, spleen, and bone marrow and may occur with either B- or T-cell lymphomas.[206] Hepatomegaly is almost always present.[206] In low-grade B-cell lymphoma, multiple small nodular tumor deposits are found in the portal tracts with variable sinusoidal penetration.[287] In high grade B-cell lymphoma, large, irregular, destructive lesions are found in the portal tracts and parenchyma (Fig. 2-23, pancreatic lymphoma).[287] MR imaging findings of secondary hepatic lymphomatous involvement are nonspecific and include single or multiple focal masses, infiltrative lesions, abnormal parenchymal SI, and hepatomegaly.[288-290]

Post-transplant Lymphoproliferative Disorder

Post-transplant lymphoproliferative disorder (PTLD) comprises a clinicopathologic spectrum of hyperplastic and neoplastic lymphoid diseases that occur in immunosuppressed transplant patients, most of whom have been infected with Epstein-Barr virus (EBV) either before or during transplantation.[291,292] Epstein-Barr virus–related PTLD arising within liver allografts occurs 4 to 12 months following transplantation.[293] PTLD spans from a reactive plasmacytic hyperplasia (similar to infectious mononucleosis) to polymorphic to monomorphic forms.[294] The polymorphic form is unique to immunocompromised patients.[294] The monomorphic form is similar to lymphoma occurring in immunocompetent patients. Most cases of PTLD are B-cell proliferations.[279] PTLD mainly infiltrates the portal tracts but may involve the hepatic parenchyma.[279]

Clinically, PTLD may manifest with an infectious mononucleosis–like syndrome, generalized lymphadenopathy with or without a mononucleosis syndrome, lymphoid tumors, or a fulminant disseminated syndrome that often includes sepsis.[291] In addition to lymph nodes, frequently involved sites are the gastrointestinal tract, central nervous system, lungs, and allograft organ.[291] The liver is the most commonly involved organ in patients with abdominal disease.[295]

Hepatic involvement in PTLD may manifest as solitary or multiple masses or diffusely infiltrative disease.[295-297] PTLD in liver transplant patients may present with periportal or porta hepatis masses with potential compromise of biliary or vascular structures.[293,298] The infectious mononucleosis and polymorphic forms of PTLD often respond to reduced immunosuppression and antiviral agents, whereas the monomorphic form or true lymphoma often requires chemotherapy and/or radiotherapy.[291]

HEPATIC METASTASES (BOX 1-12)

Metastases are the most common malignant lesion of the liver. After lymph nodes, the liver is the most common site of metastatic disease.[26] Tumor cells reach the liver through the hepatic artery, portal circulation, lymphatics, or rarely peritoneal fluid.[26] Once established, metastatic lesions are supplied by the hepatic artery, although hypovascular metastases, especially lesions smaller than 1.5 cm, may be partially supplied by the portal venous system.[26,299-303] The liver has a dual blood supply, but this factor alone does not account for its susceptibility to metastatic disease.[304] The fenestrated endothelial lining of the sinusoids allows communication with the extracellular space of Disse.[305,306] Local humoral factors may also contribute to this susceptibility.[305]

Detection of hepatic metastases is critical for staging and treatment, particularly for colorectal carcinoma, because surgical resection may prolong survival.[307-309] Metastases must not only be detected but also differentiated from benign hepatic lesions. Benign hepatic masses are common; in an autopsy series, benign hepatic masses or mass-like lesions were seen in 52%.[310] Even in oncologic patients, hepatic lesions measuring 1 cm or smaller were benign in 80%.[311] In patients with breast cancer referred to MR for suspected metastases (on the basis of other imaging studies or liver enzyme abnormalities), 32% had benign hepatic lesions.[312] MR has proved more accurate than dual- or single-phase CT for discriminating between benign and malignant hepatic lesions.[313,314] The variable conspicuity of hepatic metastases on T1- and T2-WIs and on the different phases of a dynamic CE T1-WI underscores the need for a comprehensive MR imaging examination for optimal detection and characterization.

Generally, hepatic metastases are moderately hypointense to liver parenchyma on unenhanced T1-WIs and moderately hyperintense on T2-WIs (Fig. 1-16; see Figs. 1-11, 5-1, 5-2, and 5-7).[239,315,316] The similar SI of hepatic metastases and normal splenic parenchyma on conventional SE pulse sequences has been termed the spleen-liver model and has been used to optimize contrast-to-noise ratios for improved metastatic lesion detection.[317] Significant differences, however, between liver-metastasis and liver-spleen contrast-to-noise ratios on newer, more complex, pulse sequences require that the spleen-liver model be proved for each new sequence.[317]

Although most metastases are hypointense to liver parenchyma on T1-WIs, some are hyperintense. Metastases may appear hyperintense on unenhanced T1-WIs because of intralesional substances with a short T1 relaxation time or because of relatively decreased SI of the surrounding liver parenchyma.[318] Substances that have a short T1 relaxation time or produce T1 shortening within metastases include hemorrhage, protein, mucin, melanin, fat, and Lipiodol.[318-320] Hemorrhagic hepatic metastases occur most commonly with lung carcinoma, renal carcinoma, testicular carcinoma, and melanoma (Fig. 1-17; see Fig. 5-1).[29] Hepatic metastases with high protein synthesis may be present in multiple myeloma and carcinoid.[319] Mucin produced by cystic metastases of pancreatic or ovarian mucinous neoplasms can result in hyperintense lesions.[318,319]

1-12 Hepatic Metastases

Clinical

Most common malignant lesion of the liver
High incidence of benign hepatic lesions requires accurate discrimination from metastases

Pathology

Reflect primary tumor
Most supplied by hepatic artery

MRI

T1-WI: hypointense to liver (hemorrhagic metastases may be hyperintense)
T2-WI: solid lesions hyperintense to liver, isointense to spleen (hypervascular or mucinous metastatic lesions may appear similar to benign, fluid-filled lesions on moderately or even heavily T2-WI; CE imaging is usually discriminatory)
Dynamic CE imaging
    Hypervascular metastases (e.g., breast, carcinoid, melanoma, thyroid, renal, sarcomas) best revealed on arterial-phase images with uniform peripheral rim or heterogeneous enhancement
    Hypovascular metastases (e.g., colon, lung, prostate, gastric, transitional cell) best shown on portal venous phase images when enhancement of the liver parenchyma is greatest
    Isovascular metastases (rare, e.g., colon, thyroid, endometrial) may be inconspicuous on arterial and portal venous phase images but usually detected on unenhanced T1 or T2-WI

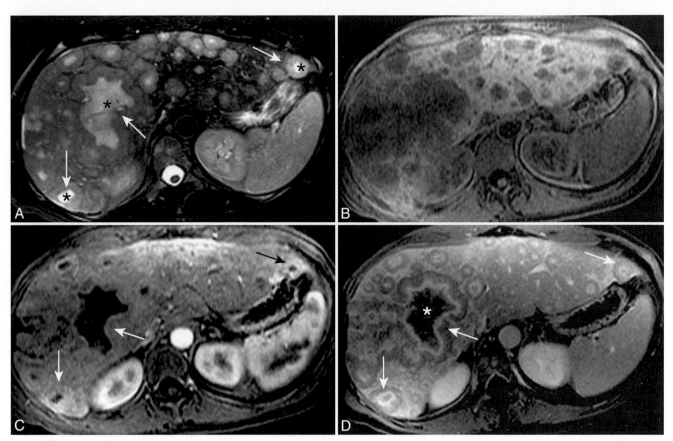

Figure 1-16 ■ MR demonstration of unresectable metastatic breast cancer. A, Fat-suppressed T2-WI shows multiple variably sized hepatic masses. The metastases have a peripheral rim *(arrows)* that is hyperintense to liver parenchyma and nearly isointense to spleen. The central portions of some of the masses are hyperintense (*) to the tumor periphery owing to the presence of necrosis or immature fibrosis. **B** and **C,** Fat-suppressed T1-WI obtained before **(B)** and after **(C)** dynamic CE show peripheral hypervascular rim enhancement *(arrows).* **D,** Delayed CE T1-WI shows the peripheral washout sign; the peripheral portions of the metastases *(arrows)* are now hypointense to liver parenchyma. Some metastases show delayed central enhancement likely due to the presence of fibrosis. The central T2 hyperintense portions of some lesions (*) do not enhance, in keeping with liquefactive necrosis or cyst formation.

Melanoma metastases may be hyperintense due to melanin, a paramagnetic substance, or hemorrhage.[318,319,321] Fat within metastases is rare but could occur with extrahepatic liposarcoma or ovarian teratoma primary lesions (Fig. 1-18).[276,322]

Hepatic metastases may also appear hyperintense on unenhanced T1-WIs owing to decreased SI of the surrounding liver parenchyma.[318] Iron overload may decrease the hepatic parenchymal SI on both T1- and T2-WIs owing to shortening of the T2 relaxation time. Hepatic edema increases the T1 relaxation time of liver. In the presence of diffuse steatosis (which results in loss of hepatic parenchymal SI on opposed-phase gradient echo images), metastases may appear isointense or hyperintense to surrounding liver parenchyma (see Fig. 1-11).[323]

On T2-WIs, hepatic metastases are hyperintense to liver, but less so than hemangiomas or cysts, and this difference is accentuated on heavily T2-WIs with a TE greater than 160 ms (see Figs. 1-11, 1-16, 5-1, and 5-7). Metastases from certain hypervascular or mucinous malignancies can appear similar to benign fluid-filled lesions on moderately T2-WIs (Fig. 1-19). Hypervascular metastases that can appear cystic or markedly hyperintense on T2-WIs include those from islet cell or neuroendocrine tumors, sarcomas, and melanoma. Factors other than hypervascularity, including interstitial water content, venous lakes, peliotic change, or fluid-filled acini, may be responsible for the T2 hyperintensity of these metastases.[237] Mucinous metastases may arise from ovarian, pancreatic, or colon primaries. Some hypovascular metastases may be inconspicuous on T2-WI and are best detected on unenhanced or CE T1-WI.[324] In the setting of hepatic steatosis, metastases may appear hypointense to surrounding liver parenchyma on fast spin echo (FSE) T2-WIs if fat suppression is not used.[325] Fat is of higher SI on FSE than SE T2-WI.[326] Wedge-shaped areas of increased SI on T2-WIs can be present peripheral to both malignant and benign hepatic masses and are likely due to edema/sinusoidal congestion.[327,328] These wedge-shaped

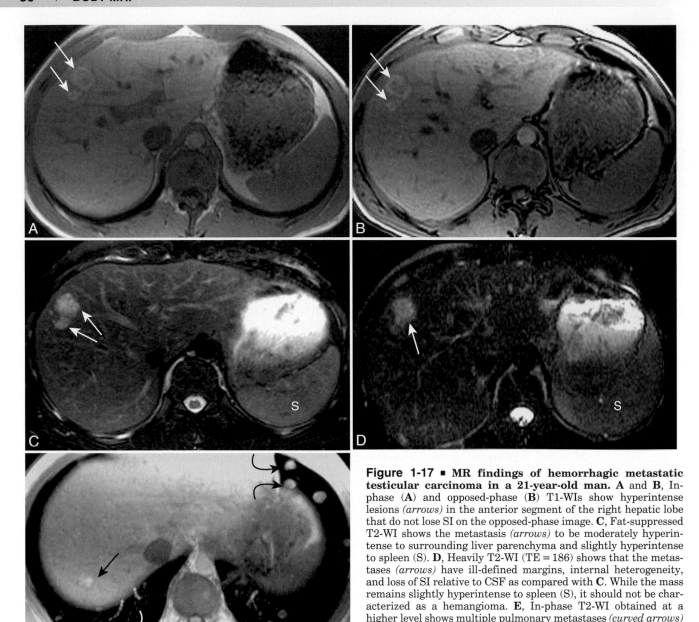

Figure 1-17 ■ MR findings of hemorrhagic metastatic testicular carcinoma in a 21-year-old man. A and **B**, In-phase (**A**) and opposed-phase (**B**) T1-WIs show hyperintense lesions *(arrows)* in the anterior segment of the right hepatic lobe that do not lose SI on the opposed-phase image. **C**, Fat-suppressed T2-WI shows the metastasis *(arrows)* to be moderately hyperintense to surrounding liver parenchyma and slightly hyperintense to spleen (S). **D**, Heavily T2-WI (TE = 186) shows that the metastases *(arrows)* have ill-defined margins, internal heterogeneity, and loss of SI relative to CSF as compared with **C**. While the mass remains slightly hyperintense to spleen (S), it should not be characterized as a hemangioma. **E**, In-phase T2-WI obtained at a higher level shows multiple pulmonary metastases *(curved arrows)* and additional metastases of the liver dome *(arrow)*.

areas may be predictive of developing or growing metastases at the apex in patients with primary tumors.[327]

Nearly half of hepatic metastases from colorectal carcinoma will show central areas of low T2 SI, particularly in larger lesions.[329] On T1-WIs, these lesions appear uniformly hypointense to liver parenchyma. Histologically, this central hypointensity corresponds to areas of desmoplastic stroma, coagulative necrosis, and mucin accumulation. The peripheral halos of T2 hyperintensity present in colorectal metastases do not reflect peritumoral edema but rather the tumor margin and variable tumor necrosis. A low T2 SI rim surrounding the metastasis corresponds to compression of hepatic

parenchyma and sinusoids, hepatocellular atrophy, and fibrosis. Some large colorectal metastases will show central areas of very high T2 SI with corresponding very low T1 SI secondary to liquefactive necrosis.

Hepatic metastases are classified into hypervascular, hypovascular, and isovascular patterns on dynamic gadolinium-enhanced MR imaging.[14,239,323] Hypervascular metastases are most easily detected on arterial-phase images and may only be detected on this phase. Arterial-phase enhancement of hypervascular metastases may be uniform, peripheral rim, or heterogeneous. The minimal enhancement of liver parenchyma during the arterial phase of enhancement increases the conspicuity of arterially

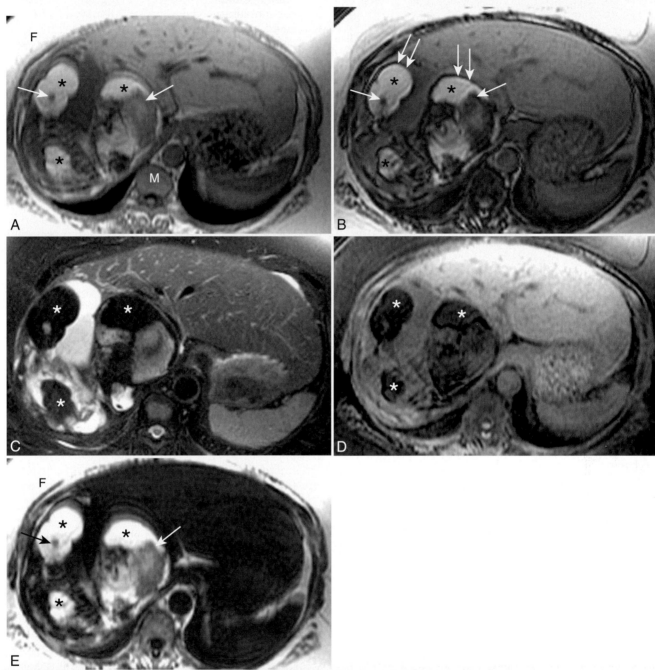

Figure 1-18 ▪ Chemical shift and fat-suppressed MR findings of lipid-containing hepatic metastases from metastatic ovarian teratoma. A, In-phase T1-WI shows multiple liver masses containing foci (*) isointense to subcutaneous fat (F). Cystic components are hypointense. Other portions of the mass have intermediate SI *(arrows)*. **B,** Opposed-phase T1-WI shows the etching artifact *(double arrows)* at the boundary between the high SI fatty components (*) and adjacent liver. Intratumoral foci that contain both lipid and water protons lose SI on the opposed-phase image *(arrows)*. Similar loss of SI is revealed within the vertebral body marrow (M). Chapter 3 discusses how this chemical shift technique is used to differentiation between lipid-containing adrenal adenomas and metastases. **C,** Fat-suppressed T2-WI shows loss of SI of the fat containing regions (*). The cystic portions of the tumor are hyperintense. **D** and **E,** Fat-suppressed T1-WI (**D**) shows loss of SI of the intratumoral fat (*), while a corresponding water-suppressed T1-WI (**E**) shows high SI intratumoral fat (*) and subcutaneous fat (F). Intratumoral voxels that contain both lipid and water protons are revealed as minimally hyperintense *(arrows)* on the water-suppressed image.

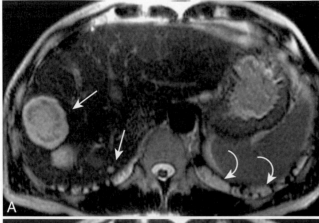

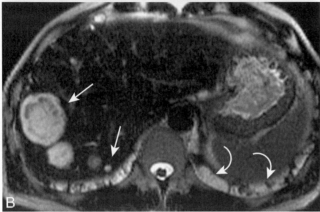

Figure 1-19 ■ **MR findings hepatic metastatic mucinous colon adenocarcinoma.** Mucin-rich adenocarcinoma can mimic nonsolid cysts and hemangiomas on T2-WIs. **A** and **B**, T2 (**A**) and heavily T2-WIs (TE = 189 ms) show multiple hyperintense heterogeneous hepatic lesions *(arrows)* that have persistent high SI in (**B**). Multiple high SI pulmonary metastases *(curved arrows)* are also present.

supplied hypervascular metastases. Hypervascular metastases include breast carcinoma, carcinoid tumors, melanoma, thyroid carcinoma, renal cell carcinoma and sarcomas. Hypovascular metastases may show thin rim enhancement on arterial-phase images but are best detected on portal venous phase images when enhancement of surrounding liver parenchyma is greatest. Hypovascular metastases include colon, lung, prostate, gastric, and transitional cell carcinomas. Rare isovascular metastases are inconspicuous on both arterial and portal venous phases of enhancement. Isovascular metastases may be easily detected on unenhanced T1- and/or T2-WIs. Metastases from colon, thyroid, or endometrial carcinomas may appear isovascular on dynamic imaging, particularly after chemotherapy.

The peripheral washout sign is a specific but insensitive sign of hepatic malignancy seen in both metastases and hepatocellular carcinoma (see Fig. 1-16).[250] This sign refers to a peripheral rim of hypointensity relative to the center of the lesion on delayed imaging. This pattern of enhancement is produced by increased vascularity within peripheral,

viable tumor and decreased vascularity and increased interstitium within the central tumor that may be fibrotic or necrotic.

Enhancement extending beyond the border of hepatic metastases as defined on unenhanced images is termed perilesional enhancement.[239,330] This perilesional enhancement may be circumferential or wedge shaped and is usually most intense on early-phase images. Perilesional enhancement of metastases is attributed to peritumoral desmoplastic reaction, inflammatory cell infiltration, and vascular proliferation.[239] Colorectal carcinoma metastases most commonly show perilesional enhancement, but this pattern has also been observed with pancreatic carcinoma, lymphoma, and breast carcinoma metastases.[323] Transient segmental enhancement could also be due to portal vein thrombosis with compensatory increased hepatic arterial flow.[166]

A cirrhosis-like pattern may develop in women with hepatic metastases from breast carcinoma who have been treated with chemotherapy.[331-334] Findings at MR imaging include decreased liver volume, lobular margins, diffuse heterogeneity, and caudate lobe enlargement.[331-334] Focal parenchymal lesions may not be identified on imaging studies.[331,332] This imaging pattern has been referred to as "pseudo-cirrhosis," but patients may develop signs of portal hypertension and encephalopathy.[331] In some women, histologic correlation reveals diffusely infiltrative, desmoplastic, poorly differentiated adenocarcinoma with distortion of the liver architecture similar to that seen in cirrhosis.[331] In other cases, pathologic examination shows residual tumor and nodular regenerative hyperplasia, without evidence of cirrhosis.[334] Development of this cirrhosis-like pattern has been attributed to the hepatotoxic effects of systemic chemotherapy.[331-334] Metastatic hepatic infiltration[331] or treatment-related tumor fibrosis may also be contributory.

HEPATIC STEATOSIS (BOX 1-13)

Lipid constitutes approximately 5% of the normal liver by weight.[206,335] Steatosis is the abnormal accumulation of lipid within hepatocytes. Histologically, macrovesicular and microvesicular forms of steatosis have been defined.[206,336] Macrovesicular steatosis is the more common form and results from a combination of increased delivery, inadequate oxygenation, and decreased secretion of lipids in the liver.[206,336] Obesity, alcohol abuse, insulin resistance and diabetes, cachexia, drugs (including steroids and tamoxifen), metabolic disorders, and hepatitis C are causes of macrovesicular steatosis.[206,336,337] Microvesicular steatosis, due to defective oxidation of free fatty acids, is often associated with severe hepatic dysfunction.[206,336] Acute fatty liver of pregnancy, Reye's syndrome, drugs, chronic alcohol abuse, urea cycle disorders, and mitochondrial cytopathies are some of the causes of microvesicular steatosis.[206,336]

1-13   Hepatic Steatosis

Clinical
Patient may be asymptomatic or have right upper
    quadrant pain, fatigue, and malaise
Hepatomegaly and elevated liver function tests

Pathology
Abnormal accumulation of lipid within hepatocytes
Macrovesicular form present in obesity, alcohol abuse,
    insulin resistance/diabetes, cachexia, drugs
    (including steroids), metabolic disorders, and
    hepatitis C
Microvesicular form can develop in patients with
    severe hepatic dysfunction such as acute fatty liver
    of pregnancy, Reye's syndrome, drugs, chronic
    alcohol abuse, urea cycle disorders, and
    mitochondrial cytopathies
Steatohepatitis, progressive inflammation, and fibrosis
    may be associated with both alcoholic and
    nonalcoholic etiologies and can progress to cirrhosis

MRI
Chemical shift MRI: loss of hepatic SI on
    opposed-phase GRE images when compared with a
    corresponding in-phase GRE images using the
    spleen as an internal reference
Steatosis may be diffuse, focal, or multifocal
Characteristic locations of focal steatosis and focal
    fatty sparing include anteromedial edge of medial
    segment, pericholecystic region, and subcapsular
    region
Focal steatosis attributed to decreased delivery of
    unknown substances from the portal vein, focal
    increase in insulin, or relative ischemia due to
    decreased portal blood flow
Focal sparing secondary to aberrant venous drainage
    or arterial supply resulting in decreased portal
    venous delivery of lipid

Macrovesicular steatosis may be associated with progressive inflammation and fibrosis, a condition termed steatohepatitis.[206,336] Steatohepatitis associated with alcohol abuse is a well-known entity. Nonalcoholic steatohepatitis (NASH) is a more recently and increasingly recognized form of chronic liver disease. The alcoholic and nonalcoholic forms of steatohepatitis show similar or identical histologic findings.[206,336] Biopsy is required for diagnosis of steatohepatitis, which by definition diffusely involves the liver.[336] NASH has two forms based on etiopathogenesis.[335] The primary form is seen in conditions associated with insulin resistance and includes diabetes mellitus (type 2), obesity, and hyperlipidemia. The secondary form is associated with certain drugs, gastrointestinal surgical procedures, and other conditions. NASH is considered the most severe nonalcoholic fatty liver disease.[335]

Clinically, some patients with hepatic steatosis are asymptomatic, whereas other patients may develop right upper quadrant pain, fatigue, and malaise.[335] Hepatomegaly is a frequent finding, and liver function tests, particularly the aminotransferases, may be elevated.[335] Steatohepatitis, alcoholic or nonalcoholic, may progress to cirrhosis. NASH is being recognized as a common cause of what was previously termed "cryptogenic" cirrhosis.[338]

Chemical shift imaging can detect and characterize the microscopic, intracellular lipid present in hepatic steatosis and within some hepatocellular neoplasms such as well-differentiated hepatocellular carcinoma or hepatic adenoma.[339-342] Visual comparison of the in-phase and opposed-phase images, using the spleen as an internal reference, is usually sufficient for detection of hepatic steatosis. Loss of SI on opposed-phase images indicates the presence of lipid. One caveat is that the TE used for the opposed-phase images should be shorter than the TE used for the in-phase images to minimize T2* effects.[343,344] In the presence of iron overload from genetic or secondary hemochromatosis, loss of SI due to susceptibility artifact may preclude imaging detection of steatosis.[342] If detection of steatosis in an iron-overloaded liver were necessary, MR spectroscopy could be performed.[342]

At MR imaging, hepatic steatosis may be diffuse, focal, or multifocal (Fig. 1-20; see Figs. 1-11, 3-4, 3-6, 3-12, and 3-13). Wedge-shaped, geographic, and nodular areas of focal steatosis have been described.[344] Nodular steatosis may mimic metastatic disease at imaging.[345,346] Focal steatosis or focal fatty sparing tends to develop in specific locations in the liver including the anteromedial edge of the medial segment, around the gallbladder, and within subcapsular portions of the liver.[342,344] Aberrant gastric venous drainage to the posterior medial segment anterior to the porta hepatis, aberrant internal thoracic arterial supply to the area around the falciform ligament, and cystic venous drainage to the pericholecystic liver all result in decreased portal venous blood flow. Focal fatty sparing can be explained by decreased delivery of lipid secondary to decreased portal venous flow (see Fig. 1-20).[347-349] Occasionally, these same areas show focal steatosis.[350] Focal sparing has also been attributed to arterioportal shunts, portal vein occlusion, and hepatic parenchymal compression by metastatic lesions.[351-354] Depending on the location, a metastasis or other mass may result in peripheral, segmental, or lobar sparing in a steatotic liver.[352]

Increased local concentration of insulin can result in focal steatosis. MR has shown focal steatosis surrounding insulinoma metastases, within the livers of patients who have received islet cell transplants injected into the portal veins, and within the subcapsular portion of liver in diabetic patients with renal failure who have insulin placed in their intraperitoneal dialysate.[355-357]

IRON DEPOSITIONAL DISEASE

There are two major forms of iron deposition disease: parenchymal and reticuloendothelial.[358-360] Parenchymal iron overload, due to increased

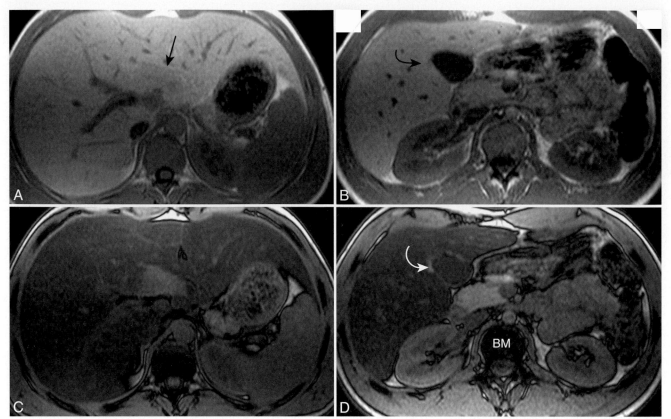

Figure 1-20 ▪ Hepatic steatosis with focal fatty sparing of the medial segment left lobe and around the gallbladder in an asymptomatic man with hypercholesterolemia. A and **B,** Two in-phase T1-WIs show accentuated high SI liver and normal low SI spleen. There are subtle areas of hypointensity relative the surrounding liver within the medial segment of the left lobe *(arrow)* and adjacent to the gallbladder wall *(curved arrow)*. Unlike metastatic disease (see Fig. 1-11) these "lesions" are hyperintense to spleen (S) and represent normal hepatocellular tissue. **C** and **D,** Corresponding opposed-phase images show marked loss of SI within the liver that establishes the diagnosis of steatosis. The areas of spared steatosis *(curved arrow)* now appear hyperintense to liver and remain hyperintense to spleen. Normal lumbar bone marrow (BM) contains both fat and water protons and thus loses SI on opposed-phase imaging.

gastrointestinal absorption of iron, occurs in genetic hemochromatosis (GH) and erythrogenic hemochromatosis. Reticuloendothelial iron overload results from multiple intravenous blood transfusions. Excess parenchymal iron results in cellular oxidative damage and potentially carcinoma.[361-363] Excess iron that is limited to the Kupffer cells of the reticuloendothelial system is benign.

GH, the most common inherited disease of Northern European descendants, is an autosomal recessive disorder characterized by a mutation on chromosome 6 (Box 1-14).[364] This genetic mutation may result in impaired detection of serum iron levels by duodenal crypt cells with resultant increased gastrointestinal absorption of iron. Defective storage of iron within the reticuloendothelial system and increased deposition in parenchymal cells is another suggested cause of GH.[365,366] Serum ferritin levels and transferrin saturation are useful screening tests, but false-positive results may occur in patients with alcoholism and infection and false-negative results may occur in young patients with GH and

very early iron overload.[360] Clinical manifestations of GH can include cirrhosis, diabetes mellitus, cardiomyopathy, endocrinopathies, arthropathy, and skin discoloration.

Genetic testing can be performed for confirmation in patients with suspected GH as well as for screening high-risk populations such as siblings of probands.[360] Genetic testing may also obviate liver biopsy in GH patients with minimally elevated serum markers and no clinical evidence of liver disease and in patients with advanced cirrhosis.[367] Liver biopsy allows quantitation of iron overload as well as detection of cirrhosis or accompanying liver disease.[367] Early detection enables treatment with phlebotomy prior to irreversible organ damage. Many centers do not allow patients with hemochromatosis to donate their blood. The rationale is that there is a financial incentive for patients with hemochromatosis to donate their blood. Patients are charged for therapeutic phlebotomy while blood donation is free of charge. An estimated 200,000 to 3 million units of phlebotomized blood from patients

1-14 Genetic Hemochromatosis

Clinical

Autosomal recessive
   Signs and symptoms usually appear in fifth or sixth decades (later in menstruating women compared with men)
      and include lethargy, arthralgia, loss of libido, glucose intolerance, abdominal pain, and heart failure
Untreated disease may progress to cirrhosis and liver failure

Pathology

Increased gastrointestinal absorption of iron results in parenchymal overload
Reticuloendothelial cell system (including the spleen and the hepatic Kupffer cells) does not accumulate excess iron
Excess hepatocyte iron results in cellular oxidative damage and, if untreated, cirrhosis and/or hepatocellular carcinoma

MRI

Susceptibility effects of iron result in decreased T2 and T2* liver SI
Iron-free liver nodules suspicious for hepatocellular carcinoma
T2-shortening effect of iron may be present in the pancreas and myocardium
Spleen and bone marrow are spared from iron overload

---

with hemochromatosis are discarded each year in the United States.[368]

Quantitation of hepatic iron overload with MR imaging is possible but requires correlation with liver biopsy samples and meticulous attention to MR technical factors.[360,369] MR imaging is useful for the noninvasive detection of iron overload in patients with GH, including organ distribution and potential complications (Figs. 1-21 and 1-22).[370] MR imaging can also be used to follow the effects of phlebotomy therapy. In GH, iron overload occurs in the liver, pancreas, myocardium,[371] pituitary gland,[372] adrenal glands, and musculoskeletal system. The magnetic susceptibility effects of iron result in decreased SI, particularly on T2- and T2*-WIs. T2*W GRE sequences, which lack a 180° refocusing pulse, are the most sensitive sequence for the detection of mild iron deposition. The TE should be at least 7 ms, and preferably greater than 15 ms, to maximize susceptibility effects and loss of SI. A flip angle of less than 30° minimizes T1 effects. Liver SI lower than that of skeletal muscle (which does not accumulate iron in GH) indicates iron overload. MR imaging also detects the potential complications of cirrhosis and hepatocellular carcinoma. Since tumor cells typically do not accumulate iron, iron-free liver nodules in patients with GH are highly suspicious for hepatocellular carcinoma.[360,373]

Patients with disorders of ineffective erythropoiesis such as thalassemia major, sideroblastic anemia, and megaloblastic anemia may develop secondary hemochromatosis because increased marrow demand incites excess gastrointestinal absorption.[360,374,375] The distribution of iron is similar to that in patients with GH.[374,376] The spleen may be spared, even in transfusion-dependent patients, possibly owing to impaired reticuloendothelial cell function. Iron deposition in bone marrow can be present in erythrogenic hemochromatosis but is not seen in GH.[374]

Another common cause of increased iron deposits is multiple blood transfusions (Box 1-15). Excess iron from transfused erythrocytes accumulates in the reticuloendothelial cells of the liver, spleen, and bone marrow (Fig. 1-23; see Figs 5-3 and 5-4). Once the storage capacity of the reticuloendothelial system is saturated (40 units of blood), excess iron will deposit in parenchymal cells, resulting in secondary hemochromatosis.[360] Patients with transfusion-dependent anemia can be given iron chelation therapy to prevent or treat parenchymal iron overload. Both GRE MR sequences and MR spectroscopy have proved accurate for measuring liver iron levels in patients with transfusional iron deposition disease and can be used to monitor therapy.[377]

1-15 Transfusional Iron Overload

Clinical

Result from multiple transfusions of erythrocytes

Pathology

Iron deposited in reticuloendothelial cells of liver, spleen, and bone marrow
Reticuloendothelial cell iron is considered benign
Once storage capacity of reticuloendothelial system is exceeded (40 units of blood), excess iron will deposit in parenchymal cells, resulting in secondary hemochromatosis

MRI

Iron in liver, spleen, and bone marrow revealed as low T2 and T2*-SI
Pancreas and myocardial SI normal except in those with severe chronic anemia

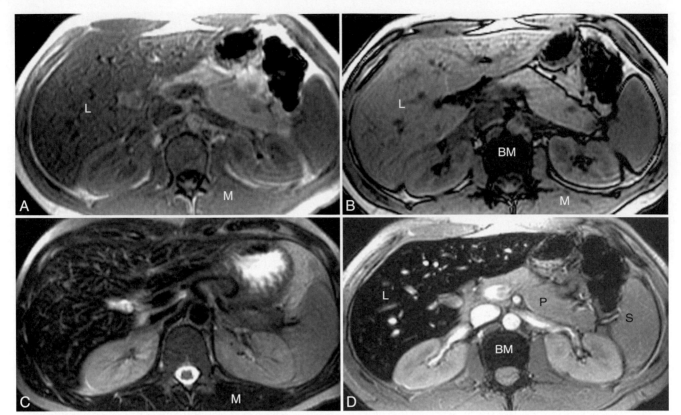

Figure 1-21 ■ MR illustration of hepatic iron overload in a 34-year-old male with genetic hemochromatosis.
A and **B**, In-phase (**A**) (TE = 4.2 ms) and opposed-phase (**B**) (TE = 2.5) T1-WIs show liver parenchyma that is isointense relative to paraspinal musculature (M) in **B** that loses SI in **A**. The longer TE of the in-phase image (**A**) allows for greater T2* susceptibility effects of the hepatic iron overload. Normal lumbar bone marrow (BM) shows loss of SI on the oppose-phase image because it contains both fat and water protons. **C**, T2-WI shows the liver parenchyma is isointense to paraspinal musculature. Fast-spin echo images are not as sensitive to the susceptibility effects of iron as "T1-weighted" in-phase GRE images or GRE images with longer echo times (see **D**). **D**, T2*-W GRE image (TR = 100, TE = 20, FA = 20°) reveals markedly hypointense liver (L). The pancreas (P) does not lose SI to indicate parenchymal iron deposition. The spleen (S) is not involved with the parenchymal iron deposition of genetic hemochromatosis. The low SI within the bone marrow is not secondary to iron deposition. Instead, susceptibility effects of bony trabeculae are responsible for the T2* effects.

Patients with cirrhosis unrelated to GH can develop diffuse hepatic iron deposition.[360,378] The reason for this iron overload is not known, but it may be due to anemia, pancreatic insufficiency, or decreased transferrin synthesis. Pancreatic iron overload is not typically seen in cirrhosis due to a cause other than GH.

VASCULAR DISEASE OF THE LIVER

Budd-Chiari Syndrome (Box 1-16)

Budd-Chiari syndrome (BCS) is a congestive liver disease consequent to obstruction of hepatic venous outflow. Obstruction may occur at the level of the hepatic veins or the inferior vena cava. Hepatic veno-occlusive disease, resulting from obliteration of the postsinusoidal venules, is considered a distinct entity. Causes of hepatic venous thrombosis and BCS can be classified into hypercoagulable states, stasis or mass lesion, vascular injury, and associations of uncertain mechanism.[379] Hypercoagulable states include hematologic and myeloproliferative disorders, pregnancy/postpartum state, and oral contraceptive medications.[380] Examples of stasis or mass lesion include membranous obstruction of the inferior vena cava and vascular invasion/compression by neoplasms such as hepatocellular, renal, or adrenal carcinomas, and metastatic disease. Vascular injury may result from trauma, catheterization, and vasculitides. The classic acute clinical triad of BCS includes right upper quadrant pain, hepatomegaly, and ascites. Subacute and chronic presentations are usually manifested as hepatic failure.

Histologically, acute hepatic venous thrombosis produces sinusoidal congestion.[379] Acute or organizing thrombi may also be present in the small hepatic and portal veins. With progression, the sinusoids become collagenized and dilated and there is hepatocellular atrophy and necrosis. The obliterated small hepatic veins produce septa interlinking the larger hepatic veins, and in venocentric cirrhosis results that relatively spares the portal triads. However, secondary

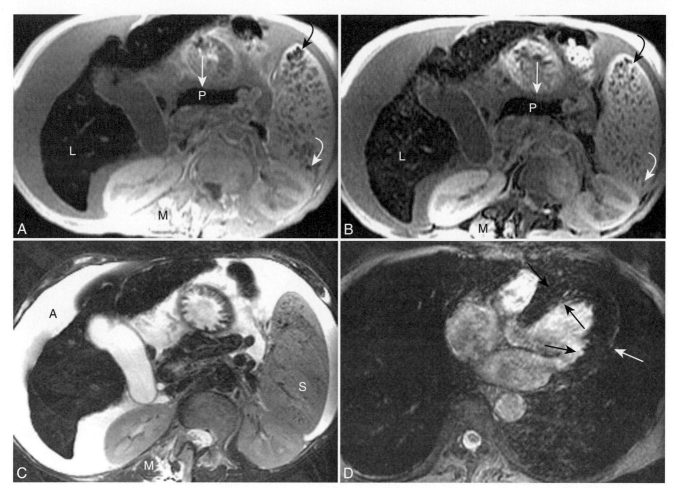

Figure 1-22 ■ MR demonstration of hepatic, pancreatic, and myocardial iron overload in a man with advanced hemochromatosis complicated by cirrhosis and portal hypertension. A and **B**, In-phase (**A**) (TE = 4.2) and opposed-phase (**B**) (TE = 2.1) T1-WIs show a cirrhotic nodular liver (L) that is of decreased SI relative to the paraspinal musculature (M). The pancreas (*arrow* P) is of abnormally low SI because of parenchymal iron deposition. The spleen reveals multiple hypointense Gamna-Gandy bodies (*curved arrows*). The T2* susceptibility effects are more pronounced on the longer TE in-phase image. **C**, Fat-suppressed T2-WI shows that the liver is hypointense to the paraspinal musculature. Ascites (A) and splenomegaly (S) also are present. **D**, Cardiac-gated GRE image (TE = 20 ms) shows decreased myocardial SI (*arrows*), indicating iron deposition.

portal vein thrombosis is common in BCS and can lead to a combined venoportal cirrhosis pattern. One, two, or all three major hepatic veins may be thrombosed.[381] The separate venous drainage of the caudate lobe into the inferior vena cava accounts for its compensatory hypertrophy in BCS.

The MR imaging appearance of BCS varies with the acute, subacute, and chronic stages.[382] In acute BCS, hepatic venous thrombosis usually is seen. The peripheral liver shows decreased T1 and increased T2 SI relative to the normal SI caudate lobe. Heterogeneously decreased enhancement is seen in the peripheral liver during the early and delayed phases on CE T1-WIs and is due to decreased inflow from the increased tissue pressure. The caudate lobe shows increased early and persistent enhancement and is of normal or moderately increased size. Hepatic congestion and edema account for the differential SI of the peripheral liver.

The unenhanced MR imaging findings of subacute and acute BCS are similar.[382] The CE T1-WIs differ, with the peripheral liver showing heterogeneous enhancement greater than the homogeneously enhancing caudate lobe. This peripheral heterogeneous enhancement becomes more homogeneous on delayed-phase imaging. Hepatic venous thrombosis typically is identified (Fig. 1-24). Intrahepatic venovenous collateral vessels can be present. The caudate lobe is moderately increased in size.

In chronic BCS there are minimal SI differences between peripheral and central liver on T1-W, T2-W, and CE T1-WIs.[382] Hepatic venous thrombosis usually is not identifiable. Extensive bridging intrahepatic and capsular venous collaterals are common in chronic BCS. The caudate lobe shows moderate to marked hypertrophy. Ascites and extrahepatic venous collateral vessels may be present in both subacute and chronic BCS.[383]

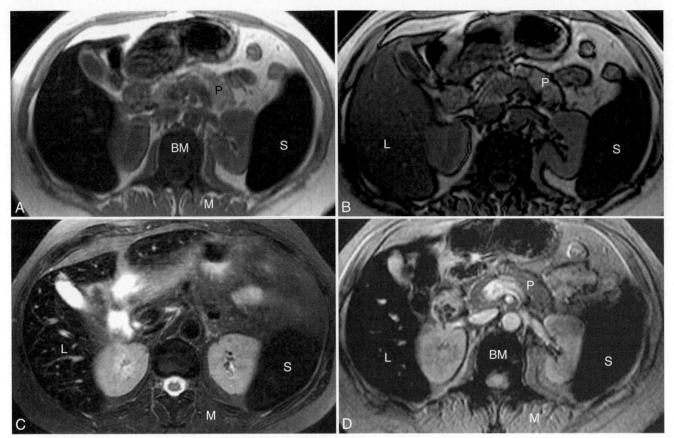

Figure 1-23 ▪ **MR findings of hepatic and splenic reticuloendothelial iron from prior transfusions in a 51-year-old female with acute myelogenous leukemia. A** and **B**, In-phase (**A**) (TE = 4.2) and opposed-phase (**B**) (TE = 2.1) T1-WIs show decreased SI of the liver (L), spleen (S), and bone marrow (BM) compared with paraspinal muscle (M). The in-phase image is more sensitive to the susceptibility effects of iron because of the longer echo time. The pancreas (P) is of normal SI. **C**, Fat-suppressed T2-WI shows decreased SI of the liver and spleen relative to muscle. **D**, T2*-W GRE image (TR = 100, TE = 20, FA = 20°) reveals markedly hypointense liver, spleen, and bone marrow. The pancreas does not lose SI, indicating absence of parenchymal iron deposition.

BCS due to a web or membranous obstruction of the inferior vena cava occurs more commonly in South Africa, Japan, and Korea.[384] Intracaval webs and membranes represent the result of prior acquired thrombosis.[385,386] MR can show either a curvilinear soft-tissue membrane or an obliterated lumen of the intrahepatic inferior vena cava. Membranous obstruction may, however, represent extension of the intrahepatic venous process rather than a primary congenital or developmental caval lesion.[379,387] Compression of the inferior vena cava due to an elevated right hemidiaphragm has also been reported as a cause of BCS.[388]

Focal hepatic masses associated with BCS include hepatocellular carcinoma and regenerative nodules. Through invasion of the hepatic veins and/or inferior vena cava, hepatocellular carcinoma can cause BCS, often with an acute or severe presentation.[387] Hepatocellular carcinoma may also result from the cirrhosis of end-stage BCS although other factors such as concomitant chronic hepatitis may be contributory.[389-391]

Large regenerative nodules may develop in BCS and other diseases that impair hepatic blood flow such as myeloproliferative and lymphoproliferative disorders; autoimmune disorders such as lupus, antiphospholipid antibodies syndrome, and scleroderma; and in patients treated with steroids or antineoplastic medications.[392] These nodules are more appropriately referred to as large regenerative or multiacinar regenerative nodules rather than nodular regenerative hyperplasia, as the latter entity is defined by absence of fibrosis in the intervening hepatic parenchyma.[393,394] Formation of regenerative nodules and other benign nodular hepatocellular lesions is attributed to abnormal hepatic perfusion with atrophy and compensatory nodule formation involving adequately perfused parenchyma.[379,392,395] Pathologically, the nodules show hyperplastic hepatocytes in plates one or two cells thick.[392] Growth is expansile with compression of the central vein.

On MR regenerative nodules vary in size from a few millimeters to 4 cm although larger lesions may occur.[391,393,396] The nodules in patients with BCS are hyperintense relative to surrounding liver on T1-WI.[391,393,396] T1-W hyperintensity may be due to the presence of copper[393,397] or to relatively decreased SI of the surrounding congested liver parenchyma[396]

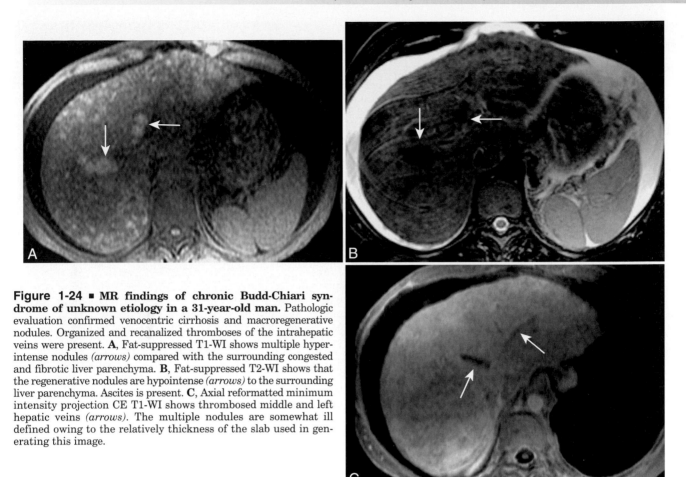

Figure 1-24 ■ MR findings of chronic Budd-Chiari syndrome of unknown etiology in a 31-year-old man. Pathologic evaluation confirmed venocentric cirrhosis and macroregenerative nodules. Organized and recanalized thromboses of the intrahepatic veins were present. **A,** Fat-suppressed T1-WI shows multiple hyperintense nodules *(arrows)* compared with the surrounding congested and fibrotic liver parenchyma. **B,** Fat-suppressed T2-WI shows that the regenerative nodules are hypointense *(arrows)* to the surrounding liver parenchyma. Ascites is present. **C,** Axial reformatted minimum intensity projection CE T1-WI shows thrombosed middle and left hepatic veins *(arrows).* The multiple nodules are somewhat ill defined owing to the relatively thickness of the slab used in generating this image.

(see Fig. 1-24). The T2 SI is more variable, with hypointense, isointense, and hyperintense lesions reported, although most are isointense.[391-393,396] Infarction may contribute to the hyperintensity seen in some regenerative nodules.[393] On dynamic CE T1-WIs regenerative nodules are usually hypervascular in the arterial phase, reflecting hepatic arterial blood supply.[391-393,396] On portal venous phase imaging, regenerative nodules remain slightly hyperintense.[392] A perinodular hypointense rim may be present on arterial phase images and reflects sinusoidal dilatation and marked congestion.[392] MR may not allow discrimination of individual regenerative nodules from hepatocellular carcinoma in chronic BCS, but the presence of greater than 10 nodules less than 4 cm in diameter is considered suggestive of benign regenerative nodules.[391]

Hepatic Veno-occlusive Disease, or Sinusoidal Obstruction Syndrome

Hepatic veno-occlusive disease (HVOD) is a congestive liver disease that results in the obliteration of hepatic venules less than 1 mm in diameter.[379] The main hepatic veins and inferior vena cava are patent. The primary site of injury is the sinusoidal endothelial cell and not the hepatic venules, and thus HVOD should be more appropriately classified as "sinusoidal obstruction syndrome."[398] Causes of HVOD include chemotherapeutic agents and radiation therapy, particularly as part of the myeloablative regime for hematopoietic stem cell transplantation. Ingestion of pyrrolizidine alkaloids in herbal teas or contaminated grain is another cause. The clinical presentation includes hepatomegaly and right upper quadrant pain, and jaundice typically develops within 30 days of stem cell transplantation.[399] Most patients recover with conservative treatment. Anticoagulation or trans-jugular intrahepatic porto-systemic shunt (TIPS) procedures have not proved effective in treating HVOD.[386]

MR findings of HVOD include hepatomegaly and attenuated but patent hepatic veins.[400,401] Additional nonspecific features of gallbladder wall thickening and T2-weighted hyperintensity, periportal cuffing, ascites, and pleural effusions are likely related to increased resistance to lymphatic and venous inflow.

Passive Hepatic Congestion

Passive hepatic congestion is seen in the setting of failure of the right side of the heart or of constrictive

1-16 Budd-Chiari Syndrome (BCS)

Clinical

Congestive hepatopathy secondary to obstruction of hepatic venous outflow
Classic triad of acute BCS: right upper quadrant pain, hepatomegaly, and ascites
Subacute and chronic presentations manifest as hepatic failure

Pathology

Causes of hepatic venous thrombosis classified into hypercoagulable states, stasis or mass lesions, vascular injury, and idiopathic mechanisms
Acute venous thrombosis produces sinusoidal congestion that progresses to hepatocellular atrophy, and necrosis ultimately results in venocentric cirrhosis
Secondary portal vein thrombosis is common and can result in combined venoportal cirrhosis
Separate venous drainage of the caudate lobe into the inferior vena cava accounts for its frequent sparing and compensatory hypertrophy

MRI

Acute Stage

Hepatic venous thrombosis
Peripheral liver decreased T1 and increased T2 SI relative to caudate lobe
Heterogeneously decreased gadolinium-enhancement in peripheral liver during early and delayed phases
Caudate lobe normal or moderately increased in size and shows increased early and persistent enhancement

Subacute Phase

Unenhanced findings similar to acute phase
Gadolinium-enhanced images differ, with peripheral liver showing heterogeneous enhancement greater than the homogeneously enhancing caudate lobe. Delayed enhancement of peripheral liver is secondary to early fibrosis or venous outflow obstruction.
Intrahepatic venovenous collateral vessels may be shown
Moderate hypertrophy of caudate lobe

Chronic Phase

Minimal SI differences between peripheral and central liver on T1, T2, and CE images
Hepatic venous thrombosis usually not identifiable
Depiction of bridging intrahepatic and capsular venous collateral vessels
Moderate to marked hypertrophy of the caudate
Ascites and extrahepatic venous collateral vessels may be present in both subacute and chronic stages

---

pericarditis.[386] In these conditions, the increased right atrial pressures are transmitted to the hepatic veins.[402] Pathologically, there is dilation of the hepatic sinusoids, atrophy of perivenular hepatocytes, and minimal focal pericellular fibrosis.[379] CE CT or MR may reveal heterogeneous or mosaic pattern of enhancement.[402] In contrast to Budd-Chiari syndrome, the hepatic veins and inferior vena cava are patent and may be distended. In addition, reflux of contrast material into the hepatic venous system can be present during arterial-phase imaging. Other findings include periportal edema, ascites, pleural effusions, and cardiomegaly.

Portal Vein Thrombosis (Box 1-17)

Causes of portal vein thrombosis include stasis and masses, hypercoagulable states, and vascular injury.[379] The most common condition leading to stasis of portal venous flow is hepatic cirrhosis and portal hypertension. Intrahepatic masses such as hepatocellular carcinoma, metastases, and cholangiocarcinoma may invade or compress the portal veins, resulting in thrombosis. Lymphadenopathy in the porta hepatis or vascular encasement by pancreatic carcinoma can also cause portal vein thrombosis. Abdominal infections such as diverticulitis or appendicitis may be complicated by mesenteric thrombophlebitis and pylephlebitis. Noninfectious, inflammatory causes of portal vein thrombosis include pancreatitis, bile leaks, and accidental or surgical trauma. Abdominal pain and gastrointestinal hemorrhage are common clinical manifestations.[403] Portal vein thrombosis can cause or exacerbate portal hypertension.

Spin-echo MR images will show portal vein thrombosis as abnormal intraluminal SI with loss of the normal flow void.[14,404] Flow-sensitive GRE images will show thrombus as intraluminal low SI and patent vessels as high SI.[404,405] Thrombus less than 5 weeks old appears hyperintense to liver parenchyma on T1- and T2-WIs, whereas thrombus between 2 and 18 months old appears hyperintense only on T2-WIs.[405] Potential pitfalls on unenhanced T1- and T2-WI include slow or turbulent flow.[14,406]

1-17   Portal Vein Thrombosis

Clinical

May manifest with abdominal pain and gastrointestinal hemorrhage

Can cause or exacerbate portal hypertension

Pathology

Causes: stasis, masses, hypercoagulable states, and vascular injury

Thrombus may be bland or malignant

MRI

Loss of normal flow void on unenhanced images

Flow-sensitive GRE images: intraluminal low SI thrombus vs. high SI flow within patent vessels

Dynamic CE imaging: confirms thrombosis and differentiates benign from malignant thrombus

Transient hepatic signal intensity difference: wedge-shaped area of increased parenchymal enhancement present on arterial-phase images with segmental portal vein thrombosis due to compensatory increase in arterial flow; becomes isointense on portal venous and delayed phase images

Cavernous transformation: development of venous collateral vessels within or around a thrombosed portal vein

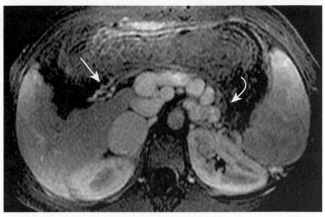

Figure 1-25 ▪ MR findings of cavernous transformation of the portal vein secondary to extrinsic compression by a (previously excised) ciliated hepatic foregut cyst. Axial maximum intensity projection (MIP) image from portal venous phase of a CE T1-WI shows replacement of the intrahepatic portal vein by numerous small collateral vessels (*arrow*). Extrahepatic portosystemic collateral vessels (*curved arrow*) are also present.

Gadolinium-enhanced MR is a highly sensitive technique for both the detection of portal vein thrombosis and the distinction between benign and malignant etiologies.[14] Benign portal vein thrombus appears as a nonenhancing filling defect. Other findings include expansion of the portal vein, enhancement of the portal vein wall, and periportal collaterals. The neovascularity of malignant portal vein thrombus causes enhancement on dynamic CE T1-WI. Additional findings of malignant portal vein thrombosis include a main portal vein diameter greater than 24 mm, enhancing vessels within the thrombus and surrounding periportal region. With segmental portal vein thrombosis, transient wedge-shaped areas of increased hepatic parenchymal enhancement can occur on hepatic arterial phase images.[166] These transient hepatic SI differences, owing to a compensatory increase in hepatic arterial flow, become isointense to surrounding liver parenchyma on portal venous and delayed images.

Development of venous collateral vessels within or around a thrombosed portal vein is termed cavernous transformation.[407] Biliary branches (cystic and paracholedochal) and gastric (left and right gastric) venous branches of the portal vein are the major collateral vessels in cavernous transformation.[408] Both portosystemic and portoportal collateralization occurs after portal vein thrombosis.[407] Cavernous transformation has been documented as early as 6 days after acute portal vein thrombosis (Fig. 1-25).[407]

COMPLICATIONS OF LIVER TRANSPLANTATION

Cadaveric and living donor liver transplantation is used for the treatment of end-stage parenchymal liver disease and for unresectable but confined hepatic tumors. Vascular, biliary, parenchymal, and extrahepatic complications are optimally detected with a comprehensive MR imaging examination that includes T1, T2, MRCP, and volumetric dynamic CE fat-suppressed T1-W sequences.[409-412] The biliary complications of liver transplantation are discussed in Chapter 2. Rejection of the liver allograft cannot be reliably detected with imaging studies and requires biopsy for diagnosis.[409]

The orthotopically transplanted liver requires four vascular anastomoses: suprahepatic and infrahepatic inferior vena cava, hepatic artery, and portal vein. A priori knowledge of both the donor's and recipient's vascular anatomy can improve surgical planning and minimize postprocedural complications.[413] Sutural calcification at the suprahepatic inferior venal caval site may appear as foci of very low SI. Periportal edema or collar is a nonspecific finding after liver transplantation that likely results from impaired lymph drainage after surgical interruption of the lymphatic channels.[414] Periportal edema does not correlate with rejection. Other normal postoperative findings include a small amount of perihepatic or intersegmental fissural fluid and a transient right pleural effusion.[411] Reactive porta hepatis or portacaval lymph nodes are frequently present, but if enlarged lymph nodes are identified between 4 and 12 months after transplantation, PTLD should be considered.[411]

Vascular complications include thrombosis and stenosis of the hepatic artery, portal vein, or inferior vena cava. Hepatic arterial thrombosis is the most common vascular complication, occurring in 3% to 12% of adult liver transplant patients.[410,411,415] Factors that may contribute to acute hepatic artery thrombosis are increased cold ischemia time of the donor liver, ABO blood group incompatibility, severe acute rejection, anatomic variants of hepatic vasculature, and discrepant size of native and donor vessels.[411,416] Hepatic artery thrombosis may result in fulminant hepatic necrosis, biliary ischemia and necrosis with bile leak, and recurrent bacteremia/sepsis due to abscess formation within infarcted parenchyma.[411,415-417] Contrast-enhanced magnetic resonance angiography (CE-MRA) can reveal an occluded hepatic artery, often at the anastomotic site.[409-412,418] False-positive diagnosis of hepatic artery thrombosis can occur with susceptibility artifact from adjacent surgical clips or low flow states.[409,410] Hepatic arterial stenosis occurs in approximately 10% of patients and may lead to thrombosis.[410,416] Suspected causes include surgical technique, clamp injury, intimal trauma from perfusion catheters, and rejection.

Other, rare arterial complications include pseudoaneurysm and arteriovenous fistula. Pseudoaneurysms usually occur at the arterial anastomosis, but intrahepatic pseudoaneurysms can develop after parenchymal biopsy, biliary interventions, or local infection.[416,419] A fistula may develop between the pseudoaneurysm and biliary ducts or portal vein. Pseudoaneurysm and fistulae may be asymptomatic or present with life-threatening hemorrhage. A pseudoaneurysm will appear as a focal enlargement of the hepatic artery on imaging.[416]

Venous complications are less common. Portal vein thrombosis or stenosis occurs in less than 5% of patients.[420] Surgical technical problems, modification of the standard end-to-end portal venous anastomosis, intraoperative splenectomy, thrombus formation around the portal venous bypass catheter, and hypercoagulable state are factors associated with portal vein complications.[416,420] Clinical manifestations of portal vein thrombosis include portal hypertension, hepatic failure, ascites, and edema.[416] Inferior venal caval thrombosis/stenosis is also rare, occurring in less than 2% of patients.[420] Surgical technical problems, incongruence of native and donor vessel size, recurrence of the underlying disease such as Budd-Chiari syndrome, and compression by adjacent fluid collections are causes of inferior vena caval complications.[410,416,420] Patients may present with hepatomegaly, pleural effusions, ascites, and lower extremity edema.[416] CE-MRA, including multiplanar and volumetric reformations, allows easy detection of venous thrombosis or stenosis.[409-412]

Hepatic parenchymal complications detectable by MR imaging include infarction, abscess, biloma, recurrent malignant tumor, and PTLD.[411] Disruption of collateral arterial supply, such as the parabiliary arteries, in the transplanted liver renders the allograft particularly susceptible to ischemia with decreased hepatic arterial flow. The resultant biliary necrosis leads to hepatic parenchymal infarcts.

Hepatic infarcts can be peripherally or centrally located and wedge-shaped or round. Periportal infarcts may be irregularly shaped. Infarcts are typically hypointense to surrounding parenchyma on T1-WIs and hyperintense on T2-WIs and do not show gadolinium enhancement (Fig. 1-26). Uncomplicated bilomas appear as irregularly shaped fluid collections without an enhancing rim, whereas abscesses show an enhancing wall.[411] Recurrent hepatocellular carcinoma has been reported in 7% to 40% of liver transplant patients.[409] PTLD is discussed earlier in this chapter.

Extrahepatic complications of liver transplantation include metastatic hepatocellular carcinoma, PTLD, and right adrenal gland hemorrhage. After liver transplantation, the most common sites of metastatic hepatocellular carcinoma are the lungs, the allograft, and local and distant lymph nodes.[421] The two causes of right-sided adrenal gland hemorrhage are venous congestion after right adrenal vein

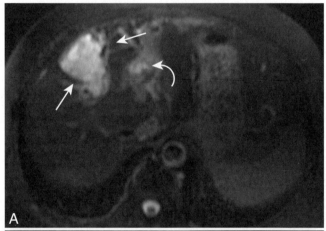

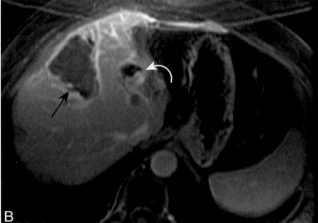

Figure 1-26 ■ Hepatic artery occlusion and liver infarction revealed on MR in a 58-year-old woman 10 years after liver transplantation. **A,** Fat-suppressed T2-WI shows a wedge-shaped high SI region of the anterior segment (arrows) and ill-defined hyperintense foci (curved arrow) of the left lobe that represent peribiliary infarcts. **B,** CE T1-WI shows peripheral rim enhancement of the infarcted region (arrow) and peribiliary infarcts (curved arrow).

ligation and coagulopathy related to preexisting liver dysfunction.[411]

HEPATIC CIRRHOSIS (BOX 1-18)

Cirrhosis is a diffuse process resulting from progressive hepatic parenchymal injury and fibrosis and the formation of parenchymal nodules.[422] Causes of cirrhosis are numerous and include toxins and drugs, infections, autoimmune disorders, genetic metabolic defects, acquired bile duct diseases, vascular disorders, and other conditions.[422] In some patients, the cause cannot be determined and the cirrhosis is termed cryptogenic. The most common toxic cause of cirrhosis is alcohol. The most common infectious etiologies are hepatitis B and C. There is increased awareness of hepatitis C infection in the United States, where the prevalence of infected individuals is almost 2%.[423] Of those who are chronically infected, 25% are expected to progress to cirrhosis. Examples of autoimmune disorders are autoimmune

---

1-18   Hepatic Cirrhosis

Clinical
Manifestations of chronic liver disease and portal hypertension
Portosystemic collateral vessels
- Esophageal and paraesophageal varices
- Paraumbilical veins and abdominal wall collateral vessels
- Retroperitoneal collateral vessels
- Superior hemorrhoidal veins (inferior mesenteric vein) to middle/inferior hemorrhoidal veins (internal iliac veins)
Splenomegaly
Ascites
Gastrointestinal wall thickening

Pathology
Causes include toxins (most commonly alcohol) and drugs, infections (most commonly hepatitis B or C), autoimmune disorders, genetic metabolic defects, acquired biliary diseases, vascular disorders, and other conditions
Hepatocellular necrosis and fibrosis
Parenchymal nodules
- Regenerative nodules: localized proliferation of hepatocytes and stroma
- Dysplastic nodules: nodular region of hepatocytes, at least 1 mm in diameter, with dysplasia but without definite malignant features; classified as low- or high-grade lesions. Diagnosis is usually made by a pathologist, not a radiologist.
- Hepatocellular carcinoma: malignant neoplasm of hepatocytes

MRI
Morphologic changes of the liver
- Segmental atrophy (right hepatic lobe and medial segment)
- Segmental hypertrophy (caudate lobe and lateral segment)
- Enlargement of the hilar periportal space between anterior wall of right portal vein and posterior edge of medial segment of left hepatic lobe
- Expanded gallbladder fossa sign
- Lobular and/or nodular contour due to atrophy/hypertrophy and parenchymal nodules
Diffuse parenchymal signal abnormalities
- Fibrosis: may be diffuse or focal, increased T2-SI. Confluent hepatic fibrosis may appear as mass-like areas or wedge-shape regions with associated capsular retraction.
- Iron: usually mild to moderate in degree, resulting in mild loss of T2-SI (in patients with cirrhosis unrelated to genetic hemochromatosis, pancreatic iron overload usually is not present)
- Steatosis: most commonly seen in alcohol-induced cirrhosis

Nodular Lesions
- Regenerative nodules: nonsiderotic nodules typically isointense on T1- and T2-WI images, with occasional hyperintensity on T1-WI and hypointensity on T2-WI images; no arterial phase enhancement and inconspicuous on portal venous phase
- Dysplastic nodules: hyperintense or hypointense on T1-WI and hypointense on T2-WI; may show arterial-phase enhancement
- Siderotic nodules (regenerative or dysplastic): hypointense on T1-weighted and T2-WI; most conspicuous on T2*-GRE images
- "Nodule within a nodule" sign: focus of hepatocellular carcinoma developing within a siderotic nodule appears hyperintense as compared with hypointense to the surrounding nodule on T2-WI
- Hepatocellular carcinoma (see Box 1-19)

hepatitis, primary biliary cirrhosis, and primary sclerosing cholangitis. Hemochromatosis and Wilson's disease are some of the genetic disorders that may cause cirrhosis. Biliary atresia, gallstone obstruction, and common bile duct stricture are acquired biliary disorders with potential for cirrhosis. Budd-Chiari syndrome, hepatic veno-occlusive disease, and chronic passive hepatic congestion are vascular disorders that may produce cirrhosis. Nonalcoholic steatohepatitis is an increasingly recognized cause of "cryptogenic" cirrhosis.[338]

Pathologically, cirrhosis is characterized by hepatocellular necrosis, fibrosis, and regeneration, with fibrosis being the critical feature.[422] Alteration of the hepatic vascular architecture by parenchymal fibrosis also is important in the cirrhotic process. The abnormal parenchymal nodules in cirrhosis are not necessarily regenerative, and regeneration is not required for the diagnosis. Fibrosis separates the parenchyma into nodules. Based on the size of parenchymal nodules, cirrhosis can be classified into micronodular, macronodular, or mixed patterns. Micronodules are defined as less than 3 mm in diameter, and macronodules are greater than 3 mm and up to several centimeters. Micronodular cirrhosis can progress to macronodular cirrhosis, which often is seen in end-stage liver disease of any cause. The micronodular pattern is exemplified by alcoholic cirrhosis. Macronodular cirrhosis is most frequently seen with chronic viral hepatitis and autoimmune hepatitis.

The terminology for nodular lesions occurring in cirrhotic livers has been standardized with a nomenclature that replaces a confusing set of older terms.[424] Regenerative nodules represent a localized proliferation of hepatocytes and their supporting stroma. Dysplastic nodules are defined as a nodular region of hepatocytes at least 1 mm in diameter with dysplasia and but no definite histologic features of malignancy. Dysplastic nodules are arbitrarily classified into low- and high-grade lesions.[425] Low-grade dysplastic nodules are characterized by minimally abnormal hepatocytes but no architectural or cytologic atypia.[424,426] Large-cell dysplasia may be present. Low-grade dysplastic nodules contain portal tracts. High-grade dysplastic nodules may show focal or diffuse architectural or cytologic atypia.[424,426] When foci of hepatocellular carcinoma develop within dysplastic nodules, they are termed dysplastic nodules with a subfocus of hepatocellular carcinoma. Hepatocellular carcinoma represents a malignant neoplasm composed of cells with hepatocellular differentiation. Thus, regenerative nodules, dysplastic nodules, and hepatocellular carcinoma can be viewed, respectively, as early, intermediate, and final steps in the hepatocarcinogenesis of cirrhosis.[427]

The MR imaging findings of cirrhosis include morphologic changes of the liver, diffuse parenchymal SI abnormalities, nodular hepatic lesions, and manifestations of portal hypertension. Segmental atrophy and hypertrophy are common in end-stage cirrhosis (see Fig. 1-13).[428] Atrophy usually involves the right hepatic lobe and medial segment, and hypertrophy usually involves the lateral segment and caudate lobe. Approximately one third of end-stage cirrhotic livers are diffusely atrophic, and approximately one quarter are of normal size and shape.[428] In patients with viral-induced cirrhosis, increasing atrophy of the right hepatic lobe and medial segment correlates with progression to decompensated cirrhosis and hypertrophy of the lateral segment and caudate lobe correlates with clinical stability.[429]

Enlargement of the hilar periportal space between the anterior wall of the right portal vein and the posterior edge of the medial segment of the left hepatic lobe is a useful indicator of early cirrhosis.[430] Thickness of the hilar periportal fat greater than 10 mm was 93% sensitive and 92% specific in one study. This enlargement was present in 98% of patients with early cirrhosis. The expanded gallbladder fossa sign refers to increasing fat in the pericholecystic space.[431] This increased fat is due to one or more of the following morphologic changes: atrophy of the medial segment, atrophy of the right hepatic lobe with counterclockwise rotation of the major interlobar fissure, hypertrophy of the caudate lobe, and hypertrophy of the lateral segment. This sign has high specificity and positive predictive value for cirrhosis (both 98%) but a lower sensitivity of 68%. The sign may not be present in early or mild cirrhosis or in advanced cirrhosis with lateral segment atrophy and preservation of the gallbladder position.

The predilection for segmental/lobar atrophy or hypertrophy in cirrhosis likely is related to alterations in portal venous blood flow that contains trophic factors.[432] The right portal vein directly enters the hepatic parenchyma after bifurcation from the main portal vein. Cirrhosis results in compression and irregular stenoses of the intrahepatic branches and consequently decreased portal venous blood flow to the right hepatic lobe. The left portal vein, which courses through the falciform ligament, remains outside the liver parenchyma prior to entering the left hepatic lobe, allowing greater portal venous blood flow. Despite receiving blood flow from the left portal vein, the medial segment also atrophies. Systemic blood flow from gastric, cystic, parabiliary, and capsular veins may drain into the medial segment and dilute or reverse portal venous perfusion, thereby promoting atrophy of this segment. In addition, circular blood flow has been reported in the umbilical portion of the left portal vein, with hepatopetal flow in the left half and hepatofugal flow in the right half.[433,434] The portal venous branches that supply the caudate lobe arise from the left portal vein and/or the bifurcation and have a short intrahepatic course. This vascular anatomy may preserve portal venous blood flow, allowing for caudate lobe hypertrophy.

In addition to distortion from segmental atrophy and hypertrophy, regenerative nodules distort the liver margin. The margin may be smooth, nodular, or grossly lobular.[428] Smooth or nodular margins may be seen with micronodular cirrhosis. A grossly lobular margin is often the result of atrophy and hypertrophy but may also be seen with one or more regenerative nodules greater than 3 cm.

Certain morphologic changes are more likely to be seen with different causes of cirrhosis. Caudate lobe hypertrophy and the presence of a right posterior hepatic notch are more commonly seen in alcoholic than viral-induced cirrhosis.[435] The right posterior hepatic notch is attributed to caudate lobe hypertrophy and right hepatic lobe atrophy. With primary sclerosing cholangitis, the lateral and posterior segments may atrophy with marked enlargement of the caudate lobe.[223,226,428] Diffuse hepatic hypertrophy is rarely seen except in patients with primary biliary cirrhosis.[428] A lobular liver margin is seen more frequently in some forms of biliary cirrhosis, such as PSC, than in other types of cirrhosis.

Diffuse fibrosis, iron, or lipid may result in parenchymal SI abnormalities at MR.[428] Fibrosis may manifest as diffuse or focal parenchymal SI abnormalities in the cirrhotic liver. Four patterns of diffuse fibrosis manifested as increased T2 SI have been described: patchy, poorly defined regions, thin perilobular bands, thick bridging bands surrounding regenerative nodules, and diffuse fibrosis causing perivascular "bull's-eye" cuffing.[428,436] Fibrosis may be less conspicuous on T1-WIs but will be of decreased SI relative to surrounding liver parenchyma.[428] Areas of fibrosis may show mild gadolinium enhancement.[436]

Confluent hepatic fibrosis may appear as mass-like areas of signal abnormality in patients with advanced cirrhosis.[437] These areas are often wedge-shaped, radiate from the porta hepatis, and are widest at the capsular surface. Involvement of the medial or anterior segments is most common and is associated with capsular retraction or lobar/lobar atrophy. Confluent hepatic fibrosis is hypointense to liver on T1-WIs and hyperintense on T2-WIs (Fig. 1-27). Confluent hepatic fibrosis does not enhance on arterial-phase imaging and becomes isointense to hyperintense to surrounding liver on delayed-phase imaging. Capsular retraction associated with confluent hepatic fibrosis is a useful discriminatory feature from hepatocellular carcinoma; the latter would be expected to show mass effect or an exophytic border.[438] SI characteristics alone cannot be used to differentiate focal confluent fibrosis from hepatocellular carcinoma.

The MR imaging periportal halo sign has been reported only in patients with primary biliary cirrhosis.[439] This sign refers to abnormal low SI surrounding the portal venous branches on both T1- and T2-WIs. The regions of signal abnormality are round, with a diameter of 5 to 10 mm, and do not produce mass effect. The lesions are present in all hepatic segments. The periportal halo sign is most conspicuous on portal venous and delayed phases of gadolinium-enhanced images. The histologic correlate may be a stellate, periportal hepatocellular parenchymal extinction encircled by a rosette of regenerating nodules.

In contrast to the lesions resulting in the periportal halo sign, regenerating nodules are usually of variable size and SI, are not centered on portal vein branches, and may show mass effect. While highly specific for primary biliary cirrhosis, the periportal halo sign had less than 50% sensitivity.

Diffuse iron deposition may occur in patient with cirrhosis, even in patients without genetic hemochromatosis or prior transfusions.[360,440] Hepatic parenchymal iron overload in cirrhotic patients without genetic hemochromatosis is usually mild to moderate in degree. On MR imaging, hepatic iron overload in cirrhosis may be evidenced by a mild, diffuse decrease in parenchymal SI or as scattered iron-containing regenerative nodules (siderotic nodules) (Fig. 1-28). In cirrhotic patients without genetic hemochromatosis, the pancreas should not depict abnormal low SI from iron deposition. Hepatic steatosis is seen most commonly in patients with alcohol-induced cirrhosis.[428] The MR imaging findings of steatosis were previously described.

Nodular lesions occurring in the cirrhotic liver include regenerative nodules, dysplastic nodules, and hepatocellular carcinoma (HCC). Iron-free regenerative nodules are usually isointense on T1- and T2-WIs with occasional T1 hyperintensity or T2 hypointensity.[427,441] In contrast to hepatocellular carcinoma, regenerative nodules are virtually never hyperintense on T2-WIs with two exceptions. Regenerative nodules in chronic Budd-Chiari syndrome and infarcted regenerative nodules with coagulative necrosis may be hyperintense on T2-WIs and simulate HCC.[391,438,442] Almost exclusively supplied by the portal vein, regenerative nodules do not show arterial-phase gadolinium enhancement.[427] Nonsiderotic regenerative nodules are usually inconspicuous on portal venous phase CE imaging owing to their histologic similarity to normal liver parenchyma.[443]

Dysplastic nodules are hyperintense or hypointense to surrounding liver on T1-WIs and hypointense on T2-WIs.[426,444,445] Dysplastic nodules may show arterial-phase enhancement at MR imaging.[444,446,447] This arterial phase enhancement likely reflects neoplastic angiogenesis evidenced by unpaired arteries at pathologic examination.[444,446,447] Unpaired arteries (isolated arteries without accompanying bile ducts) and sinusoidal capillarization progressively increase from regenerative nodules to dysplastic nodules to HCC.[446] During hepatocarcinogenesis pathologic nontriadal arteries replace the portal triads as the dominant blood supply to large dysplastic nodules and small HCCs.[438] Subtraction imaging allows detection of arterial-phase enhancement of dysplastic nodules that are hyperintense on precontrast images.[427] However, MR imaging has proved insensitive to the detection of dysplastic nodules[444,445] and HCCs that are smaller than 2 cm.[444]

Iron-containing nodules may be regenerative or dysplastic and will appear hypointense on T1- and T2-WIs. Iron-containing nodules are most conspicuous on T2*-GRE images, as the magnetic susceptibility

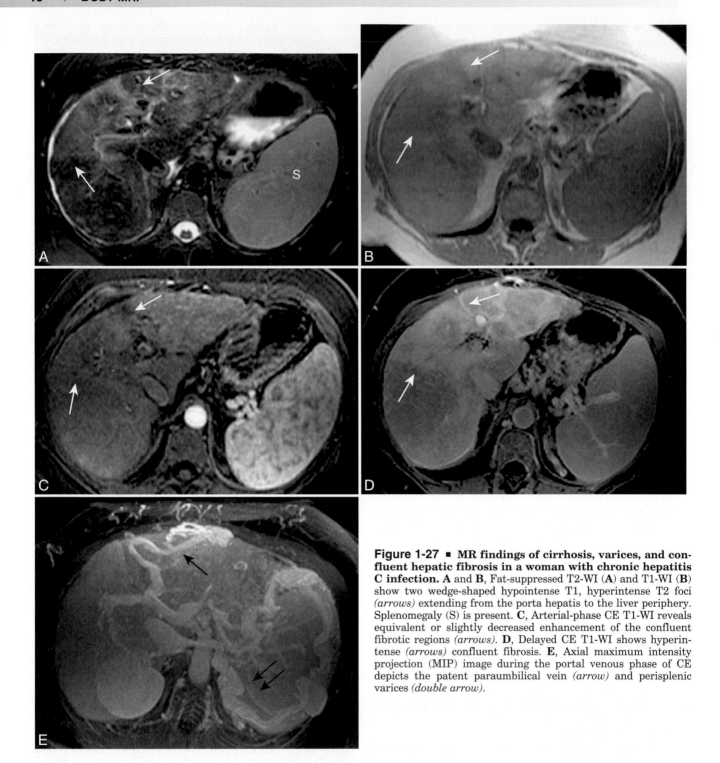

Figure 1-27 ■ **MR findings of cirrhosis, varices, and confluent hepatic fibrosis in a woman with chronic hepatitis C infection. A** and **B,** Fat-suppressed T2-WI (**A**) and T1-WI (**B**) show two wedge-shaped hypointense T1, hyperintense T2 foci *(arrows)* extending from the porta hepatis to the liver periphery. Splenomegaly (S) is present. **C,** Arterial-phase CE T1-WI reveals equivalent or slightly decreased enhancement of the confluent fibrotic regions *(arrows)*. **D,** Delayed CE T1-WI shows hyperintense *(arrows)* confluent fibrosis. **E,** Axial maximum intensity projection (MIP) image during the portal venous phase of CE depicts the patent paraumbilical vein *(arrow)* and perisplenic varices *(double arrow)*.

effect of iron results in marked hypointensity. GRE images with a TE of more than 9 ms improves sensitivity for the detection of iron-containing nodules (see Fig. 1-28).[448] Siderotic regenerative and dysplastic nodules cannot be distinguished by MR imaging, and iron-containing nodules should simply be referred to as siderotic nodules.[427,449] Iron has not been proved to

cause the dysplasia or hepatocellular carcinoma that may develop within siderotic nodules.[448]

Dysplastic nodules with a subfocus of hepatocellular carcinoma can show a characteristic appearance at MR imaging, the "nodule within a nodule" sign.[450,451] The focus of HCC will usually appear as a high T2 SI focus within a hypointense dysplastic

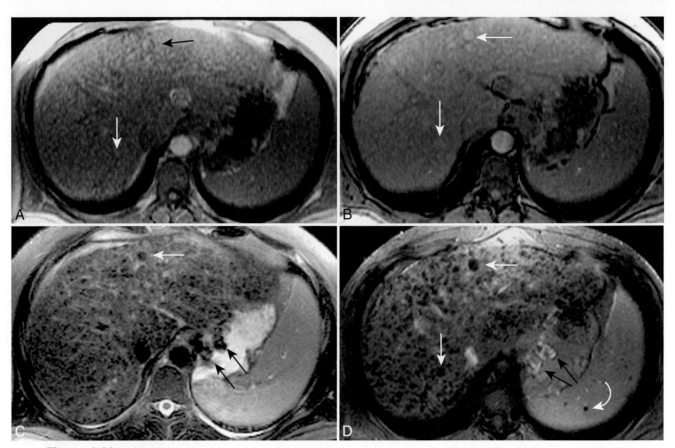

Figure 1-28 ■ MR depiction of iron-rich, siderotic, regenerative nodules and splenic Gamna-Gandy bodies in a patient with hepatitis C–induced cirrhosis. A and **B,** In-phase (**A**) and opposed-phase (**B**) T1-WIs shows multiple minimally hyperintense regenerative nodules. Some nodules *(arrows)* appear to lose SI in **A** owing to magnetic susceptibility effects that become more pronounced as the echo time is increased from 2.3 to 4.5 ms. The Gamna-Gandy bodies are not well revealed. **C,** T2-WI shows the multiple low SI siderotic nodules *(arrows)*. However, they are not as well revealed as the in-phase (**B**) or heavily T2*-W (**D**) GRE images. Flow voids are present within gastric varices *(black arrows)*. **D,** T2*- GRE image (TE = 20, FA = 20°) best shows the hypointense siderotic nodules *(arrows)* and Gamna-Gandy bodies *(curved arrow)* secondary to the T2* effects of iron. Flow-related enhancement is present within the gastric varices *(black arrows)*.

nodule (Fig. 1-29). The focus of hepatocellular carcinoma may, however, be isointense to the remainder of the dysplastic nodule.[452] In siderotic nodules, the focus of hepatocellular carcinoma appears hyperintense to the remainder of the nodule on T2*-GRE images.[450] The focus of HCC may show arterial-phase enhancement as well.[427]

Manifestations of portal hypertension detectable at MR include portosystemic collateral vessels, splenomegaly, ascites, and gastrointestinal wall thickening. Portal hypertension, an increased resistance and pressure within the portal venous system, is defined as pressure greater than 10 mm Hg.[453] Portal hypertension is classified into three major anatomic categories: prehepatic, intrahepatic, and posthepatic. Further classification based on sinusoidal pressures includes presinusoidal, intrasinusoidal, and postsinusoidal categories. Prehepatic causes include portal vein or splenic vein thrombosis. Intrahepatic portal

hypertension is usually due to cirrhosis or other chronic liver disease but may develop in severe acute hepatitis or acute fatty liver of pregnancy. Posthepatic portal hypertension results from the hepatic venous outflow obstruction that occurs in Budd-Chiari syndrome, veno-occlusive disease, and passive hepatic congestion.

Portosystemic collateral vessels allow portal venous blood to bypass the liver, but they consequently decrease delivery of hepatotropic factors to the liver, allow toxins access to the systemic circulation, and predispose to potentially life-threatening gastrointestinal hemorrhage.[453,454] Esophageal and paraesophageal varices are primarily supplied by the left gastric vein and typically drain into the azygous/hemizygous venous system.[455] Esophageal varices are the most common source of upper gastrointestinal hemorrhage.[436] Paraumbilical veins and abdominal wall collateral vessels are supplied by the left portal vein.

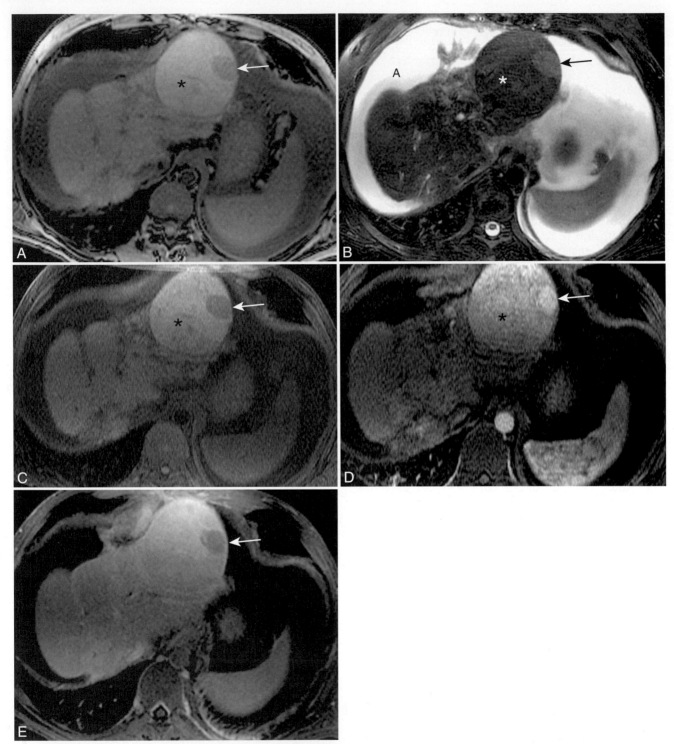

Figure 1-29 ■ **MR depiction of a hepatocellular carcinoma that shows a variation of the "nodule within a nodule" sign in a 47-year-old man with cirrhosis related to primary sclerosing cholangitis. A**, Opposed-phase T1-WI shows a hyperintense mass (∗) of the lateral segment of a cirrhotic liver. The mass did not show SI loss as compared with a corresponding in-phase image (not shown) to suggest intratumoral lipid. Along the left aspect of the mass is a hypointense nodule *(arrows)*. **B**, Fat-suppressed T2-WI shows that the mass is isointense to liver except for the internal nodule that is hyperintense *(arrow)*. Ascites (A) is present. **C** and **D**, Fat-suppressed T1-WIs obtained before (**C**) and after (**D**) the arterial phase of contrast show marked enhancement of the small internal nodule *(arrow)*. Subtraction images and SI measurements did not reveal arterial phase enhancement within the dominant mass (∗). **E**, On a delayed-phase CE T1-WI, the mass (∗) is isointense and the contrast within the nodule *(arrow)* has washed out and is now hypointense to liver. At surgery, the entire mass was moderately differentiated hepatocellular carcinoma with suspected foci of vascular invasion. The internal nodule represents a more poorly differentiated and hypervascular component. In this instance, the only specific feature of the mass that suggested hepatocellular carcinoma was its size. Lesion isointensity to liver on T2-WI and lack of arterial phase enhancement are more in keeping with a regenerative nodule. Until a nodule becomes hyperintense to liver on T2-WIs or reveals arterial-phase enhancement, a specific MR diagnosis of hepatocellular carcinoma cannot be established.

Paraumbilical veins, located within or around the ligamentum teres and falciform ligament, may anastomose with the superior epigastric or internal thoracic veins that drain into the superior vena cava or may anastomose with the inferior epigastric veins that drain into the external iliac veins and inferior vena cava.[454]

Retroperitoneal collateral vessels allow bypass of intestinal or retroperitoneal tributaries of the superior and inferior mesenteric veins into systemic veins, including the lumbar, phrenic, gonadal, and renal veins.[436,454] Two types of shunts to the left renal vein may develop: gastrorenal and splenorenal. Left gastric, posterior gastric, or short gastric veins can anastomose with the left inferior phrenic or left adrenal veins prior to draining into the left renal vein, producing a gastrorenal shunt. Other tributaries of the splenic vein may communicate with the left renal vein and produce a splenorenal shunt. Superior hemorrhoidal veins (tributaries of the inferior mesenteric vein) anastomose with middle and inferior hemorrhoidal veins that drain into the systemic internal iliac venous system. The portal venous phase of gadolinium-enhanced MR imaging is ideal for detection of portosystemic collateral vessels and varices. Multiplanar maximal intensity projection and other volume-rendering techniques are useful in depicting the tortuous course of these vessels.

Ascites represents the accumulation of serous fluid within the peritoneal space.[453] The mechanism of ascites production in cirrhosis is complex; implicated factors include portal hypertension, hypoalbuminemia, and peripheral circulatory disturbances. Development of ascites is a poor prognostic sign in cirrhosis. Ascites may be complicated by spontaneous bacterial peritonitis.

Splenomegaly and Gamna-Gandy bodies are splenic manifestations of portal hypertension. Gamna-Gandy bodies are organized foci of hemorrhage containing fibrosis, calcium, and hemosiderin.[443,456,457] Gamna-Gandy nodules are hypointense to surrounding splenic parenchyma, particularly with gradient-echo pulse sequences, because of the magnetic susceptibility effect of iron-containing hemosiderin (see Fig. 1-28). Gamna-Gandy bodies and other splenic diseases are discussed in Chapter 5.

Other abdominal imaging findings related to cirrhosis include gastrointestinal wall thickening and mesenteric, omental, and retroperitoneal edema. Portal hypertension and hypoproteinemia are suspected causes of gastrointestinal wall thickening in cirrhosis.[458] The jejunum and ascending colon are the most commonly involved segments.[459] An interesting observation in patients with cirrhosis is that mural thickening of small bowel without jejunal involvement or of colonic segments without ascending colonic involvement implies that the cause of the bowel wall thickening is a condition other than cirrhosis.[459] Haustral thickening of the colon is more common than mural thickening.[459] The decreased number of potential collateral pathways related to the superior mesenteric venous drainage of the small intestine and right colon compared with the inferior mesenteric drainage of the left colon is a suspected cause of this differential involvement.[458] The presence of pneumatosis or a pancolitis involving the entire colon and rectum implies an ischemic or infectious etiology.[458] Mesenteric, omental, and retroperitoneal edema is a common finding in patients with cirrhosis.[460] This edema correlates with volume expansion and hypoproteinemia, rather than portal hypertension, and is associated with subcutaneous edema, pleural effusions, and ascites.

HEPATOCELLULAR CARCINOMA (BOX 1-19)

Hepatocellular carcinoma (HCC) is the most common primary malignancy of the liver.[461] HCC arises from the hepatocyte, usually in association with chronic liver disease. The incidence of HCC varies considerably with geographic location.[25] HCC is the

---

1-19   Hepatocellular Carcinoma

Clinical

Most common primary malignant neoplasm of the liver
Incidence varies with prevalence of chronic hepatitis and exposure to aflatoxin
Higher incidence in males
Symptoms include right upper quadrant pain, weight loss, and fever
Serum α-fetoprotein tumor marker

Pathology

Malignant hepatocytes
Hepatic artery is the dominant blood supply
Frequent microscopic portal venous or hepatic venous invasion

MRI

T1-WI: variable SI
　Lesions < 1.5 cm often isointense to liver
　Lesions < 3.0 cm may be hyperintense to liver owing to presence of intratumoral lipid, copper, or glycogen
T2-WI: most lesions hyperintense or isointense to liver (hypointensity or isointensity correlated with better differentiated tumors)
Dynamic CE imaging
　Arterial phase: small lesions (< 1.5 to 2.0 cm) usually show homogeneous, intense enhancement; larger lesions show heterogeneous enhancement
　Portal venous phase: small lesions may be isointense; larger lesions usually hypointense
　Tumor capsule: more common in larger lesions, hypointense on arterial phase with delayed enhancement
Two findings on MR highly suspicious for hepatocellular carcinoma
　Isointensity to spleen on T2-WI
　Arterial-phase enhancement of a nodule that is also visible on other pulse sequences

third most common cause of morbidity and mortality in developing countries and is the eighth most common cancer worldwide.[462] The highest incidence occurs in Southeast Asia and tropical Africa, where HCC is the most common or one of the most common malignancies. Intermediate-risk regions include Japan, the Middle East, and the Mediterranean. The lowest incidence is found in Western countries, South America, and Australia. This variable incidence is largely related to the prevalence of chronic hepatitis B and C infections and exposure to aflatoxin. Increasing rates of HCC in the West and Japan have been attributed to the rising rate of chronic hepatitis C infection.[463] From 25% to 30% of individuals with both hepatitis C and cirrhosis develop HCC. Patients with concurrent hepatitis B and C infections have the highest risk of developing HCC.[464] Regardless of geographic location, risk factors include male gender, increasing age, and the presence of cirrhosis. The age peak is inversely related to the incidence of the tumor, occurring in younger patients in high-risk regions and older patients in low-risk regions. The male predominance, which varies from 4:1 in low-risk areas to 8:1 in high-risk areas, is incompletely understood. Suspected contributory factors include androgenic hormones or receptors, increased use of tobacco and alcohol, increased incidence of cirrhosis, and higher DNA synthesis rate in the livers of men.[25] Numerous metabolic disorders are associated with an increased incidence of hepatocellular carcinoma and include genetic hemochromatosis, chronic tyrosinemia, glycogen storage diseases types I and IIIb, α_1-antitrypsin deficiency, and Wilson's disease.

The clinical manifestations of HCC are nonspecific. Symptoms may include right upper quadrant pain, weight loss, and fever.[25,26] Jaundice, ascites and hepatic encephalopathy reflect hepatic decompensation. A more fulminant clinical presentation, similar to that of hepatic abscess, is often reported in tropical Africa.[25] Tumoral rupture with intraperitoneal hemorrhage also is common in Africa and Southeast Asia. Serum α-fetoprotein is elevated in HCC. The macroscopic pathologic appearance of hepatocellular carcinoma has been classified as expanding, spreading, multifocal and diffuse, and indeterminate forms.[25,26,463] The hepatic artery supplies HCC. Frequent invasion of the portal or hepatic veins contributes to intrahepatic and metastatic spread (Fig. 1-30). Biliary invasion may result in obstructive jaundice.

HCC may be hypointense, isointense, or hyperintense to surrounding liver parenchyma on T1-WIs. Most HCCs are hypointense on T1-WIs.

HCCs smaller than 1.5 cm are often isointense.[465] T1 hyperintensity is particularly common in lesions less than 3 cm[466] and has been correlated with degree of tumoral differentiation, the presence of intratumoral lipid, copper or glycogen, and the presence of zinc in surrounding liver parenchyma.[465-467] Intratumoral copper results in T1 hyperintensity via a paramagnetic effect. Lipid tends to be diffusely distributed in smaller HCCs, whereas focal accumulations of lipid are identified in

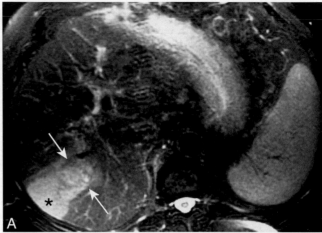

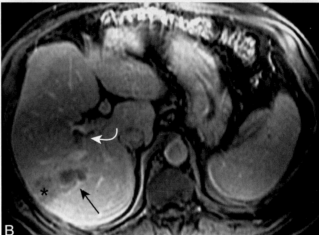

Figure 1-30 ■ **Hepatocellular carcinoma with portal vein invasion shown by MR in a man with hepatitis C. A**, Fat-suppressed T2-WI shows a heterogeneous high SI mass of the posterior segment of the right hepatic lobe (*arrows*). The wedge-shaped area of increased SI peripheral to the tumor represents peritumoral edema (*). **B**, Delayed CE T1-WI shows the hypointense hepatocellular carcinoma (*arrow*), enhancement of the tumoral pseudocapsule, and hypointense tumor thrombus in the posterior division of the right portal vein (*curved arrow*). The wedge-shaped area of edema shows decreased enhancement (*), indicating decreased portal venous blood supply.

larger tumors.[468] Chemical shift imaging allows detection of microscopic lipid in HCC (Fig. 1-31; see Fig. 5-5).[340,469] Lipiodol, used in hepatic chemoembolization, may be retained in hepatocellular carcinoma and appears hyperintense on T1-WIs owing to its fatty acid component.[318]

Most HCCs are either hyperintense or isointense to liver parenchyma on T2-WIs (see Figs. 1-31 and 5-5).[465] T2 hypointensity or isointensity has been correlated with better differentiated tumors.[426,466] HCC is more conspicuous on T2-WIs obtained with relatively shorter TR and TE.[470] Because many HCCs can be difficult to discern on T2-WIs,[471] it is important that MR examinations in cirrhotic patients include high-quality breath-hold T1-WIs and dynamic CE imaging.

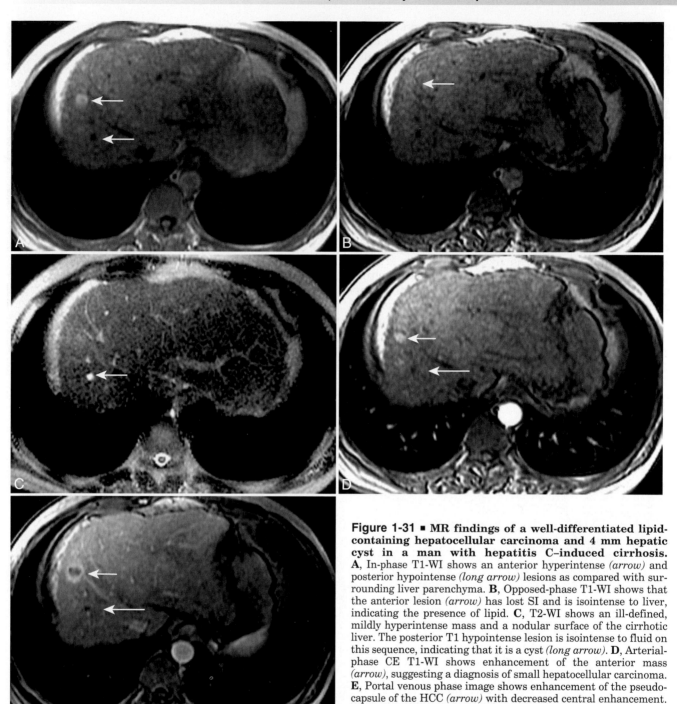

Figure 1-31 ■ MR findings of a well-differentiated lipid-containing hepatocellular carcinoma and 4 mm hepatic cyst in a man with hepatitis C–induced cirrhosis. A, In-phase T1-WI shows an anterior hyperintense *(arrow)* and posterior hypointense *(long arrow)* lesions as compared with surrounding liver parenchyma. **B**, Opposed-phase T1-WI shows that the anterior lesion *(arrow)* has lost SI and is isointense to liver, indicating the presence of lipid. **C**, T2-WI shows an ill-defined, mildly hyperintense mass and a nodular surface of the cirrhotic liver. The posterior T1 hypointense lesion is isointense to fluid on this sequence, indicating that it is a cyst *(long arrow)*. **D**, Arterial-phase CE T1-WI shows enhancement of the anterior mass *(arrow)*, suggesting a diagnosis of small hepatocellular carcinoma. **E**, Portal venous phase image shows enhancement of the pseudocapsule of the HCC *(arrow)* with decreased central enhancement. The subcentimeter cyst shows no enhancement *(long arrow)*.

In addition to the fibrolamellar variant of hepatocellular carcinoma, HCC may develop in patients without cirrhosis or other identifiable risk factors.[472,473] In some patients, viral hepatitis or excessive alcohol use may cause HCC prior to the development of cirrhosis. Even in the absence of cirrhosis, many of these "de novo" HCCs occur in a histologic background of nonspecific liver injury including inflammation, steatosis, and fibrosis.[472]

In contrast to patients with the fibrolamellar variant, most of these patients are older, are male, and have elevated serum α-fetoprotein.

In patients without cirrhosis, HCC is more likely to be unifocal than multifocal. Two factors are suspected to contribute to the multifocality of HCC in cirrhosis.[473] One factor is the field effect of multiple nodular lesions predisposed to the hepatocarcinogenic pathway. The other factor is the predilection of cirrhosis-related HCC for portal/hepatic venous invasion with consequent intrahepatic metastatic dissemination. HCC in noncirrhotic patients is often larger than in cirrhotic patients. More frequent imaging surveillance of cirrhotic patients and the increased hepatic functional reserve of noncirrhotic patients may account for the size difference at detection.[473] Central necrosis is very common in HCC occurring in noncirrhotic livers.[472]

The gadolinium-enhancement pattern of HCC is dependent on the size and differentiation of the lesion.[465,474] Small HCCs (< 2.0 cm) usually show homogeneous, intense, arterial-phase enhancement (Fig. 1-32).[465,474] Approximately 10% to 15% of small HCCs are identified only on arterial-phase imaging and will appear isointense on unenhanced images and the later phases of gadolinium-enhanced imaging.[438,465] During the progression of a dysplastic nodule to HCC, the intranodular decrease in portal venous flow precedes the increase in hepatic arterial flow, and some small HCCs may lack enhancement in arterial and portal venous phases and thus appear hypointense on portal venous phase images.[475]

The sinusoidal spaces of moderately and poorly differentiated HCCs are larger than those of well-differentiated tumors.[476] The larger sinusoidal spaces result in greater contrast enhancement. Some small, well-differentiated HCCs show minimal enhancement on arterial-phase images and appear hypointense on portal venous images. Larger HCCs show heterogeneous enhancement on arterial-phase imaging. Necrosis, fat, and hemorrhage may contribute to the heterogeneous enhancement of larger lesions.[476] A nodule in a cirrhotic liver that shows both arterial-phase enhancement and venous washout is very specific for HCC; the absence of either enhancement excludes a diagnosis of HCC with a high degree of certainty.[477]

The fibrous tumoral capsule or "pseudocapsule" is a characteristic finding of HCC at MR imaging and is more often identified in lesions larger than 1.5

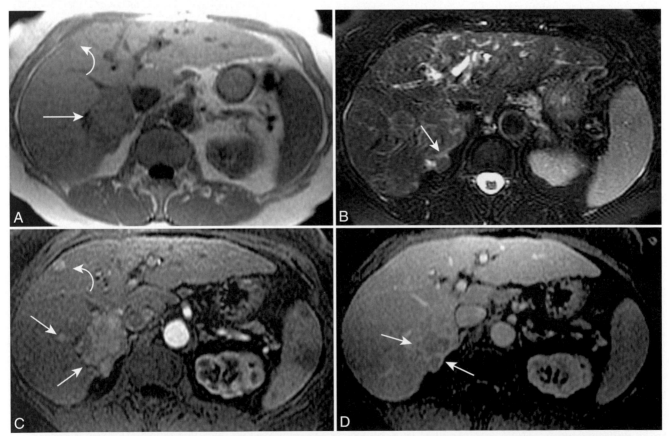

Figure 1-32 ■ MR depiction of multifocal hepatocellular carcinoma in a woman with hepatitis C–related cirrhosis. A, In-phase T1-WI shows a heterogeneously hypointense mass in the anterior and posterior segments *(arrow)* of the right lobe. A hypointense nodule is also revealed in the subcapsular medial segment *(curved arrow).* **B,** Fat-suppressed T2-WI shows the mass is isointense to liver parenchyma. An exophytic satellite nodule protrudes from the medial surface of the liver and is outlined by a rim of high SI *(arrow).* **C,** Dynamic CE T1-WI shows a hypervascular mass with adjacent hypervascular nodules *(arrows).* The medial segment left-lobe nodule *(curved arrow)* also enhances, indicating that it too represents HCC. **D,** Delayed-phase gadolinium-enhanced image no longer depicts the smaller nodules. Some small hepatocellular carcinomas may only be detected on arterial-phase imaging. The larger mass shows enhancement of the pseudocapsule *(arrows).*

to 2.0 cm.[474,478,479] The presence of a capsule correlates with tumoral differentiation.[480] The capsule contains inflammatory and stromal cells, vascular structures, and frequently bile ducts.[480] On T1- and T2-WI, the capsule is hypointense to surrounding liver.[474,480] Capsules thicker than 4 mm may show an outer T2 hyperintense ring.[474] On dynamic CE imaging, the capsule first shows enhancement during the portal venous phase and increases into the delayed phase (see Figs. 1-30 and 1-31).[480] Extracapsular invasion of HCC manifests either as a tumor nodule protruding through the capsule or as adjacent satellite nodules.[481]

Venous invasion is a frequent complication of HCC, with the portal venous system more commonly involved than the hepatic venous system.[14] Microscopic invasion is more common than macroscopic invasion.[482] Tumors invasive of the veins are more likely to be larger, produce higher levels of α-fetoprotein, and lack encapsulation.[482] Venous invasion is best detected on CE imaging (see Fig. 1-30).[14] Tumor thrombus shows enhancement on the arterial phase and appear as a filling defect with venous expansion on portal or delayed phases.[14,474]

Extrahepatic metastases usually occur in patients with advanced intrahepatic tumor (stage IVA).[483] The most common sites are the lungs, regional and distant lymph nodes, bone, adrenal glands, and peritoneum/omentum. Lymphadenopathy occurs frequently in patients with all forms of end-stage cirrhosis,[484] and benign and malignant lymphadenopathy cannot be differentiated by size criteria alone.[483] Imaging features that may help in diagnosing malignant lymphadenopathy include arterial phase enhancement or increasing size.[483] By providing a comprehensive evaluation of the bile ducts, hepatic arteries, portal and hepatic veins, and size and distribution of any HCCs, MR can help determine what therapies may be of greatest benefit to the patient (including potential liver transplantation).[485]

Several lesions that may simulate HCC at MR include incidental masses (hemangiomas, cysts, and focal nodular hyperplasia), vascular abnormalities (arteriovenous shunts, pseudoaneurysms, and transient hepatic intensity differences), focal confluent hepatic fibrosis, and infarcted regenerative nodules. Hepatic hemangiomas can show "flash-filling" on arterial-phase imaging. Persistent enhancement of hemangioma during the later phases of dynamic imaging allows differentiation from HCC.[486] Small arterioportal shunts and pseudoaneurysms, usually related to prior biopsy, may mimic HCC. HCC will show washout of contrast material, whereas the enhancement pattern of arterioportal shunts and pseudoaneurysms will follow that of the blood pool. Transient areas of arterial-phase enhancement may result from nontumorous arterioportal shunts or obstruction of portal venules and can simulate HCC.[438,487] The wedge shape and preservation of internal vasculature may allow discrimination of transient hepatic SI differences from HCC. Alternatively, a "double contrast" MR examination could be performed in which a superparamagnetic iron oxide contrast agent is injected before the gadolinium. Pseudolesions that are composed of normal hepatic parenchyma would be expected to incorporate the iron agent and thus allow potential distinction from HCC.[488] However, approximately 10% of HCCs will also enhance with iron oxide, and thus the presence of iron uptake does not completely exclude HCC.[489,490] On follow-up imaging, true HCCs would be expected to grow while pseudo-lesions would either be stable or resolve.[487]

REFERENCES

1. Campeau NG, Johnson CD, Felmlee JP, et al. MR imaging of the abdomen with a phased-array multicoil: prospective clinical evaluation. Radiology 1995;195:769-776.
2. Cameron IL, Ord VA, Fullerton GD. Characterization of proton NMR relaxation times in normal and pathological tissues by correlation with other tissue parameters. Magn Reson Imaging 1984;2:97-106.
3. Morrin MM, Rofsky NM. Techniques for liver MR imaging. Magn Reson Imaging Clin N Am 2001;9:675-696, v.
4. Keogan MT, Spritzer CE, Paulson EK, et al. Liver MR imaging: comparison of respiratory triggered fast spin echo with T2-weighted spin-echo and inversion recovery. Abdom Imaging 1996;21:433-439.
5. Pauleit D, Textor J, Bachmann R, et al. Improving the detectability of focal liver lesions on T2-weighted MR images: ultrafast breath-hold or respiratory-triggered thin-section MRI? J Magn Reson Imaging 2001;14:128-133.
6. Ito K, Mitchell DG, Outwater EK, Szklaruk J, Sadek AG. Hepatic lesions: discrimination of nonsolid, benign lesions from solid, malignant lesions with heavily T2-weighted fast spin-echo MR imaging. Radiology 1997;204:729-737.
7. McFarland EG, Mayo-Smith WW, Saini S, Hahn PF, Goldberg MA, Lee MJ. Hepatic hemangiomas and malignant tumors: improved differentiation with heavily T2-weighted conventional spin-echo MR imaging. Radiology 1994;193:43-47.
8. Kiryu S, Okada Y, Ohtomo K. Differentiation between hemangiomas and cysts of the liver with single-shot fast-spin echo image using short and long TE. J Comput Assist Tomogr 2002;26:687-690.
9. Helmberger T, Semelka RC. New contrast agents for imaging the liver. Magn Reson Imaging Clin N Am 2001;9:745-766, vi.
10. Oksendal AN, Hals PA. Biodistribution and toxicity of MR imaging contrast media. J Magn Reson Imaging 1993;3:157-165.
11. Hendrick RE, Haacke EM. Basic physics of MR contrast agents and maximization of image contrast. J Magn Reson Imaging 1993;3:137-148.
12. Lee VS, Lavelle MT, Krinsky GA, Rofsky NM. Volumetric MR imaging of the liver and applications. Magn Reson Imaging Clin N Am 2001;9:697-716, v-vi.
13. Yu JS, Rofsky NM. Dynamic subtraction MR imaging of the liver: advantages and pitfalls. AJR Am J Roentgenol 2003;180:1351-1357.
14. Low RN. MR imaging of the liver using gadolinium chelates. Magn Reson Imaging Clin N Am 2001;9:717-743.
15. Hussain HK, Londy FJ, Francis IR, et al. Hepatic arterial phase MR imaging with automated bolus-detection three-dimensional fast gradient-recalled-echo sequence: comparison with test-bolus method. Radiology 2003;226:558-566.
16. Abdou N, Napoli AM, Hynes MR, Allen JC, Jr., Wible JH, Jr. Safety assessment of gadoversetamide (OptiMARK) administered by power injector. J Magn Reson Imaging 2004;19:133-140.
17. Earls JP, Rofsky NM, DeCorato DR, Krinsky GA, Weinreb JC. Hepatic arterial-phase dynamic gadolinium-enhanced MR imaging: optimization with a test examination and a power injector. Radiology 1997;202:268-273.
18. Kopka L, Vosshenrich R, Rodenwaldt J, Grabbe E. Differences in injection rates on contrast-enhanced breath-hold three-dimensional MR angiography. AJR Am J Roentgenol 1998;170:345-348.
19. Edmondson HA, Henderson B, Benton B. Liver-cell adenomas associated with use of oral contraceptives. N Engl J Med 1976;294:470-472.
20. Tao LC. Oral contraceptive-associated liver cell adenoma and hepatocellular carcinoma: cytomorphology and mechanism of malignant transformation. Cancer 1991;68:341-347.
21. Soe KL, Soe M, Gluud C. Liver pathology associated with the use of anabolic-androgenic steroids. Liver 1992;12:73-79.
22. Labrune P, Trioche P, Duvaltier I, Chevalier P, Odievre M. Hepatocellular adenomas in glycogen storage disease type I

and III: a series of 43 patients and review of the literature. J Pediatr Gastroenterol Nutr 1997;24:276-279.

23. Ichikawa T, Federle MP, Grazioli L, Nalesnik M. Hepatocellular adenoma: multiphasic CT and histopathologic findings in 25 patients. Radiology 2000;214:861-868.

24. Paulson EK, McClellan JS, Washington K, Spritzer CE, Meyers WC, Baker ME. Hepatic adenoma: MR characteristics and correlation with pathologic findings. AJR Am J Roentgenol 1994;163:113-116.

25. Anthony PP. 1. Tumours and tumour-like lesions of the liver and biliary tract: aetiology, epidemiology, and pathology. In: MacSween RNM, Burt AD, Portmann BC, Ishak KG, Scheuer PJ, Anthony PP, eds. Pathology of the Liver, 4th ed. Churchill Livingstone, 2002, pp 711-776.

26. Craig JR, Peters RL, Edmondson HA. Tumors of the liver and intrahepatic bile ducts. Washington, D.C.: Armed Forces Institute of Pathology, 1989.

27. Grazioli L, Federle MP, Brancatelli G, Ichikawa T, Olivetti L, Blachar A. Hepatic adenomas: imaging and pathologic findings. Radiographics 2001;21:877-892; discussion 892-874.

28. Arrive L, Flejou JF, Vilgrain V, et al. Hepatic adenoma: MR findings in 51 pathologically proved lesions. Radiology 1994;193:507-512.

29. Casillas VJ, Amendola MA, Gascue A, Pinnar N, Levi JU, Perez JM. Imaging of nontraumatic hemorrhagic hepatic lesions. Radiographics 2000;20:367-378.

30. Foster JH, Berman MM. The malignant transformation of liver cell adenomas. Arch Surg 1994;129:712-717.

31. Leese T, Farges O, Bismuth H. Liver cell adenomas: a 12-year surgical experience from a specialist hepato-biliary unit. Ann Surg 1988;208:558-564.

32. Ito M, Sasaki M, Wen CY, et al. Liver cell adenoma with malignant transformation: a case report. World J Gastroenterol 2003;9:2379-2381.

33. Kerlin P, Davis GL, McGill DB, Weiland LH, Adson MA, Sheedy PF Jr. Hepatic adenoma and focal nodular hyperplasia: clinical, pathologic, and radiologic features. Gastroenterology 1983;84:994-1002.

34. Flowers BF, McBurney RP, Vera SR. Ruptured hepatic adenoma: a spectrum of presentation and treatment. Am Surg 1990;56:380-383.

35. Aseni P, Sansalone CV, Sammartino C, et al. Rapid disappearance of hepatic adenoma after contraceptive withdrawal. J Clin Gastroenterol 2001;33:234-236.

36. Kawakatsu M, Vilgrain V, Erlinger S, Nahum H. Disappearance of liver cell adenoma: CT and MR imaging. Abdom Imaging 1997;22:274-276.

37. Chung KY, Mayo-Smith WW, Saini S, Rahmouni A, Golli M, Mathieu D. Hepatocellular adenoma: MR imaging features with pathologic correlation. AJR Am J Roentgenol 1995;165:303-308.

38. Ault GT, Wren SM, Ralls PW, Reynolds TB, Stain SC. Selective management of hepatic adenomas. Am Surg 1996;62:825-829.

39. Flejou JF, Barge J, Menu Y, et al. Liver adenomatosis: an entity distinct from liver adenoma? Gastroenterology 1985;89:1132-1138.

40. Ribeiro A, Burgart LJ, Nagorney DM, Gores GJ. Management of liver adenomatosis: results with a conservative surgical approach. Liver Transpl Surg 1998;4:388-398.

41. Grazioli L, Federle MP, Ichikawa T, Balzano E, Nalesnik M, Madariaga J. Liver adenomatosis: clinical, histopathologic, and imaging findings in 15 patients. Radiology 2000;216:395-402.

42. Chiche L, Dao T, Salame E, et al. Liver adenomatosis: reappraisal, diagnosis, and surgical management: eight new cases and review of the literature. Ann Surg 2000;231:74-81.

43. Buetow PC, Pantongrag-Brown L, Buck JL, Ros PR, Goodman ZD. Focal nodular hyperplasia of the liver: radiologic-pathologic correlation. Radiographics 1996;16:369-388.

44. Hussain SM, Terkivatan T, Zondervan PE, et al. Focal nodular hyperplasia: findings at state-of-the-art MR imaging, US, CT, and pathologic analysis. Radiographics 2004;24:3-17; discussion 18-19.

45. Nguyen BN, Flejou JF, Terris B, Belghiti J, Degott C. Focal nodular hyperplasia of the liver: a comprehensive pathologic study of 305 lesions and recognition of new histologic forms. Am J Surg Pathol 1999;23:1441-1454.

46. Mathieu D, Kobeiter H, Maison P, et al. Oral contraceptive use and focal nodular hyperplasia of the liver. Gastroenterology 2000;118:560-564.

47. Leconte I, Van Beers BE, Lacrosse M, et al. Focal nodular hyperplasia: natural course observed with CT and MRI. J Comput Assist Tomogr 2000;24:61-66.

48. Mahfouz AE, Hamm B, Taupitz M, Wolf KJ. Hypervascular liver lesions: differentiation of focal nodular hyperplasia from malignant tumors with dynamic gadolinium-enhanced MR imaging. Radiology 1993;186:133-138.

49. Mortele KJ, Praet M, Van Vlierberghe H, Kunnen M, Ros PR. CT and MR imaging findings in focal nodular hyperplasia of the liver: radiologic-pathologic correlation. AJR Am J Roentgenol 2000;175:687-692.

50. Dill-Macky M, Frazer C, de Boer WB. Magnetic resonance features of focal nodular hyperplasia of the liver. Australas Radiol 1999;43:315-320.

51. Mitchell DG, Palazzo J, Hann HW, Rifkin MD, Burk DL, Jr., Rubin R. Hepatocellular tumors with high signal on T1-weighted MR images: chemical shift MR imaging and histologic correlation. J Comput Assist Tomogr 1991;15:762-769.

52. Mortele KJ, Praet M, Van Vlierberghe H, de Hemptinne B, Zou K, Ros PR. Focal nodular hyperplasia of the liver: detection and characterization with plain and dynamic-enhanced MRI. Abdom Imaging 2002;27:700-707.

53. Attal P, Vilgrain V, Brancatelli G, et al. Telangiectatic focal nodular hyperplasia: US, CT, and MR imaging findings with histopathologic correlation in 13 cases. Radiology 2003;228:465-472.

54. Soyer P, Dufresne AC, Somveille E, Scherrer A. Focal nodular hyperplasia of the liver: assessment of hemodynamic and angioarchitectural patterns with gadolinium chelate-enhanced 3D spoiled gradient-recalled MRI and maximum intensity projection reformatted images. J Comput Assist Tomogr 1996;20:898-904.

55. Charny CK, Jarnagin WR, Schwartz LH, et al. Management of 155 patients with benign liver tumours. Br J Surg 2001;88:808-813.

56. Herman P, Pugliese V, Machado MA, et al. Hepatic adenoma and focal nodular hyperplasia: differential diagnosis and treatment. World J Surg 2000;24:372-376.

57. Ba-Ssalamah A, Schima W, Schmook MT, et al. Atypical focal nodular hyperplasia of the liver: imaging features of nonspecific and liver-specific MR contrast agents. AJR Am J Roentgenol 2002;179:1447-1456.

58. McLarney JK, Rucker PT, Bender GN, Goodman ZD, Kashitani N, Ros PR. Fibrolamellar carcinoma of the liver: radiologic-pathologic correlation. Radiographics 1999;19:453-471.

59. Ichikawa T, Federle MP, Grazioli L, Madariaga J, Nalesnik M, Marsh W. Fibrolamellar hepatocellular carcinoma: imaging and pathologic findings in 31 recent cases. Radiology 1999;213:352-361.

60. Pinna AD, Iwatsuki S, Lee RG, et al. Treatment of fibrolamellar hepatoma with subtotal hepatectomy or transplantation. Hepatology 1997;26:877-883.

61. Ichikawa T, Federle MP, Grazioli L, Marsh W. Fibrolamellar hepatocellular carcinoma: pre- and posttherapy evaluation with CT and MR imaging. Radiology 2000;217:145-151.

62. Stevens WR, Johnson CD, Stephens DH, Nagorney DM. Fibrolamellar hepatocellular carcinoma: stage at presentation and results of aggressive surgical management. AJR Am J Roentgenol 1995;164:1153-1158.

63. Lee WJ, Lim HK, Jang KM, et al. Radiologic spectrum of cholangiocarcinoma: emphasis on unusual manifestations and differential diagnoses. Radiographics 2001;21 Spec No:S97-S116.

64. Lim JH. Cholangiocarcinoma: morphologic classification according to growth pattern and imaging findings. AJR Am J Roentgenol 2003;181:819-827.

65. Ros PR, Buck JL, Goodman ZD, Ros AM, Olmsted WW. Intrahepatic cholangiocarcinoma: radiologic-pathologic correlation. Radiology 1988;167:689-693.

66. Soyer P, Bluemke DA, Reichle R, et al. Imaging of intrahepatic cholangiocarcinoma: 1. Peripheral cholangiocarcinoma. AJR Am J Roentgenol 1995;165:1427-1431.

67. Vilgrain V, Van Beers BE, Flejou JF, et al. Intrahepatic cholangio-carcinoma: MRI and pathologic correlation in 14 patients. J Comput Assist Tomogr 1997;21:59-65.

68. Soyer P, Bluemke DA, Sibert A, Laissy JP. MR imaging of intrahepatic cholangiocarcinoma. Abdom Imaging 1995;20:126-130.

69. Nakajima T, Kondo Y, Miyazaki M, Okui K. A histopathologic study of 102 cases of intrahepatic cholangiocarcinoma: histologic classification and modes of spreading. Hum Pathol 1988;19:1228-1234.

70. Maetani Y, Itoh K, Watanabe C, et al. MR imaging of intrahepatic cholangiocarcinoma with pathologic correlation. AJR Am J Roentgenol 2001;176:1499-1507.

71. Murakami T, Nakamura H, Tsuda K, et al. Contrast-enhanced MR imaging of intrahepatic cholangiocarcinoma: pathologic correlation study. J Magn Reson Imaging 1995;5:165-170.

72. Fan ZM, Yamashita Y, Harada M, et al. Intrahepatic cholangiocarci-noma: spin-echo and contrast-enhanced dynamic MR imaging. AJR Am J Roentgenol 1993;161:313-317.

73. Powers C, Ros PR, Stoupis C, Johnson WK, Segel KH. Primary liver neoplasms: MR imaging with pathologic correlation. Radiographics 1994;14:459-482.

74. Worawattanakul S, Semelka RC, Noone TC, Calvo BF, Kelekis NL, Woosley JT. Cholangiocarcinoma: spectrum of appearances on MR images using current techniques. Magn Reson Imaging 1998;16:993-1003.

75. Adjei ON, Tamura S, Sugimura H, et al. Contrast-enhanced MR imaging of intrahepatic cholangiocarcinoma. Clin Radiol 1995;50:6-10.

76. Hayashi M, Matsui O, Ueda K, et al. Imaging findings of mucinous type of cholangiocellular carcinoma. J Comput Assist Tomogr 1996;20:386-389.

77. Gabata T, Matsui O, Kadoya M, et al. Delayed MR imaging of the liver: correlation of delayed enhancement of hepatic tumors and pathologic appearance. Abdom Imaging 1998;23:309-313.

78. Kim TK, Choi BI, Han JK, Jang HJ, Cho SG, Han MC. Peripheral cholangiocarcinoma of the liver: two-phase spiral CT findings. Radiology 1997;204:539-543.

79. Zhang Y, Uchida M, Abe T, Nishimura H, Hayabuchi N, Nakashima Y. Intrahepatic peripheral cholangiocarcinoma: comparison of dynamic CT and dynamic MRI. J Comput Assist Tomogr 1999;23:670-677.

80. Blachar A, Federle MP, Brancatelli G. Hepatic capsular retraction: spectrum of benign and malignant etiologies. Abdom Imaging 2002;27:690-699.

81. Yang DM, Kim HS, Cho SW. Pictorial review: various causes of hepatic capsular retraction: CT and MR findings. Br J Radiol 2002;75:994-1002.

82. Yamashita Y, Takahashi M, Kanazawa S, Charnsangavej C, Wallace S. Parenchymal changes of the liver in cholangiocarcinoma: CT evaluation. Gastrointest Radiol 1992;17:161-166.

83. Jinzaki M, Tanimoto A, Suzuki K, et al. Liver metastases from colon cancer with intra-bile duct tumor growth: radiologic features. J Comput Assist Tomogr 1997;21:656-660.

84. Shirabe K, Shimada M, Harimoto N, et al. Intrahepatic cholangiocarcinoma: its mode of spreading and therapeutic modalities. Surgery 2002;131:S159-164.

85. Ishak KG, Willis GW, Cummins SD, Bullock AA. Biliary cystadenoma and cystadenocarcinoma: report of 14 cases and review of the literature. Cancer 1977;39:322-338.

86. Buetow PC, Buck JL, Pantongrag-Brown L, et al. Biliary cystadenoma and cystadenocarcinoma: clinical-imaging-pathologic correlations with emphasis on the importance of ovarian stroma. Radiology 1995;196:805-810.

87. Lauffer JM, Baer HU, Maurer CA, Stoupis C, Zimmerman A, Buchler MW. Biliary cystadenocarcinoma of the liver: the need for complete resection. Eur J Cancer 1998;34:1845-1851.

88. Wheeler DA, Edmondson HA. Cystadenoma with mesenchymal stroma (CMS) in the liver and bile ducts: a clinicopathologic study of 17 cases, 4 with malignant change. Cancer 1985; 56:1434-1445.

89. Devaney K, Goodman ZD, Ishak KG. Hepatobiliary cystadenoma and cystadenocarcinoma. A light microscopic and immunohisto-chemical study of 70 patients. Am J Surg Pathol 1994;18:1078-1091.

90. Chamberlain RS, Blumgart LH. Mucobilia in association with a biliary cystadenocarcinoma of the caudate duct: a rare cause of malignant biliary obstruction. HPB Surg 2000;11:345-351.

91. Kokubo T, Itai Y, Ohtomo K, Itoh K, Kawauchi N, Minami M. Mucin-hypersecreting intrahepatic biliary neoplasms. Radiology 1988;168:609-614.

92. Matsumoto S, Miyake H, Mori H. Case report: biliary cystadenoma with mucin-secretion mimicking a simple hepatic cyst. Clin Radiol 1997;52:316-318.

93. Kawashima A, Fishman EK, Hruban RH, Tempany CM, Kuhlman JE, Zerhouni EA. Biliary cystadenoma with intratumoral bleeding: radiologic-pathologic correlation. J Comput Assist Tomogr 1991;15:1035-1038.

94. Soyer P, Bluemke DA, Fishman EK, Rymer R. Fluid-fluid levels within focal hepatic lesions: imaging appearance and etiology. Abdom Imaging 1998;23:161-165.

95. Korobkin M, Stephens DH, Lee JK, et al. Biliary cystadenoma and cystadenocarcinoma: CT and sonographic findings. AJR Am J Roentgenol 1989;153:507-511.

96. Singh Y, Winick AB, Tabbara SO. Multiloculated cystic liver lesions: radiologic-pathologic differential diagnosis. Radiographics 1997;17:219-224.

97. Balci NC, Sirvanci M. MR imaging of infective liver lesions. Magn Reson Imaging Clin N Am 2002;10:121-135.

98. Agildere AM, Aytekin C, Coskun M, Boyvat F, Boyacioglu S. MRI of hydatid disease of the liver: a variety of sequences. J Comput Assist Tomogr 1998;22:718-724.

99. Agildere AM, Haliloglu M, Akhan O. Biliary cystadenoma and cystadenocarcinoma. AJR Am J Roentgenol 1991;156:1113.

100. Wee A, Nilsson B, Kang JY, Tan LK, Rauff A. Biliary cystadenocar-cinoma arising in a cystadenoma: report of a case diagnosed by fine needle aspiration cytology. Acta Cytol 1993;37:966-970.

101. Woods GL. Biliary cystadenocarcinoma: Case report of hepatic malignancy originating in benign cystadenoma. Cancer 1981;47:2936-2940.

102. Lewis WD, Jenkins RL, Rossi RL, et al. Surgical treatment of bil-iary cystadenoma: a report of 15 cases. Arch Surg 1988;123:563-568.

103. Iemoto Y, Kondo Y, Fukamachi S. Biliary cystadenocarcinoma with peritoneal carcinomatosis. Cancer 1981;48:1664-1667.

104. Nakajima T, Sugano I, Matsuzaki O, et al. Biliary cystadenocarcinoma of the liver: a clinicopathologic and histochemical evaluation of nine cases. Cancer 1992;69:2426-2432.

105. Wolf HK, Garcia JA, Bossen EH. Oncocytic differentiation in intrahepatic biliary cystadenocarcinoma. Mod Pathol 1992;5:665-668.

106. Desmet VJ. Congenital diseases of intrahepatic bile ducts: variations on the theme "ductal plate malformation." Hepatology 1992;16:1069-1083.

107. Desmet VJ. Ludwig symposium on biliary disorders. 1. Pathogenesis of ductal plate abnormalities. Mayo Clin Proc 1998;73:80-89.

108. Chung EB. Multiple bile-duct hamartomas. Cancer 1970;26:287-296.

109. Lev-Toaff AS, Bach AM, Wechsler RJ, Hilpert PL, Gatalica Z, Rubin R. The radiologic and pathologic spectrum of biliary hamartomas. AJR Am J Roentgenol 1995;165:309-313.

110. Gallego JC, Suarez I, Soler R. Multiple bile duct hamartomas: US, CT, and MR findings. A case report. Acta Radiol 1995; 36:273-275.

111. Maher MM, Dervan P, Keogh B, Murray JG. Bile duct hamartomas (von Meyenburg complexes): value of MR imaging in diagnosis. Abdom Imaging 1999;24:171-173.

112. Martinoli C, Cittadini G, Jr., Rollandi GA, Conzi R. Case report: imaging of bile duct hamartomas. Clin Radiol 1992;45:203-205.

113. Cheung YC, Tan CF, Wan YL, Lui KW, Tsai CC. MRI of multiple biliary hamartomas. Br J Radiol 1997;70:527-529.

114. Semelka RC, Hussain SM, Marcos HB, Woosley JT. Biliary hamartomas: solitary and multiple lesions shown on current MR techniques including gadolinium enhancement. J Magn Reson Imaging 1999;10:196-201.

115. Slone HW, Bennett WF, Bova JG. MR findings of multiple biliary hamartomas. AJR Am J Roentgenol 1993;161:581-583.

116. Wei SC, Huang GT, Chen CH, et al. Bile duct hamartomas: a report of two cases. J Clin Gastroenterol 1997;25:608-611.

117. Wohlgemuth WA, Bottger J, Bohndorf K. MRI, CT, US and ERCP in the evaluation of bile duct hamartomas (von Meyenburg complex): a case report. Eur Radiol 1998;8:1623-1626.

118. Mortele B, Mortele K, Seynaeve P, Vandevelde D, Kunnen M, Ros PR. Hepatic bile duct hamartomas (von Meyenburg Complexes): MR and MR cholangiography findings. J Comput Assist Tomogr 2002;26:438-443.

119. Everson GT. Hepatic cysts in autosomal dominant polycystic kidney disease. Mayo Clin Proc 1990;65:1020-1025.

120. Itai Y, Ebihara R, Eguchi N, et al. Hepatobiliary cysts in patients with autosomal dominant polycystic kidney disease: prevalence and CT findings. AJR Am J Roentgenol 1995;164:339-342.

121. Gabow PA, Johnson AM, Kaehny WD, Manco-Johnson ML, Duley IT, Everson GT. Risk factors for the development of hepatic cysts in autosomal dominant polycystic kidney disease. Hepatology 1990;11:1033-1037.

122. Mortele KJ, Ros PR. Cystic focal liver lesions in the adult: differential CT and MR imaging features. Radiographics 2001;21:895-910.

123. Levine E, Cook LT, Grantham JJ. Liver cysts in autosomal-dominant polycystic kidney disease: clinical and computed tomographic study. AJR Am J Roentgenol 1985;145:229-233.

124. van Erpecum KJ, Janssens AR, Terpstra JL, Tjon ATRT. Highly symptomatic adult polycystic disease of the liver: a report of fifteen cases. J Hepatol 1987;5:109-117.

125. Telenti A, Torres VE, Gross JB, Jr., Van Scoy RE, Brown ML, Hattery RR. Hepatic cyst infection in autosomal dominant polycystic kidney disease. Mayo Clin Proc 1990;65:933-942.

126. Kida T, Nakanuma Y, Terada T. Cystic dilatation of peribiliary glands in livers with adult polycystic disease and livers with solitary nonparasitic cysts: an autopsy study. Hepatology 1992;16:334-340.

127. Terada T, Nakanuma Y. Pathological observations of intrahepatic peribiliary glands in 1,000 consecutive autopsy livers. 3. Survey of necroinflammation and cystic dilatation. Hepatology 1990; 12:1229-1233.

128. Baron RL, Campbell WL, Dodd GD III. Peribiliary cysts associated with severe liver disease: imaging—pathologic correlation. AJR Am J Roentgenol 1994;162:631-636.

129. Krause D, Cercueil JP, Dranssart M, Cognet F, Piard F, Hillon P. MRI for evaluating congenital bile duct abnormalities. J Comput Assist Tomogr 2002;26:541-552.

130. Itai Y, Ebihara R, Tohno E, et al. Hepatic peribiliary cysts: multiple tiny cysts within the larger portal tract, hepatic hilum, or both. Radiology 1994;191:107-110.

131. Dranssart M, Cognet F, Mousson C, Cercueil JP, Rifle G, Krause D. MR cholangiography in the evaluation of hepatic and biliary abnormalities in autosomal dominant polycystic kidney disease: study of 93 patients. J Comput Assist Tomogr 2002;26:237-242.

132. Vilgrain V, Silbermann O, Benhamou JP, Nahum H. MR imaging in intracystic hemorrhage of simple hepatic cysts. Abdom Imaging 1993;18:164-167.

133. Mosetti MA, Leonardou P, Motohara T, Kanematsu M, Armao D, Semelka RC. Autosomal dominant polycystic kidney disease: MR imaging evaluation using current techniques. J Magn Reson Imaging 2003;18:210-215.

134. vanSonnenberg E, Wroblicka JT, D'Agostino HB, et al. Symptomatic hepatic cysts: percutaneous drainage and sclerosis. Radiology 1994;190:387-392.

135. Ferris JV. Serial ethanol ablation of multiple hepatic cysts as an alternative to liver transplantation. AJR Am J Roentgenol 2003;180:472-474.

136. Gaines PA, Sampson MA. The prevalence and characterization of simple hepatic cysts by ultrasound examination. Br J Radiol 1989;62:335-337.

137. Cook JR, Dehner LP, Collins MH, et al. Anaplastic lymphoma kinase (ALK) expression in the inflammatory myofibroblastic tumor: a comparative immunohistochemical study. Am J Surg Pathol 2001;25:1364-1371.

138. Coffin CM, Humphrey PA, Dehner LP. Extrapulmonary inflammatory myofibroblastic tumor: a clinical and pathological survey. Semin Diagn Pathol 1998;15:85-101.

139. Narla LD, Newman B, Spottswood SS, Narla S, Kolli R. Inflammatory pseudotumor. Radiographics 2003;23:719-729.

140. Dehner LP. The enigmatic inflammatory pseudotumours: the current state of our understanding, or misunderstanding. J Pathol 2000;192:277-279.

141. Coffin CM, Dehner LP, Meis-Kindblom JM. Inflammatory myofibroblastic tumor, inflammatory fibrosarcoma, and related lesions: an historical review with differential diagnostic considerations. Semin Diagn Pathol 1998;15:102-110.

142. Sakai T, Shiraki K, Yamamoto N, et al. Diagnosis of inflammatory pseudotumor of the liver. Int J Mol Med 2002;10:281-285.

143. Yan FH, Zhou KR, Jiang YP, Shi WB. Inflammatory pseudotumor of the liver: 13 cases of MRI findings. World J Gastroenterol 2001;7:422-424.

144. Mortele KJ, Wiesner W, de Hemptinne B, Elewaut A, Praet M, Ros PR. Multifocal inflammatory pseudotumor of the liver: dynamic gadolinium-enhanced, ferumoxides-enhanced, and mangafodipir trisodium-enhanced MR imaging findings. Eur Radiol 2002;12:304-308.

145. Torzilli G, Inoue K, Midorikawa Y, Hui AM, Takayama T, Makuuchi M. Inflammatory pseudotumors of the liver: prevalence and clinical impact in surgical patients. Hepatogastroenterology 2001;48:1118-1123.

146. Abehsera M, Vilgrain V, Belghiti J, Flejou JF, Nahum H. Inflammatory pseudotumor of the liver: radiologic-pathologic correlation. J Comput Assist Tomogr 1995;19:80-83.

147. Flisak ME, Budris DM, Olson MC, Zarling EJ. Inflammatory pseudotumor of the liver: appearance on MRI. Clin Imaging 1994;18:1-3.

148. Materne R, Van Beers BE, Gigot JF, Horsmans Y, Lacrosse M, Pringot J. Inflammatory pseudotumor of the liver: MRI with mangafodipir trisodium. J Comput Assist Tomogr 1998;22:82-84.

149. Ijuin H, Ono N, Koga K, et al. Inflammatory pseudotumor of the liver—MR imaging findings. Kurume Med J 1997;44:305-313.

150. Kelekis NL, Warshauer DM, Semelka RC, Eisenberg LB, Woosley JT. Inflammatory pseudotumor of the liver: appearance on contrast enhanced helical CT and dynamic MR images. J Magn Reson Imaging 1995;5:551-553.

151. Levy S, Sauvanet A, Diebold MD, Marcus C, Da Costa N, Thiefin G. Spontaneous regression of an inflammatory pseudotumor of the liver presenting as an obstructing malignant biliary tumor. Gastrointest Endosc 2001;53:371-374.

152. Nakanuma Y, Tsuneyama K, Masuda S, Tomioka T. Hepatic inflammatory pseudotumor associated with chronic cholangitis: report of three cases. Hum Pathol 1994;25:86-91.

153. Voss SD, Kruskal JB, Kane RA. Chronic inflammatory pseudotumor arising in the hepatobiliary-pancreatic system: progressive multisystemic organ involvement in four patients. AJR Am J Roentgenol 1999;173:1049-1054.

154. Venkataraman S, Semelka RC, Braga L, Danet IM, Woosley JT. Inflammatory myofibroblastic tumor of the hepatobiliary system: report of MR imaging appearance in four patients. Radiology 2003;227:758-763.

155. Gollapudi P, Chejfec G, Zarling EJ. Spontaneous regression of hepatic pseudotumor. Am J Gastroenterol 1992;87:214-217.

156. Barreda R, Ros PR. Diagnostic imaging of liver abscess. Crit Rev Diagn Imaging 1992;33:29-58.

157. Mergo PJ, Ros PR. MR imaging of inflammatory disease of the liver. Magn Reson Imaging Clin N Am 1997;5:367-376.

158. Oto A, Akhan O, Ozmen M. Focal inflammatory diseases of the liver. Eur J Radiol 1999;32:61-75.

159. Ralls PW. Focal inflammatory disease of the liver. Radiol Clin North Am 1998;36:377-389.

160. Chou FF, Sheen-Chen SM, Chen YS, Chen MC. Single and multiple pyogenic liver abscesses: clinical course, etiology, and results of treatment. World J Surg 1997;21:384-388; discussion 388-389.

161. Lee KT, Sheen PC, Chen JS, Ker CG. Pyogenic liver abscess: multivariate analysis of risk factors. World J Surg 1991;15:372-376; discussion 376-377.

162. Balci NC, Semelka RC, Noone TC, et al. Pyogenic hepatic abscesses: MRI findings on T1- and T2-weighted and serial gadolinium-enhanced gradient-echo images. J Magn Reson Imaging 1999;9:285-290.

163. Mendez RJ, Schiebler ML, Outwater EK, Kressel HY. Hepatic abscesses: MR imaging findings. Radiology 1994;190:431-436.

164. Jeffrey RB, Jr., Tolentino CS, Chang FC, Federle MP. CT of small pyogenic hepatic abscesses: the cluster sign. AJR Am J Roentgenol 1988;151:487-489.

165. Gabata T, Kadoya M, Matsui O, et al. Dynamic CT of hepatic abscesses: significance of transient segmental enhancement. AJR Am J Roentgenol 2001;176:675-679.

166. Schlund JF, Semelka RC, Kettritz U, Eisenberg LB, Lee JK. Transient increased segmental hepatic enhancement distal to portal vein obstruction on dynamic gadolinium-enhanced gradient echo MR images. J Magn Reson Imaging 1995;5:375-377.

167. Miller FJ, Ahola DT, Bretzman PA, Fillmore DJ. Percutaneous management of hepatic abscess: a perspective by interventional radiologists. J Vasc Interv Radiol 1997;8:241-247.

168. vanSonnenberg E, Wittich GR, Goodacre BW, Casola G, D'Agostino HB. Percutaneous abscess drainage: update. World J Surg 2001;25:362-369; discussion 370-372.

169. Semelka RC, Kelekis NL, Sallah S, Worawattanakul S, Ascher SM. Hepatosplenic fungal disease: diagnostic accuracy and spectrum of appearances on MR imaging. AJR Am J Roentgenol 1997;169:1311-1316.

170. Talbot GH, Provencher M, Cassileth PA. Persistent fever after recovery from granulocytopenia in acute leukemia. Arch Intern Med 1988;148:129-135.

171. Tashjian LS, Abramson JS, Peacock JE, Jr. Focal hepatic candidiasis: a distinct clinical variant of candidiasis in immunocompromised patients. Rev Infect Dis 1984;6:689-703.

172. Thaler M, Pastakia B, Shawker TH, O'Leary T, Pizzo PA. Hepatic candidiasis in cancer patients: the evolving picture of the syndrome. Ann Intern Med 1988;108:88-100.

173. Rossetti F, Brawner DL, Bowden R, et al. Fungal liver infection in marrow transplant recipients: prevalence at autopsy, predisposing factors, and clinical features. Clin Infect Dis 1995;20:801-811.

174. Grois N, Mostbeck G, Scherrer R, et al. Hepatic and splenic abscesses—a common complication of intensive chemotherapy of acute myeloid leukemia (AML) a prospective study. Ann Hematol 1991;63:33-38.

175. Anttila VJ, Lamminen AE, Bondestam S, et al. Magnetic resonance imaging is superior to computed tomography and ultrasonography in imaging infectious liver foci in acute leukaemia. Eur J Haematol 1996;56:82-87.

176. Semelka RC, Shoenut JP, Greenberg HM, Bow EJ. Detection of acute and treated lesions of hepatosplenic candidiasis: comparison of dynamic contrast-enhanced CT and MR imaging. J Magn Reson Imaging 1992;2:341-345.

177. Kelekis NL, Semelka RC, Jeon HJ, Sallah AS, Shea TC, Woosley JT. Dark ring sign: finding in patients with fungal liver lesions and transfusional hemosiderosis undergoing treatment with antifungal antibiotics. Magn Reson Imaging 1996;14:615-618.

178. Anttila VJ, Ruutu P, Bondestam S, et al. Hepatosplenic yeast infection in patients with acute leukemia: a diagnostic problem. Clin Infect Dis 1994;18:979-981.

179. Fitzgerald EJ, Coblentz C. Fungal microabscesses in immuno-suppressed patients—CT appearances. Can Assoc Radiol J 1988;39:10-12.

180. Kimura K, Stoopen M, Reeder MM, Moncada R. Amebiasis: modern diagnostic imaging with pathological and clinical correlation. Semin Roentgenol 1997;32:250-275.

181. Juimo AG, Gervez F, Angwafo FF. Extraintestinal amebiasis. Radiology 1992;182:181-183.

182. Haque R, Huston CD, Hughes M, Houpt E, Petri WA, Jr. Amebiasis. N Engl J Med 2003;348:1565-1573.

183. Maltz G, Knauer CM. Amebic liver abscess: a 15-year experience. Am J Gastroenterol 1991;86:704-710.

184. Mondragon-Sanchez R, Cortes-Espinoza T, Alonzo-Fierro Y, Labra-Villalobos MI, Bernal Maldonado R. Amebic liver abscess: a 5 year Mexican experience with a multimodality approach. Hepatogastroenterology 1995;42:473-477.

185. Elizondo G, Weissleder R, Stark DD, et al. Amebic liver abscess: diagnosis and treatment evaluation with MR imaging. Radiology 1987;165:795-800.

186. Ralls PW, Henley DS, Colletti PM, et al. Amebic liver abscess: MR imaging. Radiology 1987;165:801-804.

187. Radin DR, Ralls PW, Colletti PM, Halls JM. CT of amebic liver abscess. AJR Am J Roentgenol 1988;150:1297-1301.

188. Ralls PW, Barnes PF, Johnson MB, De Cock KM, Radin DR, Halls J. Medical treatment of hepatic amebic abscess: rare need for percutaneous drainage. Radiology 1987;165:805-807.

189. Alvarez SZ. Hepatobiliary tuberculosis. J Gastroenterol Hepatol 1998;13:833-839.

190. Gulati MS, Sarma D, Paul SB. CT appearances in abdominal tuberculosis: a pictorial essay. Clin Imaging 1999;23:51-59.

191. Proctor DD, Chopra S, Rubenstein SC, Jokela JA, Uhl L. Mycobacteremia and granulomatous hepatitis following initial intravesical bacillus Calmette-Guérin instillation for bladder carcinoma. Am J Gastroenterol 1993;88:1112-1115.

192. Alcantara-Payawal DE, Matsumura M, Shiratori Y, et al. Direct detection of *Mycobacterium tuberculosis* using polymerase chain reaction assay among patients with hepatic granuloma. J Hepatol 1997;27:620-627.

193. Murata Y, Yamada I, Sumiya Y, Shichijo Y, Suzuki Y. Abdominal macronodular tuberculomas: MR findings. J Comput Assist Tomogr 1996;20:643-646.

194. Balci NC, Tunaci A, Akinci A, Cevikbas U. Granulomatous hepatitis: MRI findings. Magn Reson Imaging 2001;19:1107-1111.

195. Kawamori Y, Matsui O, Kitagawa K, Kadoya M, Takashima T, Yamahana T. Macronodular tuberculoma of the liver: CT and MR findings. AJR Am J Roentgenol 1992;158:311-313.

196. Wilde CC, Kueh YK. Case report: Tuberculous hepatic and splenic abscess. Clin Radiol 1991;43:215-216.

197. Jadvar H, Mindelzun RE, Olcott EW, Levitt DB. Still the great mimicker: abdominal tuberculosis. AJR Am J Roentgenol 1997;168:1455-1460.

198. Tritou I, Prassopoulos P, Daskalogiannaki M, Charoulakis N, Papakonstantinou O, Gourtsoyiannis N. Miliary hepatic tuberculosis not associated with splenic or lung involvement: a case report. Acta Radiol 2000;41:479-481.

199. Pedrosa I, Saiz A, Arrazola J, Ferreiros J, Pedrosa CS. Hydatid disease: radiologic and pathologic features and complications. Radiographics 2000;20:795-817.

200. von Sinner W. Advanced medical imaging and treatment of human cystic echinococcosis. Semin Roentgenol 1997;32:276-290.

201. Marani SA, Canossi GC, Nicoli FA, Alberti GP, Monni SG, Casolo PM. Hydatid disease: MR imaging study. Radiology 1990;175:701-706.

202. Kalovidouris A, Gouliamos A, Vlachos L, et al. MRI of abdominal hydatid disease. Abdom Imaging 1994;19:489-494.

203. Kodama Y, Fujita N, Shimizu T, et al. Alveolar echinococcosis: MR findings in the liver. Radiology 2003;15:15.

204. Sayek I, Onat D. Diagnosis and treatment of uncomplicated hydatid cyst of the liver. World J Surg 2001;25:21-27.

205. Akhan O, Ozmen MN. Percutaneous treatment of liver hydatid cysts. Eur J Radiol 1999;169:32-76-85.

206. Burt AD, Portmann BC, MacSween RNM. Liver pathology associated with diseases of other organs or systems. In: MacSween RNM, Burt AD, Portmann BC, Ishak KG, Scheuer PJ, Anthony PP, eds. Pathology of the Liver, 4th ed. Churchill Livingstone, 2002, pp 827-884.

207. Moreno-Merlo F, Wanless IR, Shimamatsu K, Sherman M, Greig P, Chiasson D. The role of granulomatous phlebitis and thrombosis in the pathogenesis of cirrhosis and portal hypertension in sarcoidosis. Hepatology 1997;26:554-560.

208. Warshauer DM, Lee JK. Imaging manifestations of abdominal sarcoidosis. AJR Am J Roentgenol 2004;182:15-28.

209. Ishak KG. Sarcoidosis of the liver and bile ducts. Mayo Clin Proc 1998;73:467-472.

210. Warshauer DM, Dumbleton SA, Molina PL, Yankaskas BC, Parker LA, Woosley JT. Abdominal CT findings in sarcoidosis: radiologic and clinical correlation. Radiology 1994;192:93-98.

211. Warshauer DM, Semelka RC, Ascher SM. Nodular sarcoidosis of the liver and spleen: appearance on MR images. J Magn Reson Imaging 1994;4:553-557.

212. Kessler A, Mitchell DG, Israel HL, Goldberg BB. Hepatic and splenic sarcoidosis: ultrasound and MR imaging. Abdom Imaging 1993;18:159-163.

213. Charnsangavej C, Cinqualbre A, Wallace S. Radiation changes in the liver, spleen, and pancreas: imaging findings. Semin Roentgenol 1994;29:53-63.

214. Lawrence TS, Robertson JM, Anscher MS, Jirtle RL, Ensminger WD, Fajardo LF. Hepatic toxicity resulting from cancer treatment. Int J Radiat Oncol Biol Phys 1995;31:1237-1248.

215. Onaya H, Itai Y, Yoshioka H, et al. Changes in the liver parenchyma after proton beam radiotherapy: evaluation with MR imaging. Magn Reson Imaging 2000;18:707-714.

216. Unger EC, Lee JK, Weyman PJ. CT and MR imaging of radiation hepatitis. J Comput Assist Tomogr 1987;11:264-268.

217. Yankelevitz DF, Knapp PH, Henschke CI, Nisce L, Yi Y, Cahill P. MR appearance of radiation hepatitis. Clin Imaging 1992;16:89-92.

218. Cutillo DP, Swayne LC, Fasciano MG, Schwartz JR. Absence of fatty replacement in radiation damaged liver: CT demonstration. J Comput Assist Tomogr 1989;13:259-261.

219. Yamasaki SA, Marn CS, Francis IR, Robertson JM, Lawrence TS. High-dose localized radiation therapy for treatment of hepatic malignant tumors: CT findings and their relation to radiation hepatitis. AJR Am J Roentgenol 1995;165:79-84.

220. Lee YM, Kaplan MM. Primary sclerosing cholangitis. N Engl J Med 1995;332:924-933.

221. Portmann BC, Nakanuma Y. Diseases of the bile ducts. In: MacSween RNM, Burt AD, Portmann BC, Ishak KG, Scheuer PJ, Anthony PP, eds. Pathology of the Liver, 4th ed. Churchill Livingstone, 2002, pp 435-506.

222. Revelon G, Rashid A, Kawamoto S, Bluemke DA. Primary sclerosing cholangitis: MR imaging findings with pathologic correlation. AJR Am J Roentgenol 1999;173:1037-1042.

223. Ito K, Mitchell DG, Outwater EK, Blasbalg R. Primary sclerosing cholangitis: MR imaging features. AJR Am J Roentgenol 1999;172:1527-1533.

224. Gabata T, Matsui O, Kadoya M, et al. Segmental hyperintensity on T1-weighted MRI of the liver: indication of segmental cholestasis. J Magn Reson Imaging 1997;7:855-857.

225. Muramatsu Y, Takayasu K, Furukawa Y, et al. Hepatic tumor invasion of bile ducts: wedge-shaped sign on MR images. Radiology 1997;205:81-85.

226. Dodd GD III, Baron RL, Oliver JH III, Federle MP. End-stage primary sclerosing cholangitis: CT findings of hepatic morphology in 36 patients. Radiology 1999;211:357-362.

227. Bader TR, Beavers KL, Semelka RC. MR imaging features of primary sclerosing cholangitis: patterns of cirrhosis in relationship to clinical severity of disease. Radiology 2003;226:675-685.

228. Zagoria RJ, Roth TJ, Levine EA, Kavanagh PV. Radiofrequency ablation of a symptomatic hepatic cavernous hemangioma. AJR Am J Roentgenol 2004;182:210-212.

229. Vilgrain V, Boulos L, Vullierme MP, Denys A, Terris B, Menu Y. Imaging of atypical hemangiomas of the liver with pathologic correlation. Radiographics 2000;20:379-397.

230. Leifer DM, Middleton WD, Teefey SA, Menias CO, Leahy JR. Follow-up of patients at low risk for hepatic malignancy with a characteristic hemangioma at US. Radiology 2000;214:167-172.

231. Choi BI, Han MC, Park JH, Kim SH, Han MH, Kim CW. Giant cavernous hemangioma of the liver: CT and MR imaging in 10 cases. AJR Am J Roentgenol 1989;152:1221-1226.

232. Hotokezaka M, Kojima M, Nakamura K, et al. Traumatic rupture of hepatic hemangioma. J Clin Gastroenterol 1996;23:69-71.

233. Nghiem HV, Bogost GA, Ryan JA, Lund P, Freeny PC, Rice KM. Cavernous hemangiomas of the liver: enlargement over time. AJR Am J Roentgenol 1997;169:137-140.

234. Semelka RC, Brown ED, Ascher SM, et al. Hepatic hemangiomas: a multi-institutional study of appearance on T2-weighted and serial gadolinium-enhanced gradient-echo MR images. Radiology 1994;192:401-406.

235. Tung GA, Vaccaro JP, Cronan JJ, Rogg JM. Cavernous hemangioma of the liver: pathologic correlation with high-field MR imaging. AJR Am J Roentgenol 1994;162:1113-1117.

236. Motohara T, Semelka RC, Nagase L. MR imaging of benign hepatic tumors. Magn Reson Imaging Clin N Am 2002;10:1-14.

237. McNicholas MM, Saini S, Echeverri J, et al. T2 relaxation times of hypervascular and non-hypervascular liver lesions: do hypervascular lesions mimic haemangiomas on heavily T2-weighted MR images? Clin Radiol 1996;51:401-405.

238. Danet IM, Semelka RC, Braga L, Armao D, Woosley JT. Giant hemangioma of the liver: MR imaging characteristics in 24 patients. Magn Reson Imaging 2003;21:95-101.

239. Danet IM, Semelka RC, Leonardou P, et al. Spectrum of MRI appearances of untreated metastases of the liver. AJR Am J Roentgenol 2003;181:809-817.

240. Lee SH, Park CM, Cheong IJ, et al. Hepatic capsular retraction: unusual finding of cavernous hemangioma. J Comput Assist Tomogr 2001;25:231-233.

241. Lim PS, Nazarian LN, Wechsler RJ, Lev-Toaff AS. Hepatic capsular retraction secondary to involuting cavernous hemangioma. J Comput Assist Tomogr 2001;25:234-235.

242. Yang DM, Yoon MH, Kim HS, Chung JW. Capsular retraction in hepatic giant hemangioma: CT and MR features. Abdom Imaging 2001;26:36-38.

243. Coumbaras M, Wendum D, Monnier-Cholley L, Dahan H, Tubiana JM, Arrive L. CT and MR imaging features of pathologically proven atypical giant hemangiomas of the liver. AJR Am J Roentgenol 2002;179:1457-1463.

244. Yamashita Y, Ogata I, Urata J, Takahashi M. Cavernous hemangioma of the liver: pathologic correlation with dynamic CT findings. Radiology 1997;203:121-125.

245. Yu JS, Kim MJ, Kim KW. Intratumoral blood flow in cavernous hemangioma of the liver: radiologic-pathologic correlation. Radiology 1998;208:549-550.

246. Outwater EK, Ito K, Siegelman E, Martin CE, Bhatia M, Mitchell DG. Rapidly enhancing hepatic hemangiomas at MRI: distinction from malignancies with T2-weighted images. J Magn Reson Imaging 1997;7:1033-1039.

247. Berger JF, Laissy JP, Limot O, et al. Differentiation between multiple liver hemangiomas and liver metastases of gastrinomas: value of enhanced MRI. J Comput Assist Tomogr 1996;20:349-355.

248. Mitchell DG, Saini S, Weinreb J, et al. Hepatic metastases and cavernous hemangiomas: distinction with standard- and triple-dose gadoteridol-enhanced MR imaging. Radiology 1994;193:49-57.

249. Whitney WS, Herfkens RJ, Jeffrey RB, et al. Dynamic breath-hold multiplanar spoiled gradient-recalled MR imaging with gadolinium enhancement for differentiating hepatic hemangiomas from malignancies at 1.5 T. Radiology 1993;189:863-870.

250. Mahfouz AE, Hamm B, Wolf KJ. Peripheral washout: a sign of malignancy on dynamic gadolinium-enhanced MR images of focal liver lesions. Radiology 1994;190:49-52.

251. Awaya H, Ito K, Honjo K, Fujita T, Matsumoto T, Matsunaga N. Differential diagnosis of hepatic tumors with delayed enhancement at gadolinium-enhanced MRI: a pictorial essay. Clin Imaging 1998;22:180-187.

252. Peterson MS, Murakami T, Baron RL. MR imaging patterns of gadolinium retention within liver neoplasms. Abdom Imaging 1998;23:592-599.

253. Jeong MG, Yu JS, Kim KW. Hepatic cavernous hemangioma: temporal peritumoral enhancement during multiphase dynamic MR imaging. Radiology 2000;216:692-697.

254. Kim KW, Kim TK, Han JK, Kim AY, Lee HJ, Choi BI. Hepatic hemangiomas with arterioportal shunt: findings at two-phase CT. Radiology 2001;219:707-711.

255. Li CS, Chen RC, Chen WT, Lii JM, Tu HY. Temporal peritumoral enhancement of hepatic cavernous hemangioma: findings at multiphase dynamic magnetic resonance imaging. J Comput Assist Tomogr 2003;27:854-859.

256. Kato H, Kanematsu M, Matsuo M, Kondo H, Hoshi H. Atypically enhancing hepatic cavernous hemangiomas: high-spatial-resolution gadolinium-enhanced triphasic dynamic gradient-recalled-echo imaging findings. Eur Radiol 2001;11:2510-2515.

257. Hanafusa K, Ohashi I, Himeno Y, Suzuki S, Shibuya H. Hepatic hemangioma: findings with two-phase CT. Radiology 1995;196:465-469.

258. Cheng HC, Tsai SH, Chiang JH, Chang CY. Hyalinized liver hemangioma mimicking malignant tumor at MR imaging. AJR Am J Roentgenol 1995;165:1016-1017.

259. Aibe H, Hondo H, Kuroiwa T, et al. Sclerosed hemangioma of the liver. Abdom Imaging 2001;26:496-499.

260. Mathieu D, Rahmouni A, Vasile N, et al. Sclerosed liver hemangioma mimicking malignant tumor at MR imaging: pathologic correlation. J Magn Reson Imaging 1994;4:506-508.

261. Brancatelli G, Federle MP, Blachar A, Grazioli L. Hemangioma in the cirrhotic liver: diagnosis and natural history. Radiology 2001;219:69-74.

262. Jang HJ, Kim TK, Lim HK, et al. Hepatic hemangioma: atypical appearances on CT, MR imaging, and sonography. AJR Am J Roentgenol 2003;180:135-141.

263. Nonomura A, Mizukami Y, Kadoya M. Angiomyolipoma of the liver: a collective review. J Gastroenterol 1994;29:95-105.

264. Carmody E, Yeung E, McLoughlin M. Angiomyolipomas of the liver in tuberous sclerosis. Abdom Imaging 1994;19:537-539.

265. Tsui WM, Colombari R, Portmann BC, et al. Hepatic angiomyolipoma: a clinicopathologic study of 30 cases and delineation of unusual morphologic variants. Am J Surg Pathol 1999;23:34-48.

266. Ahmadi T, Itai Y, Takahashi M, et al. Angiomyolipoma of the liver: significance of CT and MR dynamic study. Abdom Imaging 1998;23:520-526.

267. Hooper LD, Mergo PJ, Ros PR. Multiple hepatorenal angiomyolipomas: diagnosis with fat suppression, gadolinium-enhanced MRI. Abdom Imaging 1994;19:549-551.

268. Irie H, Honda H, Kuroiwa T, et al. Hepatic angiomyolipoma: report of changing size and internal composition on follow-up examination in two cases. J Comput Assist Tomogr 1999;23:310-313.

269. Yeh HC, Klion FM, Thung SN, Worman HJ. Angiomyolipoma: ultrasonographic signs of lipomatous hepatic tumors. J Ultrasound Med 1996;15:337-342.

270. Bergeron P, Oliva VL, Lalonde L, et al. Liver angiomyolipoma: classic and unusual presentations. Abdom Imaging 1994;19:543-545.

271. Hogemann D, Flemming P, Kreipe H, Galanski M. Correlation of MRI and CT findings with histopathology in hepatic angiomyolipoma. Eur Radiol 2001;11:1389-1395.

272. Chang JC, Lee YW, Kim HJ. Preoperative diagnosis of angiomyolipoma of the liver. Abdom Imaging 1994;19:546-548.

273. Nonomura A, Mizukami Y, Shimizu K, Kadoya M, Matsui O. Angiomyolipoma mimicking true lipoma of the liver: report of two cases. Pathol Int 1996;46:221-227.

274. Worawattanakul S, Semelka RC, Kelekis NL, Woosley JT. Hepatic angiomyolipoma with minimal fat content: MR demonstration. Magn Reson Imaging 1996;14:687-689.

275. Murakami T, Nakamura H, Hori S, et al. Angiomyolipoma of the liver. Ultrasound, CT, MR imaging and angiography. Acta Radiol 1993;34:392-394.

276. Ros PR. Hepatic angiomyolipoma: is fat in the liver friend or foe? Abdom Imaging 1994;19:552-553.

277. Bruneton JN, Kerboul P, Drouillard J, Menu Y, Normand F, Santini N. Hepatic lipomas: ultrasound and computed tomographic findings. Gastrointest Radiol 1987;12:299-303.

278. Garant M, Reinhold C. Residents' corner. Answer to case of the month #36: hepatic lipoma. Can Assoc Radiol J 1996;47:140-142.

279. Sasaki M, Harada K, Nakanuma Y, Watanabe K. Pseudolipoma of Glisson's capsule: report of six cases and review of the literature. J Clin Gastroenterol 1994;19:75-78.

280. Karhunen PJ. Hepatic pseudolipoma. J Clin Pathol 1985; 38:877-879.

281. Baschinsky DY, Weidner N, Baker PB, Frankel WL. Primary hepatic anaplastic large-cell lymphoma of T-cell phenotype in acquired immunodeficiency syndrome: a report of an autopsy case and review of the literature. Am J Gastroenterol 2001;96:227-232.

282. Memeo L, Pecorello I, Ciardi A, Aiello E, De Quarto A, Di Tondo U. Primary non-Hodgkin's lymphoma of the liver. Acta Oncol 1999;38:655-658.

283. Mohler M, Gutzler F, Kallinowski B, Goeser T, Stremmel W. Primary hepatic high-grade non-Hodgkin's lymphoma and chronic hepatitis C infection. Dig Dis Sci 1997;42:2241-2245.

284. Sato S, Masuda T, Oikawa H, et al. Primary hepatic lymphoma associated with primary biliary cirrhosis. Am J Gastroenterol 1999;94:1669-1673.

285. Scoazec JY, Degott C, Brousse N, et al. Non-Hodgkin's lymphoma presenting as a primary tumor of the liver: presentation, diagnosis and outcome in eight patients. Hepatology 1991;13:870-875.

286. Sans M, Andreu V, Bordas JM, et al. Usefulness of laparoscopy with liver biopsy in the assessment of liver involvement at diagnosis of Hodgkin's and non-Hodgkin's lymphomas. Gastrointest Endosc 1998;47:391-395.

287. Dargent JL, De Wolf-Peeters C. Liver involvement by lymphoma: identification of a distinctive pattern of infiltration related to T-cell/histiocyte-rich B-cell lymphoma. Ann Diagn Pathol 1998;2:363-369.

288. Weissleder R, Stark DD, Elizondo G, et al. MRI of hepatic lymphoma. Magn Reson Imaging 1988;6:675-681.

289. Gazelle GS, Lee MJ, Hahn PF, Goldberg MA, Rafaat N, Mueller PR. US, CT, and MRI of primary and secondary liver lymphoma. J Comput Assist Tomogr 1994;18:412-415.

290. Kelekis NL, Semelka RC, Siegelman ES, et al. Focal hepatic lymphoma: magnetic resonance demonstration using current techniques including gadolinium enhancement. Magn Reson Imaging 1997;15:625-636.

291. Nalesnik MA. Posttransplantation lymphoproliferative disorders (PTLD): current perspectives. Semin Thorac Cardiovasc Surg 1996;8:139-148.

292. Hübscher SG, Portmann BC. Transplantation Pathology. In: MacSween RNM, Burt AD, Portmann BC, Ishak KG, Scheuer PJ, Anthony PP, eds. Pathology of the Liver, 4th ed. Churchill Livingstone, 2002, pp 885-941.

293. Strouse PJ, Platt JF, Francis IR, Bree RL. Tumorous intrahepatic lymphoproliferative disorder in transplanted livers. AJR Am J Roentgenol 1996;167:1159-1162.

294. Harris NL, Jaffe ES, Diebold J, et al. The World Health Organization classification of neoplastic diseases of the haematopoietic and lymphoid tissues. Histopathology 2000;36:69-86.

295. Pickhardt PJ, Siegel MJ. Abdominal manifestations of posttransplantation lymphoproliferative disorder. AJR Am J Roentgenol 1998;171:1007-1013.

296. Pena CS, Chew FS, Keel SB. Posttransplantation lymphoproliferative disorder of the liver. AJR Am J Roentgenol 1998;171:192.

297. Kaushik S, Fulcher AS, Frable WJ, May DA. Posttransplantation lymphoproliferative disorder: osseous and hepatic involvement. AJR Am J Roentgenol 2001;177:1057-1059.

298. Moody AR, Wilson SR, Greig PD. Non-Hodgkin lymphoma in the porta hepatis after orthotopic liver transplantation: sonographic findings. Radiology 1992;182:867-870.

299. Lin G, Lunderquist A, Hagerstrand I, Boijsen E. Postmortem examination of the blood supply and vascular pattern of small liver metastases in man. Surgery 1984;96:517-526.

300. Lin G, Hagerstrand I, Lunderquist A. Portal blood supply of liver metastases. AJR Am J Roentgenol 1984;143:53-55.

301. Sica GT, Ji H, Ros PR. Computed tomography and magnetic resonance imaging of hepatic metastases. Clin Liver Dis 2002;6:165-179.

302. Haugeberg G, Strohmeyer T, Lierse W, Bocker W. The vascularization of liver metastases. Histological investigation of gelatine-injected liver specimens with special regard to the vascularization of micrometastases. J Cancer Res Clin Oncol 1988;114:415-419.

303. Kan Z, Ivancev K, Lunderquist A, et al. In vivo microscopy of hepatic tumors in animal models: a dynamic investigation of blood supply to hepatic metastases. Radiology 1993;187:621-626.

304. Killion JJ, Fidler IJ. The biology of tumor metastasis. Semin Oncol 1989;16:106-115.

305. Baker ME, Pelley R. Hepatic metastases: basic principles and implications for radiologists. Radiology 1995;197:329-337.

306. Wisse E, De Zanger RB, Charels K, Van Der Smissen P, McCuskey RS. The liver sieve: considerations concerning the structure and function of endothelial fenestrae, the sinusoidal wall and the space of Disse. Hepatology 1985;5:683-692.

307. Scheele J, Stang R, Altendorf-Hofmann A, Paul M. Resection of colorectal liver metastases. World J Surg 1995;19:59-71.

308. Fong Y, Cohen AM, Fortner JG, et al. Liver resection for colorectal metastases. J Clin Oncol 1997;15:938-946.

309. Bramhall SR, Gur U, Coldham C, et al. Liver resection for colorectal metastases. Ann R Coll Surg Engl 2003;85:334-339.

310. Karhunen PJ. Benign hepatic tumours and tumour like conditions in men. J Clin Pathol 1986;39:183-188.

311. Schwartz LH, Gandras EJ, Colangelo SM, Ercolani MC, Panicek DM. Prevalence and importance of small hepatic lesions found at CT in patients with cancer. Radiology 1999;210:71-74.

312. Noone TC, Semelka RC, Balci NC, Graham ML. Common occurrence of benign liver lesions in patients with newly diagnosed breast cancer investigated by MRI for suspected liver metastases. J Magn Reson Imaging 1999;10:165-169.

313. Semelka RC, Martin DR, Balci C, Lance T. Focal liver lesions: comparison of dual-phase CT and multisequence multiplanar MR imaging including dynamic gadolinium enhancement. J Magn Reson Imaging 2001;13:397-401.

314. Semelka RC, Worawattanakul S, Kelekis NL, et al. Liver lesion detection, characterization, and effect on patient management: comparison of single-phase spiral CT and current MR techniques. J Magn Reson Imaging 1997;7:1040-1047.

315. Imam K, Bluemke DA. MR imaging in the evaluation of hepatic metastases. Magn Reson Imaging Clin N Am 2000;8:741-756.

316. Lewis KH, Chezmar JL. Hepatic metastases. Magn Reson Imaging Clin N Am 1997;5:319-330.

317. Turkenburg JL, Pijl ME, van Persijn van Meerten EL, Hermans J, Bloem JL. MRI of liver metastases: limitation of spleen-liver model in optimizing pulse sequences. J Magn Reson Imaging 1999;9:369-372.

318. Lee MJ, Hahn PF, Saini S, Mueller PR. Differential diagnosis of hyperintense liver lesions on T1-weighted MR images. AJR Am J Roentgenol 1992;159:1017-1020.

319. Kelekis NL, Semelka RC, Woosley JT. Malignant lesions of the liver with high signal intensity on T1-weighted MR images. J Magn Reson Imaging 1996;6:291-294.

320. Sica GT, Ji H, Ros PR. CT and MR imaging of hepatic metastases. AJR Am J Roentgenol 2000;174:691-698.

321. Premkumar A, Sanders L, Marincola F, Feuerstein I, Concepcion R, Schwartzentruber D. Visceral metastases from melanoma: findings on MR imaging. AJR Am J Roentgenol 1992;158:293-298.

322. Esensten ML, Shaw SL, Pak HY, Gildenhorn HL. CT demonstration of multiple intraperitoneal teratomatous implants. J Comput Assist Tomogr 1983;7:1117-1118.

323. Pedro MS, Semelka RC, Braga L. MR imaging of hepatic metastases. Magn Reson Imaging Clin N Am 2002;10:15-29.

324. Semelka RC, Bagley AS, Brown ED, Kroeker MA. Malignant lesions of the liver identified on T1- but not T2-weighted MR images at 1.5 T. J Magn Reson Imaging 1994;4:315-318.

325. Kanematsu M, Hoshi H, Kunieda K, Nandate Y, Kato M, Yokoyama R. Metastases in fatty liver: appearance on conventional spin-echo, fast-spin-echo, and echo-planar T2-weighted MR images. Radiat Med 1998;16:175-177.

326. Outwater EK, Mitchell DG, Vinitski S. Abdominal MR imaging: evaluation of a fast spin-echo sequence. Radiology 1994;190:425-429.

327. Giovagnoni A, Terilli F, Ercolani P, Paci E, Piga A. MR imaging of hepatic masses: diagnostic significance of wedge-shaped areas of increased signal intensity surrounding the lesion. AJR Am J Roentgenol 1994;163:1093-1097.

328. Lee MJ, Saini S, Compton CC, Malt RA. MR demonstration of edema adjacent to a liver metastasis: pathologic correlation. AJR Am J Roentgenol 1991;157:499-501.

329. Outwater E, Tomaszewski JE, Daly JM, Kressel HY. Hepatic colorectal metastases: correlation of MR imaging and pathologic appearance. Radiology 1991;180:327-332.

330. Itai Y, Irie T. Metastatic liver tumor: circumferential versus wedge-shaped perilesional enhancement and quantitative image and pathologic correlation. Radiology 2001;219:298-300.

331. Nascimento AB, Mitchell DG, Rubin R, Weaver E. Diffuse desmoplastic breast carcinoma metastases to the liver simulating cirrhosis at MR imaging: report of two cases. Radiology 2001;221:117-121.

332. Schreiner SA, Gorman B, Stephens DH. Chemotherapy-related hepatotoxicity causing imaging findings resembling cirrhosis. Mayo Clin Proc 1998;73:780-783.

333. Shirkhoda A, Baird S. Morphologic changes of the liver following chemotherapy for metastatic breast carcinoma: CT findings. Abdom Imaging 1994;19:39-42.

334. Young ST, Paulson EK, Washington K, Gulliver DJ, Vredenburgh JJ, Baker ME. CT of the liver in patients with metastatic breast carcinoma treated by chemotherapy: findings simulating cirrhosis. AJR Am J Roentgenol 1994;163:1385-1388.

335. Falck-Ytter Y, Younossi ZM, Marchesini G, McCullough AJ. Clinical features and natural history of nonalcoholic steatosis syndromes. Semin Liver Dis 2001;21:17-26.

336. Brunt EM. Nonalcoholic steatohepatitis: definition and pathology. Semin Liver Dis 2001;21:3-16.

337. Nishino M, Hayakawa K, Nakamura Y, Morimoto T, Mukaihara S. Effects of tamoxifen on hepatic fat content and the development of hepatic steatosis in patients with breast cancer: high frequency of involvement and rapid reversal after completion of tamoxifen therapy. AJR Am J Roentgenol 2003;180:129-134.

338. Clark JM, Diehl AM. Nonalcoholic fatty liver disease: an underrecognized cause of cryptogenic cirrhosis. Jama 2003;289:3000-3004.

339. Martin J, Puig J, Falco J, et al. Hyperechoic liver nodules: characterization with proton fat-water chemical shift MR imaging. Radiology 1998;207:325-330.

340. Martin J, Sentis M, Zidan A, et al. Fatty metamorphosis of hepatocellular carcinoma: detection with chemical shift gradient-echo MR imaging. Radiology 1995;195:125-130.

341. Mathieu D, Paret M, Mahfouz AE, et al. Hyperintense benign liver lesions on spin-echo T1-weighted MR images: pathologic correlations. Abdom Imaging 1997;22:410-417.

342. Siegelman ES, Rosen MA. Imaging of hepatic steatosis. Semin Liver Dis 2001;21:71-80.

343. Tsushima Y, Dean PB. Characterization of adrenal masses with chemical shift MR imaging: how to select echo times. Radiology 1995;195:285-286.

344. Venkataraman S, Braga L, Semelka RC. Imaging the fatty liver. Magn Reson Imaging Clin N Am 2002;10:93-103.

345. Kroncke TJ, Taupitz M, Kivelitz D, et al. Multifocal nodular fatty infiltration of the liver mimicking metastatic disease on CT: imaging findings and diagnosis using MR imaging. Eur Radiol 2000;10:1095-1100.

346. Kemper J, Jung G, Poll LW, Jonkmanns C, Luthen R, Moedder U. CT and MRI findings of multifocal hepatic steatosis mimicking malignancy. Abdom Imaging 2002;27:708-710.

347. Matsui O, Kadoya M, Takahashi S, et al. Focal sparing of segment IV in fatty livers shown by sonography and CT: correlation with aberrant gastric venous drainage. AJR Am J Roentgenol 1995;164:1137-1140.

348. Ohashi I, Ina H, Gomi N, et al. Hepatic pseudolesion in the left lobe around the falciform ligament at helical CT. Radiology 1995;196:245-249.

349. Matsui O, Takashima T, Kadoya M, et al. Staining in the liver surrounding gallbladder fossa on hepatic arteriography caused by increased cystic venous drainage. Gastrointest Radiol 1987;12:307-312.

350. Siegelman ES. MR imaging of diffuse liver disease. Hepatic fat and iron. Magn Reson Imaging Clin N Am 1997;5:347-365.

351. Arita T, Matsunaga N, Honma Y, Nishikawa E, Nagaoka S. Focally spared area of fatty liver caused by arterioportal shunt. J Comput Assist Tomogr 1996;20:360-362.

352. Grossholz M, Terrier F, Rubbia L, et al. Focal sparing in the fatty liver as a sign of an adjacent space-occupying lesion. AJR Am J Roentgenol 1998;171:1391-1395.

353. Itai Y. Peritumoral sparing of fatty liver: another important instance of focal sparing caused by a hepatic tumor. AJR Am J Roentgenol 2000;174:868-870.

354. Chung JJ, Kim MJ, Kim JH, Lee JT, Yoo HS. Fat Sparing of Surrounding Liver From Metastasis in Patients with Fatty Liver: MR Imaging with Histopathologic Correlation. AJR Am J Roentgenol 2003;180:1347-1350.

355. Sohn J, Siegelman E, Osiason A. Unusual patterns of hepatic steatosis caused by the local effect of insulin revealed on chemical shift MR imaging. AJR Am J Roentgenol 2001;176:471-474.

356. Khalili K, Lan FP, Hanbidge AE, Muradali D, Oreopoulos DG, Wanless IR. Hepatic Subcapsular Steatosis in Response to Intraperitoneal Insulin Delivery: CT Findings and Prevalence. AJR Am J Roentgenol 2003;180:1601-1604.

357. Markmann JF, Rosen M, Siegelman ES, et al. Magnetic resonance-defined periportal steatosis following intraportal islet transplantation: a functional footprint of islet graft survival? Diabetes 2003;52:1591-1594.

358. Siegelman ES, Mitchell DG, Rubin R, et al. Parenchymal versus reticuloendothelial iron overload in the liver: distinction with MR imaging. Radiology 1991;179:361-366.

359. Siegelman ES, Mitchell DG, Semelka RC. Abdominal iron deposition: metabolism, MR findings, and clinical importance. Radiology 1996;199:13-22.

360. Pomerantz S, Siegelman ES. MR imaging of iron depositional disease. Magn Reson Imaging Clin N Am 2002;10:105-120.

361. Chapoutot C, Esslimani M, Joomaye Z, et al. Liver iron excess in patients with hepatocellular carcinoma developed on viral C cirrhosis. Gut 2000;46:711-714.

362. Andrews NC. Disorders of iron metabolism. N Engl J Med 1999;341:1986-1995.

363. Deugnier Y, Turlin B. Iron and hepatocellular carcinoma. J Gastroenterol Hepatol 2001;16:491-494.

364. Feder JN, Gnirke A, Thomas W, et al. A novel MHC class I-like gene is mutated in patients with hereditary haemochromatosis. Nat Genet 1996;13:399-408.

365. Flanagan PR, Lam D, Banerjee D, Valberg LS. Ferritin release by mononuclear cells in hereditary hemochromatosis. J Lab Clin Med 1989;113:145-150.

366. Fillet G, Beguin Y, Baldelli L. Model of reticuloendothelial iron metabolism in humans: abnormal behavior in idiopathic hemochromatosis and in inflammation. Blood 1989;74:844-851.

367. Niederau C, Erhardt A, Haussinger D, Strohmeyer G. Haemochromatosis and the liver. J Hepatol 1999;30:6-11.

368. Voelker R. Hemochromatosis patients are untapped source of blood as war, shortages loom. Jama 2003;289:1364-1366.

369. Alustiza JM, Artetxe J, Castiella A, et al. MR Quantification of Hepatic Iron Concentration. Radiology 2004;230:479-484.

370. Siegelman ES, Mitchell DG, Semelka RC. Abdominal iron deposition: metabolism, MR findings, and clinical importance. Radiology 1996;199:13-22.

371. Anderson LJ, Holden S, Davis B, et al. Cardiovascular T2-star (T2*) magnetic resonance for the early diagnosis of myocardial iron overload. Eur Heart J 2001;22:2171-2179.

372. Wahid S, Ball S. The pituitary gland and hereditary haemochromatosis. Lancet 2001;357:115.

373. Guyader D, Gandon Y, Sapey T, et al. Magnetic resonance iron-free nodules in genetic hemochromatosis. Am J Gastroenterol 1999;94:1083-1086.

374. Yoon DY, Choi BI, Han JK, Han MC, Park MO, Suh SJ. MR findings of secondary hemochromatosis: transfusional vs erythropoietic. J Comput Assist Tomogr 1994;18:416-419.

375. Turlin B, Deugnier Y. Iron overload disorders. Clin Liver Dis 2002;6:481-496, viii.

376. Westwood M, Anderson LJ, Firmin DN, et al. A single breath-hold multiecho T2* cardiovascular magnetic resonance technique for diagnosis of myocardial iron overload. J Magn Reson Imaging 2003;18:33-39.

377. Wang ZJ, Haselgrove JC, Martin MB, et al. Evaluation of iron overload by single voxel MRS measurement of liver T2. J Magn Reson Imaging 2002;15:395-400.

378. Siegelman ES, Mitchell DG, Outwater E, Munoz SJ, Rubin R. Idiopathic hemochromatosis: MR imaging findings in cirrhotic and precirrhotic patients. Radiology 1993;188:637-641.

379. Wanless IR. Vascular disorders. In: MacSween RNM, Burt AD, Portmann BC, Ishak KG, Scheuer PJ, Anthony PP, eds. Pathology of the Liver, 4th ed. Churchill Livingstone, 2002, pp 539-573.

380. Titton RL, Coakley FV. Case 51: paroxysmal nocturna hemoglobinuria with thrombotic Budd-Chiari syndrome and renal cortical hemosiderin. Radiology 2002;225:67-70.

381. Kane R, Eustace S. Diagnosis of Budd-Chiari syndrome: comparison between sonography and MR angiography. Radiology 1995;195:117-121.

382. Noone TC, Semelka RC, Siegelman ES, et al. Budd-Chiari syndrome: spectrum of appearances of acute, subacute, and chronic disease with magnetic resonance imaging. J Magn Reson Imaging 2000;11:44-50.

383. Erden A, Erden I, Karayalcin S, Yurdaydin C. Budd-Chiari syndrome: evaluation with multiphase contrast-enhanced three-dimensional MR angiography. AJR Am J Roentgenol 2002;179:1287-1292.

384. Park JH, Han JK, Choi BI, Han MC. Membranous obstruction of the inferior vena cava with Budd-Chiari syndrome: MR imaging findings. J Vasc Interv Radiol 1991;2:463-469.

385. Okuda K. Inferior vena cava thrombosis at its hepatic portion (obliterative hepatocavopathy). Semin Liver Dis 2002;22:15-26.

386. Desser TS, Sze DY, Jeffrey RB. Imaging and intervention in the hepatic veins. AJR Am J Roentgenol 2003;180:1583-1591.

387. Valla D, Benhamou JP. Obstruction of the hepatic veins or suprahepatic inferior vena cava. Dig Dis 1996;14:99-118.

388. Kim PN, Mitchell DG, Outwater EK. Budd-Chiari syndrome: hepatic venous obstruction by an elevated diaphragm. Abdom Imaging 1999;24:267-271.

389. Takayasu K, Muramatsu Y, Moriyama N, et al. Radiological study of idiopathic Budd-Chiari syndrome complicated by hepatocellular carcinoma. A report of four cases. Am J Gastroenterol 1994;89:249-253.

390. Okuda H, Yamagata H, Obata H, et al. Epidemiological and clinical features of Budd-Chiari syndrome in Japan. J Hepatol 1995;22:1-9.

391. Vilgrain V, Lewin M, Vons C, et al. Hepatic nodules in Budd-Chiari syndrome: imaging features. Radiology 1999;210:443-450.

392. Brancatelli G, Federle MP, Grazioli L, Golfieri R, Lencioni R. Benign regenerative nodules in Budd-Chiari syndrome and other vascular disorders of the liver: radiologic-pathologic and clinical correlation. Radiographics 2002;22:847-862.

393. Brancatelli G, Federle MP, Grazioli L, Golfieri R, Lencioni R Large regenerative nodules in Budd-Chiari syndrome and other vascular disorders of the liver: CT and MR imaging findings with clinicopathologic correlation. AJR Am J Roentgenol 2002;178:877-883.

394. Arvanitaki M, Adler M. Nodular regenerative hyperplasia of the liver: a review of 14 cases. Hepatogastroenterology 2001;48:1425-1429.

395. Kondo F. Benign nodular hepatocellular lesions caused by abnormal hepatic circulation: etiological analysis and introduction of a new concept. J Gastroenterol Hepatol 2001;16:1319-1328.

396. Maetani Y, Itoh K, Egawa H, et al. Benign hepatic nodules in Budd-Chiari syndrome: radiologic-pathologic correlation with emphasis on the central scar. AJR Am J Roentgenol 2002;178:869-875.

397. Soler R, Rodriguez E, Pombo F, Gonzalez J, Pombo S, Prada C. Benign regenerative nodules with copper accumulation in a case of chronic Budd-Chiari syndrome: CT and MR findings. Abdom Imaging 2000;25:486-489.

398. DeLeve LD, Shulman HM, McDonald GB. Toxic injury to hepatic sinusoids: sinusoidal obstruction syndrome (veno-occlusive disease). Semin Liver Dis 2002;22:27-42.

399. Richardson P, Guinan E. Hepatic veno-occlusive disease following hematopoietic stem cell transplantation. Acta Haematol 2001;106:57-68.

400. van den Bosch MA, van Hoe L. MR imaging findings in two patients with hepatic veno-occlusive disease following bone marrow transplantation. Eur Radiol 2000;10:1290-1293.

401. Mortele KJ, Van Vlierberghe H, Wiesner W, Ros PR. Hepatic veno-occlusive disease: MRI findings. Abdom Imaging 2002;27:523-526.

402. Gore RM, Mathieu DG, White EM, Ghahremani GG, Panella JS, Rochester D. Passive hepatic congestion: cross-sectional imaging features. AJR Am J Roentgenol 1994;162:71-75.

403. Spritzer CE. Vascular diseases and MR angiography of the liver. Magn Reson Imaging Clin N Am 1997;5:377-396.

404. Parvey HR, Raval B, Sandler CM. Portal vein thrombosis: imaging findings. AJR Am J Roentgenol 1994;162:77-81.

405. Kawamoto S, Soyer PA, Fishman EK, Bluemke DA. Nonneoplastic liver disease: evaluation with CT and MR imaging. Radiographics 1998;18:827-848.

406. Matsuo M, Kanematsu M, Nishigaki Y, et al. Pseudothrombosis with T2-weighted fast spin-echo MR images caused by static portal venous flow in severe cirrhosis. J Magn Reson Imaging 2002;15:199-202.

407. De Gaetano AM, Lafortune M, Patriquin H, De Franco A, Aubin B, Paradis K. Cavernous transformation of the portal vein: patterns of intrahepatic and splanchnic collateral circulation detected with Doppler sonography. AJR Am J Roentgenol 1995;165:1151-1155.

408. Song B, Min P, Oudkerk M, et al. Cavernous transformation of the portal vein secondary to tumor thrombosis of hepatocellular carcinoma: spiral CT visualization of the collateral vessels. Abdom Imaging 2000;25:385-393.

409. Pandharipande PV, Lee VS, Morgan GR, et al. Vascular and extravascular complications of liver transplantation: comprehensive evaluation with three-dimensional contrast-enhanced volumetric MR imaging and MR cholangiopancreatography. AJR Am J Roentgenol 2001;177:1101-1107.

410. Glockner JF, Forauer AR, Solomon H, Varma CR, Perman WH. Three-dimensional gadolinium-enhanced MR angiography of vascular complications after liver transplantation. AJR Am J Roentgenol 2000;174:1447-1453.

411. Ito K, Siegelman ES, Stolpen AH, Mitchell DG. MR imaging of complications after liver transplantation. AJR Am J Roentgenol 2000;175:1145-1149.

412. Stafford-Johnson DB, Hamilton BH, Dong Q, et al. Vascular complications of liver transplantation: evaluation with gadolinium-enhanced MR angiography. Radiology 1998;207:153-160.

413. Erbay N, Raptopoulos V, Pomfret EA, Kamel IR, Kruskal JB. Living donor liver transplantation in adults: vascular variants important in

surgical planning for donors and recipients. AJR Am J Roentgenol 2003;181:109-114.

414. Lang P, Schnarkowski P, Grampp S, et al. Liver transplantation: significance of the periportal collar on MRI. J Comput Assist Tomogr 1995;19:580-585.

415. Hanto DW. A 50-year-old man with hepatitis C and cirrhosis needing liver transplantation. Jama 2003;290:3238-3246.

416. Hussain HK, Nghiem HV. Imaging of hepatic transplantation. Clin Liver Dis 2002;6:247-270.

417. Bhattacharjya S, Gunson BK, Mirza DF, et al. Delayed hepatic artery thrombosis in adult orthotopic liver transplantation—a 12-year experience. Transplantation 2001;71:1592-1596.

418. Kim BS, Kim TK, Jung DJ, et al. Vascular complications after living related liver transplantation: evaluation with gadolinium-enhanced three-dimensional MR angiography. AJR Am J Roentgenol 2003;181:467-474.

419. Zajko AB, Tobben PJ, Esquivel CO, Starzl TE. Pseudoaneurysms following orthotopic liver transplantation: clinical and radiologic manifestations. Transplant Proc 1989;21:2457-2459.

420. Settmacher U, Nussler NC, Glanemann M, et al. Venous complications after orthotopic liver transplantation. Clin Transplant 2000;14:235-241.

421. Ferris JV, Baron RL, Marsh JW, Jr., Oliver JH III, Carr BI, Dodd GD III. Recurrent hepatocellular carcinoma after liver transplantation: spectrum of CT findings and recurrence patterns. Radiology 1996;198:233-238.

422. Crawford JM. Liver Cirrhosis. In: MacSween RNM, Burt AD, Portmann BC, Ishak KG, Scheuer PJ, Anthony PP, eds. Pathology of the Liver, 4th ed. Churchill Livingstone, 2002, pp 575-619.

423. Flamm SL. Chronic hepatitis C virus infection. Jama 2003;289:2413-2417.

424. International WP. Terminology of Nodular Hepatocellular Lesions. Hepatology 1995;22:983-993.

425. Theise ND, Park YN, Kojiro M. Dysplastic nodules and hepatocarcinogenesis. Clin Liver Dis 2002;6:497-512.

426. Earls JP, Theise ND, Weinreb JC, et al. Dysplastic nodules and hepatocellular carcinoma: thin-section MR imaging of explanted cirrhotic livers with pathologic correlation. Radiology 1996;201:207-214.

427. Krinsky GA, Lee VS. MR imaging of cirrhotic nodules. Abdom Imaging 2000;25:471-482.

428. Dodd GD III, Baron RL, Oliver JH III, Federle MP. Spectrum of imaging findings of the liver in end-stage cirrhosis: part I, gross morphology and diffuse abnormalities. AJR Am J Roentgenol 1999;173:1031-1036.

429. Ito K, Mitchell DG, Hann HW, et al. Progressive viral-induced cirrhosis: serial MR imaging findings and clinical correlation. Radiology 1998;207:729-735.

430. Ito K, Mitchell DG, Gabata T. Enlargement of hilar periportal space: a sign of early cirrhosis at MR imaging. J Magn Reson Imaging 2000;11:136-140.

431. Ito K, Mitchell DG, Gabata T, Hussain SM. Expanded gallbladder fossa: simple MR imaging sign of cirrhosis. Radiology 1999; 211:723-726.

432. Ito K, Mitchell DG, Hann HW, et al. Viral-induced cirrhosis: grading of severity using MR imaging. AJR Am J Roentgenol 1999;173:591-596.

433. Rosenthal SJ, Harrison LA, Baxter KG, Wetzel LH, Cox GG, Batnitzky S. Doppler US of helical flow in the portal vein. Radiographics 1995;15:1103-1111.

434. Lafortune M, Matricardi L, Denys A, Favret M, Dery R, Pomier-Layrargues G. Segment 4 (the quadrate lobe): a barometer of cirrhotic liver disease at US. Radiology 1998;206:157-160.

435. Okazaki H, Ito K, Fujita T, Koike S, Takano K, Matsunaga N. Discrimination of alcoholic from virus-induced cirrhosis on MR imaging. AJR Am J Roentgenol 2000;175:1677-1681.

436. Ito K, Mitchell DG, Siegelman ES. Cirrhosis: MR imaging features. Magn Reson Imaging Clin N Am 2002;10:75-92.

437. Ohtomo K, Baron RL, Dodd GD III, Federle MP, Ohtomo Y, Confer SR. Confluent hepatic fibrosis in advanced cirrhosis: evaluation with MR imaging. Radiology 1993;189:871-874.

438. Baron RL, Peterson MS. From the RSNA refresher courses: screening the cirrhotic liver for hepatocellular carcinoma with CT and MR imaging: opportunities and pitfalls. Radiographics 2001;21 Spec No: S117-132.

439. Wenzel JS, Donohoe A, Ford KL III, Glastad K, Watkins D, Molmenti E. Primary biliary cirrhosis: MR imaging findings and description of MR imaging periportal halo sign. AJR Am J Roentgenol 2001;176:885-889.

440. Kim MJ, Mitchell DG, Ito K, Hann HW, Park YN, Kim PN. Hepatic iron deposition on MR imaging in patients with chronic liver disease: correlation with serial serum ferritin concentration. Abdom Imaging 2001;26:149-156.

441. Krinsky GA, Israel G. Nondysplastic nodules that are hyperintense on T1-weighted gradient-echo MR imaging: frequency in cirrhotic patients undergoing transplantation. AJR Am J Roentgenol 2003;180:1023-1027.

442. Kim T, Baron RL, Nalesnik MA. Infarcted regenerative nodules in cirrhosis: CT and MR imaging findings with pathologic correlation. AJR Am J Roentgenol 2000;175:1121-1125.

443. Vitellas KM, Tzalonikou MT, Bennett WF, Vaswani KK, Bova JG. Cirrhosis: spectrum of findings on unenhanced and dynamic gadolinium-enhanced MR imaging. Abdom Imaging 2001;26:601-615.

444. Krinsky GA, Lee VS, Theise ND, et al. Hepatocellular carcinoma and dysplastic nodules in patients with cirrhosis: prospective diagnosis with MR imaging and explantation correlation. Radiology 2001;219:445-454.

445. Dodd GD III, Baron RL, Oliver JH III, Federle MP. Spectrum of imaging findings of the liver in end-stage cirrhosis. 2. Focal abnormalities. AJR Am J Roentgenol 1999;173:1185-1192.

446. Park YN, Yang CP, Fernandez GJ, Cubukcu O, Thung SN, Theise ND. Neoangiogenesis and sinusoidal "capillarization" in dysplastic nodules of the liver. Am J Surg Pathol 1998;22:656-662.

447. Krinsky GA, Theise ND, Rofsky NM, Mizrachi H, Tepperman LW, Weinreb JC. Dysplastic nodules in cirrhotic liver: arterial phase enhancement at CT and MR imaging—a case report. Radiology 1998;209:461-464.

448. Krinsky GA, Lee VS, Nguyen MT, et al. Siderotic nodules in the cirrhotic liver at MR imaging with explant correlation: no increased frequency of dysplastic nodules and hepatocellular carcinoma. Radiology 2001;218:47-53.

449. Krinsky GA, Lee VS, Nguyen MT, et al. Siderotic nodules at MR imaging: regenerative or dysplastic? J Comput Assist Tomogr 2000;24:773-776.

450. Mitchell DG, Rubin R, Siegelman ES, Burk DL, Jr., Rifkin MD. Hepatocellular carcinoma within siderotic regenerative nodules: appearance as a nodule within a nodule on MR images. Radiology 1991;178:101-103.

451. Sadek AG, Mitchell DG, Siegelman ES, Outwater EK, Matteucci T, Hann HW. Early hepatocellular carcinoma that develops within macroregenerative nodules: growth rate depicted at serial MR imaging. Radiology 1995;195:753-756.

452. Krinsky GA, Lee VS, Theise ND. Focal lesions in the cirrhotic liver: high resolution ex vivo MRI with pathologic correlation. J Comput Assist Tomogr 2000;24:189-196.

453. Burt AD, Day CP. Pathophysiology of the liver. In: MacSween RNM, Burt AD, Portmann BC, Ishak KG, Scheuer PJ, Anthony PP, eds. Pathology of the Liver, 4th ed. Churchill Livingstone, 2002, pp 67-105.

454. Kim M, Mitchell DG, Ito K. Portosystemic collaterals of the upper abdomen: review of anatomy and demonstration on MR imaging. Abdom Imaging 2000;25:462-470.

455. Matsuo M, Kanematsu M, Kim T, et al. Esophageal Varices: Diagnosis with Gadolinium-Enhanced MR Imaging of the Liver for Patients with Chronic Liver Damage. AJR Am J Roentgenol 2003;180:461-466.

456. Sagoh T, Itoh K, Togashi K, et al. Gamna-Gandy bodies of the spleen: evaluation with MR imaging. Radiology 1989;172:685-687.

457. Minami M, Itai Y, Ohtomo K, et al. Siderotic nodules in the spleen: MR imaging of portal hypertension. Radiology 1989;172: 681-684.

458. Guingrich JA, Kuhlman JE. Colonic wall thickening in patients with cirrhosis: CT findings and clinical implications. AJR Am J Roentgenol 1999;172:919-924.

459. Karahan OI, Dodd GD III, Chintapalli KN, Rhim H, Chopra S. Gastrointestinal wall thickening in patients with cirrhosis: frequency and patterns at contrast-enhanced CT. Radiology 2000;215:103-107.

460. Chopra S, Dodd GD III, Chintapalli KN, Esola CC, Ghiatas AA. Mesenteric, omental, and retroperitoneal edema in cirrhosis: frequency and spectrum of CT findings. Radiology 1999;211:737-742.

461. Szklaruk J, Silverman PM, Charnsangavej C. Imaging in the diagnosis, staging, treatment, and surveillance of hepatocellular carcinoma. AJR Am J Roentgenol 2003;180:441-454.

462. Liang TJ, Ghany M. Hepatitis B e Antigen—the dangerous endgame of hepatitis B. N Engl J Med 2002;347:208-210.

463. Lee KH, O'Malley ME, Kachura JR, Haider M, Hanbidge A. Pictorial essay—hepatocellular carcinoma: imaging and imaging-guided intervention. AJR Am J Roentgenol 2003;180:1015-1022.

464. Benvegnu L, Fattovich G, Noventa F, et al. Concurrent hepatitis B and C virus infection and risk of hepatocellular carcinoma in cirrhosis: a prospective study. Cancer 1994;74:2442-2448.

465. Kelekis NL, Semelka RC, Worawattanakul S, et al. Hepatocellular carcinoma in North America: a multiinstitutional study of appearance on T1-weighted, T2-weighted, and serial gadolinium-enhanced gradient-echo images. AJR Am J Roentgenol 1998;170:1005-1013.

466. Ebara M, Fukuda H, Kojima Y, et al. Small hepatocellular carcinoma: relationship of signal intensity to histopathologic findings and metal content of the tumor and surrounding hepatic parenchyma. Radiology 1999;210:81-88.

467. Koushima Y, Ebara M, Fukuda H, et al. Small hepatocellular carcinoma: assessment with T1-weighted spin-echo magnetic resonance imaging with and without fat suppression. Eur J Radiol 2002;41:34-41.

468. Yoshikawa J, Matsui O, Takashima T, et al. Fatty metamorphosis in hepatocellular carcinoma: radiologic features in 10 cases. AJR Am J Roentgenol 1988;151:717-720.

469. Sugihara E, Murakami T, Kim T, et al. Detection of hypervascular hepatocellular carcinoma with dynamic magnetic resonance imaging with simultaneously obtained in-phase and opposed-phase echo images. J Comput Assist Tomogr 2003;27:110-116.

470. Fujita T, Ito K, Honjo K, Okazaki H, Matsumoto T, Matsunaga N. Detection of hepatocellular carcinoma: comparison of T2-weighted breath-hold fast spin-echo sequences and high-resolution dynamic MR imaging with a phased-array body coil. J Magn Reson Imaging 1999;9:274-279.

471. Hussain HK, Syed I, Nghiem HV, et al. T2-weighted MR imaging in the assessment of cirrhotic liver. Radiology 2004.

472. Brancatelli G, Federle MP, Grazioli L, Carr BI. Hepatocellular carcinoma in noncirrhotic liver: CT, clinical, and pathologic findings in 39 U.S. residents. Radiology 2002;222:89-94.

473. Winston CB, Schwartz LH, Fong Y, Blumgart LH, Panicek DM. Hepatocellular carcinoma: MR imaging findings in cirrhotic livers and noncirrhotic livers. Radiology 1999;210:75-79.

474. Hussain SM, Semelka RC, Mitchell DG. MR imaging of hepatocellular carcinoma. Magn Reson Imaging Clin N Am 2002;10:31-52.

475. Efremidis SC, Hytiroglou P. The multistep process of hepatocarcinogenesis in cirrhosis with imaging correlation. Eur Radiol 2002;12:753-764.

476. Yamashita Y, Fan ZM, Yamamoto H, et al. Spin-echo and dynamic gadolinium-enhanced FLASH MR imaging of hepatocellular carcinoma: correlation with histopathologic findings. J Magn Reson Imaging 1994;4:83-90.

477. Carlos RC, Kim HM, Hussain HK, Francis IR, Nghiem HV, Fendrick AM. Developing a prediction rule to assess hepatic malignancy in patients with cirrhosis. AJR Am J Roentgenol 2003;180:893-900.

478. Fujita T, Honjo K, Ito K, Matsumoto T, Matsunaga N, Hamm B. High-resolution dynamic MR imaging of hepatocellular carcinoma with a phased-array body coil. Radiographics 1997;17:315-331; discussion 332-315.

479. Kajiwara M. MR imaging of small hepatocellular carcinoma (≤20 mm): correlation with vascularity and histological features. Kurume Med J 1997;44:327-338.

480. Grazioli L, Olivetti L, Fugazzola C, et al. The pseudocapsule in hepatocellular carcinoma: correlation between dynamic MR imaging and pathology. Eur Radiol 1999;9:62-67.

481. Imaeda T, Kanematsu M, Mochizuki R, Goto H, Saji S, Shimokawa K. Extracapsular invasion of small hepatocellular carcinoma: MR and CT findings. J Comput Assist Tomogr 1994;18:755-760.

482. Tsai TJ, Chau GY, Lui WY, et al. Clinical significance of microscopic tumor venous invasion in patients with resectable hepatocellular carcinoma. Surgery 2000;127:603-608.

483. Katyal S, Oliver JH III, Peterson MS, Ferris JV, Carr BS, Baron RL. Extrahepatic metastases of hepatocellular carcinoma. Radiology 2000;216:698-703.

484. Dodd GD III, Baron RL, Oliver JH III, Federle MP, Baumgartel PB. Enlarged abdominal lymph nodes in end-stage cirrhosis: CT-histopathologic correlation in 507 patients. Radiology 1997; 203:127-130.

485. Eubank WB, Wherry KL, Maki JH, Sahin H, Funkhouser CP, Schmiedl UP. Preoperative evaluation of patients awaiting liver transplantation: Comparison of multiphasic contrast-enhanced 3D magnetic resonance to helical computed tomography examinations. J Magn Reson Imaging 2002;16:565-575.

486. Jeong MG, Yu JS, Kim KW, Jo BJ, Kim JK. Early homogeneously enhancing hemangioma versus hepatocellular carcinoma: differentiation using quantitative analysis of multiphasic dynamic magnetic resonance imaging. Yonsei Med J 1999;40: 248-255.

487. Shimizu A, Ito K, Koike S, Fujita T, Shimizu K, Matsunaga N. Cirrhosis or chronic hepatitis: evaluation of small (≤2 cm) early-enhancing hepatic lesions with serial contrast-enhanced dynamic MR imaging. Radiology 2003;226:550-555.

488. Bhartia B, Ward J, Guthrie JA, Robinson PJ. Hepatocellular carcinoma in cirrhotic livers: double-contrast thin-section MR imaging with pathologic correlation of explanted tissue. AJR Am J Roentgenol 2003;180:577-584.

489. Vogl TJ, Hammerstingl R, Schwarz W, et al. Superparamagnetic iron oxide–enhanced versus gadolinium-enhanced MR imaging for differential diagnosis of focal liver lesions. Radiology 1996;198: 881-887.

490. Kato H, Kanematsu M, Kondo H, et al. Ferumoxide-enhanced MR imaging of hepatocellular carcinoma: correlation with histologic tumor grade and tumor vascularity. J Magn Reson Imaging 2004;19:76-81.

491. Yoshimitsu K, Varma DG, Jackson EF. Unsuppressed fat in the right anterior diaphragmatic region on fat-suppressed T2-weighted fast spin-echo MR images. J Magn Reson Imaging 1995;5:145-149.

MRI of the Bile Ducts, Gallbladder, and Pancreas

Saroja Adusumilli, MD

Evan S. Siegelman, MD

MAGNETIC RESONANCE CHOLANGIOPANCREATOGRAPHY (MRCP)

MRCP Principles and Techniques

Magnetic resonance cholangiopancreatography (MRCP) was introduced in 1991 as a noninvasive method of imaging the biliary tree.[1] Although endoscopic retrograde cholangiopancreatography (ERCP) has been the mainstay for diagnosing and treating pancreaticobiliary disease, complications such as pancreatitis, cholangitis, hemorrhage, and duodenal perforation have limited its use as a routine diagnostic test.[2] MRCP can replace diagnostic ERCP in settings where the latter would be difficult or impossible to perform. Clinical examples include patients with severe biliary obstruction (which may prohibit the physician's ability to cannulate the duct or evaluate the ducts proximal to an obstruction)[3,4] and those with biliary-enteric reconstruction, gastrojejunostomy, or obstructive lesions of the esophagus and stomach.

MRCP exploits the inherent differences in T2-W contrast between fluid-filled structures in the abdomen and adjacent soft tissue and does not require intravenous contrast agents.[5] It is recommended that patients fast for 3-4 hours before undergoing an MRCP in order to reduce fluid content within the stomach, decrease duodenal peristalsis, and promote gallbladder filling.[6,7] Negative oral contrast agents can improve the depiction of the pancreaticobiliary tree by eliminating the high signal intensity (SI) of fluid in the gastrointestinal tract but are not required, since thin-section tomographic imaging allows for the evaluation of ductal structures without these structures being obscured by adjacent bowel.[8]

The principle of MRCP is that static or slow-moving fluids such as bile and pancreatic secretions within the biliary tree and pancreatic duct have a much longer T2 than solid tissue does and have high SI on heavily T2-weighted images (T2-WIs), whereas background soft tissues have very low SI. MRCP routinely is performed in the axial and coronal planes, while the oblique coronal plane can be used to evaluate anatomic variants suspected on other images.[6,7,9] Commonly used MRCP techniques include two- or three-dimensional (2D or 3D) breathing-averaged T2-W sequences and breath-hold T2-W sequences such as single-shot fast spin-echo (SSFSE) or half-Fourier acquisition single-shot turbo spin-echo (HASTE).[10-16] Breathing-averaged T2-W sequences are limited by respiratory motion and bowel peristalsis.[6,7,10]

Because of subsecond scan times, SSFSE and HASTE sequences can be performed as a breath-hold or a free-breathing technique for patients who are uncooperative or unable to suspend respiration. The signal-to-noise ratio (SNR) and contrast-to-noise ratio (CNR) of SSFSE and HASTE sequences are decreased compared with breathing-averaged T2-W sequences because the former techniques are acquired in only a single acquisition and use very long echo trains. However, this limitation is overcome by the subsecond acquisition time, which "freezes" physiologic motion.[12,14,17]

MRCP can be performed two ways that provide complementary information (Box 2-1). One method uses breath-hold sequences that acquire a single slab of data (typically 30-80 mm) in a 1- to 2-second breath-hold that displays fluid-containing structures as having high SI.[12,13,15] These thick collimation images can be performed in the coronal, axial, and oblique coronal planes. An extremely long echo time (TE; 600-1,000 ms) is used to effectively suppress the background soft tissue and overcome partial volume averaging effect.[13,17] Postprocessing is not required, because only a single image is obtained that represents the average of the data contained in the entire imaging volume. Thick-slab images are similar to the projection images acquired by ERCP and, although useful for depicting the entire pancreaticobiliary tree and nondilated ducts, are not sensitive for the detection of intraductal filling defects that may be obscured by hyperintense bile.[12]

Thick collimation slabs are supplemented by the second MRCP method that acquires multiple thin collimation slices (3-5 mm) that can be postprocessed on an imaging workstation.[12,15] Postprocessing typically uses a maximum intensity projection (MIP) algorithm in which only the pixel with the highest SI along a ray perpendicular to the plane of projection is displayed, thus highlighting bile and fluid-filled structures. Multislice source images can be acquired in a single breath-hold sequence or as a 4- to 7-minute 2D or 3D breathing-averaged T2-W sequence obtained in the axial (best for the pancreatic duct) and coronal planes (best for the biliary tree).[11-13,15] The use of a longer TE (≥180 ms) effectively minimizes signal from most extraductal structures, and the elimination of fat saturation allows for better delineation of the boundaries of the parenchymal organs.[7,10,11,16,18] The source images from a thin collimation multislice acquisition should be reviewed in addition to the MIP reconstructions in order to demonstrate small stones or other intraductal pathology that may be obscured by partial volume averaging effects (Fig. 2-1).[12]

MRCP: Technical and Diagnostic Pitfalls

Technical and interpretative pitfalls can mask or simulate pathologic conditions of the pancreaticobiliary system. Some of these pitfalls are discussed with specific disease entities later in this chapter. The entire biliary tree and pancreatic duct often are not shown on a single MRCP image. A specific ductal segment may not be depicted, resulting in nonvisualization of a stone or stricture.[19] Unlike ERCP and percutaneous transhepatic cholangiography (PTC), MRCP provides static images that may show normal physiologic changes of the duct that can simulate disease. For example, physiologic contraction of the distal common bile duct can simulate a stenosis.[19] Extraductal material (surgical clips, gas in the gastrointestinal tract, and pulsatile flow in adjacent arteries) and intraductal material (air or blood) can decrease the SI of bile on T2-WIs and mimic biliary obstruction or intraductal pathology.[19,20] MRCP provides less spatial resolution than does ERCP, thereby limiting its ability to detect early peripheral duct abnormalities, and cannot always distinguish benign from malignant disease.[9,21] MRCP, in general, should be supplemented with other MR pulse sequences (T1, T2-W, contrast enhanced T1-W) for a more complete evaluation of ductal and extraductal soft tissues.[22]

MR OF THE BILE DUCTS

MR Technique and Normal Appearance of the Biliary Tree

The main MR technique for evaluating the biliary tree is MRCP, as discussed above. The intra- and extrahepatic ductal system are hyperintense; normal-sized intrahepatic ducts measure less than 3 mm and the common bile duct measures less than 7 mm (<10 mm after cholecystectomy). Biliary ducts are part of the portal triad (portal vein, bile duct, and hepatic artery) and can be depicted on MRCP in the peripheral third of the liver when they are dilated. MRCP cannot routinely depict nondilated intrahepatic bile ducts.

2-1 MRCP Imaging Protocol Suggestion

Single Thick-Collimation Slab
- TR = infinite (single-shot technique)
- TE = 600–1,000 ms
- Slab thickness: 20–60 mm
- FOV: 28–38 cm; NEX: 1
- Bandwidth: 32 kHz; matrix: 256 × (160–256)
- Image acquisition time: 2 s for each slab
- Plane of imaging: axial, coronal and/or oblique coronal (35° to 45° angled slabs)

Thin-Collimation Multislice
- 2D/3D breath-hold or breathing-averaged T2-W sequences
- TE = 180 ms
- Slice thickness: 3–5 mm
- FOV: 30–38 cm, NEX: 1 for breath-hold, 2–4 for breathing averaged
- Bandwidth: 32 kHz; matrix: 256 × (160–256)
- Plane of imaging: axial and coronal

± Fat saturation

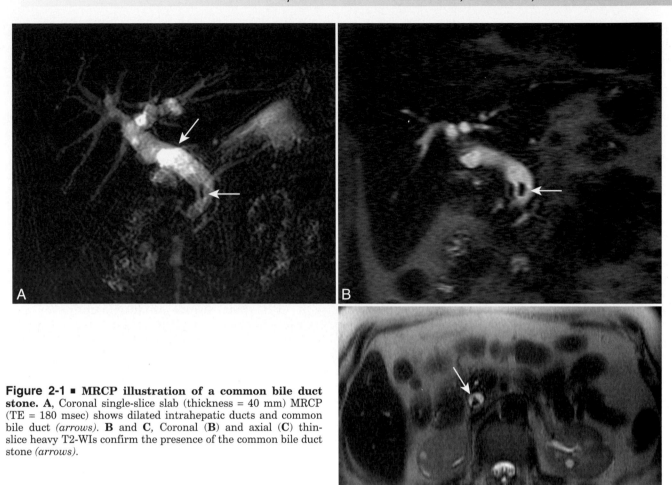

Figure 2-1 ▪ **MRCP illustration of a common bile duct stone. A**, Coronal single-slice slab (thickness = 40 mm) MRCP (TE = 180 msec) shows dilated intrahepatic ducts and common bile duct *(arrows)*. **B** and **C**, Coronal (**B**) and axial (**C**) thin-slice heavy T2-WIs confirm the presence of the common bile duct stone *(arrows)*.

MRCP is not as sensitive as ERCP and PTC, which can depict the biliary tree with a 70% to 90% success rate regardless of the degree of dilatation.[23,24]

For this reason, MR contrast agents with hepatobiliary excretion can be used to obtain functional cholangiograms of both the dilated and the nondilated biliary tree.[25] Mangafodopir trisodium (manganese dipyridoxyl diphosphate; Teslascan), Gd-EOB-DTPA (gadoxetic acid disodium, Eovist), and Gd-BOPTA (gadobenate dimeglumine, MultiHance) are lipophilic paramagnetic agents that result in hyperintense bile on delayed contrast-enhanced (CE) T1-WI.[26-28] The gallbladder and biliary tree appear hyperintense owing to biliary excretion 10 to 20 minutes after contrast injection.[24,26,28-30] Potential uses of CE T1-W functional MRCP include defining intrahepatic ductal anatomy in liver transplant donor candidates or in patients under evaluation for hepatectomy; evaluating stenoses and mural irregularities in patients with primary sclerosing cholangitis; and showing bile leaks in postcholecystectomy patients.[24,29,30]

Bile is hypointense on T1-WI because of its fluid content but can be slightly higher in SI if it is concentrated.[31] Fat-saturated CE T1-WIs are useful for evaluating the duct walls and adjacent liver parenchyma. Findings such as duct wall thickness, degree of wall enhancement, and infiltration into adjacent tissue are best assessed on enhanced imaging.

Congenital Anomalies and Anatomic Variants

ANOMALOUS PANCREATICOBILIARY JUNCTION

Congenital anomalies of the biliary tree may be contributory etiologic factors in patients with recurrent pancreatitis, cholangitis, or choledocholithiasis or in those who have nonspecific symptoms such as abdominal pain, jaundice, and nausea. The two major congenital anomalies of the biliary tree include an anomalous pancreaticobiliary junction (APBJ) and congenital biliary cystic disease. Normally, the common bile duct and pancreatic duct join with a short 4- to 5-mm common channel that is encircled by sphincter muscle fibers before entering the duodenum.

Less common configurations include an elongated 8- to 10-mm common channel or separate entrances into the duodenum.[32]

APBJ, also known as the "long common channel," is an uncommon entity (prevalence of 1.5% to 3.2%) in which the common bile duct and main pancreatic duct are joined outside the duodenal wall with the common channel being greater than 1.5 cm.[33-35] Because the junction is proximal to the sphincter of Oddi, pancreatic exocrine secretions may reflux into the common bile duct or bile may reflux into the pancreatic duct.[32] APBJ predisposes such patients to choledochal cysts (Fig. 2-2), cholangitis, stones, and pancreatitis. APBJ is present in up to 60% of patients with choledochal cysts in the U. S. and in more than 90% of patients in Japan[36,37] and can be associated with biliary tract malignancy in up to one third of affected individuals.[33,35] When APBJ is associated with a choledochal cyst, the carcinoma often arises in the cyst wall, whereas in the absence of a cyst, the carcinoma usually originates in the gallbladder.[33]

Early diagnosis of APBJ can help decrease the risk of malignancy when surgical excision of the extrahepatic common bile duct and gallbladder is performed in patients with a choledochal cyst or cholecystectomy in the absence of a choledochal cyst.[35] ERCP the procedure of choice for diagnosing APBJ. MRCP has been reported to have sensitivity of approximately 75% and specificity of 100% in the detection of APBJ.[34,35] MRI-MRCP can depict the long common channel greater than 15 mm, a coexisting choledochal cyst, and complications such as stones and masses.[33-35] Evaluating both the source images and MIP reconstructions is important for diagnosing a long common channel, especially in the

setting of a large choledochal cyst that can overlap with the common channel.[35]

CONGENITAL BILIARY CYSTIC DISEASE: CHOLEDOCHAL CYSTS

Choledochal cysts are uncommon congenital anomalies that represent cystic or fusiform dilatation of the extrahepatic or intrahepatic biliary tree and encompass the following lesions: choledochal cyst, diverticula, choledochocele, and Caroli's disease. Eighty percent of lesions are diagnosed in infancy and childhood (<10 years of age) and have a female predilection (F:M = 3–4:1).[37-39] The classic triad of symptoms of right upper quadrant pain, abdominal mass, and jaundice are present in one third.[39,40] Twenty percent of adult patients have nonspecific abdominal pain or sequelae of bile stasis such as stones, sludge, or cholangitis.[40] As described above, there is a high association of choledochal cysts with APBJ that results in chronic reflux of pancreatic enzymes into the biliary tree, thereby weakening the ductal wall and causing cyst formation.[37,41] Complications arising from the cysts include cholelithiasis, choledocholithiasis, carcinoma, pancreatitis, cholangitis, and cyst rupture. The incidence of carcinoma ranges from 2.5% to 26% and more commonly occurs in the cyst wall but can also occur in extracystic locations such as the gallbladder and biliary tree.[40,42] Cyst excision and biliary-enteric reconstruction eliminates a potential source of cancer and prevents recurrent cholangitis and pancreatitis. However, the possibility of carcinoma developing in the intrahepatic ducts necessitates long-term follow-up.[39-42]

When a choledochal cyst is very large and round and is not associated with intrahepatic dilatation, its

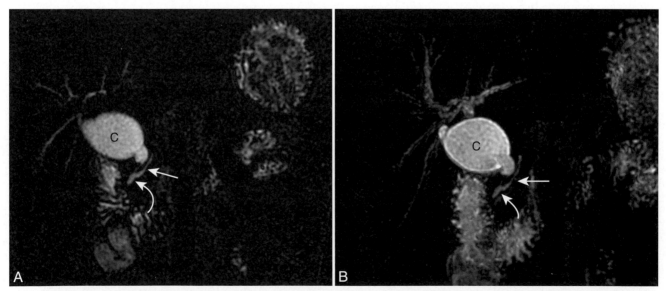

Figure 2-2 ■ **MR depiction of a choledochal cyst and aberrant junction of the pancreatic and common bile duct in a woman with right-sided pain. A** and **B,** Single thin-slice (**A**) and slab (**B**) MRCP reveals cystic dilation of the proximal common bile duct (C). The pancreatic duct *(arrow)* has a high insertion into to the common bile duct *(curved arrow)*. No solid tissue or suspect enhancement was revealed on other sequences, and an uncomplicated choledochal cyst was removed at surgery.

biliary origin can be difficult to determine by imaging. The differential diagnosis includes pancreatic pseudocyst and mesenteric, renal, adrenal, or hepatic cyst.[39] Documenting a communication between the cyst and biliary tree can establish a diagnosis. Direct cholangiography, MRCP, and ERCP provide similar results in evaluating choledochal cysts.[38,43] MRCP is used to define the extent of the cyst, determine the presence of an APBJ, and evaluate for associated complications of the pancreaticobiliary tree such as stone disease, cholangitis, and carcinoma (see Fig. 2-2).[44] For surgical planning, coronal images are the most useful, whereas for detection of stones, axial source images are the most accurate.[41] MRCP routinely detects a coexisting APBJ in adults but has a lower sensitivity in children.[41,45]

The Todani classification system subdivides the cystic lesions into five main categories (Box 2-2).[46] Type I choledochal cysts (cystic or fusiform dilatation of the common bile duct) represent 80% to 90% of lesions,[37,39] and yield the highest predisposition to cancer.[40] Type II cysts are true diverticula of the extrahepatic duct, account for 2% of lesions, and have the second highest risk of cancer.[40] A type III cyst is a choledochocele that is a focal dilatation of the intraduodenal segment of the common bile duct analogous to an ureterocele and comprises 1.4% to 5% of lesions.[47] Although usually 1- to 2-cm, they can become large enough to cause duodenal obstruction and have a higher association with choledocholithiasis.[32,37] The differential diagnosis of a choledochocele includes pancreatic pseudocyst, mucinous cystic neoplasm of the pancreas, duodenal duplication cyst, and intraluminal duodenal diverticulum.[47] A change in the size and shape of the choledochocele with duodenal peristalsis may help establish the diagnosis. Type IV disease accounts for 19% of lesions and affects either the extrahepatic biliary tree (type IVB), resulting in a "string of beads" appearance, or both the intra- and extrahepatic ducts (type IVA), resulting in saccular dilatation of the common bile and common hepatic ducts and cystic dilatation of the intrahepatic ducts.

Caroli's disease (type V) consists of multiple saccular or fusiform segmental dilatations of intrahepatic ducts affecting all or part of the liver. The more common form of the disease is associated with congenital hepatic fibrosis but not with cholangitis or stone disease. The hepatic fibrosis can progress to cirrhosis and portal hypertension with ensuing liver failure. The rare, "pure" form is associated with intrahepatic bilirubin stones and bacterial cholangitis.[48] Caroli's disease can simulate advanced biliary stone disease, polycystic liver disease, recurrent pyogenic cholangitis, hepatic abscesses, and primary sclerosing cholangitis.[48,49] Showing the communications between the saccules and bile ducts distinguishes Caroli's disease from polycystic liver disease and hepatic abscesses.[48,49] ERCP and PTC have traditionally been the accepted methods of diagnosis but MRCP can show similar findings.[49,50]

ANATOMIC VARIANTS OF THE BILIARY TREE

Anatomic variants of the biliary tree have become clinically important with the evolution of laparoscopic cholecystectomy because they may increase the risk of bile duct injury.[51] There is a twofold increase in bile duct injury with laparoscopic techniques over open cholecystectomy (0.1%). The common bile duct can be misidentified as the cystic duct and result in inadvertent ligation or resection.[51] Specific anatomic variants associated with an increased risk of injury include an aberrant right hepatic duct that inserts low into the common hepatic duct (below the bifurcation) or inserts into the cystic duct (5% of the population), a cystic duct that has a long (>2 cm) parallel course to the common hepatic duct (1.5% to 25%), a cystic duct that enters the medial surface of the common bile duct (10% to 15%), a short cystic duct (<5 mm), or a cystic duct that has a low insertion into the distal third of the common bile duct (9%).[6,52,53] MRCP is as accurate as ERCP and contrast-enhanced direct cholangiography in the diagnosis of these variants.[6,54] Clip artifact and partial volume averaging with overlapping hepatic ducts and duodenum can limit the MRCP evaluation of aberrant ducts (Fig. 2-3).[6,55] Evaluation of the source images and MIP reconstructions facilitates accurate determination of the duct insertions.[6]

2-2	Todani Classification System of Congenital Cystic Disease *(Adapted from reference 46)*	
IA	Cystic dilatation of the common bile duct (marked dilatation of part or all of the CBD; gallbladder arises from the cyst; intrahepatic ducts are normal)	
IB	Focal segmental dilatation of the CBD (usually distal); normal CBD is present between the cyst and cystic duct; biliary tree proximal to gallbladder is normal	
IC	Fusiform dilatation of common bile duct and common hepatic duct (gallbladder arises from dilated CBD; intrahepatic ducts are normal)	
II	Diverticula of the extrahepatic ducts	
III	Choledochocele	
IVA	Dilatation of the intra- and extrahepatic ducts (segmental cysts)	
IVB	Multiple segments of dilatation (segmental cysts) of the extrahepatic ducts only	
V	Caroli's disease (multiple saccular or cystic dilatations of the intrahepatic bile ducts; normal extrahepatic ducts)	

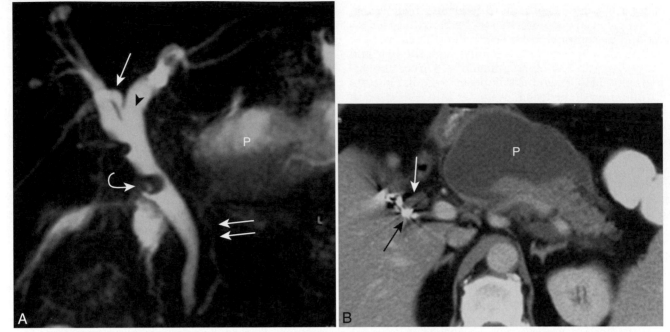

Figure 2-3 ■ **MRCP demonstration of aberrant intrahepatic ductal anatomy and false-positive diagnosis of a duct stricture secondary to adjacent surgical clips in a 57-year-old man with pancreatitis and a prior cholecystectomy. A,** Single-slab MRCP image (thickness = 40 mm, TE = 600) shows that the ducts draining the anterior segment of the right lobe *(arrow)* empty into the central segment of the left bile duct *(black arrowhead)*. This ductal variant would be of great clinical importance if this patient were a potential partial liver donor, since resection of the right lobe would be prohibitive. Focal narrowing of the right side of the bile duct *(curved arrow)* is secondary to clip artifacts from prior cholecystectomy. A large pancreatic pseudocyst (P) obscures visualization of the pancreatic duct *(double arrows)* within the pancreatic body. The pseudocyst shows decreased SI compared with bile secondary to intracystic hemorrhage and debris that was better revealed on other images. **B,** Enhanced CT scan shows multiple clips in the gallbladder fossa *(arrows)* and the pancreatic pseudocyst (P).

Biliary Obstruction

MRCP has been documented as having sensitivity of 91% to 96% and specificity of 99% to 100% for the diagnosis of biliary obstruction.[56,57] MRCP can depict the level, degree, and extent of biliary obstruction and reveal an etiology that might suggest whether the obstruction is due to an intrinsic abnormality of the ducts or extrinsic involvement of the ducts from adjacent organs and lymph nodes.[58-61] However, T1, T2-W, or CE T1-W sequences should supplement MRCP so that both ducts and extraductal abnormalities that are necessary for tumor staging, such as periductal masses, tumor extension, vascular involvement, lymphadenopathy, and metastases, can be evaluated.[22,62]

The etiology of malignant biliary obstruction can be suggested by the location of the obstruction. At the level of the porta hepatis, obstruction can be secondary to cholangiocarcinoma (Figs. 2-4 and 2-5), liver metastases, malignant lymphadenopathy, or locally invasive gallbladder and hepatocellular carcinomas. Extrahepatic suprapancreatic biliary obstruction can be secondary to lymphadenopathy or direct extension of cancer from the gallbladder, pancreas, stomach, and colon. Obstruction of the intrapancreatic segment of the common bile duct can be due to pancreatic head adenocarcinoma, ampullary carcinoma, or cholangiocarcinoma.[59] Most malignant lesions cause abrupt narrowing of the bile duct with shouldered margins

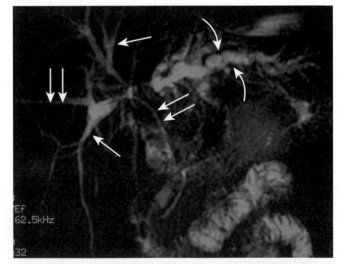

Figure 2-4 ■ **MRCP illustration of malignant obstruction at the level of the liver hilum secondary to a Klatskin tumor.** Single-projection heavily T2-W MRCP shows dilated left and right intrahepatic ducts. Other pulse sequences confirmed the diagnosis of unresectable Klatskin tumor. MRCP demonstration of a hilar cholangiocarcinoma in a 69-year-old woman with a remote history of cholecystectomy that presents with painless jaundice. Before the MR examination a right-sided biliary drain was placed. The MRCP projection image reveals the partially decompressed right-sided ducts *(arrows)*, the markedly dilated left-sided ductal system *(curved arrow)*, and the indwelling stent *(double arrows)*. Revelation of involvement of both right and left ductal systems usually indicates unresectable disease in the setting of cholangiocarcinoma.

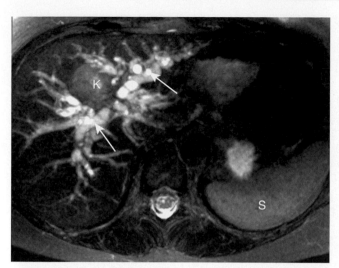

Figure 2-5 ▪ MRCP depiction of unresectable Klatskin tumor. Axial thick-section MRCP shows dilated left and right hepatic ducts *(arrows)* that terminate in a mass of the porta hepatitis (K) that is isointense to spleen (S).

and mucosal irregularities, resulting in a "rat tail" appearance.[23,59]

The most common causes of benign biliary obstruction include postsurgical or posttraumatic stricture, choledocholithiasis, chronic pancreatitis, and infectious or primary sclerosing cholangitis.[63] Benign lesions such as ampullary stenosis, stones, or benign stricture cause smooth and gradually tapered narrowing although some degree of overlap exists between benign and malignant lesions.[23,59]

Choledocholithiasis

Choledocholithiasis accounts for most cases of biliary obstruction and has become an important diagnosis in the setting of laparoscopic cholecystectomy.[63] Patients who have symptomatic cholelithiasis or acute cholecystitis complicated by jaundice, cholangitis, gallstone pancreatitis, common bile duct diameter greater than 6-7 mm on sonography, or abnormal bilirubin levels (>1.5) are considered at high risk for choledocholithiasis.[64,65] Individuals with choledocholithiasis benefit from ERCP-guided sphincterotomy and stone extraction prior to laparoscopic cholecystectomy.[64,65]

MRCP could be used to determine which subset of patients would benefit from stone extraction.[2,66,67] MRCP has the greatest utility in patients with a low suspicion of choledocholithiasis and in patients who cannot undergo ERCP because of pancreatitis, gastric surgery, or biliary-enteric reconstruction.[68] MRCP has sensitivity of 81% to 93% and specificity of 91% to 98% in the evaluation of common bile duct stones.[57,64,65,69-75] MRCP has higher sensitivity than do sonography and computed tomography (CT) in detecting common bile duct and intrahepatic stones.[71,74,76,77] MRCP has comparable sensitivity and specificity to ERCP for the evaluation of common bile duct stones[57,64,73,78] and is superior to ERCP for

diagnosing intrahepatic calculi.[78] Comparison studies are limited by the lack of a true gold standard, as ERCP and intraoperative cholangiography may not reveal small stones obscured by air bubbles or contrast material.

On MRCP, calculi appear as low SI filling defects within the high SI bile irrespective of their composition (see Figs. 1-10C and 2-1).[71,79] Axial and coronal breath-held thin-section multislice or thick-section slab projection sequences have high contrast to noise and less respiratory motion artifact and are probably the best MRCP technique for stone detection.[68,72,74,77] Breathing-averaged 2D or 3D heavily T2-WI can be performed in patients unable to hold their breath and are equally good in the detection of biliary ductal dilatation and stones.[57,69,70,72,73,80] Stone size is ultimately the most important criterion for detection by MRCP. Detection of stones on thick-slab MRCP depends on stone size, as larger calculi will be readily detected whereas 1- to 4-mm stones may be obscured by adjacent high SI bile. Thus, thick-slab MRCP techniques alone should not be relied on for common bile duct stone detection.[69,74,77,80,81] Axial source images from a multislice acquisition provide the best images for detecting small stones.[69-71,74]

There are several potential sources of misdiagnosis of common bile duct stones. The differential diagnosis of filling defects in the biliary tree includes calculus, neoplasm, blood clot, air bubble, and sludge. Stones have a round, oval, or angular shape and are located in the dependent portion of the duct. Air bubbles are present in the nondependent portion of the bile duct and may form part of an air-fluid level.[20,82] Blood clots and carcinoma may be indistinguishable from calculi on MRCP alone but are more likely to have irregular margins and are more readily characterized with T1-, T2-, and CE-MR sequences.[22] Small impacted stones in the ampulla may be either missed or misdiagnosed as ampullary stenosis, a prominent sphincter of Oddi, or neoplasm owing to the paucity of fluid in this region.[68,69,71] Signal voids from surgical clips, gas in the gastrointestinal tract, and arterial flow of the gastroduodenal artery or superior pancreaticoduodenal artery as it crosses the common bile duct can all mimic a stone or focal structure. Susceptibility artifacts from clips can be established by correlating the MRCP with radiographs, CT, or gradient echo (GRE) images. When comparing in-phase and opposed-phase GRE images, a longer TE in-phase sequence will reveal increased blooming from susceptibility artifact and suggest the presence of gas or clips (Fig. 2-6). CE–magnetic resonance angiography (MRA) can confirm the presence of an adjacent artery.[20,68,82]

Evaluation of the Postsurgical Biliary Tree

BILIARY-ENTERIC ANASTOMOSIS

Most biliary-enteric reconstructions take the form of a hepaticojejunostomy or choledochojejunostomy. Long-term complications occur with an incidence of 10% to 20% in patients with biliary-enteric anastomoses and

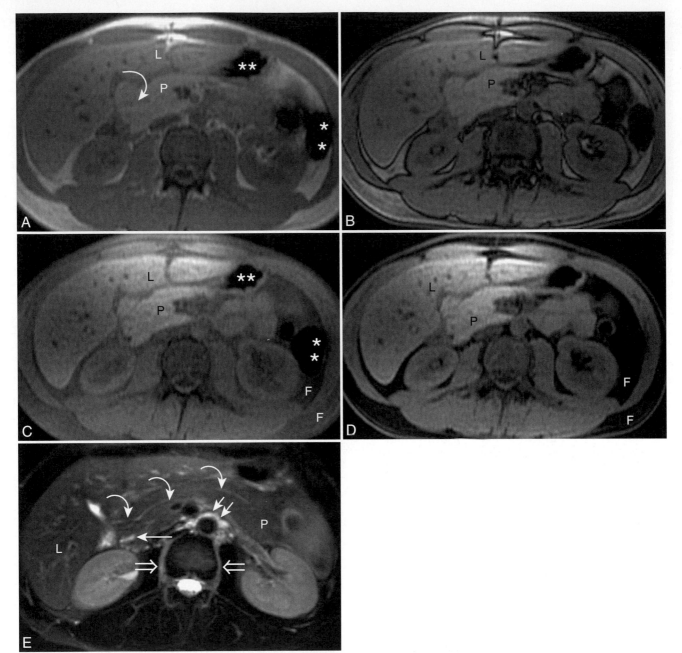

Figure 2-6 ▪ **An outside CT examination (not shown) revealed an enlarged pancreatic head, and an occult pancreatic neoplasm could not be excluded. A** and **B,** In-phase (**A**) and opposed-phase (**B**) T1-WIs show normal, hyperintense pancreatic parenchyma. Even though the pancreatic head is enlarged (which has been described in pancreatic divisum),[433] the normal SI pancreas excludes an infiltrative neoplasm. The distal segment of the accessory duct of Santorini is revealed *(curved arrow).* Normal, intermediate-to-high SI liver (L), and normal SI renal parenchyma (with renal cortex being of higher SI than renal medulla) are also present. **C** and **D,** Fat-suppressed in-phase (**C**) and opposed phase (**D**) T1-WIs acquired at the same time and location as **B** show similar normal, high SI pancreas. There is increased susceptibility artifact within gas-containing bowel segments (∗∗) in **A** and **C** compared with **B** and **D** secondary to the longer echo time. Note incomplete suppression of both the subcutaneous and retroperitoneal fat (F) in **C** compared with **D**. The choice of TE makes a difference in the degree of fat suppression when fat-suppressed GRE sequences are utilized. One reason is that the fat-suppression pulse is imperfect and the signal from some fat protons is not suppressed. If an opposed-phase sequence is then performed, the signal of the remaining fat protons cancels the signal of adjacent water protons (which are present in the membranes and lysosomes of adipocytes) to further decrease the resultant SI. Therefore, one should consider performing opposed-phase imaging when using fat-suppressed gradient echo sequences in order to optimize macroscopic fat suppression and dynamic range.[434,435] At 1.5 T it is fortuitous that the opposed-phase TE is shorter than the corresponding in-phase TE, thereby minimizing susceptibility effects. **E,** Axial fat-suppressed T2-WI shows normal, low-to-intermediate SI pancreatic parenchyma (P), normal, low-to-intermediate SI liver (L), and normal renal parenchymal SI (with renal cortex being iso- to hypointense to renal medulla). High SI within paraspinal veins *(open arrows)* and small retroperitoneal veins *(double arrows)* is secondary to slow flow that mimics the long T2 relaxation values of static fluid.[436] On fat-suppressed T2-WIs it can be difficult to determine where a normal, low-to-intermediate SI organ ends (i.e., liver, pancreas, and kidney) and the suppressed adjacent fat begins. The dorsal pancreatic duct of Santorini *(curved arrows)* drains directly into the minor papilla and does not communicate with the common bile duct *(arrow, revealed in cross section).*

2-3	Bismuth Classification of Traumatic Bile Duct Injury *(Adapted from references 84, 87)*	
	Location of Injury	**Treatment**
Type I	Injury of the common hepatic or bile duct >2 cm distal to the confluence of the right and left hepatic ducts	Hepaticojejunostomy or choledochojejunostomy
Type II	Injury of the common hepatic duct <2 cm from the confluence	Hepaticojejunostomy or choledochojejunostomy
Type III	Injury involves the entire common hepatic duct but spares the confluence	Hepaticojejunostomy
Type IV	Injury includes partial or complete destruction of the confluence (right) and left ducts are separated	Hepaticojejunostomy and reconstruction of hilar confluence

include recurrent obstruction secondary to anastomotic stenosis/stricture, cholangitis, intrahepatic stones, and dilated bile ducts.[59,83] MR-MRCP can evaluate the biliary-enteric anastomosis in patients with unexplained fever, right upper quadrant pain, or suspected cholangitis.[83]

Evaluation of the biliary-enteric anastomosis with ERCP can be technically difficult or impossible (10% to 50% failure rate) because of altered bowel anatomy (gastrojejunostomy or anastomosis beyond the level of the duodenum).[59] MRCP can show the site of anastomosis, status of the intrahepatic ducts, and any of the above complications.[59,83] Isolated biliary duct dilatation is not specific for obstruction, since some patients have a patent anastomosis with dilated ducts. However, duct dilatation in the setting of anastomotic narrowing suggests functional obstruction that could be confirmed by MRCP that uses a contrast agent with biliary excretion.[24,26,59] The MIP images alone can overestimate the stricture or not depict the actual anastomosis between bowel and the biliary tree because of adjacent bile or bowel contents. Thin-section source images should thus be inspected for complete evaluation.[83]

POSTSURGICAL BILIARY COMPLICATIONS

Most benign biliary strictures are secondary to stone disease or surgeries such as laparoscopic cholecystectomy, common bile duct exploration, liver transplantation (see next section), biliary-enteric reconstruction, pancreatic surgery, gastrectomy, and hepatic resection. Other less common etiologies include ischemia, primary sclerosing cholangitis, infectious cholangitis, chronic pancreatitis, and trauma.[84] Specific causes of injury include clip placement on a duct, ischemia from injury of adjacent arteries, and inadvertent duct ligation.

MRCP provides more information than ERCP or conventional cholangiography because it can depict the entire biliary tree proximal and distal to the stenosis regardless of whether it is high grade or complete.[85] Postsurgical strictures tend to be smooth with gradually tapered narrowing. Postoperative bile duct injury can be classified as a leak, stricture, or complete transection with possible biliary obstruction. Pertinent findings to assess on MRCP include presence or absence of biliary duct dilatation, stricture, free fluid, fluid collection, and nonvisualization of a bile duct segment that may suggest injury.[86] The Bismuth classification of traumatic bile duct injury (Box 2-3) is helpful for surgical planning because the length of the intact common duct distal to the bifurcation dictates whether the patient requires choledochojejunostomy, hepaticojejunostomy, or additional reconstruction.[84,87,88] Roux-en-Y hepaticojejunostomy is the most commonly performed surgical procedure with the best long-term results for treatment of posttraumatic bile duct stricture.[88,89]

MRCP EVALUATION AFTER LIVER TRANSPLANTATION

A variety of biliary-related complications can occur after liver transplantation (13% to 35% of patients) and require prompt diagnosis and treatment to ensure allograft survival (Box 2-4).[90,91] In addition to being able to reveal a biliary-enteric anastomosis, MRI and MRCP can accurately depict stone and sludge disease, biliary stricture and obstruction, and bile leaks.[90,92,93] The patient's T-tube or plastic biliary stent does not result in artifact on MRCP.[90]

Biliary obstruction is the second most common cause of liver dysfunction after rejection and is usually secondary to a stricture.[92] Most strictures occur after 1-3 months following transplant surgery and affect between 5% and 15% of allografts.[90] Nonanastomotic strictures are usually due to ischemia-related biliary changes such as those occurring with hepatic artery occlusion. MRCP can depict the level and degree of

2-4	Biliary Complications of Orthotopic Liver Transplantation Detected on MRI

Anastomotic Leak; Biloma (Most Common)
- Biliary duct obstruction (15%)
- Biliary stricture (5%–15%)
  Anastomotic (extrahepatic biliary tree) (most common)
  Nonanastomotic (confluence or right and left donor ducts)
  Inflammatory ampullary stenosis (rare)
- Bile duct sludge lithiasis (casts) (10%–15%)
- Bile duct stones (5%–10%)
- Sphincter of Oddi dysfunction (5%)

obstruction and also the ducts above and below the stricture. In cases of end-to-end anastomoses, the diameter of the donor common bile duct is normally twice that of the recipient common bile duct and should not be interpreted as a stricture.[93] Intrahepatic ducts greater than 2 mm and extrahepatic ducts greater than 7 mm are considered dilated. MRCP tends to overestimate anastomotic strictures and cannot always characterize the stricture although this is less of an issue in the setting of liver transplantation since strictures generally are not malignant.[90,93] Distinguishing between dilation and functional obstruction can be challenging. A CE-MRCP or follow-up MRCP may be of value to assess for progressive ductal dilatation.[93]

Anastomotic leaks and bilomas are common complications that occur within the first 30 days following transplantation. Bilomas are subhepatic fluid collections that are usually secondary to an anastomotic leak. Small amounts of peri-anastomotic ascites without an active leak are common 3 months after surgery, but the presence of bile leakage cannot be definitively diagnosed on MRI and requires further evaluation if there is strong clinical suspicion.[93] CE-MRCP that uses an agent with biliary excretion can document the presence and location of bile leaks in patients who have undergone cholecystectomy.[29] This same technique can be used to evaluate for a suspected anastomotic leak after liver transplantation. Biliary sludge and stones are precipitated by altered bile composition (cyclosporine-induced) and mechanical factors (dysfunctional T-tube; untreated obstruction of larger bile ducts) and are more common in the common bile duct and proximal intrahepatic ducts.[90,94]

MIRIZZI SYNDROME

Mirizzi syndrome is a complication of stone disease that can increase the risk of bile duct injury by obscuring the visualization of ductal structures during laparoscopic cholecystectomy and is considered by some surgeons to be a contraindication to using laparoscopic technique.[95] The syndrome refers to a partial mechanical obstruction of the common hepatic duct caused by a stone impacted in the adjacent cystic duct. The presence of a long parallel cystic duct predisposes patients to this syndrome. The common bile duct can then be mistaken for the cystic duct and transected. Preoperative identification of this entity changes the surgical approach during cholecystectomy to avoid bile duct injury.[95] MRCP can noninvasively assess the location of the gallstone, level of ductal obstruction, and presence of inflammatory changes around the gallbladder.[96]

Cholangitis

PRIMARY SCLEROSING CHOLANGITIS (BOX 2-5)

Primary sclerosing cholangitis (PSC) is a chronic and progressive disease of the biliary tree characterized by inflammation, destruction, and fibrosis of the intra- and extrahepatic bile ducts. Seventy percent of

---

2-5 Features of Primary Sclerosing Cholangitis

Clinical

M > F, fourth to fifth decades
75% of patients have inflammatory bowel disease (usually ulcerative colitis)
2%–10% of patients with ulcerative colitis have PSC
Progresses to cirrhosis after a median period of ≈12 years after diagnosis
5%–15% develop cholangiocarcinoma

Pathology

Chronic and progressive disease characterized by inflammation, destruction, and fibrosis of the intra- and extrahepatic ducts

MRI

Dilatation of intra- and extrahepatic ducts
Multifocal irregular strictures that alternate with normal ducts, giving a "beaded" appearance
"Pruning" of peripheral ducts
Isolated peripheral ducts have no visible connection to the central ducts
Periportal and portocaval lymph nodes common and reactive
Complicating cholangiocarcinoma difficult to diagnose when early

---

patients are men and are diagnosed in the fourth to fifth decades. Seventy-five percent of patients with PSC have inflammatory bowel disease (80% to 90% ulcerative colitis; 10% to 20% Crohn's disease).[97] Conversely, 2% to 10% of patients with ulcerative colitis have PSC.[98] Most patients with PSC are asymptomatic at the time of diagnosis but eventually develop signs and symptoms attributable to cholestasis such as jaundice and pruritus. Bile ducts do not regenerate, and the inflammation ultimately progresses to cirrhosis, portal hypertension, and liver failure. Cirrhosis develops after a median period of 10-12 years after diagnosis.[99] Treatment is usually palliative with medical therapy and dilatation of strictures, but the only curative therapy is liver transplantation.[97] Cholangiocarcinoma occurs with an incidence of 5% to 15% in patients with PSC, is unpredictable, and is difficult to diagnose.[97,100]

ERCP is considered the gold standard in evaluating the duct changes in patients with PSC[101]; however, MRCP displays similar cholangiographic findings with sensitivity and specificity of 88% and 97%, respectively, and along with conventional MRI may be useful in following disease status.[102,103] While ERCP depicts more ductal stenoses, MRCP can better depict dilated intrahepatic ducts peripheral to high-grade strictures that may not be revealed on ERCP.[101,103-105] MRI can also add information regarding hepatic lobar atrophy, cirrhosis, splenomegaly, and other sequelae of portal hypertension. The most common MRCP finding is dilatation of the intra- and extrahepatic ducts, while the second most common findings are multifocal, irregular strictures of the intra- and extrahepatic ducts that are out of proportion to the degree of proximal dilatation (Fig. 2-7).[101,105] If the ducts proximal to the strictures are very dilated, coexisting ascending cholangitis or cholangiocarcinoma must be considered.[106] The strictures of PSC are short and tend to alternate with normal or dilated ducts, giving a "beaded" appearance.[105] Isolated peripheral dilated ducts without a visible connection to the dilated central ducts are another suggestive finding.[105] "Pruning" refers to the presence of dilated intrahepatic ducts without dilated side branches; the latter are not shown because they are obliterated by fibrosis, thereby giving the appearance that the peripheral biliary tree is truncated.[105,106]

Since MRCP evaluates only abnormalities of the duct lumen, T1, T2, and CE-MR are used to evaluate the duct wall and hepatic parenchymal changes of PSC.[105,107] The extrahepatic ducts often show wall thickening greater than 2 mm and wall enhancement greater than that of muscle or pancreas.[105] Hepatic parenchymal abnormalities include peripheral wedge-shaped areas of increased SI relative to adjacent liver and a fine reticular pattern of increased SI on T2-WI thought to be secondary to vascular or lymphatic involvement by periductal inflammation.[105,107] Periportal edema is depicted as hyperintense T2 SI present alongside portal venous branches.[105] CE-MR imaging shows peripheral areas of increased enhancement that can persist on delayed imaging owing to a combination of increased arterial blood flow from inflammation and fibrosis.[105,107] Frequently seen morphologic changes include hypertrophy of the caudate lobe (up to 70% of patients; see Fig. 1-12) and segmental atrophy of the right or left

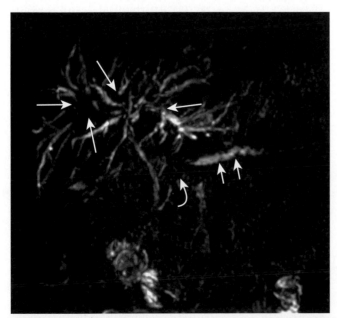

Figure 2-7 ▪ Axial slab MRCP image in a patient with primary sclerosing cholangitis reveals mild irregular intrahepatic duct dilation *(arrows)*. A structure of the pancreatic duct *(curved arrow)* with peripheral duct dilation *(small arrows)* is also present.

hepatic lobes (up to 60% of patients).[105] Periportal and portocaval lymphadenopathy is present in three fourths of patients and is not necessarily a sign of malignancy.[105,108]

Inflammatory strictures of PSC can be difficult to distinguish from malignant strictures secondary to cholangiocarcinoma. Potential malignant imaging features include progressive biliary duct dilatation on serial examinations and the presence of an enhancing ductal-periductal mass with adjacent liver invasion.[109] Neither ERCP nor MRCP can always differentiate between PSC and secondary cholangitis caused by infection, AIDS, and ischemic bile duct damage. Other potential limitations of MRCP include artifact from biliary stents, inability to accurately characterize bile ducts in their physiologic nondistended state (which may overestimate the extent of a stricture if it is collapsed peripheral to a high-grade stricture), inability to provide detailed information on the morphology of a stricture, difficulty in making the diagnosis of PSC in the setting of cirrhosis, and poor spatial resolution that may not allow for the detection of early changes of PSC such as minimal irregularity of the duct contour or subtle strictures.[102-106]

INFECTIOUS CHOLANGITIS

Infectious or ascending bacterial cholangitis is caused by partial or complete biliary obstruction of benign or malignant etiology in conjunction with an ascending infection from the bowel.[110,111] Predisposing conditions include choledocholithiasis, stricture, hepaticojejunostomy, choledochojejunostomy, and ERCP. Symptoms of abdominal pain, jaundice, and sepsis are present in 70% of patients, who may have mild disease that can be treated with antibiotics or a fulminant infection that requires biliary drainage.[110] Imaging is helpful in evaluating the level and etiology of obstruction and evaluating for the presence of complicating peribiliary abscess (see Fig. 1-9). MRCP can evaluate for the presence of extrahepatic biliary duct dilatation (>7 mm or >10 mm postcholecystectomy), intrahepatic duct dilatation (>3 mm), and stones (see Figs. 1-9 and 2-1).[111] The most consistent finding is biliary ductal dilatation in the central liver as opposed to dilatation in the peripheral third of the liver as occurs in PSC. The "beading" and "pruning" of the intrahepatic bile ducts that occur with PSC usually are absent.[111]

T2-WI reveals periportal high SI and wedge-shaped areas hyperintense to liver, reflecting parenchymal edema secondary to the inflammation. CE-MR imaging depicts corresponding wedge-shaped areas of increased enhancement in the liver parenchyma, hepatic abscesses (see Fig. 1-9), smooth and symmetric intrahepatic bile duct wall thickening (>2 mm), and duct wall enhancement.[111] Biliary obstruction and cholangitis can occur prior to visible duct dilatation. Therefore, the absence of ductal dilatation does not exclude mechanical obstruction or cholangitis and the degree of ductal dilatation does not correlate with symptom severity.[110]

RECURRENT PYOGENIC CHOLANGITIS

Recurrent pyogenic cholangitis, also known as oriental cholangiohepatitis or hepatolithiasis, is characterized by intrahepatic bile duct strictures and bile-pigmented stones. Patients have signs and symptoms of recurrent abdominal pain, jaundice, and fever and require removal of the stones and debris from the biliary tract to help treat the infection and restore normal bile flow.[112,113] The cause of recurrent pyogenic cholangitis is unclear; epidemiologic studies have implicated chronic infestation with intrahepatic parasites such as *Clonorchis sinensis* and *Ascaris lumbricoides*. *Clonorchis* is a flatworm endemic to Asia that enters the human body via ingestion of raw or undercooked fish and migrates to the intrahepatic ducts.[114,115] Fibrosis of the bile duct walls and inflammation of the portal tracts result in calculi and periductal abscesses.[112,113] Bile duct strictures may be related to the fibrosis that results from transmural ductal injury and portal venous sepsis.

The MRCP-MRI imaging hallmark of recurrent pyogenic cholangitis is complete obstruction of the intrahepatic ducts secondary to a stricture or impacted stone.[112,113] Unlike PTC and ERCP, MRCP can localize the level of the obstruction and depict the biliary tree proximal and distal to the level of obstruction.[113] An "arrowhead" appearance has been described in which there is abrupt tapering of the peripheral duct secondary to stenosis. Another suggestive imaging feature of recurrent pyogenic cholangitis is a disproportionately severe degree of extrahepatic bile duct dilatation proximal and distal to the stones.[112] Bile-pigmented stones are present in 80% of patients with recurrent pyogenic cholangitis and are hypointense on MRCP and have variable SI on T1-WI.[112]

AIDS CHOLANGIOPATHY

Acquired immunodeficiency syndrome (AIDS) can affect the biliary tree in one of two ways: infectious cholangiopathy or biliary obstruction secondary to extrinsic compression by periportal lymph nodes from AIDS-related lymphoma.[116] AIDS cholangiopathy is usually the result of bile infection by either *Cytomegalovirus* or *Cryptosporidium*. The imaging features of AIDS cholangiopathy include moderate biliary duct dilatation with irregular mural thickening and nodules, ampullary stenosis, and gallbladder sludge.[116] Intrahepatic duct findings such as focal stenoses with segmental dilatation ("beaded" appearance) simulate primary sclerosing cholangitis. The extrahepatic duct abnormalities present in PSC such as saccules and high-grade strictures are not present in AIDS cholangiopathy.[116]

Cholangiocarcinoma

Cholangiocarcinoma is a biliary carcinoma that arises from the intra- and extrahepatic bile ducts and accounts for 2% of all cancers. In 2004 it is estimated that 6,950 people in the U. S. will develop cancer of the gallbladder and extrahepatic bile ducts, resulting in 3,540 deaths.[117] Cholangiocarcinoma affects men and women equally. Most patients with cholangiocarcinoma are diagnosed over age 65 years (peak in the eighth decade)[118] Symptoms at presentation include abdominal pain, anorexia, weight loss, pruritus, and jaundice secondary to biliary obstruction. Superimposed cholangitis is uncommon at the time of initial diagnosis unless the patient has had prior biliary intervention.[118]

Several biliary tract diseases are associated with an increased incidence of cholangiocarcinoma. There is a 5% to 15% incidence of cholangiocarcinoma in patients with PSC that may be multifocal. Medical or surgical treatment of coexisting ulcerative colitis does not alter the subsequent risk for developing biliary carcinoma.[118-120] There is also an increased risk of cholangiocarcinoma in patients with congenital biliary cystic disease such as choledochal cyst or Caroli's disease. The incidence can increase to 20% in patients not treated until after 20 years of age or previously treated with cyst drainage rather than excision.[118,119] In far eastern countries, 5% to 10% of patients with recurrent pyogenic cholangitis (hepatolithiasis) and chronic infestation with biliary parasites such as *Clonorchis* (liver fluke) develop cholangiocarcinoma.[118,119]

Cholangiocarcinoma can be classified as three subtypes based on anatomic location. Peripheral tumors that arise from intrahepatic bile ducts distal to the second order branches account for 10% of cholangiocarcinomas and are discussed in Chapter 1 (see Fig. 1-5). Hilar (Klatskin) cholangiocarcinomas originate from the right and left first order ducts or their confluence and comprise 60% of tumors (see Figs. 2-4 and 2-5). Extrahepatic cholangiocarcinomas of the common hepatic or common bile ducts account for the remaining 30% of lesions.[118,119,121] More than 90% of cholangiocarcinomas are adenocarcinomas of the sclerosing subtype.[118] Infiltrative (circumferential) longitudinal spread along the duct wall and periductal soft tissue is a pathologic hallmark of hilar and extrahepatic tumors. The full extent of tumor may be underestimated by imaging studies, necessitating frozen section analysis during resection.[118,119,121]

Hilar and extrahepatic cholangiocarcinoma spreads circumferentially along the bile ducts and can be difficult to delineate on unenhanced T1- and T2-WIs. Less commonly, a hilar or extrahepatic cholangiocarcinoma will present as a small (<5 cm) mass-like lesion (see Fig. 2-5).[121,122] On MRCP, hilar and extrahepatic cholangiocarcinomas are indirectly revealed as an abrupt biliary obstruction with progressive dilatation of the ducts proximal to the tumor (see Figs. 2-4 and 2-5).[123] MRCP can show the morphology and length of the stricture, presence of hepatolithiasis, degree of ductal dilatation, and ducts both caudal and cephalad to the stricture.[123-125]

However, MRCP alone will not show subtle asymmetry of the duct wall, mural irregularities, extraductal tumor extension, vascular encasement, and nodal/distant metastases. These entities require the addition of T1- and T2-WI as well as CE images. Cholangiocarcinoma appears hypointense to isointense to hepatic parenchyma on T1-WI and isointense to mildly hyperintense to liver on T2-WI.[59,120-123] Similarly to peripheral cholangiocarcinomas, Klatskin tumors usually are hypovascular on immediate postcontrast images and show progressive heterogeneous enhancement on delayed (1- to 5-min) imaging (see Fig. 1-5). Extrahepatic circumferential tumors show the greatest degree of enhancement and conspicuity on 1- to 5-minute delayed scans.[59,121,122] Delayed enhancement corresponds to intratumoral fibrosis and is suggestive of a diagnosis of cholangiocarcinoma.[120,122,126]

Duct wall thickness greater than 5 mm has traditionally been used to determine the presence of malignancy.[120,121] However, cholangiocarcinoma can present with ductal wall thickness of less than 5 mm and cholangitis can manifest with ductal enhancement and wall thickness of more than 5 mm. The presence of mild duct wall thickening in the setting of disproportionate intrahepatic biliary dilatation is more suggestive of cholangiocarcinoma.[121] Enlarged lymph nodes (especially hepatoduodenal ligament and portocaval) are present in 70% of patients with cholangiocarcinoma and are best depicted on fat-suppressed T2-WI and CE T1-WI.[121] However, the presence of lymphadenopathy should not be considered malignancy unless proven histologically, because enlarged inflammatory lymph nodes are present in patients with biliary stents and PSC.[108,118,119,127]

Most patients with cholangiocarcinoma will have unresectable disease at diagnosis or at laparotomy.[128] MR should be used in conjunction with MRCP to assess the four major determinants of resectability: extent of tumor in the biliary tree, vascular invasion, hepatic lobar atrophy, and metastatic disease.[118,121,128] Boxes 2-6 and 2-7 provide the TNM staging for cholangiocarcinoma and the accepted criteria for unresectable disease, many of which are based on imaging findings. Vascular invasion is defined as tumor abutting and either distorting or focally narrowing the vessel or causing encasement or occlusion of the vessel.[127-129]

Hepatic lobar atrophy ipsilateral to the tumor is characterized by a small, often hypoperfused lobe with crowding of dilated intrahepatic ducts and may be secondary to either central lobar obstruction or portal vein occlusion.[118,127] When lobar atrophy is present, the apex should be evaluated to determine whether the etiology is a cholangiocarcinoma, benign stricture, or portal vein occlusion. The presence of regional lymphadenopathy on imaging is not a contraindication for exploration unless there is

---

2-6   TNM Classification of Cholangiocarcinoma *(Adapted from Cancer UIUA. TNM Classification of Malignant Tumors, 5th ed, 1997)*

T—Primary Tumor

Tis	Carcinoma in situ
T1	Tumor invades subepithelial connective tissue or fibromuscular layer
T1a	Tumor invades subepithelial connective tissue
T1b	Tumors invades fibromuscular layer
T2	Tumor invades perifibromuscular connective tissue
T3	Tumor invades adjacent structures: liver, pancreas, duodenum, gallbladder, colon, or stomach

N—Regional Lymph Nodes

N0	No regional lymph node metastasis
N1	Metastasis in cystic duct, pericholedochal, and/or hilar lymph nodes (in the hepatoduodenal ligament)
N2	Metastasis in peripancreatic (head only), periduodenal, periportal, celiac, superior mesenteric, posterior peripancreaticoduodenal lymph nodes

M—Distant Metastasis

M0	No distant metastasis
M1	Distant metastasis

Stage Groupings

Stage 0	Tis	N0	M0
Stage I	T1	N0	M0
Stage II	T2	N0	M0
Stage III	T1	N1, N2	M0
	T2	N1, N2	M0
Stage IVA	T3	Any N	M0
Stage IVB	Any T	Any N	M1

2-7   Criteria for Unresectable Cholangiocarcinoma *(Adapted from references 118, 127, 129)*

Local Disease (Stage IVA)

- Bilateral tumor extension into second order intrahepatic biliary radicles
- Encasement or occlusion of main portal vein proximal to its bifurcation or occlusion of proper hepatic artery
- Involvement of both branches of the portal vein or simultaneous involvement of one side of hepatic artery and other side of portal vein
- Atrophy of hepatic lobe with encasement of contralateral portal vein branch
- Atrophy of hepatic lobe with contralateral secondary biliary radicle involvement

N2 Lymph Node Disease (Stage III)

Distant Metastatic Disease (Stage IVB)

2-8   Bismuth-Corlette Classification of Cholangiocarcinoma *(Adapted from reference 133)*

Type I	Lesions involve only the common bile duct
Type II	Lesions involve the primary hepatic duct bifurcation and the right and left ducts but do not extend beyond
Type IIIa	Lesions involve the right secondary confluence and biliary radicles
Type IIIb	Lesions involve the left secondary confluence and biliary radicles
Type IV*	Lesions involve both the right and left secondary confluence and secondary biliary radicles

*Type IV is considered unresectable

histopathologic proof of tumor involvement of the N2 level lymph nodes that are considered unresectable. Peritoneal spread of cholangiocarcinoma can appear as enhancing nodular masses or sheet-like areas of soft tissue in the greater omentum and along the peritoneum.[127,130]

Five-year survival rates for cholangiocarcinoma are very low and depend on the TNM stage.[131] Prognostic factors that predict long-term survival include absence of multifocal disease, negative proximal bile duct margins, and a Bismuth type I or II lesion.[132] The Bismuth-Corlette system stratifies patients based on the extent of biliary ductal involvement but does not account for lobar atrophy or vascular invasion (Box 2-8).[133] Untreated cancer results in a 10-month median survival secondary to hepatic failure or complications of biliary obstruction.[118,128]

The range of treatment for cholangiocarcinoma extends from curative liver resection (and possibly liver transplantation) to palliative therapies such as surgical biliary bypass or percutaneous/surgical biliary stent placement.[118,132] Five-year survival even after potentially curative resection ranges from 0% to 30% and ultimately depends on the stage of disease and the presence of negative surgical margins.[118,131,134,135] More extensive surgery including extended right or left lobectomy, caudate lobectomy and hepaticojejunostomy is suggested in the setting of vascular involvement.[118,131] Left-sided tumors almost always involve the major caudate lobe ducts that drain into the left hepatic ducts system and require caudate lobectomy.[118] No data support the routine use of adjuvant chemotherapy or radiotherapy.[135,136]

Ampullary Lesions

DISORDERS OF THE SPHINCTER OF ODDI

Papillary dysfunction and ampullary (papillary) stenosis are disorders centered at the ampulla of Vater that can cause symptoms of intermittent biliary obstruction. Ampullary stenosis results from acute or chronic inflammation of the ampulla of Vater and is most commonly due to passage of bile duct stones. Sphincteric Oddi (papillary) dysfunction results in a functional stenosis at the ampulla that may be related to spasm of the sphincter and abnormal frequency of sphincteric peristalsis.[17] Clinical findings include upper abdominal pain and abnormal liver function tests. Common bile duct dilatation and delayed drainage of contrast from the common bile duct are present on ERCP.[17]

MRCP can depict duct dilatation with the transition point in the region of the ampulla as well as the presence or absence of a distal common bile duct stone. Additional MR sequences can exclude an ampullary mass as a cause of the biliary obstruction. Dynamic MRCP (kinematic imaging) with secretin can depict the range of contraction of the sphincter of Oddi.[17,137] The lack of relaxation of the sphincteric segment of the distal common bile duct on kinematic MRCP has sensitivity of 88% and specificity of 100% for ampullary and periampullary lesions and indicates the need for intervention to relieve the biliary obstruction.[138]

AMPULLARY NEOPLASMS

Ampullary carcinomas are adenocarcinomas that arise from the glandular epithelium of the ampulla of Vater within the medial wall of the second portion of the duodenum, where the common bile duct and main pancreatic duct drain.[139,140] Patients are usually male (2:1) in the sixth to seventh decades of life. Patients with familial adenomatous polyposis syndromes or with adenocarcinomas elsewhere in the gastrointestinal tract are at increased for the development of ampullary tumors.[139] Almost all patients are symptomatic due to either biliary obstruction or intestinal bleeding, resulting in an early diagnosis when tumor size is small (<3 cm).[141]

Cross-sectional imaging will depict pancreaticobiliary duct dilatation but not necessarily the mass itself. When an ampullary lesion becomes enlarged and extends into the duodenal lumen, it will often be revealed at imaging against the distended fluid or air-filled duodenum.[139,140] MRCP can depict dilatation of both the common bile duct and pancreatic duct to the level of the ampulla (double duct sign); however, the pancreatic duct need not be dilated if the mass is small and does not obstruct the duct orifice or if there are ductal variants such as a persistent accessory duct or pancreas divisum[59,139] (Fig. 2-8). If there is dilation of side branches of the pancreatic duct, this favors a low pancreatic head primary cancer over a primary ampullary tumor.[142] If no mass is revealed, it may not be possible to distinguish ampullary carcinoma from ampullary stricture, stone, or inflammation. Discernible ampullary carcinomas are usually of low SI (relative to pancreas) on T1- and T2-WIs, are hypoenhancing to pancreatic parenchyma on immediate enhanced images, and show heterogeneous enhancement with variable rim enhancement on delayed postcontrast sequences.[140] The decreased T2 SI and delayed enhancement reflect the desmoplastic nature of these carcinomas.

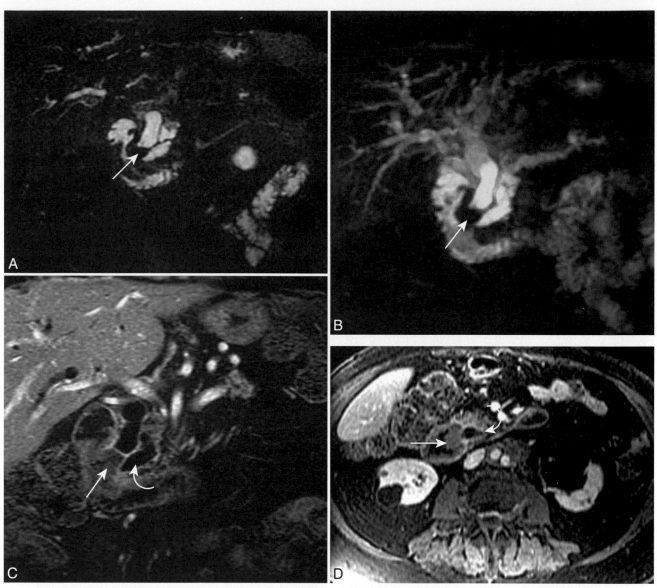

Figure 2-8 ■ **MR-MRCP illustration of an ampullary carcinoma in a man with obstructive jaundice.**
A and **B**, Single-slice thin-section (**A**) and thick-section slab (**B**) MRCP show a "double duct" sign that terminates in the region of an ampullary mass *(arrow)*. **C** and **D**, Coronal (**C**) and axial (**D**) CE T1-WIs show a hypoenhancing ampullary tumor *(arrow)* that protrudes into the duodenum. A segment of the dilated pancreatic duct *(curved arrow)* is also present.

The differential diagnosis of an ampullary mass includes ampullary adenoma and other peri-ampullary lesions such as pancreatic carcinoma, cholangiocarcinoma, villous adenomas, primary duodenal adenocarcinoma, leiomyoma, and carcinoid.[139,142] Small tumors may be difficult to distinguish from impacted stones, ampullary fibrosis, and dysfunction of the sphincter of Oddi.[59] The diagnosis of small ampullary carcinomas can be difficult with MRCP because of the difficulty in evaluating the short transmural segment of the pancreatico-biliary tree that contains little or no fluid. It has been suggested that ERCP should still be performed after a negative MRCP when there is a high suspicion of

ampullary carcinoma because early detection allows for curative resection.[143] The standard operation is the Whipple procedure (pancreaticoduodenectomy) and results in overall 5-year survival rates approaching 50%, which is better than for the more common pancreatic adenocarcinoma.[141]

MR OF THE GALLBLADDER

MR Technique

MR sequences used to evaluate the gallbladder are similar to other abdominal MR imaging protocols and include axial T1-W breath-hold GRE chemical

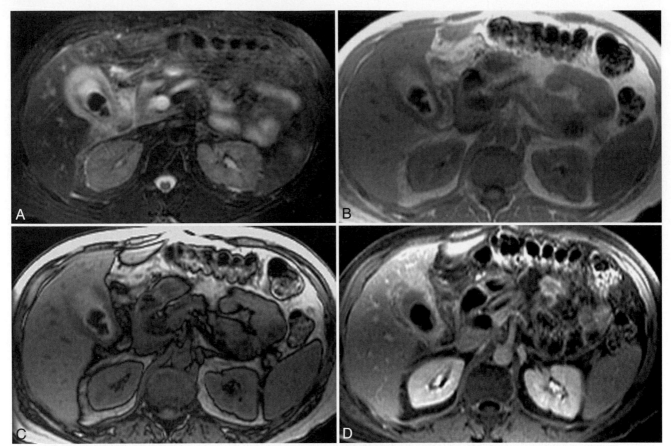

Figure 2-9 ■ MR findings of acute cholecystitis and gallstones. A, Axial T2-WI shows two gallstones and a thickened hyperintense gallbladder wall. **B** and **C,** In-phase (**B**) and opposed-phase (**C**) T1-WIs show hypointense gallstones and hyperintense bile. The bile does not lose SI on chemical shift imaging, indicating a paucity of lipid-containing cholesterol. **D,** CE T1-WI shows diffuse mural enhancement of the gallbladder wall.

shift imaging, T2-WIs, MRCP, and if needed CE T1-W sequences. It is recommended that patients fast for a minimum of 4 hours prior to the MRI in order to promote gallbladder filling and gastric emptying.[6,144] The ability of chemical shift imaging to exploit differences in behavior between lipid and water protons (see Chapter 3) allows for the evaluation of the relative concentration of bile (concentrated vs. dilute).[31] Gallstones may be revealed on T1-WIs depending on the SI of the surrounding bile.

Both T2-W and MRCP sequences yield important information about the gallbladder and related structures.[145] Gallstones including even small calculi appear as low SI foci against the higher SI of bile (Fig. 2-9; see Fig. 5-12). Gallbladder wall edema and pericholecystic fluid are hyperintense on both sequences because of their fluid content. MRCP can better depict the cystic duct and potential anatomic variants because nonfluid soft tissues have very low SI on heavily T2-WI, thereby highlighting bile-containing structures.[146] Lymph nodes and tumor extension into the liver are better depicted on T2-WI.[31]

CE breath-hold fat-suppressed T1-WI are well suited to the evaluation of the gallbladder and adjacent hepatic parenchyma.[147] Dynamic gadolinium-enhanced MR imaging may also play a role in differentiating benign and malignant gallbladder masses based on early and delayed enhancement patterns.[148,149] Enhanced MRI cannot be used to evaluate gallbladder function, because standard extracellular gadolinium agents are distributed exclusively in the intravascular and interstitial space and cleared from the body by glomerular filtration with very little biliary excretion. Several liver-specific T1-shortening agents have biliary excretion.[26,27] By providing information on the temporal course of hepatobiliary excretion, MR hepatobiliary contrast agents may potentially be used like cholescintigraphic agents.[28] Lack of excretion into the gallbladder lumen would imply cystic duct obstruction, which in conjunction with other morphologic abnormalities, could be used to diagnose cholecystitis.

Normal Appearance of the Gallbladder (Box 2-9)

Gallbladder contents show high SI on T2- and heavily T2-WIs (MRCP) because of the static fluid content of bile. The SI of bile on T1-WI varies according to

2-9	Normal Gallbladder
Bile on T1-WI	Variable SI
Concentrated bile	Hyperintense to liver and fat
Dilute bile	Hypointense to liver and fat; "layering effect" may be seen
Bile on T2-WI	High SI
Normal wall thickness	≤3 mm
Cystic duct	High SI on T2; normal diameter 1–5 mm

the patient's fasting state, bile viscosity, and bile salt and protein concentration. In the fasting state, 90% of water is removed from the bile as a solution of inorganic electrolytes with a resultant increase in the concentration of phospholipids, cholesterol, and bile salts.[150] The concentrated bile can be hyperintense to liver and fat on T1-WI due to T1 shortening from an increased fraction of water molecules bound to macromolecules (see Fig. 2-9).[150,151] After stimulation with food, dilute bile enters the gallbladder that has since emptied much of its concentrated bile into the duodenum. The low T1 SI dilute bile floats upon the residual high SI contents of the gallbladder, causing a "layering effect."[151] On chemical shift imaging, the loss of bile SI from an in-phase to out-of-phase image establishes the presence of lipid in the bile and is indicative of normal gallbladder function in a fasting patient (see Figs. 2-32 and 5-12). The lack of change in SI could reflect recent ingestion of food especially if associated with a contracted gallbladder. The normal gallbladder wall is of low SI on T1- and T2-WIs and can be imperceptible or measure up to 3 mm in thickness.[152,153]

The cystic duct connects the gallbladder to the extrahepatic common bile duct and usually enters from the right halfway between the porta hepatis and the ampulla of Vater (Figs. 2-10 and 2-11).[146] The cystic duct insertion separates the common hepatic duct proximally from the common bile duct distally. The cystic duct is 2 to 4 cm in length, has a normal

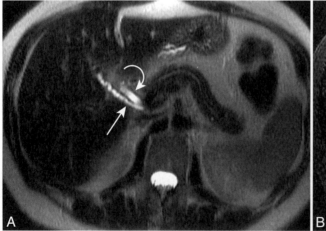
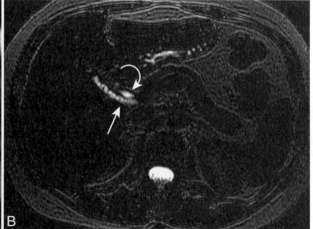
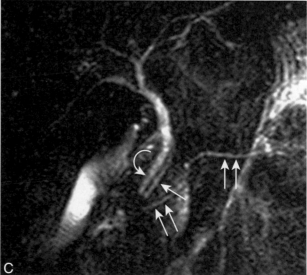

Figure 2-10 ▪ MR illustrations of the cystic duct. A and **B**, Normal cystic duct remnant in a patient after cholecystectomy. Two axial heavily T2-WIs with echo times of 180 (**A**) and 600 (**B**) show the cystic duct in long axis *(arrows)*. The cystic duct courses medial to the common hepatic duct *(curved arrow)*. It inserts medially on lower images (not shown). On the longer TE image, there is little remaining SI from the surrounding soft tissues. **C**, Single 40-mm projection MRCP in another patient reveals low medial insertion of the cystic duct *(arrow)* into the bile duct *(curved arrow)*. The distal pancreatic duct also is revealed *(double arrows)*.

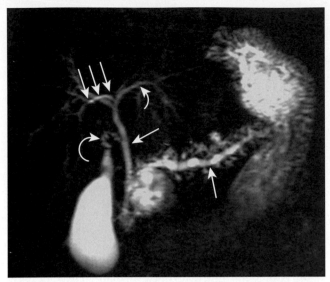

Figure 2-11 ▪ Coronal MRCP slab image (slice thickness = 40 mm) shows a cystic pancreatic head mass that results in extrinsic compression on the common bile duct *(arrow)* **and pancreatic duct** *(arrow)*. There are dilated pancreatic side branches in keeping with chronic pancreatitis. A normal cystic duct is present *(curved arrow)*. There is aberrant hepatic duct anatomy; the posterior segment right hepatic duct *(triple arrow)* drains into the left hepatic duct *(small curved arrow)*. On the basis of this single image alone it is difficult to differentiate among pseudocyst, cystic pancreatic mass, and side branch intraductal papillary mucinous tumor.

diameter of 1 to 5 mm, and often has a tortuous course. The duct contains spiral valves of Heister, which are crescent-shaped folds of mucosa that project into the lumen.[146] The cystic duct is best depicted on MRCP and T2-WIs because of its high SI bile content.[146] The coronal plane is helpful in showing the course of the cystic duct and its insertion into the common bile duct.

Hepatic steatosis with focal fatty sparing around the gallbladder fossa should not be mistaken for a space-occupying lesion. The focal fatty sparing in the liver surrounding the gallbladder is attributed to the decreased portal blood supply to the pericholecystic hepatocytes that results in decreased delivery of lipids. The regional decrease of portal blood flow is a response to increased tissue blood pressure that occurs when a cystic vein or artery carries blood from the gallbladder wall directly to the liver parenchyma.[154] This region of liver may present as a high SI pseudolesion adjacent to the gallbladder on out-of-phase T1-W GRE images. However, this same region will not be visible on in-phase images and will follow normal liver SI on T2-WIs. A more complete discussion of hepatic steatosis and focal fatty sparing is presented in Chapter 1.

Cholelithiasis

Cholelithiasis has a prevalence of 10% in the U. S. and Western Europe and is symptomatic in 20% to 30% of individuals.[155] The risk of developing stones is

related to gallbladder hypomotility and hypersecretion of cholesterol-laden bile.[156] Women are affected more commonly than men although the prevalence increases with age in both sexes.[157] A history of obesity and multiparity are correlated with cholelithiasis. The most common symptom of cholelithiasis is biliary colic that results from transient obstruction of the cystic duct by a gallstone.[157] Complications with asymptomatic gallstones are uncommon (<1%/yr) and include acute cholecystitis, acute pancreatitis, and choledocholithiasis and the less common biliary fistula, gallstone ileus, and Mirizzi syndrome.[155,157] Although MR is as sensitive as ultrasound for the detection of gallstones, it is not used as a primary modality for the diagnosis of cholelithiasis, since sonography is the imaging modality of choice.[157,158]

Cholesterol is the main component in 80% of stones and makes up less than 25% of bilirubin pigment stones.[157] MR can depict calculi independently of their composition. MR reveals gallstones by their characteristic low SI on T1- and T2-WIs compared with surrounding bile (Fig. 2-12; see Fig. 2-9).[31] Calculi may be difficult to detect on T1-WIs if the bile is of low SI but are conspicuous on T2-WIs or on T1-WIs of a fasting patient who has high SI concentrated bile. Even small stones are identified on thin-section MRCP because of the high contrast between the calculi and surrounding high SI bile.[31]

In vitro T2-WI of gallstones at 1.5 T reveals central high SI fluid-filled clefts. Additionally, portions of calcium bilirubinate and black pigment gallstones show high SI on T1-WI secondary to the paramagnetic properties of concentrated copper, iron, and manganese within the stones.[159] High SI stones on T1-WI have also been attributed to a high fatty acid

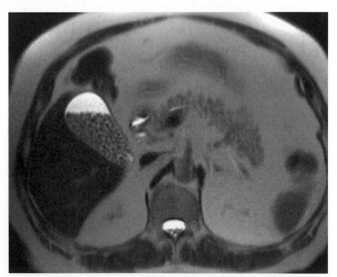

Figure 2-12 ▪ MR illustration of uncomplicated gallstones. Axial breath-hold T2-WI (TE = 180) shows multiple small gallstones without gallbladder wall thickening or pericholecystic edema. Because this image was acquired in less than 1 s, motion artifact is minimal. The gallstones are depicted without motion-induced blurring.

content[147] or concentrated bilirubin[160]; thus, the presence of high T1 SI structures in the gallbladder lumen does not necessarily exclude a diagnosis of cholelithiasis.

Cholecystitis

ACUTE CHOLECYSTITIS (BOX 2-10)

Acute cholecystitis occurs when outflow of bile is prevented by occlusion of the cystic duct, often by a gallstone impacted in the gallbladder neck or cystic duct. If the obstruction is unrelieved, the bile will cause mucosal inflammation and gallbladder wall edema that can progress to empyema, gangrene, and perforation.[161] A diagnosis of acute cholecystitis is first suspected on the basis of clinical findings and usually confirmed by sonography or cholescintigraphy.[162]

Although not used as a screening test for acute cholecystitis, MRI may be used as a primary modality for diagnosis in certain patients with a confusing clinical presentation or equivocal sonographic or cholescintigraphic findings. Early diagnosis of cholecystitis is important so that appropriate treatment, such as cholecystectomy, can be performed. In high-risk patients with comorbidities, percutaneous cholecystostomy is a feasible temporizing nonsurgical intervention.[163]

Morphologic features are used to establish the MR diagnosis of acute cholecystitis. The presence of

---

2-10   Features of Acute Cholecystitis

Clinical
Complications: empyema, gangrene, perforation

Pathology
Acute inflammation of the gallbladder secondary to
    occlusion of the cystic duct

MRI
Cholelithiasis
Gallbladder wall thickening (>3 mm)
Pericholecystic fluid
    Specific example: "C-sign" of fluid between liver
        and right hemidiaphragm
Gallbladder wall edema
Hyperemia of gallbladder wall
Transient hyperenhancement of adjacent liver
    parenchyma

Subtypes of Acute Cholecystitis
Ischemic (chemical)
    Pain 1–2 weeks after chemoembolization
    Usually self-limited
Acalculous
    Treatable cause of sepsis in critically ill patients
    Percutaneous cholecystostomy can be diagnostic
        and therapeutic
Hemorrhagic
    Severe cholecystitis with complicating hemorrhagic
        necrosis of gallbladder wall
    High SI subacute blood on T1-WI within wall
        and lumen

---

cholelithiasis, pericholecystic fluid in the absence of ascites, gallbladder wall thickening (>3 mm), and gallbladder wall edema on T2-WI suggest a diagnosis of acute cholecystitis (see Fig. 2-9).[153,164] However, wall thickening and pericholecystic fluid in themselves are nonspecific findings and can also occur in the setting of hypoalbuminemia, hepatitis, chronic cholecystitis, cirrhosis, and renal disease.

CE-MR imaging can help confirm a diagnosis of acute cholecystitis by showing hyperemia (>80% enhancement) of the gallbladder wall and transient hyperenhancement of the adjacent hepatic parenchyma.[152] Pericholecystic enhancement is present in greater than 70% of patients with acute cholecystitis and may extend into the medial segment of the left hepatic lobe. Pericholecystic enhancement is secondary to increased hepatic arterial flow in response to local inflammation of the gallbladder and should not be mistaken for a hypervascular neoplasm.[152,165] The MR finding of pericholecystic enhancement differs from the "rim sign" of cholescintigraphy in which increased radiotracer activity adjacent to an acutely inflamed gallbladder results from delayed clearance secondary to impaired hepatocyte function from the spread of inflammation.[166] Functional MR cholangiography that utilizes contrast agents which are excreted into the biliary tree could provide similar information as biliary scintigraphy to confirm functional obstruction in a patient with suspected acute cholecystitis.[167]

Gangrenous cholecystitis can be present in up to 30% of patients who present with acute cholecystitis. Older men with cardiovascular disease are at increased risk of developing gangrene in the setting of acute cholecystitis and are more likely to require an open cholecystectomy. The MR finding of segmental absence of mucosal enhancement on CE-MR imaging can suggest a diagnosis of complicating gangrene in patients with suspected acute cholecystitis.[168]

CHRONIC CHOLECYSTITIS

Chronic cholecystitis can present as a small and irregularly shaped gallbladder with a thickened gallbladder wall.[147,152] Fibrosis in the gallbladder wall shows delayed enhancement.[147,148] However, the degree of wall enhancement is significantly lower than that present in acute cholecystitis. Transient pericholecystic enhancement is not present in chronic cholecystitis, a feature that can help differentiate between the two disorders.[152]

ISCHEMIC-CHEMICAL CHOLECYSTITIS

One subtype of acute cholecystitis is ischemic or chemical cholecystitis, a potential complication of chemoembolization of liver tumors. The cystic artery originates from the right hepatic artery in more than 95% of patients; thus, the gallbladder can be subjected to high-dose chemotherapeutic agents that reflux from the hepatic artery into the cystic artery.[169,170] Most patients with this entity are asymptomatic, but some have nonspecific abdominal pain 1 to 2 weeks after intra-arterial chemotherapy. Fortunately, chemical cholecystitis is self-limited and cholecystectomy is rarely indicated. MR imaging reveals gallbladder distension, marked wall edema with increased enhancement, and transient pericholecystic hepatic enhancement.[31,147]

ACALCULOUS CHOLECYSTITIS

Acalculous cholecystitis is another subtype of acute cholecystitis that typically occurs in critically ill patients and in patients recovering from trauma or major surgery. Patients often have persistent unexplained sepsis and can have a more fulminant course of cholecystitis, including the development of gallbladder empyema, gangrene, and perforation. The pathogenesis of acalculous cholecystitis is multifactorial but is attributed to systemic sepsis, ischemia, and biliary stasis.[171] Imaging findings include gallbladder wall thickening, marked gallbladder distension, pericholecystic fluid, subserosal edema, and pericholecystic abscess.[171] The diagnosis of acalculous cholecystitis can be challenging because the clinical and imaging findings are nonspecific. Percutaneous cholecystostomy can confirm a diagnosis of acalculous cholecystitis in the setting of unexplained sepsis when patients exhibit a dramatic improvement in clinical status (defervescence and decrease in white blood count) following the procedure. Percutaneous gallbladder aspiration and bile cultures are not so useful in establishing the diagnosis, because many of these patients are on antibiotic therapy that renders bile cultures negative for microorganisms.[163]

HEMORRHAGIC CHOLECYSTITIS

Hemorrhagic cholecystitis is a rare subtype, usually associated with cholelithiasis and high mortality. The mechanism is thought to be gallstone-induced mucosal ulceration, inflammation, and necrosis that progress to hemorrhage and clot formation in the gallbladder wall and lumen. Sonography reveals heterogeneous, echogenic bile that can mimic pus, thick sludge, or even a mass.[172] Although blood is of high attenuation on CT, the differential diagnosis of high-density bile also includes vicarious excretion of contrast and milk of calcium bile.[172] MRI can more specifically reveal the presence of blood degradation products in the gallbladder lumen and wall because subacute hemorrhage appears as high SI methemoglobin on T1-WI.[31,147] Fat-saturated T1-WI or chemical shift imaging can readily distinguish between blood and lipid-rich bile.

Gallbladder Varices

Gallbladder varices are venous collaterals located within the gallbladder wall and pericholecystic bed that represent portosystemic shunts linking the cystic vein branch of the portal vein to systemic anterior abdominal veins or to intrahepatic portal venous branches.[173] Although an unusual manifestation of portal hypertension, gallbladder varices can develop in the setting of extrahepatic portal vein thrombosis, where they form collateral pathways around the thrombosed portal vein.[174,175] Dilation of the parabiliary venous plexus also occurs when the extrahepatic portal vein is thrombosed and is referred to as "cavernous transformation."[174] The incidence of gallbladder varices ranges from 12% to 30% in patients with portal hypertension, cirrhosis, or portal vein thrombosis.[173,175]

On CE-MR imaging these varices appear as contrast-filled, serpiginous, dilated venous structures in and around the gallbladder wall (Fig. 2-13) that vary in diameter from 1 to 8 mm and can extend from the gallbladder to the anterior abdominal wall.[173,176] Pericholecystic collaterals do not impair gallbladder function or contractility. A priori knowledge of these varices is important to the surgeon in order to minimize intra-operative blood loss if the patient is to

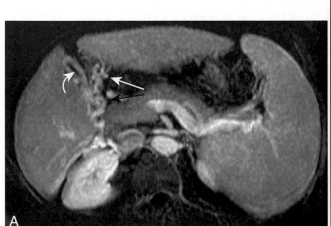
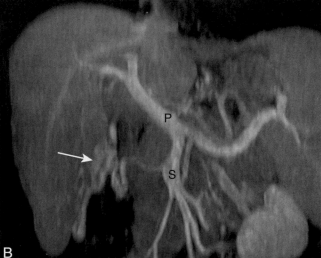

Figure 2-13 ■ **Enhanced MR appearance of gallbladder varices in a man with portal hypertension. A** and **B,** Axial (**A**) and coronal (**B**) MIP images show enhancing serpiginous varices *(arrows)* around the gallbladder *(curved arrow)* and liver capsule. Patent superior mesenteric (S) and portal (P) veins are present in **B**.

2-11   Features of Adenomyomatosis

Clinical

Female > male; age 20–70 years (mean 50 years)
Incidentally revealed in up to 20% of patients with
biliary symptoms

Pathology

Overgrowth of gallbladder mucosa
Hypertrophy of the muscular layer
Extension of mucosa into the thickened
gallbladder wall forming intramural diverticula
(Rokitansky-Aschoff sinuses)
Three subtypes
Localized: fundal location common
Diffuse
Segmental
No malignant potential: few reports of coexistent
gallbladder cancer
Management: periodic surveillance sufficient

MRI

Rokitansky-Aschoff sinuses
Diverticula in gallbladder wall
Isointense to bile on T2-WI and MRCP
No enhancement
Thickened gallbladder wall
Low SI on T2-WI
Variable enhancement on CE T1-WI

undergo cholecystectomy or liver transplantation.[173]
Gallbladder varices can be a rare cause of recurrent
and massive gastrointestinal bleeding in the setting
of portal hypertension and may require surgery or
enteroscopic sclerotherapy.[177]

Adenomyomatosis (Box 2-11)

Gallbladder adenomyomatosis is characterized by
overgrowth of mucosa, hypertrophy of the muscularis

layer, and extension of mucosa into the thickened gallbladder wall, forming intramural diverticula known as
Rokitansky-Aschoff sinuses.[178] Adenomyomatosis is
present more often in women than in men, has a mean
age of presentation of 50 years, and is revealed incidentally in up to 20% of patients who undergo
cholecystectomy for biliary symptoms such as right
upper quadrant pain.[179,180]

The etiology of the hyperplasia and intramural
diverticula is unknown but may represent an abnormality of muscle contraction.[181] The resulting
increased intracystic pressure results in invagination
of the mucosa through the muscularis as intramural
diverticula. Adenomyomatosis is classified into three
subtypes: localized (most common and usually
located in the gallbladder fundus), diffuse (thickened
wall throughout the gallbladder), and segmental
(segmental stricture composed of a thickened wall
that divides the gallbladder lumen into separate
interconnected compartments).[178,182]

Segmental or localized adenomyomatosis can
be difficult to distinguish from gallbladder carcinoma
on imaging, since the presence of gallbladder wall
thickening, intraluminal mass, and gallstones can
be present with both entities.[178] MR diagnosis of
adenomyomatosis is based on demonstration of
Rokitansky-Aschoff sinuses (Fig. 2-14). The thickened gallbladder wall appears hypointense on T2-WI,
while the intramural diverticula are revealed as discrete, linearly arranged, smoothly marginated,
intramural cyst-like structures that are isointense to
bile on T2-WI and MRCP.[183,184] The appearance of the
ring-like distribution of intramural cysts has been
termed the "pear necklace sign."[185] Breath-hold or
breathing-independent T2-WI minimizes motion artifact and can better depict small intramural diverticula
compared with breathing-averaged T2-WI. On CE
T1-WI, the gallbladder wall is segmentally thickened
and hyperintense, whereas the Rokitansky-Aschoff
sinuses do not enhance.[183,184] A study of 20 patients
comparing the accuracy of ultrasound (US), CT, and

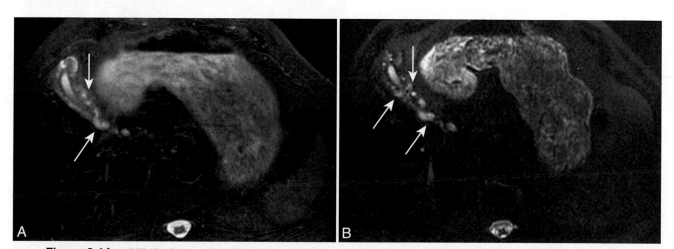

Figure 2-14 ■ MR findings of gallbladder adenomyomatosis. A and **B**, Fat-suppressed T2-WI (**A**) and heavily
T2-WI (**B**; TE = 180) show a thickened gallbladder wall. Multiple hyperintense foci *(arrows)* that remain of high SI in
B represent the intramural diverticula.

MRI in the preoperative diagnosis of adenomyomatosis revealed that MRI had a higher accuracy (93%) than did CT (75%) or US (66%).[186]

Adenomyomatosis does not show malignant potential,[187] and cholecystectomy has not been recommended in asymptomatic patients. However, coexistent gallbladder carcinoma has been associated with both the segmental and localized forms of adenomyomatosis.[182] Thus, close imaging follow-up or prophylactic cholecystectomy is suggested if the diagnosis of adenomyomatosis is equivocal or if coexistent carcinoma cannot be excluded.[183] Since it is impractical to recommend cholecystectomy for all patients with adenomyomatosis detected "by chance,"[180] sonographic surveillance could be performed every 6 months as has been suggested for gallbladder polyps.[188]

Gallbladder Polyps

Polypoid lesions of the gallbladder correspond to any elevated lesion of the mucosal surface of the gallbladder wall and often are incidental findings on imaging evaluation of abdominal pain. The differential diagnosis of polypoid lesions is large and has resulted in the establishment of a classification system (Box 2-12).[189] The prevalence of gallbladder polyps on sonography in healthy patients is 4% to 7%[190,191] while the range in cholecystectomy specimens is 1% to 12%.[192] Polyps are more common in women in the fourth to sixth decades.[188] The majority (60% to 70%) of resected lesions are cholesterol polyps that have no malignant potential.[188,192,193]

The clinical significance of an incidentally discovered gallbladder polyp is difficult to predict. However, if a lesion cannot be proved to be a cholesterol polyp on imaging, it could potentially represent a premalignant adenomatous polyp or cancer. Polyp size is a significant predictor of malignant potential with a 40% to 88% prevalence of malignancy in polyps greater than 10 mm.[192] Asymptomatic patients with gallbladder polyps that are less than 10 mm have a low likelihood of malignant transformation.[190,193]

Sonography is the preferred imaging test for polyp diagnosis and evaluation. Sonographic findings of a cholesterol polyp include a round, pedunculated, nonshadowing, hyperechoic, immobile mass that is attached to the gallbladder wall.[190,194] On MRI, polyps are depicted as focal lesions that arise from the gallbladder wall and are contrasted against the high SI bile on T2-WI. They enhance after contrast because they are vascularized,[195] a finding best depicted on fat-suppressed T1-WI. Polyps are distinguished from gallstones by their fixation to the gallbladder wall, location (can be on the nondependent wall), and enhancement.[147] Chemical shift imaging may help establish the diagnosis of a cholesterol polyp by showing loss of SI on out-of-phase T1-WI relative to in-phase images, reflecting the presence of lipid-laden macrophages within the polyp.[196]

Factors that increase the chances of a gallbladder polyp being malignant include size greater than 10 mm, presence of a solitary polyp, age greater than 60 years, sessile lesion (regardless of size), coexistence of gallstones, and rapid growth rate.[188,192,194,195] Based on these findings, several recommendations for the management of gallbladder polyps have been established (Box 2-13).[188,193,197]

Gallbladder Carcinoma

Gallbladder carcinoma is an uncommon aggressive malignancy, with an estimated 6,950 new cases (including carcinomas of the extrahepatic bile ducts) and 3,540 deaths occurring in 2004.[117] The disease predominantly affects females (3:1 over males) with a mean age of 65.[156,198] Tumors are asymptomatic in early stages[199,200] and revealed incidentally during cholecystectomy for presumed benign disease.[198,201] Symptoms are present in the setting of advanced disease and include anorexia, weight loss, abdominal pain, and jaundice.[200,201]

Although less than 1% of patients with cholelithiasis develop gallbladder cancer, gallstones are present in up to 90% of patients with cancer.[156,201,202] There is increased risk for patients who have chronic

---

2-12   Differential Diagnosis of Polypoid Lesions of the Gallbladder

Benign
True neoplasm
    Adenoma (uncommon)
    Leiomyoma (rare)
    Lipoma (rare)
Pseudotumors
    Cholesterol polyp (very common)
    Adenomyomatosis (common)
    Heterotopia (uncommon)

Malignant
Adenocarcinoma (uncommon)
Metastases (rare)

2-13   Management of Gallbladder Polyps

Indications for Cholecystectomy
Symptomatic polyps
Right upper quadrant pain
Epigastric pain or tenderness that may be referable
    to the gallbladder
Polyp size >10 mm
Sessile polyps, independent of size
Interval growth on follow-up imaging

Polyps That Can Be Followed with Imaging (Preferably Sonography)
Asymptomatic polyps <10 mm
Polyps that have been stable for 18 months do not
    need additional imaging

cholelithiasis because long-standing inflammation results in mucosal dysplasia that can progress to carcinoma.[201,203,204] Cancer is associated with the presence of larger gallstones ($\cong$3 cm) because of a greater risk of mucosal irritation.[156,205] Other associations include gallbladder polyps (as previously discussed), segmental adenomyomatosis, and anomalous junction of the pancreaticobiliary junction (APBJ).[36,156,198,206] Porcelain gallbladder (calcification in the wall of a chronically inflamed gallbladder) has been associated with 10% to 25% of gallbladder cancers[156,198,207]; however, other studies have shown no association, making this a controversial risk factor.[208]

More than 90% of primary gallbladder cancers are moderate to well-differentiated adenocarcinomas.[199,201,209] Because of the advanced stage at the time of initial diagnosis, the prognosis for gallbladder carcinoma, is poor with an overall 5-year survival of less than 5%.[156,201] For patients with disease confined to the gallbladder, the 5-year survival is 35% to 45% but decreases to 15% for regional disease and to 3% for distant metastases.[156,200] The most important prognostic factors are histologic grade and tumor stage, which determine treatment options.[156,199,201] The TNM staging predicts patient outcome because of the importance of extent of disease at the time of diagnosis (Box 2-14).[136,156,200]

The most common mode of spread is direct invasion into the liver, which is facilitated by the gallbladder's thin wall and discontinuous muscular layer and by the gallbladder's attachment to the undersurface of hepatic segments IVa and V.[209-213] Tumor can also directly invade the duodenum, colon, and pancreas.[201] Other pathways of spread include lymphatic invasion (second most common route of spread) and hematogenous and peritoneal dissemination.[201,212,213] The presence of lymph node metastases is strongly correlated with the depth of invasion of the primary tumor with nodal metastases present in 60% to 70% of patients with T3 lesions and more than 80% of patients with T4 lesions.[210,214] Tumor extension to the aortocaval and para-aortic lymph nodes is considered M1 disease.[215] The most common sites of hematogenous spread in advanced disease are the liver, lung, and brain and less frequently the kidney, adrenal gland, pancreas, and bones.[201,212]

Three patterns of gallbladder carcinoma are revealed with imaging (Box 2-15).[201,213,216,217] Whether it is an infiltrative mass, irregular wall thickening, or polypoid mass extending into the gallbladder lumen, a primary gallbladder cancer is hypointense to liver on T1-WI and slightly hyperintense to liver on T2-WI (Fig. 2-15).[213,217] T2-W and MRCP images may depict gallstones surrounded by the tumor mass.[217]

2-14 TNM Classification of Gallbladder Carcinoma (Adapted from Cancer UIUA. TNM Classification of Malignant Tumors, 5th ed, 1997)

T—Primary Tumor

T1	Tumor invades lamina propria or muscle layer
T1a	Tumor invades lamina propria
T1b	Tumor invades muscle layer
T2	Tumor invades perimuscular connective tissue; no extension beyond serosa or into liver
T3	Tumor perforates serosa (visceral peritoneum) or directly invades into one adjacent organ or both (extension 2 cm or less into liver)
T4	Tumor extends more than 2 cm into liver and/or into two or more adjacent organs (stomach, duodenum, colon, pancreas, omentum, extrahepatic bile ducts, any involvement of liver)

N—Regional Lymph Nodes

N0	No regional lymph node metastasis
N1	Metastasis in cystic duct, pericholedochal, and/or hilar lymph nodes
N2	Metastasis in peripancreatic (head only), periduodenal, periportal, celiac, and/or superior mesenteric lymph nodes

M—Distant Metastasis

M0	No distant metastasis
M1	Distant metastasis

Stage Grouping

Stage 0	Tis	N0	M0
Stage I	T1	N0	M0
Stage II	T2	N0	M0
Stage III	T1	N1	M0
	T2	N1	M0
	T3	N0, N1	M0
Stage IVA	T4	N0, N1	M0
Stage IVB	Any T	N2	M0
	Any T	Any N	M1

2-15 Imaging Patterns of Gallbladder Carcinoma (Adapted from references 201, 149)

Differential Diagnosis of Mass Filling or Replacing Gallbladder (40%–60%)

Gallbladder carcinoma (most common)
Hepatocellular carcinoma (uncommon)
Pericholecystic abscess (uncommon)

Differential Diagnosis of Irregular Thickening of Gallbladder Wall (20%–30%)

Acute or chronic cholecystitis (most common)
Noninflammatory conditions (hepatitis, low albumin, renal failure) (very common)
Adenomyomatosis (common)
Carcinoma (uncommon)

Differential Diagnosis of Polypoid Mass Protruding into Gallbladder Lumen (10%)

Polyp (cholesterol, hyperplastic, inflammatory; most common)
Adenomyomatosis (common)
Carcinoma (uncommon)
Abscess (uncommon)
Blood clot (rare)

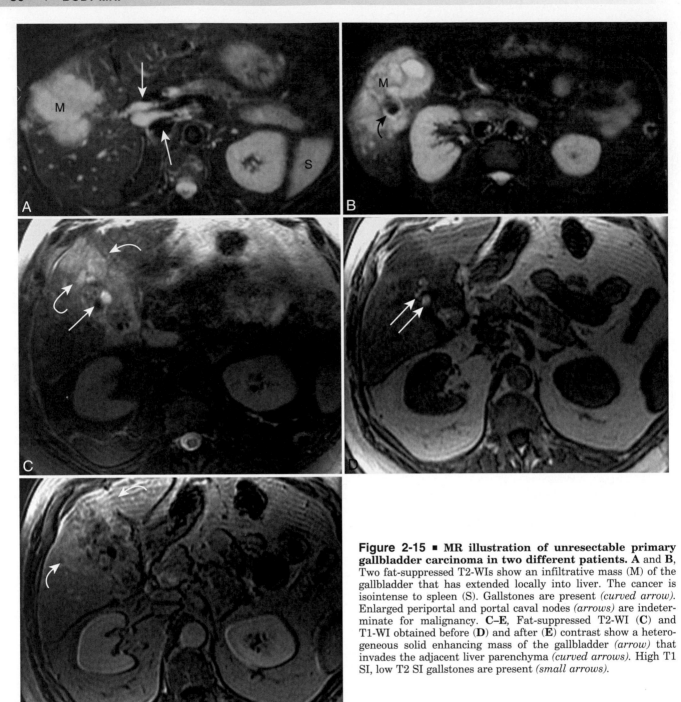

Figure 2-15 ■ **MR illustration of unresectable primary gallbladder carcinoma in two different patients. A** and **B,** Two fat-suppressed T2-WIs show an infiltrative mass (M) of the gallbladder that has extended locally into liver. The cancer is isointense to spleen (S). Gallstones are present *(curved arrow).* Enlarged periportal and portal caval nodes *(arrows)* are indeterminate for malignancy. **C–E,** Fat-suppressed T2-WI (**C**) and T1-WI obtained before (**D**) and after (**E**) contrast show a heterogeneous solid enhancing mass of the gallbladder *(arrow)* that invades the adjacent liver parenchyma *(curved arrows).* High T1 SI, low T2 SI gallstones are present *(small arrows).*

Calcification in the wall of the gallbladder (porcelain gallbladder) may be difficult to discern on MRI and is better depicted on CT (Fig. 2-16) or radiography. Direct liver invasion appears as an ill-defined tumor mass of the adjacent hepatic parenchyma contiguous with the primary tumor. Both direct liver invasion and distant liver metastases have the same SI as the primary tumor and are best depicted on T2-WI and CE T1-WI.[147,217] Tumor extension into the hepatoduodenal ligament and para-aortic region appears as nodular or infiltrative masses that are hypointense to fat and best delineated on T1-WI, where there is excellent tissue contrast between tumor, fat, vessels, and pancreas.[217]

Dynamic CE-MR imaging can demonstrate whether a lesion invades the serosa, thus defining

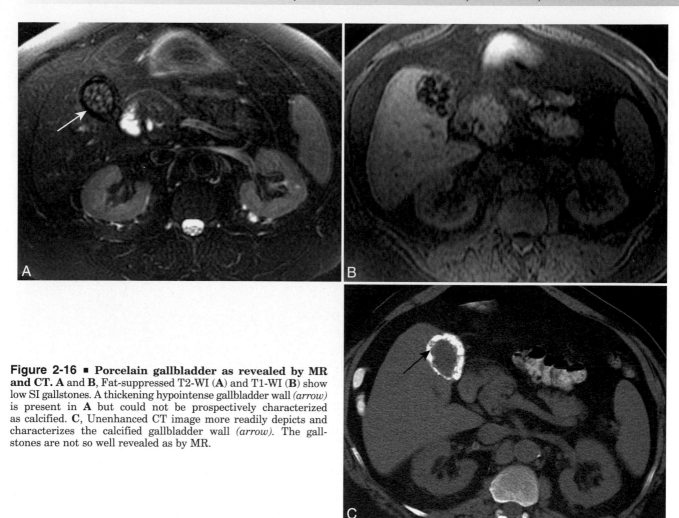

Figure 2-16 ■ **Porcelain gallbladder as revealed by MR and CT. A** and **B**, Fat-suppressed T2-WI (**A**) and T1-WI (**B**) show low SI gallstones. A thickening hypointense gallbladder wall *(arrow)* is present in **A** but could not be prospectively characterized as calcified. **C**, Unenhanced CT image more readily depicts and characterizes the calcified gallbladder wall *(arrow).* The gallstones are not so well revealed as by MR.

whether a tumor is T2 or T3. Arterial-phase enhancement that extends beyond the gallbladder wall correlates with the pathologic finding of serosal invasion. Enhancement limited to the gallbladder wall suggests invasion of the subserosa but not into or beyond the serosa.[148] MRI can also depict portal vein encasement and biliary duct dilation at the level of the porta hepatis, a common finding due to extrinsic compression by lymphadenopathy or to direct spread of tumor along the cystic duct to the common bile duct.[201,217,218] CT and MRI are not reliable in depicting all histologically proved regional lymph node metastases; however, the identification of lymph nodes greater than 10 mm in AP diameter with ring-like or heterogeneous enhancement suggests lymphatic spread.[215]

The increased use of laparoscopic cholecystectomy has resulted in a larger number of patients with incidentally discovered gallbladder cancers that may recur owing to the increased risk of rupture of the gallbladder during the procedure, which results in inadvertent dissemination of tumor. The recurrence can present as peritoneal carcinomatosis or as an anterior abdominal wall mass located along the trocar sites with extension into the subjacent omental fat (Fig. 2-17).[212,219]

The imaging differential diagnosis of gallbladder cancer can be quite extensive because of the nonspecific appearance of many gallbladder lesions (see Box 2-15).[149,201] Malignant polypoid lesions show early and persistent enhancement, whereas benign lesions show early enhancement with immediate washout. In cases of diffuse wall thickening, malignant lesions show early and prolonged enhancement, while benign lesions show late and prolonged enhancement.[149] Dynamic CE-MR imaging may distinguish between cancer and chronic cholecystitis. Chronic cholecystitis demonstrates smoothly delineated arterial enhancement of a thickened gallbladder wall, whereas tumors show irregular areas of arterial enhancement.[148,213] In general, gallbladder wall thickening that is irregular and greater than 10 mm raises concern for malignancy or complicated cholecystitis.[201] Although infiltrating gallbladder carcinoma can sometimes be difficult to distinguish from hepatocellular carcinoma, metastases, and complicated cholecystitis,[220]

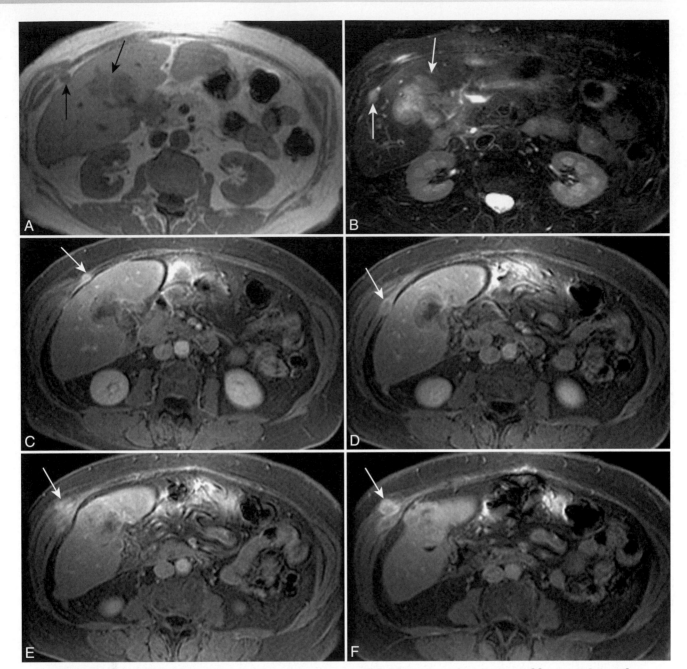

Figure 2-17 ■ **MR findings of residual and recurrent gallbladder cancer in a 71-year-old woman 2 months after invasive cholecystectomy. A** and **B,** T1-WI (**A**) and fat-suppressed T2-WI (**B**) show residual infiltrating gallbladder cancer within the surgical bed. A peritoneum-based nodule is present adjacent to the liver *(arrows)*. **C–F,** Four consecutive CE fat-suppressed T1-WIs show heterogeneous enhancing tumor within the gallbladder fossa and also within abdominal wall at site of prior laparoscopic port incisions *(arrows)*.

it should be suspected in the setting of a focal gallbladder mass with associated lymphadenopathy, hepatic metastases, and biliary obstruction at the porta hepatis.

Therapeutic options for gallbladder cancer are limited because most patients are at an advanced stage of the disease at diagnosis. Although surgery is considered the mainstay of treatment, there is

controversy over the extent of resection for each stage. The most potentially curable neoplasms are those found incidentally during cholecystectomy for symptomatic gallstones.[199] Radical re-resection is recommended when T2 or T3 tumors are discovered incidentally at cholecystectomy and involves resection of the adjacent liver and regional lymph nodes.[212,221] If the patient has undergone laparoscopic cholecystectomy, re-exploration must also include assessment and resection of the laparoscopic port sites, since gallbladder carcinoma has a great propensity for seeding these tracts.[212,219]

In patients with localized disease, complete surgical resection is performed for long-term control.[200] Simple cholecystectomy is adequate for stage 0. Radical resection is recommended for stage II disease because of improved survival[222,223] and includes cholecystectomy; wedge resection of adjacent liver; en bloc resection of regional lymph nodes including those in the hepatoduodenal ligament, those in the porta hepatis, and those adjacent to the posterosuperior aspect of the pancreatic head; and occasionally resection of the suprapancreatic segment of the extrahepatic bile duct.[222,223] The extent of hepatic resection depends on the extent of hepatic invasion and degree of vascular involvement (portal vein or hepatic artery invasion) and may range from resection of hepatic segments IVa and V to lobectomy or even trisegmentectomy.[212] The presence of N1 and N2 nodes (see Box 2-14) is a poor prognostic factor but not a contraindication to radical resection, which is also advocated for stages III and IVA disease.[210,212,224] However, the presence of discontiguous liver metastases, vascular or biliary involvement not amenable to reconstruction, distant nodal metastases (para-aortic or aortocaval), peritoneal metastases, or pulmonary metastases classifies these tumors as unresectable.[212]

Gallbladder carcinoma was originally thought to be radioresistant, but studies have shown that there is slight improvement in survival with stage IVA disease (9% to 10% 3-year survival versus 0% to 3% with surgery alone) when radiotherapy is combined with radical surgery.[224] Although advanced cancer usually is unresponsive to chemotherapy, preliminary studies have shown some response to gemcitabine and 5-fluorouracil and to trimodality therapy that combines surgery with adjuvant chemotherapy and radiotherapy.[214]

Other Gallbladder Malignancies

Gallbladder involvement by malignancies other than primary gallbladder carcinoma is rare. The gallbladder can be a target site for melanoma and breast metastases with malignant melanoma being the most common cause of metastasis.[225] Melanoma can present as a focal mass that may have high SI on T1-WI depending on its melanin content and the presence of intratumoral hemorrhage.[147] Primary non-Hodgkin's lymphoma (NHL) of the gallbladder is a rare entity characterized by a poor prognosis[226,227] and presents as nonspecific circumferential thickening of the gallbladder wall with moderate wall enhancement.[147]

MR OF THE PANCREAS

MR Appearance of the Normal Pancreas

The pancreas is a nonencapsulated retroperitoneal organ composed of a head, uncinate process, neck, body, and tail. On T1-WI, the normal pancreas reveals higher SI than does other nonfatty tissue such as liver and muscle (see Fig. 2-6).[228,229] The relative hyperintensity of normal pancreas is secondary to aqueous proteins in the glandular elements of the pancreas, intracellular paramagnetic substances such as manganese, and abundant endoplasmic reticulum in the pancreatic exocrine cells.[229,230] The relative SI of the pancreas increases on fat-suppressed T1-WI owing to reduced motion and chemical shift artifact and an increase in the dynamic range of remaining SIs. Normal pancreatic parenchyma is only slightly hyperintense to muscle on T2-WI. On fat-suppressed T2-WI, there is minimal contrast between the normal pancreas and the surrounding suppressed fat (see Figs. 2-6 and 2-22).[229,230]

The pancreas is a highly vascular organ and shows maximum enhancement 30-45 seconds after a bolus contrast injection.[231-235] Maximal pancreatic parenchymal enhancement occurs 15 seconds after gadolinium arrival in the abdominal aorta. Normal pancreatic parenchyma shows a homogeneous capillary blush on arterial-phase images (see Fig. 1-14D)[229,231] that is hyperintense to liver and fat and shows diminished SI by 3 minutes.

The main pancreatic duct is normally 2–3 mm in diameter and increases slightly in caliber from the tail to the head.[21,236] Short side branches (20–35) enter the main duct at right angles but usually are not revealed on MRCP unless dilated.[236] Although there are great variations in the course of the duct, in 50% of cases it courses cephalad from the pancreatic head, takes a 45° to 90° turn in the neck, and continues horizontally in the body and tail.[21,236] In 90% of individuals, the main drainage route of the exocrine pancreas is a result of the fusion that occurs at 7 weeks of gestation between the duct draining the pancreatic body and tail and the duct draining the inferior pancreatic head and uncinate process (duct of Wirsung). The duct of Wirsung then joins the common bile duct at the ampulla of Vater to drain into the duodenum. In approximately 40% of individuals, the accessory duct (duct of Santorini) persists and drains through the minor papilla with primary drainage still occurring through the duct of Wirsung. In 10%, the duct of Santorini provides the sole drainage of the pancreatic body and tail (see Figs. 1-5 and 2-6).

The main pancreatic duct is routinely visualized as high SI on T2-WI and MRCP because of its high fluid content.[236,237] The pancreatic duct may not always be depicted in its entirety on a single MRCP image owing to its curvilinear course. Reviewing the source images or creating an MIP image aids in the visualization and evaluation of the entire duct.[21,236] The delineation of the pancreatic duct on MRCP is also improved by the exogenous administration of secretin, an enzyme that stimulates the pancreatic secretion of fluid and bicarbonate, thereby increasing the volume of fluid in the duct and transiently increasing duct caliber. The normal pancreatic duct enlarges during the first minute after secretin administration, reaches a maximum diameter at

23 minutes, and returns to baseline after 5 minutes as pancreatic juices drain into the duodenum.[238-240]

MR Techniques for Imaging the Pancreas

The pancreas is best imaged on a high–field strength system (=1.0 T) with an adequate fat-water frequency shift for chemically selective fat suppression[229] and high-performance gradients that enable the use of fast MR sequences. An optimized protocol for imaging the pancreas includes axial T1-WI with and without fat suppression that can take the form of a breath-hold GRE or breathing-averaged SE sequences.[241,242] Fat-suppressed T1-WIs provide the greatest contrast between high SI normal parenchyma and low SI abnormal pancreatic tissue (see Fig. 2-6) that increases the sensitivity of detecting small pancreatic neoplasms or focal pancreatitis.[229,230] T1-WIs without fat suppression are ideal for showing extrapancreatic extension of inflammatory and neoplastic diseases and are useful for determining vessel encasement by malignant tumors (see Fig. 2-17).[230,243] Fat-suppressed T2-WIs are useful for depicting ducts, peripancreatic fluid collections, liver metastases, cystic lesions, and islet cell tumors.[243]

Two- or three-dimensional fat-suppressed dynamic CE-MR imaging aids in the evaluation of the pancreas and peripancreatic tissues.[234,244] CE-MRA provides information about vascular encasement or thrombosis by malignant tumors, whereas the "pancreatic" phase of CE helps detect and characterize mass lesions and assess diffuse inflammatory processes such as pancreatitis. Imaging at 15 and 35-45 seconds after the arrival of contrast in the abdominal aorta is an effective method of obtaining high-quality images of the pancreatic parenchyma and peripancreatic vessels.[234] The time required for contrast to reach the abdominal aorta can be determined by test-bolus injection, MR fluoroscopy, or triggering software (see Chapter 11). These are preferred methods of obtaining arterial-phase images of the pancreas over arbitrarily imaging 20 to 40 seconds after contrast injection,[233,244,245] since aortic transit time is dependent on a patient's cardiac output and circulation time and can vary by as much as 9 to 29 seconds. Maximum enhancement of the liver and peripancreatic vessels (superior mesenteric artery and vein) occurs 25 seconds or later after contrast arrival in the aorta.[234]

The addition of MRCP helps evaluate ductal anomalies or obstruction of the pancreaticobiliary tree that can occur with pancreatic neoplasms and inflammatory disease. MR pancreatography uses heavily T2-WI that exploits the fluid content of the pancreatic duct[236,240] and can take the form of a 2D or 3D breathing-averaged[21,237] or breath-hold FSE sequence.[240] Because the pancreatic duct is susceptible to respiratory motion, breath-hold imaging is preferred and data can be acquired in the axial, coronal, and oblique coronal planes as a thick-slab projection image or as a thin-section multislice acquisition (see above).[236] Breath-hold MRCP can also depict the multilocular nature of cystic pancreatic lesions to better advantage because of the elimination of blurring from respiratory motion.[246]

Secretin-enhanced MRCP can improve the visualization of the normal pancreatic duct and anatomic variants and assess pancreatic exocrine function and may be most helpful in patients with suspected pancreatic disease who have no abnormalities revealed on standard MRCP. Breath-hold thick-slab 2D projection sequences are preferred for acquiring data with good temporal resolution that will depict the pancreatic duct, common bile duct, and duodenum on one image. Once the appropriate coronal or oblique coronal position has been determined, images are acquired before secretin administration and then every 15 to 30 seconds for 10 to 15 minutes after a dose of 1 mL/10 kg body weight is administered intravenously.[240] A T2 negative oral contrast agent can be used to mask high SI fluid in the bowel that may overlap with the pancreatic duct. In the absence of obstruction, stricture, stone, or mass, prolonged dilation of the main duct or side branches and reduced duodenal filling are some of the findings that can suggest impairment of pancreatic exocrine function.[240,247]

Congenital/Developmental Anomalies

ANNULAR PANCREAS

Annular pancreas is a rare congenital anomaly characterized by a ring of normal pancreatic tissue that partially or completely encircles the duodenum. Annular pancreas results from abnormal migration and rotation of the ventral anlagen of the pancreatic head during embryogenesis.[248,249] Most patients with annular pancreas present during infancy with signs or symptoms of gastric outlet obstruction. Infants with symptomatic annular pancreas can have associated anomalies such as trisomy 21, duodenal atresia, and tracheoesophageal fistula. Adults with annular pancreas may present with peptic ulcer disease and pancreatitis.[248,249]

The diagnosis of annular pancreas can be established on ERCP by showing an aberrant pancreatic duct that encircles the duodenum and joins the main pancreatic duct. These findings have also been reported using MRCP.[250] Demonstration of a ring of high SI pancreatic tissue that surrounds the duodenum on fat-suppressed T1-WI is another method of establishing an MR diagnosis.[228,251] Treatment of symptomatic annular pancreas consists of gastro- or duodenojejunostomy in order to bypass the obstructed duodenal segment. Primary resection of the annulus is not performed because of the high incidence of complications such as fistula formation and pancreatic laceration.[248,249]

PANCREAS DIVISUM

Pancreas divisum is the most common congenital variant of the pancreatic duct, affecting 5% to 14% of the population, and represents the failure of fusion of the ducts of the dorsal and ventral pancreas.[236,252]

In most patients, absence of fusion is complete and there is no connection between the ducts. The clinical relevance of pancreas divisum is controversial, since most patients are asymptomatic. However, in a subset of patients with recurrent pancreatitis or abdominal pain, the pathogenesis is thought to be a functional stenosis at the minor papilla with an outflow obstruction of exocrine juices that results in high intraductal pressure, ductal distension, and pancreatitis.[253] This theory has been supported by the detection of a "Santorinicele" in some patients with pancreas divisum and recurrent pancreatitis.[253,254] The "Santorinicele" (analogous to ureterocele or choledochocele) is a focal dilatation of the terminal portion of the dorsal duct just proximal to the minor papilla that results from a combination of relative obstruction and weakness of the duct wall.[253,254] Such patients may benefit from endoscopic or surgical drainage of the minor papilla.[255]

Evaluation of the ducts is limited on ERCP because only the ventral duct is opacified during cannulation of the major papilla. MRCP can noninvasively depict the two independent ductal systems: the dorsal duct (Santorini), which is anterior and superior to the ventral duct (Wirsung) (see Figs. 1-6 and 2-6). The dominant dorsal duct extends from the pancreatic tail to the head and crosses anterior to the common bile duct to empty into the duodenum at the minor (accessory) papilla, while the ventral duct joins the common bile duct to empty into the major papilla.[21,236,237,252] Using the axial plane improves the visualization of the pancreatic ducts and increases the diagnostic accuracy of MRCP.[252] Administration of secretin during MRCP can improve the detection of pancreas divisum and may also reveal the presence of an occult "Santorinicele."[256,257]

Solid Neoplasms of the Pancreas

PANCREATIC ADENOCARCINOMA

Adenocarcinoma of the exocrine pancreas is the most common pancreatic malignancy (95% of all pancreatic malignant tumors) and is estimated to account for 2% of new cancers diagnosed in 2004 and 5% to 6% of cancer deaths.[117] In 2003, 31,860 individuals were estimated to develop pancreatic adenocarcinoma and 31,270 to die of the disease.[117] The disease predominantly affects the elderly population, with 80% of patients diagnosed above age 60 years and the peak age occurring between 70 and 79 years.[258-260] Of the tumors 70% are located in the pancreatic head, 20% in the pancreatic body, and 10% in the tail.[261,262] Symptoms and signs of pancreatic head tumors include jaundice, weight loss, pain, and nausea. Tumors of the body and tail tend to present late with symptoms of weight loss, abdominal pain radiating to the back, and anorexia.[263] Serum tumor markers such as CA 19-9 (carbohydrate antigen 19-9) and CEA (carcinoembryonic antigen) are being used increasingly in the diagnosis of pancreatic cancer owing to their improved sensitivity and specificity (75% and 96%, respectively).[263,264]

Obstruction of the main pancreatic duct is one of the most common findings in adenocarcinoma. Contiguous obstruction of the pancreatic and common bile ducts by a pancreatic head mass is known as the "double duct" sign and is highly suggestive of malignancy.[265] Pancreatic adenocarcinomas are typically hypointense to pancreatic parenchyma on T1-WI (Figs. 2-18 and 2-19).[265-267] Fat suppression helps increase the conspicuity of the low SI tumor against the higher SI of the normal parenchyma.[268] Tumors have variable SI on T2-WI depending on the degree of hemorrhage, necrosis, and inflammatory changes. In general, T2-WIs are less helpful, since there is poor contrast between the mass and normal pancreas in most patients.[266,267,269-271] Pancreatic cancer is usually hypovascular to the normal glandular tissue on arterial-phase imaging and then shows gradual enhancement on delayed imaging, reflecting its desmoplastic content.[266,267] Immediate CE imaging is the most sensitive for detecting adenocarcinomas, especially non–border deforming lesions.[228,267]

When adenocarcinoma is superimposed on underlying chronic pancreatitis, the tumor can be difficult to detect because both the tumor and surrounding pancreas may have similar low SI (see Fig. 2-19).[229,272] However, immediate CE images may still be able to delineate the size and extent of cancers that tend to enhance less than adjacent chronically inflamed tissue.[267] In general, the diagnosis of pancreatic adenocarcinoma is straightforward and the role of imaging is to determine resectability. In some patients, an inflammatory mass cannot be distinguished from a pancreatic adenocarcinoma because both processes can result in focal pancreatic enlargement, distortion of the normal contour, ductal dilatation, and abnormal enhancement.[273]

The overall 5-year survival rate is 24% for patients receiving surgical therapy compared with 5% for those not receiving any cancer-directed treatment.[258] The presence of positive surgical margins is a significant factor in overall survival.

Therapeutic options for pancreatic adenocarcinoma depend on the stage (Box 2-16) and resectability at the time of diagnosis. Complete surgical resection is the only treatment associated with long-term survival and possibility of cure. Only 10% to 20% of patients are candidates for resection, and 60% of patients have metastatic disease at presentation.[260] Criteria for unresectable tumor (Box 2-17) include invasion of adjacent tissues other than the duodenum, vascular encasement, lymph node metastases, liver metastases, and omental or peritoneal implants.

The five major vessels that are evaluated for vascular invasion are celiac artery, superior mesenteric artery (SMA), hepatic artery, portal vein, and superior mesenteric vein (SMV). Splenic artery and vein involvement does not preclude resection, because splenectomy can be performed along with resection of a pancreatic body or tail tumor. The absence of invasion is defined as tumor confined to the pancreas with preservation of the perivascular fat planes.[274,275]

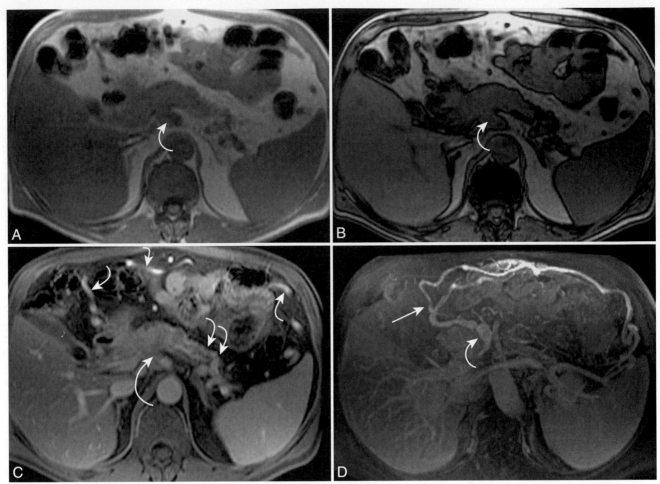

Figure 2-18 ■ MR demonstration of unresectable pancreatic adenocarcinoma with superior mesenteric artery encasement and a thrombosed splenic vein in a man with abdominal pain. A and **B,** Axial in-phase (**A**) and opposed-phase (**B**) T1-WIs show normal SI liver and spleen. There is an infiltrative process involving the pancreatic neck that extends posteriorly to encase the right side of the superior mesenteric artery *(curved arrow).* **C,** Axial fat-suppressed CE T1-WI obtained at a slightly higher level reconfirms an infiltrative hypovascular adenocarcinoma that extends to superior mesenteric artery *(long curved arrow).* Other images (not shown) identified encasement of the splenic artery. Mildly atrophic, enhancing pancreatic parenchymal tissue is present peripheral to the mass *(double curved arrow)* and surrounds a nonenhancing dilated distal pancreatic duct. Segments of a collateral vessel are revealed in cross section *(curved arrows).* **D,** MIP image from the venous phase of a fat-suppressed 3D CE T1-W sequence shows that the collateral vessel represents an enlarged gastrocolic trunk *(arrow)* that drains into the superior mesenteric vein *(curved arrow).* No flow is identified in the expected location of the splenic vein, indicating encasement and/or thrombosis.

A vessel is considered encased when tumor has obliterated the fat plane within 5 mm of the vessel and surrounds greater than half its circumference or demonstrates focal reduction in caliber.[274-278] Mere contiguity of tumor to vessel does not automatically signify vascular invasion.[274,275] For example, the anterior and lateral margins of the SMV may be directly contiguous with normal pancreatic tissue, and tumor involving this part of the pancreas can be contiguous with the vein without invasion (see Fig. 2-19). Traditionally, portal or superior mesenteric vein involvement was considered a contraindication to tumor resection. However, some surgeons perform segmental resection of the involved venous segments

at the time of the primary tumor removal without significant morbidity or decrease in overall survival.[279]

Lymph nodes are best shown on fat-suppressed T2-WI, where they reveal moderately high SI compared with suppressed fat and low SI pancreatic parenchyma.[280] Lymph nodes measuring greater than 10 mm in short axis are considered suspicious for malignancy.[266] Nodal staging of pancreatic cancer with imaging is inaccurate because even 1- to 2-mm peripancreatic nodes can contain metastases. The liver should also be included in the field-of-view in order to evaluate for liver metastases. Peritoneal implants are the most difficult to detect on preoperative imaging but are best revealed on CE

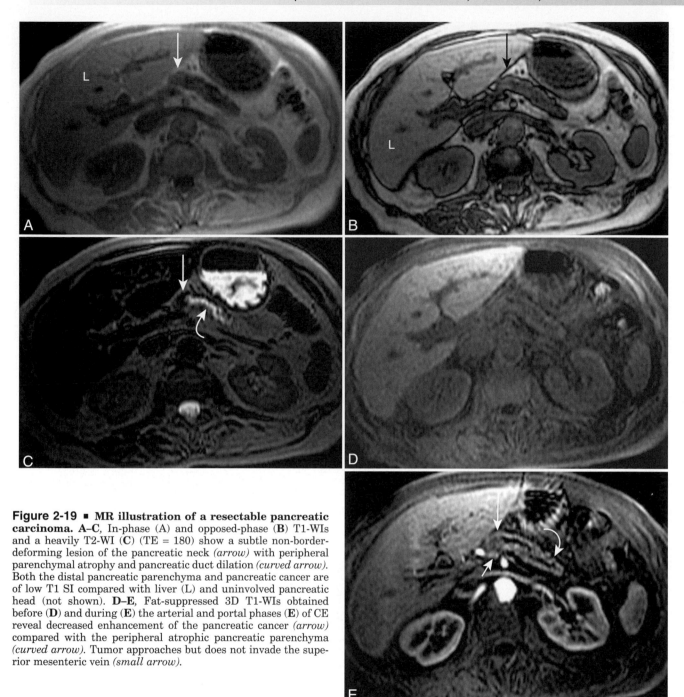

Figure 2-19 ■ MR illustration of a resectable pancreatic carcinoma. A–C, In-phase (A) and opposed-phase (**B**) T1-WIs and a heavily T2-WI (**C**) (TE = 180) show a subtle non-border-deforming lesion of the pancreatic neck *(arrow)* with peripheral parenchymal atrophy and pancreatic duct dilation *(curved arrow)*. Both the distal pancreatic parenchyma and pancreatic cancer are of low T1 SI compared with liver (L) and uninvolved pancreatic head (not shown). **D–E,** Fat-suppressed 3D T1-WIs obtained before (**D**) and during (**E**) the arterial and portal phases (**E**) of CE reveal decreased enhancement of the pancreatic cancer *(arrow)* compared with the peripheral atrophic pancreatic parenchyma *(curved arrow)*. Tumor approaches but does not invade the superior mesenteric vein *(small arrow)*.

fat-suppressed T1-WI.[281,282] To date the greatest limitations of staging pancreatic cancer with state-of-the-art MR and multidetector CT is in the false negative findings of small liver metastases, the presence of cancer in normal sized nodes, and small peritoneal implants.[283]

The standard operative technique for pancreatic head lesions is the Whipple procedure, also known as pancreaticoduodenectomy. The surgery involves resection of at least the head and neck of the pancreas, most or all of the duodenum, common bile duct,

and regional lymph nodes, followed by reanastomosis of the stomach or duodenal bulb, pancreas, and biliary tract to the jejunum.[139,284] Lesions in the body and tail undergo resection of the involved pancreas but sometimes may require total pancreatectomy.[262]

Of patients with pancreatic adenocarcinoma 80% to 90% have advanced disease that is not amenable to resection (35% to 40% have locally advanced disease and 50% have distant metastases).[259,261] Locally advanced pancreatic adenocarcinoma is defined as tumor confined to the pancreas (including involvement

2-16 TNM Classification of Pancreatic Carcinoma (Adapted from Cancer UIUA, TNM Classification of Malignant Tumors, 5th ed, 1997)

Anatomic Subcategory

Head of pancreas	Tumors arising to the right of the left border of the superior mesenteric vein; the uncinate process is part of the head
Body of pancreas	Tumors arising between the left border of the superior mesenteric vein and left border of the aorta
Tail of pancreas	Tumors arising between the left border of the aorta and the hilum of the spleen

T—Primary Tumor

T0	No evidence of primary tumor
Tis	Carcinoma in situ
T1	Tumor limited to the pancreas, 2 cm or less in greatest dimension
T2	Tumor limited to the pancreas, more than 2 cm in greatest dimension
T3	Tumor extends directly into any of the following: duodenum, bile duct (includes involvement of the ampulla of Vater), peripancreatic tissues (retroperitoneal fat; mesentery, or mesenteric fat; mesocolon; greater and lesser omentum; and peritoneum)
T4	Tumor extends directly into any of the following: stomach, spleen, colon, adjacent large vessels (portal vein, celiac artery, superior mesenteric and common hepatic arteries and veins (not splenic vessels)

N—Regional Lymph Nodes*

N0	No regional lymph node metastasis	
N1	Regional lymph node metastasis	
	N1a	Metastasis in a single regional lymph node
	N1b	Metastasis in multiple regional lymph nodes

M—Distant Metastasis

M0	No distant metastasis
M1	Distant metastasis

Stage Grouping

Stage 0	Tis	N0	M0
Stage I	T1	N0	M0
	T2	N0	M0
Stage II	T3	N0	M0
Stage III	T1	N1	M0
	T2	N1	M0
	T3	N1	M0
Stage IVA	T4	Any N	M0
Stage IVB	Any T	Any N	M1

*Regional lymph nodes are peripancreatic lymph nodes subdivided as follows:

Superior	Superior to head and body
Inferior	Inferior to head and body
Anterior	Anterior pancreaticoduodenal, pyloric (for tumors of the head only), and proximal mesenteric
Posterior	Posterior pancreaticoduodenal, common bile duct, and proximal mesenteric
Splenic	Hilum of spleen and tail (for tumors of body and tail only)
Celiac	(for tumors of the head only)

2-17 Criteria for Unresectable Pancreatic Adenocarcinoma

- Invasion of peripancreatic vessels
  - Celiac artery, SMA, common hepatic/proper hepatic artery
  - Portal vein*, SMV*
- Invasion of the neural plexus around the celiac axis and SMA
- Invasion of local contiguous structures other than the duodenum
- Distant metastases
  - Lymph nodes outside the margin of resection
  - Liver metastases
  - Omental and peritoneal metastases

*See text

of the superior mesenteric artery and vein), adjacent regional lymph nodes, and contiguous organs, or disease that can be included in a 10 cm × 10 cm radiation field.[285] Treatment usually consists of chemotherapy and radiation therapy and is associated with a median survival of approximately 9 months.[285] The current standard therapy for patients with metastatic disease to distant sites such as the liver, distant lymph nodes, pleura, peritoneum, and omentum is the use of a systemic chemotherapeutic agent such as gemcitabine that results in a 1-year survival rate of 20% to 25%.[286] Palliative strategies for patients with unresectable or metastatic disease include pain control (percutaneous celiac blockade), biliary decompression for obstructive jaundice, and possible gastric bypass for patients with mechanical gastric outlet obstruction.[261]

PANCREATIC NEUROENDOCRINE TUMORS

Neuroendocrine (islet cell) tumors are uncommon, slow-growing pancreatic or peripancreatic masses that either result in symptomatic hormonal overproduction (functional) or show no clinical findings of hormone secretion (nonfunctional). The overall incidence of pancreatic neuroendocrine tumors is 1-1.5 per 100,000 in the general population.[287] Islet cell tumors are well depicted on MRI because of the high contrast between normal high SI pancreas and the hypointense tumors on T1-WI and because of their typical hypervascular enhancement (Figs. 2-20 and 2-21).[229,288,289] Fat-suppressed T2-WIs often reveal high SI components within pancreatic neuroendocrine tumors compared with adjacent pancreas (see Fig. 2-21).[290,291] Less commonly, tumors may have T2 hypointense or iso-intense to pancreas because of increased fibrous tissue content.[288,289]

Functioning neuroendocrine tumors manifest early owing to symptoms of hormone overproduction and are named according to the hormone they produce. Insulinoma is the most common functional islet cell tumor and manifests as symptomatic hypoglycemia secondary to insulin secretion (Box 2-18).[292,293] Insulinomas are usually solitary (90%), smaller than 2 cm, and distributed uniformly throughout the pancreas.[292,294,295]

Insulinomas show homogeneous low SI on fat-suppressed T1-WI, homogenous high SI on T2-WI, and intense enhancement (greater than that of pancreas) on dynamic CE images (see Fig. 2-20).[229,280,290,291,296,297] Preoperative localization of some insulinomas can be

difficult owing to their small size and lack of both mass effect and duct dilation. However, most insulinomas can be revealed during surgical exploration with the aid of intraoperative ultrasound. Ninety percent of insulinomas are benign. Treatment for cure consists of surgical resection.[287,293]

Gastrinomas are the second most common functional islet cell tumor (Box 2-19). The increase in gastrin secretion results in fulminant peptic ulcer disease known as Zollinger-Ellison syndrome.[287] Of gastrinomas 70% to 75% are sporadic and 20% to 25% occur as part of the multiple endocrine neoplasia (MEN)-1 syndrome. Tumors generally are small

2-18   Features of Insulinomas

Clinical

50% of pancreatic neuroendocrine tumors
Most common hyperfunctioning neuroendocrine tumor
Present with symptomatic hypoglycemia

Pathology

Homogenous masses, mean size 2 cm
90% are benign
90% are single lesions

MRI

Low SI on T1-WI relative to pancreas
High SI on T2-WI relative to pancreas
Homogenous and hyperintense after dynamic CE

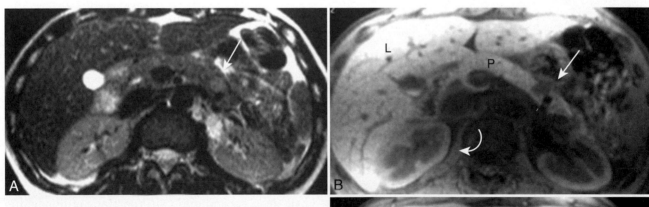
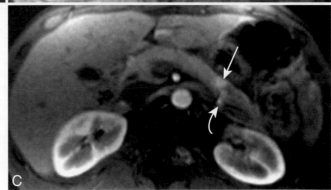

Figure 2-20 ■ MR illustration of a functioning insulinoma in a woman with signs and symptoms of insulin excess. **A,** Axial T2-WI shows a subtle mass of the pancreas *(arrow)* that has slightly higher SI than adjacent parenchyma. No peripheral pancreatic atrophy or duct dilation is present. **B,** Axial fat-suppressed T1-WI shows a well-circumscribed low SI lesion *(arrow)* of the pancreatic body. There is normal, high SI within the liver (L), pancreas (P) and renal cortex *(curved arrow)*. **C,** Arterial-phase CE T1-WI shows homogeneous intense tumoral enhancement *(arrow)* that is hyperintense to both pancreas and liver. The enhancing structure posterior to the insulinoma *(curved arrow)* is the splenic artery imaged in short axis. The splenic artery showed a low SI flow void in **A** and **B**.

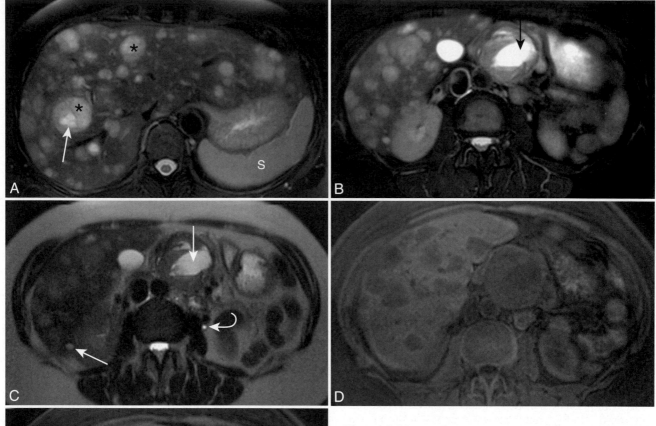

Figure 2-21 ■ **MR findings of metastatic nonfunctioning neuroendocrine tumor of the pancreas. A** and **B**, T2-WIs through the liver (**A**) and lower pancreas (**B**) reveal the presence of multiple liver metastases (∗) that are isointense to spleen (S). A heterogeneous low pancreatic head mass is present with similar T2 SI. Intratumoral cystic necrosis is present within the primary tumor and one of the liver metastases *(arrows)*. The primary tumor was hyperintense to the remainder of the pancreas (not shown). **C**, Heavily T2-WI (TE = 180) shows that the liver metastases are poorly visualized. Fluid-containing structures such as the intratumoral cystic necrosis *(vertical arrow)*, left ureter *(curved arrow)*, and <10 mm right renal cyst *(arrow)* are better revealed on this image. **D** and **E**, 3D fat-suppressed T1-WI obtained before (**D**) and after (**E**) contrast shows moderate to marked enhancement of the solid components of the primary tumor and of some of the liver metastases *(arrows)*.

2-19 Features of Gastrinomas

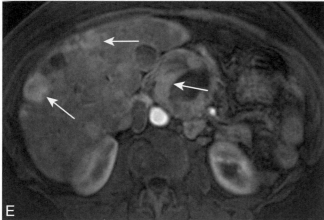

Clinical

30% of pancreatic neuroendocrine tumors
Second most common hyperfunctioning
    neuroendocrine tumor
Associated with Zollinger-Ellison syndrome,
    MEN-1 (duodenal and periduodenal gastrinomas)

Pathology

Homogenous masses, mean size 4 cm
60%–80% lesions are malignant

MRI

Low SI on T1-WI relative to pancreas
High SI on T2-WI relative to pancreas
Rim enhancement after dynamic CE

(<4 cm), and up to 50% are not localized preoperatively.[287,296] Most gastrinomas are located in the "gastrinoma triangle" that is bounded by the cystic duct, second and third portions of duodenum, and neck of pancreas. Of sporadic gastrinomas 50% to 60% occur in the pancreas, 35% to 40% are localized to the duodenal wall (Fig. 2-22), and the remainder are located within the stomach and lymph nodes.[287,292,298]

Gastrinomas typically show low SI on T1-WI, high SI on T2-WI, and rim enhancement with smooth margins on CE images (see Fig. 2-22).[229,291,296,299,300] Sixty to eighty percent of gastrinomas are malignant but follow a protracted and indolent course.[295] Sporadic pancreatic gastrinomas are treated by enucleation or partial pancreatectomy. Intraoperative endoscopy and duodenotomy are performed to detect

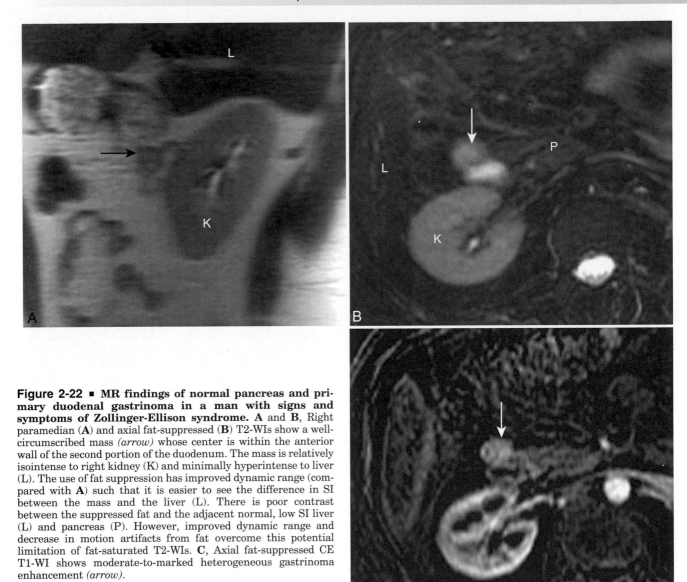

Figure 2-22 ▪ MR findings of normal pancreas and primary duodenal gastrinoma in a man with signs and symptoms of Zollinger-Ellison syndrome. A and **B**, Right paramedian (**A**) and axial fat-suppressed (**B**) T2-WIs show a well-circumscribed mass (*arrow*) whose center is within the anterior wall of the second portion of the duodenum. The mass is relatively isointense to right kidney (K) and minimally hyperintense to liver (L). The use of fat suppression has improved dynamic range (compared with **A**) such that it is easier to see the difference in SI between the mass and the liver (L). There is poor contrast between the suppressed fat and the adjacent normal, low SI liver (L) and pancreas (P). However, improved dynamic range and decrease in motion artifacts from fat overcome this potential limitation of fat-saturated T2-WIs. **C**, Axial fat-suppressed CE T1-WI shows moderate-to-marked heterogeneous gastrinoma enhancement (*arrow*).

duodenal lesions, which are then locally resected. Approximately 40% of patients with MEN-1 syndrome have multiple gastrinomas and are less likely to achieve a biochemical cure after resection. The gastrinomas that develop in patients with MEN-1 are almost always duodenal in origin and spread to adjacent lymph nodes.[301] The pancreatic neuroendocrine tumors that are present in MEN-1 patients are usually nonhyperfunctioning[298]; these individuals are managed nonsurgically unless they have a clearly depicted mass greater than 3 cm on imaging.[287,293]

Glucagonomas, VIPomas (from vasoactive intestinal polypeptide), and somatostatinomas are functional neuroendocrine tumors that manifest late in the disease course, in part because the signs and symptoms of hormonal overproduction can be nonspecific. Glucagonomas secrete glucagon, which results in diabetes, dermatitis, and painful glossitis.[287,292] VIPomas result in a syndrome of watery diarrhea, hypokalemia, and achlorhydria (WDHA), and individuals with somatostatinomas have symptoms of abdominal pain, diarrhea, cholelithiasis, and diabetes.[287] The majority (50% to 70%) of these less common functional neuroendocrine tumors are malignant and have a mean diameter of 3-5 cm at the time of diagnosis; this makes preoperative localization less of a challenge.[287,293] Of glucagonomas larger than 5 cm, 60% to 80% are malignant and most of these

2-20 Features of Nonfunctioning Neuroendocrine Tumors

Clinical

15% of pancreatic neuroendocrine tumors
Asymptomatic, or present with symptoms of mass effect

Pathology

Heterogeneous masses, mean size 6–10 cm
>50% are malignant

MRI

Low SI on T1-WI relative to pancreas
Foci of high SI necrosis and cystic degeneration on T2-WI relative to pancreas
Heterogeneous and hyperintense after dynamic CE

patients have metastatic disease at the time of imaging.[287,295] These three tumors show similar T1 and T2 imaging features and reveal heterogeneous solid enhancement after contrast.[229,291,302] Surgery may be the only chance for cure and requires resection of the primary tumor and liver and lymph node metastases if possible.[293]

Nonfunctioning islet cell tumors may be discovered incidentally, or the patient may have abdominal pain secondary to mass effect or metastatic disease[292] (Box 2-20). Nonhyperfunctioning neuroendocrine tumors are typically large (6–10 cm) and show foci of cystic degeneration and necrosis on T2-WI with associated heterogeneous enhancement (see Fig. 2-21).[289,303] Greater than 50% of tumors are malignant, show local invasion and distant metastases, and have a poorer prognosis than hyperfunctioning tumors.[294,295]

Most patients with functioning islet cell tumors are diagnosed on clinical grounds, and the role of imaging is to localize and stage the lesion. However, larger nonfunctioning tumors can be shown in asymptomatic patients and have a wide differential diagnosis that includes adenocarcinoma, mucinous cystic tumor, metastases, and solid pseudopapillary tumor of the pancreas (SPT). Certain distinguishing imaging and clinical features of the tumors may help characterize such lesions.[292,304-309]

Islet cell tumors most commonly metastasize to the liver, bones, and adjacent lymph nodes.[310,311] Variables associated with a poorer prognosis include liver metastases (most significant factor), lack of complete resection of the primary tumor, lymph node metastases, local invasion of the tumor, primary tumor size of 3 cm, and nonfunctioning tumor.[295] Patients without metastatic disease are medically stabilized prior to undergoing surgery. Initial management for patients with metastatic disease is expectant observation and control of hormonal symptoms.[287] The primary tumor and hepatic metastases in asymptomatic patients are followed with serial imaging every 3 to 6 months. Hepatic artery embolization, surgical resection, radiotherapy, and chemotherapy can be considered for patients with uncontrollable pain, hormonal symptoms, or rapid tumor progression.[287,293,312]

PANCREATIC ACINAR CELL CARCINOMA

Acinar cell carcinoma of the pancreas is a rare malignancy, accounting for 1% of pancreatic exocrine tumors and occurring predominantly in men.[313] The neoplasm is occasionally associated with a syndrome of subcutaneous and intraosseous fat necrosis and polyarthralgia secondary to the release of lipase that results in hydrolysis of fat.[313-315] Osseous lesions of metastatic fat necrosis manifest as multiple lytic foci of the distal extremities.[314] Imaging findings of the primary tumor are nonspecific and can range from a large mass with an enhancing capsule and areas of necrosis to a hyperenhancing mass similar to a functioning neuroendocrine tumor.[316,317] Acinar cell carcinomas are aggressive but survival rates are slightly better than those of ductal adenocarcinoma.[313]

PRIMARY PANCREATIC LYMPHOMA

Unlike Hodgkin's disease, which rarely spreads outside the lymphatic system, non-Hodgkin's lymphoma (NHL) frequently involves extranodal sites such as the gastrointestinal tract. In 30% of NHL patients with extranodal disease, the pancreas is secondarily involved in the setting of confluent retroperitoneal and periaortic lymphadenopathy (Fig. 2-23). Isolated primary pancreatic lymphoma is rare and accounts for less than 1% of extranodal non-Hodgkin's lymphomas arising in the pancreas.[318] Diagnostic criteria for primary pancreatic lymphoma include predominantly a pancreatic mass, no hepatic or splenic involvement, no mediastinal or superficial palpable lymphadenopathy, and a normal leukocyte count.[319]

The most common MR finding of pancreatic lymphoma is that of extensive abdominal lymphadenopathy with direct extension and infiltration of the pancreas. The lymph nodes and infiltrated pancreas have similar SI and enhancement patterns, showing lower SI than normal pancreas on T1-W, variable SI on T2-W, and less enhancement than normal pancreatic parenchyma (see Fig. 2-23).[229,319,320] Both tumors can cause ductal obstruction and involve the fat around the celiac and superior mesenteric arteries.[320] However, the degree of ductal dilation is not so marked in lymphoma,[319] and lymphadenopathy below the level of the renal veins is more indicative of pancreatic lymphoma.[319,320]

Distinguishing between an intrinsic pancreatic lymphoma and pancreatic invasion from adjacent lymphadenopathy can be challenging but is not an important clinical distinction because treatment is similar for both.[320] However, differentiating between lymphoma and pancreatic adenocarcinoma is clinically relevant, since lymphoma has a better prognosis; almost one third of patients with pancreatic lymphoma have a successful response to chemotherapy.[319] Nonsurgical biopsy is ideal to establish a diagnosis of pancreatic lymphoma because, unlike adenocarcinoma, lymphoma does not require surgical staging or a Whipple procedure.[318,319]

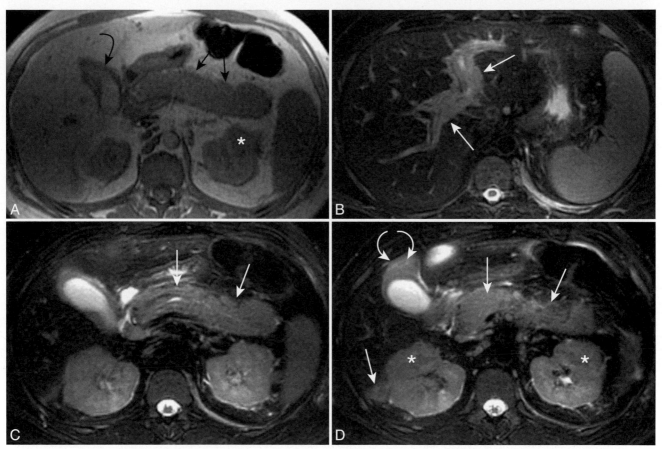

Figure 2-23 ■ **MR findings of lymphomatous infiltration of the pancreas, liver, gallbladder, and kidneys in a 28-year-old man. A**, Axial in-phase T1-WI shows mild diffuse enlargement of the pancreas *(arrows)* that has abnormal, low SI. Abnormal soft tissue also is present anterior to the gallbladder *(curved arrow)* and within the anterior aspect of the left kidney (*). **B–D**, Three axial fat-suppressed T2-WIs show diffuse high SI of the portal veins and periportal soft issues *(arrows in **B**)*, pancreas, *(arrows in **C** and **D**)*, pericholecystic soft tissues *(curved arrows)* and right perirenal fat, and anterior aspect of the parenchyma of both left and right kidneys (* in **D**). This patient also had disseminated lymphoma of bone marrow and central nervous system.

PANCREATIC METASTASES

Metastatic lesions to the pancreas are uncommon and may appear long after the primary malignancy is diagnosed. The most frequently involved tumors are those with hematogenous spread such as renal cell carcinoma (30% of cases); bronchogenic, breast, and colon carcinoma; and melanoma.[305,321] Solitary metastases are more characteristic of renal cell carcinoma, whereas lung cancer and melanoma tend to diffusely involve the pancreas.[321] Distinguishing between metastasis and primary adenocarcinoma is important because the former has a better prognosis. Metastases tend to enhance homogeneously or heterogeneously, whereas primary pancreatic adenocarcinomas are relatively hypovascular due to their desmoplastic content. Arterial encasement from extrapancreatic extension of metastatic tumor is also relatively uncommon compared with primary pancreatic carcinoma.[305]

Certain metastases have MR imaging findings that are highly suggestive of the diagnosis especially in the setting of a known primary malignancy.

Melanoma lesions can reveal high T1 SI owing to the presence of intratumoral hemorrhage or the paramagnetic properties of melanin (see Fig. 5-1).[322] Metastases from clear cell renal carcinoma may show loss of SI on opposed-phase GRE images compared with corresponding in-phase images, indicating the presence of intracellular lipid, which can be present in primary or metastatic clear cell renal cancer but not in primary pancreatic malignancies (Fig. 2-24).[306] Pancreatic renal cell cancer metastases reveal high T2 SI, show hyperintensity on dynamic MR imaging, and may be difficult to distinguish from nonfunctioning neuroendocrine tumors.[304] However, the presence of a hypervascular pancreatic tumor (especially with loss of SI on chemical shift MRI) in a patient with a history of renal cell cancer should be considered metastasis until proved otherwise.

Cystic Lesions of the Pancreas

Cystic lesions of the pancreas are frequently revealed on abdominal MR examinations (Box 2-21).

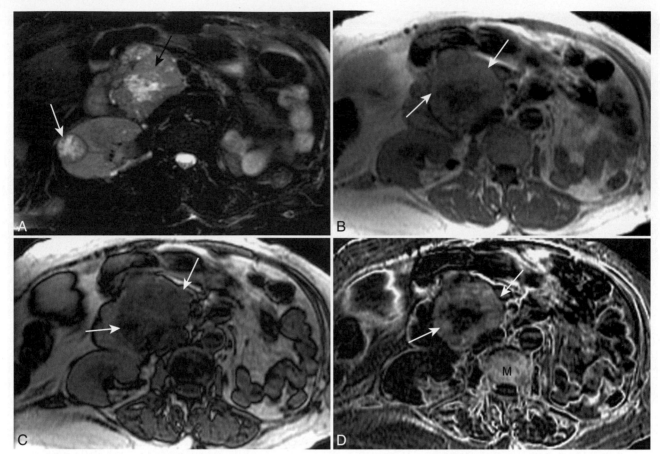

Figure 2-24 ■ **Chemical shift MR findings of metastatic clear cell carcinoma of the pancreas in a woman with prior left nephrectomy and established metastatic renal cell carcinoma at other sites (same patient as in Fig. 3-8). A**, Fat-suppressed T2-WI shows a large heterogeneous pancreatic head mass *(black arrow)* and a similar-appearing right renal mass *(white arrow)*. The pancreatic tumor has a similar appearance to a neuroendocrine tumor (see Fig. 2-21). **B** and **C**, In-phase and opposed-phase T1-WIs show the loss of SI within the mass *(arrows)* in **C**. This establishes the presence of the intratumoral lipid. On adjacent images (not shown), the renal lesion also showed loss of SI, in keeping with clear cell renal cell carcinoma. **D**, Postprocessed subtraction image (in phase – opposed phase) provides a map of those voxels that contain both water and lipid protons. High SI is present within the solid portions of the pancreatic metastases *(arrows)* and within bone marrow (M).

2-21	Differential Diagnosis of Cystic Pancreatic Lesions

Nonneoplastic Cysts

Pseudocysts (very common; 80%–90% of all
   pancreatic cysts)
Hydatid cyst (rare)

Cystic Neoplasms: 10%–15% of Pancreatic "Cysts"

Serous cystadenoma
Mucinous cystic neoplasms
Intraductal papillary mucinous tumor (IPMT)
Solid and papillary epithelial neoplasm (SPEN):
   cystic subtype
Cystic neuroendocrine neoplasm

True Cysts and Associated Diseases

Von Hippel–Lindau disease
Adult polycystic disease
Cystic fibrosis

Other

Duodenal diverticula

The prevalence of small (<10 mm) pancreatic cysts present on heavily T2-WI is 20% and is higher in patients with pancreatitis.[323] The most common cystic mass of the pancreas is a pseudocyst that accounts for 75% to 85% of pancreatic cysts.[324-326] Congenital true cysts (having true epithelium lining the inner surface) tend to be multiple and are associated with hereditary disorders.[324] Cystic neoplasms are less common and account for only 10% to 15% of all cystic pancreatic masses. While not a pancreatic lesion, duodenal diverticula occasionally mimic a cystic pancreatic mass.[327] The presence of intralesional gas and typical paraduodenal location allow distinction from a pancreatic cyst in most instances.

SEROUS CYSTADENOMA (BOX 2-22)

Serous cystadenomas (microcystic adenomas) are benign pancreatic neoplasms composed of a central fibrous scar and multiple predominantly small (<2 cm), thin-walled cysts lined by glycogen-rich serous cells.[328,329] Serous cystadenomas comprise approximately 25% of cystic neoplasms and mainly affect

2-22   Features of Serous Cystadenoma of the Pancreas

Clinical/Pathology

F:M = 1.5:1
Age range: 50–80 yr
Size range: 1-13 cm, median size 5–6 cm
Located in all pancreatic segments; slight
   predominance in pancreatic head
Multiple cysts (>6), most <2 cm
Multiple thin septa
Consider observation if small in size and asymptomatic

MRI

Serous cysts follow fluid SI and do not enhance
Septa and central scar do enhance
Central calcification (better revealed by CT)

older women although an association does exist with von Hippel–Lindau disease.[325,328,330,331] Eighty percent of patients are 60 years of age or older at the time of diagnosis. The majority are asymptomatic. However, some may have signs or symptoms such as abdominal pain, weight loss, or palpable abdominal mass.[246,328] Tumors are well circumscribed and range in size from 1 to 13 cm (average 5 cm).[246] Serous cystadenomas are distributed throughout the pancreas with a slight predilection for the pancreatic head.[328] They are hypervascular secondary to a rich subepithelial capillary network and show no arterial encasement.[332] While uncommon,[333] the pancreaticobiliary tree can be displaced or obstructed by the tumor secondary to mass effect.[328]

The MR appearance of a typical serous cystadenoma is that of a round, well-circumscribed pancreatic mass that is composed of more than six cysts, each less than 2 cm, with very high T2 and low T1 SI (Figs. 2-25 and 2-26; see also cover of text).[324,334-336] Spontaneous hemorrhage within some of the cysts is uncommon but may result in foci of high SI on T1-WI.[336] The small cysts and intervening septa look like a "cluster of grapes" on T2-WI. The intratumoral septa are most clearly depicted on breathing-independent T2-WI owing to the elimination of blurring that can occur with breathing-averaged T2-W sequences.[246] The tumor septations and cyst wall usually show minimal enhancement on early and delayed gadolinium-enhanced images. The central fibrous scar is hypointense on T1-WI and shows variable enhancement that can persist on delayed (3-5 min) CE imaging.[335,336] Calcification within the central scar is present in 25% of tumors and is better depicted by CT than MR.[246,337,338]

Patients with a serous cystadenoma who develop symptoms such as abdominal pain, jaundice, or recurrent pancreatitis should probably undergo surgical resection.[329] A serous cystadenocarcinoma is rare and cannot be differentiated from its more common benign counterpart unless local invasion or distant metastases are present. Thus, some suggest that typical serous cystadenomas on imaging be surgically removed if the patient is an operative candidate.[339] Others suggest that serous cystadenomas that are well characterized on imaging studies be followed with imaging if the patient is asymptomatic.[329,340]

MUCINOUS CYSTIC NEOPLASM (BOX 2-23)

Mucinous cystic neoplasms are uncommon primary cystic tumors of the pancreas that are considered potentially malignant and surgically treated lesions. Histologically, they represent a continuum ranging from benign mucinous cystadenoma to borderline tumor with malignant potential to frankly malignant mucinous cystadenocarcinoma. They are composed of mucin-producing columnar cells and an overlying ovarian-type stroma that can have thick fibrous walls with papillary projections.[332,341-343] Mucinous cystic neoplasms predominantly affect women (>95% of cases) at an earlier age (fourth to sixth decades) than do serous cystadenomas.[246,325,329,341] Mucinous cystic neoplasms have an average diameter of 6 to 10 cm and three fourths of lesions are located in the pancreatic body or tail.[246,329,332,341-344] Patients can be asymptomatic or have symptoms of mass effect that include abdominal pain, fullness, and anorexia. Some patients have a history of pancreatitis, resulting in misdiagnosis of the neoplasm as a pseudocyst.[345,346]

On MR a mucinous cystic tumor appears as a unilocular cyst (Fig. 2-27) or a multilocular cystic mass with individual cysts measuring greater than 2 cm (Fig. 2-28).[246,334] T1-WIs show variable SI with simple fluid showing low SI while hemorrhagic or proteinaceous/mucinous fluid reveals varying degrees of higher SI.[332,335,336,341] T2-WIs depict the cysts as high SI and internal septations and papillary projections as lower in SI.[332,336] Just as for serous cystadenomas, the septations of mucinous tumors are best visualized on breathing-independent T2-WI.[246] MRCP can show that mucinous cystic neoplasms do not communicate with the pancreatic duct.[343,347,348] The septa, cyst wall, papillary projections, and solid mural nodules enhance.[246,332,336,346]

If calcification is present, it is located peripherally in the wall or septa of the lesion and is better shown on CT.[335,341,342] Certain imaging features are more predictive of malignancy and include a thick wall or septa, calcifications in the wall or septa, and solid mural nodules.[337,344,349] Obstruction of the pancreatic duct is more common with malignant cystic lesions.[333] Adjacent organ invasion or hepatic metastases are more specific for malignancy.[346] A large unilocular or multilocular cystic mass in the pancreatic body or tail in a middle-aged woman without a history of pancreatitis is characteristic of a mucinous cystic neoplasm (see Figs. 2-27 and 2-28).

The differential diagnosis of mucinous cystic neoplasm includes all cystic masses of the pancreas, but the most important diagnostic consideration is a pseudocyst that represents up to 85% of all cystic pancreatic lesions. Pseudocysts usually change in

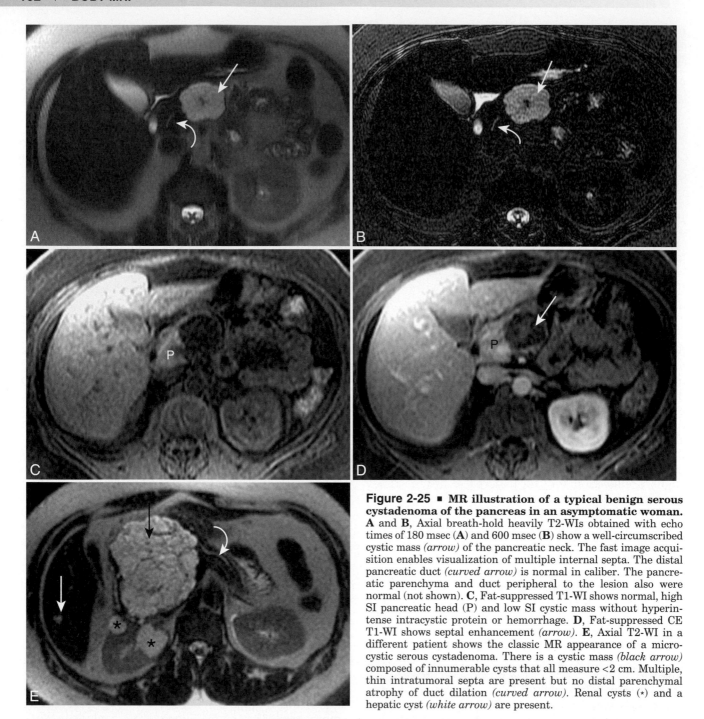

Figure 2-25 ▪ **MR illustration of a typical benign serous cystadenoma of the pancreas in an asymptomatic woman.** **A** and **B**, Axial breath-hold heavily T2-WIs obtained with echo times of 180 msec (**A**) and 600 msec (**B**) show a well-circumscribed cystic mass *(arrow)* of the pancreatic neck. The fast image acquisition enables visualization of multiple internal septa. The distal pancreatic duct *(curved arrow)* is normal in caliber. The pancreatic parenchyma and duct peripheral to the lesion also were normal (not shown). **C**, Fat-suppressed T1-WI shows normal, high SI pancreatic head (P) and low SI cystic mass without hyperintense intracystic protein or hemorrhage. **D**, Fat-suppressed CE T1-WI shows septal enhancement *(arrow)*. **E**, Axial T2-WI in a different patient shows the classic MR appearance of a microcystic serous cystadenoma. There is a cystic mass *(black arrow)* composed of innumerable cysts that all measure <2 cm. Multiple, thin intratumoral septa are present but no distal parenchymal atrophy of duct dilation *(curved arrow)*. Renal cysts (∗) and a hepatic cyst *(white arrow)* are present.

appearance over time and are associated with peripancreatic inflammatory changes and characteristic ductal abnormalities, but these ancillary findings can coexist with mucinous tumors.[236,237,343,346] If misdiagnosed as a pseudocyst and drained, a mucinous cystic neoplasm will recur or metastasize.[344]

If imaging or serum tumor markers (e.g., CA 19-9, which has sensitivity of 75% and specificity of 96% in detecting mucinous tumors and pancreatic adenocarcinoma) cannot establish a diagnosis, then cyst aspiration may help differentiate a mucinous cystic neoplasm from other lesions.[264,329,334,350] Cytologic assessment of mucin-containing epithelium has sensitivity of 48% and specificity of 100% in distinguishing a mucinous cystic tumor from a pseudocyst and often is accompanied by cyst fluid biochemical analysis.[264] The presence of mucin, high relative viscosity (compared with that of serum), and

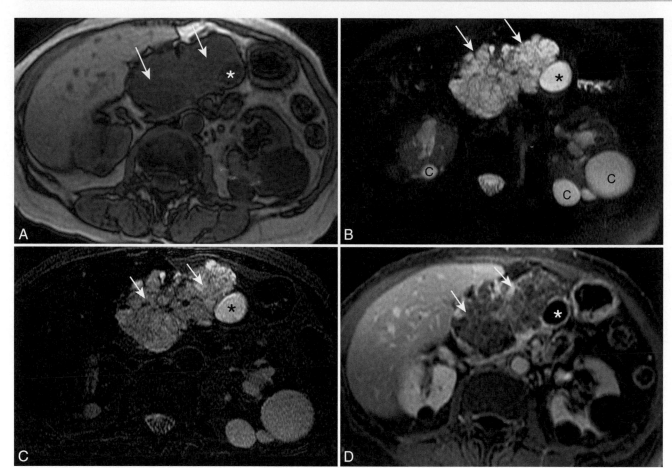

Figure 2-26 ■ MR findings of a microcystic adenoma in an 84-year-old woman. Diagnosis was established by aspiration cytologic study. Surgical excision was avoided. **A**, T1-WI shows a multilocular mass of the pancreatic body *(arrows)*. The lowest SI component is present along the lateral margin (*). Renal cysts are present. **B** and **C**, Axial breath-hold heavily T2-WIs (TE = 180 msec in **B** and 500 msec in **C**) reveal a cystic mass *(arrows)* of the pancreatic body that contains innumerable cysts measuring <2 cm and multiple internal septations. The adjacent "cyst" (*) along the lateral margin of the mass represents a dilated peripheral pancreatic duct (confirmed on other images). The duct dilation is due to extrinsic compression and is not secondary to communication with the duct. Bilateral renal cysts (C) are present. **D**, CE fat-suppressed T1-WI shows internal septal enhancement of the septa. The close approximation of the internal septa *(arrows)* explains why serous microcystic adenomas may appear solid on sonography or CT.

2-23 Features of Mucinous Cystic Neoplasm of the Pancreas

Clinical/Pathology

F:M = 4:1
Age range: fourth to sixth decades
Size range: 3–36 cm, median size 6–10 cm
Body and tail: 75% of lesions
Unilocular or multilocular with individual cysts >2 cm
All are potentially malignant and require surgical resection

MRI

Variable SI on T1-W due to protein/mucin or hemorrhage
Septa, cyst wall, papillary projections, solid nodules enhance
Peripheral calcification (better revealed by CT)

high levels of CEA and CA 72-4 in cyst fluid can be useful in differentiating mucinous lesions with sensitivities of 40% to 100% for CEA and 80% for CA 72-4 from pseudocysts and serous cystadenomas.[264,334,350] Once the diagnosis of a mucinous cystic neoplasm of the pancreas is suggested, complete operative resection is indicated because of the known malignant potential of mucinous neoplasms.[246,325,341,342]

INTRADUCTAL PAPILLARY MUCINOUS TUMOR OF THE PANCREAS (BOX 2-24)

Intraductal papillary mucinous tumor of the pancreas (IPMT) is a spectrum of neoplasms composed of mucinous cells lining the main pancreatic duct or side branches. It is a premalignant disorder that is also called mucinous ductal ectasia, ductectatic cystadenoma, and intraductal mucin-hypersecreting tumor.[329,351] However, the term IPMT is thought to reflect its main morphologic features of intraductal

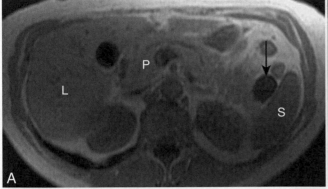

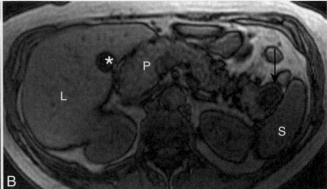

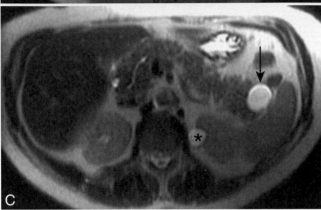

Figure 2-27 ■ MR findings of a unilocular mucinous cystadenoma. Neither pathologic studies nor follow-up imaging suggest malignant disease. **A** and **B**, Axial opposed-phase (**A**) and in-phase (**B**) T1-WIs show normal SI liver (L), spleen (S), and pancreas (P). There is susceptibility artifact from surgical clips in the gallbladder fossa (*white ⋆*). A unilocular cyst *(arrow)* is present in the pancreatic tail without internal hyperintensity, solid components, or adjacent abnormalities of the pancreatic parenchyma. **C**, Breath-hold T2-WI reveals a nonaggressive unilocular cyst *(arrow)* without internal debris or solid components. No solid or suspect enhancement was revealed after contrast (not shown). Microscopic mucinous cell and ovarian stroma were present in the lining of the cyst at subsequent surgery. Because there were no imaging findings of acute or chronic pancreatitis, pseudocyst was not diagnosed at imaging. A renal cyst (*black ⋆*) is present.

papillomatous growth and excess mucin secretion.[352,353] IPMT has two subtypes: main duct IPMT and side branch IPMT.

IPMT of the main pancreatic duct can be difficult to diagnose because it mimics the clinical and imaging findings of chronic pancreatitis. There is no gender predilection, and the peak age is in the sixth decade. Patients may have abdominal pain or recurrent episodes of acute pancreatitis secondary to duct obstruction by thick mucin or tumor.[354] The main pancreatic duct can be diffusely or segmentally involved with progressive duct dilation and parenchymal atrophy. ERCP findings include a bulging or patulous orifice of the papilla of Vater with secretion of mucin through this orifice, mucinous filling defects, and dilated main duct and side branches in the absence of an obstructing stricture.[352,355,356] Thick mucous can prevent adequate evaluation of the ducts on ERCP.

MRCP-MRI has been shown to be more effective than ERCP and CT in depicting the entire ductal system and demonstrating septa and mural nodules in patients with IPMT (Fig. 2-29).[347,354,357-362] The enlarged major papilla may be shown to protrude into the duodenal lumen on MRI.[363] The mucin-filled, dilated ducts show high T2 and variable T1 SI that depends on the hydration of the mucin.[336] Main duct tumors can result in moderate dilation of the entire pancreatic duct to the level of the ampulla.[336,359] Low SI filling defects on MRCP sequences represent papillary projections or mural nodules (see Fig. 2-29); extracellular mucin tends to have SI similar to that of pancreatic juice.[359,360,362,364,365] Contrast is useful because mural nodules enhance whereas mucin does not (see Fig. 2-29).[365] The detection of the mural nodules

2-24 Intraductal Papillary Mucinous Tumor of the Pancreas (IPMT)

Main Duct

M = F

Peak age in sixth decade

MRI/MRCP

   Moderate dilatation of mucin-filled main pancreatic duct

   Enhancing papillary projections and mural nodules

   Mural nodules and duct diameter >15 mm suggest malignancy

Treatment: surgical resection

Side Branch

M > F

Peak in sixth to seventh decades

Microcystic or macrocystic pattern

MRI/MRCP

   Communicates with normal caliber duct

   Mural nodule, cyst > 3 cm, and main duct dilation suggest malignancy; requires surgery

   Lesion <2.5 cm with thin wall, no solid component, and normal main duct can be followed with imaging

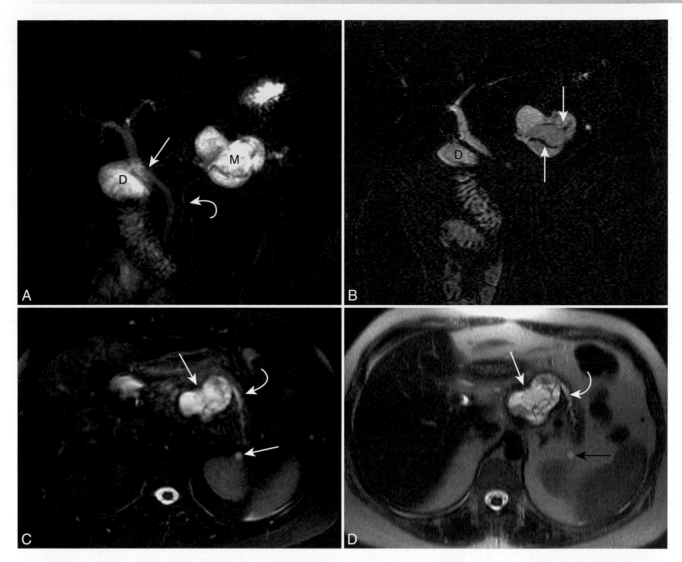

Figure 2-28 ▪ **MR illustration of a multilocular mucinous cystadenocarcinoma of the pancreas in a 41-year-old woman with abdominal pain.** This cystic pancreatic lesion required surgery for the following reasons: <6 loculi, thick enhancing septa, peripheral pancreatic duct dilation, and presence of pain. **A,** Coronal thick-slab single-slice MRCP shows a cystic mass of the pancreatic body (M) with peripheral pancreatic duct dilation *(curved arrow)*. The cystic structure adjacent to the duodenum was shown to represent a duodenal diverticulum (D) on other images and did not represent an additional cystic pancreatic mass. The central pancreatic duct *(arrow)* and common bile duct are normal. **B,** Thin-slice MRCP better reveals the internal architecture of the cyst, showing thick septa *(arrows)* and cyst SI that is hypointense to fluid within the common bile duct and the adjacent duodenal diverticulum. **C,** Fat-suppressed T2-WI redemonstrates the multilocular pancreatic cyst *(arrow)* and peripheral duct dilation *(curved arrow)*. There is poor contrast between the normal pancreatic parenchyma and adjacent suppressed fat. A subcentimeter left renal cyst is present *(arrow)*. **D,** Corresponding heavily T2-WI (TE = 180) obtained without fat saturation shows that the cyst contents do not follow the SI of normal fluid. There is better contrast between normal pancreas and surrounding fat, since fat suppression was not used. Volume averaging of an exophytic 3-mm renal cyst is present *(arrow).*   *(Continued)*

can help distinguish IPMT from focal duct dilation of chronic pancreatitis.[354]

At the time of diagnosis, 30% to 40% of patients with main duct IPMT have invasive malignancy and the remainder have atypia, dysplasia, or carcinoma in situ.[329,355,366] Any suspected main branch IPMT should be resected. Specifically, the presence of mural nodules, size larger than 3 cm, interval growth, or main pancreatic duct dilation greater than 7 mm within any IPMT is suspicious for malignancy and necessitates surgical excision.[367,368]

Side branch IPMTs appear as cystic masses that are frequently located in the pancreatic head/uncinate process and demonstrate a macrocystic or microcystic pattern (Fig. 2-30).[358,369] Mucin distends the side branch duct to create the cystic lesion, and the adjacent parenchyma atrophies to become the capsule of the mass.[343] IPMTs occur more commonly in men aged 60 to 70 years.[348] The microcystic pattern consists of a cluster of 1- to 2-mm cysts separated by thin septa, resembling a serous cystadenoma. Demonstrating a communication between the mass and the main duct suggests a diagnosis of an IPMT.[359] The macrocystic form has a unilocular or multilocular architecture that can mimic a mucinous cystic neoplasm or pseudocyst (see Fig. 2-30). An IPMT, however, communicates with the main pancreatic duct, which distinguishes it from a mucinous cystic tumor, and may contain enhancing papillary projections, which differentiates it from a pseudocyst.[363]

In the early stages of disease, the mass is small and lobulated and often eccentric in position with respect to the visualized or expected location of the main pancreatic duct.[370] If the lesion seeds the main duct, the typical findings of main duct IPMT develop including diffuse main and side branch duct dilation and bulging of the papilla into the duodenum. In general, the side branch lesions are associated with less aggressive histologic features.[371]

With the advent of high-resolution cross-sectional imaging, small (<25 mm) cystic pancreatic lesions are not uncommonly detected when imaging is performed for clinical indications not referable to the pancreas.

Although the differential diagnosis of a cystic lesion can be extensive, it has been suggested that the majority of these small lesions represent side branch IPMTs.[370,372,373] However, a history of acute or chronic pancreatitis should be elicited to ensure that a lesion does not represent a small pseudocyst. An IPMT smaller than 2.5 cm with a thin wall and normal-appearing main pancreatic duct can be monitored safely by serial imaging.[363,370,374-376] In one series of resected IPMTs, all side branch lesions that were less than 3 cm and lacked mural nodules were benign.[377] If follow-up imaging shows growth, solid components, or main duct involvement, then surgical resection should be considered.[370]

SOLID-PSEUDOPAPILLARY TUMOR OF THE PANCREAS (BOX 2-25)

Solid-pseudopapillary tumor of the pancreas (SPT) is an uncommon low-grade malignant neoplasm found predominantly in young women (especially African American and Asian).[309,378,379] The mean age of presentation is 25 years of age with 85% of lesions presenting by 30 years.[309,379,380] Macroscopically, the tumor is a large (3-17 cm, mean of 9 cm), well-encapsulated mass with an internal architecture that varies from solid to a mixture of solid and cystic to a

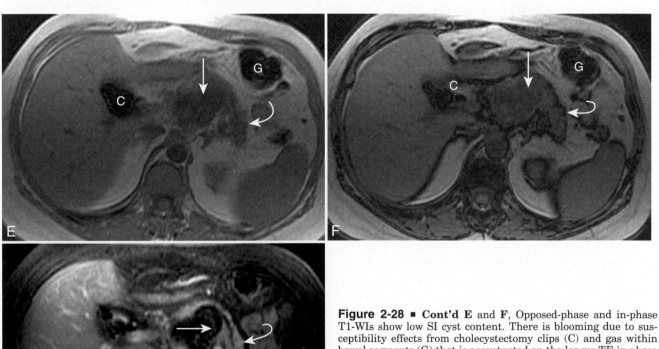

Figure 2-28 ▪ Cont'd E and **F**, Opposed-phase and in-phase T1-WIs show low SI cyst content. There is blooming due to susceptibility effects from cholecystectomy clips (C) and gas within bowel segments (G) that is accentuated on the longer TE in-phase image. There is decreased T1 SI of the pancreas peripheral to the mass, in keeping with obstructive pancreatopathy. **G,** CE fat-suppressed T1-WI shows enhancing internal septa within the lesion (*horizontal arrow*).

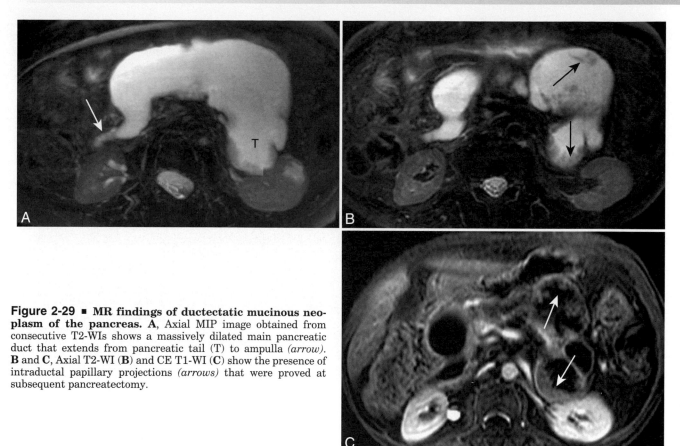

Figure 2-29 ■ MR findings of ductectatic mucinous neoplasm of the pancreas. A, Axial MIP image obtained from consecutive T2-WIs shows a massively dilated main pancreatic duct that extends from pancreatic tail (T) to ampulla *(arrow)*. **B** and **C**, Axial T2-WI (**B**) and CE T1-WI (**C**) show the presence of intraductal papillary projections *(arrows)* that were proved at subsequent pancreatectomy.

thick-walled cyst.[309,378] A suggestive imaging and histologic feature is that of intratumoral hemorrhage followed by cystic degeneration secondary to disruption of a delicate intratumoral vascular network.[309,378]

MR imaging shows the complex internal architecture of an SPT and depicts areas of hemorrhagic necrosis in either the solid or cystic component of the

mass as being of high SI on T1-WI and of variable SI on T2-WI, reflecting the presence of blood degradation products such as methemoglobin.[309,378-380] Hemorrhagic cystic degeneration can also present as a fluid-debris level (hematocrit effect).[309] The tumor is surrounded by a fibrous capsule that is of low SI on T1- and T2-WI.[308,309,378] Infrequent peripheral calcification is better shown on CT.[309,378,380] These tumors have no preferential location in the pancreas.

The most common imaging and gross histologic finding of SPT is that of a mixed solid and cystic lesion with areas of hemorrhagic necrosis (Fig. 2-31). The primary differential diagnostic consideration is a nonfunctioning cystic islet tumor. While both entities are managed surgically, an SPT is favored in a young African American woman.[309,378] Complete surgical resection can ensure cure before potential malignant transformation.[380]

Hereditary Conditions Involving the Pancreas

CYSTIC FIBROSIS

Cystic fibrosis is an autosomal recessive disease characterized by exocrine gland dysfunction that results in pulmonary infections and progressive pancreatic insufficiency in 85% of affected children.[381] Precipitation of secretions in the small pancreatic ducts result in fatty and fibrous degeneration that

---

2-25   Features of Solid-pseudopapillary Tumor of the Pancreas (SPT)

Clinical/Pathology

Predominantly affects young women, aged 20–30 yr
African American and Asian > white
Classic pattern of mixed solid and cystic mass;
    mean size 9 cm
Treatment; surgical resection, since tumor is a
    low-grade malignancy

MRI

Areas of high SI on T1-WI = hemorrhage necrosis
Fluid-debris or fluid-fluid levels
Fibrous capsule of low SI on T1 and T2-WI

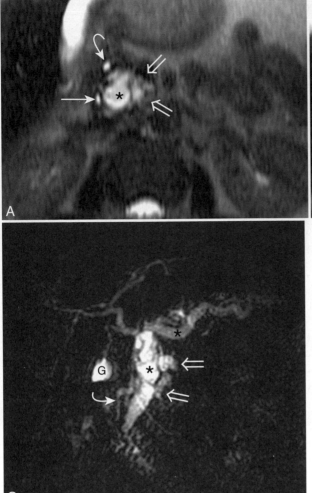

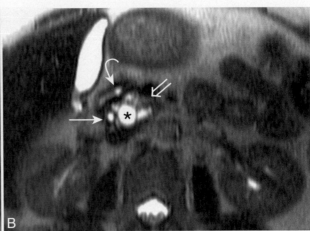

Figure 2-30 ■ **MR illustration of a side branch intrapapillary mucinous tumor. A** and **B,** Two axial T2-WIs (TE = 188) show a multilocular cystic mass of the medial aspect of the low pancreatic head *(arrows)* that communicates with a dilated pancreatic duct depicted in cross section (*). A patent accessory duct also is present *(curved arrow).* **C,** Projection MRCP (slice thickness = 40 mm, TE = 780) shows the diffuse dilated pancreatic duct (*), accessory duct *(curved arrow),* and separate cystic low pancreatic head mass *(open arrows).* Fluid is present within the gallbladder (G). A cystic mucinous neoplasm or microcystic cystadenoma was considered less likely because of the communication with the pancreatic duct. The lack of intracystic protein, hemorrhage, or debris and lack of interval change for 1 year (prior study not shown) argue against a pseudocyst. Because the patient had pain and neoplasm could not be excluded, surgery was performed that confirmed a side branch IPMT. The remainder of the pancreas revealed chronic pancreatitis. No neoplastic seeding was seen within the main pancreatic duct.

leads to the exocrine dysfunction.[381] The resultant T1 SI of the pancreas depends on the proportions of fat (which has a short T1) and mature fibrosis (which has a long T1) that have replaced the parenchyma. The most common pattern is that of diffuse fatty replacement in an enlarged, lobulated pancreas (Fig. 2-32).[381-383] Rarely, the pancreas is markedly enlarged by multiple nodular fatty masses, an entity referred to as lipomatous pseudohypertrophy.[382,384]

Pancreatic cysts are common in cystic fibrosis and tend to be small (1-3 mm). Small calcific concretions present within dilated ducts are better depicted on CT.[384] Associated abnormalities involving the biliary system include bile duct strictures, cystic duct stenosis or atresia, and microgallbladder.[384]

HEMOCHROMATOSIS

Hemochromatosis is an autosomal recessive disorder of iron storage in which there is progressive accumulation of iron in parenchymal organs, such as the liver (hepatocytes) and pancreas, and to a lesser extent in the endocrine glands and myocardium,

resulting in organ dysfunction (see Chapter 1).[385] The reticuloendothelial system of the liver (Kupffer cells), spleen, and bone marrow are normal and do not accumulate excess iron. This is in contrast to transfusional iron overload in which there is reticuloendothelial iron deposition and sparing of the parenchymal organs.

Just as in the liver, the pancreas can show decreased SI (less than that of skeletal muscle) on T2- or T1-WI secondary to the paramagnetic effects of iron. The presence of iron can be confirmed as low SI in the gland on an iron-sensitive T2*-weighted GRE sequence (see Fig. 1-22B).[386,387] In patients with genetic hemochromatosis, the iron is deposited in the beta cells of the pancreas and can result in glucose intolerance and overt diabetes.[388] The spleen, however, is of normal SI because the reticuloendothelial cells do not accumulate iron, even in the setting of total body iron overload.[386] A pancreas of low SI, cirrhotic liver of low SI, and spleen of normal SI on T2-WI are suggestive of genetic hemochromatosis (see Fig. 1-22).[385,387]

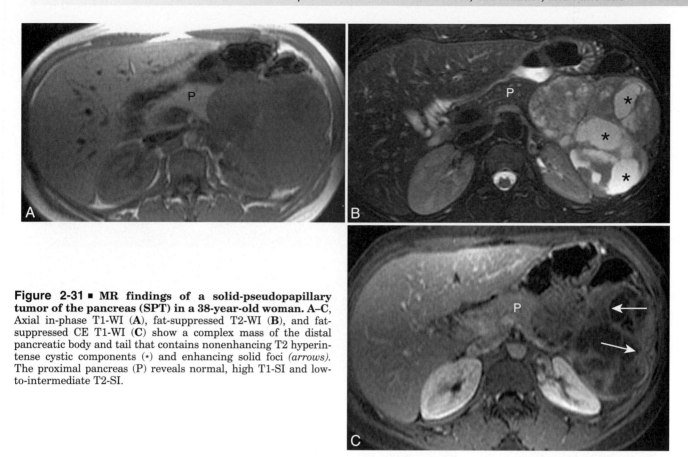

Figure 2-31 ■ **MR findings of a solid-pseudopapillary tumor of the pancreas (SPT) in a 38-year-old woman. A–C,** Axial in-phase T1-WI (**A**), fat-suppressed T2-WI (**B**), and fat-suppressed CE T1-WI (**C**) show a complex mass of the distal pancreatic body and tail that contains nonenhancing T2 hyperintense cystic components (∗) and enhancing solid foci *(arrows).* The proximal pancreas (P) reveals normal, high T1-SI and low-to-intermediate T2-SI.

Von Hippel–Lindau Disease

Von Hippel–Lindau (VHL) disease is an autosomal dominant disease characterized by central nervous system hemangioblastomas and visceral tumors including renal cell carcinomas (see Chapter 4), pheochromocytomas (see Chapter 3), solid and cystic pancreatic lesions, and epididymal cystadenomas.[331] Most pancreatic lesions are asymptomatic and discovered during screening of family members and may precede any other manifestation of VHL disease by several years.[389,390] The two most common pancreatic lesions in patients with VHL disease are benign and include true cysts (single or multiple), and serous cystadenomas (discussed above). Less common pancreatic neoplasms include neuroendocrine tumors[330,331,390,391] and metastatic renal cell carcinoma. Multiple pancreatic cysts are highly suggestive of VHL disease, especially in light of a positive family history, and occur in more than 70% of affected patients.[392] The pancreatic cysts in VHL disease can replace or enlarge the gland (Fig. 2-33).

Nonfunctional neuroendocrine tumors occur in approximately 15% of patients with VHL disease. A solid, enhancing pancreatic mass in a patient with VHL disease is likely to be a neuroendocrine neoplasm.[330,392] The most common imaging findings of neuroendocrine tumors in the patient with VHL disease is that of a less than 3 cm solid, enhancing mass

of the pancreatic head.[391] Although the cystic pancreatic disease of VHL is benign, the solid islet cell tumors can exhibit malignant behavior when larger than 3 cm.[331,392] Presumed pancreatic neuroendocrine tumors in patients with VHL disease that are about 1 cm are followed every 12 months by cross-sectional imaging. Lesions between 1 and 3 cm are managed depending on location (pancreatic head lesions are removed if they reach 2 cm and body/tail lesions can be resected when they reach 2-3 cm). Masses greater than 3 cm and symptomatic lesions undergo resection with an enucleation procedure when possible.[392]

Pancreatitis

Acute Pancreatitis

Pancreatitis is the most common benign disease affecting the pancreas and is classified as acute or chronic on the basis of clinical, morphologic, and histologic criteria. Acute pancreatitis is a complex disease with a clinical spectrum varying from mild inflammation to fulminant disease that may be complicated by necrosis, hemorrhage, and infection. Abdominal pain and elevated serum amylase and lipase suggest the diagnosis. There are a variety of causes but the most common include alcohol abuse and cholelithiasis.

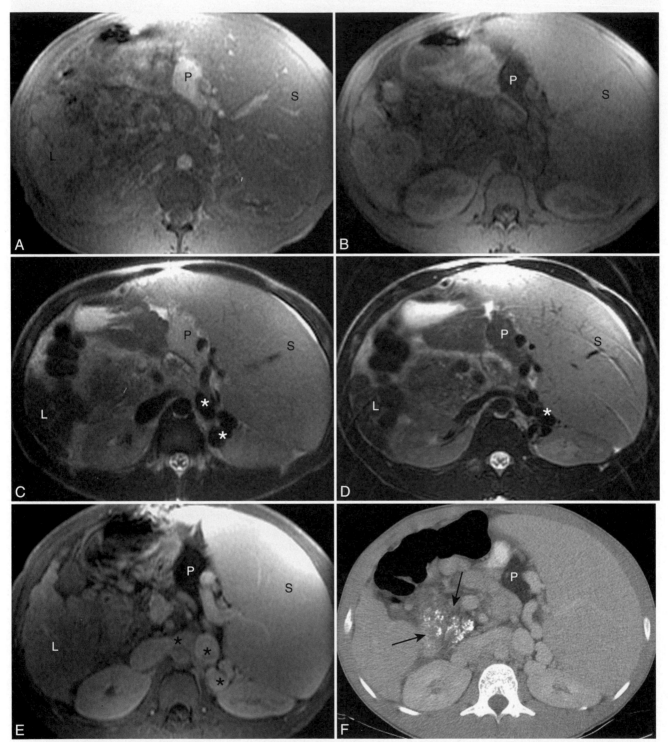

Figure 2-32 ■ MR findings of fat replacement of the pancreas, focal pancreatitis, and splenic varices in a 25-year-old man with cystic fibrosis. A–D, T1-WIs (**A** and **B**) and T2-WIs (**C** and **D**) obtained without (**A** and **C**) and with (**B** and **D**) fat saturation show moderate-to-marked splenomegaly (S), a nodular cirrhotic liver (L), and flow voids within splenic varices (∗). The pancreatic body (P) shows high SI before fat saturation and low SI after fat saturation, in keeping with fatty replacement. The pancreatic head *(arrow)* is poorly defined and not well depicted. It has low SI on all images. **E**, CE T1-WI shows enhancing splenic varices (∗) that formed a spontaneous spleno-renal shunt. **F**, Nonenhanced CT scan also shows the fat-replaced pancreatic body (P) and better reveals the enlarged calcified pancreatic head *(arrows)*. CT is superior to MR for detection and characterization of calcium.

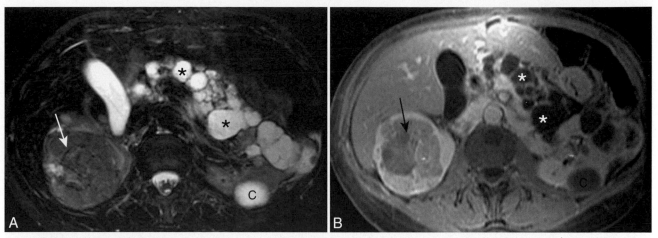

Figure 2-33 ▪ MR illustration of multiple pancreatic cysts, renal cell carcinoma, and renal cysts in a woman with von Hippel–Lindau disease. A and **B,** Axial T2-WI (**A**) and CE fat-suppressed T1-WI (**B**) show multiple nonenhancing pancreatic cysts (*). A large, infiltrative right renal cell carcinoma *(arrow)* and portion of a left renal cyst (C) are present.

The role of imaging is not so much to diagnose acute pancreatitis as to detect a possible cause or complication. For example, MRCP can be used to detect gallstones or choledocholithiasis and, in patients with recurrent acute idiopathic pancreatitis, can evaluate for an etiology such as pancreas divisum or congenital anomaly.[236,393] Occasionally, the diagnosis of pancreatitis may initially be made on imaging studies if the cause of abdominal pain is unclear. However, the presence of a normal-appearing pancreas on CT or MR does not exclude the diagnosis of acute pancreatitis, especially in light of abnormal laboratory data. Complications of acute pancreatitis include pancreatic necrosis, acute peripancreatic fluid collections, pseudocyst, pancreatic abscesses, pseudoaneurysm, and venous thrombosis.

Acute pancreatitis is classified as mild or severe based on clinical and laboratory findings as well as severity of pathologic changes (Atlanta classification system).[394] Assessing the presence and degree of pancreatic and peripancreatic inflammation, fluid collections, and pancreatic necrosis on imaging studies provides additional prognostic information. In very mild pancreatitis, the gland may maintain its normal shape and SI characteristics.[395] In more advanced cases of acute pancreatitis, thickening of the left anterior pararenal fascial plane and enlargement of the gland are present. The inflamed pancreas shows decreased SI on fat-suppressed T1-WI.[396,397] Peripancreatic edema is better revealed on T1-WI as low SI strands within the high SI retroperitoneal fat or on fat-suppressed T2-WI as areas of high SI.[397,398] In severe pancreatitis, the pancreas shows enlargement, heterogeneous decreased enhancement, and loss of definition of its normal boundaries on CE imaging (Fig. 2-34).[228,395,396,398]

In more than half of cases of moderate to severe pancreatitis, acute fluid collections develop in the pancreas, peripancreatic region, lesser sac, and paracolic gutters and represent a serous or exudative reaction to pancreatic inflammation. Acute fluid collections tend to be multiple, are irregular in shape, do not communicate with the pancreatic duct, and lack a well-defined wall of granulation tissue or sharp interface with adjacent organs. While more than 50% of these acute fluid collections regress spontaneously in 4 to 6 weeks, 10% to 15% of these fluid collections that persist for more than 3 weeks may develop a capsule and eventually form a pseudocyst.[399]

Approximately 75% to 85% of cystic pancreatic lesions are pseudocysts that are localized fluid collections within or adjacent to the pancreas enclosed by a well-defined nonepithelialized cyst wall. Pseudocysts are round or oval and often communicate with the pancreatic duct.[399] T2-WIs are sensitive in showing fluid collections and are more accurate than CT for discriminating between fluid and solid debris; the presence of the latter occurs more frequently in complicated pseudocysts that require percutaneous drainage.[396,398,400]

Uncomplicated pseudocysts are of low T1 SI, high T2 SI, and do not enhance.[395] Up to 40% of pseudocysts smaller than 6 cm and without communication with the pancreatic duct will spontaneously regress. Complicated pseudocysts are heterogeneous on MR because of hemorrhage and proteinaceous material and show high SI on fat-suppressed T1-WI and variable T2 SI (Figs. 2-35 and 2-36).[401] Indications for drainage of a pseudocyst includes mass effect, enlargement of the cyst, and complications such as infection or hemorrhage.[399] The presence of solid necrotic debris in a fluid collection can result in secondary infection if endoscopic or percutaneous drainage procedures are performed and instead requires an open surgical approach. T2-WI and MRCP techniques are superior to CT in identifying solid debris and can help assess the drainability of a pseudocyst.[400]

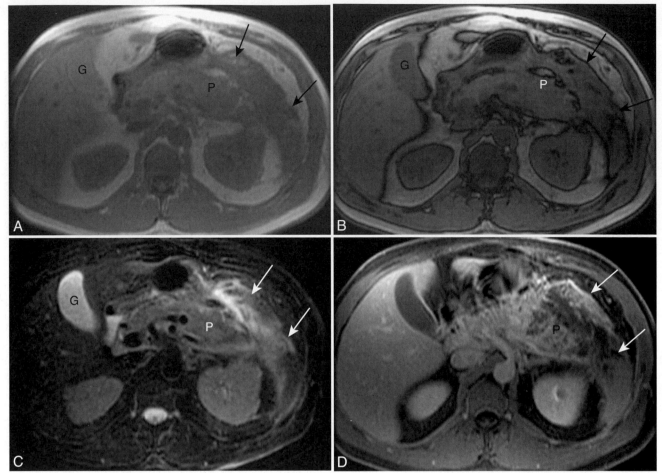

Figure 2-34 ■ MR findings of acute pancreatitis. A and **B**, In-phase (**A**) and opposed-phase (**B**) T1-WIs show low SI of the distal pancreas (P) and more normal SI pancreas proximally. There is abnormal, low SI of the fat in the left anterior pararenal space *(arrows)* that represents peripancreatic edema and phlegmon. The normal loss of SI of gallbladder bile (G) in **B** indicates lipid content. **C** and **D**, Fat-suppressed T2-WI (**C**) and CE T1-WI (**D**) show high SI edematous distal pancreas (P) that enhances less than the adjacent proximal pancreas. Patchy enhancement of the edematous peripancreatic fat *(arrows)* is present.

Pancreatic necrosis is a complication of severe acute pancreatitis in which there are focal or diffuse areas of nonviable parenchyma. Necrosis occurs in 20% of patients with pancreatitis who fail to respond to medical treatment. Pancreatic necrosis usually requires surgical débridement to prevent abscess formation, which can increase mortality from 20% to as much as 60%.[396,402,403] Ductal disruption with leakage of pancreatic enzymes into the gland and adjacent tissue can occur with severe necrosis and contributes to high morbidity.[395] Patients with greater than 75% necrosis or progression of necrosis on serial imaging are more likely to require necrosectomy because of the high mortality rate.[402] Percutaneous drainage also is possible if there has been complete liquefaction without remaining solid necrotic debris.[400]

CE-CT is the traditional test of choice to diagnose pancreatic necrosis. Necrotic parenchyma shows decreased or absent enhancement and is usually sharply demarcated from the normally enhancing viable pancreas. Necrosis tends to affect the body and tail, sparing the pancreatic head because of its abundant vascular supply.[402] Necrotic tissue eventually

liquefies and forms an intrapancreatic fluid collection or pseudocyst that can become secondarily infected.[399] CE-MR imaging detects the presence and extent of necrosis as well as CT does and shows nonviable parenchyma as having absent enhancement that is sharply demarcated from normal pancreas (see Fig. 2-35).[396,398,401] The administration of gadolinium is important in detecting necrosis because the SI of necrosis on unenhanced MRI may not significantly differ from that of inflamed pancreas (see Fig. 2-35).[404] MR can also characterize peripancreatic fat necrosis with hemorrhage. Persistent high SI within the peripancreatic fat on a fat-suppressed T1-WI suggests a diagnosis of hemorrhagic fat necrosis and is more likely to be present in patients with more severe inflammatory changes.[405]

An uncommon but potentially fatal cause of gastrointestinal and intraperitoneal bleeding is rupture of a pseudoaneurysm caused by pancreatitis. The frequency of pseudoaneurysm formation has been reported to be as high as 10% in patients with pancreatitis, with a mortality rate of up to one third if rupture and hemorrhage occur.[406] Leakage of pancreatic

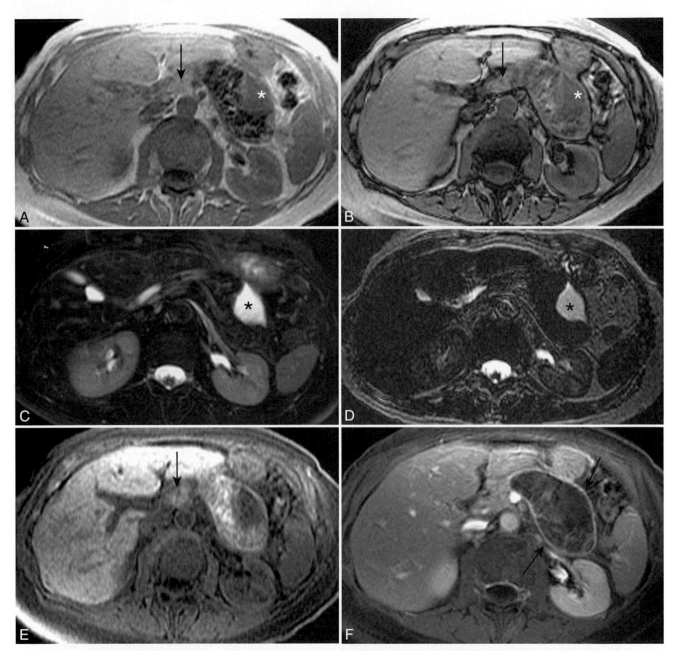

Figure 2-35 ▪ MR illustration of an evolving, complicated pseudocyst: pancreatic necrosis in a woman that developed after endoscopic retrograde cholangiopancreatography. Chronic pain necessitated distal pancreatectomy, which confirmed necrotic and hemorrhagic debris without viable parenchymal tissue. **A** and **B**, Opposed-phase (**A**) and in-phase (**B**) T1-WIs show replacement of the pancreatic body and tail by a process with two separate components. Low SI is present anteriorly (*). The dependent portion of the pseudocyst shows intermediate-to-high SI in **A** (TE = 2.3) and low SI in **B** (TE = 4.6). The loss of SI is secondary to susceptibility effects due to hemorrhage. The adjacent pancreatic parenchyma *(arrows)* is hypointense to liver, in keeping with pancreatitis. **C** and **D**, Fat-suppressed T2-WI (**C**) and heavily T2-WI (**D**) show simple fluid (*) within the anterior component and low SI-dependent hemorrhage/debris. **E** and **F**, Fat-suppressed 3D T1-WIs obtained before (**E**) and after (**F**) contrast show no pseudocyst enhancement. The use of fat suppression and a short TE (0.8 msec) provide ideal T1 contrast to reveal the hyperintense proteinaceous and hemorrhage components within the pseudocyst.

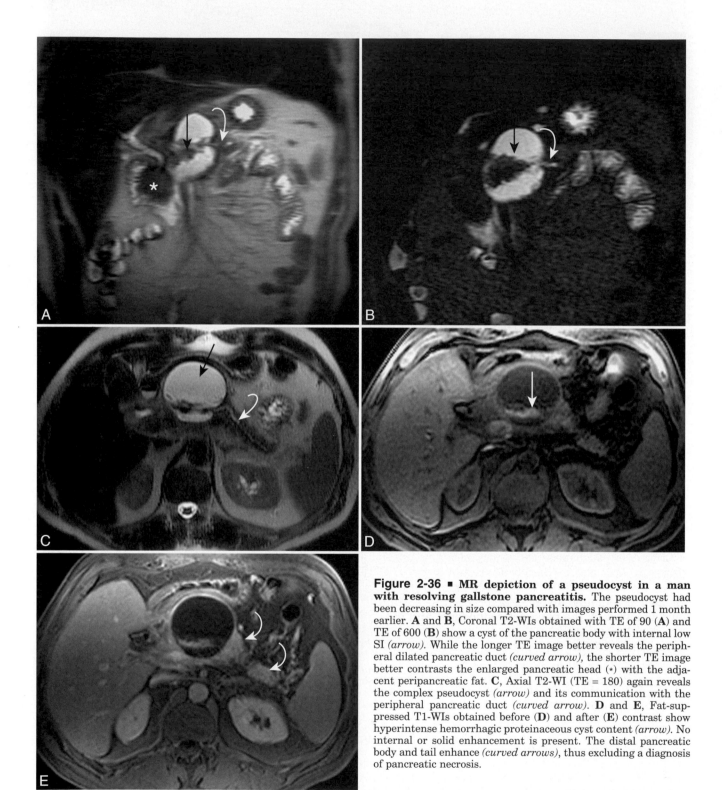

Figure 2-36 ■ **MR depiction of a pseudocyst in a man with resolving gallstone pancreatitis.** The pseudocyst had been decreasing in size compared with images performed 1 month earlier. **A** and **B,** Coronal T2-WIs obtained with TE of 90 (**A**) and TE of 600 (**B**) show a cyst of the pancreatic body with internal low SI *(arrow)*. While the longer TE image better reveals the peripheral dilated pancreatic duct *(curved arrow)*, the shorter TE image better contrasts the enlarged pancreatic head (∗) with the adjacent peripancreatic fat. **C,** Axial T2-WI (TE = 180) again reveals the complex pseudocyst *(arrow)* and its communication with the peripheral pancreatic duct *(curved arrow)*. **D** and **E,** Fat-suppressed T1-WIs obtained before (**D**) and after (**E**) contrast show hyperintense hemorrhagic proteinaceous cyst content *(arrow)*. No internal or solid enhancement is present. The distal pancreatic body and tail enhance *(curved arrows)*, thus excluding a diagnosis of pancreatic necrosis.

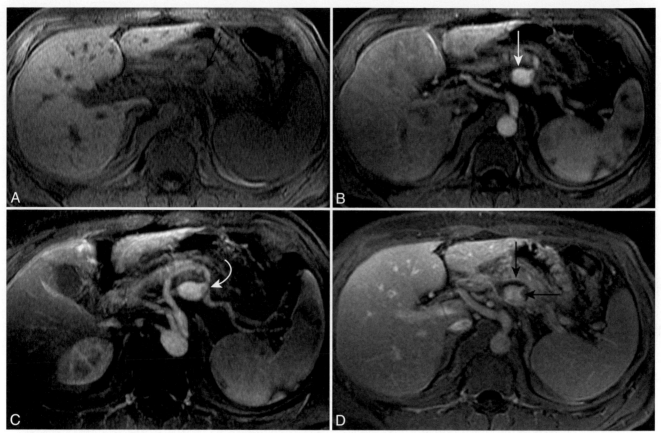

Figure 2-37 ▪ **MR depiction of a splenic artery pseudoaneurysm as a complication of pancreatitis. A** and **B**, Fat-suppressed T1-WIs obtained before (**A**) and after (**B**) contrast show a focal hyperenhancing mass *(arrow)*. The surrounding pancreas in *A* shows abnormal, low SI, in keeping with pancreatitis. **C** and **D**. Axial MIP image obtained during the MRA (**C**) better depicts the aneurysm neck *(curved arrow)* and the remainder of the splenic artery, while the delayed image (**D**) reveals nonenhancing mural thrombus *(black arrow)*.

enzymes from an inflamed pancreas can cause autodigestion of arterial walls, with a resultant perivascular blood leak and pseudoaneurysm formation.[407] Pancreatic pseudocysts may also erode into a visceral artery and convert a pseudocyst into a pseudoaneurysm.[408] The most commonly involved artery is the splenic artery, followed by the pancreaticoduodenal and gastroduodenal arteries.[402]

During the arterial phase of an enhanced MR, a pseudoaneurysm will appear as a circumscribed oval or round structure lying outside the normal confines of a vessel in the peripancreatic region and display enhancement that may approach that of the abdominal aorta.[402,406] Three-dimensional MRA techniques (see Chapter 11) allow for multiplanar reformations that can readily locate the vessel of origin (Fig. 2-37). Percutaneous angiographic embolization is advocated as the initial treatment for pseudoaneurysms in hemodynamically stable patients.[408]

Venous thrombosis is the most common venous complication of acute pancreatitis and may be related to spasm or to mass effect from adjacent inflammatory pancreatic and peripancreatic tissue. The splenic vein is most commonly affected because of its proximity to the pancreatic body and tail, but the superior mesenteric, splenoportal confluence, and portal veins also can be involved.[406,409] Venous thrombosis is diagnosed when an enhanced vessel wall surrounds a central, low SI clot on CE T1-WI.[410] A diagnosis of splenic vein thrombosis can be inferred when there is enlargement of the gastroepiploic and gastrocolic collateral veins (see Fig. 1-27), which drain into the SMV.[411] Isolated superior mesenteric venous thrombosis is rare in acute pancreatitis but does not necessarily indicate a poor prognosis as it often resolves without sequelae.[409]

CHRONIC PANCREATITIS

Chronic pancreatitis represents a continuing inflammatory disease of the pancreas characterized by irreversible morphologic changes in the parenchyma and pancreatic duct that cause pain or permanent loss of exocrine and endocrine function.[412,413] Alcohol abuse is the main cause of chronic pancreatitis, but 30% of cases have no clear etiology and are classified as idiopathic. In the recent literature, additional variants such as autoimmune pancreatitis and nonalcoholic

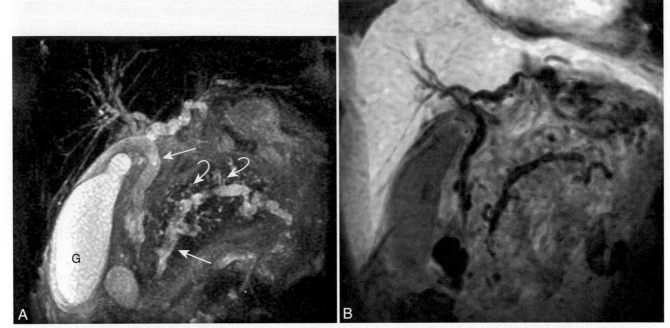

Figure 2-38 ■ MRCP findings of chronic pancreatitis. A Whipple procedure performed for chronic pain confirmed the diagnosis and excluded a neoplasm. **A,** Single-slice MIP T2-W MRCP shows dilated pancreatic duct side branches *(curved arrows),* main pancreatic duct *(arrow),* common bile duct *(upper arrow),* and gallbladder (G). **B,** MIP image obtained on 3D fat-suppressed T1-WI after contrast shows "black bile" cholangiography. The unenhanced bile and pancreatic secretions are well contrasted with enhancing adjacent liver and pancreatic parenchyma.

duct-destructive chronic pancreatitis have been described as having specific pathogenesis and imaging features.[414,415] Fibrosis and atrophy of the gland are hallmarks of chronic pancreatitis and decrease the proteinaceous fluid content of the gland, which results in low SI on fat-suppressed T1-WI. Fibrosis attenuates the vascularity of the pancreas and results in decreased enhancement on immediate CE imaging.[228,272,273,416] Parenchymal calcification is the most pathognomonic feature of chronic pancreatitis, occurs late in the disease, and is better revealed on CT.

Pancreatic duct changes in chronic pancreatitis include dilation of the main pancreatic duct and side branches, stenoses, stricture formation, intraductal calculi, and in severe cases marked dilation of the side branches, resulting in a "chain of lakes" or "string of pearls" appearance.[18,236,237] MRCP has moderate to high diagnostic accuracy as compared with ERCP in depicting pancreatic duct dilation, strictures, and filling defects such as calculi (Fig. 2-38).[18,417] Stenoses associated with pancreatitis are shorter, smoother, and more symmetrical than those secondary to neoplasms.[21] MRCP can also depict the number, size, and location of pseudocysts and confirm their continuity to the pancreatic duct, which is helpful in planning appropriate intervention.[21,237]

MRCP has limited application in the early stages of chronic pancreatitis because of its inability to show subtle side branch involvement and irregularity of the wall of the main pancreatic duct, which

can be detected at ERCP.[18,21] Secretin stimulation during dynamic MRCP improves visualization of the main pancreatic duct and side branches and assesses duodenal filling, which allows for an earlier and more accurate MR diagnosis of chronic pancreatitis in patients with suspected pancreatic disease.[239,418]

Focal chronic pancreatitis can be difficult to differentiate from pancreatic adenocarcinoma because both demonstrate low SI on T1-WI, are associated with ductal obstruction, and show more gradual progressive enhancement on dynamic MR imaging than does normal pancreas. The similar imaging findings are attributed to the large amounts of fibrosis present in both disease processes.[273,419] When fibrosis is distributed uniformly throughout the gland, no discrete mass is seen and the diagnosis of chronic pancreatitis is usually evident.[419] When fibrosis occurs in a mass-like distribution, distinction between focal pancreatitis and resectable adenocarcinoma can be difficult and may require biopsy.

Other Lesions of the Pancreas

PANCREATIC LIPOMA

A pancreatic lipoma is a benign mesenchymal neoplasm usually discovered as an incidental finding. The mass is well circumscribed and composed almost entirely of fat with a few scattered vessels or septa. The lipoma is isointense to peripancreatic fat on T1- and

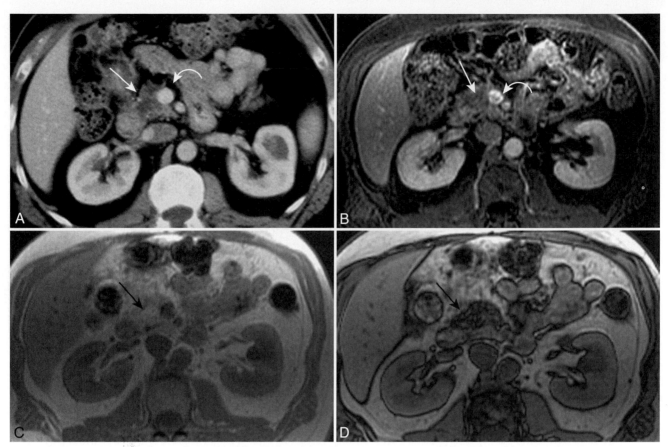

Figure 2-39 ▪ MR illustration of focal fatty change of the pancreas as revealed on chemical shift MR. MR was requested to confirm the diagnosis of pancreatic tumor of the low pancreatic head, which was depicted as a hypoattenuating mass on CT. Focal fatty change or focal fatty sparing of the pancreas can mimic a mass on imaging. **A** and **B**, Enhanced CT (**A**) and fat-suppressed CE (**B**) T1-WIs show hypoattenuating (**A**), hypointense (**B**) pancreatic tissue *(arrow)* that abuts the lateral margin of the superior mesenteric vein *(curved arrow)*. On the basis of these images alone it would be difficult to exclude an occult neoplasm. **C** and **D**, In-phase (**C**) and opposed-phase (**D**) T1-WIs show normal, hyperintense pancreas (**C**) that loses SI on opposed-phase imaging (**D**) *(arrow)*. Pancreatic cancer does not appear hyperintense on T1-WIs and does not reveal lipid on chemical shift imaging.

T2-WI.[420] The key to establishing a definitive diagnosis of macroscopic fat within the lipoma is to compare T1-WI performed with and without fat saturation (see Figs. 1-19A, 1-19D, and 3-1).[241] These MR techniques are discussed in greater detail in Chapter 3. Complete fatty replacement diffusely affects the gland, and localized lipomatosis (focal fatty infiltration) does not appear as a round, encapsulated mass.[421] Pancreatic lipomas are managed conservatively if there is no mass effect on the pancreaticobiliary tree.

FATTY CHANGES OF THE PANCREAS

Diffuse fatty infiltration or replacement of the pancreatic parenchyma is a common process in older individuals and appears as a heterogeneous decrease in SI of the pancreatic parenchyma on opposed-phase T1-W GRE images (Fig 2-39).[422] The lipid is confined to the interstitial stroma of the pancreas and is of no clinical import, since the endocrine and exocrine cells are not affected.[423] Complete fatty replacement has also been associated with cystic fibrosis (see Fig. 2-32), obesity, corticosteroid therapy, diabetes mellitus, and chronic pancreatitis.[424,425] Occasionally, focal fatty change can mimic a hypoattenuating neoplasm on CE-CT. Focal fatty change more commonly occurs in the posterior pancreatic head and uncinate process owing to differences in fat content between the dorsal (body, tail, and anterior and superior pancreatic head) and ventral (posterior and inferior pancreatic head and uncinate process) pancreatic anlagen.[424,425] Chemical shift MR imaging can establish a diagnosis of fatty change and exclude malignancy by depicting the lesion as having normal or high SI on in-phase imaging and loss of SI on a corresponding opposed-phase image.[423] Based on similar pathogenetic mechanisms, fatty change of the pancreas can spare a segment of parenchyma. Focal fatty sparing can be characterized using similar chemical shift techniques as for focal fatty change.

Pancreas Transplantation

Pancreas transplantation is used to manage certain cases of complicated type 1 diabetes mellitus.

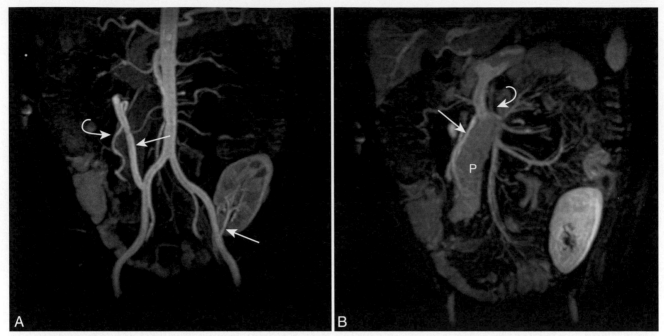

Figure 2-40 ▪ **Normal pancreatic transplant vasculature as revealed by CE-MRA. A**, MIP-MRA (magnetic resonance angiography) image depicts normal arterial graft segments of a donor iliac *(arrow)* and splenic artery *(curved arrow)* to supply a right-sided pancreatic transplant. A normal-appearing left lower quadrant renal transplant and artery *(lower arrow)* are present. **B**, MIP-MRV (magnetic resonance venography) shows a normal segment of splenic vein *(arrow)* that drains into the superior mesenteric vein *(curved arrow)*. Normal pancreatic parenchymal enhancement is present (P).

Traditional surgery employs systemic diversion of pancreatic venous outflow and drainage of exocrine secretions into the bladder (systemic-bladder) but can be complicated by hyperinsulinemia.[426] A newer technique employs portal venous drainage of the allograft and enteric drainage of the exocrine secretions (portal-enteric) to promote physiologic glucose metabolism.[426,427] Both techniques use a similar method of arterial reconstruction in which the splenic and superior mesenteric arteries of the donor pancreas are anastomosed to the internal and external branches of a donor iliac artery Y-graft. The allograft is implanted in the recipient through an end-to-side anastomosis between the common iliac portion of the Y-graft and the recipient's common or external iliac artery (Fig. 2-40).[427]

The systemic-bladder technique places the allograft in the pelvis and diverts venous drainage into the systemic circulation through an anastomosis between the portal vein of the allograft and the recipient's common or external iliac vein. Exocrine secretions are drained through a segment of donor duodenum that communicates with the bladder. The portal-enteric technique places the allograft vertically and intraperitoneally in the right side of the abdomen and establishes venous drainage through an anastomosis between the portal vein of the allograft and the recipient's superior mesenteric vein[428]

(see Fig 2-40). Exocrine secretions drain into the donor duodenum that is anastomosed to a Roux-en-Y limb formed from the recipient's jejunum.[427]

The pancreas transplant is enlarged and inhomogeneous in the immediate postoperative period but decreases in size after 4 weeks.[429] Subsequently, normal parenchyma is hyperintense to adjacent organs and fat on T1-WI with fat suppression and enhances avidly and uniformly, similarly to native pancreas.[428,430] The allograft is susceptible to a variety of postoperative complications the most common of which are arterial and venous thrombosis, allograft rejection, and transplant pancreatitis. Vascular thrombosis is suspected when a patient has rising serum glucose and a normal creatinine, reflecting impaired venous drainage of insulin from the allograft.[428] Venous or arterial thrombosis is diagnosed when the transplant vessel shows absent enhancement, stenosis, or a central, low SI clot surrounded by enhanced vessel wall. Absent enhancement of the allograft in the setting of thrombosis represents graft infarction and necessitates explantation to prevent superinfection (Fig 2-41).[410,428,431] Imaging diagnosis of graft rejection is difficult but is suggested by abnormally low SI on T1-WI and decreased enhancement.[432] Transplant pancreatitis is no different from native pancreatitis and manifests as pancreatic enlargement and peripancreatic edema.[428,430]

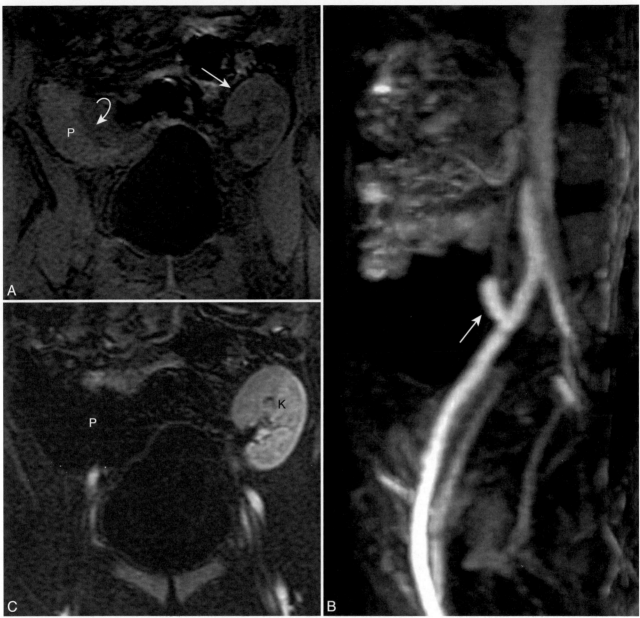

Figure 2-41 ■ **Pancreatic transplant artery thrombosis and pancreatic necrosis as revealed by MR.** **A**, Coronal fat-suppressed T1-WI shows a left lower quadrant renal *(arrow)* and right lower quadrant pancreatic transplant (P, *curved arrow*). Normal pancreatic parenchyma should be hyperintense to muscle on T1-WIs. **B**, MIP image during an arterial-phase MR shows occlusion of the proximal segment of the iliac arterial graft *(arrow)*. **C**, Subtraction image of a venous-phase CE T1-WI shows normal renal enhancement but absent pancreatic parenchymal enhancement.

REFERENCES

1. Wallner B, Schumacher K, Weidenmaier W, Friedrich J. Dilated biliary tract: evaluation with MR cholangiography with a T2-weighted contrast-enhanced fast sequence. Radiology 1991;181:805-808.
2. Loperfido S, Angelina G, Benedetti G. Major early complications from diagnostic and therapeutic ERCP: a prospective multicenter study. Gastrointest Endosc 1998;48:1-10.
3. Varghese J, Farrell M, Courtney G, Osborne H, Murray F, Lee M. Role of MR cholangiopancreatography in patients with failed or inadequate ERCP. Am J Roentgenol 1999;173:1527-1533.
4. Soto J, Yucel E, Barish M, Chuttani R, Ferrucci J. MR cholangiopancreatography after unsuccessful or incomplete ERCP. Radiology 1996;199:91-98.
5. Outwater E, Mitchell D. MR imaging techniques for evaluation of the pancreas. Top Magn Reson Imaging 1996;8:248-264.
6. Taourel P, Bret PM, Reinhold C, Barkun AN, Atri M. Anatomic variants of the biliary tree: diagnosis with MR cholangiopancreatography. Radiology 1996;199:521-527.
7. Vitellas K, Keogan M, Spritzer C, Nelson R. MR cholangiopancreatography of bile and pancreatic duct abnormalities with emphasis on the single-shot fast spin-echo technique. Radiographics 2000;20: 939-957.
8. Chan J, Tsui E, Yuen M, et al. Gadopentetate dimeglumine as an oral negative gastrointestinal contrast agent for MRCP. Abdom Imaging 2000;25:405-408.
9. Barish M, Soto J. MR cholangiopancreatography: techniques and clinical applications. Am J Roentgenol 1997;169:1295-1303.
10. Macaulay S, Schulte S, Sekijima J, et al. Evaluation of a non-breath-hold MR cholangiography technique. Radiology 1995;196:227-232.

11. Barish M, Yucel E, Soto J, Chuttani R, Ferrucci J. MR cholangio-pancreatography: efficacy of three-dimensional turbo spin-echo technique. Am J Roentgenol 1995;165:295-300.

12. Yamashita Y, Abe Y, Tang Y, Urata J, Sumi S, Takahashi M. In vitro and clinical studies of image acquisition in breath-hold MR cholangiocreateography: single-shot projection technique versus multislice technique. Am J Roentgenol 1997;168:1449-1454.

13. Holzknecht N, Gauger J, Sackmann M, et al. Breath-hold MR cholangiography with snapshot techniques: prospective comparison with endoscopic retrograde cholangiography. Radiology 1998;206:657-664.

14. Ichikawa T, Nitatori T, Hachiya J, Mizutani Y. Breath-held MR cholangiopancreatography with half-averaged single shot hybrid rapid acquisition with relaxation enhancement sequence: comparison of fast GRE and SE sequences. J Comput Assist Tomogr 1996;20:798-802.

15. Miyazaki T, Yamashita Y, Tsuchigame T, Yamamoto H, Urata J, Takahashi M. MR cholangiopancreatography using HASTE (half-Fourier acquisition single-shot turbo spin-echo) sequences. Am J Roentgenol 1996;166:1297-1303.

16. Kim T, Han J, Kim S, Bae S, Choi B. MR cholangiopancreatography: comparison between half-Fourier acquisition single-shot turbo spin-echo and two-dimensional turbo spin-echo pulse sequences. Abdom Imaging 1998;23:398-403.

17. Takehara Y. Fast MR imaging for evaluating the pancreaticobiliary system. Eur J Radiol 1999;29:211-232.

18. Takehara Y, Ichijo K, Tooyama N, et al. Breath-hold MR cholangiopancreatography with a long-echo-train fast spin-echo sequence and a surface coil in chronic pancreatitis. Radiology 1994;192:73-78.

19. Fulcher A, Turner M. Pitfalls of MR cholangiopancreatography (MRCP). J Comput Assist Tomogr 1998;22:845-850.

20. Watanabe Y, Dohke M, Ishimori T, et al. Diagnostic pitfalls of MR cholangiopancreatography in the evaluation of the biliary tract and gallbladder. Radiographics 1999;19:415-429.

21. Larena J, Astigarraga E, Saralegui I, Merino A, Capelastegui A, Calvo M. Magnetic resonance cholangiopancreatography in the evaluation of pancreatic duct pathology. Br J Radiol 1998;71: 1100-1104.

22. Kim M-J, Mitchell DG, Ito K, Outwater EK. Biliary dilatation: Differentiation of benign from malignant causes: value of adding conventional MR imaging to MR cholangiopancreatography. Radiology 2000;214:173-181.

23. Takehara Y. Can MRCP replace ERCP? J Magn Reson Imaging 1998;8:517-534.

24. Lee V, Rofsky N, Morgan G, et al. Volumetric mangafodipir trisodium-enhanced cholangiography to define intrahepatic biliary anatomy. Am J Roentgenol 2001;176:906-908.

25. Fayad LM, Holland GA, Bergin D, et al. Functional magnetic resonance cholangiography (fMRC) of the gallbladder and biliary tree with contrast-enhanced magnetic resonance cholangiography. J Magn Reson Imaging 2003;18:449-460.

26. Mitchell D, Alam F. Mangafodipir trisodium: effects on T2- and T1-weighted MR cholangiography. J Magn Reson Imaging 1999;9:366-368.

27. Runge V. A comparison of two MR hepatobiliary gadolinium chelates: Gd-BOPTA and Gd-EOB-DTPA. J Comput Assist Tomogr 1998;22:643-650.

28. Bollow M, Taupitz M, Hamm B, Staks T, Wolf K, Weinmann H. Gadolinium-ethoxybenzyl-DTPA as a hepatobiliary contrast agent for use in MR cholangiography: results of an in vivo phase-I clinical evaluation. Eur Radiol 1997;7:126-132.

29. Vitellas K, El-Dieb A, Vaswani K, et al. Using contrast-enhanced MR cholangiography with IV mangafodipir trisodium (Teslascan) to evaluate bile duct leaks after cholecystectomy: a prospective study of 11 patients. Am J Roentgenol 2002;179:409-416.

30. Carlos R, Hussain H, Song J, Francis I. Gadolinium-ethoxybenzyl-diethylenetriamine pentaacetic acid as an intrabiliary contrast agent: preliminary assessment. Am J Roentgenol 2002;179:87-92.

31. Adusumilli S, Siegelman E. MR imaging of the gallbladder. J Magn Reson Imaging Clin North Am 2002;10:165-184.

32. Rizzo RJ, Szucs RA, Turner MA. Congenital anomalies of the pancreas and biliary tree in adults. Radiographics 1995;15:49-68.

33. Dohke M, Watanabe Y, Okumura A, et al. Anomalies and anatomic variants of the biliary tree revealed by MR cholangiopancreatography. Am J Roentgenol 1999;173:1251-1254.

34. Tang Y, Yamashita Y, Abe Y, Namimoto T, Tsuchigame T, Takahashi M. Congenital anomalies of the pancreaticobiliary tract: findings on MR cholangiopancreatography (MRCP) using haf-Fourier-acquistion single-shot turbo spin-echo sequence (HASTE). Comput Med Imaging Graph 2001;25:423-431.

35. Sugiyama M, Baba M, Atomi Y, Hanaoka H, Mizutani Y, Hachiya J. Diagnosis of anomalous pancreaticobiliary junction: value of magnetic resonance cholangiopancreatography. Surgery 1998; 123:391-397.

36. Sugiyama M, Atomi Y. Anomalous pancreaticobiliary junction without congenital choledochal cyst. Br J Surg 1998;85:911-916.

37. Savader SJ, Benenati JF, Venbrux AC, et al. Choledochal cysts: classification and cholangiographic appearance. Am J Roentgenol 1991;156:327-331.

38. Matos C, Nicaise N, Deviere J, et al. Choledochal cysts: comparison of findings at MR cholangiopancreatography and endoscopic retrograde cholangiopancreatography in eight patients. Radiology 1998;209:443-448.

39. Kim OH, Chung HJ, Choi B, Gil. Imaging of the choledochal cyst. Radiographics 1995;15:69-88.

40. Weyant MJ, Maluccio MA, Bertagnolli MM, Daly JM. Choledochal cysts in adults: a report of two cases and review of the literature. Am J Gastroenterol 1998;93:2580-2583.

41. Irie H, et al. Value of MR cholangiopancreatography in evaluating choledochal cysts. Am J Roentgenol 1998;171:1381-1385.

42. Fieber SS, Nance FC. Choledochal cyst and neoplasm: a comprehensive review of 106 cases and presentation of two original cases. Am Surg 1997;63:982-987.

43. Kim S, Lim J, Yoon H, Han B, Lee S, Kim Y. Choledochal cyst: comparison of MR and conventional cholangiography. Clin Radiol 2000;55:378-383.

44. Brine D, Soulen R. Pancreaticobiliary carcinoma associated with a large choledochal cyst: role of MRI and MR cholangiopancreatography in diagnosis and preoperative assessment. Abdom Imaging 1999;24:292-294.

45. Kim M, Han S, Yoon C, et al. Using MR cholangiopancreatography to reveal anomalous pancreaticobiliary ductal union in infants and children with choledochal cysts. Am J Roentgenol 2002;179:209-214.

46. Todani T, Watanabe Y, Narusue M, Tabuchi K, Okajima K. Congenital bile duct cysts: classification, operative procedures, and review of thirty-seven cases including cancer arising from choledochal cyst. Am J Surg 1977;134:263-269.

47. De Backer A, Van den Abbeele K, De Schepper A, Van Baarle A. Choledochocele: diagnosis by magnetic resonance imaging. Abdom Imaging 2000;25:508-510.

48. Miller WJ, Sechtin AG, Campbell WL, Pieters PC. Imaging findings in Caroli's disease. Am J Roentgenol 1995;165:333-337.

49. Asselah T, Ernst O, Sergent G, l'Herminé C, Paris J-C. Caroli's disease: a magnetic resonance cholangiopancreatography diagnosis. Am J Gastroenterol 1998;93:109-110.

50. Guy F, Cognet F, Dranssart M, Cercueil JP, Conciatori L, Krause D. Caroli's disease: magnetic resonance imaging features. Eur Radiol 2002;12:2730-2736.

51. Davidoff AM, Pappas TN, Murray EA, et al. Mechanisms of major biliary injury during laparoscopic cholecystectomy. Ann Surg 1992;215:196-202.

52. Martin RF, Rossi RL. Bile duct injuries: spectrum, mechanisms of injury, and their prevention. Surg Clin North Am 1994;74:781-803.

53. Mortele K, Ros PR. Anatomic variants of the biliary tree: MR cholangiographic findings and clinical applications. Am J Roentgenol 2001;177:389-394.

54. Vanbeckevoort D, Van Hoe L, Ponette E, et al. Imaging of gallbladder and biliary tract before laparoscopic cholecystectomy: comparison of intravenous cholangiography and the combined use of HASTE and single-shot MR imaging. J Belge Radiol 1997;80:6-8.

55. Hirao K, Miyazaki A, Fujimoto T, Isomoto I, Hayashi K. Evaluation of aberrant bile ducts before laparoscopic cholecystectomy: helical CT cholangiography versus MR cholangiography. Am J Roentgenol 2000;175:713-720.

56. Magnuson T, Bender J, Duncan M. MRCP in biliary obstruction: a useful test? Am J Gastroenterol 2000;95:3646-3649.

57. Guibaud L, Bret PM, Reinhold C, Atri M, Barkun AN. Bile duct obstruction and choledocholithiasis: diagnosis with MR cholangiopancreatography. Radiology 1995;197:109-115.

58. Schwartz LH, Coakley FV, Sun Y, Blumgart LH, Fong Y, Panicek DM. Neoplastic pancreaticobiliary duct obstruction: evaluation with breath-hold MR cholangiopancreatography. Am J Roentgenol 1998;170:1491-1495.

59. Soto JA, Alvarez O, Lopera JE, Munera F, Restrepo JC, Correa G. Biliary obstruction: findings at MR cholangiography and cross-sectional MR imaging. Radiographics 2000;20:353-366.

60. Schwartz LH, Lefkowitz RA, Panicek DM, et al. Breath-hold magnetic resonance cholangiopancreatography in the evaluation of malignant pancreaticobiliary obstruction. J Comput Assist Tomogr 2003;27:307-314.

61. Courbiere M, Pilleul F, Henry L, Ponchon T, Touzet S, Valette PJ. Value of magnetic resonance cholangiography in benign and malignant biliary stenosis: comparative study with direct cholangiography. J Comput Assist Tomogr 2003;27:315-320.

62. Adamek HE, Albert J, Breer H, Weitz M, Schilling D, Riemann JF. Pancreatic cancer detection with magnetic resonance cholangiopancreatography and endoscopic retrograde cholangiopancreatography: a prospective controlled study. Lancet 2000;356:190-193.

63. Materne R, Van Beers B, Gigot J, et al. Extrahepatic biliary obstruction: Magnetic resonance imaging compared with endoscopic ultrasonography. Endoscopy 2000;32:3-9.
64. Liu TH, Consorti ET, Kawashima A, et al. The efficacy of magnetic resonance cholangiography for the evaluation of patients with suspected choledocholithiasis before laparoscopic cholecystectomy. Am J Surg 1999;178:480-484.
65. Dwerryhouse S, Brown E, Vipond M. Prospective evaluation of magnetic resonance cholangiography to detect common bile duct stones before laparoscopic cholecystectomy. Br J Surg 1998;85:1364-1366.
66. Cohen S, Siegel J, Kasmin F. Complications of diagnostic and therapeutic ERCP. Abdom Imaging 1996;21:285-394.
67. Kim J, Kim M, Park S, et al. MR cholangiography in symptomatic gallstones: diagnostic accuracy according to clinical risk group. Radiology 2002;224:410-416.
68. Gallix B, Régent D, Bruel J. Use of magnetic resonance cholangiography in the diagnosis of choledocholithiasis. Abdom Imaging 2001;26:21-27.
69. Becker CD, Grossholz M, Becker M, Mentha G, de Peyer R, Terrier F. Choledocholithiasis and bile duct stenosis: Diagnostic accuracy of MR cholangiopancreatography. Radiology 1997; 205:523-530.
70. Boraschi P, Neri E, Braccini G, et al. Choledocholithiasis: Diagnostic accuracy of MR cholangiopancreatography. Three-year experience. Magnetic Resonance Imaging 1999;17:1245-1253.
71. Varghese J, Liddell R, Farrell M, Murray F, Osborne D, Lee M. Diagnostic accuracy of magnetic resonance cholangiopancreatography and ultrasound compared with direct cholangiography in the detection of choledocholithiasis. Clin Radiol 2000;55:25-35.
72. Soto JA, Barish MA, Alvarez O, Medina S. Detection of choledocholithiasis with MR cholangiography: comparison of three-dimensional fast spin-echo and single- and multisection half-Fourier rapid acquisition with relaxation enhancement sequences. Radiology 2000;215:737-745.
73. Reinhold C, Taourel P, Bret PM, et al. Choledocholithiasis: evaluation of MR cholangiography for diagnosis. Radiology 1998;209:435-442.
74. Sugiyama M, Atomi Y, Hachiya J. Magnetic resonance cholangiography using half-Fourier acquisition for diagnosing choledocholithiasis. Am J Gastroenterol 1998;93:1886-1890.
75. Stiris M, Tennoe B, Aadland E, Lunde O. MR cholangiopanc reaticography and endoscopic retrograde cholangiopancreaticography in patients with suspected common bile duct stones. Acta Radiologica 2000;41:269-272.
76. Soto JA, Alvarez O, Munera F, Valez SM, Valencia J, Ramirez N. Diagnosing bile duct stones: comparison of unenhanced helical CT, oral contrast-enhanced CT cholangiography, and MR cholangiography. Am J Roentgenol 2000;175:1127-1134.
77. Regan F, Fradin J, Khazan R, Bohlman M, Magnuson T. Choledocholithiasis: Evaluation with MR cholangiography. Am J Roentgenol 1996;167:1441-1445.
78. Kim T, Kim B, Kim J, et al. Diagnosis of intrahepatic stones: superiority of MR cholangiopancreatography over endoscopic retrograde cholangiopancreatography. Am J Roentgenol 2002;179:429-434.
79. Chan Y, Lam W, Metreweli C, Chung S. Detectability and appearance of bile duct calculus on MR imaging of the abdomen using axial T1- and T2-weighted sequences. Clin Radiol 1997;52:351-355.
80. Chan Y-l, Chan AC, Lam WW, et al. Choledocholithiasis: comparison of MR cholangiography and endoscopic retrograde cholangiography. Radiology 1996;200:85-89.
81. Fulcher A, Turner M, Capps G, Zfass A, Baker K. Half-Fourier RARE MR cholangiopancreatography: experience in 300 subjects. Radiology 1998;207:21-32.
82. Irie H-J, Honda H, Kuroiwa T, et al. Pitfalls in MR cholangio-pancreatographic interpretation. Radiographics 2001;21:23-37.
83. Pavone P, Laghi A, Catalano C, et al. MR cholangiography in the examination of patients with biliary-enteric anastomoses. Am J Roentgenol 1997;169:807-811.
84. Lillemoe KD, Pitt HA, Cameron JL. Current management of benign bile duct strictures. Adv Surg 1992;25:119-173.
85. Yeh T, Jan Y, Tseng J, Hwang T, Jeng L, Chen M. Value of magnetic resonance cholangiopancreatography in demonstrating major bile duct injuries following laparoscopic cholecystectomy. Br J Surg 1999;86:181-184.
86. Khalid TR, Casillas VJ, Montalvo BM, Centeno R, Levi JU. Using MR cholangiopancreatography to evaluate iatrogenic bile duct injury. Am J Roentgenol 2001;177:1347-1352.
87. Chartrand-Lefebvre C, Dufresne M, Lafortune M, Lapointe R, Dagenais M, Roy A. Iatrogenic injury to the bile duct: a working classification for radiologists. Radiology 1994;193:523-526.
88. Moossa A, Mayer A, Stabile B. Iatrogenic injury to the bile duct: who, how, where? Arch Surg 1990;125:1028-1030.
89. Lillemoe K, Martin S, Cameron J, et al. Major bile duct injuries during laparoscopic cholecystectomy: follow-up after combined surgical and radiological management. Ann Surg 1997;225:459-468.
90. Laghi A, Pavone P, Catalano C, et al. MR cholangiography of late biliary complications after liver transplantation. Am J Roentgenol 1999;172:1541-1546.
91. Greif F, Bronsther O, Van Thiel D, et al. The incidence, timing, and management of biliary tract complications after orthotopic liver transplantation. Ann Surg 1994;219:40-45.
92. Fulcher AS, Turner MA. Orthotopic liver transplantation: evaluation with MR cholangiography. Radiology 1999;211:715-722.
93. Boraschi P, Braccini G, Gigoni R, et al. Detection of biliary complications after orthotopic liver transplantation with MR cholangiography. Magnetic Resonance Imaging 2001;19:1097-1105.
94. Starzl TE, Putnam CW, Hansbrough JF, Porter KA, Reid H. Biliary complications after liver transplantation: With special reference to the biliary cast syndrome and techniques of secondary duct repair. Surgery 1977;81:212-221.
95. Matthews BD, Sing RF, Heniford BT. Magnetic resonance cholangiopancreatographic diagnosis of Mirizzi's syndrome. J Am Coll Surg 2000;190:630.
96. Kim PN, Outwater EK, Mitchell DG. Mirizzi syndrome: evaluation by MR imaging. Am J Gastroenterol 1999;94:2546-2550.
97. Lee Y-M, Kaplan MM. Primary sclerosing cholangitis. N Engl J Med 1995;331:924-933.
98. Olsson R, Danielsson A, Jarnerot G, et al. Prevalence of primary sclerosing cholangitis in patients with ulcerative colitis. Gastroenterology 1991;100:1319-1323.
99. Ponsioen C, Tytgat G. Primary sclerosing cholangitis: a clinical review. Am J Gastroenterol 1998;93:515-523.
100. Chalasani N, Baluyut A, Ismail A, et al. Cholangiocarcinoma in patients with primary sclerosing cholangitis: a multi-center case-control study. Hepatology 2000;31:7-11.
101. Ernst O, Asselah T, Sergent G, et al. MR cholangiography in primary sclerosing cholangitis. Am J Roentgenol 1998;171:1027-1030.
102. Vitellas KM, Enns RA, Keogan MT, et al. Comparison of MR cholangiopancreatographic techniques with contrast-enhanced cholangiography in the evaluation of sclerosing cholangitis. Am J Roentgenol 2002;178:327-334.
103. Fulcher AS, Turner MA, Franklin KJ, et al. Primary sclerosing cholangitis: evaluation with MR cholangiography: a case-control study. Radiology 2000;215:71-80.
104. Angulo P, Pearce DH, Johnson CD, et al. Magnetic resonance cholangiography in patients with biliary disease: its role in primary sclerosing cholangitis. J Hepatology 2000;33:520-527.
105. Ito K, Mitchell D, Outwater E, Blasbalg R. Primary sclerosing cholangitis: MR imaging features. Am J Roentgenol 1999; 172:1527-1533.
106. Vitellas KM, Keogan MT, Freed KS, et al. Radiologic manifestations of sclerosing cholangitis with emphasis on MR cholangio-pancreatography. Radiographics 2000;20:959-975.
107. Revelon G, Rashid A, Kawamoto S, Bluemke DA. Primary sclerosing cholangitis: MR imaging findings with pathologic correlation. Am J Roentgenol 1999;173:1037-1042.
108. Outwater E, Kaplan MM, Bankoff MS. Lymphadenopathy in sclerosing cholangitis: pitfall in the diagnosis of malignant biliary obstruction. Gastrointest Radiol 1992;17:157-160.
109. Campbell WL, Peterson MS, Federle MP, Sigueira ES, et al. Using CT and cholangiography to diagnose biliary tract carcinoma complicating primary sclerosing cholangitis. Am J Roentgenol 2001;177:1095-1100.
110. Balthazar EJ, Birnbaum BA, Naidich M. Acute cholangitis: CT evaluation. J Comput Assist Tomogr 1993;17:283-289.
111. Bader TR, Braga L, Beavers KL, Semelka RC. MR imaging findings of infectious cholangitis. Magn Reson Imaging 2001;19:781-788.
112. Kim M-J, Cha S-W, Mitchell DG, Chung J-J, Park S, Chung JB. MR imaging findings in recurrent pyogenic cholangitis. Am J Roentgenol 1999;173:1545-1549.
113. Park M-S, Yu J-S, Kim KW, Kim M-J, et al. Recurrent pyogenic cholangitis: comparison between MR cholangiography and direct MR cholangiography. Radiology 2001;220:677-682.
114. Seel D, Park Y. Oriental infestational cholangitis. Am J Surg 1983;146:366-370.
115. Lim J. Oriental cholangiohepatitis: pathologic, clinical, and radiologic features. Am J Roentgenol 1991;157:1-8.
116. Miller FH, Gore RM, Nemcek AA, Fitzgerald SW. Pancreaticobiliary manifestations of AIDS. Am J Roentgenol 1996;166:1269-1274.
117. Jemal A, Tiwari RC, Murray T, et al. Cancer Statistics, 2004. CA Cancer J Clin 2004;54:8-29.
118. Jarnagin WR, Fong Y, Blumgart LH. The current management of hilar cholangiocarcinoma. Adv Surg 1999;33:345-373.
119. Lee WF, Kim HK, Fang KM, et al. Radiologic spectrum of cholangiocarcinoma: emphasis on unusual manifestations and differential diagnosis. Radiographics 2001;21:S97-S116.

120. Campbell WL, Ferris JV, Holbert BL, Thaete FL, Baron RL. Biliary tract carcinoma complicating primary sclerosing cholangitis: evaluation with CT, cholangiography, US, and MR imaging. Radiology 1998;207:41-50.

121. Worawattanakul S, Semelka RC, Noone TC, Calvo BF, Kelekis NL, Woosley JT. Cholangiocarcinoma: spectrum of appearances on MR images using current techniques. Magn Reson Imaging 1998;16:993-1003.

122. Guthrie JA, Ward J, Robinson PJ. Hilar cholangiocarcinomas: T2-weighted spin-echo and gadolinium-enhanced FLASH MR imaging. Radiology 1996;201:347-335.

123. Pavone P, Laghi A, Passariello R. MR cholangiopancreatography in malignant biliary obstruction. Semin Ultrasound CT MR 1999;20:317-323.

124. Fulcher AS, Turner MA. HASTE MR cholangiography in the evaluation of hilar cholangiocarcinoma. Am J Roentgenol 1997;169:1501-1505.

125. Yeh T-S, Jan Y-Y, Tseng J-H, et al. Malignant perihilar biliary obstruction: Magnetic resonance cholangiopancreatographic findings. Am J Gastroenterol 2000;95:432-440.

126. Keogan MT, Seabourn JT, Paulson EK, McDermott VG, Delong DM, Nelson DR. Contrast-enhanced CT of intrahepatic and hilar cholangiocarcinoma: delay time for optimal imaging. Am J Roentgenol 1997;169:1493-1499.

127. Burke EC, Jarnagin WR, Hochwald SN, Pisters PW, Fong Y, Blumgart LH. Hilar cholangiocarcinoma: patterns of spread, the importance of hepatic resection for curative operation, and a presurgical clinical staging system. Ann Surg 1998;228:385-394.

128. Jarnagin WR, Fong Y, DeMatteo RP, et al. Staging, resectability, and outcome in 225 patients with hilar cholangiocarcinoma. Ann Surg 2001;234:507-519.

129. Cha J, Han J, Kim T, et al. Preoperative evaluation of Klatskin tumor: accuracy of spiral CT in determining vascular invasion as a sign of unresectability. Abdom Imaging 2000;25:500-507.

130. Tillich M, Mischinger H-J, Preisegger K-H, Rabl H, Szolar DH. Multiphasic helical CT in diagnosis and staging of hilar cholangiocarcinoma. Am J Roentgenol 1998;171:651-658.

131. Launois B, Terblanche J, Lakehal M, et al. Proximal bile duct cancer: high resectability rate and 5-year survival. Ann Surg 1999;230:266-275.

132. Gerhards MF, van Gulik TM, Bosma A, et al. Long-term survival after resection of proximal bile duct carcinoma (Klatskin tumors). World J Surg 1999;23:91-96.

133. Bismuth H, Corlette M. Intrahepatic cholangioenteric anastomosis in carcinoma of the hilus of the liver. Surg Gynecol Obstet 1975;140:170-178.

134. Zidi S, Prat F, Le Guen O, Rondeau Y, Pelletier G. Performance characteristics of magnetic resonance cholangiography in the staging of malignant hilar strictures. Gut 2000;46:103-106.

135. Lillemoe K, Cameron J. Surgery for hilar cholangiocarcinoma: the Johns Hopkins approach. J Hepatobiliary Pancreat Surg 2000;7:115-121.

136. Anderson CD, Pinson CW, Berlin J, Chari RS. Diagnosis and treatment cholangiocarcinoma. Oncologist 2004;9:43-57.

137. Koike S, Ito K, Honjo K, Takano K, Yasui M, Matsunaga N. Oddi sphincter and common channel: evaluation with pharmaco-dynamic MR cholangiopancreatography using fatty meal and secretin stimulation. Radiat Med 2000;18:115-122.

138. Kim J, Kim M, Park S, et al. Using kinematic MR cholangio-pancreatography to evaluate biliary dilatation. Am J Roentgenol 2002;178:909-914.

139. Buck JL, Elsayed AM. Ampullary tumors: radiologic-pathologic correlation. Radiographics 1993;13:193-212.

140. Semelka RC, Kelekis NL, Gesine J, Ascher SM, Burdeny D, Siegelman ES. Ampullary carcinoma: demonstration by current MR techniques. J Magn Reson Imaging 1997;7:153-156.

141. Karl R, Carey L. Staging of pancreatic cancer: impact on treatment. Endoscopy 1993;25:69-74.

142. Kim JH, Kim MJ, Chung JJ, Lee WJ, Yoo HS, Lee JT. Differential diagnosis of periampullary carcinomas at MR imaging. Radiographics 2002;22:1335-1352.

143. Geier A, Nguyen H, Matern S. MRCP and ERCP to detect small ampullary carcinoma. Lancet 2000;356:1607-1608.

144. Cohen-Solal C, Parquet M, Tiffon B, Volk A, Laurent M, Lutton C. Magnetic resonance imaging for the visualization of cholesterol gallstones in hamster fed a new high sucrose lithogenic diet. J Hepatol 1995;22:486-494.

145. Fulcher AS, Turner MA, Capps GW. MR cholangiography: technical advances and clinical applications. Radiographics 1999;19:25-41.

146. Turner MA, Fulcher AS. The cystic duct: normal anatomy and disease processes. Radiographics 2001;21:3-22.

147. Kelekis N, Semelka R. MR imaging of the gallbladder. Top Magn Reson Imaging 1996;8:312-320.

148. Demachi H, Matsui O, Hoshiba K, et al. Dynamic MRI using a surface coil in chronic cholecystitis and gallbladder carcinoma: radiologic and histopathologic correlation. J Comput Assist Tomogr 1997;21:643-651.

149. Yoshimitsu K, Honda H, Kaneko K, et al. Dynamic MRI of the gallbladder lesions: differentiation of benign from malignant. J Magn Reson Imaging 1997;7:696-701.

150. Demas B, Hricak H, Moseley M, et al. Gallbladder bile: an experimental study in dogs using MR imaging and proton MR spectroscopy. Radiology 1985;157:453-455.

151. Hricak H, Filly R, Margulis A, Moon K, Crooks L, Kaufman L. Work in progress: nuclear magnetic resonance imaging of the gallbladder. Radiology 1983;147:481-484.

152. Loud P, Semelka R, Kettritz U, Brown J, Reinhold C. MRI of acute cholecystitis: comparison with the normal gallbladder and other entities. Magn Reson Imaging 1996;14:349-355.

153. Hakansson K, Leander P, Ekberg O, Hakansson H. MR imaging in clinically suspected acute cholecystitis: a comparison with ultrasonography. Acta Radiologica 2000;41:322-328.

154. Tochio H, Kudo M, Okabe Y, Morimoto Y, Tomita S. Association between a focal spared area in the fatty liver and intrahepatic efferent blood flow from the gallbladder wall: evaluation with color Doppler sonography. Am J Roentgenol 1999;172:1249-1253.

155. Abou-Saif A, Al-Kawas F. Complications of gallstone disease: Mirizzi syndrome, cholecystocholedochal fistula, and gallstone ileus. Am J Roentgenol 2002;97:249-254.

156. Lazcano-Ponce E, Miquel J, Munoz N, et al. Epidemiology and molecular pathology of gallbladder cancer. CA Cancer J Clin 2001;51:349-364.

157. Bortoff G, Chen M, Ott D, Wolfman N, Routh W. Gallbladder stones: imaging and intervention. Radiographics 2000;20:751-766.

158. Calvo M, Bujanda L, Heras I, et al. Magnetic resonance cholangiography versus ultrasound in the evaluation of the gallbladder. J Clin Gastroenterol 2002;34:233-236.

159. Ukaji M, Ebara M, Tsuchiya Y, et al. Diagnosis of gallstone composition in magnetic resonance imaging: in vitro analysis. Eur J Radiol 2002;41:49-56.

160. Gabata T, Kadoya M, Matsui O, Kobayashi T, Sanada J, Mori A. Intrahepatic biliary calculi: correlation of unusual MR findings with pathologic findings. Abdom Imaging 2000;25:266-268.

161. Park M, Yu J, Kim Y, et al. Acute cholecystitis: comparison of MR cholangiography and US. Radiology 1998;209:781-785.

162. Trowbridge RL, Rutkowski NK, Shojania KG. Does this patient have acute cholecystitis? JAMA 2003;289:80-86.

163. Patel M, Miedema B, James M, Marshall J. Percutaneous cholecystostomy is an effective treatment for high-risk patients with acute cholecystitis. Am Surg 2000;66:33-37.

164. Regan F, Schaefer D, Smith D, Petronis J, Bohlman M, Magnuson T. The diagnostic utility of HASTE MRI in the evaluation of acute cholecystitis: half-Fourier acquisition single-shot turbo SE. J Comput Assist Tomogr 1998;22:638-642.

165. Yamashita K, Jin M, Hirose Y, et al. CT finding of transient focal increased attenuation of the liver adjacent to the gallbladder in acute cholecystitis. Am J Roentgenol 1995;164:343-346.

166. Brachman M, Goodman M, Waxman A. The rim sign in acute cholecystitis. Comparison of radionuclide, surgical, and pathologic findings. Clin Nucl Med 1993;18:863-866.

167. Kim KW, Park MS, Yu JS, et al. Acute cholecystitis at T2-weighted and manganese-enhanced T1-weighted MR cholangiography: preliminary study. Radiology 2003;13:13.

168. Pedrosa I, Guarise A, Goldsmith J, Procacci C, Rofsky NM. The interrupted rim sign in acute cholecystitis: a method to identify the gangrenous form with MRI. J Magn Reson Imaging 2003;18:360-363.

169. Ottery F, Scupham R, Weese J. Chemical cholecystitis after intrahepatic chemotherapy: the case for prophylactic cholecystectomy during pump placement. Dis Colon Rectum 1986;29:187-190.

170. Carrasco C, Freeny P, Chuang V, Wallace S. Chemical cholecystitis associated with hepatic artery infusion chemotherapy. Am J Roentgenol 1983;141:703-706.

171. Kalliafas S, Ziegler D, Flancbaum L, Choban P. Acute acalculous cholecystitis: incidence, risk factors, diagnosis, and outcome. Am Surg 1998;64:471-475.

172. Jenkins M, Golding R, Cooperberg P. Sonography and computed tomography of hemorrhagic cholecystitis. Am J Roentgenol 1983;140:1197-1198.

173. West M, Garra B, Horii S, et al. Gallbladder varices: imaging findings in patients with portal hypertension. Radiology 1991;179:179-182.

174. Gabata T, Matsui O, Kadoya M, et al. Gallbladder varices: demonstration of direct communication to intrahepatic portal veins by color doppler sonography and CT during arterial portography. Abdom Imaging 1997;22:82-84.

175. Chawla Y, Dilawari J, Katariya S. Gallbladder varices in portal vein thrombosis. Am J Roentgenol 1994;162:643-645.

176. Malkan G, Bhatia S, Bashir K, et al. Cholangiopathy associated with portal hypertension: diagnostic evaluation and clinical implications. Gastrointest Endosc 1999;49:344-348.
177. Getzlaff S, Benz C, Schilling D, Riemann J. Enteroscopic cyanoacrylate sclerotherapy of jejunal and gallbladder varices in a patient with portal hypertension. Endoscopy 2001;33:462-464.
178. Hwang J, Chou Y, Tsay S, et al. Radiologic and pathologic correlation of adenomyomatosis of the gallbladder. Abdom Imaging 1998;23:73-77.
179. Ram M, Midha D. Adenomyomatosis of the gallbladder. Surgery 1975;78:224-229.
180. Aldridge M, Gruffaz F, Castaing D, Bismuth H. Adenomyomatosis of the gallbladder: a premalignant lesion? Surgery 1991;109:107-110.
181. Williams I, Slavin G, Cox A, Simpson P, de Lacey G. Diverticular disease (adenomyomatosis) of the gallbladder: a radiological-pathological survey. Br J Radiol 1986;59:29-34.
182. Ootani T, Shirai Y, Tsukada K, Muto T. Relationship between gallbladder carcinoma and the segmental type of adenomyomatosis of the gallbladder. Cancer 1992;69:2645-2652.
183. Kim M, Oh Y, Park Y, et al. Gallbladder adenomyomatosis: findings on MRI. Abdom Imaging 1999;24:410-413.
184. Yoshimitsu K, Honda H, Jimi M, et al. MR diagnosis of adenomyomatosis of the gallbladder and differentiation from gallbladder carcinoma: importance of showing Rokitansky-Aschoff sinuses. Am J Roentgenol 1999;172:1535-1540.
185. Haradome H, Ichikawa T, Sou H, et al. The pearl necklace sign: an imaging sign of adenomyomatosis of the gallbladder at MR cholangiopancreatography. Radiology 2003;227:80-88.
186. Yoshimitsu K, Honda H, Aibe H, et al. Radiologic diagnosis of adenomyomatosis of the gallbladder: comparative study among MRI, helical CT, and transabdominal US. J Comput Assist Tomogr 2001;25:843-850.
187. Berk R, van der Vegt J, Lichtenstein J. The hyperplastic cholecystoses: cholesterolosis and adenomyomatosis. Radiology 1983;146:593-601.
188. Mainprize K, Gould S, Gilbert J. Surgical management of polypoid lesions of the gallbladder. Br J Surg 2000;87:414-417.
189. Christensen A, Ishak K. Benign tumors and pseudotumors of the gallbladder: report of 180 cases. Arch Pathol Lab Med 1970;90:423-432.
190. Collett J, Allan R, Chisholm R, Wilson I, Burt M, Chapman B. Gallbladder polyps: prospective study. J Ultrasound Med 1998;17:207-211.
191. Jorgensen T, Jensen K. Polyps in the gallbladder: a prevalence study. Scand J Gastroenterol 1990;25:3.
192. Terzi C, Sokmen S, Seckin S, Albayrak L, Ugurlu M. Polypoid lesions of the gallbladder: report of 100 cases with special reference to operative indications. Surgery 2000;127:622-627.
193. Csendes A, Burgos A, Csendes P, Smok G, Rojas J. Late follow-up of polypoid lesions of the gallbladder smaller than 10 mm. Ann Surg 2001;234:657-660.
194. Sugiyama M, Atomi Y, Kuroda A, Muto T, Wada N. Large cholesterol polyps of the gallbladder: diagnosis by means of US and endoscopic US. Radiology 1995;196:493-497.
195. Furukawa H, Kosuge T, Shimada K, et al. Small polypoid lesions of the gallbladder: differential diagnosis and surgical indications by helical computed tomography. Arch Surg 1998;133:735-739.
196. Levy A, Murakata L, Abbott R, Rohrmann CJ. From the archives of the AFIP: benign tumors and tumorlike lesions of the gallbladder and extrahepatic bile ducts: radiologic-pathologic correlation. Armed Forces Institute of Pathology. Radiographics 2002;22:387-413.
197. Tublin M. Question and answer. Sonographic follow-up of patients with gallbladder polyps. Am J Roentgenol 2001;177:467.
198. Sheth S, Bedford A, Chopra S. Primary gallbladder cancer: recognition of risk factors and the role of prophylactic cholecystectomy. Am J Gastroenterol 2000;95:1402-1410.
199. Donohue J, Stewart A, Menck H. The National Cancer Data Base report on carcinoma of the gallbladder, 1989-1995. Cancer 1998;83:2618-2628.
200. North JJ, Pack M, Hong C, Rivera D. Prognostic factors for adenocarcinoma of the gallbladder: an analysis of 162 cases. Am Surg 1998;64:437-440.
201. Levy A, Murakata L, Rohrmann CJ. Gallbladder carcinoma: radiologic-pathologic correlation. Radiographics 2001;21:295-314.
202. Moerman C, Lagerwaard F, Bueno de Mesquita H, van Dalen A, van Leeuwen M, Schrover P. Gallstone size and the risk of gallbladder cancer. Scand J Gastroenterol 1993;28:482-486.
203. Yamaguchi K, Enjoji M. Carcinoma of the gallbladder: a clinico-pathology of 103 patients and a newly proposed staging. Cancer 1988;62:1425-1432.
204. Okamoto M, Okamoto H, Kitahara F, et al. Ultrasonographic evidence of association of polyps and stones with gallbladder cancer. Am J Gastroenterol 1999;94:446-450.
205. Lowenfels A, Walker A, Althaus D, Townsend G, Domellof L. Gallstone growth, size, and risk of gallbladder cancer: an interracial study. Int J Epidemiol 1989;18:50-54.
206. Sasatomi E, Tokunaga O, Miyazaki K. Precancerous conditions of gallbladder carcinoma: overview of histopathologic characteristics and molecular genetic findings. J Hepatobiliary Pancreat Surg 2000;7:556-567.
207. Roa I, Araya J, Villaseca M, et al. Preneoplastic lesions and gallbladder cancer: an estimate of the period required for progression. Gastroenterology 1996;111:232-236.
208. Towfigh S, McFadden D, Cortina G, et al. Porcelain gallbladder is not associated with gallbladder carcinoma. Am Surg 2001;67:7-10.
209. Levin B. Gallbladder carcinoma. Ann Oncol 1999;10:129-130.
210. Tsukada K, Hatakeyama K, Kurosaki I, et al. Outcome of radical surgery for carcinoma of the gallbladder according to the TNM stage. Surgery 1996;120:816-821.
211. Yoshimitsu K, Honda H, Kuroiwa T, et al. Liver metastasis from gallbladder carcinoma: anatomic correlation with cholecystic venous drainage demonstrated by helical computed tomography during injection of contrast medium in the cholecystic artery. Cancer 2001;92:340-348.
212. Fong Y, Malhotra S. Gallbladder cancer: recent advances and current guidelines for surgical therapy. Adv Surg 2001;35:1-20.
213. Schwartz L, Black J, Fong Y, et al. Gallbladder carcinoma: findings at MR imaging with MR cholangiopancreatography. J Comput Assist Tomogr 2002;26:405-410.
214. Sasson A, Hoffman J, Ross E, et al. Trimodality therapy for advanced gallbladder cancer. Am Surg 2001;67:277-283.
215. Ohtani T, Shirai Y, Tsukada K, Muto T, Hatakeyama K. Spread of gallbladder carcinoma: CT evaluation with pathologic correlation. Abdom Imaging 1996;21:195-201.
216. Pandey M, Sood B, Shukla R, Aryya N, Singh S, Shukla V. Carcinoma of the gallbladder: role of sonography in diagnosis and staging. J Clin Ultrasound 2000;28:227-232.
217. Sagoh T, Itoh K, Togashi K, et al. Gallbladder carcinoma: evaluation with MR imaging. Radiology 1990;174:131-136.
218. Kim JH, Kim TK, Eun HW, et al. Preoperative evaluation of gallbladder carcinoma: efficacy of combined use of MR imaging, MR cholangiography, and contrast-enhanced dual-phase three-dimensional MR angiography. J Magn Reson Imaging 2002;16:676-684.
219. Winston C, Chen J, Fong Y, Schwartz L, Panicek D. Recurrent gallbladder carcinoma along laparoscopic cholecystectomy port tracks: CT demonstration. Radiology 1999;212:439-444.
220. Wilbur A, Sagireddy P, Aizenstein R. Carcinoma of the gallbladder: color Doppler ultrasound and CT findings. Abdom Imaging 1997;22:187-189.
221. Bartlett D, Fong Y, Fortner J, Brennan M, Blumgart L. Long-term results after resection for gallbladder cancer. Implications for staging and management. Ann Surg 1996;224:639-646.
222. Muratore A, Polastri R, Capussotti L. Radical surgery for gallbladder cancer: current options. Eur J Surg Oncol 2000;26:438-443.
223. Shirai Y, Yoshida K, Tsukada K, Muto T, Watanabe H. Radical surgery for gallbladder carcinoma: long-term results. Ann Surg 1992;216:565-568.
224. Todoroki T, Kawamoto T, Otsuka M, et al. Benefits of combining radiotherapy with aggressive resection for stage IV gallbladder cancer. Hepatogastroenterology 1999;46:1585-1591.
225. Holloway B, King D. Ultrasound diagnosis of metastatic melanoma of the gallbladder. Br J Radiol 1997;70:1122-1125.
226. Mitropoulos F, Angelopoulou M, Siakantaris M, et al. Primary non-Hodgkin's lymphoma of the gall bladder. Leuk Lymphoma 2000;40:123-131.
227. Chatila R, Fiedler P, Vender R. Primary lymphoma of the gallbladder: case report and review of the literature. Am J Gastroenterol 1996;91:2242-2244.
228. Semelka RC, Kroeker MA, Shoenut JP, Kroeker R, Yaffe CS, Micflikier AB. Pancreatic disease: prospective comparison of CT, ERCP, and 1.5-T MR imaging with dynamic gadolinium enhancement and fat suppression. Radiology 1991;181:785-791.
229. Semelka RC, Ascher SM. MR imaging of the pancreas. Radiology 1993;188:593-602.
230. Winston CB, Mitchell DG, Outwater EK, Ehrlich SM. Pancreatic signal intensity on T1-weighted fat saturation MR images: clinical correlation. J Magn Reson Imaging 1995;5:267-271.
231. Hamed MM, Hamm B, Ibrahim ME, Taupitz M, Mahfouz AE. Dynamic MR imaging of the abdomen with gadopentetate dimeglumine: normal enhancement of the liver, spleen, stomach, and pancreas. Am J Roentgenol 1992;158:303-307.
232. Brailsford J, Ward J, Chalmers A, Ridgway J, Robinson P. Dynamic MRI of the pancreas-gadolinium enhancement in normal tissue. Clin Radiol 1994;49:104-108.
233. Lu DS, Vedantham S, Krasny RM, Kadell B, Berger W, Reber HA. Two-phase helical CT for pancreatic tumors: pancreatic versus

hepatic phase enhancement of tumor, pancreas, and vascular structures. Radiology 1996;199:697-701.

234. Kanematsu M, Shiratori Y, Hoshi H, Kondo H, Matsuo M, Moriwaka H. Pancreas and peripancreatic vessels: effect of imaging delay on gadolinium enhancement at dynamic gradient-recalled-echo MR imaging. Radiology 2000;215:95-102.

235. McNulty NJ, Francis IR, Platt JF, Cohan RH, Korobkin M, Gebremariam A. Multi-detector row helical CT of the pancreas: effect of contrast-enhanced multiphasic imaging on enhancement of the pancreas, peripancreatic vasculature, and pancreatic adenocarcinoma. Radiology 2001;220:97-102.

236. Fulcher AS, Turner MA. MR pancreatography: a useful tool for evaluating pancreatic disorders. Radiographics 1999;19:5-24.

237. Soto JA, Barish MA, Yucel EK, et al. Pancreatic duct: MR cholangiopancreatography with a three-dimensional fast spin-echo technique. Radiology 1995;196:459-464.

238. Matos C, Metens T, Deviere J, et al. Pancreatic duct: morphologic and functional evaluation with dynamic MR pancreatography after secretin stimulation. Radiology 1997;203:435-441.

239. Cappeliez O, Delhaye M, Deviere J, et al. Chronic pancreatitis: evaluation of pancreatic exocrine function with MR pancreatography after secretin stimulation. Radiology 2000;215:358-364.

240. Matos C, Winant C, Deviere J. Magnetic resonance pancreatography. Abdom Imaging 2001;26:243-253.

241. Siegelman E, Outwater E, Vinitski S, Mitchell D. Fat suppression by saturation/opposed-phase hybrid technique: spin echo versus gradient echo imaging. Magn Reson Imaging 1995;13:545-548.

242. Chan T, Listerud J, Kressel H. Combined chemical-shift and phase-selective imaging for fat suppression: theory and initial clinical experience. Radiology 1991;181:41-47.

243. Mitchell DG, Winston CB, Outwater EK, Ehrlich SM. Delineation of pancreas with MR imaging: Multiobserver comparison of five pulse sequences. J Magn Reson Imaging 1995;5:193-199.

244. Gohde SC, Toth J, Krestin GP, Debatin JF. Dynamic contrast-enhanced FMPSPGR of the pancreas: Impact on diagnostic performance. Am J Roentgenol 1997;168:689-696.

245. Hollet M, Jorgensen M, Jeffrey RJ. Quantitative evaluation of pancreatic enhancement during dual-phase helical CT. Radiology 1995;195:359-361.

246. Balci NC, Semelka RC. Radiologic features of cystic, endocrine, and other pancreatic neoplasms. Eur J Radiol 2001;38:113-119.

247. Khalid A, Peterson M, Slivka A. Secretin-stimulated magnetic resonance pancreaticogram to assess pancreatic duct outflow obstruction in evaluation of idiopathic acute recurrent pancreatitis: a pilot study. Dig Dis Sci 2003;48:1475-1481.

248. Urayama S, Kozarek R, Ball T, et al. Presentation and treatment of annular pancreas in an adult population. Am J Gastroenterol 1995;90:995-999.

249. Jadvar H, Mindelzun R. Annular pancreas in adults: imaging features in seven patients. Abdom Imaging 1999;24:174-177.

250. Hidaka T, Hirohashi S, Uchida H, et al. Annular pancreas diagnosed by single-shot MR cholangiopancreatography. Magn Reson Imaging 1998;16:441-444.

251. Desai MB, Mitchell DG, Munoz SJ. Asymptomatic annular pancreas: detection by magnetic resonance imaging. Magn Reson Imaging 1994;12:683-685.

252. Bret PM, Reinhold C, Taourel P, Guibaud L, Atri M, Barkun AN. Pancreas divisum: evaluation with MR cholangiopancreatography. Radiology 1996;199:99-103.

253. Seibert DG, Matulis SR. Santorinicele as a cause of chronic pancreatic pain. Am J Gastroenterol 1995;90:121-123.

254. Eisen G, Schutz S, Metzler D, Baillie J, Cotton PB. Santorinicele: new evidence for obstruction in pancreas divisum. Gastrointest Endosc 1994;40:73-76.

255. Boerma D, Huibregtse K, Gulik T, Rauws E, Obertop H, Gouma D. Long-term outcome of endoscopic stent placement for chronic pancreatitis associated with pancreas divisum. Endoscopy 2000;32:452-455.

256. Manfredi R, Costamagna G, Brizi MG, et al. Pancreas divisum and "Santorinicele": Diagnosis with dynamic MR cholangiopancreatography with secretin stimulation. Radiology 2000;217:403-408.

257. Matos C, Metens T, Deviere J, Delhaye M, Le Monie O, Cremer M. Pancreas divisum: evaluation with secretin-enhanced magnetic resonance cholangiopancreatography. Gastrointest Endosc 2001;53:728-733.

258. Sener SF, Fremgen A, Menck HR, Winchester DP. Pancreatic cancer: a report of treatment and survival trends for 100,313 patients diagnosed from 1985-1995 using the National Cancer Database. J Am Coll Surg 1999;189:1-7.

259. Delcore R, Rodriguez FJ, Forster J, Hemreck AS, Thomas JH. Significance of lymph node metastases in patients with pancreatic cancer undergoing curative resection. Am J Surg 1996;172:463-469.

260. Tamm EP, Silverman PM, Charnsangavej C, Evans DB. Diagnosis, staging, and surveillance of pancreatic cancer. AJR Am J Roentgenol 2003;180:1311-1323.

261. Molinari M, Helton W, Espat NJ. Palliative strategies for locally advanced unresectable and metastatic pancreatic cancer. Surg Clin North Am 2001;81:651-665.

262. Brennan MF, Moccia RD, Klimstra D. Management of adenocarcinoma of the body and tail of the pancreas. Ann Surg 1996;223:506-512.

263. Balci NC, Semelka RC. Radiologic diagnosis and staging of pancreatic ductal adenocarcinoma. Eur J Radiol 2001;38:105-112.

264. Sperti C, Pasquali C, Guolo P, Polverosi R, Liessi G, Pedrazzoli S. Serum tumor markers and cyst fluid analysis are useful for the diagnosis of pancreatic cystic tumors. Cancer 1996;78:237-243.

265. Catalano C, Pavone P, Laghi A, et al. Pancreatic adenocarcinoma: combination of MR imaging, MR angiography, and MR cholangiopancreatography for the diagnosis and assessment of resectability. Eur Radiol 1998;8:428-434.

266. Obuz F, Dicle O, Coker A, Ozgül S, Karademir S. Pancreatic adenocarcinoma: detection and staging with dynamic MR imaging. Eur J Radiol 2001;38:146-150.

267. Gabata T, Matsui O, Kadoya M, et al. Small pancreatic adenocarcinomas: efficacy of MR imaging with fat suppression and gadolinium enhancement. Radiology 1994;193:683-688.

268. Semelka RC, Simm FC, Recht MP, Deimling M, Lenz G, Laub GA. MR imaging of the pancreas at high field strength: comparison of six sequences. J Comput Assist Tomogr 1991;15:966-971.

269. Ichikawa T, Haradome H, Hachiya J, et al. Pancreatic ductal adenocarcinoma: Preoperative assessment with helical CT versus dynamic MR imaging. Radiology 1997;202:655-662.

270. Vellet AD, Romano W, Bach DB, Passi RB, Taves DH, Munk PL. Adenocarcinoma of the pancreatic ducts: comparative evaluation with CT and MR imaging at 1.5 T. Radiology 1992;183:87-95.

271. Piironen A, Kivasaari R, Laippala P, Poutanen V-P, Kivasaari L. Pancreatic carcinoma and fast MR imaging: technical considerations for signal intensity difference measurements. Eur J Radiol 2001;38:137-145.

272. Semelka RC, Shoenut JP, Kroeker MA, Micflikier AB. Chronic pancreatitis: MR imaging features before and after administration of gadopentetate dimeglumine. J Magn Reson Imaging 1993;3:79-82.

273. Johnson PT, Outwater EK. Pancreatic carcinoma versus chronic pancreatitis: dynamic MR imaging. Radiology 1999;212:213-218.

274. Lu DS, Reber HA, Krasny RM, Kadell BM, Sayre J. Local staging of pancreatic cancer: criteria for unresectability of major vessels as revealed by pancreatic-phase, thin-section helical CT. Am J Roentgenol 1997;168:1439-1443.

275. Sironi S, De Cobelli F, Zerbi A, Balzano G, Di Carlo V, Del Maschio A. Pancreatic carcinoma: MR assessment of tumor invasion of the peripancreatic vessels. J Comput Assist Tomogr 1995;19:739-744.

276. Imbriaco M, Megibow AJ, Camera L, et al. Dual-phase versus single-phase helical CT to detect and assess resectability of pancreatic carcinoma. Am J Roentgenol 2002;178:1473-1479.

277. Valls C, Andía E, Sanchez A, et al. Dual-phase helical CT of pancreatic adenocarcinoma: assessment of resectability before surgery. Am J Roentgenol 2002;178:821-826.

278. Nakayama Y, Yamashita Y, Kadota M, et al. Vascular encasement by pancreatic cancer: correlation of CT findings with surgical and pathologic results. J Comput Assist Tomogr 2001;25:337-342.

279. van Greenen RC, ten Kate FJ, de Wit LT, van Gulik TM, Obertop H, Gouma DJ. Segmental resection and wedge excision of the portal or superior mesenteric vein during pancreatoduodenectomy. Surgery 2001;129:158-163.

280. Low RN, Semelka RC, Worawattanakul S, Alzate GD. Extrahepatic abdominal imaging in patients with malignancy: comparison of MR imaging and helical CT in 164 patients. J Magn Reson Imaging 2000;12:269-277.

281. Low RN, Semelka RC, Worawattanakul S, Alzate GD, Sigeti JS. Extrahepatic abdominal imaging in patients with malignancy: comparison of MR imaging and helical CT with subsequent surgical correlation. Radiology 1999;210:625-632.

282. Chou C, Liu G, Su J, Chen L, Sheu R, Jaw T. MRI demonstration of peritoneal implants. Abdom Imaging 1994;19:95-101.

283. Vargas R, Nino-Murcia M, Trueblood W, Jeffrey RB, Jr. MDCT in pancreatic adenocarcinoma: prediction of vascular invasion and resectability using a multiphasic technique with curved planar reformations. AJR Am J Roentgenol 2004;182:419-425.

284. Di Carlo V, Zerbi A, Balzano G, Corso V. Pylorus-sparing pancreaticoduodenectomy versus conventional Whipple operation. World J Surg 1999;23:920-925.

285. Kozuch P, Petryk M, Evans A, Bruckner HW. Therapy for regionally unresectable pancreatic cancer. Surg Clin North Am 2001;81:691-697.

286. Kozuch P, Petryk M, Evans A, Bruckner HW. Treatment of metastatic pancreatic adenocarcinoma. Surg Clin North Am 2001;81:683-690.

287. Brentjens R, Saltz L. Islet cell tumors of the pancreas: the medical oncologist's perspective. Surg Clin North Am 2001;81:527-542.

288. Thoeni RF, Mueller-Lisse UG, Chan R, Do NK, Shyn PB. Detection of small, functional islet cell tumors in the pancreas: selection of MR imaging sequences for optimal sensitivity. Radiology 2000;214:483-490.

289. Owen N, Sohaib S, Peppercorn P, et al. MRI of pancreatic neuroendocrine tumours. Br J Radiol 2001;74:968-973.

290. Mori H, Fukuda T, Nagayoshi K, et al. Insulinoma: correlation of short-TI inversion-recovery (STIR) imaging and histopathologic findings. Abdom Imaging 1996;21:337-341.

291. Semelka RC, Custodio CM, Balci NC, Woosley JT. Neuroendocrine tumors of the pancreas: spectrum of appearances on MRI. J Magn Reson Imaging 2000;11:141-148.

292. Buetow PC, Miller DL, Parrino TV, Buck JL. Islet cell tumors of the pancreas: clinical, radiologic, and pathologic correlation in diagnosis and localization. Radiographics 1997;17:453-472.

293. Azimuddin K, Chamberlain RS. The surgical management of pancreatic neuroendocrine tumors. Surg Clin North Am 2001;81:511-525.

294. Buetow PC, Parrino TV, Buck JL, et al. Islet cell tumors of the pancreas: pathologic-imaging correlation among size, necrosis, and cysts, calcification, malignant behavior, and functional status. Am J Roentgenol 1995;165:1175-1179.

295. Madeira I, Terris B, Voss M, et al. Prognostic factors in patients with endocrine tumors of the duodenopancreatic area. Gut 1998;43:422-427.

296. Semelka RC, Cumming MJ, Shoenut JP, et al. Islet cell tumors: comparison of dynamic contrast-enhanced CT and MR imaging with dynamic gadolinium enhancement and fat suppression. Radiology 1993;186:799-802.

297. Catalano C, Pavone P, Laghi A, et al. Localization of pancreatic insulinomas with MR imaging at 0.5 T. Acta Radiologica 1999;39:644-648.

298. Pipeleers-Marichal M, Donow C, Heitz P, Kloppel G. Pathologic aspects of gastrinomas in patients with Zollinger-Ellison syndrome with and without multiple endocrine neoplasia type I. World J Surg 1993;17:481-488.

299. Tham RTT, Falke TH, Jansen JB, Lamers CB. CT and MR imaging of advanced Zollinger-Ellison syndrome. J Comput Assist Tomogr 1989;13:821-828.

300. Mitchell DG, Cruvella M, Eschelman DJ, Miettinen MM, Vernick JJ. MRI of pancreatic gastrinomas. J Comput Assist Tomogr 1992;16:583-585.

301. Mignon M, Ruszniewski P, Podevin P, et al. Current approach to the management of gastrinoma and insulinoma in adults with multiple endocrine neoplasia type I. World J Surg 1993;17:489-497.

302. Tham RTT, Jansen JB, Falke TH, Lamers CB. Imaging features of somatostatinoma: MR, CT, US, and angiography. J Comput Assist Tomogr 1994;18:427-431.

303. Moore N, Rogers C, Britton B. Magnetic resonance imaging of endocrine tumours of the pancreas. Br J Radiol 1995;68:341-347.

304. Kelekis NL, Semelka RC, Siegelman ES. MRI of pancreatic metastases from renal cancer. J Comput Assist Tomogr 1996;20:249-253.

305. Klein KA, Stephens DH, Welch TJ. CT characteristics of metastatic disease of the pancreas. Radiographics 1998;18:369-378.

306. Carucci LR, Siegelman ES, Feldman MD. Pancreatic metastasis from clear cell renal carcinoma: diagnosis with chemical shift MRI. J Comput Assist Tomogr 1999;23:934-936.

307. Takeshita K, Furui S, Makita K, et al. Cystic islet cell tumors: radiologic findings in three cases. Abdom Imaging 1994;19:225-228.

308. Procacci C, Graziani R, Bicego E, et al. Papillary cystic neoplasm of the pancreas: radiological findings. Abdom Imaging 1995;20:554-558.

309. Buetow PC, Buck JL, Pantongrag-Brown L, Beck KG, Ros PR, Adair CF. Solid and papillary epithelial neoplasm of the pancreas: imaging-pathologic correlation in 56 cases. Radiology 1996;199:707-711.

310. Carlson B, Johnson CD, Stephens DH, Ward EM, Kvols LK. MRI of pancreatic islet cell carcinoma. J Comput Assist Tomogr 1993;17:735-740.

311. Debray M, Geoffroy O, Laissy J, et al. Imaging appearances of metastases from neuroendocrine tumours of the pancreas. Br J Radiol 2001;74:1065-1070.

312. Henn AR, Levine EA, McNulty W, Zagoria RJ. Percutaneous radiofrequency ablation of hepatic metastases for symptomatic relief of neuroendocrine syndromes. AJR Am J Roentgenol 2003;181:1005-1010.

313. Klimstra DS, Heffess CS, Oertel JE, Rosai J. Acinar cell carcinoma of the pancreas. A clinicopathologic study of 28 cases. Am J Surg Pathol 1992;16:815-837.

314. Radin DR, Colletti PM, Forrester DM, Tang WW. Pancreatic acinar cell carcinoma with subcutaneous and intraosseous fat necrosis. Radiology 1986;158:67-68.

315. Ashley SW, Lauwers GY. Case records of the Massachusetts General Hospital, Weekly Clinicopathological Exercises, Case 37-2002: a 69-year-old man with painful cutaneous nodules, elevated lipase levels, and abnormal results on abdominal scanning. N Engl J Med 2002;347:1783-1791.

316. Lim J, Chung K, Cho O, Cho K. Acinar cell carcinoma of the pancreas: ultrasonography and computed tomography findings. Clin Imaging 1990;14:301-304.

317. Mustert BR, Stafford-Johnson DB, Francis IR. Appearance of acinar cell carcinoma of the pancreas on dual-phase CT. Am J Roentgenol 1998;171:1709.

318. Bouvet M, Staerkel GA, Spitz FR, et al. Primary pancreatic lymphoma. Surgery 1998;123:382-390.

319. Merkle EM, Bender GN, Brambs H-J. Imaging findings in pancreatic lymphoma: differential aspects. Am J Roentgenol 2000;174:671-675.

320. Van Beers B, Lalonde L, Soyer P, et al. Dynamic CT in pancreatic lymphoma. J Comput Assist Tomogr 1993;17:94-97.

321. Boudghene FP, Deslandes PM, LeBlanche AF, Bigot JMR. US and CT imaging features of intrapancreatic metastases. J Comput Assist Tomogr 1994;18:905-910.

322. Enochs W, Petherick P, Bogdanova A, Mohr U, Weissleder R. Paramagnetic metal scavenging by melanin: MR imaging. Radiology 1997;204:417-423.

323. Zhang X-M, Mitchell DG, Dohke M, Holland GA, Parker L. Pancreatic cysts: Depiction on single-shot fast spin-echo MR images. Radiology 2002;223:547-553.

324. Ros PR, Hamrick-Turner JE, Chiechi MV, Ros LH, Gallego P, Burton SS. Cystic masses of the pancreas. Radiographics 1992;12:673-686.

325. Box JC, Douglass HO. Management of cystic neoplasms of the pancreas. Am J Surg 2000;66:495-501.

326. Demos TC, Posniak HV, Harmath C, Olson MC, Aranha G. Cystic lesions of the pancreas. AJR Am J Roentgenol 2002;179:1375-1388.

327. Macari M, Lazarus D, Israel G, Megibow A. Duodenal diverticula mimicking cystic neoplasms of the pancreas: CT and MR imaging findings in seven patients. AJR Am J Roentgenol 2003;180:195-199.

328. Buck JL, Hayes WS. Microcystic adenoma of the pancreas. Radiographics 1990;10:313-322.

329. Sarr MG, Kendrick ML, Nagorney DM, Thompson GB, Farley DR, Farnell MB. Cystic neoplasms of the pancreas: benign to malignant epithelial neoplasms. Surg Clin North Am 2001;81:497-509.

330. Binkovitz L, Johnson C, Stephens D. Islet cell tumors in von Hippel-Lindau disease: increased prevalence and relationship to the multiple endocrine neoplasias. Am J Roentgenol 1990;155:501-505.

331. Choyke PL, Glenn GM, Walther MM, Patronas NJ, Linehan WM, Zbar B. von Hippel-Lindau disease: genetic, clinical, and imaging features. Radiology 1995;194:629-642.

332. Minami M, Itai Y, Ohtomo K, Yoshida H, Yoshikawa K, Iio M. Cystic neoplasms of the pancreas: comparison of MR imaging with CT. Radiology 1989;171:53-56.

333. Gazelle GS, Mueller PR, Raafat N, Halpern EF, Cardenosa G, Warshaw AL. Cystic neoplasms of the pancreas: evaluation with endoscopic retrograde pancreatography. Radiology 1993;188:633-636.

334. Iselin C, Meyer P, Hauser H, Kurt A, Vermeulen B, Rohner A. Computed tomography and fine-needle aspiration cytology for preoperative evaluation of cystic tumours of the pancreas. Br J Surg 1993;80:1166-1169.

335. Itai Y, Ohtomo K. Cystic tumours of the pancreas. Eur Radiol 1996;6:844-850.

336. Mergo PJ, Helmberger TK, Buetow PC, Helmberger RC, Ros PR. Pancreatic neoplasms: MR imaging and pathologic correlation. Radiographics 1997;17:281-301.

337. Soyer P, Rabenandrasana A, Van Beers B, et al. Cystic tumors of the pancreas: dynamic CT studies. J Comput Assist Tomogr 1994;18:420-426.

338. Procacci C, Graziani R, Bicego E, et al. Serous cystadenoma of the pancreas: report of 30 cases with emphasis on the imaging findings. J Comput Assist Tomogr 1997;21:373-382.

339. Strobel O, Z'Graggen K, Schmitz-Winnenthal FH, et al. Risk of malignancy in serous cystic neoplasms of the pancreas. Digestion 2003;68:24-33.

340. Nodell CG, Freent PC, Dale DH, Ryan JA. Serous cystadenoma of the pancreas with a metachronous adenocarcinoma. Am J Roentgenol 1994;162:1352-1354.

341. Buetow PC, Rao P, Thompson LD. Mucinous cystic neoplasms of the pancreas: radiologic-pathologic correlation. Radiographics 1998;18:433-449.

342. Thompson LD, Becker RC, Przygodzki RM, Adair CF, Heffess CS. Mucinous cystic neoplasm (mucinous cystadenocarcinoma of low-grade malignant potential) of the pancreas: a clinicopathologic study of 130 cases. Am J Surg Pathol 1999;23:1-16.

343. Grogan JR, Saeian K, Taylor AJ, Quiroz F, Demeure MJ, Komorowski RA. Making sense of mucin-producing pancreatic tumors. Am J Roentgenol 2001;176:921-929.

344. Le Borgne J, de Calan L, Partensky C, Association FS. Cystadenomas and cystadenocarcinomas of the pancreas: a multiinstitutional retrospective study of 398 cases. Ann Surg 1999;230:152-161.

345. Shyr Y-M, Su C-H, Tsay S-H, Lui W-Y. Mucin-producing neoplasms of the pancreas: intraductal papillary and mucinous cystic neoplasms. Ann Surg 1996;223:141-146.

346. Scott J, Martin I, Redhead D, Hammond P, Garden O. Mucinous cystic neoplasms of the pancreas: imaging features and diagnostic difficulties. Clin Radiol 2000;55:187-192.

347. Koito K, Namieno T, Ichimura T, et al. Mucin-producing pancreatic tumors: comparison of MR cholangiopancreatography with endoscopic retrograde cholangiopancreatography. Radiology 1998;208: 231-237.

348. Albert J, Schilling D, Breer H, Jungius K, Riemann J, Adamek H. Mucinous cystadenomas and intraductal papillary mucinous tumors of the pancreas in magnetic resonance cholangiopancreatography. Endoscopy 2000;32:472-476.

349. Procacci C, Carbognin G, Accordini S, et al. CT features of malignant mucinous cystic tumours of the pancreas. Eur Radiol 2001;11:1626-1630.

350. Lewandrowski KB, Southern JF, Pins MR, Compton CC, Warshaw AL. Cyst fluid analysis in the differential diagnosis of pancreatic cysts. Ann Surg 1993;217:41-47.

351. Warshaw AL, Brugge WR, Lewandrowski KB, Pitman MB. Case records of the Massachusetts General Hospital, Weekly Clinicopathological Exercises, Case 35-2003: a 75-year-old man with a cystic lesion of the pancreas. N Engl J Med 2003;349:1954-1961.

352. Azar C, Van de Stadt J, Devière J, et al. Intraductal papillary mucinous tumours of the pancreas: clinical and therapeutic issues in 32 patients. Gut 1996;39:457-464.

353. Procacci C, Megibow AJ, Carbognin G, et al. Intraductal papillary mucinous tumor of the pancreas: a pictorial essay. Radiographics 1999;19:1447-1463.

354. Taouli B, Vilgrain V, O'Toole D, Vullierme M-P, Terris B, Menu Y. Intraductal papillary mucinous tumors of the pancreas: features with multimodality imaging. J Comput Assist Tomogr 2002;26:223-231.

355. Tenner S, Carr-Locke DL, Banks PA, et al. Intraductal mucin-hypersecreting neoplasm "mucinous ductal ectasia": endoscopic recognition and management. Am J Gastroenterol 1996;91:2548-2554.

356. Pavone E, Mehta SN, Hilzenrat N, et al. Role of ERCP in the diagnosis of intraductal papillary mucinous neoplasms. Am J Gastroenterol 1997;92:887-890.

357. Fukukura Y, Fujiyoshi F, Hamada H, et al. Intraductal papillary mucinous tumors of the pancreas: comparison of helical CT and MR imaging. Acta Radiol 2003;44:464-471.

358. Sugiyama M, Atomi Y, Kuroda A. Two types of mucin-producing cystic tumors of the pancreas: diagnosis and treatment. Surgery 1997;122:617-625.

359. Sugiyama M, Atomi Y, Hachiya J. Intraductal papillary tumors of the pancreas: evaluation with magnetic resonance cholangiopancreatography. Am J Gastroenterol 1998;93:156-159.

360. Fukukura Y, Fujiyoshi F, Sasaki M, et al. HASTE MR cholangiopancreatography in the evaluation of intraductal papillary-mucinous tumors of the pancreas. J Comput Assist Tomogr 1999;23:301-305.

361. Arakawa A, Yamashita Y, Namimoto T, et al. Intraductal papillary tumors of the pancreas. Histopathologic correlation of MR cholangiopancreatography findings. Acta Radiologica 2000;41:343-347.

362. Silas AM, Morrin MM, Raptopoulos V, Keogan MT. Intraductal papillary mucinous tumors of the pancreas. Am J Roentgenol 2001;176:179-185.

363. Procacci C, Biasiutti C, Carbognin G, et al. Characterization of cystic tumors of the pancreas: CT accuracy. J Comput Assist Tomogr 1999;23:906-912.

364. Onaya H, Itai Y, Niitsu M, Chiba T, Michishita N, Saida Y. Ductectatic mucinous cystic neoplasms of the pancreas: evaluation with MR cholangiopancreatography. Am J Roentgenol 1998; 171:171-177.

365. Irie H, Honda H, Aibe H, et al. MR cholangiopancreatographic differentiation of benign and malignant intraductal mucin-producing tumors of the pancreas. Am J Roentgenol 2000;174:1403-1408.

366. Loftus EVJ, Olivares-Pakzad BA, Batts KP, et al. Intraductal papillary-mucinous tumors of the pancreas: clinicopathologic features, outcome, and nomenclature. Gastroenterology 1996;110:1909-1918.

367. Seki M, Yanagisawa A, Ohta H, et al. Surgical treatment of intraductal papillary-mucinous tumor (IPMT) of the pancreas: operative indications based on surgico-pathologic study focusing on invasive carcinoma derived from IPMT. J Hepatobiliary Pancreat Surg 2003;10:147-155.

368. Sugiyama M, Izumisato Y, Abe N, Masaki T, Mori T, Atomi Y. Predictive factors for malignancy in intraductal papillary-mucinous tumours of the pancreas. Br J Surg 2003;90:1244-1249.

369. Procacci C, Graziani R, Bicego E, et al. Intraductal mucin-producing tumors of the pancreas: imaging findings. Radiology 1996;198: 249-257.

370. Megibow A, Lombardo F, Guarise A, et al. Cystic pancreatic masses: cross-sectional imaging observations and serial follow-up. Abdom Imaging 2001;26:640-647.

371. Terris B, Ponsot P, Paye F, et al. Intraductal papillary mucinous tumors of the pancreas confined to secondary ducts show less aggressive pathologic features as compared with those involving the main pancreatic duct. Am J Surg Pathol 2000;24:1372-1377.

372. Krinsky G. Letter to the editor. N Engl J Med 2001;344:141.

373. Anon. Case records of the Massachusetts General Hospital, Weekly Clinicopathological Exercises, Case 26-2000: a 47-year-old man was admitted to the hospital because of recurrent abdominal pain and a pancreatic lesion. N Engl J Med 2000;343:563-570.

374. Irie H, Yoshimitsu K, Aibe H, et al. Natural history of pancreatic intraductal papillary mucinous tumor of branch duct type. J Comput Assist Tomogr 2004;28:117-122.

375. Wakabayashi T, Kawaura Y, Morimoto H, et al. Clinical management of intraductal papillary mucinous tumors of the pancreas based on imaging findings. Pancreas 2001;22:370-377.

376. Obara T, Maguchi H, Saitoh Y, et al. Mucin-producing tumor of the pancreas: natural history and serial pancreatogram changes. Am J Gastroenterol 1993;88:564-569.

377. Bernard P, Scoazec JY, Joubert M, et al. Intraductal papillary-mucinous tumors of the pancreas: predictive criteria of malignancy according to pathological examination of 53 cases. Arch Surg 2002;137:1274-1278.

378. Ohtomo K, Furui S, Onoue M, et al. Solid and papillary epithelial neoplasm of the pancreas: MR imaging and pathologic correlation. Radiology 1992;184:567-570.

379. Coleman KM, Doherty MC, Bigler SA. Solid-pseudopapillary tumor of the pancreas. Radiographics 2003;23:1644-1648.

380. Savci G, Kilicturgay S, Sivri Z, Parlak M, Tuncel E. Solid and papillary epithelial neoplasm of the pancreas: CT and MR findings. Eur Radiol 1996;6:86-88.

381. Murayama S, Robinson A, Mulvihill D, et al. MR imaging of pancreas in cystic fibrosis. Pediatr Radiol 1990;20:536-539.

382. Tham RTT, Heyerman HG, Falke TH, et al. Cystic fibrosis: MR imaging of the pancreas. Radiology 1991;179:183-186.

383. Ferrozzi F, Bova D, Campodonico F, et al. Cystic fibrosis: MR assessment of pancreatic damage. Radiology 1996;198:875-879.

384. King LJ, Scurr ED, Murugan N, Williams SG, Westaby D, Healy JC. Hepatobiliary and pancreatic manifestations of cystic fibrosis: MR imaging appearances. Radiographics 2000;20:767-777.

385. Jager H, Mehring U, Gotz G, et al. Radiologic features of the visceral and skeletal involvement of hemochromatosis. Eur Radiol 1997;7:1199-1206.

386. Siegelman ES, Mitchell DG, Outwater E, Munoz SJ, Rubin R. Idiopathic hemochromatosis: MR imaging findings in cirrhotic and precirrhotic patients. Radiology 1993;188:637-641.

387. Siegelman ES, Mitchell DG, Semelka RC. Abdominal iron deposition: metabolism, MR findings, and clinical importance. Radiology 1996;199:13-22.

388. Lu J, Hayashi K. Selective iron deposition in pancreatic islet B cells of transfusional iron-overloaded autopsy cases. Pathol Int 1994;44: 194-199.

389. Hough DM, Stephens DH, Johnson CD, Binkovitz LA. Pancreatic disease in von Hippel-Lindau disease: Prevalence, clinical significance, and CT findings. Am J Roentgenol 1994;162:1091-1094.

390. Hammel PR, Vilgrain V, Terris B, Penfornis A, et al. Pancreatic involvement in von Hippel-Lindau disease. Gastroenterology 2000;119:1087-1095.

391. Marcos HB, Libutti SK, Alexander HR, et al. Neuroendocrine tumors of the pancreas in von Hippel-Lindau disease: spectrum of appearances at CT and MR imaging with histopathologic comparison. Radiology 2002;225:751-758.

392. Libutti SK, Choyke PL, Bartlett DL, et al. Pancreatic neuroendocrine tumors associated with von Hippel-Lindau disease: Diagnostic and management recommendations. Surgery 1998;124:1153-1159.

393. Levy MJ, Geenen JE. Idiopathic acute recurrent pancreatitis. Am J Gastroenterol 2001;96:2540-2555.

394. Bradley EL III. A clinically based classification system for acute pancreatitis: summary of the International Symposium on Acute Pancreatitis, Atlanta, GA, Sept 11-13, 1992. Arch Surg 1993;128:586-590.

395. Piironen A. Severe acute pancreatitis: contrast-enhanced CT and MRI features. Abdom Imaging 2001;26:225-233.

396. Ward J, Chalmers A, Guthrie A, Larvin M, Robinson P. T2-weighted and dynamic enhanced MRI in acute pancreatitis: comparison with contrast enhanced CT. Clin Radiol 1997;52:109-114.
397. Amano Y, Oishi T, Takahashi M, Kumazaki T. Nonenhanced magnetic resonance imaging of mild acute pancreatitis. Abdom Imaging 2001;26:59-63.
398. Saifuddin A, Ward J, Ridgway J, Chalmers A. Comparison of MR and CT scanning in severe acute pancreatitis: initial experiences. Clin Radiol 1993;48:111-116.
399. Pitchumoni C, Agarwal N. Pancreatic pseudocysts: when and how should drainage be performed? Gastroenterol Clin North Am 1999;28:615-639.
400. Morgan DE, Baron TH, Smith JK, Robbin ML, Kenney PJ. Pancreatic fluid collections prior to intervention: evaluation with MR imaging compared with CT and US. Radiology 1997;203:773-778.
401. Lecesne R, Taourel P, Bret PM, Atri M, Reinhold C. Acute pancreatitis: interobserver agreement and correlation of CT and MR cholangiopancreatography with outcome. Radiology 1999;211:727-735.
402. Paulson EK, Vitellas KM, Keogan MT, Low VH, Nelson RC. Acute pancreatitis complicated by gland necrosis: spectrum of findings on contrast-enhanced CT. Am J Roentgenol 1999;172:609-613.
403. Vitellas KM, Paulson EK, Enns RA, Keogan MT, Pappas TN. Pancreatitis complicated by gland necrosis: evolution of findings on contrast-enhanced CT. J Comput Assist Tomogr 1999;23:898-905.
404. Piironen A, Kivasaari L, Pitkaranta P, et al. Contrast-enhanced magnetic resonance imaging for the detection of acute haemorrhagic necrotizing pancreatitis. Eur Radiol 1997;7:17-20.
405. Martin DR, Karabulut N, Yang M, McFadden DW. High signal peripancreatic fat on fat-suppressed spoiled gradient echo imaging in acute pancreatitis: preliminary evaluation of the prognostic significance. J Magn Reson Imaging 2003;18:49-58.
406. Waslen T, Wallace K, Burbridge B, Kwauk S. Pseudoaneurysm secondary to pancreatitis presenting as GI bleeding. Abdom Imaging 1998;23:318-321.
407. Stabile B, Wilson S, Debas HT. Reduced mortality from bleeding pseudocysts and pseudoaneurysms caused by pancreatitis. Arch Surg 1983;118:45-51.
408. Carr JA, Cho J-S, Shepard AD, Nypaver TJ, Reddy DJ. Visceral pseudoaneurysms due to pancreatic pseudocysts: rare buth lethal complications of pancreatitis. J Vascular Surg 2000;32:722-730.
409. Crowe P, Sagar G. Reversible superior mesenteric vein thrombosis in acute pancreatitis: the CT appearance. Clin Radiol 1995;50:628-633.
410. Eubank WB, Schmiedl UP, Levy AR, Marsh CL. Venous thrombosis and occlusion after pancreas transplantation: evaluation with breath-hold gadolinium-enhanced three-dimensional MR imaging. Am J Roentgenol 2000;175:381-385.
411. Marn CS, Glazer GM, Williams DM, Francis IR. CT-angiographic correlation of collateral venous pathways in isolated splenic vein occlusion: new observations. Radiology 1990;175:375-380.
412. Fernandez-del Castillo CF, Sahani DV, Lauwers GY. Case records of the Massachusetts General Hospital, Weekly Clinicopathological Exercises, Case 27-2003: a 36-year-old man with recurrent epigastric pain and elevated amylase levels. N Engl J Med 2003;349:893-901.
413. Etemad B, Whitcomb DC. Chronic pancreatitis: diagnosis, classification, and new genetic developments. Gastroenterology 2001;120:682-707.
414. Irie H, Honda H, Baba S, et al. Autoimmune pancreatitis: CT and MR characteristics. AJR Am J Roentgenol 1998;170:1323-1327.
415. Van Hoe L, Gryspeerdt S, Ectors N, et al. Nonalcoholic duct-destructive chronic pancreatitis: imaging findings. Am J Roentgenol 1998;170:643-647.
416. Zhang XM, Shi H, Parker L, Dohke M, Holland GA, Mitchell DG. Suspected early or mild chronic pancreatitis: enhancement patterns on gadolinium chelate dynamic MRI. J Magn Reson Imaging 2003;17:86-94.
417. Sica GT, Braver J, Cooney MJ, Miller FH, Ch JL, Adams DF. Comparison of endoscopic retrograde cholangiopancreatography with MR cholangiopancreatography in patients with pancreatitis. Radiology 1999;210:605-610.
418. Manfredi R, Costamagna G, Brizi MG, et al. Severe chronic pancreatitis versus suspected pancreatic disease: dynamic MR cholangiopancreatography after secretin stimulation. Radiology 2000;214:849-855.
419. Kim T, Murakami T, Takamura M, et al. Pancreatic mass due to chronic pancreatitis: correlation of CT and MR imaging features with pathologic findings. Am J Roentgenol 2001;177:367-371.
420. Katz DS, Nardi PM, Hines J, et al. Lipomas of the pancreas. Am J Roentgenol 1998;170:1485-1487.
421. Di Maggio EM, Solcia M, Dore R, et al. Intrapancreatic lipoma: first case diagnosed with CT. Am J Roentgenol 1996;167:56-57.
422. Ito K, Koike S, Matsunaga N. MR imaging of pancreatic diseases. Eur J Radiol 2001;38:78-93.
423. Isserow JA, Siegelman ES, Mammone J. Focal fatty infiltration of the pancreas: MR characterization with chemical shift imaging. Am J Roentgenol 1999;173:1263-1265.
424. Jacobs JE, Coleman BG, Arger PH, Langer JE. Pancreatic sparing of focal fatty infiltration. Radiology 1994;190:437-439.
425. Matsumoto S, Mori H, Miyake H, et al. Uneven fatty replacement of the pancreas: evaluation with CT. Radiology 1995;194:453-458.
426. Gaber AO, Shokouh-Amiri MH, Hathaway DK, et al. Results of pancreas transplantation with portal venous and enteric drainage. Ann Surg 1995;221:613-624.
427. Shokouh-Amiri M, Gaber AO, Gaber L, et al. Pancreas transplantation with portal venous drainage and enteric exocrine diversion: a new technique. Transplant Proc 1992;24:776-777.
428. Heyneman LE, Keogan MT, Tuttle-Newhall JE, Porte RJ, Leder RA, Nelson RC. Pancreatic transplantation using portal venous and enteric drainage: the postoperative appearance of a new surgical procedure. J Comput Assist Tomogr 1999;23:283-290.
429. Yuh WT, Hunsicker LG, Nghiem DD, et al. Pancreatic transplants: evaluation with MR imaging. Radiology 1989;170:171-177.
430. Dachman AH, Newmark GM, Thistlethwaite JR, Oto A, Bruce DS, Newell KA. Imaging of pancreatic transplantation using portal venous and enteric exocrine drainage. Am J Roentgenol 1998;171:157-263.
431. Krebs TL, Daly B, Wong JJ, Chow CC, Bartlett ST. Vascular complications of pancreatic transplantation: MR evaluation. Radiology 1995;196:793-798.
432. Krebs TL, Daly B, Cheong JJ, Carroll K, Bartlett ST. Acute pancreatic transplant rejection: evaluation with dynamic contrast-enhanced MR imaging compared with histopathologic analysis. Radiology 1999;210:437-442.
433. Soulen MC, Zerhouni EA, Fishman EK, Gayler BW, Milligan F, Siegelman SS. Enlargement of the pancreatic head in patients with pancreas divisum. Clin Imaging 1989;13:51-57.
434. Chan TW, Listerud J, Kressel HY. Combined chemical-shift and phase-selective imaging for fat suppression: theory and initial clinical experience. Radiology 1991;181:41-47.
435. Siegelman ES, Outwater EK, Vinitski S, Mitchell DG. Fat suppression by saturation/opposed-phase hybrid technique: spin echo versus gradient echo imaging. Magn Reson Imaging 1995;13:545-548.
436. Bluemke DA, Wolf RL, Tani I, Tachiki S, McVeigh ER, Zerhouni EA. Extremity veins: evaluation with fast-spin-echo MR venography. Radiology 1997;204:562-565.

MRI of the Adrenal Glands

Evan S. Siegelman, MD

NORMAL ANATOMY OF THE ADRENAL GLAND

The adrenals are paired retroperitoneal endocrine glands composed of an outer cortex and inner medulla. The adrenal cortex is derived from the mesoderm and is responsible for the secretion of aldosterone, cortisol, and androgens, while the adrenal medulla is derived from neural crest cells and secretes norepinephrine and epinephrine.[1] The normal adrenal medulla and cortex are not routinely distinguished on routine MR imaging. On high-resolution T2-W ex vivo images, the adrenal medulla is a hyperintense band compared with the adrenal cortex.[2]

CHEMICAL SHIFT IMAGING TECHNIQUES

The two most common neoplasms involving the adrenal gland are adrenocortical adenomas and metastatic disease. The adrenocortical cells that comprise adenomas contain intracellular lipid. The ability to detect and characterize intracellular lipid makes chemical shift MR an ideal imaging technique for evaluating adrenal masses and distinguishing between metastatic disease and benign cortical adenomas. The following is a brief discussion of chemical shift methods.

The term "chemical shift" when applied to clinical MR imaging refers to the difference in behavior of lipid and water protons when placed in a magnetic field. The chemical shift of lipid and water protons is 3.5 parts per million (ppm); water protons precess at a slightly higher frequency. According to the Larmor equation, at 1.5 tesla (T) protons precess at approximately 63 million times per second. Therefore, the chemical shift difference between lipid and water protons at

1.5 T is approximately 220 hertz (Hz; 63×3.5 ppm). Thus, at 1.5 T, lipid protons precess at a frequency of 63 million times per second and water protons precess at 63 million 220 times per second. A 220-Hz frequency corresponds to a period of once every 4.2 msec.

Imagine the precessing lipid and water protons within a voxel of tissue in a 1.5 T magnet as individuals running around a racetrack. Every 4.2 msec both the lipid and water protons would cross the finish line at the same instant, even though they were running (precessing) at different speeds (frequencies). At 1.5 T gradient echo (GRE) sequences with echo times of 4.2 msec result in the addition of signal intensities (SIs) from lipid and water protons contained within the same voxel ("in phase"). With an echo time of 2.1 msec (and odd multiples of 2.1) the SIs of lipid and water protons are at opposite sides of the racetrack; thus, their SIs will be destructive, not additive. These GRE sequences are termed "opposed phase."

Spin-echo (SE) and fast spin-echo (FSE) sequences are in-phase techniques because they use 180° refocusing pulses that are applied halfway before an echo is sampled. For example, a T1 SE sequence with an echo time of 10 msec employs a 180° refocusing pulse at 5 msec. Thus, any "lead" that the water protons have accumulated at 5 msec is converted to an equivalent "loss" because the 180° refocusing pulse places the water protons on the opposite side of the racetrack. Conversely, the slower lipid protons are given an equivalent "head start" at the beginning of the second half of the echo time. During the second half of the race (the second 5 msec), the water protons catch up to the lipid protons so that at 10 msec, when the echo is sampled, there is a "photo finish" and the protons are in phase. GRE sequences lack 180° refocusing pulses and thus this difference in behavior between water protons and lipid can be exploited to generate both in-phase and opposed-phase images by selection of the appropriate echo times to sample.[3]

Another type of chemical shift effect is to some extent present on all MR images and is secondary to the inherent difference in precessional frequency between lipid and water protons (e.g., 220 Hz at 1.5 T). When acquiring GRE or SE sequences there is a frequency encoding and phase encoding direction that allows the MR system to reconstruct an image using Fourier transformation. A gradient is applied across the frequency-encoding axis during the read-out period. This enables the magnet's receiver to determine what column (assuming the frequency encoding direction was the x-y plane) of tissue protons originate based on its precessional frequency. However, since water protons precess faster than lipid protons, the signal from water protons is shifted by a few pixels because the receiver cannot determine if a change in precessional frequency is due to lipid-water chemical shift differences or to gradient-induced changes in the frequency-encoding axis. This type of chemical shift (Fig. 3-1) is more accentuated when low bandwidth techniques (which are commonly used

on low-field-strength magnets as a method of increasing signal to noise) are used. Before the implementation of chemical shift and fat saturation methods, identification of this chemical shift band was used to establish that a boundary between two tissues was a fat-water interface.

NEOPLASMS OF THE ADRENAL CORTEX

Adrenocortical Adenomas

Adrenocortical adenomas are benign neoplasms of the adrenal cortex. Between 2% and 9% of autopsies reveal adrenal tumors[4] and 1% to 2% of patients have incidental adrenal masses discovered at cross-sectional imaging.[5-7] The majority of these masses are nonhyperfunctioning adrenocortical adenomas that are benign and require no treatment. Demonstration of loss of signal intensity (SI) within an adrenal mass on an opposed-phase image when compared with a corresponding in-phase image establishes the presence of intracellular lipid and a presumptive diagnosis of adrenal adenoma[8,9] (Figs. 3-2 and 3-3 and Box 3-1; see Fig. 3-1).[10] If one wanted to use quantitative

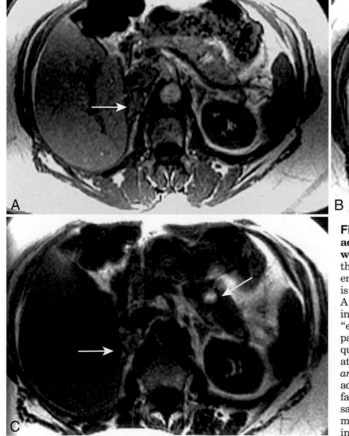

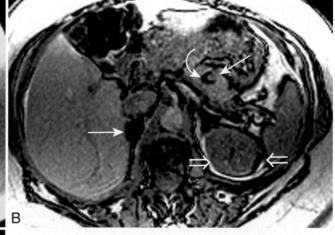

Figure 3-1 ▪ Chemical shift imaging findings of a right adrenal adenoma and pancreatic lipoma in an asymptomatic woman. A and **B,** In-phase (**A**) and opposed-phase (**B**) T1-WIs show that a right adrenal mass *(arrow)* loses SI in **B,** indicating the presence of lipid and water protons within the same voxel. The loss of SI is secondary to the presence of intracellular lipid within an adenoma. A pancreatic body mass *(arrow in* **B***)* is present that is isointense to fat in **A** and minimally loses SI in **B.** There is a low SI "India ink" or "etching" artifact along the right border of the mass and the adjacent pancreatic parenchyma *(curved arrow).* From right to left (the frequency-encoding axis of this image), the etching artifact is prominent at water-fat interfaces and absent at fat-water interfaces (see *open arrows* on the medial and lateral aspects of the left kidney). Since the adjacent pancreas is composed of water, the mass must be composed of fat. This chemical shift phenomenon is explained in the text. **C,** Water-saturated T1-WI shows very high SI within the pancreatic lipoma and mild-high SI within the adrenal adenoma, reflecting the difference in appearance between macroscopic fat and intracellular lipid.

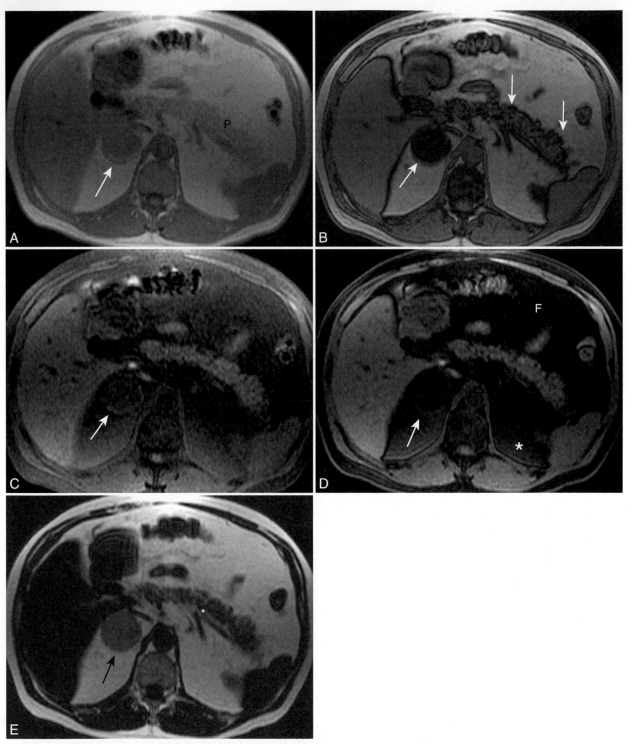

Figure 3-2 ■ **Chemical shift imaging characterization of an adrenal adenoma in an asymptomatic man.**
A and **B**, In-phase (**A**) and opposed-phase (**B**) T1-WIs show a 4.5 cm right adrenal mass *(arrow)* that loses SI in **B**, indicating the presence of intracellular lipid. Normal high SI pancreas is present (P) on the in-phase imaging. In **A**, the
heterogeneous regions of low and high SI in and around the border of the pancreas *(arrows)* is from opposed-phase effects
secondary to the presence of pancreatic parenchyma and peripancreatic fat within the same voxels. **C** and **D**, Corresponding
fat-suppressed in-phase (**C**) and opposed-phase (**D**) T1-WIs shows fair suppression of the fat anterior to the pancreas (F)
but poor saturation of the fat posterior to the adrenal glands (*). Incomplete fat saturation of the posterior superior
retroperitoneum is secondary to susceptibility effects from the adjacent lung base. There is moderate loss of signal within
the right adrenal mass *(arrow)*. The fat-suppressed opposed-phase image (**D**) better suppresses SI within adipose tissue
when compared with fat-suppressed in-phase sequences. The moderate SI loss within the adenoma on this image is potentially misleading. In typical adrenal adenomas, greater SI loss is expected on opposed-phase images compared with
fat-suppressed opposed-phase images. Had the resultant fat suppression been optimal, no signal from lipid protons within
the adenoma would have been present to oppose the signal from water protons within the mass. In this case, the incomplete fat saturation resulted in residual lipid signal within the adenoma that was available to cancel the signal from
adjacent intratumoral water protons. **E**, Water-suppressed T1-WI reveals subtle residual signal within the adenoma
(arrow), indicating the presence of intracellular lipid. This technique is ideal for demonstrating small amounts of macroscopic fat (such as in myelolipomas, angiomyelolipomas, and cystic teratomas). In-phase and opposed-phase imaging
(**A** and **B**) are best for characterizing intracellular lipid within lesions such as adrenal adenoma.

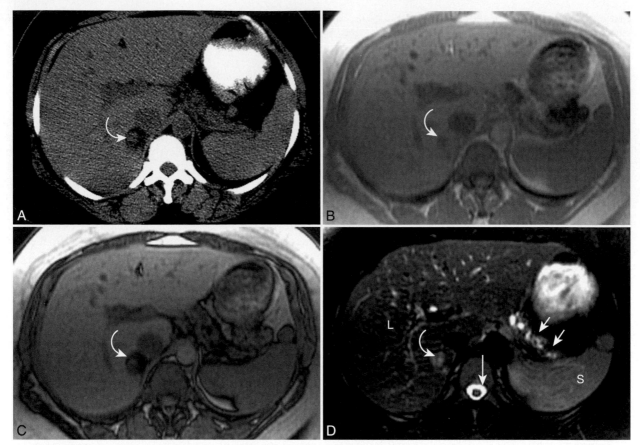

Figure 3-3 ▪ **MR illustration of an adrenal adenoma with lipid-rich and lipid-poor components in a 37-year-old woman. A,** Noncontrast CT obtained through the right adrenal gland shows two zones: a subcentimeter focus of higher attenuation *(curved arrow)* surrounded by lower attenuation adenoma. **B and C,** Corresponding in-phase (**B**) and opposed-phase (**C**) T1-WIs obtained at a similar level as in **A** show a similar two-zone adrenal gland with a subcentimeter focus of lower SI tissue *(curved arrow)* in **B** that does not lose SI in **C**. The apparent decrease in SI of this lipid-poor region when comparing this opposed-phase image with the corresponding in-phase image with a longer TE of 4.6 (**B**) was not confirmed on quantitative ROI analysis and is attributable to differences in dynamic range. The remainder of the adrenal gland does lose SI in keeping with an adenoma. **D,** Fat-suppressed respiratory-triggered T2-WI shows normal soft tissue contrast with low-to-intermediate SI liver (L), intermediate to high SI spleen (S) and very high SI intensity CSF *(arrow)*. There is dilation of the pancreatic duct *(small arrows)*, in keeping with chronic pancreatitis. The SI of the lipid-rich adrenal adenoma is isointense to minimally hyperintense to liver and hypointense to spleen. Although relative isointensity of an adrenal mass to liver on T2-WI is suggestive of an adenoma (and was the MR method of choice for characterization before the clinical implementation of chemical shift imaging of the adrenal gland), it is not sufficient to establish that diagnosis. The lipid-poor segment of the adenoma is of relative high SI *(curved arrow)*. Given the lack of a known primary and the absence of signs or symptoms of pheochromocytoma, this lipid-poor focus is unlikely to represent a "collision tumor."[101]

3-1	Adrenal Adenoma vs. Adrenal Metastasis	
	Adenoma	*Metastasis*
Loss of signal with chemical shift imaging	Yes (>90%)	No
Size	Smaller, most <2 cm	Larger, most >2 cm
Known primary	Usually no	Usually yes
Tumor margin	Regular	Irregular
MR signal intensity	Homogeneous	Heterogeneous
T2 signal intensity	Isointense to liver	Isointense to spleen
Growth on follow-up	No	Yes

measurements to diagnose a cortical adenoma, a chemical shift index [(SI of adrenal lesion on in-phase image – SI on opposed-phase image)/(SI on in-phase image)] of >0.15 has high specificity and positive predictive value.[11] The amount of intracellular lipid within adenomas corresponds to the amount of SI loss on chemical shift imaging[12] and could be used to quantitate the amount of lipid within adenomas.

Certain clinical and MR imaging features are helpful in distinguishing adenomas from metastases independently of the loss of SI on chemical shift and appearance on T2-WI. Adenomas tend to be smaller, to reveal homogeneous SI on all pulse sequences, and to be well marginated, whereas adrenal metastases tend to be larger, heterogeneous, poorly marginated and occur in patients with known primary malignancies (Box 3-1). Before the widespread implementation of chemical shift imaging, both qualitative and quantitative measurements of adrenal gland SI on T2-WI were used to distinguish adenomas from nonadenomas.[13-15] Such techniques were only 80% accurate and thus cannot be used in isolation to establish the diagnosis of a benign adrenal mass. T2-WIs are still of value to detect and characterize potential metastatic disease elsewhere in the abdomen.

Chemical shift imaging and unenhanced CT are not complimentary in the characterization of adrenal adenomas, since both examinations will likely characterize the same subset of lipid-rich adenomas (see Fig. 3-3).[7] Thus, if chemical shift MR cannot establish the lipid content of an adrenal mass, it would be unlikely that a nonenhanced CT would reveal an HU value of less than 10, which is the accepted CT criterion for characterizing an adenoma.[16]

HYPERSECRETING ADRENOCORTICAL ADENOMAS

Referring physicians should perform a patient history and physical examination in an attempt to elicit signs or symptoms of hormonal hypersecretion in individuals who have an adrenal adenoma detected at imaging.[4,17] In a 1990 *New England Journal of Medicine* article, Ross and Aron suggested keeping additional laboratory and imaging studies to a minimum. However, subsequent literature indicates an increasing prevalence of cortisol- and aldosterone-secreting adenomas in patients who do not present with classic signs and symptoms of Cushing's or Conn's syndromes (see next sections).

Cushing's syndrome. MR cannot accurately distinguish between hypersecreting and nonhypersecreting adrenocortical adenomas in most patients. One imaging clue, which is present only in some patients with Cushing's syndrome, is relative atrophy of the contralateral adrenal gland secondary to feedback inhibition of pituitary ACTH secretion by a hyperfunctioning adrenal adenoma.[18] In the absence of this imaging sign, one must again rely on the history and physical examination.

The absence of obesity and hypertension excludes a diagnosis of Cushing's syndrome with a high specificity, and thus additional testing is not necessary.[17] However, given the presence of hypertension, obesity, or type 2 diabetes, a dexamethasone suppression test should be performed to determine whether there is autonomous cortisol production by the adrenal gland.[19]

Subclinical Cushing's syndrome is more common than classic Cushing's syndrome and may be present in up to 25% of patients who have adrenocortical adenomas detected at imaging.[20] Even though such patients do not have overt signs and symptoms of classic Cushing's syndrome, they may still benefit from adrenalectomy. One author considers surgery for younger patients (<50 yr) and for those with recent onset of weight gain, obesity, hypertension,

diabetes, or osteopenia.[19] Affected patients are treated with perioperative hormones in order to prevent a postoperative addisonian crisis. A prospective study has yet to be performed to determine whether medical therapy or adrenalectomy is the optimal therapy in patients with subclinical Cushing's syndrome.

Conn's syndrome. Primary hyperaldosteronism is the most common etiology of secondary renal hypertension.[21] Two thirds of patients with hyperaldosteronism have a single aldosterone-secreting adrenocortical adenoma; these patients would benefit from adrenalectomy. The remaining third of patients have forms of adrenal hyperplasia that do not benefit from surgery and are best treated medically.[22] If an imaging study detects a single adrenal adenoma in a patient with clinically suspected Conn's syndrome, then adrenalectomy can be performed with the expectation that most patients wall benefit.[23-25] A patient with primary aldosteronism who has enlarged adrenal glands without a focal mass is likely to have hyperplasia and not a single, hypersecreting adenoma.[26] In equivocal patients, adrenal vein renin sampling is recommended to detect an occult unilateral aldosterone-producing adenoma.[21]

Previously it was advocated that only those hypertensive patients with hypokalemia be further evaluated for Conn's syndrome when an adrenocortical adenoma was detected at imaging. However, more than half of patients with Conn's syndrome have normal potassium levels.[27] Thus, hypertensive patients with an adrenocortical adenoma should have laboratory evaluation of aldosterone and plasma renin activity in order to identify a greater number of individuals who may benefit from adrenalectomy or targeted antihypertensive therapy.[28] Selective adrenal artery embolization is an alternative treatment to surgery in the management of unilateral aldosteronomas.[29] When MR is performed for renal artery stenosis, chemical shift imaging should be included to detect an adrenal mass that may be a cause of the hypertension. In a series of 77 patients referred for MR angiography, four had adrenal masses that were the cause of the hypertension.[30]

NONHYPERSECRETING ADRENOCORTICAL ADENOMAS

Even with the recent insights into subclinical Cushing's syndrome and hypertensive patients with normal serum potassium that have aldosterone-producing adenomas, the nonhypersecreting adrenocortical adenoma is still the most commonly encountered adrenal mass at cross-sectional imaging.[7] Although recent reviews have emphasized the importance of excluding a pheochromocytoma,[31,32] such an evaluation is unnecessary if MR has demonstrated the presence of lipid within an adrenal mass. Pheochromocytomas originate from the adrenal medulla and do not lose SI on chemical shift imaging.

If MR does not demonstrate loss of SI on chemical shift imaging, then follow-up imaging can be considered (primary malignancies are discussed in later sections; see Fig. 3-3). The physician could obtain a contrast-enhanced CT as a means of evaluating a lipid-poor or nonlipid-containing adrenal mass revealed at MRI.[7] CT studies have shown that lipid-poor adenomas (as well as the more common lipid-containing adenomas) show a greater degree of washout of iodinated contrast at 15 minutes compared with nonadenomas.[33-35] Similar MR gadolinium washout patterns have been described.[36,37] However, a quantitative analysis has not been standardized, and measurements of adrenal SI depend on the type of T1-W pulse sequence used. The CT washout sign should not be considered pathognomonic of a cortical adenoma. Pheochromocytomas that exhibit similar washout curves as cortical adenomas have been reported.[38]

If a chemical shift MR or CT examination establishes a diagnosis of a cortical adenoma and initial testing does not reveal signs, symptoms, or laboratory findings of cortical hyperfunction, then conservative observation can be performed. Some recommend "ignoring" the lesion and not obtaining follow-up imaging.[31] A study that followed 75 patients with adrenal incidentaloma found that an initial size of more than 3 cm was associated with an increased probability that an adenoma would become hyperfunctioning.[39]

Adrenocortical Carcinoma

Adrenocortical carcinoma is a rare aggressive malignancy with an estimated annual incidence of one per million (Box 3-2).[40] There is a bimodal age distribution of adrenocortical carcinomas with an initial peak in the pediatric population and a second peak in the fourth to fifth decades of life.[40,41] Patients with hyperfunctioning cancers present with signs and symptoms of cortisol or androgen excess. Nonhypersecreting tumors either are discovered incidentally or are found secondary to localized mass effect or symptomatic metastatic disease.

Three pathologic features that predict poor prognosis include large tumor size (>12 cm), intratumoral hemorrhage, and high mitotic rates.[42] There are conflicting data concerning the prognostic implications of the functional status of the tumor, with centers reporting both a poorer prognosis[41] and improved survival.[43]

3-2	Adrenal Cortical Carcinoma	
Rare	Incidence = 1/million/yr
Size	Hyperfunctioning: 9 cm
	Not hyperfunctioning: 13 cm
Chemical shift imaging	Loss of signal within small portion of mass in some cases
Poor prognosis	Best survival in those who have complete resection

Patients who have successful resection of a localized tumor have the best long-term outcome.[41,43,44] Individuals who have a complete resection have a median survival rate of 74 months, while those who have an incomplete primary resection have a median survival of only 12 months.[45]

MR can often detect adrenocortical carcinomas, localize the masses to the adrenal gland, and evaluate for local extension and metastatic disease (Figs. 3-4 and 3-5). On T1, T2, and contrast-enhanced scans, adrenocortical carcinomas appear aggressive and infiltrative. High SI on T1-WIs that persists on fat-saturated T1-WIs represents intratumoral hemorrhage. MR can detect growth of adrenocortical carcinoma tumor thrombus into the left renal vein, inferior vena cava, or right atrium (see Fig. 3-5).[46]

Chemical shift imaging of adrenocortical carcinomas reveals that some masses may focally lose SI.[47,48] This finding reflects the tumor's origin from the adrenal cortex. This should not create confusion with an adrenal adenoma because adrenocortical carcinomas are usually large (>5 cm), are heterogeneous, and have only small foci of lipid. Unusual examples of degenerated large adrenocortical adenomas have been described[49,50] that are indistinguishable from adrenocortical carcinoma on imaging. Fortunately, these benign adrenocortical neoplasms with atypical imaging findings are uncommon. Surgical removal is still required, with the determination of benignancy vs. malignancy to be made by the pathologist.

METASTASES TO THE ADRENAL GLAND

The adrenal gland is a common site of metastatic disease. Approximately one fourth of patients with epithelial malignancies have adrenal metastases at autopsy.[51] Primary tumors that commonly metastasize to the adrenal gland include lung, breast, and renal cell carcinomas and melanoma.[51,52] Benign adrenal masses are common not only in the general population[7] but also in patients with cancer. For example, in patients with lung cancer, fewer than half of adrenal masses are metastases.[53] It is important to differentiate adrenal metastases from benign adrenal masses, as this may determine whether patients can undergo curative resection of their primary tumor.

Adrenal adenomas and metastatic adrenal lesions have different MR imaging features (as described above and outlined in Box 3-1). Most adrenocortical adenomas lose SI on chemical shift imaging, whereas metastatic lesions do not (Figs. 3-6 and 3-7). Clear cell renal cell carcinoma is the one primary tumor that can develop metastatic adrenal masses containing intracellular lipid (Fig. 3-8). These cases are rare and reportable[54] and usually coexist with other imaging findings of metastatic renal cell carcinoma.

If a patient has other findings of metastatic disease, then the characterization of an adrenal mass usually does not alter therapy. However, in patients with bilateral adrenal metastases signs or symptoms of Addison's disease should be identified and treated with

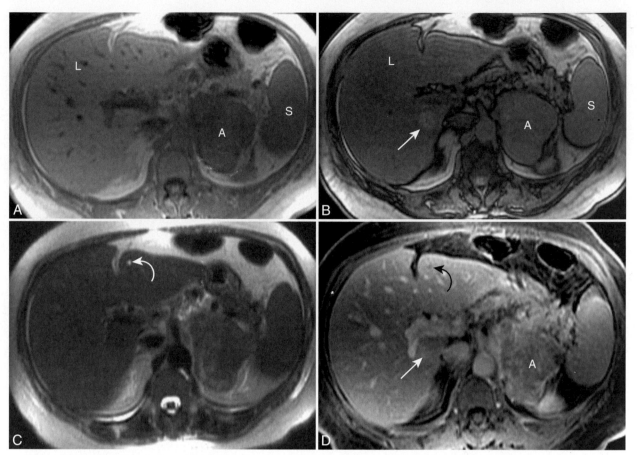

Figure 3-4 ▪ **MR depiction of a left adrenocortical carcinoma in a 55-year-old woman with signs and symptoms of hyperaldosteronism.** Hepatic steatosis, focal nodular hyperplasia, and a 3-mm liver cyst are also present. **A** and **B**, In-phase (**A**) and opposed-phase (**B**) T1-WIs show a large left adrenal mass (A) that is isointense to spleen (S) and does not lose SI on chemical shift imaging. The liver loses SI on opposed-phase imaging, indicating hepatic steatosis. There is a well-circumscribed lesion of the right lobe of the liver (L) that is hyperintense to liver on the opposed-phase image *(arrow)* and isointense to liver on the in-phase image. The isointensity to liver indicates that it is hepatocellular in origin. A low SI central scar is present. Focal nodular hyperplasia (FNH) is the most common hepatocellular lesion that has a central scar. **C**, Breath-hold heavily T2-WI (TE = 185 msec) shows low SI liver and spleen because of the long echo time. The liver shows minimal SI because fat suppression was not used and the patient has steatosis. The adrenal mass is heterogeneous and shows foci of intermediate SI. The lack of high SI does not exclude pheochromocytoma, but this was excluded at surgery. The FNH is relatively isointense to liver. A 3-mm high SI lesion *(curved arrow)* of the lateral segment of the left lobe that is isointense to cerebral spinal fluid represents a benign cyst. Liver metastases would be expected to be isointense to spleen. The fact that this liver lesion is visualized on this sequence is supportive of a non-solid benign lesion such as a cyst or hemangioma. **D**, Delayed CE fat-suppressed T1-WI (slice thickness = 8 mm) shows heterogeneous enhancement of the adrenal mass (A) and enhancement of the central scar of the FNH *(arrow)*. The SI within the 3-mm cyst *(curved arrow)* is from volume averaging with adjacent enhanced liver parenchyma. Heavily T2-WIs often outperform enhanced T1-WIs in both detecting and characterizing subcentimeter renal, pancreatic, and hepatic cysts.

hormone replacement.[55] How should the physician approach a patient with a known primary and no metastatic disease who has an adrenal mass that does not lose SI on chemical shift imaging? Documenting lesion stability by obtaining prior cross-sectional imaging studies is the most cost-effective method. If an adrenal lesion has not grown for more than 6 months, an occult metastasis with high negative predictive value is excluded.[35] Interval growth of a lesion is suspicious for metastatic disease (see Fig. 3-6). If prior imaging studies are not available, the physician can consider obtaining an enhanced CT scan with delayed imaging. Lipid-poor adenomas show similar washout CT kinetics to lipid-containing adenomas.[33,34] Alternatively one can consider performing an image-guided needle biopsy[56-58] or laparoscopic adrenelectomy[59] in order to prove a diagnosis of metastatic disease and thus guide appropriate therapy. In patients who have isolated adrenal metastases, laparoscopic removal may be therapeutic.[60]

ADRENAL PHEOCHROMOCYTOMA

Pheochromocytomas are catecholamine-producing neoplasms that originate from the sympathetic

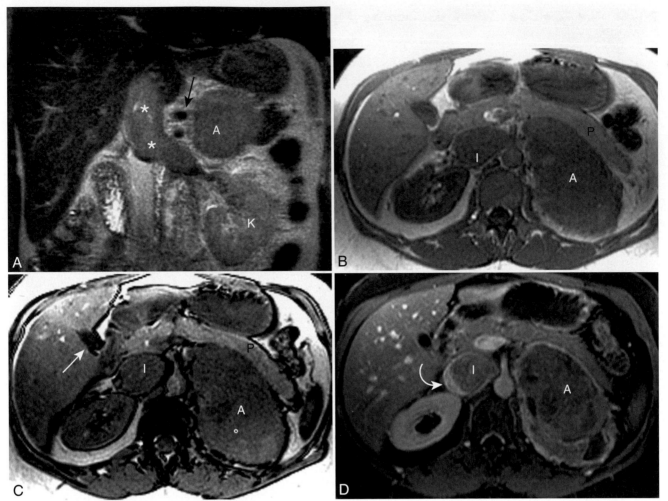

Figure 3-5 ■ **MR depiction of left renal vein and inferior vena cava (IVC) tumor thrombus in two different patients with left adrenal cortical carcinomas. A**, Coronal T2-WI depicts a left adrenal mass (A) that displaces the left kidney (K) inferiorly. Tumor thrombus (∗) is present within the visualized segment of left renal vein and intrahepatic IVC. Normal flow voids are present within the celiac *(black arrow)* and superior mesenteric arteries. **B** and **C**, In-phase (**B**) and opposed-phase (**C**) axial T1-WIs shows no change in SI within the left adrenal mass (A) posterior to the pancreas (P). The tumor thrombus within the IVC (I) and the primary tumor has similar SI. There is loss of SI within the gall-bladder bile *(arrow)* because of its cholesterol content. **D**, Fat-suppressed CE T1-WI shows heterogenous enhancement within the primary adrenal cancer and the tumor thrombus. Some flow is revealed within the IVC as high SI *(curved arrow)*.
(Continued)

nervous system. Patients can present with signs or symptoms of excess catecholamines. If a clinician suspects a pheochromocytoma, the initial screening test of choice is measurement of the plasma free metanephrines.[61] Approximately 85% to 90% of pheochromocytomas are located within the adrenal medulla (Box 3-3) and 10% to 15% outside of the adrenal gland. Extra-adrenal pheochromocytomas, termed paragangliomas, can occur anywhere from the bladder to the brain.[62-64] These tumors are more aggressive and are malignant in 40% of cases, whereas orthotopic pheochromocytomas are malignant in 10% to 15%. Often it is the radiologist and not the pathologist who determines whether the primary tumor is benign or malignant based on the presence or absence of metastatic disease.

Pheochromocytomas can occur sporadically or a part of a hereditary syndrome (Box 3-4). Hereditary pheochromocytoma is associated with four syndromes: multiple endocrine neoplasia (MEN) type IIA (Fig. 3-9), von Hippel–Lindau disease,[65] neurofibromatosis, and isolated familial pheochromocytoma.[66] A hereditary syndrome should be suspected when bilateral pheochromocytomas are revealed, since this may be the initial finding in patients with von Hippel–Lindau disease and MEN type IIA. Twenty-five percent (and not the widely quoted 10%) of patients with sporadic pheochromocytomas are found to have one of four responsible genetic mutations.[67,68] Although it is not feasible to perform genetic testing on all individuals with suspected pheochromocytoma, a detailed family history should be obtained and first-degree relatives evaluated.

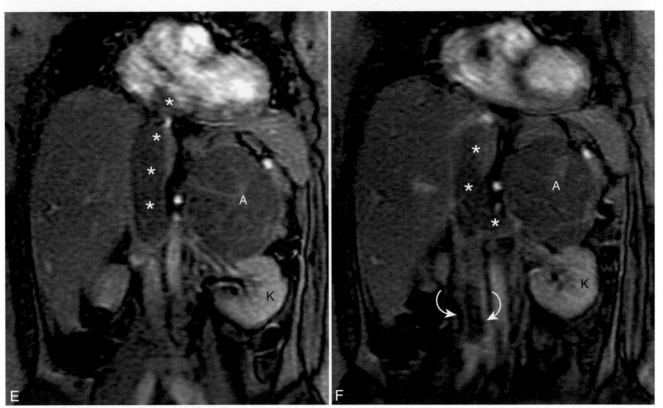

Figure 3-5 ▪ Cont'd E and **F,** Two sequential coronal CE T1-WIs (TR = 12, TE = 2.5, flip angle = 30°) in a different patient show a hypoenhancing left adrenal mass (A) that inferiorly displaces the left kidney (K). Thrombus within the intrahepatic IVC (∗) has similar SI as the primary tumor and represents tumor thrombus. Lower SI nonenhancing thrombus located peripherally within the IVC *(curved arrow)* represents bland thrombus.

The treatment of choice for pheochromocytoma is laparoscopic adrenalectomy.[69,70] Before surgery, patients are treated with alpha blockers to prevent a potential hypertensive crisis. Intra-operative control of the adrenal vein prior to manipulation-removal of the tumor itself is important to prevent hypertensive complications during surgery.[71] In a patient with hereditary pheochromocytoma and an identifiable unilateral adrenal mass, prophylactic contralateral adrenalectomy is not recommended because of the long interval for those individuals who do develop a second pheochromocytoma. In patients who have bilateral adrenalectomy, heterotopic autotransplantation of medullary free adrenocortical tissue can preclude steroid replacement therapy and a potential postprocedural addisonian crisis.[72] Preserving adrenocortical tissue in an orthotopic location is not recommended because it is associated with a higher rate of recurrent disease.[66]

The MR appearance of pheochromocytomas was initially described as a "light bulb" because lesions revealed homogeneous high SI on T2-WIs (Fig. 3-10).[73,74] However, with refined MR techniques most pheochromocytomas show heterogeneous low, intermediate, and high SI on T2-WIs and the light bulb sign is neither sensitive nor specific (see Fig. 3-10).[75,76] Tumor heterogeneity is, in part, secondary to intratumoral hemorrhage and cyst formation. Some pheochromocytomas are mostly cystic (Fig. 3-11).[77]

Almost all pheochromocytomas do not contain intracellular lipid and do not reveal loss of SI on chemical shift MR. One pheochromocytoma has been reported to have intracellular lipid within the neoplastic medullary cells[38]; however, this should be considered a rare exception. Given a patient with signs or symptoms of a pheochromocytoma, MR is an ideal imaging modality for pheochromocytoma detection and localization, with detection rates approaching 100%.[78]

ADRENAL MYELOLIPOMA

Myelolipomas are uncommon, benign encapsulated neoplasms composed of variable amounts of mature fat and bone marrow elements.[79] Most myelolipomas originate within the adrenal gland. Unusual extraadrenal myelolipomas have been reported in the retroperitoneum and liver on MR.[80,81] Most myelolipomas are asymptomatic and are followed conservatively when a diagnosis can be established with imaging.[82-84] Symptomatic myelolipomas are secondary to localized mass effect or extracapsular hemorrhage[85] and are treated with surgical excision. Some advocate elective surgical resection of larger myelolipomas because of the unknown risk of catastrophic hemorrhage.[86]

Detection and characterization of macroscopic fat within an adrenal mass establishes a diagnosis of

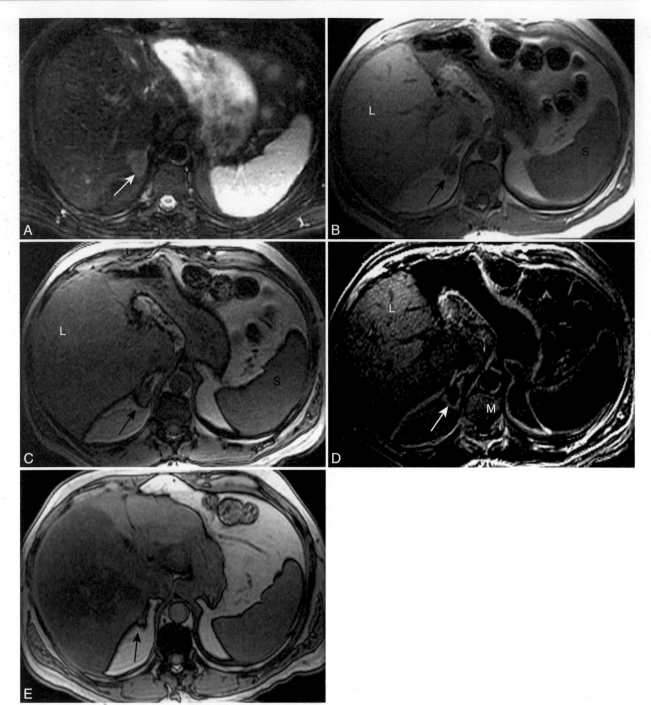

Figure 3-6 ▪ **MR findings of metastatic colon cancer to the right adrenal gland and hepatic steatosis.**
A, Axial fat-suppressed T2-WI shows a poorly marginated right adrenal mass *(arrow)* that is closely associated with the adjacent right lobe of the liver. The mass is intermediate in SI between liver and spleen. On the basis of this image alone, no specific diagnosis is possible. **B** and **C**, In-phase (**B**) and opposed-phase (**C**) T1-WIs show that the adrenal mass *(arrow)* remains isointense to spleen and thus does not contain detectable intracellular lipid. The liver (L) loses SI compared with spleen (S) on the opposed-phase image (**C**), indicating the presence of hepatic steatosis. When performing qualitative visual analysis of change in SI of the adrenal gland on chemical shift imaging, the adrenal gland should be compared with the adjacent spleen. Comparing the SI of an adrenal mass and liver could potentially result in a false-negative diagnosis of an adenoma if there was greater loss of hepatic SI secondary to steatosis. The spleen does not develop fatty change and thus is a suitable reference tissue. Alternatively, when duel-echo GRE images are obtained, direct comparison of adrenal mass SI without reference to other tissues is possible. A subtraction image could be processed (in phase – opposed phase; **D**) that would display a map of voxels that contained both lipid and water protons. **D**, Subtraction image confirms the presence of signal within the liver, indicating hepatic steatosis. Normal marrow (M) of the lumbar spine also contains lipid. Because "pure fat" such as the posterior pararenal fat and the fat within the gastrohepatic interval contains water protons (e.g., within membranes and lysosomes), these tissues show some signal on this image. The adrenal metastasis does not contain lipid and thus shows no signal. **E**, Opposed-phase T1-WI performed 3 months earlier reveals a 4-mm mass *(arrow)* of the lateral limb of the right adrenal gland. The presence of prior imaging examinations is invaluable in the evaluation of an indeterminate adrenal mass. The interval enlargement of the mass over 3 months without the presence of intratumoral hemorrhage is very suggestive of metastatic disease.

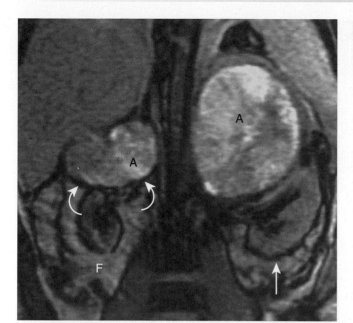

Figure 3-7 ■ MR depiction of bilateral hemorrhagic adrenal metastases secondary to melanoma in a 35-year-old woman. Coronal opposed-phase T1-WI shows heterogeneous high SI adrenal masses (A). The left kidney is being displaced and rotated inferiorly *(arrow)*. Two findings indicate that these masses are not fat-containing myelolipomas: (1) the SI within the lesions is hyperintense to adjacent retroperitoneal fat (F) and (2) an etching artifact is present at the interface between the right adrenal mass and the right perinephric fat *(curved arrows)*, indicating a fat-water interface. Thus, the high SI within the mass must be derived from water protons, in this instance from the T1-shortening effects of methemoglobin and/or melanin.

myelolipoma with high diagnostic certainty.[76,87] Macroscopic fat can be revealed on MR by showing loss of SI on a fat-suppressed sequence when compared with an identical sequence obtained without fat saturation (Figs. 3-12 and 3-13). It is not unusual to see adipocyte-rich and adipocyte-poor regions

---

3-3   Clinical and MR Imaging Findings of Pheochromocytoma

Signs and symptoms of adrenal medulla hyperfunction
Elevated catecholamines in 24-hour urine
90% adrenal, 10% extra-adrenal
90% benign, 10% malignant (higher percentage in extra-adrenal lesions)
   Malignancy diagnosed more by radiologists than pathologists
Size: mean size approximately 4–6 cm
No loss of signal intensity on chemical shift imaging
Heterogeneous high SI on T2-WI
   Intratumoral necrosis
   Intratumoral cyst formation
Hypervascular on contrast enhancement—contrast not often needed

---

3-4   Conditions Associated with Pheochromocytoma

- Neurofibromatosis
- Von Hippel–Lindau disease
- Multiple endocrine neoplasia (MEN) type IIA
- Familial pheochromocytoma

---

within the same myelolipoma. Adipocyte-rich regions reveal similar SI changes on chemical shift imaging when compared with the "pure fat" within the adjacent retroperitoneum. Adipocyte-poor regions (where adipocytes and marrow elements are contained within the same voxel) can have identical chemical shift imaging findings to those of an adrenal adenoma. Alternatively, a water-suppressed gradient echo image can be used to depict the presence of fat.[88,89] Large foci of macroscopic fat show very high SI, while smaller amounts of fat and intracellular lipid show some SI but are not so hyperintense (see Figs. 3-1, 3-2, and 3-13). The unusual complication of peritumoral hemorrhage will appear as high SI on T1-WIs that persists with fat saturation secondary to the T1-shortening effects of methemoglobin.[81,90]

ADRENAL HEMATOMA

Adrenal hemorrhage/hematoma can have either traumatic or nontraumatic etiologies. Traumatic causes include severe abdominal trauma, right-sided hepatic surgery, and child abuse.[91,92] Nontraumatic causes include disorders of coagulation (Fig. 3-14), stress, and hemorrhage into an underlying adrenal neoplasm (see Fig. 3-7).[93] When hematomas are bilateral, the physician should evaluate for signs and symptoms of adrenal failure (Addison's disease), which often is not diagnosed, resulting in unnecessary morbidity and mortality.[94]

The specific MR imaging finding of a subacute hematoma is the presence of a high SI rim sign, indicating the presence of methemoglobin within the periphery of the hematoma (see Fig. 3-14).[95,96] In the absence of a known primary tumor, it is very unusual to detect an adrenal hematoma as the initial finding of occult metastatic disease. In questionable cases, follow-up imaging should reveal a decrease in size of a benign hematoma (see Fig. 3-14).

ADRENAL CYSTS

Adrenal cysts are rare and have been categorized as endothelial, epithelial, parasitic, and pseudocystic.[7,97] The majority are asymptomatic and can be managed with observation[98] or aspiration.[99] Symptomatic adrenal cysts or cysts larger than 5 cm can be removed laparoscopically.[100] Adrenal pseudocysts are the result of prior hemorrhage into either a normal adrenal

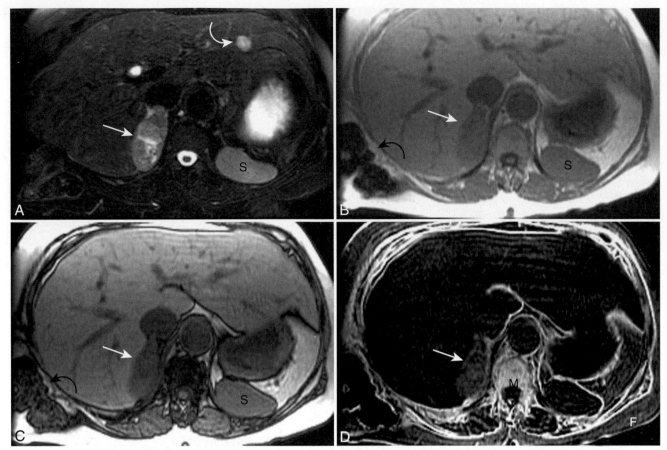

Figure 3-8 ▪ MR illustration of metastatic clear cell renal carcinoma to the adrenal gland that reveals loss of SI on chemical shift imaging. Metastatic lesions of clear cell carcinoma may contain intracellular lipid, similarly to the primary tumor. **A,** Fat-suppressed T2-WI shows a heterogeneous right adrenal mass *(arrow)* that has SI similar to that of the spleen (S). A liver metastasis *(curved white arrow)* is also present. **B** and **C,** In-phase and opposed-phase T1-WIs show that the right adrenal mass *(arrow)* loses SI on the opposed-phase image relative to the spleen. There is an incisional hernia that contains right-sided colon segments *(curved black arrows)*. Gas-containing colon has lower SI on the longer TE in-phase image secondary to susceptibility effects. **D,** Postprocessed subtraction image (in phase–opposed phase) shows the highest SI within the lumbar marrow (M). The subcutaneous fat (F) and the adrenal metastases *(arrow)* have equal SI. The subcutaneous fat has approximately 90% lipid and 10% water, while the clear cell carcinoma metastasis is comprised of 10% lipid and 90% water. Because both tissues lose approximately 20% of their SI, they have a similar appearance on this subtraction image.

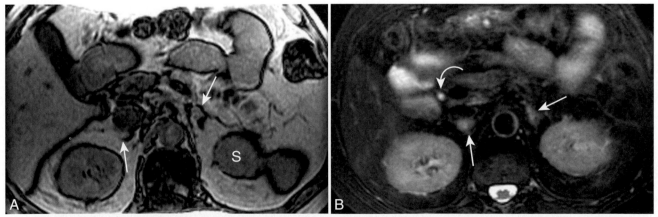

Figure 3-9 ▪ MR findings of proven bilateral subcentimeter pheochromocytomas in a man with multiple endocrine neoplasia type IIA. A, Opposed-phase T1-WI shows bilateral small adrenal masses *(arrows)*. Neither adrenal mass lost SI relative to spleen (S) when compared with the corresponding in-phase image (not shown). **B,** Fat-suppressed T2-WI shows that both the masses *(arrows)* are hyperintense to liver (L) but hypointense to adjacent bile in the common bile duct *(curved arrow)*.

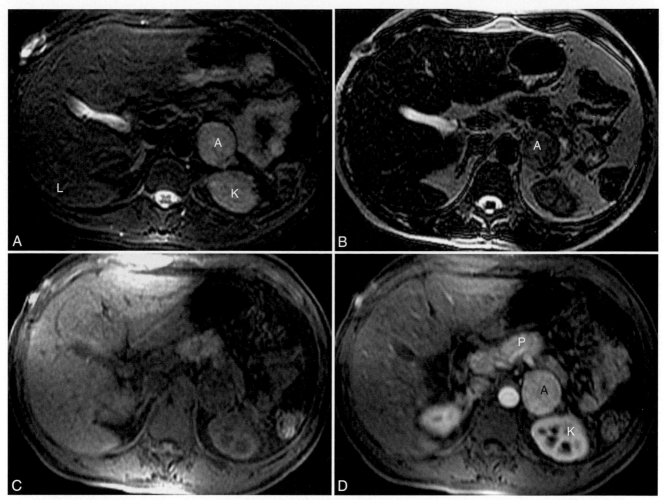

Figure 3-10 ■ **MR illustration of a surgically proven left adrenal pheochromocytoma in a 36-year-old man with episodic hypertension and headaches. A**, Fat-suppressed T2-WI shows a left adrenal mass (A) that is hyperintense to liver (L) and isointense to adjacent left kidney (K). The term "MR light bulb sign" was used in the past to describe the relative high SI of pheochromocytoma on moderately T2-WIs. **B**, Corresponding heavily T2-WI (TE = 240) shows no high SI within the adrenal mass, thus excluding the diagnosis of an adrenal cyst or intratumoral cyst formation/liquefactive necrosis. Chemical shift imaging (not shown) did not reveal intratumoral lipid. **C** and **D**, T1-WIs obtained before (**C**) and dynamically after (**D**) contrast show moderate-to-marked adrenal mass enhancement. Note the normal arterial enhancement of the pancreas (P) and renal cortex (K). Although the relative T2 SI, lack of intratumoral lipid, and hyperenhancement all suggest pheochromocytoma, the diagnosis has to be confirmed by correlating with clinical signs and symptoms and analysis of urinary catecholamines.

gland or a gland that contained a benign neoplasm.[87] MR reveals an adrenal mass with fluid SI content. Wall calcification is better revealed by CT than by MR (Fig. 3-15).

SUMMARY

MR imaging can detect adrenal masses and potentially characterize many subtypes of adrenal masses. The presence of intracellular lipid within an adrenal mass revealed with chemical shift imaging techniques establishes a diagnosis of adrenocortical neoplasm. Most of these lesions will be nonhyperfunctioning cortical adenomas. Hyperfunctioning cortisol and aldosterone-producing adenomas are diagnosed more on the basis of clinical evaluation than of MR findings. Pure fat within an adrenal mass is diagnostic for a myelolipoma. MR imaging findings are not diagnostic for pheochromocytoma, and an imaging and clinical diagnosis must be confirmed by metanephrine measurements. An adrenal mass in a patient with a primary malignancy can be either a metastasis or a cortical adenoma. If chemical shift imaging cannot show the presence of intratumoral lipid, then an enhanced CT with washout images or tissue sampling should be considered when patient management is affected.

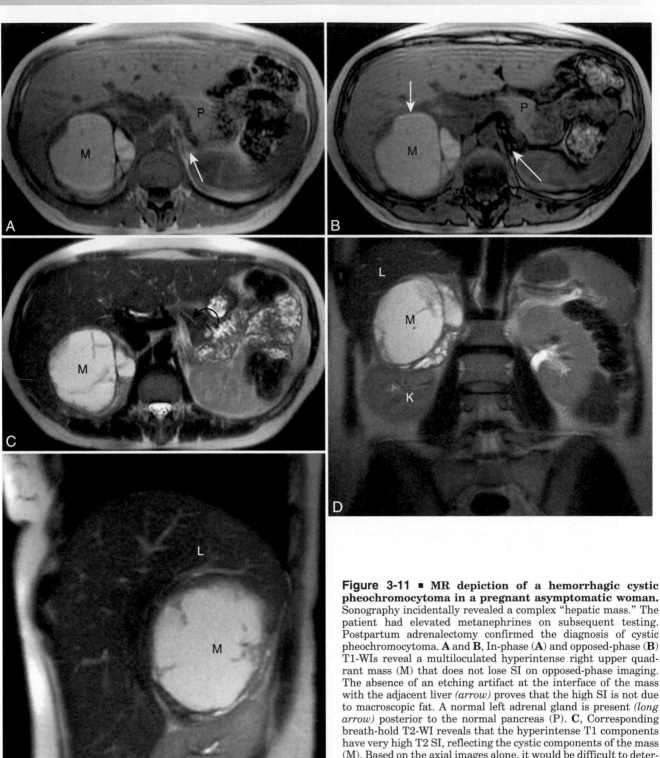

Figure 3-11 ▪ MR depiction of a hemorrhagic cystic pheochromocytoma in a pregnant asymptomatic woman. Sonography incidentally revealed a complex "hepatic mass." The patient had elevated metanephrines on subsequent testing. Postpartum adrenalectomy confirmed the diagnosis of cystic pheochromocytoma. **A** and **B**, In-phase (**A**) and opposed-phase (**B**) T1-WIs reveal a multiloculated hyperintense right upper quadrant mass (M) that does not lose SI on opposed-phase imaging. The absence of an etching artifact at the interface of the mass with the adjacent liver *(arrow)* proves that the high SI is not due to macroscopic fat. A normal left adrenal gland is present *(long arrow)* posterior to the normal pancreas (P). **C**, Corresponding breath-hold T2-WI reveals that the hyperintense T1 components have very high T2 SI, reflecting the cystic components of the mass (M). Based on the axial images alone, it would be difficult to determine whether this mass arises from the liver, adrenal gland, or kidney. The use of breath-hold techniques minimizes motion-induced artifacts. Note the clear depiction of the normal, 1-mm pancreatic duct *(curved arrow)*. **D** and **E**, Coronal (**D**) and sagittal (**E**) breath-hold T2-WIs show inferior displacement of the right kidney (K) and anterior displacement of the liver (L). A normal right adrenal gland was not depicted.

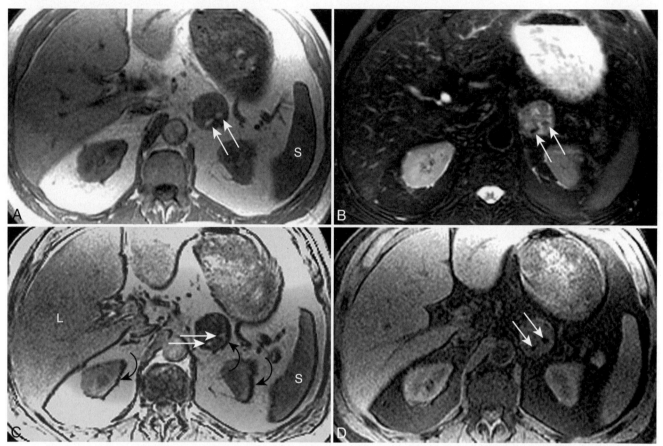

Figure 3-12 ▪ **MR demonstration of the varying lipid content within an asymptomatic myelolipoma and hepatic steatosis in a 70-year-old man. A**, In-phase T1-WI shows normal SI liver (L) and spleen (S). A left adrenal mass shows components with two different SIs. Most of the mass is isointense to liver. Two 3-mm foci of higher SI *(arrows)* are isointense to surrounding retroperitoneal fat. **B**, Fat-suppressed T2-WI shows that most of the mass has heterogeneous low-to-intermediate SI and the two 3 mm foci are of very low SI *(white arrows)*. On the basis of this image and the in-phase image, a diagnosis of macroscopic fat cannot definitely be established, since protein or hemorrhage could have a similar appearance on both T1- and T2-WIs. **C**, Opposed-phase T1-WI shows moderate-to-marked loss of SI within the right adrenal mass, indicating its lipid content. There also is loss of signal within the liver (L) secondary to hepatic steatosis. There has been no appreciable loss of SI within the two subcentimeter hyperintense adrenal foci. However, there is an "India ink," or "etching," artifact at the right-sided interface of these foci and the adjacent adrenal gland, indicating a fat-water interface *(arrows)*. Similar etching artifacts *(curved arrows)* are present at the left-sided border of the left adrenal gland and both kidneys with the perinephric fat. Thus, the residual SI within the adrenal gland is from water protons and the high SI foci represent the macroscopic fat within the myelolipoma. [See the text for an explanation of the asymmetric etching artifact in the frequency-encoding axis that appears wider on the left side of the spleen and left kidney *(curved arrow)* and is not perceptible on the right-sided interface.] **D**, Opposed-phase, fat-saturated T1-WI shows two types of lipid suppression. In the voxels of the two intratumoral foci that are entirely composed of adipocytes there is marked loss of SI *(arrows)*, similar to the drop in SI of the adjacent perinephric fat. There is a lower degree of lipid suppression within the remainder of the myelolipoma, where both lipid and nonlipid protons are present within the same voxels.

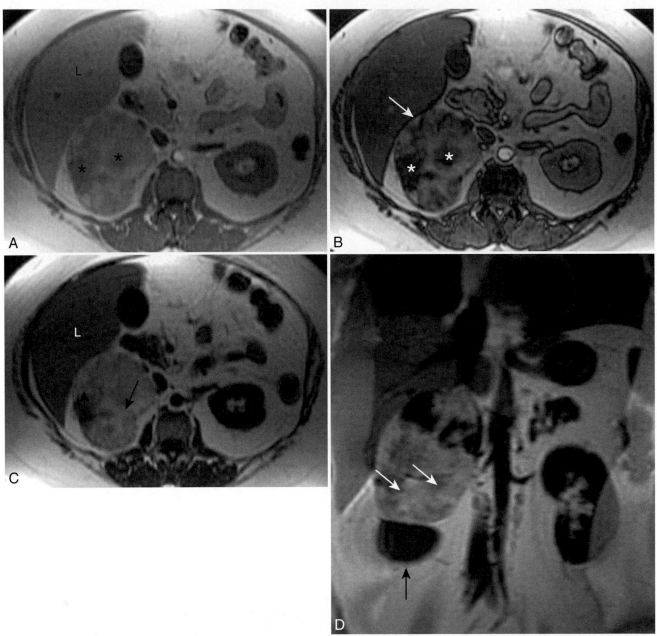

Figure 3-13 ■ **MR depiction of a fat-containing myelolipoma and hepatic steatosis revealed with chemical shift and water saturation techniques in an asymptomatic 44-year-old woman.** An outside CT scan had suggested an angiomyelolipoma of the upper pole of the right kidney. **A** and **B**, In-phase (**A**) and opposed-phase (**B**) T1-WIs show a right retroperitoneal mass that focally loses SI with chemical shift imaging (∗), indicating its lipid content. Other portions of the tumor do not lose SI. There is loss of SI of the liver (L) secondary to hepatic steatosis. There is an "India ink," or "etching," artifact *(arrow)* at the interface of the right side of the mass (which has persistent high SI) and the adjacent liver. Thus, the intratumoral foci of high SI represent macroscopic fat. **C**, Water-suppressed T1-WI shows varying degrees of high SI within the mass, indicating the various lipid components. The highest SI foci represent regions of fat *(arrows)*. Hepatic steatosis (L) shows less SI. It is easier to establish the presence of steatosis by comparing the in-phase and opposed-phase images. **D**, Water-suppressed coronal T1-WI shows that the mass displaces the right kidney *(black arrow)* inferiorly. Thus, the mass represents a right adrenal myelolipoma and not a renal angiomyelolipoma. The hyperintense components within the mass *(white arrows)* indicate macroscopic fat.

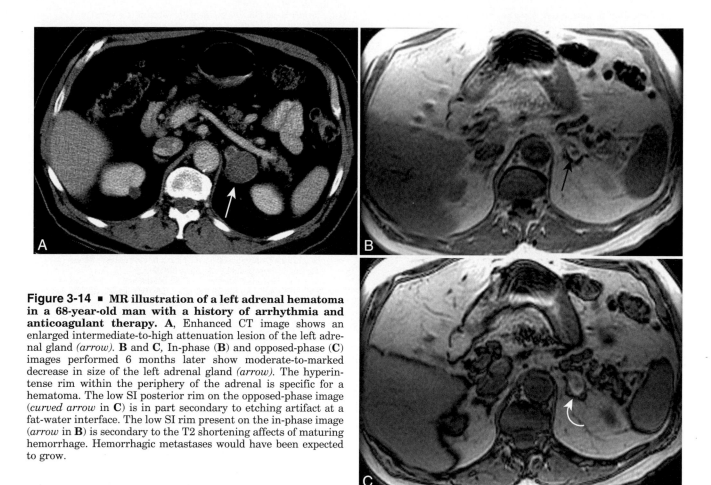

Figure 3-14 ■ **MR illustration of a left adrenal hematoma in a 68-year-old man with a history of arrhythmia and anticoagulant therapy. A**, Enhanced CT image shows an enlarged intermediate-to-high attenuation lesion of the left adrenal gland *(arrow)*. **B** and **C**, In-phase (**B**) and opposed-phase (**C**) images performed 6 months later show moderate-to-marked decrease in size of the left adrenal gland *(arrow)*. The hyperintense rim within the periphery of the adrenal is specific for a hematoma. The low SI posterior rim on the opposed-phase image *(curved arrow* in **C**) is in part secondary to etching artifact at a fat-water interface. The low SI rim present on the in-phase image *(arrow* in **B**) is secondary to the T2 shortening affects of maturing hemorrhage. Hemorrhagic metastases would have been expected to grow.

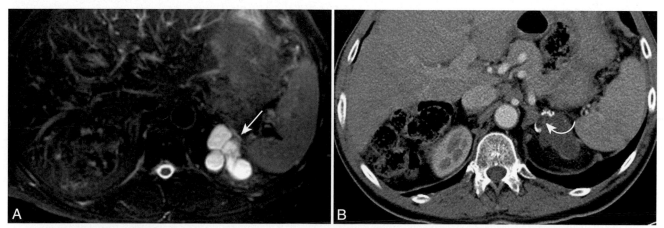

Figure 3-15 ■ **MR illustration of an adrenal pseudocyst in a man with treated thyroid cancer.** The lesion has been stable on cross-sectional imaging for >5 years. **A**, Axial T2-WI shows a lobulated cyst *(arrow)* that was localized to the adrenal gland. **B**, Enhanced CT scan better illustrates segmental calcification of the cyst wall *(curved arrow)*. Since this patient was asymptomatic, surgical excision was not performed.

REFERENCES

1. Mayo-Smith WW, Boland GW, Noto RB, Lee MJ. State-of-the-art adrenal imaging. Radiographics 2001;21:995-1012.
2. Mitchell DG, Nascimento AB, Alam F, Grasel RP, Holland G, O'Hara BJ. Normal adrenal gland: in vivo observations, and high-resolution in vitro chemical shift MR imaging-histologic correlation. Acad Radiol 2002;9:430-436.
3. Wehrli FW, Perkins TG, Shimakawa A, Roberts F. Chemical shift-induced amplitude modulations in images obtained with gradient refocusing. Magn Reson Imaging 1987;5:157-158.
4. Allolio B. Adrenal incidentalomas. In: Margioris AN, Chrousos GP (eds). Comptemporary Endocrinology: Adrenal Disorders. Totowa, NJ: Humana Press, 2001;249-261.
5. Murai M, Baba S, Nakashima J, Tachibana M. Management of incidentally discovered adrenal masses. World J Urol 1999;17:9-14.
6. Abecassis M, McLoughlin MJ, Langer B, Kudlow JE. Serendipitous adrenal masses: prevalence, significance, and management. Am J Surg 1985;149:783-788.
7. Dunnick NR, Korobkin M. Imaging of adrenal incidentalomas: current status. AJR Am J Roentgenol 2002;179:559-568.
8. Outwater EK, Siegelman ES, Huang AB, Birnbaum BA. Adrenal masses: correlation between CT attenuation value and chemical shift ratio at MR imaging with in-phase and opposed-phase sequences [erratum in Radiology Dec 1996;201:880]. Radiology 1996;200:749-752.
9. Mitchell DG, Crovello M, Matteucci T, Petersen RO, Miettinen MM. Benign adrenocortical masses: diagnosis with chemical shift MR imaging [see comments]. Radiology 1992;185:345-351.
10. Namimoto T, Yamashita Y, Mitsuzaki K, et al. Adrenal masses: quantification of fat content with double-echo chemical shift in-phase and opposed-phase FLASH MR images for differentiation of adrenal adenomas. Radiology 2001;218:642-646.
11. Fujiyoshi F, Nakajo M, Fukukura Y, Tsuchimochi S. Characterization of adrenal tumors by chemical shift fast low-angle shot MR imaging: comparison of four methods of quantitative evaluation. AJR Am J Roentgenol 2003;180:1649-1657.
12. Korobkin M, Giordano TJ, Brodeur FJ, et al. Adrenal adenomas: relationship between histologic lipid and CT and MR findings. Radiology 1996;200:743-747.
13. Doppman JL, Reinig JW, Dwyer AJ, et al. Differentiation of adrenal masses by magnetic resonance imaging. Surgery 1987;102:1018-1026.
14. Baker ME, Blinder R, Spritzer C, Leight GS, Herfkens RJ, Dunnick NR. MR evaluation of adrenal masses at 1.5 T. AJR Am J Roentgenol 1989;153:307-312.
15. Glazer GM, Woolsey EJ, Borrello J, et al. Adrenal tissue characterization using MR imaging. Radiology 1986;158:73-79.
16. Boland GW, Lee MJ, Gazelle GS, Halpern EF, McNicholas MM, Mueller PR. Characterization of adrenal masses using unenhanced CT: an analysis of the CT literature. AJR Am J Roentgenol 1998;171:201-204.
17. Ross NS, Aron DC. Hormonal evaluation of the patient with an incidentally discovered adrenal mass [see comments]. N Engl J Med 1990;323:1401-1405.
18. Choyke PL, Doppman JL. Case 18: adrenocorticotropic hormone-dependent Cushing syndrome. Radiology 2000;214:195-198.
19. Reincke M. Subclinical Cushing's syndrome. Endocrinol Metab Clin North Am 2000;29:43-56.
20. Rossi R, Tauchmanova L, Luciano A, et al. Subclinical Cushing's syndrome in patients with adrenal incidentaloma: clinical and biochemical features. J Clin Endocrinol Metab 2000;85:1440-1448.
21. Young WF, Jr. Primary aldosteronism: a common and curable form of hypertension. Cardiol Rev 1999;7:207-214.
22. Ganguly A. Primary aldosteronism. N Engl J Med 1998;339:1828-1834.
23. Sohaib SA, Peppercorn PD, Allan C, et al. Primary hyperaldosteronism (Conn syndrome): MR imaging findings. Radiology 2000;214:527-531.
24. Wang JH, Wu HM, Sheu MH, Tseng HS, Chiang JH, Chang CY. High resolution MRI of adrenal glands in patients with primary aldosteronism. Chung Hua I Hsueh Tsa Chih 2000;63:475-481.
25. Doppman JL, Gill JR, Jr., Miller DL, et al. Distinction between hyperaldosteronism due to bilateral hyperplasia and unilateral aldosteronoma: reliability of CT [see comments]. Radiology 1992;184:677-682.
26. Lingam RK, Sohaib SA, Vlahos I, et al. CT of primary hyperaldosteronism (Conn's syndrome): the value of measuring the adrenal gland. AJR Am J Roentgenol 2003;181:843-849.
27. Gordon RD, Stowasser M, Rutherford JC. Primary aldosteronism: are we diagnosing and operating on too few patients? World J Surg 2001;25:941-947.
28. Stowasser M. Primary aldosteronism: rare bird or common cause of secondary hypertension? Curr Hypertens Rep 2001;3:230-239.
29. Hokotate H, Inoue H, Baba Y, Tsuchimochi S, Nakajo M. Aldosteronomas: experience with superselective adrenal arterial embolization in 33 cases. Radiology 2003;227:401-406.
30. Tello R, Chaoui A, Hymphrey M, et al. Incidence of adrenal masses in patients referred for renal artery stenosis screening MR. Invest Radiol 2001;36:518-520.
31. Kievit J, Haak HR. Diagnosis and treatment of adrenal incidentaloma: a cost-effectiveness analysis. Endocrinol Metab Clin North Am 2000;29:69-90.
32. Higgins JC, Fitzgerald JM. Evaluation of incidental renal and adrenal masses. Am Fam Physician 2001;63:288-294, 299.
33. Caoili EM, Korobkin M, Francis IR, Cohan RH, Dunnick NR. Delayed enhanced CT of lipid-poor adrenal adenomas. AJR Am J Roentgenol 2000;175:1411-1415.
34. Pena CS, Boland GW, Hahn PF, Lee MJ, Mueller PR. Characterization of indeterminate (lipid-poor) adrenal masses: use of washout characteristics at contrast-enhanced CT. Radiology 2000;217:798-802.
35. Caoili EM, Korobkin M, Francis IR, et al. Adrenal masses: characterization with combined unenhanced and delayed enhanced CT. Radiology 2002;222:629-633.
36. Slapa RZ, Jakubowski W, Januszewicz A, et al. Discriminatory power of MRI for differentiation of adrenal non-adenomas vs adenomas evaluated by means of ROC analysis: can biopsy be obviated? Eur Radiol 2000;10:95-104.
37. Chung JJ, Semelka RC, Martin DR. Adrenal adenomas: characteristic postgadolinium capillary blush on dynamic MR imaging. J Magn Reson Imaging 2001;13:242-248.
38. Blake MA, Krishnamoorthy SK, Boland GW, et al. Low-density pheochromocytoma on CT: a mimicker of adrenal adenoma. AJR Am J Roentgenol 2003;181:1663-1668.
39. Barzon L, Scaroni C, Sonino N, Fallo F, Paoletta A, Boscaro M. Risk factors and long-term follow-up of adrenal incidentalomas. J Clin Endocrinol Metab 1999;84:520-526.
40. Schulick RD, Brennan MF. Adrenocortical carcinoma. World J Urol 1999;17:26-34.
41. Wajchenberg BL, Albergaria Pereira MA, Medonca BB, et al. Adrenocortical carcinoma: clinical and laboratory observations. Cancer 2000;88:711-736.
42. Harrison LE, Gaudin PB, Brennan MF. Pathologic features of prognostic significance for adrenocortical carcinoma after curative resection. Arch Surg 1999;134:181-185.
43. Tritos NA, Cushing GW, Heatley G, Libertino JA. Clinical features and prognostic factors associated with adrenocortical carcinoma: Lahey Clinic Medical Center experience. Am Surg 2000;66:73-79.
44. Demeure MJ, Somberg LB. Functioning and nonfunctioning adrenocortical carcinoma: clinical presentation and therapeutic strategies. Surg Oncol Clin N Am 1998;7:791-805.
45. Schulick RD, Brennan MF. Long-term survival after complete resection and repeat resection in patients with adrenocortical carcinoma. Ann Surg Oncol 1999;6:719-726.
46. Siegelbaum MH, Moulsdale JE, Murphy JB, McDonald GR. Use of magnetic resonance imaging scanning in adrenocortical carcinoma with vena caval involvement. Urology 1994;43:869-873.
47. Schlund JF, Kenney PJ, Brown ED, Ascher SM, Brown JJ, Semelka RC. Adrenocortical carcinoma: MR imaging appearance with current techniques. J Magn Reson Imaging 1995;5:171-174.
48. Yamada T, Saito H, Moriya T, et al. Adrenal carcinoma with a signal loss on chemical shift magnetic resonance imaging. J Comput Assist Tomogr 2003;27:606-608.
49. Masugi Y, Kameyama K, Aiba M, et al. Non-functional adrenocortical adenoma with extensive degeneration. Pathol Int 2003;53:241-245.
50. Newhouse JH, Heffess CS, Wagner BJ, Imray TJ, Adair CF, Davidson AJ. Large degenerated adrenal adenomas: radiologic-pathologic correlation. Radiology 1999;210:385-391.
51. Abrams HL, Spiro R, Goldstein N. Metastases in carcinoma. Cancer 1950;3:74-85.
52. Dunnick NR, Korobkin M, Francis I. Adrenal radiology: distinguishing benign from malignant adrenal masses. AJR Am J Roentgenol 1996;167:861-867.
53. Pope RJ, Hansell DM. Extra-thoracic staging of lung cancer. Eur J Radiol 2003;45:31-38.
54. Shinozaki K, Yoshimitsu K, Honda H, et al. Metastatic adrenal tumor from clear-cell renal cell carcinoma: a pitfall of chemical shift MR imaging. Abdom Imaging 2001;26:439-442.
55. Efremidis SC, Harsoulis F, Douma S, Zafiriadou E, Zamboulis C, Kouri A. Adrenal insufficiency with enlarged adrenals. Abdom Imaging 1996;21:168-171.
56. Kocijancic K, Kocijancic I, Guna F. Role of sonographically guided fine-needle aspiration biopsy of adrenal masses in patients with lung cancer. J Clin Ultrasound 2004;32:12-16.
57. Arellano RS, Harisinghani MG, Gervais DA, Hahn PF, Mueller PR. Image-guided percutaneous biopsy of the adrenal gland: review of indications, technique, and complications. Curr Probl Diagn Radiol 2003;32:3-10.
58. Mody MK, Kazerooni EA, Korobkin M. Percutaneous CT-guided biopsy of adrenal masses: immediate and delayed complications. J Comput Assist Tomogr 1995;19:434-439.

59. Heniford BT, Arca MJ, Walsh RM, Gill IS. Laparoscopic adrenalectomy for cancer. Semin Surg Oncol 1999;16:293-306.
60. Kebebew E, Siperstein AE, Clark OH, Duh QY. Results of laparoscopic adrenalectomy for suspected and unsuspected malignant adrenal neoplasms. Arch Surg 2002;137:948-951; discussion 952-953.
61. Lenders JW, Pacak K, Walther MM, et al. Biochemical diagnosis of pheochromocytoma: which test is best? JAMA 2002;287:1427-1434.
62. Whalen RK, Althausen AF, Daniels GH. Extra-adrenal pheochromocytoma. J Urol 1992;147:1-10.
63. Atiyeh BA, Barakat AJ, Abumrad NN. Extra-adrenal pheochromocytoma. J Nephrol 1997;10:25-29.
64. Saurborn DP, Kruskal JB, Stillman IE, Parangi S. Best cases from the AFIP: paraganglioma of the organs of Zuckerkandl. Radiographics 2003;23:1279-1286.
65. Taouli B, Ghouadni M, Correas JM, et al. Spectrum of abdominal imaging findings in von Hippel–Lindau disease. AJR Am J Roentgenol 2003;181:1049-1054.
66. Inabnet WB, Caragliano P, Pertsemlidis D. Pheochromocytoma: inherited associations, bilaterality, and cortex preservation. Surgery 2000;128:1007-1011; discussion 1011-1012.
67. Neumann HP, Bausch B, McWhinney SR, et al. Germ-line mutations in nonsyndromic pheochromocytoma. N Engl J Med 2002;346:1459-1466.
68. Dluhy RG. Pheochromocytoma—death of an axiom. N Engl J Med 2002;346:1486-1488.
69. Kenady DE, McGrath PC, Sloan DA, Schwartz RW. Diagnosis and management of pheochromocytoma. Curr Opin Oncol 1997;9:61-67.
70. Jaroszewski DE, Tessier DJ, Schlinkert RT, et al. Laparoscopic adrenalectomy for pheochromocytoma. Mayo Clin Proc 2003;78:1501-1504.
71. Salomon L, Rabii R, Soulie M, et al. Experience with retroperitoneal laparoscopic adrenalectomy for pheochromocytoma. J Urol 2001;165:1871-1874.
72. Lee JE, Curley SA, Gagel RF, Evans DB, Hickey RC. Cortical-sparing adrenalectomy for patients with bilateral pheochromocytoma. Surgery 1996;120:1064-1070; discussion 1070-1071.
73. Quint LE, Glazer GM, Francis IR, Shapiro B, Chenevert TL. Pheochromocytoma and paraganglioma: comparison of MR imaging with CT and I-131 MIBG scintigraphy. Radiology 1987;165:89-93.
74. Beland SS, Vesely DL, Arnold WC, et al. Localization of adrenal and extra-adrenal pheochromocytomas by magnetic resonance imaging. South Med J 1989;82:1410-1413.
75. Varghese JC, Hahn PF, Papanicolaou N, Mayo-Smith WW, Gaa JA, Lee MJ. MR differentiation of phaeochromocytoma from other adrenal lesions based on qualitative analysis of T2 relaxation times. Clin Radiol 1997;52:603-606.
76. Krebs TL, Wagner BJ. MR imaging of the adrenal gland: radiologic-pathologic correlation. Radiographics 1998;18:1425-1440.
77. Lee TH, Slywotzky CM, Lavelle MT, Garcia RA. Best cases from the AFIP: cystic pheochromocytoma. Radiographics 2002;22:935-940.
78. Lucon AM, Pereira MA, Mendonca BB, Halpern A, Wajchenberg BL, Arap S. Pheochromocytoma: study of 50 cases. J Urol 1997;157:1208-1212.
79. Yildiz L, Akpolat I, Erzurumlu K, Aydin O, Kandemir B. Giant adrenal myelolipoma: case report and review of the literature. Pathol Int 2000;50:502-504.
80. Savoye-Collet C, Goria O, Scotte M, Hemet J. MR imaging of hepatic myelolipoma. AJR Am J Roentgenol 2000;174:574-575.
81. Kammen BF, Elder DE, Fraker DL, Siegelman ES. Extraadrenal myelolipoma: MR imaging findings. AJR American Journal of Roentgenology 1998;171:721-723.
82. Rao P, Kenney PJ, Wagner BJ, Davidson AJ. Imaging and pathologic features of myelolipoma. Radiographics 1997;17:1373-1385.
83. Hoeffel CC, Kowalski S. Giant myelolipoma of the adrenal gland: natural history. Clin Radiol 2000;55:402-404.
84. Han M, Burnett AL, Fishman EK, Marshall FF. The natural history and treatment of adrenal myelolipoma. J Urol 1997;157:1213-1216.
85. Russell C, Goodacre BW, vanSonnenberg E, Orihuela E. Spontaneous rupture of adrenal myelolipoma: spiral CT appearance. Abdom Imaging 2000;25:431-434.
86. El-Mekresh MM, Abdel-Gawad M, El-Diasty T, El-Baz M, Ghoneim MA. Clinical, radiological and histological features of adrenal myelolipoma: review and experience with a further eight cases. Br J Urol 1996;78:345-350.
87. Otal P, Escourrou G, Mazerolles C, et al. Imaging features of uncommon adrenal masses with histopathologic correlation. Radiographics 1999;19:569-581.
88. Kier R, Smith RC, McCarthy SM. Value of lipid- and water-suppression MR images in distinguishing between blood and lipid within ovarian masses. AJR Am J Roentgenol 1992;158:321-325.
89. Kier R, Mason BJ. Water-suppressed MR imaging of focal fatty infiltration of the liver. Radiology 1997;203:575-576.
90. Bradley WG, Jr. MR appearance of hemorrhage in the brain [see comments]. Radiology 1993;189:15-26.
91. Nimkin K, Teeger S, Wallach JC, DuVally JC, Spevak MR, Kleinman PK. Adrenal hemorrhage in abused children: imaging and postmortem findings. AJR Am J Roentgenol 1994;162:661-663.
92. Gouliamos AD, Metafa A, Ispanopoulou SG, Stamatelopoulou F, Vlahos LJ, Papadimitriou JD. Right adrenal hematoma following hepatectomy. Eur Radiol 2000;10:583-585.
93. Kawashima A, Sandler CM, Ernst RD, et al. Imaging of nontraumatic hemorrhage of the adrenal gland. Radiographics 1999;19:949-963.
94. Ten S, New M, Maclaren N. Clinical review 130: Addison's disease 2001. J Clin Endocrinol Metab 2001;86:2909-2922.
95. Hahn PF, Saini S, Stark DD, Papanicolaou N, Ferrucci JT Jr. Intraabdominal hematoma: the concentric-ring sign in MR imaging. AJR Am J Roentgenol 1987;148:115-119.
96. Siegelman ES, Outwater EK. The concentric-ring sign revisited. AJR Am J Roentgenol 1996;166:1493.
97. Cheema P, Cartagena R, Staubitz W. Adrenal cysts: diagnosis and treatment. J Urol 1981;126:396-399.
98. de Bree E, Schoretsanitis G, Melissas J, Christodoulakis M, Tsiftsis D. Cysts of the adrenal gland: diagnosis and management. Int Urol Nephrol 1998;30:369-376.
99. Neri LM, Nance FC. Management of adrenal cysts. Am Surg 1999;65:151-163.
100. Bellantone R, Ferrante A, Raffaelli M, Boscherini M, Lombardi CP, Crucitti F. Adrenal cystic lesions: report of 12 surgically treated cases and review of the literature. J Endocrinol Invest 1998;21:109-114.
101. Schwartz LH, Macari M, Huvos AG, Panicek DM. Collision tumors of the adrenal gland: demonstration and characterization at MR imaging. Radiology 1996;201:757-760.

4

Renal MRI

E. Scott Pretorius, MD
Evan S. Siegelman, MD

RENAL MR IMAGING TECHNIQUES

MRI protocols for evaluation of patients with known or suspected renal disease have evolved, with advancements in pulse sequences, surface coils, and gradients.[1,2] Renal MR examinations are best performed on high-field systems, using a phased-array surface coil centered at the level of the kidneys. The use of surface coils enhances the signal-to-noise ratio (SNR) and allows for the use of smaller fields of view to obtain high-resolution renal images (Box 4-1).

Initial coronal and sagittal breath-hold T2-W sequences allow selection of an appropriate center and field of view for the remainder of the examination. The localizer sequences may reveal findings (e.g., solitary kidney, metastatic disease) that would change the focus or modify the techniques used for the subsequent MR examination. T1-W gradient echo (GRE) images can replace T1-WSE images for MR imaging of the liver and are also ideal for imaging extrahepatic abdominal structures. The repetition time (TR) is adjusted based on the patient's ability to breath-hold. The field of view is adjusted based on body habitus and the focus of the examination. Both in-phase and opposed-phase T1-WIs are acquired in order to obtain chemical shift imaging (see Chapter 3) information that enables detection of lipid and fat in renal or adrenal lesions (Figs. 4-1 to 4-4).

For T2-WI, an axial, fat-suppressed, respiratory-triggered fast spin-echo (FSE) sequence provides high SNR images with reasonable acquisition times. The field of view and slice thickness are similar to those of the T1-WI. Additional precontrast sequences can be performed. If, for example, an angiomyolipoma is suspected, frequency selective fat-saturated T1-GRE or water-saturated T1-GRE images can be obtained, maintaining the TR of the original in-phase and opposed-phase T1-WIs. These sequences allow definitive detection and characterization of the macroscopic fat present in most angiomyolipomas (see Fig. 4-4 and Box 4-1).

The coronal plane is generally chosen for the CE images because it allows dynamic evaluation of kidneys, renal vessels, inferior vena cava (IVC), and spine in the smallest number of slices or slabs. Exophytic polar lesions that are not well depicted on axial images generally are well displayed on coronal images (see Fig. 4-4). For characterization of a specific renal mass, the plane that best displays the lesion should be chosen; for exophytic anterior and posterior lesions, this may be the sagittal or axial plane.

The CE portion of the examination may be performed as either a two-dimensional (2D) or three-dimensional (3D) sequence. 3D images allow for simultaneous evaluation of renal parenchyma and the renal vessels. When primarily evaluating the renal parenchyma, a flip angle of 10° to 12° is used to minimize soft tissue saturation and optimize renal mass detection and characterization. When primarily evaluating the renal arteries, the flip angle is increased to 30° to 60° to increase soft tissue saturation and optimize the contrast between enhanced vessels and adjacent renal parenchyma.[3]

4-1 Protocol for MR Evaluation of a Potential Renal Mass (1.5 T)

	Sequence	Plane	TR	TE	Flip	FOV (cm)	Thickness (mm)	Skip (mm)
Localizer	T2	Coronal Sagittal	Infinite	90 and 180		26–38	7	1
Chemical shift	T1-GRE	Axial	100–300 msec	2.1 and 4.2 msec	90°	26–38	6	1
Respiratory triggered, fat-saturated T2	T2 FSE	Axial	4000–6000	80–110		26–38	7	1
Pre/post Gd 3D	T1-GRE	Coronal	min	min	10°	26–36	4 interpolated to 2	0
Delayed/ post Gd	T1-GRE	Axial	68–280	4.2	90°	26–38	6	1

Optional sequences to characterize fat within an angiomyolipoma

	Sequence	Plane	TR	TE	Flip	FOV (cm)	Thickness (mm)	Skip (mm)
Fat-saturated	T1-GRE	Axial	100–300	2.1	90°	26–38	6	1
Water-saturated	T1-GRE	Axial	100–300	4.2	90°	26–38	6	1

CE MRU (1.5 T)

	Sequence	Plane	TR	TE	Flip	FOV	Thickness	Skip
Pre/post Gd 3D	T1-GRE	Coronal	min	min	10	36	2 interpolated to 1	0

TR = repetition time, TE = echo time, Flip = flip angle, FOV = field of view, Skip = interslice gap, Gd = gadolinium.

3D sequences are postprocessed to generate projection images of the renal arteries, renal veins, and IVC. Analogous to the 2D examination, a breath-hold precontrast set of images and three CE sequences are acquired to evaluate the renal vasculature in both arterial and venous phases and to depict the renal parenchyma in both corticomedullary and nephrographic phases. The patient's arms are elevated above the head to decrease phase wrap when imaging in the coronal plane. Delayed, axial, 2D, fat-saturated T1-WIs are then obtained as the final sequence, imaging from the top of the hemidiaphragms to the iliac crests.

MR urography (MRU) is unnecessary in the routine evaluation of a renal mass although it can be very useful in the evaluation of suspected transitional cell carcinoma, for renal donor evaluation, and for imaging of renal transplants (see Box 4-1).[4,5] For enhanced, T1-weighted MRU, 10 mg of furosemide is injected with the gadolinium chelate.[6,7] Dynamic enhanced 2D or 3D images of the kidneys are acquired as above, and then the field of view is increased in the z plane to include the kidneys, ureters, and urinary bladder. Coronal 3D, breath-hold, thin-slab (2 mm interpolated to 1 mm) fat-suppressed T1-GRE images are then acquired after a delay of several minutes. The delay optimizes washout of the contrast from the vasculature and parenchymal tissues and wash-in of the contrast into the collecting systems (Figs. 4-5 to 4-7).[8]

A second MRU technique for evaluating the collecting system is MR hydrography with heavily T2-WIs (see Fig. 4-7).[7-10] This sequence is identical to that used in the liver to characterize hepatic cysts and hemangiomas and, when combined with contrast-enhanced images, can be used to characterize subcentimeter renal cysts and demonstrate hydronephrosis. T2-W MRU can be useful in depicting an obstructed collecting system in a nonfunctioning kidney. If renal excretory function is still present, 3D T1-WIs of the excreted gadolinium are preferred for MR detection and characterization of ureteral calculi and urothelial neoplasms.

Renal transplants can be evaluated using sequences similar to those outlined above, with an appropriately placed pelvic surface coil.[11] Axial and coronal T2-WIs are helpful in evaluating for hydronephrosis and demonstrating the relationship between the transplant and possible pelvic fluid collections. Coronal or oblique coronal 3D CE MR angiography (MRA) imaging is useful, since the transplant renal vessels are most commonly anastomosed to the native external iliac vessels and the anastomoses are often oriented in the coronal plane. In the future, MR techniques will be increasingly used to obtain functional renal information including glomerular filtration rate, blood flow, oxygenation, and tubular concentration and transit.[12]

RENAL NEOPLASMS

Renal Cell Carcinoma (RCC)

EPIDEMIOLOGY

In 2004 in the United States, approximately 35,710 new cases of renal cell carcinoma (RCC) will be diagnosed

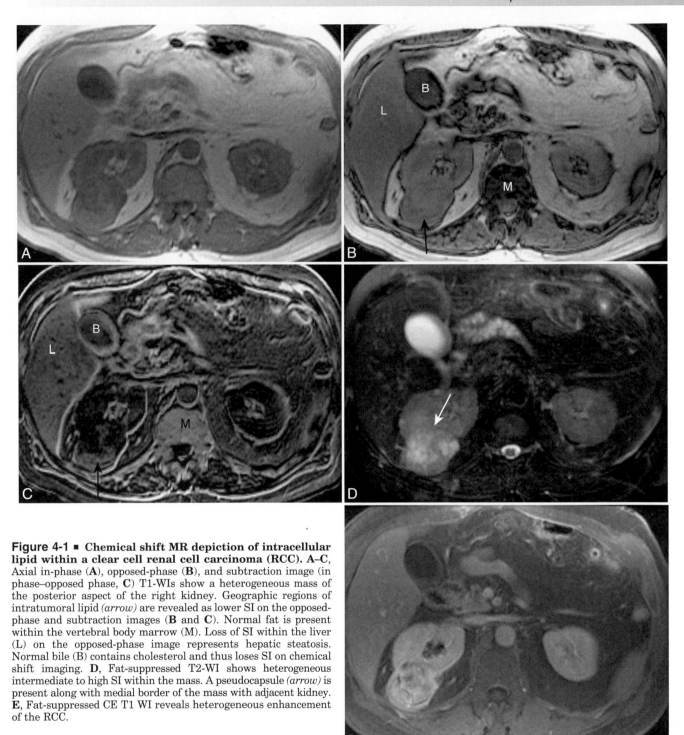

Figure 4-1 ▪ **Chemical shift MR depiction of intracellular lipid within a clear cell renal cell carcinoma (RCC). A–C,** Axial in-phase (**A**), opposed-phase (**B**), and subtraction image (in phase–opposed phase, **C**) T1-WIs show a heterogeneous mass of the posterior aspect of the right kidney. Geographic regions of intratumoral lipid *(arrow)* are revealed as lower SI on the opposed-phase and subtraction images (**B** and **C**). Normal fat is present within the vertebral body marrow (M). Loss of SI within the liver (L) on the opposed-phase image represents hepatic steatosis. Normal bile (B) contains cholesterol and thus loses SI on chemical shift imaging. **D,** Fat-suppressed T2-WI shows heterogeneous intermediate to high SI within the mass. A pseudocapsule *(arrow)* is present along with medial border of the mass with adjacent kidney. **E,** Fat-suppressed CE T1 WI reveals heterogeneous enhancement of the RCC.

and 12,480 people will die of the disease.[13] In 2004 RCC will account for 3% of new cancers diagnosed in American men and result in 3% of cancer-related deaths.[13] Although less common than prostate or bladder carcinoma, RCC is more commonly fatal than other urinary tract neoplasms. More than one third of affected individuals die of their disease.[14]

Known risk factors for RCC include cigarette smoking, exposure to petroleum products or asbestos, hypertension, and obesity.[15] RCC is approximately twice as common in men as in women and slightly more common in African Americans than in people of European descent. Most affected patients are more than 40 years of age, and persons in the seventh and

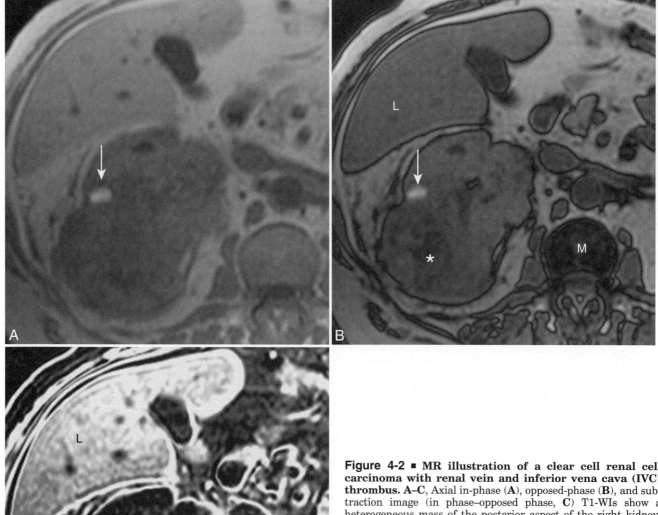

Figure 4-2 ■ MR illustration of a clear cell renal cell carcinoma with renal vein and inferior vena cava (IVC) thrombus. A–C, Axial in-phase (**A**), opposed-phase (**B**), and subtraction image (in phase–opposed phase, **C**) T1-WIs show a heterogeneous mass of the posterior aspect of the right kidney. Focal high SI *(arrow)* represents introtumoral hemorrhage in **A** and **B**. Foci of intratumoral lipid are revealed as lower SI (∗) on the opposed-phase (**B**) and high SI *(arrows in* **C**) on the subtraction image (**C**). Normal fat is present within the vertebral body marrow (**M**). Loss of SI within the liver (**L**) on the opposed-phase image represents hepatic steatosis. *(Continued)*

eighth decades of life are most commonly affected. Individuals with acquired cystic kidney disease (ACKD) and hereditary conditions including von Hippel–Lindau syndrome (VHL), hereditary papillary renal cancer (HPRC), tuberous sclerosis (TS), and sickle cell trait are also at increased risk.

RENAL LESION DETECTION

Improved imaging detection of renal masses by ultrasound (US), CT, and MRI has led to smaller average size of neoplasm at time of initial detection,[16] and most of these incidentally discovered renal cell carcinomas are of low stage and tumor grade.[17] In prior decades, nearly all patients with RCC had hematuria or other signs and symptoms related to the renal tumor. Currently, however, approximately 30% of all renal cell carcinomas are incidentally identified on imaging studies performed for other purposes.[18]

Sonography detects the vast majority of renal masses larger than 2.5 cm. The sensitivity of

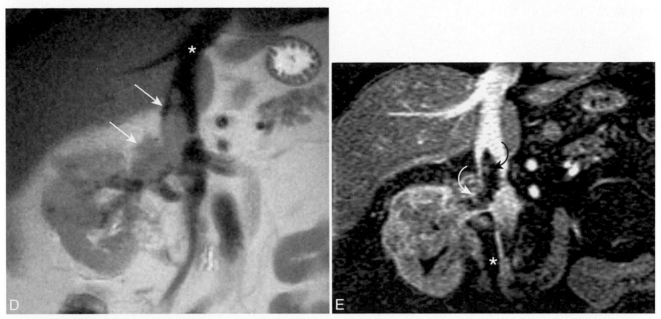

Figure 4-2 ▪ Cont'd D and **E,** Coronal T2 (**D**) and fat-suppressed (**E**) CE T1-WIs reveal intermediate T2-SI thrombus in the right renal vein and infrahepatic IVC *(white arrows)*. The superior segment of the intrahepatic IVC shows normal flow void (∗). Benign thrombus located within the infrarenal IVC does not enhance (∗), whereas tumor thrombus does enhance *(curved arrows)*.

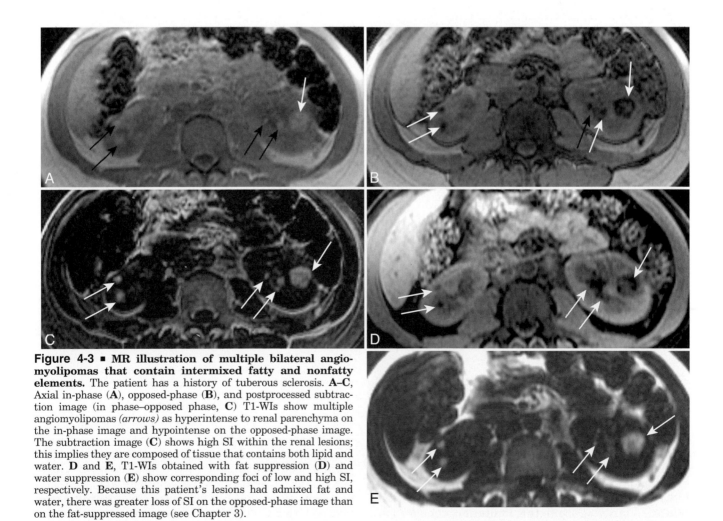

Figure 4-3 ▪ MR illustration of multiple bilateral angiomyolipomas that contain intermixed fatty and nonfatty elements. The patient has a history of tuberous sclerosis. **A–C,** Axial in-phase (**A**), opposed-phase (**B**), and postprocessed subtraction image (in phase–opposed phase, **C**) T1-WIs show multiple angiomyolipomas *(arrows)* as hyperintense to renal parenchyma on the in-phase image and hypointense on the opposed-phase image. The subtraction image (**C**) shows high SI within the renal lesions; this implies they are composed of tissue that contains both lipid and water. **D** and **E,** T1-WIs obtained with fat suppression (**D**) and water suppression (**E**) show corresponding foci of low and high SI, respectively. Because this patient's lesions had admixed fat and water, there was greater loss of SI on the opposed-phase image than on the fat-suppressed image (see Chapter 3).

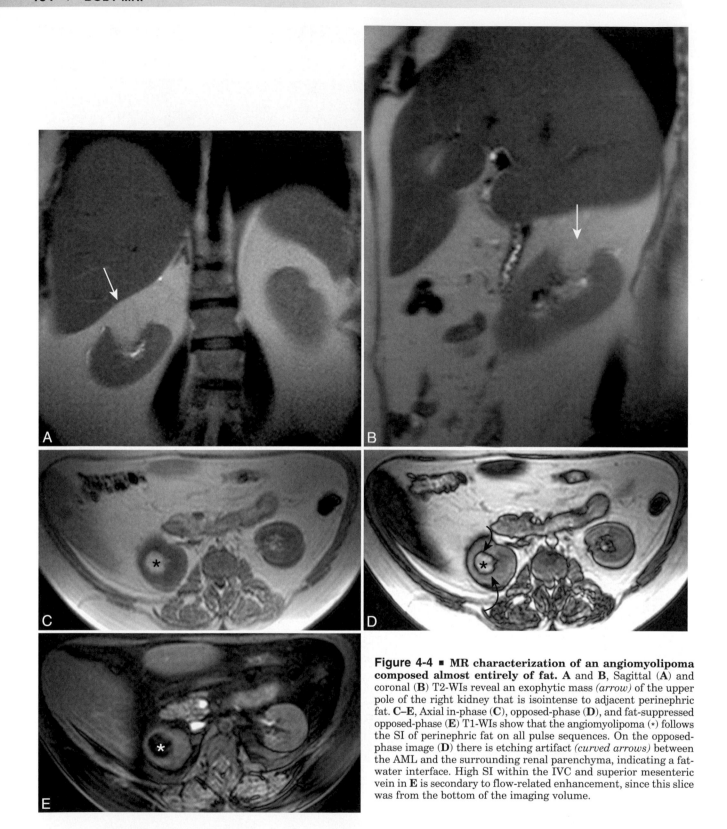

Figure 4-4 ▪ MR characterization of an angiomyolipoma composed almost entirely of fat. A and **B**, Sagittal (**A**) and coronal (**B**) T2-WIs reveal an exophytic mass *(arrow)* of the upper pole of the right kidney that is isointense to adjacent perinephric fat. **C–E**, Axial in-phase (**C**), opposed-phase (**D**), and fat-suppressed opposed-phase (**E**) T1-WIs show that the angiomyolipoma (⋆) follows the SI of perinephric fat on all pulse sequences. On the opposed-phase image (**D**) there is etching artifact *(curved arrows)* between the AML and the surrounding renal parenchyma, indicating a fat-water interface. High SI within the IVC and superior mesenteric vein in **E** is secondary to flow-related enhancement, since this slice was from the bottom of the imaging volume.

sonography, however, greatly decreases for smaller masses, and only 25% of masses 10 to 15 mm in size are detectable by US.[19] Sonography is excellent at detecting and characterizing simple cysts, but its ability to differentiate benign from malignant solid masses is limited. Despite this limitation, sonography

is a mainstay of pediatric renal imaging owing to the absence of ionizing radiation and lack of need for patient sedation.

CT with thin-section (5 mm or thinner), pre- and postcontrast images can characterize most renal neoplasms larger than 1 cm. Many renal masses detected

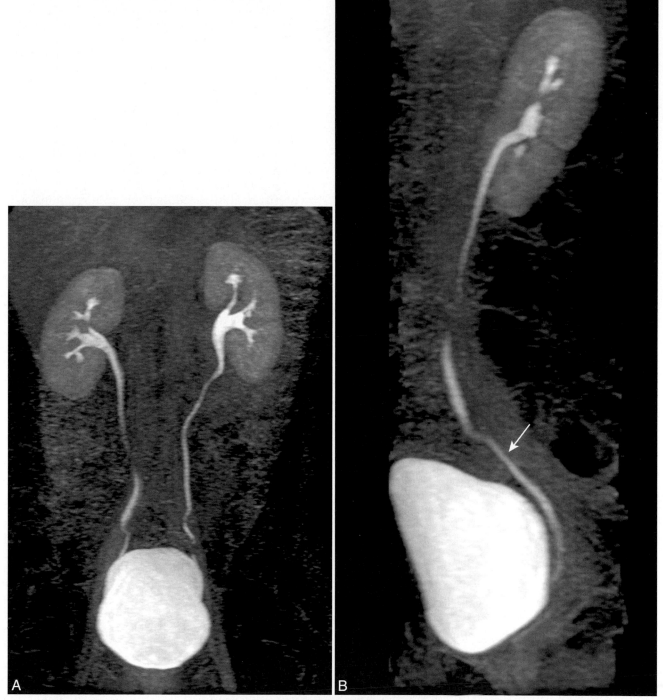

Figure 4-5 ■ Normal contrast-enhanced T1-W MR urogram (CE MRU) in a potential renal donor. **A**, Coronal maximum intensity projection (MIP) reformatted image of an excretory phase, 3D T1-WI shows normal collecting systems and solitary bilateral ureters. **B**, Right anterior oblique projection optimizes depiction of the distal left ureter *(arrow)*.

on CT, however, will be found on enhanced studies performed for nonrenal indications when precontrast images were not carried out. As such, many of these masses will not be adequately characterized, because the degree of renal enhancement cannot be assessed. Further evaluation with dedicated renal CT or MRI may be required.

The ability of dedicated renal CT and MRI to detect and characterize renal lesions greater than 1 cm is similar although MRI is superior in the detection of small polar lesions owing to its ability to image directly in nonaxial planes.[20] MRI is the examination of choice for the characterization of renal masses in patients with limited renal function

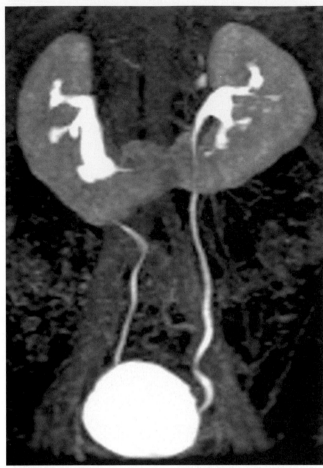

Figure 4-6 ▪ MR urography depiction of a collection system in a potential renal donor. Coronal MIP reformatted image of an excretory phase, 3D CE MRU reveals normal excretion from both moieties of a horseshoe kidney. Enhancing renal parenchymal tissue is present within the isthmus that connects the lower poles of both kidneys.

(creatinine >2.0 mg/dL) and severe allergy to iodinated contrast or for masses not adequately characterized by other imaging modalities.

RENAL LESION CHARACTERIZATION

Ideally, diagnostic imaging would unequivocally separate malignant renal lesions from benign ones. Unfortunately, this is not entirely possible, since oncocytomas and lipid-poor angiomyolipomas may have imaging appearances that may be indistinguishable from RCC (Box 4-2). The realistic goal of renal lesion characterization by CT or MRI, then, is to separate surgical lesions (renal cell carcinoma, cystic renal cell carcinoma, oncocytoma) from nonsurgical lesions (cyst, hemorrhagic cyst, angiomyolipoma, pseudotumor) (Boxes 4-3 and 4-4).

RCC has a highly variable appearance on MR imaging owing to the existence of multiple RCC histologic features[21] and to variability in internal necrosis, hemorrhage, or intratumoral lipid. On MRI, RCC most commonly appears hypointense or isointense to renal parenchyma on T1-WI, heterogeneously hyperintense

on T2-WI, and enhanced following contrast administration. Variability is the rule, however, and lesions may be primarily hyperintense, hypointense, or isointense to normal renal parenchyma on both T1- and T2-WIs. RCCs tend to enhance less than normal renal parenchyma and are often most easily identified on postcontrast dynamic T1-WI.[22] If quantitative criteria are used, it has been suggested that any mass that enhances by greater than 15% should be considered a solid renal neoplasm.[23]

A subset of clear cell RCCs, the most common subtype of RCC, may focally lose signal on opposed-phase GRE images because of the presence of microscopic intratumoral lipid (see Figs. 4-1 and 4-2).[24,25] Thus, the presence of intracellular lipid in a renal lesion is not diagnostic of an angiomyolipoma (AML). The presence of macroscopic fat within a renal lesion, however, remains very specific for AML. It is only the extremely rare and reportable renal cell carcinoma that contains fat[26,27] and often is secondary to osseous metaplasia.[28]

Differentiation between adrenal cortical adenomas and adrenal metastases is discussed in Chapter 2. Rarely, clear cell renal cell carcinoma can metastasize to an adrenal gland or other organs and reveal loss of SI on chemical shift imaging (see Figs. 2-24 and 3-8).[29,30] In the authors' experience, this uncommon subtype of patients usually has findings of metastatic disease elsewhere and so clinical care is not affected.

A thin pseudocapsule, a compressed band of normal renal parenchyma surrounding an expansile mass, surrounds some renal neoplasms. MRI is superior to CT for detection of pseudocapsules, and T2-WIs are the most sensitive for pseudocapsule detection (see Fig. 4-1D).[31] However, pseudocapsules are not specific for RCC and can surround any slow-growing solid mass. When a pseudocapsule is revealed in association with RCC, the tumor is generally of lower grade and lower stage at time of detection.[15,32]

Individuals with RCC may occasionally have a spontaneous perirenal hematoma and have pain or hematuria. This finding is not specific, however, as patients with angiomyolipomas, autosomal dominant polycystic kidney disease (ADPCKD), trauma (Fig. 4-8), and coagulopathies may also develop perinephric hemorrhage. The presence of perirenal blood, however, should prompt an evaluation for an underlying lesion.[33]

STAGING OF RCC BY MRI

Since RCC is relatively resistant to both radiotherapy and chemotherapy, surgical procedures have long been the mainstay of therapy. Accurate staging is critical in directing appropriate approach and resection for maximal disease control. Staging also is critical in determining prognosis, as tumor stage at time of diagnosis correlates directly with average survival. RCC is most commonly staged using the Robson classification,[34] although the TNM system may also be employed (Box 4-5).

Both CT and MRI are 80% to 90% accurate in staging RCC.[35,36] MRI appears to be superior for evaluation of tumor involvement of the perinephric

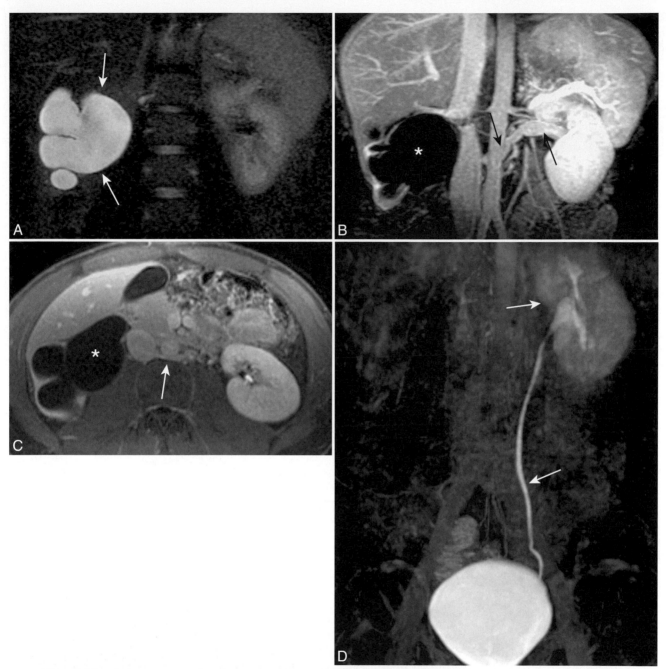

Figure 4-7 ■ MR illustration of developmental right-sided ureteropelvic (UPJ) obstruction and retroaortic left renal vein. A, Coronal heavily T2-WI (TE = 180 msec) reveals dilated right calyces and renal pelvis *(white arrows)*. The normal undistended left-sided collecting system and ureter are not visualized. T2-W MR urography is ideally suited to evaluate dilated or obstructed urinary tracks but poorly depicts normal ureters. (**B** and **C**), Coronal MIP (**B**) and axial (**C**) CE T1-WIs show a retroaortic left renal vein *(arrows)*, marked right renal parenchymal atrophy, and absent contrast within the right renal pelvis (∗). **D**, Delayed CE T1-W MR urogram shows the normal left renal pelvis and ureters *(arrows)* and nonvisualization of the right collecting system.

fat, renal vein, IVC, and adjacent organs.[37] Sonography is limited in its ability to stage RCC because of difficulty in assessing retroperitoneal lymphadenopathy.[38] High accuracy for staging of advanced RCC has also been reported for 18F-fluorodeoxyglucose positron emission tomography (FDG PET),[39] although few such investigations have been performed. Cross-sectional imaging of the pelvis is not cost effective for staging patients with known RCC.[40]

CT cannot reliably differentiate Robson stage I disease (tumor confined by the renal capsule) from Robson stage II disease (tumor spread to the perinephric fat). Historically this distinction has not been critical, since the perinephric fat is excised as part of a radical nephrectomy.[41] If, however, partial nephrectomy is contemplated, the presence of tumor in the adjacent perinephric fat might affect the surgical approach. The negative predictive value of MRI appears to be

4-2 Differential Diagnosis of a Solid Enhancing Renal Lesion

- Renal cell carcinoma—most common
- Transitional cell carcinoma
- Angiomyolipoma (usually has macroscopic fat)
- Oncocytoma—difficult to distinguish from RCC
- Lymphoma
- Renal leiomyoma

4-3 "Don't Touch" Renal Lesions

- Simple cyst (Bosniak I)
- Proteinaceous or hemorrhagic cyst (Bosniak II)
- AML <4 cm (>4 cm treated with embolization)
- Renal pseudotumor – prominent column of Bertin

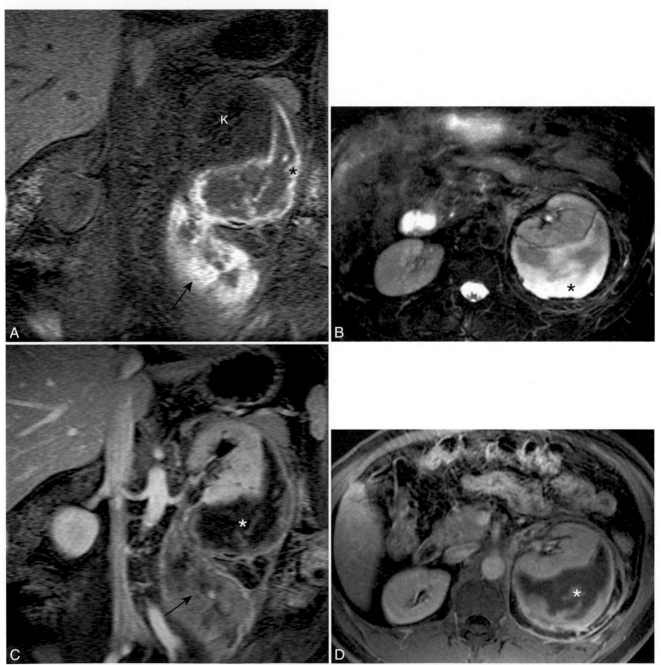

Figure 4-8 ▪ MR illustration of a perinephric hematoma in a 52-year-old man with flank pain following trauma. A and **B**, Coronal fat-suppressed T1-WI (**A**) and axial (**B**) T2-WI show soft tissue (∗) in a subcapsular portion of the left kidney that extends inferiorly *(arrow)* along the plane of the psoas muscle. The T1 hyperintense rim of the hematoma is secondary to methemoglobin. **C** and **D**, CE fat-suppressed coronal (**C**) and axial (**D**) T1-WIs show no enhancement within the hematoma or an occult adjacent renal parenchymal neoplasm. Follow-up imaging documented resolution of the hematoma (∗).

4-4   Renal Lesions Requiring Treatment

* Renal cell carcinoma
* Thickly septated (≥3 mm) cystic lesion (Bosniak III)
* Cystic lesion with mural nodule or enhancing solid tissue (Bosniak IV cystic RCC)
* Transitional cell carcinoma
* Oncocytoma
* Multilocular cystic nephroma (MLCN)

high; in 38/38 cases (100%) in which the perinephric fat was thought to be uninvolved by tumor on MRI, this finding was confirmed at pathologic sectioning.[42]

Although tumor thrombus may be suspected on T1- and T2-WI, CE MRA can be used to confirm the presence of renal vein or IVC thrombus (see Fig. 4-2).[43] Venous phase CE MRA is 88% to 100% sensitive in detection of a malignant tumor renal vein thrombus.[43,44] RCC involves the IVC in 5% to 10% of patients. In evaluation of the IVC, the second or third set of enhanced coronal images is ideal for detection and characterization of the extent of thrombus within the renal veins and IVC. In general, tumor thrombus enhances whereas benign thrombus does not (see Figs. 3-4 and 6-7).[45,46]

MRI is the modality of choice for the determination of the superior extent of IVC thrombus. The cephalad extent of tumor thrombus does not appear to affect expected survival, but it has a significant impact on surgical approach.[47,48] Level I thrombus extends into the IVC, no more than 2 cm above the renal vein confluence with the IVC, and can be removed through either a standard flank approach or an anterior approach. Level II thrombus extends more than 2 cm above the renal veins but remains inferior to the hepatic veins and requires an anterior approach through bilateral subcostal transperitoneal or thoracoabdominal incisions. Level III thrombus involves the intrahepatic IVC but remains below the diaphragm; the surgical approach is transperitoneal and thoracoabdominal, similarly to level 2 thrombus, but may additionally require cardiac bypass and hypothermic circulatory arrest. Level IV thrombus involves the supradiaphragmatic IVC or right atrium. Excision of level 4 thrombus requires a median sternotomy, cardiac bypass, and hypothermic circulatory arrest, in addition to a transabdominal incision.

DISEASES ASSOCIATED WITH RCC

Patients with acquired cystic kidney disease (ACKD) and several hereditary syndromes (Box 4-6) are at increased risk for development of RCC.[49] The high prevalence of both benign and malignant renal lesions in patients with these conditions presents a challenge for the diagnostic imager. No increased risk of renal cell carcinoma has been reported in patients with autosomal dominant or autosomal recessive polycystic kidney disease, provided they do not have ACKD. Hepatic findings in patients with autosomal dominant polycystic kidney disease are discussed in Chapter 1.

Acquired cystic kidney disease. Patients with ACKD generally are receiving dialysis or have end-stage renal disease and have small kidneys to with numerous cysts (see front cover).[50] Hemorrhage within cysts is not uncommon and may cause flank pain or hematuria. Affected patients are at approximately six times baseline risk for development of renal cell carcinoma,[51] and tumors are frequently bilateral (9%) and multicentric (50%).[52] The limited or absent renal function of these individuals and the presence of numerous simple and complex cysts make MRI an excellent modality for evaluation of potential renal malignancies, although CE CT may also be used if patients are receiving dialysis.

Screening those with ACKD for RCC is controversial because many of these individuals have short expected life spans on dialysis, are poor surgical candidates, and are asymptomatic from their renal tumors.[53] Annual imaging surveillance has not been shown to have a significant effect on patient outcome.[50] Some authors have advocated screening only

4-5   Staging of Renal Cell Carcinoma

Robson Stage	Description		TNM	TNM Stage
I	Tumor confined to renal capsule			
		Tumor <2.5 cm	T1	I
		Large tumor >2.5 cm	T2	II
II	Tumor spread to perinephric fat or adrenal		T3a	III
IIIA	Venous tumor thrombus			
		Renal vein thrombus only	T3b	III
		IVC thrombus	T3c	III
IIIB	Regional lymph node metastases		N1–N3	III/IV
IIIC	Venous tumor thrombus and regional nodes		T3b/c, N1–N3	III/IV
IVA	Direct invasion of adjacent organs outside Gerota's fascia		T4	IV
IVB	Distant metastases		M1	IV

4-6 Abdominal Imaging Findings of Autosomal Dominant Renal Diseases

Autosomal Dominant Polycystic Kidney Disease (ADPCKD)

Variable nephromegaly
Multiple bilateral renal cysts—both simple and
  complex
Liver cysts in 60% (see Chapter 1)
Pancreatic cysts in 10% (see Chapter 2)

Tuberous Sclerosis (TS)

Renal Cysts
Renal angiomyolipomas (AML), as compared with
  sporadic
    More often bilateral and multiple
    Present at younger age
    Grow faster and more likely to require treatment
Solid renal mass without macroscopic fat
    Lipid-poor AML
    Renal leiomyoma
    Possible RCC (at some increased risk)

Von Hippel–Lindau (VHL) Disease

Renal cysts
Renal cell carcinoma
    Clear cell subtype
    Multifocal and bilateral
Pancreatic manifestations (see Chapter 2)
    Pancreatic cysts—most common
    Microcystic cystadenoma
    Islet cell tumor
    Metastatic RCC
Pheochromocytoma—can be bilateral (see
  Chapter 3)
Metastatic hemangioblastoma in spinal canal

Hereditary Papillary Renal Cell Carcinoma (HPRC)

Rare; Multiple papillary RCCs
No renal cysts, AML, or extrarenal imaging findings

---

the youngest and healthiest dialysis patients, who are most likely to realize survival benefit from tumor excision.[54]

Hereditary renal cancers. Multiple syndromes are associated with hereditary renal cancers (see Box 4-6).[49,55] These syndromes are more likely to present at a younger age and to be multifocal compared with sporadic tumors (Box 4-7). The four most common hereditary syndromes are described here. Several less common hereditary syndromes are detailed elsewhere.[49,55]

Von Hippel–Lindau (VHL) disease. Von Hippel–Lindau (VHL) disease (see Box 4-6) is autosomal dominant, with near 100% penetrance (see Box 4-10). VHL affects approximately 1 in 40,000 to 50,000 individuals in the U. S.[56,57] Cysts are the most common renal manifestation of the syndrome, but approximately 25% to 45% of affected patients will develop clear cell RCC (Figs. 4-9 and 4-10; see Fig. 2-33).[49,58] Patients with

VHL tend to develop RCC in the fourth or fifth decade of life, younger than the average for sporadic cases.[59] Patients with VHL and HPRC are also likely to develop synchronous or metachronous RCC, and imaging surveillance with CT or MRI at 6- to 12-month intervals, depending on tumor growth rate, is warranted.[60] Since patients with VHL and HPRC tend to develop multiple low-grade RCCs in the course of their life, they are managed, when possible, with multiple partial nephrectomy or other nephron-sparing therapy in order to preserve renal function for as long as possible.[61] A threshold of 3 cm usually is used for resection, as distant metastases from RCCs smaller than this are rare.[60,61]

Hereditary Papillary Renal Cancer (HPRC). HPRC (see Box 4-6) is a recently described autosomal dominant hereditary cancer syndrome caused by a single gene mutation[62,63] that results in an abnormality of the tyrosine kinase transmembrane receptor. Affected individuals develop multiple papillary renal cell carcinomas (which make up approximately 15% of all RCCs), which on both CT and MRI tend to enhance uniformly, grow slowly, and enhance less than clear cell carcinomas of similar size.[49,64] Because patients with HPRC develop well-differentiated, type 1 papillary tumors, they often present later than those with VHL and can die of other causes.[49]

Tuberous Sclerosis (TS). Tuberous sclerosis (see Box 4-6) displays autosomal dominant inheritance but with variable penetrance. Sporadic cases occur in more than half of patients.[65] The prevalence of TS is estimated to be between 1/6,000 and 1/10,000 individuals.[49] Most affected individuals develop bilateral renal cysts and angiomyolipomas (see Fig. 4-3).[66] Approximately 1% to 2% of those with TS develop RCC.[49,67,68] Failure to demonstrate macroscopic fat in an enhancing solid renal lesion in a patient with TS raises the possibility of RCC.

Medullary carcinoma of the kidney. Medullary carcinoma of the kidney is a rare, aggressive malignancy that almost exclusively develops in patients with sickle cell trait.[69] Patients often have metastatic disease at time of presentation, and the prognosis

4-7 Renal Cell Carcinoma: Sporadic vs. Hereditary

	Sporadic	*Hereditary*
Decade at presentation	6th to 8th	2nd to 5th
Gender	M > F	M ≤ F
Number of tumors	Single	Multiple
Family history of RCC	Absent	Often present
Percentage of RCCs	96%	4%

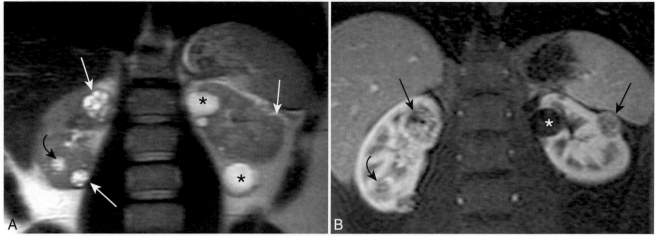

Figure 4-9 ▪ MR illustration of renal cysts and renal cell carcinomas in a 26-year-old man with von Hippel–Lindau disease. A and **B,** Coronal T2 (**A**) and fat-suppressed CE (**B**) T1-WIs reveal renal cysts (∗) and several solid RCCs *(arrows)*. One of the centrally located right renal tumors *(curved arrow)* is poorly depicted in **B** because it has similar SI as the surrounding renal medulla. This potential pitfall of dynamic enhanced imaging of RCCs has been documented in CT. The patient subsequently had 12 RCCs removed by wedge resection. Three years after surgery MR shows residual growing lesions, none of which measure >2 cm.

is poor, with a median survival of 4 months.[70] It is hypothesized that chronic hypoxia of the renal medulla contributes to tumor development. Since the frequency of medullary carcinoma in those with sickle cell trait (which affects 1 in 12 African Americans) is so low, other unknown factors must contribute to the development of this rare tumor.[49]

SURGICAL THERAPIES FOR RCC (BOX 4-8)

Radical nephrectomy, which involves resection of the entire kidney, proximal ureter, and ipsilateral adrenal gland, was for many years the sole surgical therapy offered to patients with RCC. Recently, partial nephrectomy has been performed for selected renal neoplasms, namely, those which occur in solitary kidneys, synchronously in both kidneys, or in those patients with poor renal function. Reported rates of local tumor recurrence following partial nephrectomy range from 4% to 10%,[15,71] but overall patient survival has not significantly differed from that of patients with similar stage disease who have undergone radical nephrectomy.[72,73] Many institutions now perform "elective" partial nephrectomy in patients with small renal neoplasms and normal contralateral kidneys, and studies demonstrate no

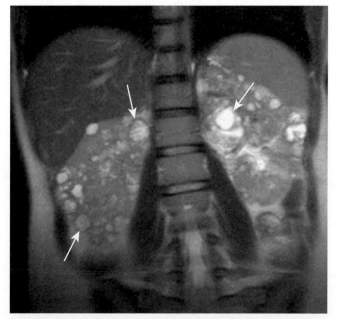

Figure 4-10 ▪ MR depiction of multiple bilateral renal cysts and renal cell carcinomas in a 23-year-old woman with von Hippel–Lindau disease. Several years prior to this examination she had undergone bilateral partial nephrectomies for RCCs. A coronal T2-WI reveals interval growth of multiple lesions *(arrows)*.

| 4-8 | Treatment of Renal Cell Carcinoma |

Surgical options
- Radical nephrectomy
- Open partial nephrectomy
- Laparoscopic partial nephrectomy

Nonsurgical therapies (evolving)
- Cryotherapy
- Radiofrequency ablation
- Focused US ablation

difference in patient 5- or 10-year survival[74,75] or in patient quality of life.[76] Open partial nephrectomy may carry a slightly lower surgical complication rate than radical nephrectomy, although both procedures have relatively low morbidity and mortality.[77]

Imaging parameters suggesting that a renal lesion can be successfully and completely removed by partial nephrectomy include small (<4 cm) tumor size; peripheral location; lack of invasion of the renal sinus fat, perinephric fat, and renal collecting system; presence of a pseudocapsule; lack of renal vein involvement; and absence of lymphadenopathy or distant metastases.[42] Larger tumors[78] and lesions that focally invade the renal sinus fat, renal collecting system, or perinephric fat may be removed by partial nephrectomy if there are compelling reasons (i.e., limited renal function, bilateral renal malignancies, or tumor in a solitary kidney). The presence of tumor thrombus or adjacent organ invasion excludes the possibility of curative partial nephrectomy.

An evolving alternative to open surgery is laparoscopic partial nephrectomy.[79,80] Although previously applied solely to benign disease such as chronic pyelonephritis or calculus disease, the technique has now been advocated for small, indeterminate renal masses.[81] This is generally performed on lesions that measure <2 cm and is associated with very low morbidity and mortality. Other minimally invasive therapies for RCC include tumor cryoablation, radiofrequency ablation, focused ultrasound, and microwave therapy.[82-87] Although technical procedural success has been reported, it has not yet been established whether these new therapies will achieve tumor cure rates similar to those of open radical and partial nephrectomies.[88]

Some institutions have performed MR-guided interventions on open configuration MR systems.[89] Advantages of combining real-time MR imaging with focused tumor ablation are the ability to show the RF electrode or cryoablation device within the tumor and potentially to confirm adequate tumor treatment by real-time imaging. As the number of interventional MR systems increases and image quality improves, the frequency of such procedures is likely to increase.

IMAGING FOLLOW-UP FOR RCC

Authors' recommendations differ for imaging follow-up of surgical treatment for RCC, although recurrence rates are related to the size, histologic grade, and stage of the primary neoplasm.[90] In a retrospective study of 200 patients with RCC treated with radical or partial nephrectomy, no patient with a T1 neoplasm smaller than 4 cm had tumor recurrence at mean follow-up of 47 months.[91] Thus, patients with such tumors may not require routine imaging follow-up. Patients with larger tumors, high tumor grade, or advanced stage may be followed with semiannual chest CT and with abdominal CT[91] or MRI. Local tumor recurrence following complete resection is less than 2% at 5 years, but it carries a poor prognosis, with 28% survival at 5 years.[92]

Few studies have been performed on imaging following focal laparoscopic ablation of renal neoplasms. The MR appearance of most cryoablated tumors (95%) is isointense to hypointense to normal parenchyma on T2-WI. A minority of lesions displays a thin hypointense rim on T2-WI. Serial imaging demonstrates interval decrease in size of the cryoablation site.[93]

Renal Cysts and Cystic Neoplasms

SIMPLE CYSTS, COMPLICATED CYSTS, AND CYSTIC RCC

Approximately 10% to 15% of RCCs display some cystic component.[94,95] The architectural features and enhancement characteristics of nonsimple cystic renal lesions are important in determining lesion management. MR features of cystic renal lesions that are highly associated with malignancy include mural irregularity, nodules, and intense mural enhancement.[96]

Although Bosniak's classification system for cystic renal lesions was described for CT,[97] the morphologic features described in the various categories can be applied to MR, with the limitation that calcification is difficult to detect on MRI (Box 4-9). Category I lesions are simple cysts. Simple renal cysts are common and are present in greater than 10% of patients who have renal sonograms and more than half of patients who have abdominal MRI.[98,99] Simple cysts are twice as common in men as in women and are more common in older patients. Simple renal cysts grow approximately 3 mm/yr if they are followed with serial imaging. Heavily T2-WI, MR hydrography[9] can both detect and characterize renal cysts as small as 1 to 2 mm.[99,100] Just as in hepatic imaging, a focal lesion that has persistent high SI on a heavily T2-W sequence should be an uncomplicated cyst.

Lesions with a single thin septation or with fine mural calcification are probably benign (category II). Also included in category II are CT "hyperdense"

4-9 Differential Diagnosis of Cystic Renal Lesions

Unilocular, Unifocal
- Simple (Bosniak I) cyst
- Hemorrhagic or proteinaceous (Bosniak II) cyst
- Thickly septated (Bosniak III) cyst
- Cystic RCC (Bosniak IV)

Unilocular, Multifocal (See Box 4-6)
- Multiple simple cysts
- Autosomal dominant polycystic kidney disease
- Von Hippel–Lindau disease
- Tuberous sclerosis

Multilocular
- Multiple simple cysts
- Multilocular cystic nephroma (see Box 4-10)
- Localized cystic disease of the kidney

cysts, which contain internal protein or hemorrhage (Fig. 4-11). The MR equivalent of the CT hyperdense cyst is hyperintense to normal renal parenchyma on T1-WI, has variable SI of T2-WI, and does not enhance after contrast (see Fig. 4-11). Cystic renal lesions with uniform wall thickening and/or thicker septa or multiple septa are indeterminate (category III) (Fig. 4-12). Approximately 60% of Bosniak category III lesions represent cystic renal cell carcinoma.[101,102] Some have suggested that biopsy of Bosniak III lesions is appropriate. Those individuals with positive biopsies can be treated and those with negative biopsies can be followed by imaging and avoid unnecessary treatment.[102] Lesions with enhancing mural solid nodules (category IV) should be excised, and the majority of these lesions will be cystic renal cell carcinomas. Surgical cure rates for cystic renal cell carcinomas are high.[103]

A fifth category of cystic lesion is termed IIF ("F" = follow-up). These renal cysts have minimal wall thickening or an increased number of septa; most are benign. If follow-up imaging shows no increase in septa or progressive wall thickening, then the patient can be managed conservatively. The optimal frequency and duration of follow-up imaging studies have yet to be determined.[104] The amount and distribution of calcification within a cystic renal mass are less predictive of malignancy than is the amount of solid enhancing tissue.[104] Thus, although calcification is more accurately revealed on CT than on MR, it is of less clinical importance in the evaluation of complex cystic renal masses.

Most cystic neoplasms that require surgery will enhance greater than 20 Hounsfield units (HU) on CT, and enhancement of less than 12 HU probably is not significant in the absence of other lesion features

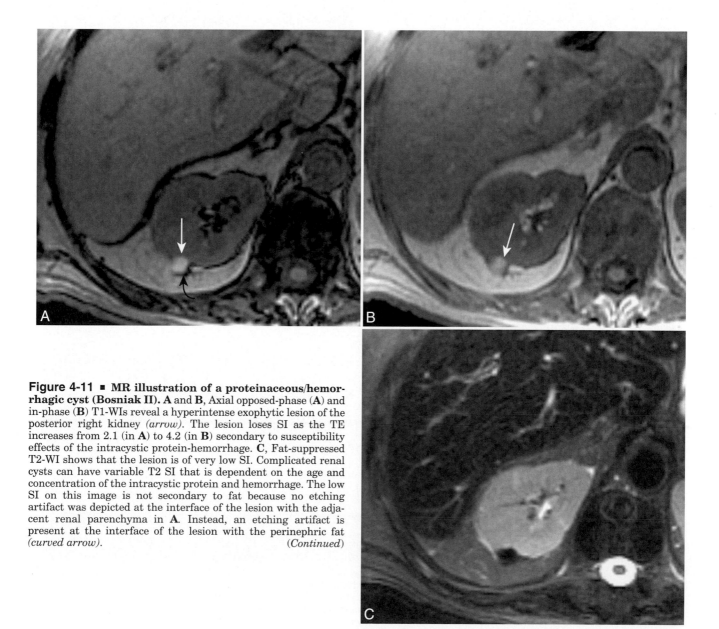

Figure 4-11 ▪ MR illustration of a proteinaceous/hemorrhagic cyst (Bosniak II). A and **B,** Axial opposed-phase (**A**) and in-phase (**B**) T1-WIs reveal a hyperintense exophytic lesion of the posterior right kidney *(arrow).* The lesion loses SI as the TE increases from 2.1 (in **A**) to 4.2 (in **B**) secondary to susceptibility effects of the intracystic protein-hemorrhage. **C,** Fat-suppressed T2-WI shows that the lesion is of very low SI. Complicated renal cysts can have variable T2 SI that is dependent on the age and concentration of the intracystic protein and hemorrhage. The low SI on this image is not secondary to fat because no etching artifact was depicted at the interface of the lesion with the adjacent renal parenchyma in **A.** Instead, an etching artifact is present at the interface of the lesion with the perinephric fat *(curved arrow).* *(Continued)*

suspicious for malignancy.[105] Many CT scanners may erroneously increase postcontrast attenuation values in simple cysts, a process termed pseudoenhancement.[106] Pseudoenhancement is most pronounced in lesions smaller than 1.5 cm, measured during maximal parenchymal enhancement on multidetector machines.[107-109] Renal cyst pseudoenhancement has not been reported on MR. However, the absence of an absolute scale of intensity in MR imaging makes it difficult to quantify degree of enhancement, although an ROI increase of greater than 15% is suspicious for malignancy.[23] Pre- and postcontrast MR images should always be obtained in the same scanning series with identical imaging parameters, so that meaningful comparisons of SI can be made (see Figs. 4-11 and 4-12).

MULTILOCULAR CYSTIC NEPHROMA (MLCN)

In the differential diagnosis of complex cystic renal lesions is the multilocular cystic nephroma (Box 4-10). This complex cystic renal lesion most commonly presents in young boys and adult women.[110] Patients may be asymptomatic or have hematuria. On MR imaging, MLCN is most commonly depicted as a multiloculated agglomeration of high SI cystic, noncommunicating spaces on T2-WI, which may herniate into the renal collecting system.[111] Individual cystic loculi may contain protein or hemorrhage, and as such may be hyperintense to renal parenchyma on T1-WI. The septa between the cystic loculi enhance, but the loculi themselves do not (Fig. 4-13). Although MLCN is considered benign, rare cases of sarcomatous

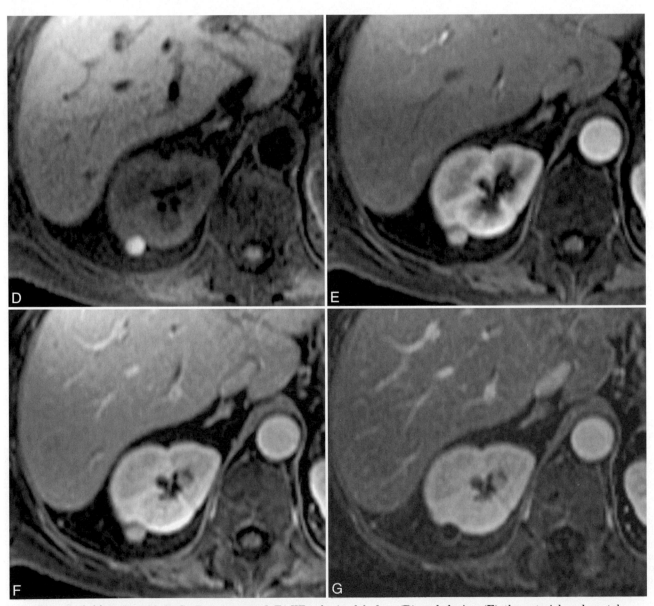

Figure 4-11 ■ Cont'd D–G, Fat-suppressed T1-WIs obtained before (**D**) and during (**E**) the arterial and portal (**F**) phases of CE show no lesion enhancement. Normal arterial and interstitial patterns of renal enhancement are revealed. The cyst shows very high SI in **D** because of the use of fat suppression (which improves the dynamic range) and shorter echo time (1.1 msec) compared with the longer echo times used in **A** and **B**. **G,** Subtraction enhanced image (image **F**–image **D**) confirms the absence of cyst enhancement.

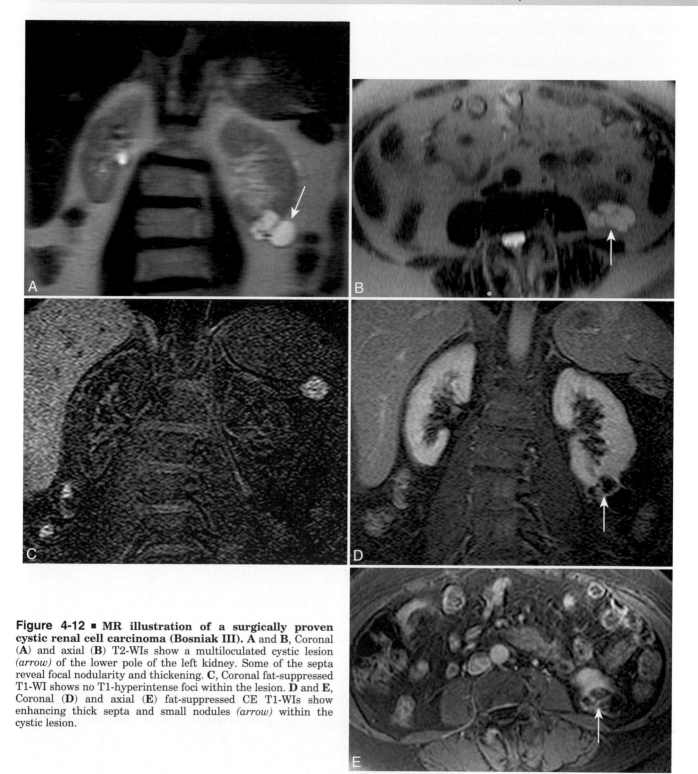

Figure 4-12 ▪ **MR illustration of a surgically proven cystic renal cell carcinoma (Bosniak III).** **A** and **B**, Coronal (**A**) and axial (**B**) T2-WIs show a multiloculated cystic lesion *(arrow)* of the lower pole of the left kidney. Some of the septa reveal focal nodularity and thickening. **C**, Coronal fat-suppressed T1-WI shows no T1-hyperintense foci within the lesion. **D** and **E**, Coronal (**D**) and axial (**E**) fat-suppressed CE T1-WIs show enhancing thick septa and small nodules *(arrow)* within the cystic lesion.

degeneration have been reported, and MLCN is therefore considered to be a surgical lesion.

AUTOSOMAL DOMINANT POLYCYSTIC KIDNEY DISEASE (ADPCKD)

Autosomal dominant polycystic kidney disease (ADPCKD; see Box 4-6) is a common hereditary disorder that results in variable enlargement of the kidneys, which contain innumerable cysts. The responsible genes (*PDK-1* and *-2*) have been identified.[112] Approximately 1 in 500 people have the disease (600,000 in the U. S.).[113,114] Most patients with ADPCKD develop renovascular hypertension and renal failure. Patients with ADPCKD make up 5% of nondiabetic patients who receive dialysis or renal transplants in the U. S. On MR, the kidneys are

4-10 Features of Multilocular Cystic Nephroma (MLCN)

Clinical
Young boys and middle-aged women
Patient usually asymptomatic, can have hematuria
Therapy: resection to exclude rare foci of sarcomatous degeneration

MRI
Multiloculated cystic mass, cysts do not communicate
Some cysts may show high T1 SI secondary to intracystic protein or hemorrhage
Invagination into renal pelvic highly suggestive but not pathognomonic

enlarged and contain numerous simple cysts and also cysts that contain varying amounts of hemorrhage or protein (Fig. 4-14).[115] Symptomatic cysts can be treated with percutaneous drainage and sclerotherapy with either ethanol or n-butyl-2-cyanoacrylate.[113,116] The hepatic and pancreatic manifestations of ADPCKD are discussed in Chapters 1 and 2, respectively.

Localized Cystic Disease of the Kidney

Non-neoplastic localized cystic disease of the kidney is a recently described condition that affects a single kidney. Pathologically and by imaging it consists of a conglomerate of cysts separated by normal renal parenchyma.[117] Since the condition is non-neoplastic, treatment is conservative[118] although differentiation from MLCN may be difficult.

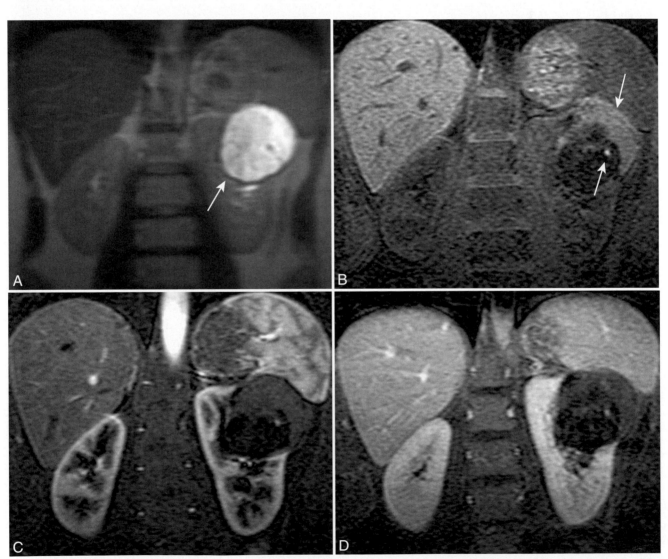

Figure 4-13 ■ **MR depiction of a multilocular cystic nephroma in a middle-aged woman. A**, Coronal T2-WI shows a multiloculated cystic lesion *(arrow)* of the mid to upper pole of the left kidney. The inferior medial aspect of the lesion approaches the left renal pelvis. **B**, Coronal fat-suppressed T1-WI shows hyperintense components *(arrows)* within the mass, in keeping with intracystic protein or hemorrhage. **C** and **D**, Arterial (**C**) and interstitial (**D**) phase CE fat-suppressed T1-WIs show no solid enhancement within the lesion. On delayed imaging (not shown), these cysts did not communicate with the collecting system.

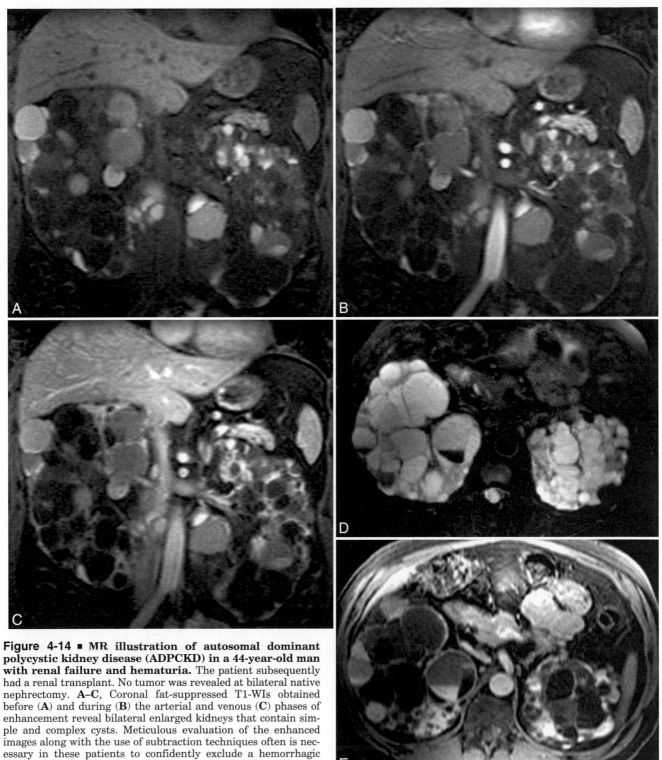

Figure 4-14 ■ MR illustration of autosomal dominant polycystic kidney disease (ADPCKD) in a 44-year-old man with renal failure and hematuria. The patient subsequently had a renal transplant. No tumor was revealed at bilateral native nephrectomy. **A–C,** Coronal fat-suppressed T1-WIs obtained before (**A**) and during (**B**) the arterial and venous (**C**) phases of enhancement reveal bilateral enlarged kidneys that contain simple and complex cysts. Meticulous evaluation of the enhanced images along with the use of subtraction techniques often is necessary in these patients to confidently exclude a hemorrhagic renal neoplasm. **D** and **E,** Axial fat-suppressed T2-WI (**D**) and CE T1-WI (**E**) also show bilateral nephromegaly and multiple simple and complex cysts.

Transitional Cell Carcinoma (TCC)

Transitional cell carcinoma (TCC) is the second most common primary renal malignancy, although it is far more common in the urinary bladder than in the upper urinary tract. Between 30% and 75% of patients with upper tract TCC will have synchronous bladder tumors and 2% to 4% of patients with bladder TCC will have synchronous upper tract disease.[119] Diagnosis of TCC, therefore, requires evaluation of the entire urothelium. Imaging evaluation of suspected upper urinary tract TCC is primarily performed with intravenous urography (IVU) and retrograde pyelography, both of which provide greater spatial resolution for detection of small urothelial abnormalities than do CT and MR.[120]

Still, cross-sectional imaging modalities can detect TCC of the upper tracts.[121] Heavily T2-W MR hydrography can evaluate dilated collecting systems even in the absence of renal function. Additionally, MR can stage upper tract TCC by showing distant metastases or tumor involvement of the renal parenchyma, perinephric fat, or periureteral fat (Box 4-11).[122] The one reported series of MR-staging of upper tract TCC found MR to be superior to CT,

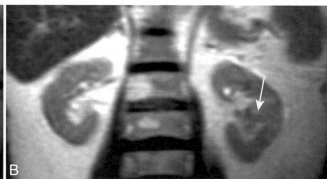

4-11 Staging of Transitional Cell Carcinoma of the Renal Pelvis[119]	
Carcinoma in situ	Tis
Tumor is epithelial (and usually papillary)	Ta
Tumor invades lamina propria	T1
Tumor invades muscularis propria	T2
Tumor invades peripelvic fat, periureteral fat, or renal parenchyma	T3
Tumor invades contiguous organs	T4
One positive regional node, 2 cm	N1
One positive node <5 cm but >2 cm, or multiple nodes <5 cm	N2
Regional nodes >5 cm	N3
Hematogenous or distant nodal metastases	M1

although one case of superficial invasion of the renal parenchyma was not shown on MR.[123]

Transitional cell carcinomas of the renal pelvis or renal collecting system are visualized on MRU or on T2-WI as filling defects, with or without proximal hydronephrosis (Fig. 4-15). In contrast to calculi,

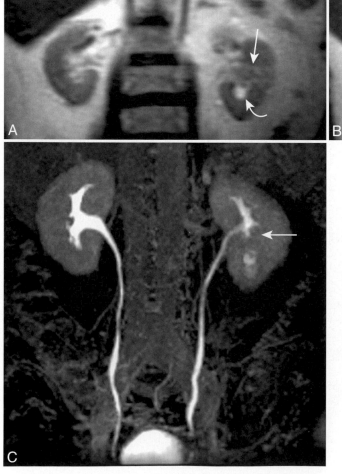

Figure 4-15 ■ Transitional cell carcinoma of the lower pole collecting system as revealed by MR in a 76-year-old woman with hematuria. A and **B,** Two consecutive coronal T2-WIs show soft tissue infiltration of the left renal pelvis *(arrow)* with a peripheral obstructed lower pole renal calyx *(curved arrow).* The mass showed mild enhancement (not shown). **C,** Coronal MIP reformatted image of an excretory phase CE T1-WI shows the tumor *(arrow)* as a low SI mass surrounded by dilute hyperintense contrast within the left lower pole collecting system.

TCCs will enhance following the administration of gadolinium chelate,[16] although tumors tend to enhance less than renal parenchyma. TCC is hypointense to urine on T2-WI. The SI of TCC on T1-WI is dependent on the concentration of excreted gadolinium in the surrounding urine.[123]

Lymphoma

Primary renal lymphoma is extremely rare.[124] Renal lymphoma usually is a manifestation of widespread systemic disease; Non-Hodgkin's B cell lymphoma is the most common cell type to involve the kidney. Renal involvement in systemic lymphoma is common, with up to two thirds of patients affected in autopsy series. The most common imaging presentation in patients with renal lymphoma is that of a large para-aortic retroperitoneal mass with extension into the renal hilum or subcapsular space (Fig. 4-16).[125,126] Rounded intraparenchymal masses most often represent recurrent lymphoma in treated patients (Box 4-12).

Untreated renal lymphoma is hypointense to renal cortex on T1-WI, hypointense or isointense to renal cortex on T2-WI, and enhances less than surrounding renal parenchyma after contrast.[127] The MR imaging characteristics of treated lymphoma are more variable[128] and the multifocal parenchymal appearance of lymphoma is more common in those patients who have recurrent disease.

Angiomyolipoma (AML)

Angiomyolipomas (AMLs) are benign renal hamartomas composed of varying amounts of blood vessels, smooth muscle, and fat. Twenty percent of AMLs occur in patients with tuberous sclerosis,[65] while the remaining 80% occur sporadically. AMLs may bleed,

---

4-12 Lymphoma of the Kidneys: Two Patterns of Disease

Pattern 1: Aggressive Infiltrative Retroperitoneal Mass
More common pattern (two thirds); initial presentation of lymphoma
Aggressive lymphomatous mass surrounds kidney
Surrounding malignant adenopathy

Pattern 2: Bilateral Multifocal Renal Masses
Less common pattern (one third); history of treated lymphoma
Hematogenous spread of recurrent disease
Low to intermediate SI on T2-WI
Hypoenhancing after contrast

---

and the risk of hemorrhage increases with increasing lesion size and the presence of intratumoral aneurysms.[129] AMLs smaller than 4 cm are followed conservatively, while those larger than 4 cm are embolized to avoid the complication of intratumoral-peritumoral hemorrhage.[130,131]

Since they are vascular lesions, AMLs may enhance and must be differentiated from RCCs. Identifying intratumoral fat establishes an MR diagnosis of AML. This is best performed by comparing T1-WIs performed with and without fat saturation (see Fig. 4-4B and E). In-phase and opposed-phase T1-W chemical shift imaging has been used to detect small amounts of fat in AMLs and will demonstrate lipid in some lesions in which fat could not be shown on CT (see Chapter 3 for chemical shift imaging techniques).[132] Some smaller AMLs may become more conspicuous on out-of-phase images owing to fat/water

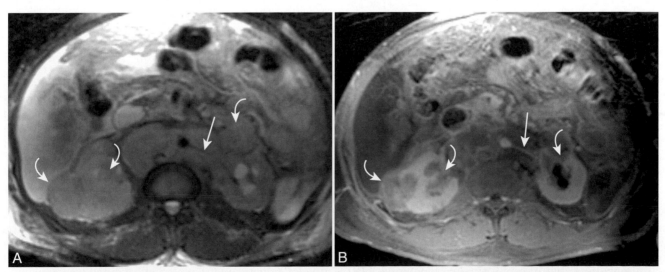

Figure 4-16 ▪ **MR illustration of primary renal lymphoma. A** and **B**, Axial T2-WI (**A**) and CE T1-WI (**B**) show an aggressive, solid, enhancing retroperitoneal mass that encases the aorta, left renal artery *(arrows),* and both kidneys. Ascites is present. Intraparenchymal renal masses *(curved arrows)* in **B** are due to direct invasion by adjacent lymphoma.

signal cancellation and resultant etching artifact at the margin between the AML and the adjacent renal parenchyma.[133] On opposed-phase images, a small AML with lipid and water admixed throughout the entire lesion will often become entirely low SI as a result of intratumoral lipid-water signal cancellation (see Fig. 4-3).

Signal loss on chemical shift imaging within a solid renal neoplasm is not specific for AML because some clear cell RCCs may contain intracellular lipid[25] (see Figs. 4-1 and 4-2). The presence of signal loss on chemical shift imaging in a renal lesion can therefore not by itself be used to diagnose AML. If an AML is suspected after the acquisition of in-phase and opposed-phase T1-WIs, then the diagnosis is confirmed by obtaining either a fat- or water-saturated T1-WI. Macroscopic intratumoral fat will follow the SI of perinephric and subcutaneous fat and will be hypointense on the fat-saturated T1-WI and hyperintense on the water-saturated T1-WI (see Fig. 4-4D and E). The presence of macroscopic fat in a renal lesion is specific for AML. The presence of fat within a renal cell carcinoma is extremely rare and secondary either to renal sinus fat invasion or to fat or cholesterol necrosis.[27]

Some AMLs contain little or no fat and thus may not be definitively characterized with MR or other imaging techniques. The renal leiomyoma, a benign neoplasm that is not uncommon in patients with tuberous sclerosis, is thought to represent an angiomyolipoma devoid of fat.[134] A renal leiomyoma–lipid poor angiomyolipoma appears as a well-circumscribed, solid, homogeneously enhancing exophytic mass. A suggestive imaging feature of some exophytic AMLs is the absence of a "claw" sign because many are choristomas that arise from the renal capsule and not the renal parenchyma.[135] In general, though, renal leiomyomas are generally considered to be indistinguishable from other solid renal neoplasms and thus may require excision.

Oncocytoma

Oncocytomas represent approximately 3% of renal neoplasms[49,136] and are considered to be indistinguishable from RCC on all imaging modalities, including MRI. Features that suggest oncocytoma include relative lesion homogeneity, well-defined lesion borders, absence of necrosis and hemorrhage, and presence of a central scar. These findings may allow the diagnosis of oncocytoma to be considered, but these findings may also be present in RCC and are therefore not diagnostic for oncocytoma.

The vast majority of oncocytomas are benign, although rare metastases have been reported.[137] On MR, they are generally isointense to hypointense to normal parenchyma on T1-WI and have variable SI on T2-WI.[138,139] Oncocytomas tend to enhance relatively homogeneously although, like many RCCs, they tend to enhance less than normal renal parenchyma. MRI is superior to CT and US in identifying the central scar of an oncocytoma,[138] but MR imaging findings are

not specific enough to provide a definitive diagnosis. Although oncocytoma may be suggested on MRI, a solid enhancing renal mass without macroscopic fat should be excised. The contribution of the MR to the management of a patient with a suspected oncocytoma may be to suggest that such a lesion may be amenable to partial nephrectomy.

Metastatic Disease of the Kidney

Renal metastases are common in patients with advanced stage malignancies. At autopsy, 5% to 15% of patients who died of malignant neoplasms of epithelial origin had renal metastases.[140,141] Many of these foci are microscopic and not detectable by MR. Renal metastases are rarely symptomatic, however, and small lesions are unlikely to produce gross hematuria, pain, or renal failure.[142] Few reports of the MRI appearance of renal metastases have been published. The most common CT appearance of metastatic disease to the kidney is that of multiple focal nodules which enhance less than the normal renal parenchyma; contain irregular, somewhat infiltrative margins; and do not respect the margins of the kidney.[142] This likely is also the most common MR appearance. However, as the cross-sectional imaging appearance of renal metastases is not pathognomonic, it can often be inferred based on the presence of a known primary and other foci of metastatic disease.

RENAL TRAUMA

CT is the imaging modality of choice for the evaluation of hematuria in the setting of acute abdominal trauma.[143] Although animal studies have shown MRI to be equal or superior to CT for the detection of renal injuries,[144] MRI's utility in the setting of trauma has been hindered by relative lack of availability at off hours, longer imaging times, and more difficult patient monitoring in the magnetic bore. At present, MRI is generally reserved for renal trauma patients who have an inconclusive CT examination or a contraindication to enhanced CT.

Both CT and MRI are capable of simultaneously evaluating renal parenchymal and renal vascular injuries (Figs. 4-17 and 4-18; see Fig. 4-8).[145] With either modality, delayed-phase images can show extravasation of excreted contrast material. MR is more accurate than CT in differentiating perirenal from intrarenal hematoma,[146] (see Fig. 4-17) as well as in depicting the extent of post-traumatic renal parenchymal injury.[147]

PYELONEPHRITIS

Most patients with suspected pyelonephritis can be diagnosed by history, physical examination, urinalysis, and, if imaging is required, CT.[148] Findings of pyelonephritis on CT include ill-defined wedge-shaped regions of decreased enhancement. On delayed-phase CT or MR, there will be a "striated nephrogram,"

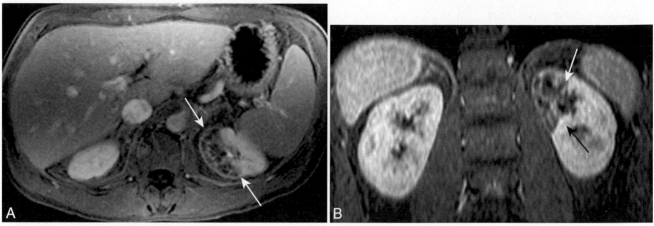

Figure 4-17 ■ **MR depiction of segmental infarction of the kidney in a man with hematuria and pain following cardiac catheterization. A** and **B,** Axial (**A**) and coronal (**B**) CE fat-saturated T1-WIs show sharp demarcation between the normal portion of the left kidney and the region of segmental infarction *(arrows).* There is preservation of capsular blood flow.

alternating linear bands of alternating attenuation or SI, respectively (Fig. 4-19).[149]

MR investigations of focal pyelonephritis in pediatric populations showed that MR has higher sensitivity and interobserver agreement than nuclear scintigraphy does.[150] Experience with MR imaging in the adult population is limited, since CT generally is preferred owing to its greater ability to demonstrate obstructing calculi or air from gas-producing organisms. Enhanced MR, however, may be useful in

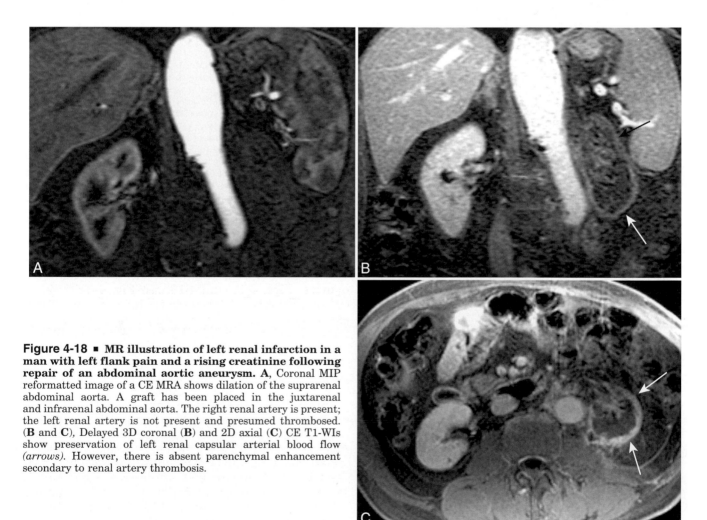

Figure 4-18 ■ **MR illustration of left renal infarction in a man with left flank pain and a rising creatinine following repair of an abdominal aortic aneurysm. A,** Coronal MIP reformatted image of a CE MRA shows dilation of the suprarenal abdominal aorta. A graft has been placed in the juxtarenal and infrarenal abdominal aorta. The right renal artery is present; the left renal artery is not present and presumed thrombosed. (**B** and **C**), Delayed 3D coronal (**B**) and 2D axial (**C**) CE T1-WIs show preservation of left renal capsular arterial blood flow *(arrows).* However, there is absent parenchymal enhancement secondary to renal artery thrombosis.

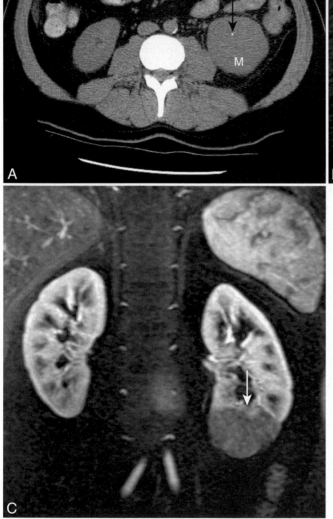

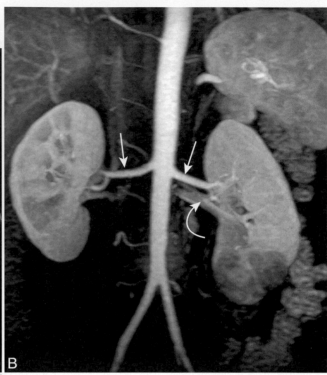

Figure 4-19 ■ MRI MRA depiction of normal renal arteries and focal pyelonephritis in a man with left flank pain, fever, and pyuria. A, Unenhanced CT shows a 1- to 2-mm calcified stone *(arrow)* and a possible mass (M) in lower pole of the left kidney. MR is insensitive and not specific for detection of small foci of calcification, and the renal stone was not identified on the subsequent MR image. B, Coronal thick section MIP CE MRA shows normal single renal arteries *(arrows)* and abdominal aorta. Early enhancement of the renal veins *(curved arrow)* does not prevent evaluation of the renal arteries for stenosis. Because this MIP image includes a large amount of renal parenchyma, the focal pyelonephritis is poorly visualized. C, Coronal arterial phase T1-WI (obtained from the source images that were used to create image B) better shows the geographic region of decreased enhancement *(arrow)* of the left lower pole.

(Continued)

patients with renal insufficiency or iodine allergy. Both CT and MRI can detect complications of pyelonephritis, including renal abscess and renal cortical scars.

MRI AND RENAL TRANSPLANTATION

Evaluation of Potential Renal Donors

Combined MRI-MRA-MRU provides a means by which to evaluate potential renal donors, as renal morphology, vasculature, and function can be evaluated in a single examination (Box 4-13).[151-153] Compared with digital subtraction angiography, MRI can result in an overall cost savings, while the potential complications of percutaneous angiography and iodinated contrast are avoided.[154] Inability to detect small renal calculi is a potential limitation of MR evaluation of renal donors, as the presence of calculi is a relative contraindication to renal donation. Unenhanced CT is superior to MR in its ability to depict small, nonobstructing renal calculi.

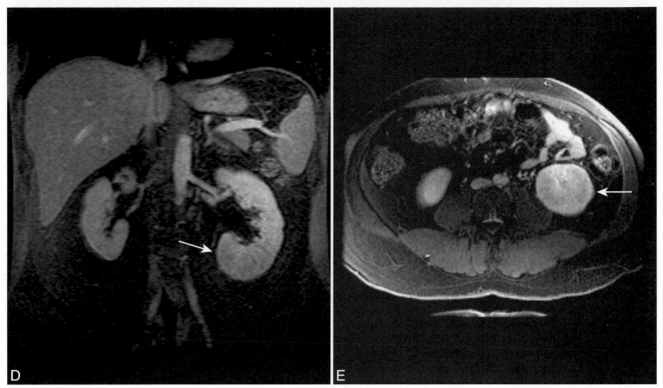

Figure 4-19 ▪ **Cont'd D** and **E**, Coronal (**D**) and axial (**E**) delayed CE T1-WI image show a striated nephrogram of pyelonephritis *(arrows)*. No abscess was revealed. The patient responded clinically to antibiotics and the appearance of the kidney improved on follow-up imaging.

Sonography has traditionally been used to screen potential living related donors for ADPCKD. Although US has a very high negative predictive value for ADPCKD in patients over age 30 years, it may not detect cysts smaller than 4 mm, which may be the only manifestation of younger individuals with ADPCKD. MR has been advocated to screen renal donors potentially affected with ADPCKD owing to the very high sensitivity of heavily T2-WIs for identifying small cysts.[100]

Both CE MRA and CT angiography (CTA) have been reported to be 100% sensitive for the detection of main renal arteries.[155,156] Accessory renal arteries are common, however, occurring in approximately 30% of kidneys,[157] and must be detected to allow successful harvest and reimplantation of all renal vessels (Figs. 4-20 and 4-21).

Earlier attempts at CE MRA were inferior to conventional angiography for detection of accessory renal arteries. However, improvements in MR gradient strengths and MRA techniques have occurred so that conventional angiography and dynamic CE MRA are comparable.[158] In addition to accessory arteries, early renal artery branching is of interest to transplant surgeons, since at least 2 cm of nonbranching renal artery is preferred to allow uncomplicated creation of the surgical anastomoses (Fig. 4-22).

CTA and CE MRA are approximately equal in their ability to demonstrate accessory renal arteries, with sensitivities of greater than 90% reported for both modalities.[155] Smaller (1 to 2 mm) accessory renal arteries are subject to higher rates of nondetection by imaging, as well as a greater likelihood of interobserver disagreement. Both CTA and CE MRA examinations of renal donors demonstrate high degrees of interobserver agreement for presence of accessory renal arteries and of early arterial bifurcations.[156]

4-13   Checklist for Renal Donor Evaluation

- Two kidneys
  Normal in size and location
  No benign or malignant renal lesions
- Renal arteries
  Single arteries bilaterally of normal caliber
  Expected origin on aorta and insertion on kidney
  No early (<2 cm) branching or polar branches
  No focal stenoses
- Left renal vein
  Not retroaortic or circumaortic
  No large draining gonadal or lumbar vein
- Ureters
  Single, without partial or complete duplication
  No obstruction

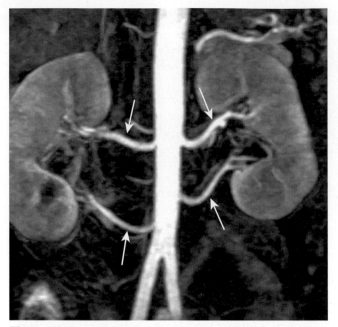

Figure 4-20 ■ **Contrast-enhanced magnetic resonance angiography (CE MRA) depiction of bilateral accessory renal arteries in a renal donor.** Coronal reformatted MIP image shows two left and two right renal arteries *(arrows)*. Inadvertent occlusion of a lower pole renal artery at the time of kidney harvest could result in ischemic necrosis of the proximal ureters or lower pole renal parenchyma.

Renal vein anatomy also is assessed in potential renal donors. Although abnormalities of the renal veins are rare in kidney donors, normal variants such as a circumaortic (0.2% to 0.3%) or retroaortic (0.5% to 3%) left renal vein may require an open surgical approach as opposed to a laparoscopic approach if the left kidney is to be harvested.[159]

Finally, renal collecting system anomalies are evaluated by MRU. Ureteral duplication can be readily identified by MR[158] and in most cases will result in the harvesting of the contralateral kidney. It is technically possible to transplant a kidney with complete ureteral duplication if there are compelling reasons to do so,[160] but in most cases the contralateral kidney will be preferred. Although MRU is capable of identifying large collecting system abnormalities, it remains inferior to conventional excretory urography in the detection of small calyceal abnormalities.[7] As such, MRU is best reserved for use in a population that is at relatively low risk for urothelial abnormalities, such as prospective renal donors.

Evaluation of Renal Transplant Complications

MRI has several advantages over other modalities in the evaluation of failing renal transplants. Anatomic, vascular, and functional data can be obtained a single examination.[161] Nuclear medicine studies and US

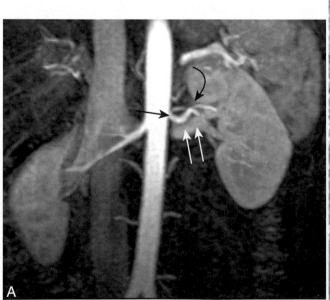

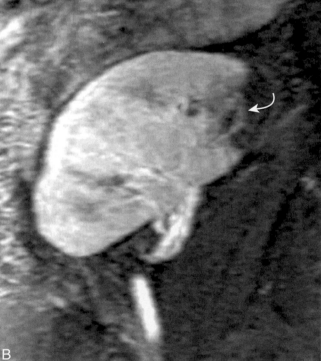

Figure 4-21 ■ **MRA depiction of a left upper pole accessory renal artery in a renal donor and subsequent segmental infarction secondary to its occlusion in the recipient. A,** Coronal MIP reformatted image of a CE MRA shows a left upper pole accessory renal artery *(curved arrow)*. The main left renal artery *(arrow)* and the vein *(double arrow)* are also depicted. **B,** Oblique sagittal MIP image from a CE MRA within the recipient shows infarction of the upper pole of the kidney *(curved arrow)* secondary to thrombosis of the accessory artery.

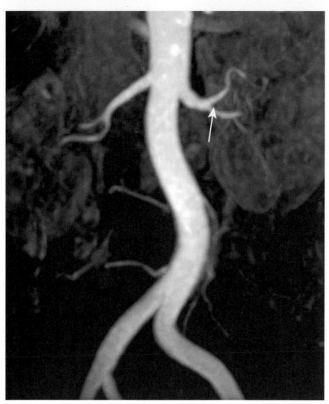

Figure 4-22 ▪ **Early branching renal artery revealed by MRA.** Coronal MIP image from a CE MRA shows early branching of the left renal artery *(arrow).*

suffer from limited spatial resolution, and CT examinations are limited by the potentially nephrotoxic iodinated contrast material. MRI can have a profound effect on the management of patients with renal transplant dysfunction (Box 4-14). In a recent

---

4-14 Complications of Renal Transplantation

Arterial in-flow stenosis
- Aortoiliac disease
- Anastomotic strictures
- Transplant artery stenosis

Renal vein thrombosis
Arteriovenous fistula
Ureteral obstruction
Peritransplant fluid collections
- Hematoma
- Urinoma
- Lymphocele

PTLD
- Benign lymphoid hyperplasia
- Malignant lymphoma

Parenchymal disease: rejection vs. acute tubular necrosis
- Difficult to establish specific MR diagnosis
- Often requires biopsy

---

study of 31 patients with transplant dysfunction, transplant physicians were asked to identify their most likely diagnosis before and after MR. MR increased physicians' diagnostic confidence, changed the most likely diagnosis in 65% of patients, and prevented invasive procedures in 39% of patients.[162]

ARTERIAL IN-FLOW STENOSIS

For pelvic renal transplants, the allograft renal artery is most commonly anastomosed to the ipsilateral external iliac artery. CE MRA can accurately evaluate the transplant renal artery, and shows high correlation with digital subtraction angiography for transplant renal artery stenosis, particularly for lesions of 50% or greater.[163,164] Approximately 2% to 10% of renal transplantations are complicated by allograft renal artery stenosis[165] (Fig. 4-23), and the differential diagnosis includes anastomotic structure due to surgical technique, intimal fibrosis secondary to rejection, vessel kinking, and external compression of the artery. Treatment of hemodynamically significant stenoses is by percutaneous angioplasty, although anastomotic stenoses may require surgical intervention.

Stenoses in the abdominal aorta, common iliac artery, or the external iliac artery can also lead to

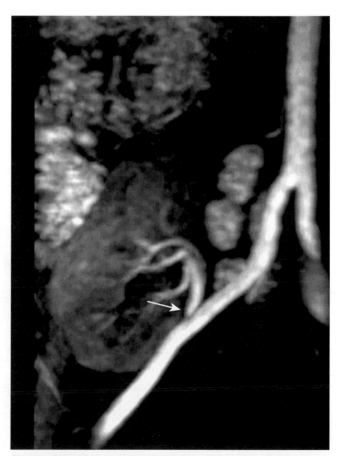

Figure 4-23 ▪ **Transplant anastomotic renal artery stenosis revealed by MRA.** Oblique sagittal MIP image from a CE MRA shows a high-grade stenosis *(arrow)* at the anastomosis of the transplanted renal artery with the native external iliac artery.

in-flow insufficiency, and the ability of CE MRA to evaluate these vessels is well established (see Chapter 11). Individuals with diabetes are particularly at risk for this complication, and usually are screened with angiography, CTA, or CE MRA prior to transplantation so that potential vascular occlusions or stenoses can be treated.

Susceptibility artifact from surgical clips is a known potential pitfall of renal transplant MRA, since the presence of a metallic clip may simulate an arterial stenosis[165] or fibromuscular dysplasia.[166] Correlation of projection MRA images with anatomic source images or radiographs should prevent this potential source of confusion.

RENAL VEIN THROMBOSIS

Thrombosis of the transplant renal vein is a rare complication of transplantation that must be promptly recognized and treated if the transplant is to remain viable. Untreated venous thrombosis will compromise arterial in-flow and lead to infarction. The diagnosis of renal transplant vein thrombosis is most commonly made on sonography,[167] but MRI can readily show this complication as well. On T2-WI, the thrombosed transplant renal vein will not show normal flow void and the transplant kidney often is enlarged.

On CE MRA, the walls of the thrombosed vein will enhance, but the luminal thrombus will not.[168]

ARTERIOVENOUS FISTULA

Arteriovenous fistula is a complication of renal transplant biopsy, but arteriovenous malformations also can be present spontaneously in native kidneys (Fig. 4-24). Both Doppler US and CE MRA[169] are useful in depicting the presence of abnormal arteriovenous communications and their relation to other vascular structures of the kidney. Arteriovenous fistulas can be treated by embolization.[170]

URETERAL ABNORMALITIES

Ureteral obstruction following transplantation is a rare complication, but one which may lead to rapid loss of transplant function. Although sonography can show the presence of hydronephrosis, MRI with MRU often can identify the cause of the obstruction. Known causes of renal transplant obstruction include anastomotic stricture of the ureter and extrinsic compression of the ureter by lymphocele.[171] It is important to differentiate between hydronephrosis due to true obstruction and pyelocaliectasis due to vesicoureteral reflux. CE MRU can often differentiate these entities through demarcating the course and

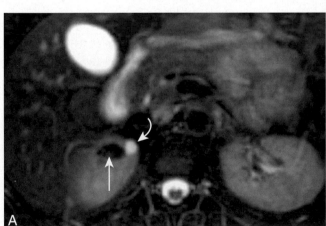
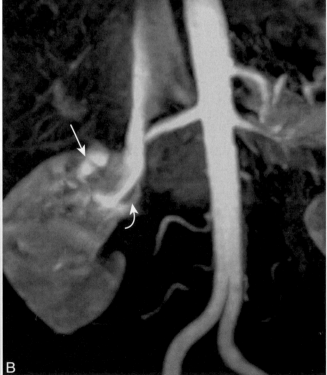

Figure 4-24 ■ **MRA depiction of a renal arteriovenous malformation.** The patient had successful embolization following MRI. **A,** Axial T2-WI shows a focal region of low SI secondary to a flow void *(arrow)*. An adjacent subcentimeter cyst is present *(curved arrow)*. **B,** Coronal MIP from an arterial-phase CE MRA shows an enhancing tubular structure *(arrow)* in the upper pole of the right kidney that corresponds to a vascular nidus. There is early filling of the right renal vein *(curved arrow)*. The vascular nidus remained enhanced on delayed imaging (not shown).

caliber of the ureter and showing the presence or absence of excreted gadolinium in the urinary bladder. Necrosis of the distal ureter can occur if the blood supply of the ureter becomes compromised, either during ureteral harvest or due to compression by the mucosal tunnel of the bladder. This complication results in urinary extravasation.

REJECTION VERSUS ACUTE TUBULAR NECROSIS

No MR findings allow for specific diagnosis of transplant rejection or acute tubular necrosis (ATN). Loss of corticomedullary differentiation on T1-WI has been reported to be a sign of transplant dysfunction, but this finding is not specific for any individual type of dysfunction (Fig. 4-25).

Serial dynamic gadolinium-enhanced images are useful in differentiating ATN from rejection[172] although MRI has not been widely adopted for this use. Normal transplants display rapid increase in SI on dynamic CE T1-WI. Postcontrast increase in cortical signal intensity has been reported to be significantly lower in cases of rejection than in normal allografts or in kidneys with ATN. Patients experiencing ATN have mildly delayed and diminished cortical enhancement relative to normal allografts.

FLUID COLLECTIONS

Lymphoceles are the most common post-transplant fluid collection and are present in up to 20% of transplanted kidneys. Lymphoceles often have internal septa and tend to be hypointense to renal cortex on T1-WI and hyperintense on T2-WI. Lymphoceles are of little clinical importance unless they cause obstruction of the ureter owing to mass effect.

Although they do not have internal septa, urinomas have similar SI to lymphoceles, and the two cannot be differentiated reliably by MR imaging unless excretion of contrast into the urinoma is identified. US-guided aspiration of the fluid is diagnostic. The presence of urinoma implies an anastomotic leak, which must be repaired surgically.

Post-transplantation Lymphoproliferative Disorder (PTLD)

Post-transplantation lymphoproliferative disorder (PTLD) is a heterogeneous group of lymphoid disorders that result from use of post-transplant immunosuppression agents such as cyclosporin. Proliferative lymphoid cell lines range from benign lymphoid hyperplasia to malignant non-Hodgkin's lymphoma. Regions involved include the central nervous system, thoracic and abdominal lymph nodes, and abdominal parenchymal organs. In renal transplantation, the hilum of the transplanted kidney is the most common site of involvement (Fig. 4-26). PTLD may encase vessels or obstruct the transplant ureter.[173,174] PTLD involving the renal transplant is isointense or hypointense to normal parenchyma on T1-WI and hypointense to normal parenchyma on T2-WI.[173]

RENAL ARTERY STENOSIS/RENOVASCULAR HYPERTENSION

Renal vascular disease accounts for 1% to 5% of cases of hypertension.[175] Atherosclerosis (Fig. 4-27) is responsible for approximately two thirds of all cases, with fibromuscular dysplasia (Fig. 4-28) accounting for most of the remaining cases (Box 4-15). Takayasu's arteritis and neurofibromatosis are less common etiologies. CE MRA is an ideal technique for imaging the renal arteries in patients with hypertension and potential renal artery stenosis (RAS).[176,177] Preliminary imaging of patients with medication-resistant hypertension and potential RAS can save more lives than immediate change to enhanced medical therapy.[178]

Compared with conventional angiography, which is the traditional gold standard diagnostic examination for suspected RAS, CE MRA is considerably less invasive and has the additional advantage of utilizing a non-nephrotoxic contrast agent that can be administered safely in patients with elevated creatinine. Compared with catheter angiography considered the gold standard, CE MRA is 88% to 100% sensitive and 83% to 98% specific in the detection of hemodynamically significant (>50% luminal diameter) renal artery stenosis.[179-181]

CTA also is an excellent examination for characterization of renal artery disease.[182] A recent meta-analysis has determined that CTA and CE MRA are comparable modalities in the evaluation of RAS and that both are superior to US and to captopril scintigraphy.[175,183] Stenting of the renal artery is effective in improving both hypertension and renal function in individuals with RAS.[184]

Known limitations of CE MRA include overestimation of the degree of stenosis in 5% to 10% of renal arteries[180] and inability to accurately evaluate a

---

4-15 Differential Diagnosis of Renal Artery Stenosis

Native renal artery
  Atherosclerosis
    Most common: two thirds of cases
    Middle aged to elderly individuals, M>F
    Ostial and proximal arterial segments
    Contrast-enhanced MRA: high diagnostic accuracy
  Fibromuscular dysplasia
    Second most common
    Younger individuals, F > M
    Middle and distal arterial segments
  Takayasu's arteritis
  Neurofibromatosis
  Transplant renal artery stenosis
    Anastomotic stricture
    Vessel kinking
    External compression
    Intimal fibrosis due to rejection

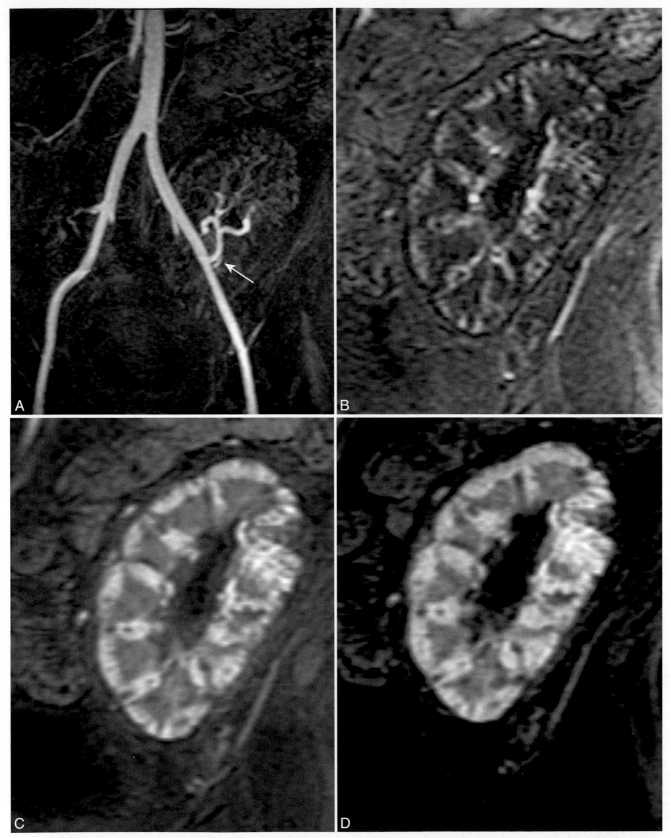

Figure 4-25 ■ **A 48-year-old transplant recipient with decreased renal function that required dialysis.** Renal biopsy confirmed the clinical diagnosis of rejection. **A,** Oblique coronal MIP reformatted image of an arterial-phase CE MRA reveals a normal transplant renal artery *(arrow)*. **B–D,** Arterial, venous, and interstitial phases from a three-phase CE MRI-MRA shows delayed enhancement of the transplant with prolonged corticomedullary differentiation. This is a nonspecific but common finding of transplant rejection.

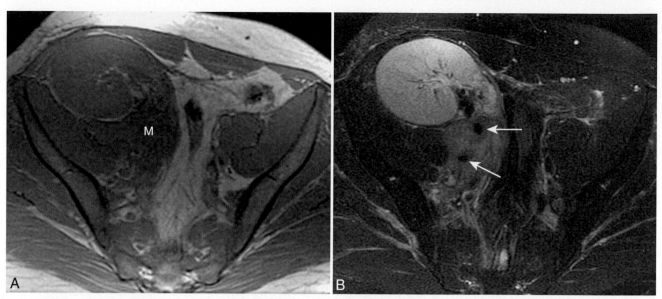

Figure 4-26 ■ **MR depiction of post-transplant lymphoproliferative disorder (PTLD) in a renal transplant recipient with rising creatinine. A** and **B**, Axial T1-WI (**A**) and T2-WI (**B**) show a soft tissue mass (M) adjacent to the hilum of the renal transplant. Flow voids in the right iliac vessels *(arrows)* are encased by this process.

vessel that has been previously stented (Fig. 4-29). Some stent devices are now available that have little if any susceptibility artifact and thus do not prohibit accurate evaluation by MR after their deployment.[185] Additionally, evaluation of small (1 to 2 mm) accessory renal arteries is limited by inadequate spatial and temporal resolution. However, the occurrence rate of

an isolated, hemodynamically significant stenosis of an accessory renal artery is less than 2%, and thus this limitation of MRA should not discourage its use for evaluating patients with suspected renovascular hypertension.[186] Because the kidneys move 2 to 3 mm/sec in a cranial-caudal dimension during a suspended respiration, techniques that shorten the acquisition time of a CE MRA sequence will improve detection of accessory renal arteries and branch vessels.[187] Finally, unlike catheter angiography, CTA and

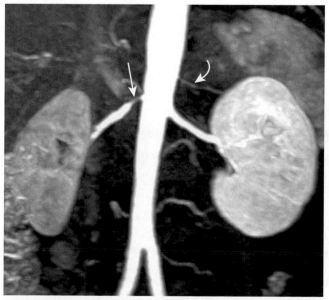

Figure 4-27 ■ **MR depiction of renal artery stenosis in a 54-year-old man with hypertension.** Coronal MIP image from a CE MRA shows high-grade ostial stenosis of the right renal artery *(arrow)*. The left renal artery reveals no stenosis. A 1.5-mm superior accessory left renal artery *(curved arrow)* directly supplies the right upper pole parenchyma.

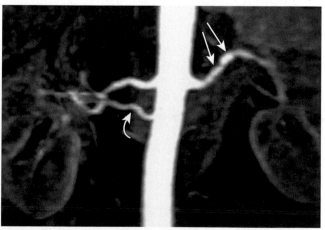

Figure 4-28 ■ **MR illustration of fibromuscular dysplasia in a 42-year-old woman.** Coronal MIP reformatted image from a CE MRA shows alternating segments of stenosis and dilation ("beading") of the left renal artery *(arrows)*, representing renal artery stenoses on the basis of fibromuscular dysplasia. Normal-appearing main and inferior accessory right renal arteries *(curved arrow)* are also present. The patient responded to angioplasty and stenting.

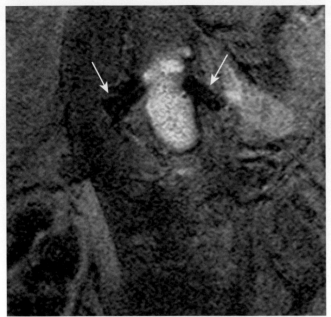

Figure 4-29 ▪ Susceptibility artifacts from bilateral renal artery stents in a patient with treated renovascular hypertension. Coronal MIP reformatted image from CE MRA shows signal voids at the ostia of the renal arteries *(arrows),* secondary to bilateral stents. Determination of patency of stented vascular segments may not be possible by CE MRA. Knowledge of prior stent placement prevents misinterpreting the artifactual signal voids as segmentally occluded vessels. Some stent models are composed of materials that minimize artifacts in such a way that MR can evaluate internal flow.

routine CE MRA are anatomic examinations; pressure gradients across stenoses cannot be measured. However, functional CE MRA could be performed by administering an angiotension-converting enzyme (ACE) inhibitor at the time of MR.[188,189] The identification of decreased medullary enhancement after ACE inhibition suggests functional renal artery obstruction.

REFERENCES

1. Keogan MT, Edelman RR. Technologic advances in abdominal MR imaging. Radiology 2001;220:310-320.
2. Israel GM, Krinsky GA. MR imaging of the kidneys and adrenal glands. Radiol Clin North Am 2003;41:145-159.
3. Rofsky NM, Lee VS, Laub G, et al. Abdominal MR imaging with a volumetric interpolated breath-hold examination. Radiology 1999;212:876-884.
4. Nolte-Ernsting CC, Staatz G, Tacke J, Gunther RW. MR urography today. Abdom Imaging 2003;28:191-209.
5. El-Diasty T, Mansour O, Farouk A. Diuretic contrast-enhanced magnetic resonance urography versus intravenous urography for depiction of nondilated urinary tracts. Abdom Imaging 2003;28:135-145.
6. Blandino A, Gaeta M, Minutoli F, et al. MR Urography of the Ureter. AJR Am J Roentgenol 2002;179:1307-1314.
7. Nolte-Ernsting CC, Adam GB, Gunther RW. MR urography: examination techniques and clinical applications. Eur Radiol 2001;11:355-372.
8. Kawashima A, Glockner JF, King BF, Jr. CT urography and MR urography. Radiol Clin North Am 2003;41:945-961.
9. Jara H, Barish MA, Yucel EK, Melhem ER, Hussain S, Ferrucci JT. MR hydrography: theory and practice of static fluid imaging. AJR Am J Roentgenol 1998;170:873-882.
10. Roy C, Saussine C, Jacqmin D. Magnetic resonance urography. BJU Int 2000;86(Suppl 1):42-47.
11. Fang YC, Siegelman ES. Complications of renal transplantation: MR findings. J Comput Assist Tomogr 2001;25:836-842.
12. Grenier N, Basseau F, Ries M, Tyndal B, Jones R, Moonen C. Functional MRI of the kidney. Abdom Imaging 2003;28:164-175.
13. Jemal A, Tiwari RC, Murray T, et al. Cancer statistics, 2004. CA Cancer J Clin 2004;54:8-29.
14. Van Poppel H, Nilsson S, Algaba F, et al. Precancerous lesions in the kidney. Scand J Urol Nephrol Suppl 2000;205:136-165.
15. Motzer RJ, Bander NH, Nanus DM. Renal-cell carcinoma. N Engl J Med 1996;335:865-875.
16. Wagner BJ. The kidney: radiologic-pathologic correlation. Magn Reson Imaging Clin N Am 1997;5:13-28.
17. Tsui KH, Shvarts O, Smith RB, Figlin R, de Kernion JB, Belldegrun A. Renal cell carcinoma: prognostic significance of incidentally detected tumors. J Urol 2000;163:426-430.
18. Bono AV, Lovisolo JA. Renal cell carcinoma—diagnosis and treatment: state of the art. Eur Urol 1997;31:47-55.
19. Jamis-Dow CA, Choyke PL, Jennings SB, Linehan WM, Thakore KN, Walther MM. Small (≤3-cm) renal masses: detection with CT versus US and pathologic correlation. Radiology 1996;198:785-788.
20. Rofsky NM, Bosniak MA. MR evaluation of small (<3.0 cm) renal masses. MR Clin North Am 1997;5:67-81.
21. Shinmoto H, Yuasa Y, Tanimoto A, et al. Small renal cell carcinoma: MRI with pathologic correlation. J Magn Reson Imaging 1998;8:690-694.
22. Yamashita Y, Miyazaki T, Hatanaka Y, Takahashi M. Dynamic MRI of small renal cell carcinoma. J Comput Assist Tomogr 1995;19:759-765.
23. Ho VB, Allen SF, Hood MN, Choyke PL. Renal masses: quantitative assessment of enhancement with dynamic MR imaging. Radiology 2002;224:695-700.
24. Yoshimitsu K, Honda H, Kuroiwa T, et al. MR detection of cytoplasmic fat in clear cell renal cell carcinoma utilizing chemical shift gradient-echo imaging. J Magn Reson Imaging 1999;9:579-585.
25. Outwater EK, Bhatia M, Siegelman ES, Burke MA, Mitchell DG. Lipid in renal clear cell carcinoma: detection on opposed-phase gradient-echo MR images [see comments]. Radiology 1997;205:103-107.
26. D'Angelo PC, Gash JR, Horn AW, Klein FA. Fat in renal cell carcinoma that lacks associated calcifications. AJR Am J Roentgenol 2002;178:931-932.
27. Lesavre A, Correas JM, Merran S, Grenier N, Vieillefond A, Helenon O. CT of papillary renal cell carcinomas with cholesterol necrosis mimicking angiomyolipomas. AJR Am J Roentgenol 2003;181:143-145.
28. Helenon O, Merran S, Paraf F, et al. Unusual fat-containing tumors of the kidney: a diagnostic dilemma. Radiographics 1997;17:129-144.
29. Shinozaki K, Yoshimitsu K, Honda H, et al. Metastatic adrenal tumor from clear-cell renal cell carcinoma: a pitfall of chemical shift MR imaging. Abdom Imaging 2001;26:439-442.
30. Muram TM, Aisen A. Fatty metastatic lesions in 2 patients with renal clear-cell carcinoma. J Comput Assist Tomogr 2003;27:869-870.
31. Yamashita Y, Honda S, Nishiharu T, Urata J, Takahashi M. Detection of pseudocapsule of renal cell carcinoma with MR imaging and CT. AJR Am J Roentgenol 1996;166:1151-1155.
32. Soyer P, Dufresne A, Klein I, Barbagelatta M, Herve JM, Scherrer A. Renal cell carcinoma of clear type: correlation of CT features with tumor size, architectural patterns, and pathologic staging. European Radiology 1997;7:224-229.
33. Brkovic D, Moehring K, Doersam J, et al. Aetiology, diagnosis and management of spontaneous perirenal haematomas. Eur Urol 1996;29:302-307.
34. Robson CJ, Churchill BM, Anderson W. The results of radical nephrectomy for renal cell carcinoma. J Urol 1969;101:297-301.
35. Ergen FB, Hussain HK, Caoili EM, et al. MRI for preoperative staging of renal cell carcinoma using the 1997 TNM classification: comparison with surgical and pathologic staging. AJR Am J Roentgenol 2004;182:217-225.
36. Reznek RH. Imaging in the staging of renal cell carcinoma. Eur Radiol 1996;6:120-128.
37. Semelka RC, Shoenut JP, Magro CM, Kroeker MA, MacMahon R, Greenberg HM. Renal cancer staging: comparison of contrast-enhanced CT and gadolinium-enhanced fat-suppressed spin-echo and gradient-echo MR imaging. J Magn Reson Imaging 1993;3:597-602.
38. Zagoria RJ, Bechtold RE. The role of imaging in staging renal adenocarcinoma. Semin Ultrasound CT MR 1997;18:91-99.
39. Ramdave S, Thomas GW, Berlangieri SU, et al. Clinical role of F-18 fluorodeoxyglucose positron emission tomography for detection and management of renal cell carcinoma. J Urol 2001;166:825-830.
40. Fielding JR, Aliabadi N, Renshaw AA, Silverman SG. Staging of 119 patients with renal cell carcinoma: the yield and cost-effectiveness of pelvic CT. AJR Am J Roentgenol 1999;172:23-25.
41. Choyke PL. Detection and staging of renal cancer. Magn Reson Imaging Clin N Am 1997;5:29-47.

42. Pretorius ES, Siegelman ES, Ramchandani P, Cangiano T, Banner MP. Renal neoplasms amenable to partial nephrectomy: MR imaging. Radiology 1999;212:28-34.
43. Choyke PL, Walther MM, Wagner JR, Rayford W, Lyne JC, Linehan WM. Renal cancer: preoperative evaluation with dual-phase three-dimensional MR angiography. Radiology 1997;205:767-771.
44. Laissy JP, Menegazzo D, Debray MP, et al. Renal carcinoma: diagnosis of venous invasion with Gd-enhanced MR venography. Eur Radiol 2000;10:1138-1143.
45. Hallscheidt P, Pomer S, Roeren T, Kauffmann GW, Staehler G. Preoperative staging of renal cell carcinoma with caval thrombus: is staging in MRI justified? [Prospective histopathological correlated study.] Urologe A 2000;39:36-40.
46. Nguyen BD, Westra WH, Zerhouni EA. Renal cell carcinoma and tumor thrombus neovascularity: MR demonstration with pathologic correlation. Abdom Imaging 1996;21:269-271.
47. Oto A, Herts BR, Remer EM, Novick AC. Inferior vena cava tumor thrombus in renal cell carcinoma: staging by MR imaging and impact on surgical treatment. AJR Am J Roentgenol 1998;171:1619-1624.
48. Aslam Sohaib SA, Teh J, Nargund VH, Lumley JS, Hendry WF, Reznek RH. Assessment of tumor invasion of the vena caval wall in renal cell carcinoma cases by magnetic resonance imaging. J Urol 2002;167:1271-1275.
49. Choyke PL, Glenn GM, Walther MM, Zbar B, Linehan WM. Hereditary renal cancers. Radiology 2003;226:33-46.
50. Levine E. Acquired cystic kidney disease. Radiol Clin North Am 1996;34:947-964.
51. Levine E. Renal cell carcinoma in uremic acquired renal cystic disease: incidence, detection, and management. Urol Radiol 1992;13:203-210.
52. Truong LD, Krishnan B, Cao JT, Barrios R, Suki WN. Renal neoplasm in acquired cystic kidney disease. Am J Kidney Dis 1995;26:1-12.
53. Mindell HJ. Imaging studies for screening native kidneys in long-term dialysis patients. AJR Am J Roentgenol 1989;153:768-769.
54. Sarasin FP, Wong JB, Levey AS, Meyer KB. Screening for acquired cystic kidney disease: a decision analytic perspective. Kidney Int 1995;48:207-219.
55. Choyke PL. Imaging of hereditary renal cancer. Radiol Clin North Am 2003;41:1037-1051.
56. Maher ER, Kaelin WG, Jr. von Hippel-Lindau disease. Medicine (Baltimore) 1997;76:381-391.
57. Taouli B, Ghouadni M, Correas JM, et al. Spectrum of abdominal imaging findings in von Hippel-Lindau disease. AJR Am J Roentgenol 2003;181:1049-1054.
58. Reichard EA, Roubidoux MA, Dunnick NR. Renal neoplasms in patients with renal cystic diseases. Abdom Imaging 1998;23:237-248.
59. Choyke PL, Glenn GM, Walther MM, Patronas NJ, Linehan WM, Zbar B. Von Hippel-Lindau disease: genetic, clinical, and imaging features. Radiology 1995;194:629-642.
60. Walther MM, Choyke PL, Glenn G, et al. Renal cancer in families with hereditary renal cancer: prospective analysis of a tumor size threshold for renal parenchymal sparing surgery. J Urol 1999;161:1475-1479.
61. Herring JC, Enquist EG, Chernoff A, Linehan WM, Choyke PL, Walther MM. Parenchymal sparing surgery in patients with hereditary renal cell carcinoma: 10-year experience. J Urol 2001;165:777-781.
62. Zbar B, Tory K, Merino M, et al. Hereditary papillary renal cell carcinoma. J Urol 1994;151:561-566.
63. Zbar B. Inherited epithelial tumors of the kidney: old and new diseases. Semin Cancer Biol 2000;10:313-318.
64. Choyke PL, Walther MM, Glenn GM, et al. Imaging features of hereditary papillary renal cancers. J Comput Assist Tomogr 1997;21:737-741.
65. Logue LG, Acker RE, Sienko AE. Best cases from the AFIP: angiomyolipomas in tuberous sclerosis. Radiographics 2003;23:241-246.
66. Torres VE, Zincke H, King BK, Bjornsson J. Renal manifestations of tuberous sclerosis complex. Contrib Nephrol 1997;122:64-75.
67. Jimenez RE, Eble JN, Reuter VE, et al. Concurrent angiomyolipoma and renal cell neoplasia: a study of 36 cases. Mod Pathol 2001;14:157-163.
68. Choyke PL. Inherited cystic diseases of the kidney. Radiol Clin North Am 1996;34:925-946.
69. Davis CJ, Jr., Mostofi FK, Sesterhenn IA. Renal medullary carcinoma: the seventh sickle cell nephropathy. Am J Surg Pathol 1995;19:1-11.
70. Swartz MA, Karth J, Schneider DT, Rodriguez R, Beckwith JB, Perlman EJ. Renal medullary carcinoma: clinical, pathologic, immunohistochemical, and genetic analysis with pathogenetic implications. Urology 2002;60:1083-1089.
71. Lau WK, Blute ML, Weaver AL, Torres VE, Zincke H. Matched comparison of radical nephrectomy vs nephron-sparing surgery in patients with unilateral renal cell carcinoma and a normal contralateral kidney. Mayo Clin Proc 2000;75:1236-1242.
72. D'Armiento M, Damiano R, Feleppa B, Perdona S, Oriani G, De Sio M. Elective conservative surgery for renal carcinoma versus radical nephrectomy: a prospective study. Br J Urol 1997;79:15-19.
73. Licht MR, Novick AC, Goormastic M. Nephron sparing surgery in incidental versus suspected renal cell carcinoma. J Urol 1994;152:39-42.
74. Ghavamian R, Zincke H. Open surgical partial nephrectomy. Semin Urol Oncol 2001;19:103-113.
75. Fergany AF, Hafez KS, Novick AC. Long-term results of nephron sparing surgery for localized renal cell carcinoma: 10-year followup. J Urol 2000;163:442-445.
76. Clark PE, Schover LR, Uzzo RG, Hafez KS, Rybicki LA, Novick AC. Quality of life and psychological adaptation after surgical treatment for localized renal cell carcinoma: impact of the amount of remaining renal tissue. Urology 2001;57:252-256.
77. Corman JM, Penson DF, Hur K, et al. Comparison of complications after radical and partial nephrectomy: results from the National Veterans Administration Surgical Quality Improvement Program. BJU Int 2000;86:782-789.
78. Russo P, Goetzl M, Simmons R, Katz J, Motzer R, Reuter V. Partial nephrectomy: the rationale for expanding the indications. Ann Surg Oncol 2002;9:680-687.
79. Kozlowski PM, Winfield HN. Laparoscopic partial nephrectomy and wedge resection for the treatment of renal malignancy. J Endourol 2001;15:369-374; discussion 375-376.
80. Gill IS, Desai MM, Kaouk JH, et al. Laparoscopic partial nephrectomy for renal tumor: duplicating open surgical techniques. J Urol 2002;167:469-467; discussion 475-476.
81. Hollenbeck BK, Wolf JS, Jr. Laparascopic partial nephrectomy. Semin Urol Oncol 2001;19:123-132.
82. Yoshimura K, Okubo K, Ichioka K, Terada N, Matsuta Y, Arai Y. Laparoscopic partial nephrectomy with a microwave tissue coagulator for small renal tumor. J Urol 2001;165:1893-1896.
83. Murphy DP, Gill IS. Energy-based renal tumor ablation: a review. Semin Urol Oncol 2001;19:133-140.
84. Gervais DA, McGovern FJ, Arellano RS, McDougal WS, Mueller PR. Renal cell carcinoma: clinical experience and technical success with radio-frequency ablation of 42 tumors. Radiology 2003;226:417-424.
85. Roy-Choudhury SH, Cast JE, Cooksey G, Puri S, Breen DJ. Early experience with percutaneous radiofrequency ablation of small solid renal masses. AJR Am J Roentgenol 2003;180:1055-1061.
86. Farrell MA, Charboneau WJ, DiMarco DS, et al. Imaging-guided radiofrequency ablation of solid renal tumors. AJR Am J Roentgenol 2003;180:1509-1513.
87. Mayo-Smith WW, Dupuy DE, Parikh PM, Pezzullo JA, Cronan JJ. Imaging-guided percutaneous radiofrequency ablation of solid renal masses: techniques and outcomes of 38 treatment sessions in 32 consecutive patients. AJR Am J Roentgenol 2003;180:1503-1508.
88. Rassweiler JJ, Abbou C, Janetschek G, Jeschke K. Laparoscopic partial nephrectomy: the European experience. Urol Clin North Am 2000;27:721-736.
89. Lewin JS, Connell CF, Duerk JL, et al. Interactive MRI-guided radiofrequency interstitial thermal ablation of abdominal tumors: clinical trial for evaluation of safety and feasibility. J Magn Reson Imaging 1998;8:40-47.
90. Blute ML, Amling CL, Bryant SC, Zincke H. Management and extended outcome of patients with synchronous bilateral solid renal neoplasms in the absence of von Hippel-Lindau disease. Mayo Clin Proc 2000;75:1020-1026.
91. Gofrit ON, Shapiro A, Kovalski N, Landau EH, Shenfeld OZ, Pode D. Renal cell carcinoma: evaluation of the 1997 TNM system and recommendations for follow-up after surgery. Eur Urol 2001;39:669-674; discussion 675.
92. Itano NB, Blute ML, Spotts B, Zincke H. Outcome of isolated renal cell carcinoma fossa recurrence after nephrectomy. J Urol 2000;164:322-325.
93. Remer EM, Weinberg EJ, Oto A, O'Malley CM, Gill IS. MR imaging of the kidneys after laparoscopic cryoablation. AJR Am J Roentgenol 2000;174:635-640.
94. Hartman DS, Davis CJ, Jr., Johns T, Goldman SM. Cystic renal cell carcinoma. Urology 1986;28:145-153.
95. Koga S, Nishikido M, Inuzuka S, et al. An evaluation of Bosniak's radiological classification of cystic renal masses. BJU Int 2000;86:607-609.
96. Balci NC, Semelka RC, Patt RH, et al. Complex renal cysts: findings on MR imaging. AJR Am J Roentgenol 1999;172:1495-1500.
97. Bosniak MA. The small (≤3.0 cm) renal parenchymal tumor: detection, diagnosis, and controversies [published erratum appears in Radiology 1991;181:189]. Radiology 1991;179:307-317.
98. Terada N, Ichioka K, Matsuta Y, Okubo K, Yoshimura K, Arai Y. The natural history of simple renal cysts. J Urol 2002;167:21-23.
99. Nascimento AB, Mitchell DG, Zhang XM, Kamishima T, Parker L, Holland GA. Rapid MR imaging detection of renal cysts: age-based standards. Radiology 2001;221:628-632.

100. Zand MS, Strang J, Dumlao M, Rubens D, Erturk E, Bronsther O. Screening a living kidney donor for polycystic kidney disease using heavily T2-weighted MRI. Am J Kidney Dis 2001;37:612-619.

101. Curry NS, Cochran ST, Bissada NK. Cystic renal masses: accurate Bosniak classification requires adequate renal CT. AJR Am J Roentgenol 2000;175:339-342.

102. Harisinghani MG, Maher MM, Gervais DA, et al. Incidence of malignancy in complex cystic renal masses (Bosniak category III): should imaging-guided biopsy precede surgery? AJR Am J Roentgenol 2003;180:755-758.

103. Corica FA, Iczkowski KA, Cheng L, et al. Cystic renal cell carcinoma is cured by resection: a study of 24 cases with long-term followup. J Urol 1999;161:408-411.

104. Israel GM, Bosniak MA. Calcification in cystic renal masses: is it important in diagnosis? Radiology 2003;226:47-52.

105. Silverman SG, Lee BY, Seltzer SE, Bloom DA, Corless CL, Adams DF. Small (≤3 cm) renal masses: correlation of spiral CT features and pathologic findings. AJR Am J Roentgenol 1994;163:597-605.

106. Maki DD, Birnbaum BA, Chakraborty DP, Jacobs JE, Carvalho BM, Herman GT. Renal cyst pseudoenhancement: beam-hardening effects on CT numbers. Radiology 1999;213:468-472.

107. Abdulla C, Kalra MK, Saini S, et al. Pseudoenhancement of simulated renal cysts in a phantom using different multidetector CT scanners. AJR Am J Roentgenol 2002;179:1473-1476.

108. Birnbaum BA, Maki DD, Chakraborty DP, Jacobs JE, Babb JS. Renal cyst pseudoenhancement: evaluation with an anthropomorphic body CT phantom. Radiology 2002;225:83-90.

109. Heneghan JP, Spielmann AL, Sheafor DH, Kliewer MA, DeLong DM, Nelson RC. Pseudoenhancement of simple renal cysts: a comparison of single and multidetector helical CT. J Comput Assist Tomogr 2002;26:90-94.

110. Madewell JE, Goldman SM, Davis CJ, Jr., Hartman DS, Feigin DS, Lichtenstein JE. Multilocular cystic nephroma: a radiographic-pathologic correlation of 58 patients. Radiology 1983;146:309-321.

111. Kettritz U, Semelka RC, Siegelman ES, Shoenut JP, Mitchell DG. Multilocular cystic nephroma: MR imaging appearance with current techniques, including gadolinium enhancement. J Magn Reson Imaging 1996;6:145-148.

112. Peters DJ, Breuning MH. Autosomal dominant polycystic kidney disease: modification of disease progression. Lancet 2001;358:1439-1444.

113. Kim SH, Moon MW, Lee HJ, Sim JS, Ahn C. Renal cyst ablation with n-butyl cyanoacrylate and iodized oil in symptomatic patients with autosomal dominant polycystic kidney disease: preliminary report. Radiology 2003;226:573-576.

114. Grantham JJ. The Jeremiah Metzger Lecture—polycystic kidney disease: old disease in a new context. Trans Am Clin Climatol Assoc 2002;113:211-224.

115. Brown JA. Images in clinical medicine: end-stage autosomal dominant polycystic kidney disease. N Engl J Med 2002;347:1504.

116. el-Diasty TA, Shokeir AA, Tawfeek HA, Mahmoud NA, Nabeeh A, Ghoneim MA. Ethanol sclerotherapy for symptomatic simple renal cysts. J Endourol 1995;9:273-276.

117. Slywotzky CM, Bosniak MA. Localized cystic disease of the kidney. AJR Am J Roentgenol 2001;176:843-849.

118. Dario Casas J, Mariscal A, Perez-Andres R. Localized renal cystic disease: imaging findings, pathologic correlation, and management approach. Comput Med Imaging Graph 2002;26:247-249.

119. Messing EM, Catalona WJ. Urothelial tumors of the urinary tract. In *Campbell's Urology*, 7th ed. Philadelphia: WB Saunders, 2000;2385-2387.

120. Jung P, Brauers A, Nolte-Ernsting CA, Jakse G, Gunther RW. Magnetic resonance urography enhanced by gadolinium and diuretics: a comparison with conventional urography in diagnosing the cause of ureteric obstruction. BJU Int 2000;86:960-965.

121. Urban BA, Buckley J, Soyer P, Scherrer A, Fishman EK. CT appearance of transitional cell carcinoma of the renal pelvis. 1. Early-stage disease. AJR Am J Roentgenol 1997;169:157-161.

122. Urban BA, Buckley J, Soyer P, Scherrer A, Fishman EK. CT appearance of transitional cell carcinoma of the renal pelvis. 2. Advanced-stage disease. AJR Am J Roentgenol 1997;169:163-168.

123. Weeks SM, Brown ED, Brown JJ, Adamis MK, Eisenberg LB, Semelka RC. Transitional cell carcinoma of the upper urinary tract: staging by MRI. Abdom Imaging 1995;20:365-367.

124. Stallone G, Infante B, Manno C, Campobasso N, Pannarale G, Schena FP. Primary renal lymphoma does exist: case report and review of the literature. J Nephrol 2000;13:367-372.

125. Urban BA, Fishman EK. Renal lymphoma: CT patterns with emphasis on helical CT. Radiographics 2000;20:197-212.

126. Sheeran SR, Sussman SK. Renal lymphoma: spectrum of CT findings and potential mimics. AJR Am J Roentgenol 1998;171:1067-1072.

127. Semelka RC, Kelekis NL, Burdeny DA, Mitchell DG, Brown JJ, Siegelman ES. Renal lymphoma: demonstration by MR imaging. AJR 1996;166:823-827.

128. Montalban C, Rodriguez-Garcia JL, Mazairas L, Ayala I, Marcos-Robles J. Magnetic resonance imaging for the assessment of residual masses after treatment of non-Hodgkin's lymphomas. Postgrad Med J 1992;68:643-647.

129. Yamakado K, Tanaka N, Nakagawa T, Kobayashi S, Yanagawa M, Takeda K. Renal Angiomyolipoma: relationships between tumor size, aneurysm formation, and rupture. Radiology 2002;225:78-82.

130. Soulen MC, Faykus MH, Jr., Shlansky-Goldberg RD, Wein AJ, Cope C. Elective embolization for prevention of hemorrhage from renal angiomyolipomas. J Vasc Interv Radiol 1994;5:587-591.

131. Dickinson M, Ruckle H, Beaghler M, Hadley HR. Renal angiomyolipoma: optimal treatment based on size and symptoms. Clin Nephrol 1998;49:281-286.

132. Kido T, Yamashita Y, Sumi S, et al. Chemical shift GRE MRI of renal angiomyolipoma. J Comput Assist Tomogr 1997;21:268-270.

133. Burdeny DA, Semelka RC, Kelekis NL, Reinhold C, Ascher SM. Small (<1.5 cm) angiomyolipomas of the kidney: characterization by the combined use of in-phase and fat-attenuated MR techniques. Magn Reson Imaging 1997;15:141-145.

134. Wagner BJ, Wong-You-Cheong JJ, Davis CJ, Jr. Adult renal hamartomas. Radiographics 1997;17:155-169.

135. Jinzaki M, Tanimoto A, Narimatsu Y, et al. Angiomyolipoma: imaging findings in lesions with minimal fat. Radiology 1997;205:497-502.

136. Kovacs G, Akhtar M, Beckwith BJ, et al. The Heidelberg classification of renal cell tumours. J Pathol 1997;183:131-133.

137. Perez-Ordonez B, Hamed G, Campbell S, et al. Renal oncocytoma: a clinicopathologic study of 70 cases. Am J Surg Pathol 1997;21:871-883.

138. De Carli P, Vidiri A, Lamanna L, Cantiani R. Renal oncocytoma: image diagnostics and therapeutic aspects. J Exp Clin Cancer Res 2000;19:287-290.

139. Harmon WJ, King BF, Lieber MM. Renal oncocytoma: magnetic resonance imaging characteristics. J Urol 1996;155:863-867.

140. Abrams HL, Spiro R, Goldstein N. Metastases in carcinoma. Cancer 1950;3:74-85.

141. Bracken RB, Chica G, Johnson DE, Luna M. Secondary renal neoplasms: an autopsy study. South Med J 1979;72:806-807.

142. Bailey JE, Roubidoux MA, Dunnick NR. Secondary renal neoplasms. Abdom Imaging 1998;23:266-274.

143. Kawashima A, Sandler CM, Corl FM, et al. Imaging of renal trauma: a comprehensive review. Radiographics 2001;21:557-574.

144. Weishaupt D, Hetzer FH, Ruehm SG, Patak MA, Schmidt M, Debatin JF. Three-dimensional contrast-enhanced MRI using an intravascular contrast agent for detection of traumatic intra-abdominal hemorrhage and abdominal parenchymal injuries: an experimental study. Eur Radiol 2000;10:1958-1964.

145. Heiss SG, Shifrin RY, Sommer FG. Contrast-enhanced three-dimensional fast spoiled gradient-echo renal MR imaging: evaluation of vascular and nonvascular disease. Radiographics 2000;20:1341-1352; discussion 1353-1354.

146. Ku JH, Jeon YS, Kim ME, Lee NK, Park YH. Is there a role for magnetic resonance imaging in renal trauma? Int J Urol 2001;8:261-267.

147. Leppaniemi A, Lamminen A, Tervahartiala P, Haapiainen R, Lehtonen T. Comparison of high-field magnetic resonance imaging with computed tomography in the evaluation of blunt renal trauma. J Trauma 1995;38:420-427.

148. Papanicolaou N, Pfister RC. Acute renal infections. Radiol Clin North Am 1996;34:965-995.

149. Kawashima A, Sandler CM, Goldman SM. Imaging in acute renal infection. BJU Int 2000;86 Suppl 1:70-79.

150. Lonergan GJ, Pennington DJ, Morrison JC, Haws RM, Grimley MS, Kao TC. Childhood pyelonephritis: comparison of gadolinium-enhanced MR imaging and renal cortical scintigraphy for diagnosis. Radiology 1998;207:377-384.

151. Israel GM, Lee VS, Edye M, et al. Comprehensive MR imaging in the preoperative evaluation of living donor candidates for laparoscopic nephrectomy: initial experience. Radiology 2002;225:427-432.

152. Hussain SM, Kock MC, JN IJ, Pattynama PM, Myriam Hunink MG, Krestin GP. MR imaging: a "one-stop shop" modality for preoperative evaluation of potential living kidney donors. Radiographics 2003;23:505-520.

153. Jha RC, Korangy SJ, Ascher SM, Takahama J, Kuo PC, Johnson LB. MR angiography and preoperative evaluation for laparoscopic donor nephrectomy. AJR Am J Roentgenol 2002;178:1489-1495.

154. Liem YS, Kock MC, Ijzermans JN, Weimar W, Visser K, Hunink MG. Living renal donors: optimizing the imaging strategy—decision- and cost-effectiveness analysis. Radiology 2003;226:53-62.

155. Rankin SC, Jan W, Koffman CG. Noninvasive imaging of living related kidney donors: evaluation with CT angiography and gadolinium-enhanced MR angiography. AJR Am J Roentgenol 2001;177:349-355.

156. Halpern EJ, Mitchell DG, Wechsler RJ, Outwater EK, Moritz MJ, Wilson GA. Preoperative evaluation of living renal donors: comparison of CT angiography and MR angiography. Radiology 2000;216:434-439.

157. Nelson HA, Gilfeather M, Holman JM, Nelson EW, Yoon HC. Gadolinium-enhanced breathhold three-dimensional time-of-flight renal MR angiography in the evaluation of potential renal donors. J Vasc Interv Radiol 1999;10:175-181.

158. Low RN, Martinez AG, Steinberg SM, et al. Potential renal transplant donors: evaluation with gadolinium-enhanced MR angiography and MR urography. Radiology 1998;207:165-172.

159. Satyapal KS, Kalideen JM, Haffejee AA, Singh B, Robbs JV. Left renal vein variations. Surg Radiol Anat 1999;21:77-81.

160. Nakatani T, Uchida J, Kim T, Yamamoto K, Kishomoto T. Modified extravesical ureterocystoneostomy of the kidney transplant allograft with completely duplicated ureters. Int J Urol 2000;7:313-315.

161. Verswijvel GA, Oyen RH, Van Poppel HP, et al. Magnetic resonance imaging in the assessment of urologic disease: an all-in-one approach. Eur Radiol 2000;10:1614-1619.

162. Omary RA, Baden JG, Becker BN, Odorico JS, Grist TM. Impact of MR angiography on the diagnosis and management of renal transplant dysfunction. J Vasc Interv Radiol 2000;11:991-996.

163. Chan YL, Leung CB, Yu SC, Yeung DK, Li PK. Comparison of non-breath-hold high resolution gadolinium-enhanced MRA with digital subtraction angiography in the evaluation on allograft renal artery stenosis. Clin Radiol 2001;56:127-132.

164. Ferreiros J, Mendez R, Jorquera M, et al. Using gadolinium-enhanced three-dimensional MR angiography to assess arterial inflow stenosis after kidney transplantation. AJR. Am J Roentgenol 1999;172: 751-757.

165. Neimatallah MA, Dong Q, Schoenberg SO, Cho KJ, Prince MR. Magnetic resonance imaging in renal transplantation. J Magn Reson Imaging 1999;10:357-368.

166. Verswijvel G, Van Hoe L, Stockx L, Oyen R. Magnetic susceptibility artifacts by titanium surgical clips mimicking fibromuscular dysplasia of the renal artery in a kidney transplant. Eur Radiol 2000;10:543.

167. Mochtar H, Anis AM, Ben Moualhi S, Mohammed C, Ben Abdallah T, Ayed M. [Thrombosis of the renal transplant vein.] Ann Urol (Paris) 2001;35:10-12.

168. Froehlich JB, Prince MR, Greenfield LJ, Downing LJ, Shah NL, Wakefield TW. "Bull's-eye" sign on gadolinium-enhanced magnetic resonance venography determines thrombus presence and age: a preliminary study. J Vasc Surg 1997;26:809-816.

169. Bagga H, Bis KG. Contrast-enhanced MR angiography in the assessment of arteriovenous fistula after renal transplant biopsy. AJR Am J Roentgenol 1999;172:1509-1511.

170. Kitajima K, Fuchinoue S, Koyama I, et al. Embolization for a rteriovenous fistula after graft biopsy in renal transplant recipients: is it essential for all cases? Transplant Proc 2000;32:1911.

171. Schubert RA, Gockeritz S, Mentzel HJ, Rzanny R, Schubert J, Kaiser WA. Imaging in ureteral complications of renal transplantation: value of static fluid MR urography. Eur Radiol 2000;10:1152-1157.

172. Szolar DH, Preidler K, Ebner F, et al. Functional magnetic resonance imaging of human renal allografts during the posttransplant period: preliminary observations. Magn Reson Imaging 1997;15:727-735.

173. Ali MG, Coakley FV, Hricak H, Bretan PN. Complex post-transplantation abnormalities of renal allografts: evaluation with MR imaging. Radiology 1999;211:95-100.

174. Lopez-Ben R, Smith JK, Kew CE, 2nd, Kenney PJ, Julian BA, Robbin ML. Focal posttransplantation lymphoproliferative disorder at the renal allograft hilum. AJR Am J Roentgenol 2000;175:1417-1422.

175. Vasbinder GB, Nelemans PJ, Kessels AG, Kroon AA, de Leeuw PW, van Engelshoven JM. Diagnostic tests for renal artery stenosis in patients suspected of having renovascular hypertension: a meta-analysis. Ann Intern Med 2001;135:401-411.

176. Dong Q, Schoenberg SO, Carlos RC, et al. Diagnosis of renal vascular disease with MR angiography. Radiographics 1999;19:1535-1554.

177. Fain SB, King BF, Breen JF, Kruger DG, Riederer SJ. High-spatial-resolution contrast-enhanced MR angiography of the renal arteries: a prospective comparison with digital subtraction angiography. Radiology 2001;218:481-490.

178. Carlos RC, Kim HM, Hussain HK, Francis IR, Nghiem HV, Fendrick AM. Developing a prediction rule to assess hepatic malignancy in patients with cirrhosis. AJR Am J Roentgenol 2003;180:893-900.

179. Volk M, Strotzer M, Lenhart M, et al. Time-resolved contrast-enhanced MR angiography of renal artery stenosis: diagnostic accuracy and interobserver variability. AJR Am J Roentgenol 2000;174:1583-1588.

180. Korst MB, Joosten FB, Postma CT, Jager GJ, Krabbe JK, Barentsz JO. Accuracy of normal-dose contrast-enhanced MR angiography in assessing renal artery stenosis and accessory renal arteries. AJR Am J Roentgenol 2000;174:629-634.

181. De Cobelli F, Venturini M, Vanzulli A, et al. Renal arterial stenosis: prospective comparison of color Doppler US and breath-hold, three-dimensional, dynamic, gadolinium-enhanced MR angiography. Radiology 2000;214:373-380.

182. Urban BA, Ratner LE, Fishman EK. Three-dimensional volume-rendered CT angiography of the renal arteries and veins: normal anatomy, variants, and clinical applications. Radiographics 2001;21:373-386; questionnaire 549-555.

183. Qanadli SD, Soulez G, Therasse E, et al. Detection of renal artery stenosis: prospective comparison of captopril-enhanced Doppler sonography, captopril-enhanced scintigraphy, and MR angiography. AJR Am J Roentgenol 2001;177:1123-1129.

184. Gill KS, Fowler RC. Atherosclerotic renal arterial stenosis: clinical outcomes of stent placement for hypertension and renal failure. Radiology 2003;226:821-826.

185. Buecker A, Spuentrup E, Ruebben A, Gunther RW. Artifact-free in-stent lumen visualization by standard magnetic resonance angiography using a new metallic magnetic resonance imaging stent. Circulation 2002;105:1772-1775.

186. Bude RO, Forauer AR, Caoili EM, Nghiem HV. Is it necessary to study accessory arteries when screening the renal arteries for renovascular hypertension? Radiology 2003;226:411-416.

187. Vasbinder GB, Maki JH, Nijenhuis RJ, et al. Motion of the distal renal artery during three-dimensional contrast-enhanced breath-hold MRA. J Magn Reson Imaging 2002;16:685-696.

188. Huang AJ, Lee VS, Rusinek H. MR imaging of renal function. Radiol Clin North Am 2003;41:1001-1017.

189. Prasad PV, Goldfarb J, Sundaram C, Priatna A, Li W, Edelman RR. Captopril MR renography in a swine model: toward a comprehensive evaluation of renal arterial stenosis. Radiology 2000;217:813-818.

5

MRI of the Spleen

Laura Carucci, MD

Evan S. Siegelman, MD

NORMAL MR APPEARANCE OF THE SPLEEN

The spleen is an intraperitoneal, left upper quadrant organ that has lower signal intensity (SI) than liver on T1-WI and higher SI than liver on T2-WI (Fig. 5-1 and Box 5-1).[1,2] The spleen is composed of two tissue types, termed white pulp and red pulp, that are indistinguishable on unenhanced MR imaging. The white pulp represents lymphatic reticuloendothelial cells and lymphoid follicles. The vascular red pulp is composed of two distinct circulatory systems. The open circulation of the spleen contains a filtration system through which abnormal and aged erythrocytes, granulocytes, and platelets are cleared from the bloodstream. This is a relatively slow flow compartment. The closed, or direct, circulation supplies the splenic parenchyma that is exposed to more rapid blood flow.

In the neonate, the normal spleen appears hypointense on T2-WI and isointense to slightly hypointense on T1-WI relative to the liver. The neonatal spleen is composed primarily of red pulp with sparse lymphoid follicles. Blood within engorged sinusoids results in the low T2 SI. As the lymphoid tissue expands and matures, the amount of white pulp gradually increases, along with a decrease in the total area of red pulp. There is a corresponding increase in T2 SI and decrease in T1 SI until 8 months of age, when the adult pattern is present.[3] Therefore, before the lymphatic system fully matures, low T2 SI within the neonatal spleen should not be considered abnormal.

Many malignant disease processes parallel the normal SI of the spleen and are hypointense on T1 and hyperintense on T2-WI relative to the liver. The T1 and T2 relaxation times of normal splenic tissue and tumor vary by only 9% and 11%, respectively.[1] Because of the similar relaxation times of normal spleen and tumor, focal splenic lesions may not be readily detected by unenhanced MR.[4,5] Since lymphatic tissue and malignancy can have similar MR characteristics, the SI of lymph nodes cannot be used reliably to determine whether a lymph node is benign or malignant. The unenhanced spleen also lacks visible internal structure, and splenic size and contour may vary considerably, making detection of focal lesions even more difficult. Occasionally, malignant lesions may be detected owing to SI changes from tumor necrosis with cystic change or to paramagnetic effects of intratumoral hemorrhage or melanin (see Fig. 5-1). However, without the benefit of contrast enhancement, some lesions may not be detected.

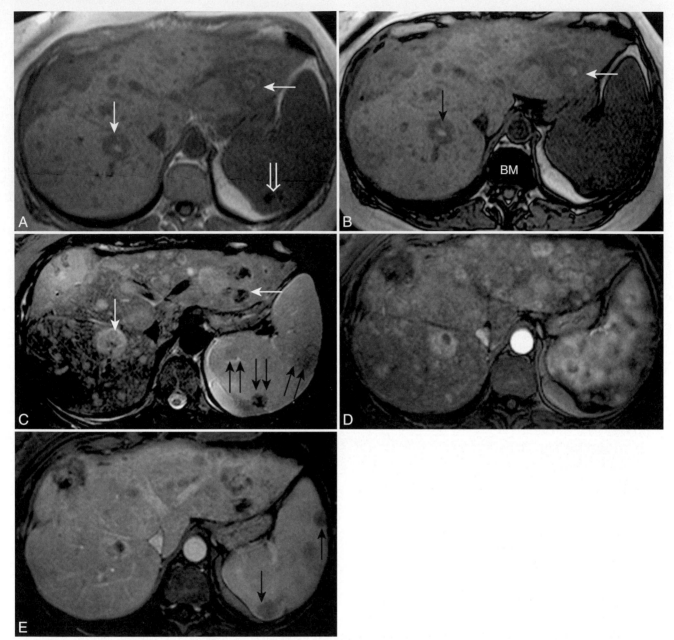

Figure 5-1 ▪ MR illustration of metastatic melanoma to the spleen and liver. A and **B,** Axial in-phase (**A**) and opposed-phase (**B**) T1-WIs show multiple liver lesions that are isointense to spleen. There are two liver lesions *(arrows)* with central high SI. This does not represent fat because no "etching artifact" is present at the periphery on the opposed-phase image to indicate a fat-water interface. One splenic lesion is suggested because of a contour abnormality and the presence of lower SI on the in-phase image *(open arrow),* suggesting chronic hemorrhage. The lumbar bone marrow (BM) loses SI in **B** because of the presence of both lipid and water within normal marrow elements. **C,** Axial T2-WI shows innumerable hepatic metastases that are isointense to spleen. The hyperintense T1 liver lesion shows low T2 SI *(arrows),* indicating the presence of intracellular methemoglobin. Subtle splenic lesions are present *(double arrows).* It may be difficult to depict metastatic disease to the spleen on unenhanced MR because the T1 and T2 of metastatic disease and of normal splenic parenchyma are similar. **D,** Arterial-phase CE T1-WI shows multiple hypervascular liver metastases and a normal arciform enhancement pattern of the spleen. **E,** Delayed CE T1-WI better reveals multiple splenic metastases *(arrows).*

Contrast-enhanced (CE) MR increases the conspicuity of splenic disease. Because the spleen is a vascular organ, it enhances intensely, with the peak at 45 seconds.[6] During the arterial phase of contrast enhancement, the spleen appears as alternating, wavy bands of high and low SI, which has been termed the arciform enhancement pattern (Fig. 5-2; see Figs. 1-17 and 1-27).[6-8] In patients with normal circulation times, arciform enhancement is present within 1 minute following contrast injection and is thought to be due to variable rates of flow within the two compartments of the red pulp.[9,10] Variation from

5-1 Normal MR Appearance of the Spleen

- T1-WI: Hypointense to liver, hyperintense to fluid
- T2-WI: Hyperintense to liver, hypointense to fluid
- Malignant tissue and normal spleen: Similar SI on T1 and T2
- Dynamic contrast: Heterogeneous/arciform pattern

this pattern is suggestive of diffuse splenic disease. CE MR increases the conspicuity of focal lesions that have differential enhancement relative to normal splenic parenchyma. After 1 minute, the distribution of contrast within the spleen rapidly equilibrates, and there is homogenous, intense enhancement (see Fig. 5-1E).[6-8]

SPLENOMEGALY

The normal spleen has a craniocaudal dimension of less than 13 cm.[11] However, as the spleen is often obliquely oriented and variable in shape, splenic volume is a more accurate measure of determining the presence and degree of splenomegaly. Adding the calculated splenic areas from each MR image and multiplying by the slice thickness can determine splenic volume. Alternatively, a splenic volume can be estimated by utilizing a formula for a prolate ellipse that incorporates measurements of the craniocaudal, anteroposterior, and transverse dimensions of the spleen.[12] Mean splenic volume in adults is approximately 215 cm.[13] Confirming the presence and determining the etiology of suspected splenomegaly is a common indication for cross-sectional imaging.

Although the causes of splenomegaly are numerous, the most common in North America and Europe is portal hypertension (see Figs. 1-22, 1-27, and 2-32).[10]

Enlargement of the spleen may be due to passive congestion, hematologic disorders, infection, inflammatory conditions, storage disorders, neoplasm, or trauma.[2,11,14] MR not only can evaluate the spleen but may reveal associated findings such as adenopathy, hepatic abnormalities, bone marrow infiltration, abdominal varices, or splenic vein occlusion, which can suggest the cause of the enlarged spleen. MR may also identify complications of splenomegaly including splenic infarction, hemorrhage, and rupture.

SPLENIC IRON DISPOSITION

MR can sensitively detect the susceptibility effects of iron deposition within the spleen. Diffuse iron deposition within the spleen is most often encountered in patients who have received blood transfusions. Focal iron deposition within the spleen can be revealed within iron-containing intraparenchymal hemorrhages (Gamna-Gandy bodies) in the setting of portal hypertension. Although genetic hemochromatosis is a condition of iron overload, the spleen is usually spared.

Hemosiderosis

Hemosiderosis is characterized by excess iron deposition within the reticuloendothelial cells of the liver, spleen, and bone marrow. Hemosiderosis is most commonly occurs secondary to blood transfusions. Hepatic and splenic iron overload from blood transfusions causes T2 shortening and results in diffusely decreased SI on T2- and T2*-W sequences (Figs. 5-3 and 5-4; see Figs. 1-11 and 1-23).[15] Splenic function is

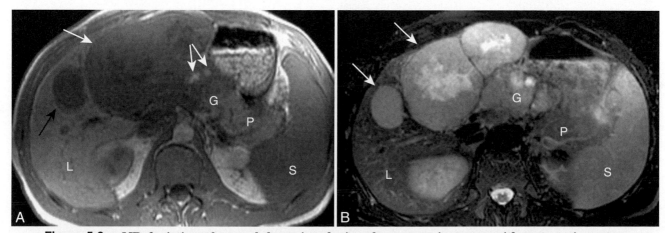

Figure 5-2 ▪ MR depiction of normal dynamic splenic enhancement in a man with metastatic gastrointestinal stromal tumor (GIST) of the stomach. A and **B,** Axial T1-WI (**A**) and T2-WI (**B**) show the primary GIST of the lesser curve of the stomach (G) and multiple liver lesions *(arrows)* that are isointense to spleen (S). Normal high T1, low T2 SI liver (L) and pancreas (P) are present. Focal increased T1 SI within the GIST *(small arrows)* reflects intratumoral hemorrhage.
(Continued)

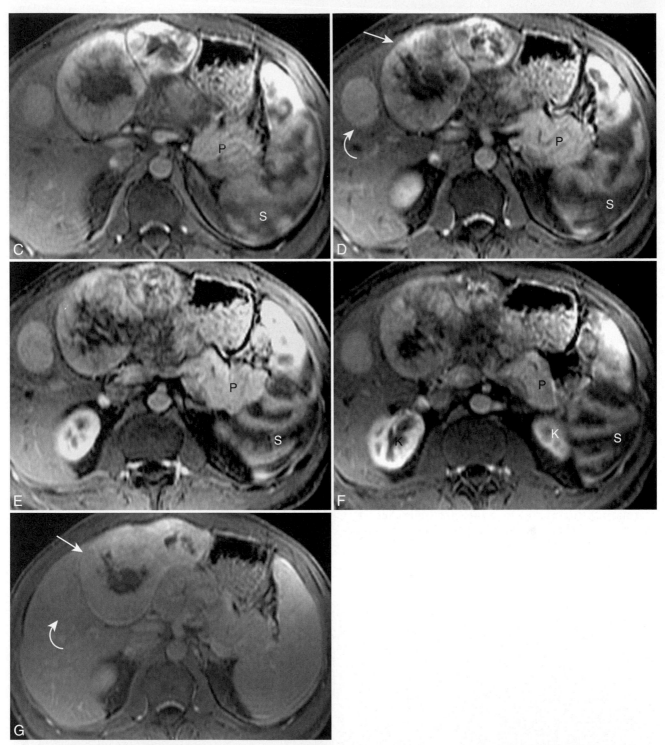

Figure 5-2 ▪ Cont'd C–F, Four consecutive dynamic CE T1-WIs show homogeneous enhancement of the small right lobe metastasis *(curved arrow)* and continuous rim enhancement of the left lobe metastasis *(arrow)*. Note the normal homogeneous pancreatic enhancement (P), heterogeneous arciform splenic enhancement (S), and corticomedullary differentiation of the kidneys (K). These are the organ enhancement features of an optimized arterial-phase CE sequence. **G,** Delayed CE T1-WI shows washout of the right lobe metastasis *(arrow)* and of the peripheral components of the dominant left lobe metastasis *(curved arrow)*. The right kidney, pancreas, and spleen are of homogenous high SI. An exophytic, necrotic, infiltrative mass lesion of the stomach is typical of GIST.[92,93] Accurate histologic diagnosis is important because patients with advanced GIST often respond to imatinib mesylate therapy.[94]

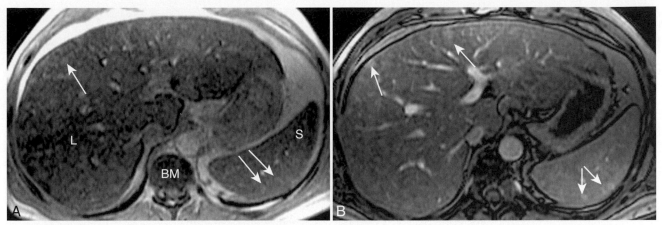

Figure 5-3 ■ **MR findings of hepatic and splenic tuberculosis and iron overload in a 46-year-old immuno-compromised man with treated leukemia. A**, In-phase T1-WI shows low SI of liver (L), spleen (S), and bone marrow (BM) secondary to iron deposition from prior transfusions. Multiple, subtle, hyperintense liver and splenic lesions are present *(arrow)*. **B**, Delayed CE T1-WI shows ill-defined enhancement of the lesions *(arrows)*. Noncaseating granulomas were revealed on liver biopsy, and acid-fast organisms were present in pulmonary lymph nodes. In this patient, the MR findings were not pathognomonic for tuberculosis. Treated leukemia or other types of infection could have a similar MR appearance.

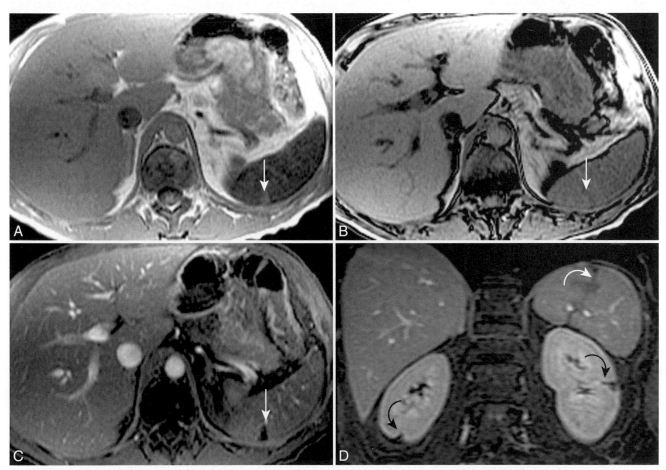

Figure 5-4 ■ **MR findings of splenic iron deposition from blood transfusions and both splenic and renal infarcts secondary to emboli in an immunosuppressed man with treated leukemia. A** and **B**, Axial in-phase (**A**) and opposed-phase (**B**) T1-WIs show a wedge-shaped region of abnormal SI involving the subcapsular portion of the spleen *(arrow)*. The spleen loses SI as the TE is increased from 2.3 in **A** to 4.6 in **B** because of prior iron deposition from transfusions. It is not uncommon to see greater T2* shortening effects in the spleen compared with the liver in patients who have received transfusions. The wedge-shaped infarct has high SI relative to surrounding spleen in **A** as it has been excluded from iron deposition because of its lack of splenic arterial supply. **C** and **D**, Axial (**C**) and coronal (**D**) fat-suppressed CE T1-WIs show no enhancement within the infarct *(arrow)* but normal enhancement of the remainder of the liver and spleen. Additional splenic and renal infarcts are revealed in **D** *(curved arrows)*.

not affected by the iron deposition of transfused blood. Focal splenic lesions are often more conspicuous in the setting of iron deposition and appear hyperintense on T2-WI relative to surrounding splenic tissue.

Genetic Hemochromatosis

Primary, or genetic, hemochromatosis (GH) is an autosomal recessive condition characterized by excess absorption of iron by the gut. Iron is deposited initially in the liver and subsequently in the pancreas, myocardium, and other organs. The cells within the reticuloendothelial system of patients with GH are dysfunctional and do not store excess iron. Thus, on T2- and T2*-WIs in patients with GH, the spleen is spared from the iron overload that is often present within the liver and other parenchymal organs (see Figs. 1-21 and 1-22).[16] MR imaging can, therefore, distinguish between GH and iron overload secondary to blood transfusions by revealing the distribution of tissue iron within the abdominal organs. A more complete discussion of GH is provided in Chapter 1.

Gamna-Gandy Bodies

Portal hypertension results in passive congestion of the spleen with enlargement of the splenic vein, perisplenic collateral vessels, and the development of small, multifocal, intrasplenic hemorrhages.[17] These subcentimeter foci of intrasplenic hemorrhage are known as Gamna-Gandy bodies (Box 5-2) and are composed of a combination of hemosiderin, fibrous tissue, and calcium.[17,18] Gamna-Gandy bodies appear as multiple subcentimeter foci of low SI especially on T2- and T2*-WIs due to "blooming" from susceptibility effects of the intralesional ferritin (Fig. 5-5; see Figs. 1-22 and 1-28). Gamna-Gandy bodies are revealed with MR in 10% to 15% of patients with portal hypertension.[17] Gamna-Gandy bodies are very suggestive but not 100% specific for portal hypertension, since they rarely may be present in other conditions such as hemolytic anemia and leukemia.[18]

Superparamagnetic Iron Oxide Contrast Agents

The reticuloendothelial cells of the spleen and the hepatic Kupffer cells phagocytose the superparamagnetic iron oxide (SPIO) contrast. "Enhancement" by iron contrast results in decreased SI of normal spleen and Kupffer cell–containing liver owing to T2 shortening, which is most pronounced on T2- and T2*-WI.[19] Malignant cells do not phagocytose SPIO contrast, and thus there is no change in SI of splenic or hepatic malignancies after contrast administration. SPIO contrast improves splenic lesion detection and conspicuity in comparison with precontrast imaging alone by 53% and 73%, respectively.[20]

5-2 Multiple Splenic Lesions: the "Spotted Spleen"[95]

Gamna-Gandy Bodies

Small, <1 cm intraparenchymal foci of hemorrhagic ischemia
Very low SI on heavily T2*-WI
Splenomegaly and other findings of portal hypertension

Lymphoma

Large, variable-sized nodules
Splenomegaly, malignant adenopathy
Subtle on T2-WI, hypoenhancing after contrast

Abscess (see Box 5-6)

Immunosuppressed patient
Smaller, more uniform nodules
High SI on T2-WI with rim enhancement
Similar-appearing liver lesions

Sarcoidosis

Spleen involved in 50% by histologic studies, <50% by imaging
Splenic lesions revealed 2–3 times as often as liver lesions
Intermediate size
Clinical history and chest radiography often confirmatory

Gaucher's Disease

Metabolic disease secondary to glucocerebrosidase deficiency
Hepatosplenomegaly, splenic lesions in 25%, intermediate in size
Abnormal bone marrow

Metastatic Disease

Spleen less common site for metastatic disease
Patient usually has known primary and other sites of metastatic disease

Hemangioma (see Box 5-5)/Lymphangioma

Patient asymptomatic, liver normal
Very high SI on T2-WI, no perilesional edema
Lymphangiomas show no enhancement or septal enhancement
Hemangiomas show delayed homogenous enhancement

CONGENITAL ABNORMALITIES OF THE SPLEEN

Polysplenia/Asplenia (Box 5-3)

Polysplenia is a rare congenital anomaly in which there are multiple (2 to 15), aberrant nodules of splenic tissue within the right or left upper quadrant of the abdomen (Fig. 5-6). Malformation within other organ systems is common and may include left isomerism, bilateral hyparterial bronchi, anomalous position of abdominal viscera with a midline liver, a hypoplastic pancreatic body and tail, abnormal bowel

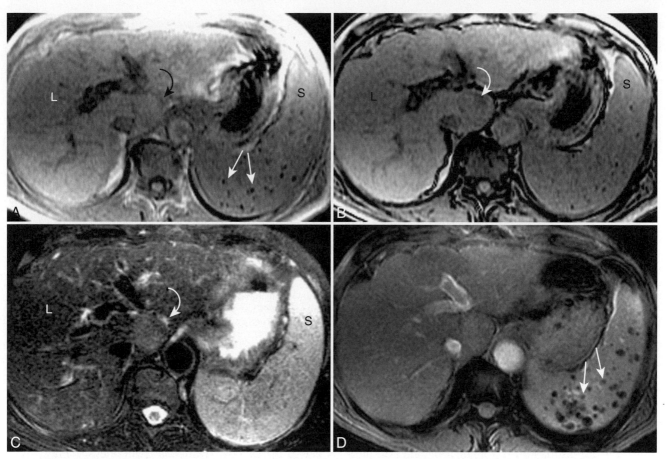

Figure 5-5 ■ **MR illustration of Gamna-Gandy bodies and a well-differentiated hepatocellular carcinoma in a 58-year-old man with hepatitis C. A** and **B,** In-phase (**A**) and opposed-phase (**B**) T1-WIs show normal SI liver (L) and spleen (S). There are multiple hypointense splenic foci that appear more distinct on the longer TE image *(arrows).* There is also a subtle encapsulated mass of the caudate lobe *(curved arrow)* that focally loses SI on the opposed-phase image. **C,** Fat-suppressed T2-WI shows normal low-to-intermediate SI liver (L) and intermediate-to-high SI spleen (S). The splenic nodules are not detectable. The hepatic mass *(curved arrow)* has SI approaching that of the spleen. Focal liver lesions within a cirrhotic liver that are isointense to spleen on T2-WIs are very suspicious for hepatocellular carcinoma, which was proved at subsequent liver transplantation. **D,** Heavily T2*-W GRE image (TE = 20, FA = 20°) shows marked "blooming" of the Gamna-Gandy bodies *(arrows).*

rotation, interruption of the inferior vena cava (IVC) with azygous continuation, and cardiac anomalies.[21]

Asplenia is characterized by congenital absence of the spleen, midline liver, right isomerism, bilateral eparterial bronchi, situs and rotational anomalies, and more severe cardiac anomalies than in polysplenia.[22] Thus, MR imaging for congenital heart disease should evaluate for the presence of either asplenia or polysplenia. Multiple spleens, a "short" pancreas, and azygous continuation can all be associated with polysplenia and should not be characterized as other pathologic conditions.[23]

Accessory Spleens

Accessory spleens, or splenuli, are present in up to 30% of individuals.[24] Splenuli are congenital, spherical masses that vary in size between 1 mm and 3 cm and are composed of tissue that is identical to normal

5-3	Congenital Cardiosplenic Syndromes	
	Polysplenia	*Asplenia*
Gender	M > F	F > M
Spleen	2 to 15 splenic nodules	Absent spleen
Liver	Midline	Midline
Gallbladder	Absent	Present
Situs	Ambiguous	Ambiguous
IVC	Interrupted with azygous continuation	Same side as aorta
Congenital heart disease	Less severe	More severe
Lungs/bronchi	Left, hyparterial	Right, eparterial

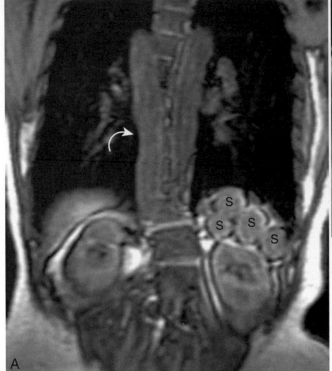

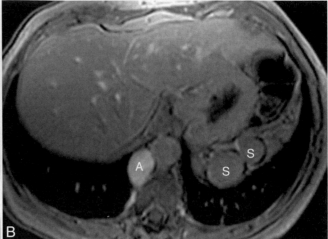

Figure 5-6 ▪ **MR findings of polysplenia in an asymptomatic 43-year-old woman. A,** Large field of view coronal T1-WI shows multiple well-circumscribed left upper quadrant soft tissue masses (S) that represent the patient's multiple spleens. The tubular structure that parallels the descending aorta is a dilated azygous vein *(curved arrow)*. **B,** Bottom image of a similar T1-W sequence shows two of the spherical spleens (S). The hyperintense azygous vein (A) is secondary to flow-related enhancement. No intrahepatic inferior vena cava is present because the patient has azygous continuation.

splenic parenchyma.[10] Splenuli are located within the embryonic dorsal mesentery of the stomach and pancreas, usually within the splenic hilum. Up to one fifth are present in or near the pancreatic tail.[24] The only clinical importance of splenuli occurs when unnecessary evaluations are performed because a splenulus is mischaracterized as a left adrenal mass, adenopathy, or a pancreatic tail mass. Splenuli appear similar to normal splenic parenchyma on T1- and T2-WIs. A specific diagnosis can be established with the use of nuclear scintigraphy. An SPIO-enhanced MR examination can confirm that an indeterminate abdominal mass is composed of functioning splenic tissue.[20]

BENIGN SPLENIC MASSES

Cyst

Splenic cysts (Box 5-4) are uncommon and are often revealed incidentally on MR and other imaging examinations.[25] There are four types of splenic cysts: congenital epidermoid cysts, post-traumatic pseudocysts, hydatid cysts due to *Echinococcus granulosus* infection, and intrasplenic pancreatic pseudocysts.[26] Most acquired splenic cysts in the U. S. (approximately 80%) are post-traumatic in etiology and likely are the sequela of an intrasplenic hematoma.[27,28] Post-traumatic splenic cysts are false cysts (pseudocysts) because they lack an endothelial lining. Epidermoid cysts (also known as mesothelial or true cysts) are congenital and constitute approximately 10% to 20% of nonparasitic splenic cysts.[10,28] It has been

suggested that lesions that have previously been classified as post-traumatic pseudocysts may represent epidermoid cysts with a denuded epithelial lining. A trabeculated appearance of the inner cyst wall at gross inspection is characteristic.[29]

5-4   Splenic Cysts

Clinical: Uncommon, most incidental
Secondary false cysts (pseudocysts)
    Secondary to prior trauma, infection, or infarct
    Intrasplenic pseudocyst: detect other findings
      of pancreatitis

Hydatid cysts
    Spleen involved in 2% of infected individuals
    Most common cause of splenic cyst worldwide;
      correlate with travel history
        Imaging clues
            Daughter cysts of spleen
            Hepatic cysts

Developmental epithelial cysts
    Develop from invagination of mesothelium into
      the spleen.
    Many may have been misdiagnosed as post-traumatic
      pseudocysts in older literature as the epithelial
      lining may not be entirely present
        MR Findings: characteristics of fluid
            Variable T1 SI—dependent on the presence
              of intracystic hemorrhage
        High T2 SI
        No enhancement

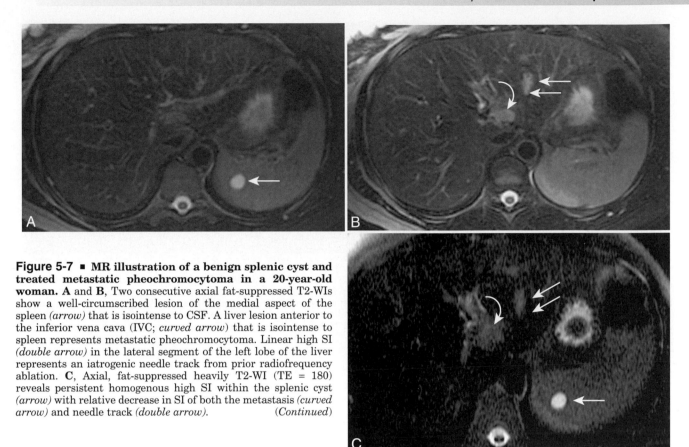

Figure 5-7 ▪ **MR illustration of a benign splenic cyst and treated metastatic pheochromocytoma in a 20-year-old woman. A** and **B,** Two consecutive axial fat-suppressed T2-WIs show a well-circumscribed lesion of the medial aspect of the spleen *(arrow)* that is isointense to CSF. A liver lesion anterior to the inferior vena cava (IVC; *curved arrow*) that is isointense to spleen represents metastatic pheochromocytoma. Linear high SI *(double arrow)* in the lateral segment of the left lobe of the liver represents an iatrogenic needle track from prior radiofrequency ablation. **C,** Axial, fat-suppressed heavily T2-WI (TE = 180) reveals persistent homogenous high SI within the splenic cyst *(arrow)* with relative decrease in SI of both the metastasis *(curved arrow)* and needle track *(double arrow).* *(Continued)*

Rarely, a pancreatic pseudocyst may extend along the splenorenal ligament into the splenic hilum and dissect into the splenic parenchyma, resulting in an intrasplenic pseudocyst.[30] Individuals with an intrasplenic pancreatic pseudocyst often have other signs, symptoms, and imaging findings of pancreatitis. Although rare in North America, hydatid cysts are the most common type of splenic cysts worldwide. The spleen is involved in 2% of cases of hydatid disease (see Chapter 1). Splenic cysts are of low intensity on T1-WI and very high intensity on T2-WI relative to the normal splenic parenchyma, and they do not enhance (Fig. 5-7). Variable SI may be identified within false splenic cysts on T1-WI owing to proteinaceous or hemorrhagic content.[8,14]

Hemangioma

Hemangiomas (Box 5-5; see Box 5-2) are the most common benign splenic neoplasm, occurring in up to 14% of autopsy cases.[31,32] Hemangiomas are believed to be congenital lesions composed of proliferative endothelium-lined vascular channels. They may be single or multiple. Most hemangiomas are less than 2 cm in size.[10] The natural course is slow growth; however, most patients with splenic hemangiomas are asymptomatic. The unenhanced MR appearance is similar to that of hepatic hemangiomas: minimally hypointense to isointense compared with liver and spleen on

T1- and hyperintense on T2-WI (Fig. 5-8).[14,32] After intravenous contrast administration, there is immediate enhancement that is most often peripheral, with centripetal progression of enhancement on delayed images. Alternatively, immediate enhancement may be homogeneous, especially in lesions smaller than 1.5 cm. There is persistent, uniform, increased enhancement on delayed images. Although the pattern of centripetal progression of enhancement is similar to that of hepatic hemangiomas, splenic hemangiomas generally do not demonstrate nodular peripheral enhancement, as do hepatic hemangiomas.[32]

Lymphangioma

Lymphangiomas (see Box 5-2) are benign neoplasms composed of endothelium-lined cystic lymphatic spaces. They may be solitary or multiple or may even replace the entire spleen. On MR, they appear as multiloculated cystic spaces of increased intensity on T2-W sequences (Fig. 5-9).[33] Internal septa may appear as thin hypointense bands on T2-WI as compared with splenic parenchyma. Lymphangiomas are typically isointense to hypointense to spleen on T1-WI. The cystic spaces do not enhance, but internal septa may enhance on delayed images.[33,34] In regions where hydatid disease is endemic, it can be difficult to differentiate a multiloculated lymphangioma from a hydatid cyst of the spleen.[35]

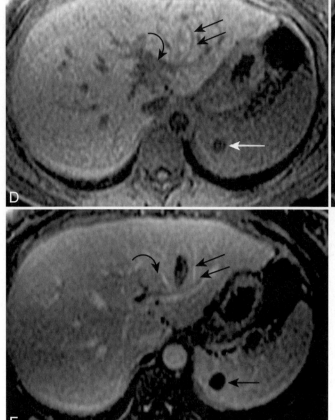

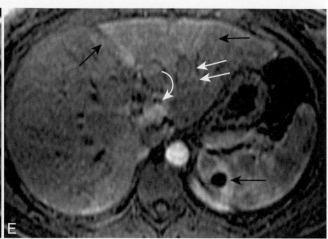

Figure 5-7 ■ **Cont'd D**, Axial fat-suppressed T1-WI shows the hypointense cyst *(arrow)* and relatively isointense metastases compared to spleen *(curved arrow)*. Relative T1 SI is not as specific as heavily T2-WIs and CE images for characterizing cystic and solid focal liver and splenic lesions. The left lobe needle track *(double arrows)* has a peripheral high SI rim that is characteristic of subacute hemorrhage. **E**, Arterial-phase CE T1-WI shows no cyst *(arrow)* or hematoma *(double arrow)* enhancement but marked enhancement of the metastasis *(curved arrow)*. There is a wedge-shaped region of hyperenhancement *(arrows)* peripheral to the metastases. Inspection of the apex of any hyper-enhancing wedge of liver parenchyma may reveal the presence of metastasis in a patient with a known primary tumor. A normal arciform appearance of the spleen is present. **F**, Delayed CE T1-WI shows persistent nonenhancement of the cyst *(arrow)* and hematoma *(double arrow)* and washout but persistent enhancement of the metastases *(curved arrow)*.

Splenic Hamartomas

Splenic hamartomas are rare, benign lesions that are usually imaged incidentally. Splenic hamartomas are not neoplasms; they are composed of a variable mixture of normal red pulp splenic elements.[32,36,37] They are important only in that they should be differentiated from lymphoma or metastatic disease to the spleen. Hamartomas may demonstrate heterogeneous hyperintensity on T2-WI.[32] Hamartomas demonstrate diffuse, heterogeneous enhancement on immediate post–gadolinium enhanced images. This pattern differs from the normal arciform arterial enhancement pattern of the spleen and from the immediate peripheral enhancement of hemangiomas. On delayed images, there is homogeneous increased enhancement relative to the normal splenic parenchyma, likely on the basis of fibrosis within the lesion.[38]

INFLAMMATORY PSEUDOTUMOR

Inflammatory pseudotumor (IPT) of the spleen is a rare reactive mass composed of inflammatory cells with abundant fibrous stroma.[39-41] IPT is thought to represent a reparative response to one or more unidentified stimuli.[37] A subset of IPT, termed inflammatory myofibroblastic tumor, is neoplastic and secondary to Epstein-Barr infection.[37] It is characterized histologically by a predominant spindle cell component and cannot be distinguished from IP by imaging. Systemic symptoms such as fever, weight loss, and abdominal pain are not uncommon. IPT of spleen is revealed on MR as a solitary, solid mass that is isointense to splenic parenchyma on T1-WI and heterogeneously hypointense on T2-WI. The T2 hypointensity is due to fibrosis within the lesion.

5-5 Splenic Hemangioma

Clinical

Most common benign neoplasm of spleen
Most <2 cm and asymptomatic

MRI

Similar T1 and T2 to liver hemangiomas:
Hypointense to spleen on T1
Hyperintense to spleen on T2
Peripheral nodular enhancement not often revealed
Centripetal enhancement with delayed homogenous
 hyperintensity

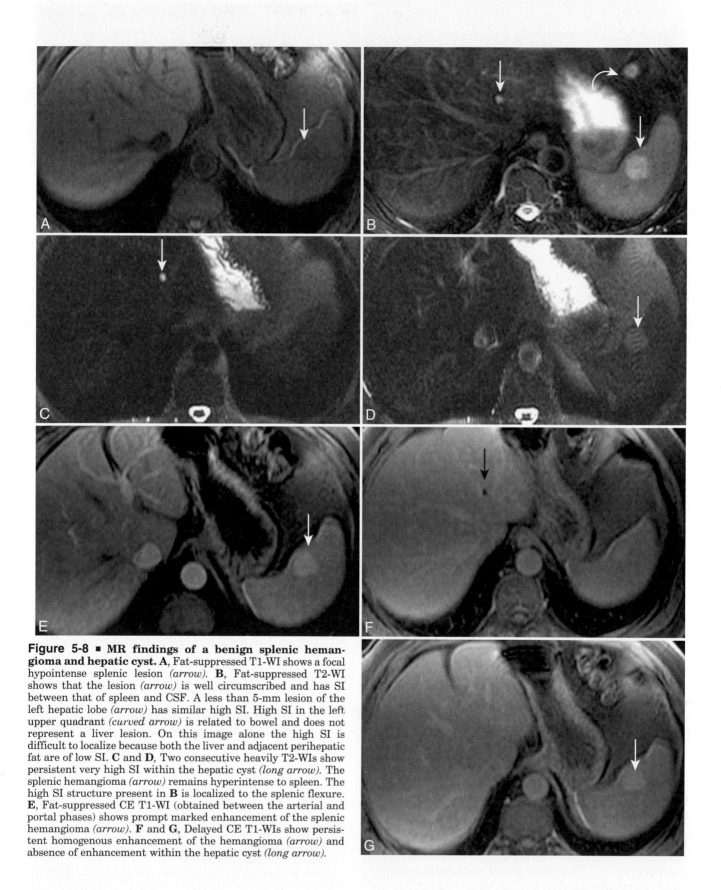

Figure 5-8 ■ **MR findings of a benign splenic hemangioma and hepatic cyst. A**, Fat-suppressed T1-WI shows a focal hypointense splenic lesion *(arrow)*. **B**, Fat-suppressed T2-WI shows that the lesion *(arrow)* is well circumscribed and has SI between that of spleen and CSF. A less than 5-mm lesion of the left hepatic lobe *(arrow)* has similar high SI. High SI in the left upper quadrant *(curved arrow)* is related to bowel and does not represent a liver lesion. On this image alone the high SI is difficult to localize because both the liver and adjacent perihepatic fat are of low SI. **C** and **D**, Two consecutive heavily T2-WIs show persistent very high SI within the hepatic cyst *(long arrow)*. The splenic hemangioma *(arrow)* remains hyperintense to spleen. The high SI structure present in **B** is localized to the splenic flexure. **E**, Fat-suppressed CE T1-WI (obtained between the arterial and portal phases) shows prompt marked enhancement of the splenic hemangioma *(arrow)*. **F** and **G**, Delayed CE T1-WIs show persistent homogenous enhancement of the hemangioma *(arrow)* and absence of enhancement within the hepatic cyst *(long arrow)*.

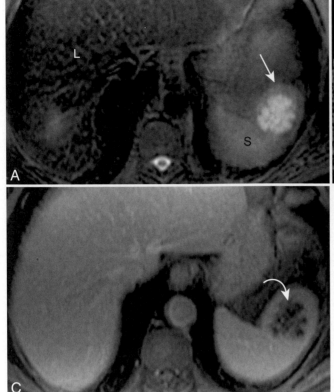

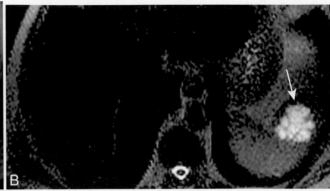

Figure 5-9 ▪ MR illustration of a benign lymphangioma that has been stable for more than 10 years by imaging. **A,** Fat-suppressed breath-hold T2-WI shows a lobulated septate mass *(arrow)* within the superior aspect of the spleen. The liver (L) and spleen (S) show normal SI. **B,** Fat-suppressed heavily T2-WI shows that the internal contents of the mass *(arrow)* are isointense to cerebral spinal fluid, indicating that it is a nonsolid lesion. **C,** Delayed fat-suppressed CE T1-WI shows septal enhancement of the lymphangioma *(arrow).*

Delayed contrast enhancement likely reflects the fibrous content of the tumor. Early peripheral enhancement following dynamic gadolinium administration is variable.[40] IPT of the liver is discussed in Chapter 1.

INFECTIOUS/INFLAMMATORY SPLENIC LESIONS

Pyogenic Abscess

Focal pyogenic disease of the spleen is uncommon; however, with the increasing prevalence of immunosuppression and immunocompromised states, the incidence is rising.[42] Splenic pyogenic infection is usually the result of hematogenous dissemination. A primary, predisposing infection elsewhere is present in two thirds of patients, most commonly endocarditis.[14] Direct spread from adjacent organs (e.g., infected pancreatitis or perinephric abscess) may also occur. Disruption of splenic parenchyma, by infarction or trauma, predisposes to subsequent infection.[43] Splenomegaly, fever and abdominal pain are present in approximately one-half of patients with splenic abscess.

On MR, a focal pyogenic splenic abscess (Box 5-6) has similar imaging findings to a liver abscess, with characteristics of necrotic tissue and inflammatory fluid: hypointense on T1-WI and predominately hyperintense on T2-WI relative to the normal splenic parenchyma. Perilesional enhancement may be identified. Early diagnosis and treatment are important because of the high associated mortality rate from complications such as splenic rupture, subphrenic abscess, and peritonitis. If the patient does not respond to antibiotics, image-guided drainage[44] or splenectomy[43,45] may be necessary.

5-6 Splenic Abscess

Clinical
Uncommon
Splenomegaly, pain, and fever in 50%
Routes of infection
    Hematogenous spread most common (endocarditis)
    Focal extension from infected pseudocyst or
      left-sided pyelonephritis
    Secondary infection of ischemic spleen from trauma
      or emboli
Immunosuppressed patients at risk, especially for
    fungal infection

MRI
T1: low SI relative to spleen
T2: high SI
Irregular rim enhancement
Multiple lesions <2 cm with liver lesions favor fungal
    over pyogenic

Fungal Abscess

Fungal microabscesses (see Box 5-6) occur primarily in immunosuppressed patients and constitute approximately 25% of splenic abscesses in this population.[42] In immunocompromised patients, *Candida albicans* is the most common organism causing hepatosplenic infection, and patients with acute myelogenous leukemia are at particular risk.[46] Infection by *Candida* is systemic, and multiple organ involvement is not uncommon.[47] Immunosuppressed leukemic patients who are febrile are often receive prophylactic treatment with antifungal agents.

Splenic fungal infection typically appears as miliary or multifocal disease. MR imaging of acute candidiasis reveals small, subcentimeter, well-defined lesions (microabscesses) of both liver and spleen (see Fig. 1-11).[48] Microabscesses are best identified on T2-WI, where they appear as multiple, small foci of increased SI. Acute lesions are more apparent in the spleen than in the liver. Since many of these patients are anemic and have received blood transfusions, microabscesses are easily revealed on T2-WI relative to the diffusely decreased SI of liver and spleen from iron deposition.[39] On post–gadolinium enhanced images, lesions may appear as small foci of decreased SI relative to the avidly enhancing spleen. Perilesional enhancement may be present. T2-W and CE MR imaging has higher sensitivity than CT in the detection of acute fungal microabscesses.[46] Since patient survival depends upon prompt antifungal therapy and because blood cultures for fungal organisms are positive in less than 50% of cases, MR may be helpful in establishing this complication of systemic fungal infection. Once infection is documented in liver and spleen, ultrasound likely is a more cost-effective modality for following the lesions with treatment.[49]

GRANULOMATOUS DISEASE OF THE SPLEEN

Granulomatous infections, such as histoplasmosis and tuberculosis, may involve the spleen in both immunocompetent and immunocompromised patients. Splenic infection with *Mycobacterium tuberculosis* usually occurs in the miliary form of hematogenous dissemination (see Fig. 5-3). In patients with disseminated tuberculosis infection, the spleen is involved in 80% to 100% of cases at autopsy.[14] Micronodular, or less commonly macronodular, granulomatous splenic foci may be found, often with associated splenomegaly. Healed granulomatous infections result in multifocal calcifications within liver and spleen. These small foci of calcification are difficult to identify with MR (Fig. 5-10). Fortunately, this is rarely of clinical importance.[2,14]

Sarcoidosis (Fig. 5-11) has been reported to involve the spleen in 25% to 75% of patients on histologic studies.[50,51] Intra-abdominal involvement is less common than involvement of the chest, skin, or eyes. The majority of patients with abdominal sarcoidosis have pulmonary parenchymal involvement or thoracic adenopathy.[52] Splenic involvement in the absence of thoracic disease on imaging examinations in unusual.[53] With splenic sarcoid, splenomegaly is present in 60%, and there often is associated subdiaphragmatic adenopathy. Granulomatous lesions of sarcoidosis are typically uniform in size, ranging from 0.5 to 1.5 cm, and have decreased SI on T1- and T2-WI relative to splenic parenchyma.[54] The focal sarcoid granulomas are most conspicuous on T2-W and early post–gadolinium enhanced images.[51] There may be enhancement on delayed images. The decreased SI of these lesions on T2-WI helps distinguish sarcoidosis from abscess. Additionally, in comparison with acute fungal infection, splenic lesions of sarcoidosis tend to be larger in size and fewer in number. Clinical history is important, since patients with splenic sarcoid usually are not immunosuppressed or febrile.

GAUCHER'S DISEASE

Gaucher's disease is a multiorgan-system hereditary disease of glucocerebrosidase deficiency. There is resultant accumulation of glycolipid (glucocerebroside) within organ macrophages. Within the abdomen, there is invariably hepatosplenomegaly. In 20% to 30% of patients, the spleen contains multiple inclusion nodules. The presence of splenic nodules is not correlated with the size of the spleen. Splenic nodules are of variable SI and size, ranging from 0.5 to 6.0 cm in diameter (Fig. 5-12).[55,56] The nodules are benign and are thought to represent Gaucher cells (reticuloendothelial cells laden with glucocerebroside), fibrosis, or infarction.[55] SI of the nodules varies, since pathologically some nodules also contain dilated sinusoids filled with blood. Focal splenic infarcts are present in up to one third of patients with Gaucher's disease and are more common in larger spleens. A potential advantage of MR imaging in patients with Gaucher disease is the use of chemical shift imaging (see Chapter 3) to evaluate marrow involvement both before and during treatment with enzyme replacement therapy.[57,58] Normal marrow contains lipid, while marrow replaced by Gaucher cells has a paucity of marrow fat.

VASCULAR DISEASE OF THE SPLEEN

Vascular phenomena that involve the spleen include passive congestion from portal hypertension or splenic vein occlusion, infarction (including venoocclusive episodes in sickle cell disease), and splenic artery aneurysm or pseudoaneurysm. The splenic artery and vein lie next to the pancreas throughout much of their course; therefore, processes within the pancreas, such as pancreatitis, may result in splenic vascular occlusion or splenic artery pseudoaneurysm secondary to autodigestion (see Fig. 2-37).[59]

Splenic Artery Aneurysm

A true splenic artery aneurysm is the most common abdominal visceral artery aneurysm, and it is associated

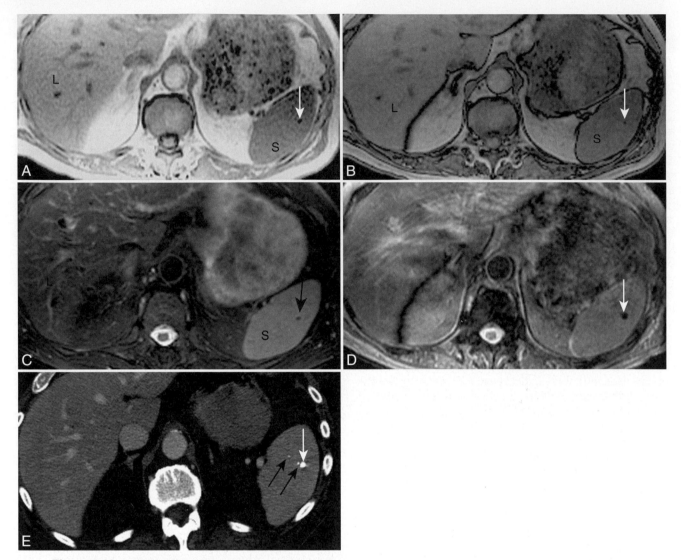

Figure 5-10 ■ MR findings of a benign calcified splenic granuloma in a 78-year-old man. MR is not sensitive in the detection of calcium, and most calcified splenic and hepatic granulomas are not shown on routine MR pulse sequences. **A** and **B**, In-phase (**A**) and opposed-phase (**B**) T1-WIs show normal SI liver (L) and spleen (S). There is a subtle 1- to 2-mm focus of low SI within the spleen *(arrow)*. **C**, Corresponding fat-suppressed T2-WI (TE = 83) shows normal low-to-intermediate SI liver (L) and intermediate-to-high SI spleen (S). A subtle, low SI 1- to 2-mm splenic lesion is present *(arrow)*. **D**, Heavily T2*-W GRE image (TE = 20, FA = 20°), a sequence not routinely performed in the abdomen but useful for detection and characterization of iron overload, shows relative "blooming" of the splenic lesion *(arrow)*. Greater blooming would be present if this lesion contained iron as in Gamna-Gandy bodies (see Figs. 1-22, 1-28, and 5-5). The spine marrow has lost SI secondary to susceptibility effects of the bony trabeculae. **E**, CT shows the calcified splenic granulomas *(white arrow)* and two smaller adjacent granulomas *(black arrows)* that were not revealed by MR.

with pregnancy and portal hypertension.[60,61] The cause is thought to be medial degeneration, often with superimposed arteriosclerosis. Rupture is associated with a high mortality rate. Splenic artery aneurysms revealed on imaging examinations of patients being considered for liver transplantation are electively repaired, since they are at increased risk of rupture postoperatively.[61]

Splenic Infarction

Splenic infarction may be focal or diffuse throughout the spleen. The most common cause in older patients is embolic, usually from cardiovascular disease, such as endocarditis or atrial fibrillation.[10] Infarction in younger patients is often due to local thrombosis from vasculitis, a hematologic disorder (e.g., myelofibrosis, sickle cell disease), leukemia, or lymphoma.[14,62] As described previously, pancreatic disease may result in splenic vascular compromise with resultant infarction.

Classically, infarcts appear as wedge-shaped regions of nonenhancing parenchyma. Less commonly, infarcts may appear round or irregular, making differentiation from splenic abscess or other mass lesions difficult (see Fig. 5-4). The SI varies with the age of the infarct and the presence of

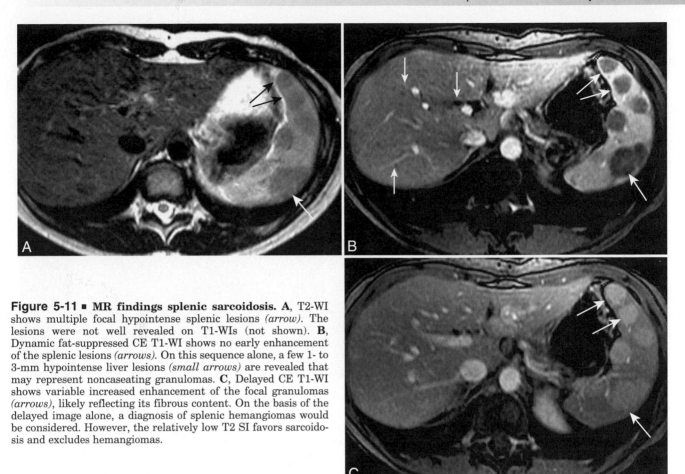

Figure 5-11 ▪ MR findings splenic sarcoidosis. A, T2-WI shows multiple focal hypointense splenic lesions *(arrow)*. The lesions were not well revealed on T1-WIs (not shown). **B**, Dynamic fat-suppressed CE T1-WI shows no early enhancement of the splenic lesions *(arrows)*. On this sequence alone, a few 1- to 3-mm hypointense liver lesions *(small arrows)* are revealed that may represent noncaseating granulomas. **C**, Delayed CE T1-WI shows variable increased enhancement of the focal granulomas *(arrows)*, likely reflecting its fibrous content. On the basis of the delayed image alone, a diagnosis of splenic hemangiomas would be considered. However, the relatively low T2 SI favors sarcoidosis and excludes hemangiomas.

blood products. When liquefied, infarcts may appear hyperintense on T2-WI.[2,14] Infarcts do not enhance; however, a rim of peripheral enhancement may be present owing to collateral flow in capsular vessels. Uncomplicated splenic infarcts can be managed medically. Infarcted spleens that are complicated by abscess or rupture are treated with splenectomy.[62,63]

Sickle Cell Anemia

In sickle cell anemia, veno-occlusive episodes result in splenic infarction with gradual loss of splenic function. Diffuse, extensive perivascular fibrosis with calcium and hemosiderin deposition results in a very small, shrunken spleen. The spleen is of very low SI on both T1- (Fig. 5-13) and T2-WI secondary to diffuse calcium and hemosiderin deposition.[64,65] Low T2 SI splenic parenchyma in patients with sickle cell disease who have not received transfusions is secondary to the sequestration of damaged red blood cells and accumulation of endogenous iron within splenic reticuloendothelial cells.[65]

Acute splenic sequestration crisis (ASSC) is a rare, life-threatening complication of sickle cell disease in adults. In ASSC, sudden, massive splenic enlargement occurs due to sequestration of red blood cells in the spleen, presumably as a result of venous obstruction at the level of small intrasplenic veins or sinusoids.[66] ASSC usually occurs in children with homozygous sickle cell disease prior to progressive splenic fibrosis. However, ASSC may occur in adults with heterozygous disease such as sickle cell–thalassemia or sickle cell–hemoglobin C disease. Imaging usually is not required to establish a diagnosis of ASSC, since patients usually have acute to subacute splenomegaly and a drop in hemoglobin.[67] In patients for whom MR was performed, massive splenomegaly was revealed along with multiple peripheral masses of increased T1 and T2 SI, consistent with subacute hemorrhage or hemorrhagic infarction.[66]

MALIGNANT MASSES OF THE SPLEEN

Lymphoma

Lymphoma (see Box 5-2) is the most common malignant tumor of the spleen.[27,68] Secondary splenic lymphoma is much more common than primary. When laparotomy with splenectomy was routinely performed in the initial staging of lymphoma, splenic involvement was revealed in approximately one third of patients with Hodgkin's and non-Hodgkin's lymphoma.[69,70]

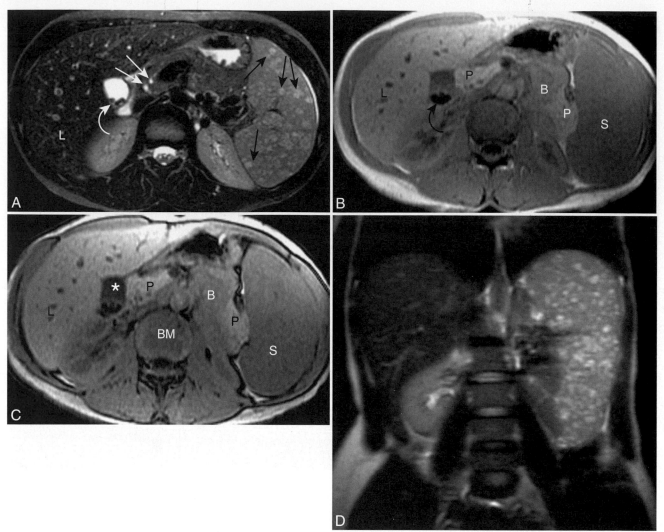

Figure 5-12 ■ **MR findings of Gaucher's disease of the spleen in a 38-year-old woman. A,** Axial fat-suppressed T2-WI shows normal SI of liver (L). Multiple, focal, hyperintense splenic lesions vary in size between 2 and 20 mm *(black arrows)*. Dependent gallstones are present *(curved arrow)*. With respiratory triggering, the fluid-containing common bile duct and pancreatic duct are revealed with minimal blurring *(arrows)*. **B** and **C,** In-phase (**B**) and opposed-phase (**C**) T1-WIs show the expected normal high SI of liver (L) and pancreas (P) and low SI of the enlarged spleen (S). No focal splenic lesions are revealed. Gallstones *(curved arrow)* are present in the dependent portion of the gallbladder. Normal small bowel segments (B) anatomically mimic the body of the pancreas. However, the lower SI should suggest that this is not pancreatic parenchyma. On the opposed-phase image (**C**) there is loss of SI within gallbladder bile (*) secondary to its cholesterol content. The marrow of the lumbar bone marrow (BM) does not lose SI, suggesting that the normal marrow fat has been replaced. Normal marrow contains lipid and reveals loss of SI on chemical shift imaging (e.g., see Fig. 5-1, **A** and **B**) Quantitative chemical shift imaging can be performed to document the degree of marrow involvement in Gaucher's disease. **D,** Coronal breath-hold T2-WI shows gallstones and an enlarged spleen containing multiple "gaucheromas."

Para-aortic lymphadenopathy is associated with splenic involvement in 70% of patients with non-Hodgkin's lymphoma.[70]

In patients with Hodgkin's disease, it is of greater clinical importance to determine splenic involvement when imaging for lymphoma. It is the histopathologic subtype of non-Hodgkin's lymphoma that often dictates prognosis and treatment, and the presence or absence of splenic involvement is less important.[10] In patients with Hodgkin's disease, splenic involvement may influence the decision to irradiate the left upper quadrant.

Splenic lymphoma often is difficult to assess with imaging studies, since microscopic specimens in 45% to 70% of cases reveal homogeneous splenic enlargement with diffuse tumor infiltration or military, subcentimeter nodules. Less commonly, solitary or multifocal lesions measuring up to 10 cm in size are present.[71] Splenic size is a poor predictor of the presence or absence of lymphomatous infiltration. Microscopic involvement is found in 30% of normal-sized spleens, while mild-to-moderate splenomegaly may occur without lymphomatous infiltration, owing to reactive hyperplasia or congestion.[72] However, markedly

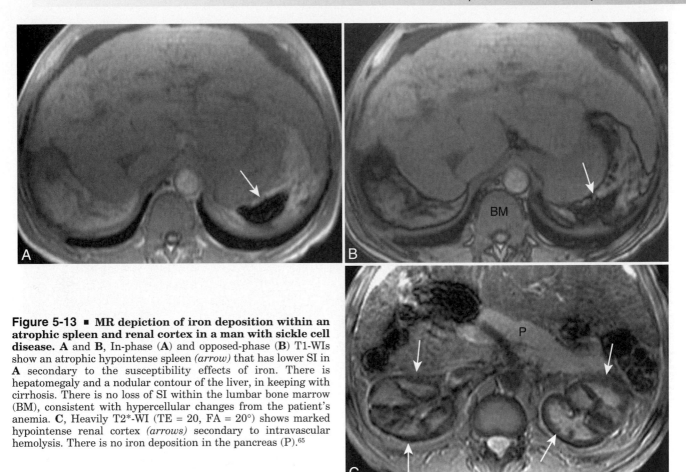

Figure 5-13 ■ **MR depiction of iron deposition within an atrophic spleen and renal cortex in a man with sickle cell disease.** **A** and **B**, In-phase (**A**) and opposed-phase (**B**) T1-WIs show an atrophic hypointense spleen *(arrow)* that has lower SI in **A** secondary to the susceptibility effects of iron. There is hepatomegaly and a nodular contour of the liver, in keeping with cirrhosis. There is no loss of SI within the lumbar bone marrow (BM), consistent with hypercellular changes from the patient's anemia. **C**, Heavily T2*-WI (TE = 20, FA = 20°) shows marked hypointense renal cortex *(arrows)* secondary to intravascular hemolysis. There is no iron deposition in the pancreas (P).[65]

enlarged spleens in patients with lymphoma invariably contain lymphoma.[73,74]

The accuracy of CT in detecting splenic lymphoma is approximately 60%.[73,74] Unenhanced MR imaging (Fig. 5-14) does not significantly improve upon this accuracy. Lymphomatous lesions are not well detected, as no significant SI changes may be present, even with a diffusely infiltrated spleen.[2,5,27,72] However, CE-MRI may be superior to CT in evaluating splenic lymphoma.[75] Diffuse splenic infiltration may appear as irregular, patchy enhancement with loss of the normal arterial phase arciform enhancement. Focal lymphomatous lesions are hypovascular relative to the spleen, and appear as lower SI foci compared with enhancing splenic parenchyma on dynamic CE MR imaging. Lymphomatous foci equilibrate early and become isointense to spleen within 2 minutes.[75] Intravenous SPIO agents (discussed earlier in this chapter) improve the accuracy of MR imaging in the diagnosis of splenic lymphoma. Focal splenic lymphoma becomes more conspicuous and is revealed as low SI foci on T2 and T2*-WI obtained after SPIO administration.[20,72]

If MR imaging cannot establish a specific diagnosis and knowledge of splenic involvement by lymphoma will alter treatment, then image-guided biopsy is a relatively safe technique and can be performed to determine the cause of a focal splenic lesion.[76,77] In staging patients with lymphoma, MR outperforms CT because MR can more accurately determine the presence or absence of marrow involvement by tumor.[78]

Metastatic Disease

Metastatic involvement of the spleen (see Box 5-2) is unusual and typically appears late in the course of malignant disease.[27] The spleen is only the tenth most frequent site of metastatic tumor and has an incidence of less than 10% in autopsy studies.[79] Splenic metastases develop most commonly secondary to hematogenous spread and are almost always present in patients with widespread metastatic disease. Solitary splenic metastases are unusual and reportable.[80] Melanoma has the highest frequency of splenic metastasis, occurring in approximately one third of patients (see Fig. 5-1).[79] However, the most common primary tumors resulting in splenic metastasis are breast and lung carcinoma, partly because these primaries are much more prevalent.[79] Splenic metastases appear most often as multiple nodules of

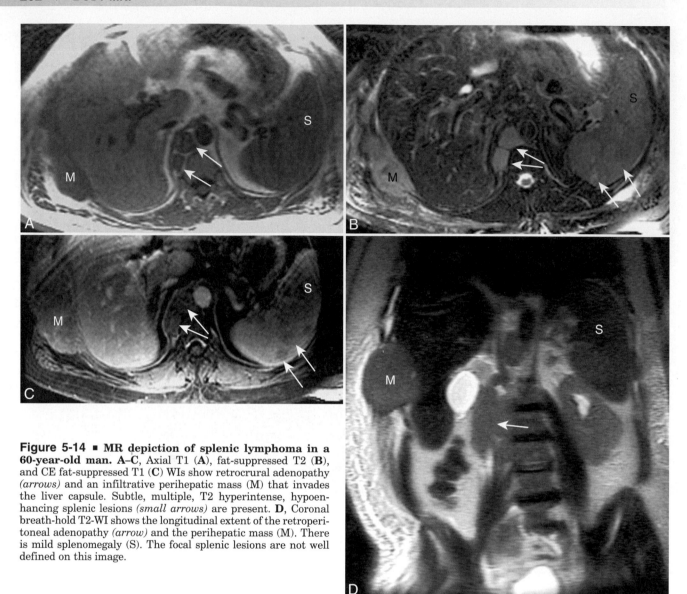

Figure 5-14 ■ MR depiction of splenic lymphoma in a 60-year-old man. A–C, Axial T1 (**A**), fat-suppressed T2 (**B**), and CE fat-suppressed T1 (**C**) WIs show retrocrural adenopathy *(arrows)* and an infiltrative perihepatic mass (M) that invades the liver capsule. Subtle, multiple, T2 hyperintense, hypoenhancing splenic lesions *(small arrows)* are present. **D,** Coronal breath-hold T2-WI shows the longitudinal extent of the retroperitoneal adenopathy *(arrow)* and the perihepatic mass (M). There is mild splenomegaly (S). The focal splenic lesions are not well defined on this image.

varying size. As for splenic lymphoma, splenic metastasis may be difficult to detect on unenhanced MR sequences, and contrast enhancement may be helpful to further characterize potential metastatic disease to the spleen, bone, and other abdominal organs.

Angiosarcoma

Angiosarcoma is a rare, aggressive, malignant neoplasm that arises from the endothelial lining of blood vessels and most commonly affects the skin, soft tissues, breast, and liver. Although splenic involvement is rare, angiosarcoma is the most common primary nonlymphoid malignant neoplasm of the spleen.[14,81] Prognosis is poor, with a 6-month survival rate of 20% and only rare instances of curative resection.[81,82] Patients with splenic angiosarcoma have splenomegaly and abdominal pain, and 25% have spontaneous

splenic rupture.[82,83] Lesions may be single or multiple, or there may be diffuse neoplastic infiltration of the spleen. The MR imaging appearance is variable owing to the various stages of hemorrhage, necrosis, cyst formation, and viable tissue present within the lesion.

SPLENIC TRAUMA

The spleen is the most commonly injured intraperitoneal organ in the setting of blunt trauma.[2,27] Types of splenic injury include subcapsular hematoma, intrasplenic hematoma secondary to contusion or laceration, devascularization, and splenic artery pseudoaneurysm. Contrast-enhanced CT remains the diagnostic study of choice in the evaluation of acute abdominal trauma. Dynamic contrast-enhanced CT is

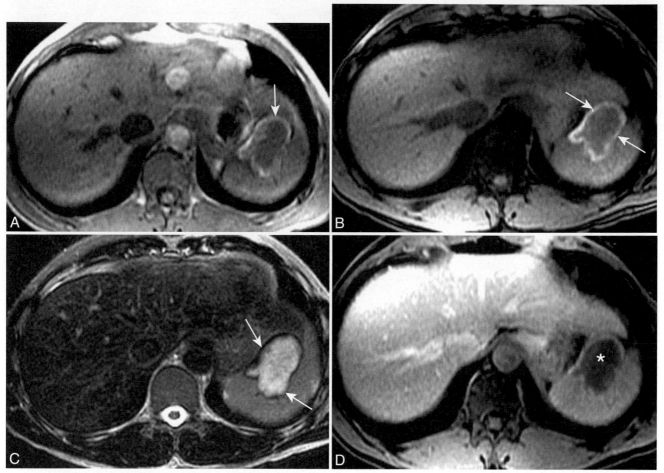

Figure 5-15 ■ MR depiction of a splenic hematoma in a 19-year-old man 2 months after a motor vehicle accident. A, In-phase T1-WI shows a focal splenic lesion with a high SI rim *(arrow).* **B,** Fat-suppressed T1-WI shows persistent high SI within the periphery of the splenic lesion, indicating that it is secondary to hemorrhage and not fat. **C,** Fat-suppressed T2 WI shows high SI centrally within the hematoma and a very low SI rim *(arrows),* representing either intracellular methemoglobin or hemosiderin. **D,** CE T1-WI shows no internal enhancement (*). In patients with hemorrhage neoplasms, CE MR usually reveals enhancing solid components.

more than 95% sensitive in the detection of splenic injury and can help determine whether patients are treated surgically or nonoperatively.[84,85] MR imaging may occasionally be performed as a follow-up evaluation. The SI of a hematoma depends on the time course following injury and the types of hemoglobin present within the hematoma. Subacute hemorrhage is revealed as high SI on T1-WI secondary to the T1-shortening effects of methemoglobin (Fig. 5-15; see Figs. 6-23 and 6-24 and Box 6-35). A rim of low T1 and T2 SI at the periphery of the hematoma may be present and is due to the superparamagnetic effects of hemosiderin within macrophages.[86,87]

Splenosis

Splenosis represents autotransplantation of splenic tissue and is the result of remote splenic rupture or splenectomy. As for accessory splenuli foci of splenosis vary in size and shape and can be present throughout the peritoneal and pleural cavities and,

rarely, the retroperitoneum. This entity is important in that splenic nodules may be confused with adenopathy or malignant implants.[88] The nodules follow all the MR imaging characteristics of the spleen,[89] but as discussed previously, malignancy may have a similar appearance on unenhanced MR sequences. However, accessory splenic tissue usually exhibits the same pattern of dynamic gadolinium enhancement as the normal spleen, with arciform arterial phase enhancement. Splenosis can also be characterized with SPIO agents, since the reticuloendothelial cells contained within islands of splenosis are still functional and can phagocytose the contrast.[90,91]

SUMMARY

MR imaging allows for direct multiplanar imaging of the spleen and is particularly useful for characterizing nonsolid lesions such as cysts, hemangiomas, lymphangiomas, and abscesses. Identification and characterization of solid splenic disease processes can be challenging, since many pathologic processes possess similar relaxation times as normal splenic parenchyma. Dynamic CE MR is often helpful for splenic lesion detection and characterization. Finally, since imaging characteristics of some solid lesions within the spleen may be nonspecific, imaging findings in the remainder of the abdomen often are helpful in determining diagnosis and therapy.

REFERENCES

1. Hahn PF, Weissleder R, Stark DD, Saini S, Elizondo G, Ferrucci JT. MR imaging of focal splenic tumors. AJR Am J Roentgenol 1988;150:823-827.
2. Torres GM, Terry NL, Mergo PJ, Ros PR. MR imaging of the spleen. Magn Reson Imaging Clin N Am 1995;3:39-50.
3. Donnelly LF, Emery KH, Bove KE, Bissett GS III. Normal changes in the MR appearance of the spleen during early childhood. AJR Am J Roentgenol 1996;166:635-639.
4. Runge VM, Williams NM. Dynamic contrast-enhanced magnetic resonance imaging in a model of splenic metastasis. Invest Radiol 1998;33:45-50.
5. Nyman R, Rhen S, Ericsson A, et al. An attempt to characterize malignant lymphoma in spleen, liver and lymph nodes with magnetic resonance imaging. Acta Radiol 1987;28:527-533.
6. Hamed MM, Hamm B, Ibrahim ME, Taupitz M, Mahfouz AE. Dynamic MR imaging of the abdomen with gadopentetate dimeglumine: normal enhancement patterns of the liver, spleen, stomach, and pancreas. AJR Am J Roentgenol 1992;158:303-307.
7. Mirowitz SA, Brown JJ, Lee JK, Heiken JP. Dynamic gadolinium-enhanced MR imaging of the spleen: normal enhancement patterns and evaluation of splenic lesions. Radiology 1991;179:681-686.
8. Ito K, Mitchell DG, Honjo K, et al. Gadolinium-enhanced MR imaging of the spleen: artifacts and potential pitfalls. AJR Am J Roentgenol 1996;167:1147-1151.
9. Groom AC. The Microcirculatory Society Eugene M. Landis award lecture. Microcirculation of the spleen: new concepts, new challenges. Microvasc Res 1987;34:269-289.
10. Robertson F, Leander P, Ekberg O. Radiology of the spleen. Eur Radiol 2001;11:80-95.
11. Taylor AJ, Dodds WJ, Erickson SJ, Stewart ET. CT of acquired abnormalities of the spleen. AJR Am J Roentgenol 1991;157:1213-1219.
12. Yetter EM, Acosta KB, Olson MC, Blundell K. Estimating Splenic Volume: Sonographic Measurements Correlated with Helical CT Determination. AJR Am J Roentgenol 2003;181:1615-1620.
13. Prassopoulos P, Daskalogiannaki M, Raissaki M, Hatjidakis A, Gourtsoyiannis N. Determination of normal splenic volume on computed tomography in relation to age, gender and body habitus. Eur Radiol 1997;7:246-248.
14. Rabushka LS, Kawashima A, Fishman EK. Imaging of the spleen: CT with supplemental MR examination. Radiographics 1994;14:307-332.
15. Siegelman ES, Mitchell DG, Semelka RC. Abdominal iron deposition: metabolism, MR findings, and clinical importance. Radiology 1996;199:13-22.
16. Siegelman ES, Mitchell DG, Outwater E, Munoz SJ, Rubin R. Idiopathic hemochromatosis: MR imaging findings in cirrhotic and precirrhotic patients. Radiology 1993;188:637-641.
17. Sagoh T, Itoh K, Togashi K, et al. Gamna-Gandy bodies of the spleen: evaluation with MR imaging. Radiology 1989;172:685-687.
18. Minami M, Itai Y, Ohtomo K, et al. Siderotic nodules in the spleen: MR imaging of portal hypertension. Radiology 1989;172:681-684.
19. Chen F, Ward J, Robinson PJ. MR imaging of the liver and spleen: a comparison of the effects on signal intensity of two superparamagnetic iron oxide agents. Magn Reson Imaging 1999;17:549-556.
20. Harisinghani MG, Saini S, Weissleder R, et al. Splenic imaging with ultrasmall superparamagnetic iron oxide ferumoxtran-10 (AMI-7227): preliminary observations. J Comput Assist Tomogr 2001;25:770-776.
21. Gayer G, Apter S, Jonas T, et al. Polysplenia syndrome detected in adulthood: report of eight cases and review of the literature. Abdom Imaging 1999;24:178-184.
22. Applegate KE, Goske MJ, Pierce G, Murphy D. Situs revisited: imaging of the heterotaxy syndrome. Radiographics 1999;19:837-852; discussion, 853-854.
23. Fulcher AS, Turner MA. Abdominal manifestations of situs anomalies in adults. Radiographics 2002;22:1439-1456.
24. Sica GT, Reed MF. Case 27: intrapancreatic accessory spleen. Radiology 2000;217:134-137.
25. Avital S, Kashtan H. A large epithelial splenic cyst. N Engl J Med 2003;349:2173-2174.
26. Urrutia M, Mergo PJ, Ros LH, Torres GM, Ros PR. Cystic masses of the spleen: radiologic-pathologic correlation. Radiographics 1996;16:107-129.
27. Ito K, Mitchell DG, Honjo K, et al. MR imaging of acquired abnormalities of the spleen. AJR Am J Roentgenol 1997;168:697-702.
28. Garvin DF, King FM. Cysts and nonlymphomatous tumors of the spleen. Pathol Annu 1981;16:61-80.
29. Morgenstern L. Nonparasitic splenic cysts: pathogenesis, classification, and treatment. J Am Coll Surg 2002;194:306-314.
30. Heider R, Behrns KE. Pancreatic pseudocysts complicated by splenic parenchymal involvement: results of operative and percutaneous management. Pancreas 2001;23:20-25.
31. Willcox TM, Speer RW, Schlinkert RT, Sarr MG. Hemangioma of the spleen: presentation, diagnosis, and management. J Gastrointest Surg 2000;4:611-613.
32. Ramani M, Reinhold C, Semelka RC, et al. Splenic hemangiomas and hamartomas: MR imaging characteristics of 28 lesions. Radiology 1997;202:166-172.
33. Ito K, Murata T, Nakanishi T. Cystic lymphangioma of the spleen: MR findings with pathologic correlation. Abdom Imaging 1995;20:82-84.
34. Bezzi M, Spinelli A, Pierleoni M, Andreoli G. Cystic lymphangioma of the spleen: US-CT-MRI correlation. Eur Radiol 2001;11:1187-1190.
35. Anadol AZ, Oguz M, Bayramoglu H, Edali MN. Cystic lymphangioma of the spleen mimicking hydatid disease. J Clin Gastroenterol 1998;26:309-311.
36. Ohtomo K, Fukuda H, Mori K, Minami M, Itai Y, Inoue Y. CT and MR appearances of splenic hamartoma. J Comput Assist Tomogr 1992;16:425-428.
37. Krishnan J, Frizzera G. Two splenic lesions in need of clarification: hamartoma and inflammatory pseudotumor. Semin Diagn Pathol 2003;20:94-104.
38. Fernandez-Canton G, Capelastegui A, Merino A, Astigarraga E, Larena JA, Diaz-Otazu R. Atypical MRI presentation of a small splenic hamartoma. Eur Radiol 1999;9:883-885.
39. Neuhauser TS, Derringer GA, Thompson LD, et al. Splenic inflammatory myofibroblastic tumor (inflammatory pseudotumor): a clinicopathologic and immunophenotypic study of 12 cases. Arch Pathol Lab Med 2001;125:379-385.
40. Irie H, Honda H, Kaneko K, et al. Inflammatory pseudotumors of the spleen: CT and MRI findings. J Comput Assist Tomogr 1996;20:244-248.
41. Narla LD, Newman B, Spottswood SS, Narla S, Kolli R. Inflammatory pseudotumor. Radiographics 2003;23:719-729.
42. Nelken N, Ignatius J, Skinner M, Christensen N. Changing clinical spectrum of splenic abscess: a multicenter study and review of the literature. Am J Surg 1987;154:27-34.
43. Smyrniotis V, Kehagias D, Voros D, et al. Splenic abscess. An old disease with new interest. Dig Surg 2000;17:354-357.
44. Thanos L, Dailiana T, Papaioannou G, Nikita A, Koutrouvelis H, Kelekis DA. Percutaneous CT-Guided Drainage of Splenic Abscess. AJR Am J Roentgenol 2002;179:629-632.
45. Green BT. Splenic abscess: report of six cases and review of the literature. Am Surg 2001;67:80-85.
46. Semelka RC, Shoenut JP, Greenberg HM, Bow EJ. Detection of acute and treated lesions of hepatosplenic candidiasis: comparison of dynamic contrast-enhanced CT and MR imaging. J Magn Reson Imaging 1992;2:341-345.
47. Kontoyiannis DP, Luna MA, Samuels BI, Bodey GP. Hepatosplenic candidiasis: a manifestation of chronic disseminated candidiasis. Infect Dis Clin North Am 2000;14:721-739.
48. Balci NC, Sirvanci M. MR imaging of infective liver lesions. Magn Reson Imaging Clin N Am 2002;10:121-135.
49. Karthaus M, Huebner G, Elser C, Geissler RG, Heil G, Ganser A. Early detection of chronic disseminated Candida infection in leukemia patients with febrile neutropenia: value of computer-assisted serial ultrasound documentation. Ann Hematol 1998;77:41-45.
50. Selroos O, Koivunen E. Usefulness of fine-needle aspiration biopsy of spleen in diagnosis of sarcoidosis. Chest 1983;83:193-195.
51. Warshauer DM, Lee JK. Imaging manifestations of abdominal sarcoidosis. AJR Am J Roentgenol 2004;182:15-28.
52. Britt AR, Francis IR, Glazer GM, Ellis JH. Sarcoidosis: abdominal manifestations at CT. Radiology 1991;178:91-94.
53. Thanos L, Zormpala A, Brountzos E, Nikita A, Kelekis D. Nodular hepatic and splenic sarcoidosis in a patient with normal chest radiograph. Eur J Radiol 2004;41:10-11.
54. Warshauer DM, Semelka RC, Ascher SM. Nodular sarcoidosis of the liver and spleen: appearance on MR images. J Magn Reson Imaging 1994;4:553-557.
55. Terk MR, Esplin J, Lee K, Magre G, Colletti PM. MR imaging of patients with type 1 Gaucher's disease: relationship between bone and visceral changes. AJR Am J Roentgenol 1995;165:599-604.

56. Hill SC, Damaska BM, Ling A, et al. Gaucher disease: abdominal MR imaging findings in 46 patients. Radiology 1992;184:561-566.
57. Maas M, Poll LW, Terk MR. Imaging and quantifying skeletal involvement in Gaucher disease. Br J Radiol 2002;75:A13-24.
58. Terk MR, Dardashti S, Liebman HA. Bone marrow response in treated patients with Gaucher disease: evaluation by T1-weighted magnetic resonance images and correlation with reduction in liver and spleen volume. Skeletal Radiol 2000;29:563-571.
59. Carr JA, Cho JS, Shepard AD, Nypaver TJ, Reddy DJ. Visceral pseudoaneurysms due to pancreatic pseudocysts: rare but lethal complications of pancreatitis. J Vasc Surg 2000;32:722-730.
60. Dave SP, Reis ED, Hossain A, Taub PJ, Kerstein MD, Hollier LH. Splenic artery aneurysm in the 1990s. Ann Vasc Surg 2000;14:223-229.
61. Lee PC, Rhee RY, Gordon RY, Fung JJ, Webster MW. Management of splenic artery aneurysms: the significance of portal and essential hypertension. J Am Coll Surg 1999;189:483-490.
62. Jaroch MT, Broughan TA, Hermann RE. The natural history of splenic infarction. Surgery 1986;100:743-750.
63. Nores M, Phillips EH, Morgenstern L, Hiatt JR. The clinical spectrum of splenic infarction. Am Surg 1998;64:182-188.
64. Adler DD, Glazer GM, Aisen AM. MRI of the spleen: normal appearance and findings in sickle-cell anemia. AJR Am J Roentgenol 1986;147:843-845.
65. Siegelman ES, Outwater E, Hanau CA, et al. Abdominal iron distribution in sickle cell disease: MR findings in transfusion and nontransfusion dependent patients. J Comput Assist Tomogr 1994;18:63-67.
66. Roshkow JE, Sanders LM. Acute splenic sequestration crisis in two adults with sickle cell disease: US, CT, and MR imaging findings. Radiology 1990;177:723-725.
67. Sheridan MB, Ward J, Guthrie JA, et al. Dynamic contrast-enhanced MR imaging and dual-phase helical CT in the preoperative assessment of suspected pancreatic cancer: a comparative study with receiver operating characteristic analysis. AJR Am J Roentgenol 1999;173:583-590.
68. Rabushka LS, Fishman EK, Goldman SM. Pictorial review: computed tomography of renal inflammatory disease. Urology 1994;44:473-480.
69. Veronesi U, Musumeci R, Pizzetti F, Gennari L, Bonadonna G. Proceedings: the value of staging laparotomy in non-Hodgkin's lymphomas (with emphasis on the histiocytic type). Cancer 1974;33:446-459.
70. Kim H, Dorfman RF. Morphological studies of 84 untreated patients subjected to laparotomy for the staging of non-Hodgkin's lymphomas. Cancer 1974;33:657-674.
71. Fishman EK, Kuhlman JE, Jones RJ. CT of lymphoma: spectrum of disease. Radiographics 1991;11:647-669.
72. Weissleder R, Elizondo G, Stark DD, et al. The diagnosis of splenic lymphoma by MR imaging: value of superparamagnetic iron oxide. AJR Am J Roentgenol 1989;152:175-180.
73. Castellino RA. Hodgkin disease: practical concepts for the diagnostic radiologist. Radiology 1986;159:305-310.
74. Castellino RA. The non-Hodgkin lymphomas: practical concepts for the diagnostic radiologist. Radiology 1991;178:315-321.
75. Semelka RC, Shoenut JP, Lawrence PH, Greenberg HM, Madden TP, Kroeker MA. Spleen: dynamic enhancement patterns on gradient-echo MR images enhanced with gadopentetate dimeglumine. Radiology 1992;185:479-482.
76. Keogan MT, Freed KS, Paulson EK, Nelson RC, Dodd LG. Imaging-guided percutaneous biopsy of focal splenic lesions: update on safety and effectiveness. AJR Am J Roentgenol 1999;172:933-937.
77. Lucey BC, Boland GW, Maher MM, Hahn PF, Gervais DA, Mueller PR. Percutaneous nonvascular splenic intervention: a 10-year review. AJR Am J Roentgenol 2002;179:1591-1596.
78. Hoane BR, Shields AF, Porter BA, Borrow JW. Comparison of initial lymphoma staging using computed tomography (CT) and magnetic resonance (MR) imaging. Am J Hematol 1994;47:100-105.
79. Berge T. Splenic metastases. Frequencies and patterns. Acta Pathol Microbiol Scand [A] 1974;82:499-506.
80. Agha-Mohammadi S, Calne RY. Solitary splenic metastasis: case report and review of the literature. Am J Clin Oncol 2001;24:306-310.
81. Vrachliotis TG, Bennett WF, Vaswani KK, Niemann TH, Bova JG. Primary angiosarcoma of the spleen—CT, MR, and sonographic characteristics: report of two cases. Abdom Imaging 2000;25:283-285.
82. Neuhauser TS, Derringer GA, Thompson LD, et al. Splenic angiosarcoma: a clinicopathologic and immunophenotypic study of 28 cases. Mod Pathol 2000;13:978-987.
83. Karakas HM, Demir M, Ozyilmaz F, Cakir B. Primary angiosarcoma of the spleen: in vivo and in vitro MRI findings. Clin Imaging 2001;25:192-196.
84. Federle MP, Courcoulas AP, Powell M, Ferris JV, Peitzman AB. Blunt splenic injury in adults: clinical and CT criteria for management, with emphasis on active extravasation. Radiology 1998;206:137-142.
85. Ochsner MG. Factors of failure for nonoperative management of blunt liver and splenic injuries. World J Surg 2001;25:1393-1396.
86. Bradley WG, Jr. MR appearance of hemorrhage in the brain [see comments]. Radiology 1993;189:15-26.
87. Siegelman ES, Outwater EK. The concentric-ring sign revisited. AJR Am J Roentgenol 1996;166:1493.
88. Foroudi F, Ahern V, Peduto A. Splenosis mimicking metastases from breast carcinoma. Clin Oncol 1999;11:190-192.
89. Lin WC, Lee RC, Chiang JH, et al. MR features of abdominal splenosis. AJR Am J Roentgenol 2003;180:493-496.
90. De Vuysere S, Van Steenbergen W, Aerts R, Van Hauwaert H, Van Beckevoort D, Van Hoe L. Intrahepatic splenosis: imaging features. Abdom Imaging 2000;25:187-189.
91. Storm BL, Abbitt PL, Allen DA, Ros PR. Splenosis: superparamagnetic iron oxide-enhanced MR imaging. AJR Am J Roentgenol 1992;159:333-335.
92. Hasegawa S, Semelka RC, Noone TC, et al. Gastric stromal sarcomas: correlation of MR imaging and histopathologic findings in nine patients. Radiology 1998;208:591-595.
93. Levy AD, Remotti HE, Thompson WM, Sobin LH, Miettinen M. From the Archives of the AFIP: Gastrointestinal stromal tumors: radiologic features with pathologic correlation. Radiographics 2003;23:283-304.
94. Demetri GD, von Mehren M, Blanke CD, et al. Efficacy and safety of imatinib mesylate in advanced gastrointestinal stromal tumors. N Engl J Med 2002;347:472-480.
95. Warshauer DM, Molina PL, Worawattanakul S. The spotted spleen: CT and clinical correlation in a tertiary care center. J Comput Assist Tomogr 1998;22:694-702.

6

MRI of the Retroperitoneum and Peritoneum

Drew A. Torigian, MD
Evan S. Siegelman, MD

RETROPERITONEUM AND PERITONEUM

The peritoneum is the largest and most complexly arranged serous membrane in the body; it is closed in men but open to the ends of the fallopian tubes in women.[1] The peritoneal cavity is the potential space surrounded by the parietal peritoneal lining of the abdominal wall and the visceral peritoneal lining that envelop the abdominal organs, and it normally contains a small amount of serous fluid.[1,2] The major function of the peritoneum is to allow unimpeded activity and mobility of the contained viscera by providing a moist smooth surface between organs although it also has absorptive and immune functions.[2] However, the peritoneal cavity, peritoneal ligaments, mesenteries, and omentum are frequently involved by disease processes and may serve as either boundaries or conduits for the spread of disease between the peritoneum and the retroperitoneum.[1,3,4] The retroperitoneum is the compartmentalized space located external to and predominantly posterior to the posterior parietal peritoneum, contains several organ systems such as the pancreaticobiliary and genitourinary systems, and is frequently also involved by pathologic processes.[1,3-6]

Although CT has higher spatial resolution than MRI, MRI has superior contrast resolution, allowing for acquisition of multiple image sequences that may each be useful for depicting different inherent characteristics of a disease process affecting either the peritoneum or retroperitoneum.[7,8] The distinction between intra- and retroperitoneal sites of disease is of clinical significance because surgery that requires opening of the peritoneal cavity carries the risk of adhesion formation.[2]

On MR, T1-WIs are useful for demonstrating high SI fat or hemorrhage, lymphadenopathy, and vascular invasion by tumors.[9] Fat-suppressed T2-WIs can depict lymphadenopathy, cystic change or necrosis, fluid collections, and dilatation or obstruction of fluid-containing structures such as the biliary tree and gallbladder, the bowel, or the genitourinary system.[9] Delayed-CE T1-WI is the single most useful MRI acquisition for rapid screening of the extra-parenchymal abdomen and pelvis owing to increased conspicuity of pathologic processes; and it can depict the solid or cystic/necrotic nature of lesions; extent of peritoneal, mesenteric, mesocolic, omental, gastrointestinal, and osseous sites of disease; and presence and nature of vascular thrombosis or tumor encasement of abdominal vessels.[7-10] The normal peritoneum is isointense with that of abdominal wall muscles on T1 and T2-WIs.[10] This chapter reviews the pathologic and MR imaging features of various diseases that may affect the peritoneum and nonparenchymal portions of the retroperitoneum.

RETROPERITONEAL SARCOMAS

Soft tissue sarcomas are rare mesenchymal neoplasms with an incidence in the U. S. of approximately 7,000 new cases per year, accounting for less than 1% of adult malignancies. Fifteen percent of sarcomas originate within the retroperitoneum (Box 6-1),[11] 45% in the lower extremity, 15% in the upper extremity, 10% in the head and neck region, and the remainder in the abdominal and chest walls.[12] Most retroperitoneal neoplasms are malignant, and one third of malignant retroperitoneal neoplasms are sarcomas, with an incidence rate of 1 to 2 cases per million per year.[13,14] Retroperitoneal sarcomas may develop at any age but most present during the sixth and seventh decades of life and are slightly more common in men. Most retroperitoneal sarcomas are of high histologic grade and tend to be large, with a mean size of 17 cm.[14,15] The most common histologic subtype of retroperitoneal sarcoma is liposarcoma (40%), followed by leiomyosarcoma (30%).[14,16] In contrast to

its occurrence in the extremities, malignant fibrous histiocytoma (MFH) is uncommonly found in the retroperitoneum and comprises only 15% of retroperitoneal sarcomas.[6,14] Sarcomas rarely develop from preexisting benign soft tissue tumors, with the exception of malignant peripheral nerve sheath tumors that can arise from neurofibromas, nearly always in patients with neurofibromatosis type 1 (NF-1).[12]

The retroperitoneal cavity can accommodate a large volume of growing tumor mass.[17] Retroperitoneal sarcomas are often very large before producing any symptoms or signs. The late presenting signs and symptoms are usually vague and nonspecific, resulting in a delay in diagnosis and contributing to a poor prognosis.[15,16,18] MR can define the extent of the primary tumor and assess for involvement of adjacent organs and vessels. MR imaging features that suggest unresectable disease include extensive vascular involvement, peritoneal implantation, and distant metastatic disease.[14] In patients with potentially resectable tumors, preoperative biopsy may be avoided.[6,19]

Although MRI is excellent for the evaluation of soft tissue, a specific histologic diagnosis often cannot be made owing to the overlap in imaging appearances of the various soft-tissue lesions. However, determination of the dominant histologic component or location may help to provide a specific histologic diagnosis.[20,21] For example, the presence of macroscopic fat within a large retroperitoneal mass favors the diagnosis of a well-differentiated liposarcoma, whereas caval involvement favors a leiomyosarcoma, particularly if cystic or necrotic intratumoral components or metastases are present.[6,21,22] Similarly, a large retroperitoneal mass that contains low SI calcifications or extensive hemorrhage but no fatty components or central necrosis favors a diagnosis of MFH.[6,21]

Grading and staging of soft tissue sarcomas are essential for determining prognosis and for planning and evaluating therapy.[12] Grading determines the degree of histologic malignancy of a sarcoma. The two most important parameters in grading soft tissue sarcomas are the number of mitotic figures and the extent of necrosis. Low-grade sarcomas rarely metastasize but can be locally aggressive, whereas higher grade sarcomas have a propensity to metastasize and show locally aggressive behavior. While the histologic examination can generally predict tumor aggressiveness, follow-up imaging is often the ultimate arbiter of whether a resected sarcoma exhibits malignant behavior.[12]

In general, the staging of soft tissue sarcomas is based on clinical, imaging, and histologic data and provides information on the state or extent of disease at a specific point in time. Retroperitoneal sarcomas are staged according to the GTNM classification (Box 6-2). According to the GTNM system, the G stage is based on the tumor grade, the T stage is assigned based on size and depth of the lesion relative to the fascia ("a" signifies that the lesion is entirely above the superficial fascia, whereas "b" means that

---

6-1 Retroperitoneal Sarcoma

- Uncommon, one third of retroperitoneal malignancies
- Peak age: 6th to 7th decades of life, M:F slightly >1:1
- Mean size at diagnosis = 17 cm
- Two most common subtypes: liposarcoma and leiomyosarcoma
- Treatment: complete surgical resection; radiation therapy and chemotherapy less effective

6-2 AJCC* GTNM Classification and Stage Grouping of Soft Tissue Sarcomas[12]

GTNM Description

Tumor Grade

G1   Well differentiated
G2   Moderately differentiated
G3   Poorly differentiated
G4   Undifferentiated

Primary Tumor

    T1   Tumor ≤5 cm in greatest diameter
    T1a   Superficial tumor
    T1b   Deep tumor
    T2   Tumor >5 cm in greatest diameter
    T2a   Superficial
    T2b   Deep

Regional Lymph Node Involvement

    N0   No known metastases to lymph nodes
    N1   Verified metastases to lymph nodes

Distant Metastasis

    M0   No known distant metastasis
    M1   Known distant metastasis

Stage System Grouping

IA   Low grade, small (G1-2, T1, N0, M0)
IB   Low grade, large, superficial (G1-2, T2a, N0, M0)
IIA   Low grade, large, deep (G1-2, T2b, N0, M0)
IIB   High grade, small (G3-4, T1, N0, M0)
IIC   High grade, large, superficial (G3-4, T2a, N0, M0)
III   High grade, large, deep (G3-4, T2b, N0, M0)
IV   Nodal or distant metastases (G1-4, T1-2,
        N1, M0 or G1-4, T1-2, N0, M1)

*American Joint Committee on Cancer

---

there is invasion of the superficial fascia or that the lesion is entirely below the superficial fascia), the N stage is based on the presence of regional lymph node metastases, and the M stage is dependent on the presence of distant metastases. Therefore, all intra-abdominal sarcomas are by definition "b" lesions. Overall, regional lymphadenopathy is uncommon in soft tissue sarcomas, with a frequency of less than 4% at presentation.[12] Furthermore, less than one third of patients have metastases at presentation. Resectability rates for retroperitoneal sarcoma range from 38% to 100%.[13]

Chemotherapy for retroperitoneal soft-tissue sarcoma is not effective, and adjuvant radiation is limited by toxicity to adjacent intra-abdominal structures.[13,14,16,23] Thus, an attempt at complete surgical resection is the treatment of choice for primary and recurrent retroperitoneal sarcoma but is often difficult or impossible to perform owing to the deep anatomic location with proximity to vital retroperitoneal structures, the frequent late presentation, and the frequent invasion of adjacent retroperitoneal structures.[14,16,19] Concomitant resection of adjacent organs that are involved by tumor is performed to ensure clear surgical margins, although this is often difficult.[17]

The median survival of patients with primary retroperitoneal sarcoma is 72 months. Those with local recurrent disease have a median survival of 28 months, while patients with metastatic disease have a median survival of 10 months. The 5-year survival rates after complete resection range from 40% to 75%. Recurrent tumor, unresectable disease, incomplete resection, and high histologic grade are significantly associated with decreased survival time. In patients who undergo complete resection, the median survival is 103 months as compared with 18 months with incomplete resection. There is no significant difference in survival in patients with unresectable disease (i.e., with distant metastases, peritoneal implants, or extensive vascular involvement) compared with those with incompletely resected disease. Thus, patients with primary disease or a local recurrence should undergo aggressive attempts at complete surgical resection if there are no imaging findings of unresectable disease. Incomplete resection should be performed only for palliative symptom relief. Overall, complete en bloc resection of retroperitoneal sarcomas including resection of involved adjacent structures is the most important independent prognostic factor for survival.[14-16]

Following complete resection of a retroperitoneal sarcoma, histologic grade is the most important prognostic factor in regard to local recurrence and overall survival.[15,19] Five-year survival rates after radical excision are on average 75% for well-differentiated tumors, compared with 30% for less well-differentiated tumors.[13] Distant metastases from retroperitoneal sarcomas are uncommon and occur mostly with high-grade tumors after a long time of primary tumor growth, with an incidence of approximately 25%.[11,13] Resection of distant metastases with curative intent is the best manner of prolonging survival. This is best performed for patients with a limited number of metastases, a long disease-free interval, and slow clinical growth and who have undergone or are undergoing complete resection of the primary tumor.[13,24]

Liposarcoma

Liposarcoma (Box 6-3) is the most common retroperitoneal sarcoma (accounting for approximately 40%), whereas primary mesenteric and primary peritoneal liposarcomas are rare.[6,14,25] Most liposarcomas occur in deep soft tissue, in contrast to lipomas, which more commonly occur in superficial soft tissue.[12] Liposarcomas originate from primitive mesenchymal cells rather than from mature fat cells.[26] Although the World Health Organization (WHO) identifies five subtypes (well-differentiated, myxoid, round cell, dedifferentiated, and pleomorphic), the liposarcomas may be conceptually divided into three subgroups. Well-differentiated and dedifferentiated liposarcomas comprise one subgroup, since over time a subset of well-differentiated liposarcomas histologically can progress to dedifferentiated sarcomas, which have metastatic potential. A second subgroup is composed of the myxoid and

6-3   Features of Liposarcoma

Clinical

Most common retroperitoneal sarcoma (40%)
Second most common adult soft tissue sarcoma (15%)
Peak age: 6th to 7th decades of life, M:F=1:1
Mean size=20 cm
5-Year survival=40–75%
The only retroperitoneal sarcoma with survival benefit
    after incomplete resection

Well-differentiated Subtype

Best prognosis, 5-year survival=60% to 90%
MRI
    Most of tumor follows appearance of fat
    Large size (>10 cm), thick septa (>2 mm), nodular
        and globular areas, nonadipose mass-like areas,
        and decreased percentage of fat composition
        (<75% fat) favor liposarcoma over lipoma

Dedifferentiated Subtype

Poor prognosis, 5-year survival=30%
MRI
    May reveal fatty components
    Larger proportion of nonfatty intratumoral tissue

Myxoid Subtype

Peak age: 5th decade of life, one decade younger than
    other subtypes
Intermediate prognosis between well-differentiated
    and dedifferentiated subtypes
MRI
    Myxoid components can mimic a cyst on T2-WI
    Contrast enhancement differentiates myxoid tissue
        from cyst/intratumoral cystic necrosis
    Intratumoral fat may be present

Pleomorphic and Round Cell Subtypes

Very aggressive with a poor prognosis
MRI
    Heterogeneous SI on T1-WI and T2-WI
    Intratumoral hemorrhage and necrosis common

---

addition to symptom palliation, particularly in patients resected for primary disease, in contradistinction to patients with other types of retroperitoneal sarcoma. Partial resection was an independent factor for increased survival as compared with exploration or biopsy alone (median survival 26 months vs. 4 months), and successful palliation of symptoms was achieved in 75% with preoperative symptoms.[11]

WELL-DIFFERENTIATED LIPOSARCOMA

Well-differentiated liposarcoma is the most common subtype of retroperitoneal liposarcoma, reaching a peak incidence during the sixth and seventh decades of life, with men and women affected equally. Together, the well-differentiated and dedifferentiated subtypes account for approximately 35% to 40% of liposarcomas. On T1-WI and T2-WI, well-differentiated liposarcomas are usually isointense to subcutaneous fat, with loss of SI on fat-suppressed imaging sequences (Figs. 6-1 and 6-2).[6,25,26,28,29] Imaging features that favor well-differentiated liposarcoma over lipoma include large lesion size (>10 cm), presence of thick septa (>2 mm), nodular or globular areas, nonadipose mass-like areas within the lesion, and decreased percentage of fat composition (<75% fat in mass). The presence of thick septa and associated nonadipose mass-like areas increase the likelihood of a well-differentiated liposarcoma over a lipoma by 9- and 32-fold, respectively.[30]

An exophytic renal angiomyolipoma may be difficult to differentiate from a well-differentiated perirenal retroperitoneal liposarcoma. Imaging features more typical of an angiomyolipoma include a renal parenchymal defect (as the kidney is its most common site of origin), enlarged internal vascularity, and presence of other fatty lesions in the ipsilateral or contralateral kidney. Features more characteristic of a perirenal retroperitoneal liposarcoma include extrinsic mass effect on the kidney with a smooth interface and without a renal parenchymal defect, lack of enlarged internal vascularity, and lack of other fatty renal lesions (Fig. 6-3). Although more aggressive liposarcomas may invade the kidney, these tend not to be the well-differentiated liposarcomas.[31] (See Chapter 4 for further discussion of renal angiomyolipomas.)

Well-differentiated liposarcomas are for the most part nonmetastasizing lesions that are grade I lesions at histology, but their rate of local recurrence in the retroperitoneum approaches 100%.[32] With local recurrence, cachexia and intestinal obstruction are common.[11] Approximately 10% of well-differentiated retroperitoneal liposarcomas can dedifferentiate, after an average of 7 to 8 years.[12]

DEDIFFERENTIATED LIPOSARCOMA

Dedifferentiated liposarcomas develop in approximately the same age group as well-differentiated liposarcomas, reaching a peak during the early seventh decade of life, with males and females affected equally.[12,33] Histologically, the lesions have areas of well-differentiated liposarcoma and a nonlipogenic

---

round cell liposarcomas, with the continuum of lesions ranging from pure myxoid liposarcoma at one extreme to round cell (poorly differentiated myxoid) liposarcomas at the other. The third subgroup exhibits unusual features or combines patterns not accounted for in the above classifications (liposarcomas of pleomorphic or mixed type).[12]

Retroperitoneal liposarcoma has a mean diameter of 20 cm and is associated with local recurrence and negatively associated with metastasis.[6,11,14,27] The rate of distant metastasis to both liver and lung is less than 10%. Local recurrence of tumor is responsible for most morbidity and mortality.[11,14] In comparison, patients with nonliposarcoma retroperitoneal tumors have an approximately fourfold higher risk of metastases.[15] In patients with unresectable retroperitoneal liposarcoma, incomplete resection or debulking can provide improvement in survival in

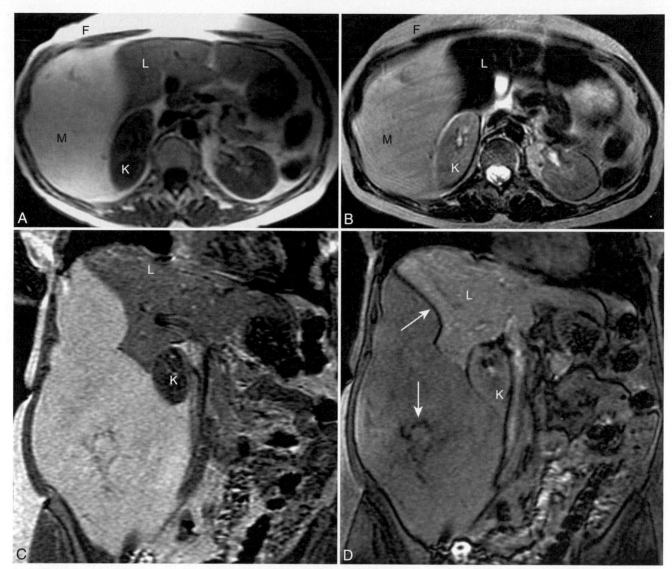

Figure 6-1 ■ **MR depiction of macroscopic fat in a well-differentiated retroperitoneal liposarcoma in a 62-year-old woman. A** and **B,** Axial T1-WI (**A**) and T2-WI (**B**) shows a right retroperitoneal lesion (M) that is isointense to subcutaneous fat (F), causes extrinsic mass effect up the lateral aspect of the right lobe of the liver (L), and displaces the right kidney (K) medially. **C** and **D,** Coronal in-phase (**C**) and out-of-phase (**D**) T1-WIs show only minimal loss of SI of the macroscopic fat within the well-differentiated tumor. Several hypointense nonfatty septa are present centrally *(vertical arrow)* that exhibit greater loss of SI owing to the phase cancellation of water and fat protons within voxels at the interfaces of the nonfatty septa and adjacent intratumoral fat. The presence of an "etching artifact" *(diagonal arrow)* at the interface of the mass with the liver in **D** indicates a fat-water interface. Because the liver is composed of water, this chemical shift feature establishes the presence of fat within the mass.

(dedifferentiated) component, which has the appearance of a high-grade fibrosarcoma or malignant fibrous histiocytoma.[12] On MRI, dedifferentiated liposarcomas have areas with SI characteristic of fat-containing well-differentiated liposarcoma, but they have more mass-like areas of nonfatty tissue with lower T1-WI and higher T2-WI SI (Fig. 6-4).[34] Those patients whose tumors reveal ossification or calcification on CT or MR have a poorer prognosis.[35] The biological behavior of dedifferentiated liposarcomas is similar to that of other pleomorphic high-grade sarcomas in adults, with a 5-year survival rate of less than 25%.[12,13,33]

MYXOID LIPOSARCOMA

Myxoid liposarcoma is the second most common subtype of retroperitoneal sarcoma.[12,26] Unlike well-differentiated liposarcomas, myxoid liposarcoma occurs in a younger age group, with a peak incidence during the fifth decade of life.[12] The myxoid subtype has an intermediate prognosis between that of the well-differentiated and dedifferentiated subtypes.[26] Histologically, myxoid liposarcomas are composed of a myxoid matrix containing mucopolysaccharides with small amounts of mature fat. A spectrum of features on MRI may be present in myxoid liposarcomas related to the fat content, amount of myxoid material, degree of cellularity and vascularity, and presence of necrosis.[26] On MRI, myxoid liposarcomas typically demonstrate SI similar to fluid with low SI on T1-WI and very high SI relative to muscle on T2-WI.[25,26] Foci of fat or low SI septa may be revealed within the predominately myxoid-containing mass.[25,26,29] Some myxoid-rich liposarcomas can mimic a cyst or cystic mass on unenhanced images.[21,26] The myxoid stroma will enhance to a variable degree depending on its degree of vascularity, and thus enhanced images can distinguish cystic and myxoid components of the neoplasm (see Fig. 6-3). Myxoid tissue may also be present within MFH, and in the absence of fat, a myxoid liposarcoma may appear similar.[21]

PLEOMORPHIC AND ROUND CELL LIPOSARCOMA

Pleomorphic liposarcoma is the least common subtype of retroperitoneal liposarcoma. Histologically, there is a disorderly growth pattern with a marked degree of cellular pleomorphism including bizarre giant cells.[12] Pleomorphic liposarcomas and round cell liposarcomas are heterogeneous nonfatty tumors with imaging characteristics indistinguishable from those of other malignant soft-tissue masses.[25] On MRI, they appear heterogeneous on T1-WI and T2-WI and commonly reveal foci of intratumoral hemorrhage and necrosis.[36] The pleomorphic and round cell subtypes are highly malignant and have a tendency toward local recurrence and metastasis.[26]

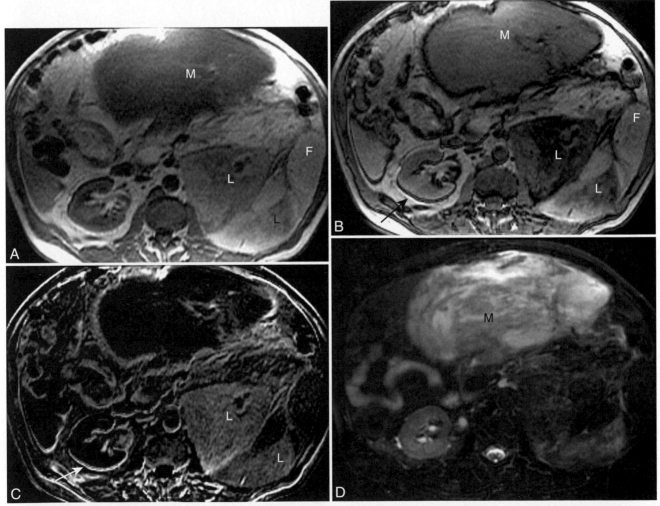

Figure 6-2 ■ **MR illustrations of both myxoid and fatty components of a liposarcoma in a 60-year-old man.** **A** and **B**, Axial in-phase (**A**) and out-of-phase (**B**) T1-WIs show a heterogeneous left retroperitoneal and anterior abdominal mass. Two regions of the tumor lose SI on chemical shift imaging (L), indicating the presence of intratumoral lipid. Posterolaterally there is peripheral hyperintense well-differentiated tumoral fat (F). Anteriorly, there is a large component of the mass that is isointense to skeletal muscle that corresponds to the myxoid component of the mass (M). Etching artifacts *(arrow)* at fat-water interfaces in B indicate that it is an opposed-phase image. **C**, Postprocessed subtraction image [in phase (**A**) – out of phase (**B**)] reveals the greatest SI within voxels that have both lipid and water protons. Thus, the intratumoral foci of microscopic lipid (L) show the greatest SI. Low SI etching artifact in **B** (e.g., at the interface of right kidney and posterior perirenal fat) appears as high SI on these subtraction images *(arrow)*. **D**, Axial fat-suppressed T2-W FSE image shows low SI of the suppressed fatty components of the tumor and high SI within the myxoid portions (M).

(Continued)

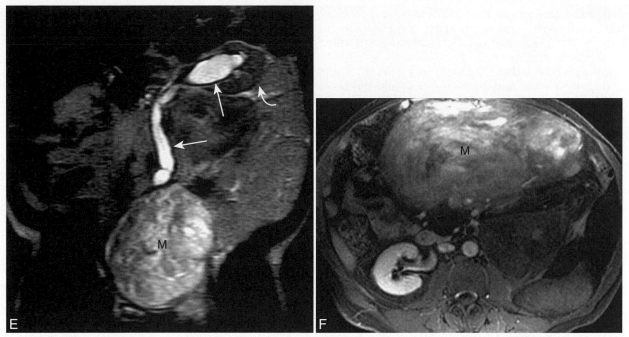

Figure 6-2 ■ Cont'd E, Coronal T2-W breath-hold FSE image shows left hydronephrosis and hydroureter *(arrows)* secondary to obstruction by a myxoid (M) component of the mass, with malrotation and superior displacement of the left kidney *(curved arrow)* by the remainder of the mass. **F**, Axial fat-suppressed CE T1-WI shows heterogeneous enhancement of the myxoid (M) and nonfatty portions of the sarcoma.

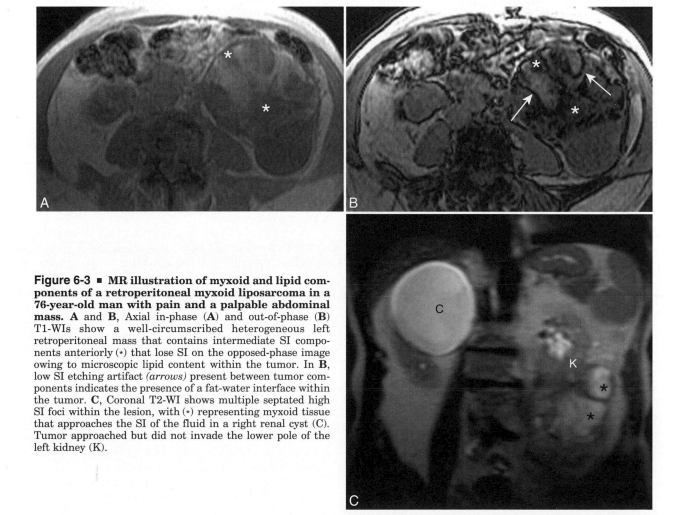

Figure 6-3 ■ MR illustration of myxoid and lipid components of a retroperitoneal myxoid liposarcoma in a 76-year-old man with pain and a palpable abdominal mass. A and **B**, Axial in-phase (**A**) and out-of-phase (**B**) T1-WIs show a well-circumscribed heterogeneous left retroperitoneal mass that contains intermediate SI components anteriorly (∗) that lose SI on the opposed-phase image owing to microscopic lipid content within the tumor. In **B**, low SI etching artifact *(arrows)* present between tumor components indicates the presence of a fat-water interface within the tumor. **C**, Coronal T2-WI shows multiple septated high SI foci within the lesion, with (∗) representing myxoid tissue that approaches the SI of the fluid in a right renal cyst (C). Tumor approached but did not invade the lower pole of the left kidney (K).

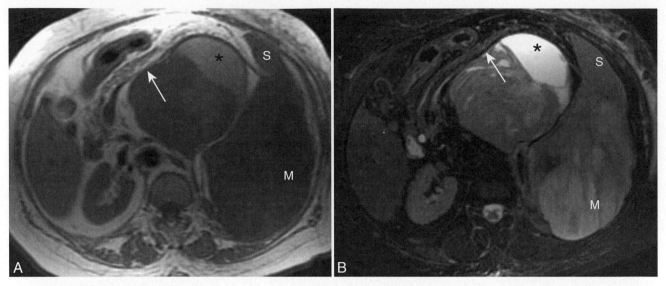

Figure 6-4 ▪ **MR illustration of an aggressive liposarcoma with dedifferentiated and myxoid components in an 81-year-old woman. A** and **B**, Axial T1-WI (**A**) and fat-suppressed T2-WI (**B**) show an infiltrative heterogeneous mass that displaces the pancreatic body and tail (*arrows*) anteriorly, confirming the retroperitoneal origin of the mass. Anteriorly within the tumor there is T1 and T2 hyperintense proteinaceous-hemorrhagic fluid (*). Low T1, high T2 SI components posterolaterally (M) adjacent to the spleen (S) likely represent myxomatous portions of the sarcoma. (*Continued*)

Leiomyosarcoma

Leiomyosarcoma (Box 6-4) is the second most common retroperitoneal sarcoma, accounting for approximately 30%.[6,14,37] Most leiomyosarcomas present in the fifth or sixth decades of life, and approximately two thirds of retroperitoneal leiomyosarcomas occur in women.[12,22] About half of all soft tissue leiomyosarcomas develop in the retroperitoneum, making it the single most common soft tissue site. Retroperitoneal leiomyosarcomas are typically well circumscribed,

have a mean diameter of 16 cm, and show intratumoral necrosis and hemorrhage. Adjacent organs are usually initially displaced without direct invasion, but commonly adjacent retroperitoneal structures do become involved by direct extension. Two thirds of retroperitoneal leiomyosarcomas are found in an extraluminal location relative to the inferior vena cava (IVC; Figs. 6-5 and 6-6), whereas approximately one third have both intraluminal and extraluminal components (Fig. 6-7). Leiomyosarcoma is the most common intraluminal venous neoplasm and is the most common primary tumor of the IVC.[22] The finding of a retroperitoneal mass which has both intraluminal and extraluminal components is highly suggestive of a leiomyosarcoma.[22]

The 5% of purely intraluminal caval leiomyosarcomas are very common in women (80% to 90% of patients) and present at a younger age (mean age of 50 years).[22,38] On imaging, the pure intracaval leiomyosarcomas are revealed as polypoid or nodular masses that are firmly attached to the vessel wall. They are smaller than those which are entirely extravascular, less likely to show intratumoral hemorrhage and necrosis, and most frequently located between the diaphragm and the renal veins (see Fig. 6-7). Leiomyosarcomas with an intraluminal component are more likely to produce early symptoms than those which are completely extraluminal. Patients with upper segment IVC involvement may develop symptoms and signs of Budd-Chiari syndrome (see Chapter 1). Lower extremity edema occurs when there is lower segment IVC involvement. Tumors that do not extend into or above the intrahepatic IVC are resectable, whereas tumors that

---

6-4   Features of Leiomyosarcoma

Clinical

Second most common retroperitoneal sarcoma (30%)
Most common intraluminal venous tumor
Peak age: 5th to 6th decades of life
M:F = 1:2–3 for retroperitoneal origin
M:F = 1:8–9 for IVC origin
Mean size = 16 cm
5-Year survival = 15%, resectable IVC tumor
    survival >50%

MRI

Solid, large, heterogeneous retroperitoneal mass
Suggestive features
    Intratumoral cystic necrosis: high T2-W SI that does
        not enhance
    Location in or around the IVC: one third of lesions
    Intratumoral hemorrhage: high T1-W SI

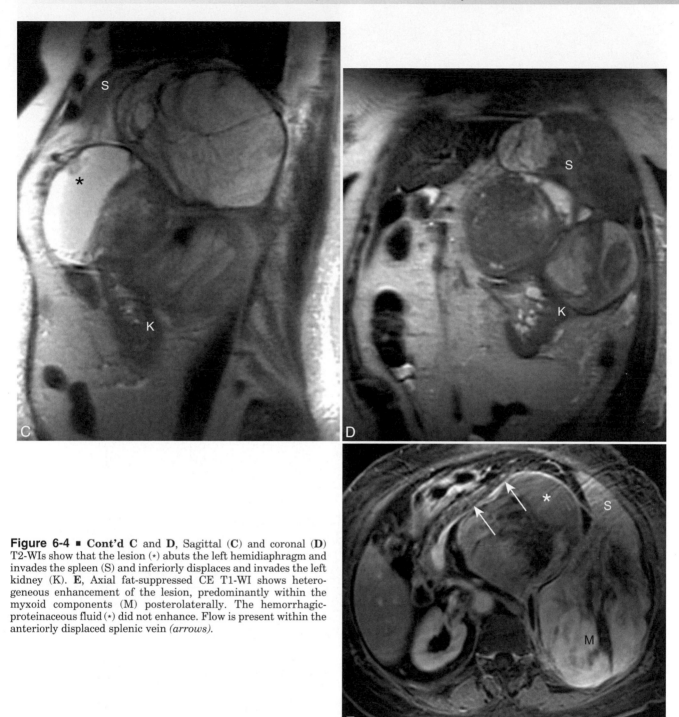

Figure 6-4 ■ Cont'd C and **D**, Sagittal (**C**) and coronal (**D**) T2-WIs show that the lesion (*) abuts the left hemidiaphragm and invades the spleen (S) and inferiorly displaces and invades the left kidney (K). **E**, Axial fat-suppressed CE T1-WI shows heterogeneous enhancement of the lesion, predominantly within the myxoid components (M) posterolaterally. The hemorrhagic-proteinaceous fluid (*) did not enhance. Flow is present within the anteriorly displaced splenic vein *(arrows)*.

infiltrate the intrahepatic IVC, hepatic veins, right atrium, and beyond are often unresectable.[7,22]

On MRI, leiomyosarcomas usually have low-intermediate SI on T1-WI and heterogeneous intermediate-high SI on T2-WI.[6,39] Foci of central liquefactive necrosis (which is more common and extensive compared with other sarcomas) show low SI on T1-WI and high SI on T2-WI (see Fig. 6-5).[6,22] Areas of hemorrhage typically appear with high SI

on T1-WI. Less commonly, a solid non-necrotic mass may be present, usually with smaller tumors. Leiomyosarcomas show variable enhancement that depends on their muscular and fibrous components and usually is delayed relative to the enhancement of the surrounding skeletal muscles.[39] Intraluminal bland thrombus and tumor thrombus can be differentiated with CE T1-WI, and findings that favor tumor thrombus include enlargement of the

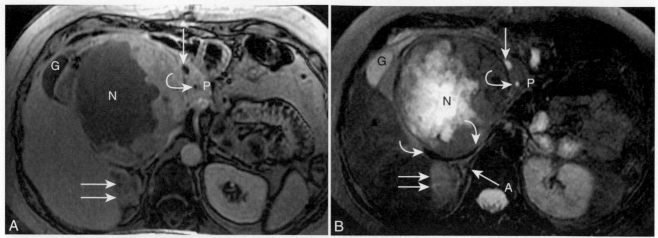

Figure 6-5 ■ **MR depiction of a high-grade retroperitoneal leiomyosarcoma with metastatic disease to the liver in a 57-year-old woman with pain and a palpable mass.** Aggressive tumors located adjacent to the IVC are suggestive of leiomyosarcoma. **A** and **B**, Axial CE T1-WI (**A**) and fat-suppressed T2-WI (**B**) show a large right retroperitoneal mass with central low T1, high T2 SI necrosis (N), and peripheral intermediate T2 SI enhancing tissue. The mass displaces the pancreatic head (P) to the left and the gallbladder (G) to the right. The common bile duct *(arrow)* and pancreatic duct *(curved arrow)* are depicted in cross-section. A second irregular enhancing mass *(double arrow)* within the posterior segment of the right lobe of the liver represents a hepatic metastasis. The IVC *(double curved white arrow)* is displaced posteriorly and extrinsically compressed but is not occluded, as revealed by a normal flow void in **B**. The right adrenal gland is present in its orthotopic location posterior to the IVC *(arrow A).* Thus, the mass does not originate from the adrenal gland.

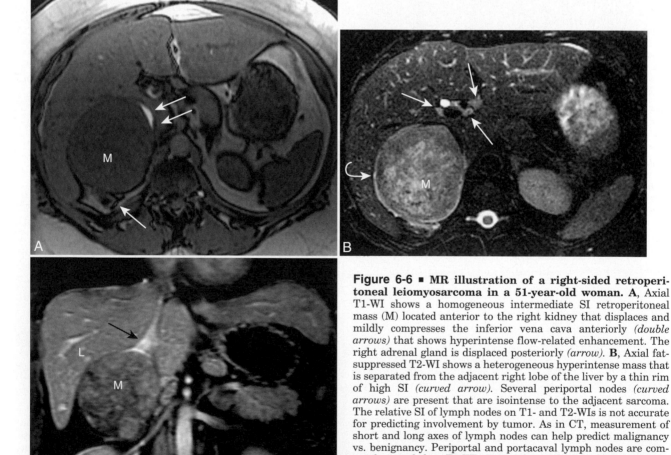

Figure 6-6 ■ **MR illustration of a right-sided retroperitoneal leiomyosarcoma in a 51-year-old woman. A,** Axial T1-WI shows a homogeneous intermediate SI retroperitoneal mass (M) located anterior to the right kidney that displaces and mildly compresses the inferior vena cava anteriorly *(double arrows)* that shows hyperintense flow-related enhancement. The right adrenal gland is displaced posteriorly *(arrow).* **B,** Axial fat-suppressed T2-WI shows a heterogeneous hyperintense mass that is separated from the adjacent right lobe of the liver by a thin rim of high SI *(curved arrow).* Several periportal nodes *(curved arrows)* are present that are isointense to the adjacent sarcoma. The relative SI of lymph nodes on T1- and T2-WIs is not accurate for predicting involvement by tumor. As in CT, measurement of short and long axes of lymph nodes can help predict malignancy vs. benignancy. Periportal and portacaval lymph nodes are commonly revealed on T2-WIs in patients with and without primary tumors. These nodes were not involved by sarcoma at surgery. **C,** Coronal fat-suppressed CE T1-WI shows that the heterogeneously enhancing mass is separate from the liver (L) and right kidney, inferiorly displaces the right kidney (K), and extrinsically compresses the inferior vena cava *(arrow).* At surgery, no hepatic or renal invasion was found.

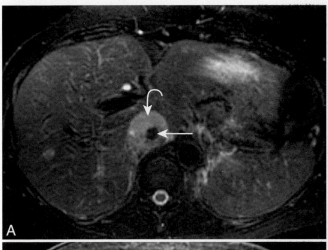

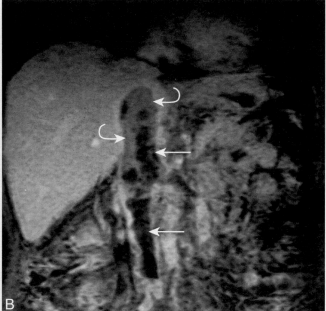

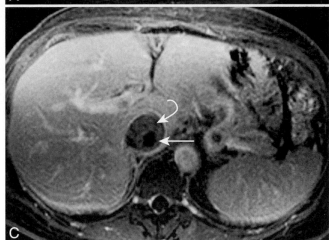

Figure 6-7 ■ **MR depiction of a primary leiomyosarcoma of the inferior vena cava (IVC) in a 62-year-old woman with abdominal pain and elevated creatinine. A,** Axial fat-suppressed T2-WI shows expansion of the intrahepatic IVC by hyperintense tumor thrombus peripherally *(curved arrow)* and intermediate SI bland thrombus centrally *(arrow).* **B** and **C,** Coronal **(B)** and axial **(C)** fat-suppressed CE T1-WIs show the cephalocaudal extent of the thrombus within both the intrahepatic and extrahepatic segments of the IVC. Tumor thrombus enhances *(curved arrows),* whereas bland thrombus does not enhance *(arrows).*

vascular lumen and enhancement of the thrombus (see Fig. 6-7).[6,22]

As for other retroperitoneal sarcomas, complete surgical removal is the treatment of choice of abdominopelvic leiomyosarcoma and is the most important factor affecting patient survival.[22,40,41] However, local recurrence after resection occurs in 40% to 75% of patients.[22] Retroperitoneal leiomyosarcomas have a poor prognosis and only an approximately 15% 5-year survival rate.[42] Many patients have either unresectable disease at the time of presentation secondary to infiltration of the intrahepatic IVC, hepatic veins, or right atrium, or metastatic disease, which is present in 40% of patients. Those women with resectable IVC leiomyosarcoma have the best outcome, with a 5-year survival rate of 68%.[43]

Malignant Fibrous Histiocytoma (MFH)

Malignant fibrous histiocytoma (MFH; Box 6-5) is the most common soft tissue sarcoma of late adult life, accounting for almost 25% of all soft-tissue sarcomas.[12,37] Only 15% arise in the retroperitoneum, and MFH is the third most common retroperitoneal

sarcoma after liposarcoma and leiomyosarcoma.[6] Most patients with MFH present between the sixth and eighth decades, and approximately two thirds of cases occur in men.[5,12]

Retroperitoneal MFH appears as a solitary, multilobulated, large mass often with hemorrhage and

---

6-5   Features of Malignant Fibrous Histiocytoma (MFH)

Clinical

Third most common retroperitoneal sarcoma (15%)
Most common adult soft tissue sarcoma
Peak age: 6th to 8th decades of life, M : F = 2 : 1

MRI

Suggestive features
Heterogeneous low, intermediate, and high SI on T2-WI ("bowl of fruit" sign) suggestive
Low SI calcifications on T2-WI, better shown on CT
Intratumoral hemorrhage: high SI on T1-WI

necrosis, sometimes with intratumoral calcification (Fig. 6-8). The most common histologic subtype is the storiform-pleomorphic MFH. The myxoid subtype of MFH is the second most common and is characterized by prominent myxoid stroma and a better prognosis.[12]

On MRI, MFH appears as a large, relatively well circumscribed mass that spreads along fascial planes and between muscle fibers, with low-intermediate SI on T1-WI and heterogeneously increased SI on T2-WI relative to muscle.[6] Intratumoral fat is absent. The "bowl of fruit" sign is a mosaic of mixed low,

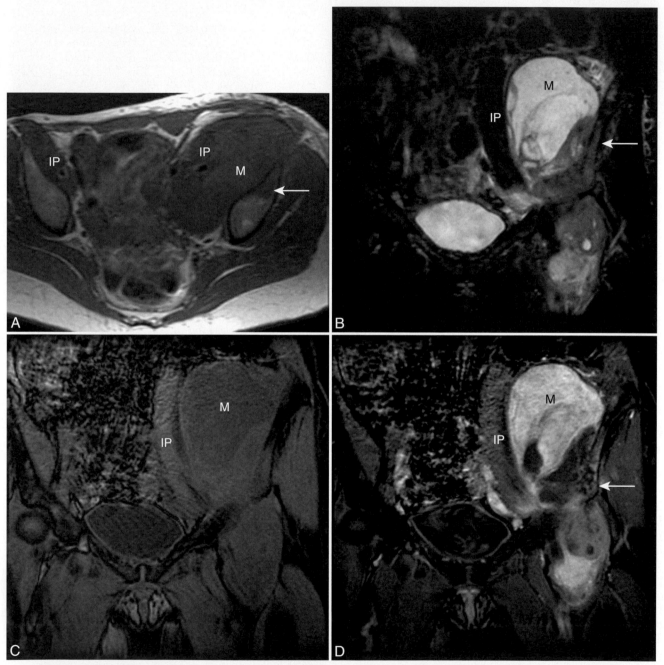

Figure 6-8 ■ MR depiction of invasive retroperitoneal malignant fibrous histiocytoma in a 50-year-old woman with pain and a palpable left lower quadrant mass. A, Axial T1-W SE image shows an infiltrative retroperitoneal mass (M) with intermediate SI relative to skeletal muscle. The mass displaces the left iliopsoas muscle (IP) and left common iliac vessels medially, and extends into the anterior aspect of the left ilio-ischial junction. Replaced fat of the left anterior acetabulum *(arrow)* suggests direct marrow infiltration by tumor. **B–D,** Coronal fat-suppressed T2-WI (**B**) and T1-WI obtained before (**C**) and after (**D**) contrast shows sarcoma extending through the femoral canal into the proximal left thigh. The superior and inferior portions of the lesion (M) are hypointense on T1, hyperintense on T2, and enhance, in keeping with myxoid tissue. The mass extrinsically displaces the left iliopsoas muscle (IP) medially. Heterogeneous T2 hyperintensity and enhancement of the left acetabulum and ilium *(arrows)* confirm marrow invasion by the sarcoma.

intermediate, and high SI on T2-WI that correlates to the presence of intratumoral solid components, cystic degeneration, hemorrhage, myxoid stroma, and fibrous tissue. While the "bowl of fruit" sign is commonly revealed in MFH, it is not specific, as it has been described in other tumors such as synovial sarcoma and Ewing's sarcoma, although these latter subtypes only very rarely occur in the retroperitoneum. Extensive intratumoral hemorrhage frequently occurs in MFH. However, most masses of MFH have nonhemorrhagic solid components, and thus most tumors can be differentiated from a bland benign hematoma. Intratumoral calcifications may be revealed in 20% of MFH lesions on CT but are more difficult to detect prospectively on MRI.[21,44]

PERITONEAL MESOTHELIOMA

Mesothelioma is a rare neoplasm that originates from mesothelial cells lining the serosal cavities of the body, with an incidence of 300 to 400 new cases per year in the U. S. The pleural lining is involved by mesothelioma two to five times more commonly than the peritoneum. Peritoneal mesothelioma (Box 6-6) is much less frequently associated with asbestosis or with tobacco use when compared with pleural mesothelioma.[12,45] As pleural mesothelioma frequently extends to the peritoneal cavity, spread from a primary pleural site must be excluded before mesothelioma of peritoneal origin is diagnosed.

On MRI, imaging findings are usually nonspecific and include peritoneal, mesenteric, or omental thickening, nodularity or mass formation, omental caking (often massive), intratumoral hemorrhage, diffuse peritoneal enhancement, adhesions, and ascites.[46-49] Tumor is present in greater amounts on the parietal peritoneal surfaces, since tumor cells are less adherent to visceral peritoneum lining peristaltic small bowel surfaces.[47] Management of malignant peritoneal mesothelioma typically involves cytoreductive surgery with extensive peritonectomy. Peri- and postoperative hyperthermic intraperitoneal chemotherapy is performed for palliation of debilitating ascites and offers some benefit for long-term survival. Patients have a median survival of 31 months, a 3-year survival rate of 56%, and a 5-year survival rate of 36%[45,50,51]

PRIMARY PERITONEAL CARCINOMA (PPC)

Primary peritoneal carcinoma (PPC; Box 6-7) is an uncommon malignancy that has an incidence of 7% in women initially thought to have ovarian cancer, and it is characterized by abdominopelvic carcinomatosis with no or minimal surface involvement of the ovaries.[52,53] PPC occurs predominantly in postmenopausal Caucasian women with a peak age in the seventh decade of life, one decade later in onset when compared with epithelial ovarian carcinoma.[54] Women with hereditary ovarian carcinoma have a 10-fold increased risk of PPC and need to be followed

---

6-6　Features of Malignant Peritoneal Mesothelioma

Clinical

Rare mesothelial neoplasm, peritoneal site 2–5 times less common than pleural site
Much less frequently associated with asbestos or tobacco use than pleural site
Peak age: 6th decade of life, F:M slightly >1:1
Treatment: cytoreductive surgery with extensive peritonectomy
Median survival of 31 months, 5-year survival = 36%

MRI

Nonspecific peritoneal, mesenteric, or omental thickening, nodularity or mass formation
Ascites and adhesions
Parietal peritoneum involvement > visceral peritoneum
Favorable prognosis
   Small tumor nodules preferentially involving greater omentum
   Free ascites
   Absent or minimal small bowel and mesenteric involvement
Poor prognosis
   Large soft tissue dissemination over peritoneal surfaces
   Entrapment and clumping of small bowel segments

6-7　Features of Primary Peritoneal Carcinoma (PPC)

Clinical

Approximately 7% of all cases of initially suspected epithelial ovarian carcinoma
Peak age: 7th decade of life, F:M >> 1:1
Histologic: papillary serous cystadenocarcinoma in >95%
Ovarian involvement is absent or minimal secondary to spread to surface
Treatment: cytoreductive surgery and combination chemotherapy (similar to ovarian cancer)
Median survival of 12–25 months, 5-year survival = 0% to 25%
Prognosis similar to or worse than for advanced ovarian carcinoma

MRI

Nonspecific imaging features
Peritoneal, mesenteric, and omental nodules or masses
Diffuse peritoneal nodular thickening and enhancement
Extensive peritoneal calcification in 85% on CT, less accurately revealed on MRI
Ascites
Ovaries of normal size
Lack of another visualized primary site of neoplasm

even after prophylactic oophorectomy.[54,55] There are two theories concerning the etiology of PPC. The tumor may originate from malignant degeneration of nests of ovarian tissue remnants left within the peritoneum during embryonic gonadal migration. Alternatively, PPC may arise from a secondary mesodermal müllerian system in the peritoneal mesothelium.[56-58]

Symptoms and signs when present tend to be nonspecific, mild, and similar to those of patients with epithelial ovarian carcinoma. Histologically, PPC is similar to the papillary serous subtype of epithelial ovarian carcinoma in more than 95% of cases.[54,58] On MRI, imaging findings include ascites; peritoneal, mesenteric, and omental nodules or masses, sometimes with omental caking; and diffuse peritoneal nodular thickening and enhancement. The presence of normal ovaries excludes a diagnosis of primary ovarian carcinoma.[52,53] The surgical staging and treatment of PPC are similar to those of epithelial ovarian carcinoma (see Chapter 7).

PSEUDOMYXOMA PERITONEI

The term pseudomyxoma peritonei, or "false mucinous tumor of the peritoneum," has been used historically as a pathologic diagnostic term to describe any benign or malignant condition that results in intraperitoneal mucin accumulation.[59,60] However, pseudomyxoma peritonei should be used strictly as a clinical descriptor for patients with mucinous ascites that originates from a primary appendiceal mucinous adenoma with pathologic features of disseminated peritoneal adenomucinosis (DPAM), as opposed to peritoneal mucinous carcinomatosis (PMCA) that originates from a mucinous adenocarcinoma from one of many potential sites.[59-61]

Pseudomyxoma peritonei (corresponding to DPAM pathologically; Box 6-8) is a rare condition that

occurs twice as often in men than in women, with a peak age in the sixth decade, and is found in approximately 2 of 10,000 laparotomies.[60-62] Pseudomyxoma peritonei has an indolent clinical course, and the peritoneal lesions only rarely change morphologically over time.[60] Although the ovaries and gastrointestinal tract were thought to be potential sites of origin, histologic and molecular genetic studies have shown that DPAM originates from mucinous adenomas of the appendix.[60] Coexistent ovarian mucinous tumor implants are often present, tend to be small and superficial, and are either bilateral or right-sided.[59,60,63]

Pseudomyxoma peritonei starts with a primary appendiceal mucinous adenoma that progressively grows within the appendiceal lumen. This eventually occludes the lumen, causing distention and eventual rupture, with subsequent spread of mucus-containing epithelial cells from the adenoma to the peritoneal cavity over time.[59] Thus, peritoneal dissemination usually occurs before lymphatic or vascular spread, and as such, lymph node metastases and parenchymal metastases are extremely unusual.[64] Moving peritoneal surfaces such as the visceral peritoneum tend to be sparsely seeded, whereas abdominal surfaces that absorb peritoneal fluid, such as the greater and lesser omenta and the undersurfaces of the hemidiaphragms, are often coated by tumor cells.[59,64] The other mechanism of tumor redistribution is gravity, and as such, free-floating intraperitoneal tumor cells tend to accumulate within the dependent aspects of the peritoneal cavity including the pouch of Douglas, Morrison's pouch (the hepatorenal space), the left abdominal gutter, and the fossa created by the ligament of Treitz.

On MRI, early pseudomyxoma peritonei may appear as loculated mucinous ascites and mucinous tumor implants in the peritoneal cavity, with intermediate SI on T1-WI, high SI on T2-WI, and relative sparing of a centrally compartmentalized normal caliber small bowel and mesentery.[59,63,65,66] An omental cake is characteristically present with small areas of residual omental fat remaining, and the undersurfaces of the hemidiaphragms (predominantly on the right) may appear greatly thickened by large cystic masses of mucinous tumor with scalloping of the contour of the liver.[59,63] Identification of the primary appendiceal mucinous adenoma usually is not possible, because it is difficult to distinguish it from the large amount of mucinous tumor in the abdomen and pelvis.[59] Metastatic lymphadenopathy and parenchymal metastases are absent.[63]

Treatment of pseudomyxoma peritonei includes peritonectomy and intraoperative intraperitoneal chemotherapy with curative intent.[59,60] Those patients with appendiceal adenoma should undergo evaluation of the entire colon, since there is a strong association with synchronous or metachronous colorectal adenoma and carcinoma.[67] Overall, the 5-year and 10-year survival rates of treated patients are up to 90% and 68%, respectively, with a mean survival of 112 months. Although pseudomyxoma peritonei is not biologically aggressive, since it does not invade or

---

| 6-8 | Features of Pseudomyxoma Peritonei |

Clinical

Old definition: mucinous ascites of benign or malignant etiology

New definition: mucinous ascites due to rupture of a benign primary mucinous appendiceal adenoma

Rare

Peak age: 5th decade of life, M:F = 2:1

Treatment: peritonectomy and intraoperative chemotherapy

5-Year and 10-year survival after successful treatment = 90% and 68%, respectively

MRI

Loculated mucinous ascites with intermediate SI on T1-WI and high SI on T2-WI

Scalloping of parenchymal organs often present

Lymphadenopathy and distant metastases absent

Primary appendiceal mucinous adenoma usually is not visualized but if revealed suggests diagnosis

metastasize, it is fatal if untreated, because the space of the abdomen and pelvis for nutritional function becomes replaced by mucinous tumor.[59]

PERITONEAL MUCINOUS CARCINOMATOSIS (PMCA)

With peritoneal mucinous carcinomatosis (PMCA), a primary mucinous adenocarcinoma most commonly originates within the ovary, appendix, colon, or small bowel, leading to intraperitoneal spread of tumor. In contradistinction to true pseudomyxoma peritonei (or DPAM), malignant metastatic implants may be adherent to peritoneal surfaces, including the visceral peritoneum of the small bowel, with frequent associated lymph node involvement, parenchymal organ infiltration, and distant metastatic disease outside the peritoneal cavity (Fig. 6-9).[59,60,62]

On imaging, the primary site of tumor should be determined and also lymphadenopathy, distant metastatic disease, and extent of small bowel or mesenteric involvement sought, since all are associated with decreased patient survival.[59,68,69]

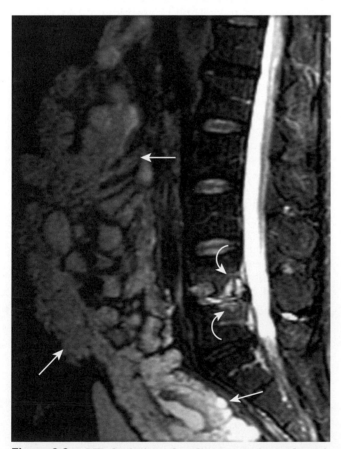

Figure 6-9 ■ MR depiction of malignant peritoneal mucinous adenocarcinomatosis. Sagittal T2-WI shows multiple loculated hyperintense peritoneal masses *(arrows)* representing metastatic mucinous adenocarcinoma of the appendix. This image also depicts diskitis of L4–L5, with adjacent endplate infection *(curved arrows)*.

Imaging findings that predict incomplete cytoreduction most reliably are tumor greater than 5 cm on the small bowel and mesentery in the jejunum and proximal ileum, and segmental obstruction of the small bowel.[59,68,69] The 5-year and 10-year survival rates for patients undergoing treatment for mucinous peritoneal carcinomatosis are 50% and 21%, respectively, with a mean survival time of 46 months.[60] (See Chapter 7 for a more detailed discussion of ovarian carcinoma.)

INTRA-ABDOMINAL DESMOPLASTIC SMALL ROUND CELL TUMOR (DSRCT)

Intra-abdominal desmoplastic small round cell tumor (DSRCT; Box 6-9) is a rare aggressive malignant neoplasm that typically involves the peritoneum, omentum, and mesentery of young men.[12,70] The exact nature and cell of origin of this tumor is still uncertain, although some believe that it originates from mesothelial or submesothelial cells.[12,71,72] Most patients with DSRCT are in the second through fourth decades of life, and men are affected five times more commonly than women.[73-75]

On MRI, the most characteristic imaging finding is that of multiple infiltrative soft-tissue masses without an organ-based primary site located within the intraperitoneal, omental, mesenteric, or perivesical sites. The lesions of DSRCT can reveal a relatively specific but insensitive pattern of hypointense masses on TI- and T2-WI that show minimal enhancement, reflecting the histologic findings of densely packed cellularity of small cells and the desmoplastic stroma.[70,71,74,76] The mean diameter of each of the soft-tissue masses is 5 cm (range of 2 to 12 cm) with a mean of four to five mass lesions occurring per patient (range of 1 to 17).[74] Ascites or distant metastatic disease is present in half of patients at the time of imaging.[71,74] The treatment of patients with DSRCT

6-9 Features of Intra-abdominal Desmoplastic Small Round Cell Tumor (DSRCT)

Clinical
Rare, highly aggressive malignant neoplasm
Peak age: 2nd to 4th decades of life, M:F = 5:1
Poor prognosis, median survival of 17-32 months

MRI
Classic appearance: multiple infiltrative soft-tissue masses of the peritoneum, omentum, and/or mesentery without an organ-based primary
Mean size of each mass = 5 cm, mean number of masses present = 4-5
Low SI masses on T1-WI and T2-WI due to densely packed, small round cells and desmoplastic stroma
High SI on T1-WI and T2-WI possibly present due to intratumoral hemorrhage or necrosis
Ascites or distant metastatic disease in 50%

typically consists of a multimodality approach, including aggressive surgical resection, combination chemotherapy, and external radiotherapy. Complete excision often is impossible owing to the extent of infiltrative disease.[12,71,77] DSRCT has an extremely poor prognosis, with a median survival of approximately 17 to 32 months.[71,72]

PRIMARY RETROPERITONEAL EXTRAGONADAL GERM CELL TUMOR (EGCT)

The primary retroperitoneal extragonadal germ cell tumor (EGCT; Box 6-10) represents from 1% to 3% of all germ cell tumors and occurs most commonly within the mediastinum and slightly less commonly within the retroperitoneum.[78,79] Primary EGCTs occur more commonly in men than women, with a peak age in the fourth and fifth decades, which is a slightly older age group than that of patients with primary testicular germ cell neoplasms.[6,78,79]

Primary retroperitoneal EGCTs are hypothesized to arise from primordial midline germ cell remnants of the genital ridge that failed to migrate properly.[6,78] An alternative etiology is that primary EGCTs are related synchronously or metachronously to an occult gonadal germ cell tumor (carcinoma in situ or "burned-out" tumor).[78,80,81] Since most retroperitoneal germ cell tumors are metastases from primary testicular tumors, careful clinical and imaging evaluation should be performed in affected men to exclude a coexistent primary testicular neoplasm.[78] Grossly, seminomas (accounting for 15% of EGCTs) are usually homogeneous lobulated masses, whereas mixed and nonseminomatous tumors are heterogeneous with solid and cystic areas, necrosis, and hemorrhage.[78,79]

Seminomatous EGCTs are not associated with elevated tumor markers, whereas most nonseminomatous EGCTs are associated with elevated levels of serum α-fetoprotein (correlating with components of yolk sac tumor or embryonal carcinoma) or human chorionic gonadotropin (correlating with components of choriocarcinoma). Serial levels of tumor markers correlate with the clinical course and therapeutic response, and high levels are associated with a poor survival rate.[78]

On MRI, primary retroperitoneal EGCTs typically appear as large (average size of 7 to 8 cm), midline retroperitoneal masses of low-intermediate SI on T1-WI and intermediate-high SI on T2-WI, sometimes with areas of central high SI on T2-WI.[6] Seminomatous EGCTs tend to be more homogeneous in SI, whereas mixed and nonseminomatous EGCTs tend to be more heterogeneous in SI, with areas of cystic necrosis or hemorrhage.[82] A midline location of a retroperitoneal mass is probably the most helpful finding to suggest this diagnosis, whereas metastatic retroperitoneal lymphadenopathy from a primary testicular neoplasm tends to be lateral and paramedian in location.[6,78] The prognosis and treatment of primary retroperitoneal EGCT are similar to those of primary testicular neoplasms with retroperitoneal metastases (see Chapter 8).[83]

6-10   Features of Primary Retroperitoneal Extragonadal Germ Cell Tumor (EGCT)

Clinical

Peak age: 4th to 5th decades of life, M:F >1:1
Less common than secondary metastatic disease from a primary gonadal tumor
Histologic classification
Seminomatous (15%); usually not associated with elevated tumor markers
Nonseminomatous and mixed (85%); associated with elevated tumor markers
Treatment and prognosis: similar to that of metastatic spread of primary testicular tumor of similar histologic features
Poor prognostic factors
Nonseminomatous histologic features
   Nonpulmonary visceral metastases
   Elevated hCG levels
Overall survival = 65% (88% vs. 63% for seminomatous vs. nonseminomatous subtypes)

MRI

Large midline retroperitoneal mass (secondary EGCT tends to be located off the midline)
Average size = 7–8 cm
Similar SI and enhancement characteristics to primary gonadal germ cell tumors
Seminomatous tumors: homogeneous
Nonseminomatous and mixed tumors
   Heterogeneous
   Cystic change/necrosis (high SI on T2-WI without enhancement)
   Intratumoral hemorrhage (high SI on T1-WI)

CARCINOID TUMOR

Carcinoid tumors (Box 6-11) are slow-growing neuroendocrine neoplasms derived from endocrine amine precursor uptake and decarboxylation (APUD) cells that comprise 2% of all gastrointestinal tumors.[84-86] Most carcinoid tumors (75% to 85%) arise in the gastrointestinal tract, with approximately 10% to 20% arising in the lungs (bronchial carcinoid) and the remainder in other organs.[84,87,88] Of gastrointestinal carcinoid tumors, the appendix is the most common site (up to 40%), the small bowel is the second most common site (up to 20%, most in the ileum), and the rectum is the third most common site (approximately 13%).[85,87,89,90] Carcinoid tumor is the second most common malignant small bowel neoplasm (30%), following adenocarcinoma, and up to one third may be multiple.[87,90] Although it is not a primary malignancy of the mesentery, the initial abdominal imaging findings of carcinoid are often those of mesenteric nodal metastases and thus are addressed in this chapter.

6-11   Features of Carcinoid Tumor

Clinical

Slow-growing neuroendocrine neoplasm with malignant potential
85% originate in gastrointestinal tract
Three most common locations in decreasing frequency:
  Appendix: often incidental diagnosis at appendectomy
  Distal small bowel
  Rectum
Second most common small bowel malignancy
Four most common types in decreasing frequency
  Adenocarcinoma
  Carcinoid
  Lymphoma

Malignant Gastrointestinal Stromal Tumor

Peak age: 5th to 6th decades of life
M:F = 1:1 (1:2 for appendiceal carcinoid tumors)
Most are asymptomatic

Carcinoid Syndrome

Develops in 10% due to circulation of serotonin or other humoral substances beyond the portal vein
Associated with hepatic metastases, large volume disease, or large small bowel primary tumor
Carcinoid heart occurs in one third to two thirds, with a mortality rate of approximately 50%

Metastases

Mesenteric lymph nodes, most common
Liver, second most common
Rare in tumors <1 cm, common in tumors >2 cm
Treatment
  Surgical resection of primary tumor and resectable lymphadenopathy and hepatic metastases
  Palliative hepatic chemoembolization or cryoablation of unresectable hepatic metastases
  Octreotide or ^{131}I-MIBG for symptomatic carcinoid syndrome
5-Year survival
  >90% for localized disease
  20% to 30% for unresectable disease, hepatic metastases, or carcinoid syndrome
  Appendiceal and rectal primary sites have the best prognosis

MRI

Primary tumor: two patterns
  Well-defined nodular mass, intermediate SI on T1-WI, intermediate-high SI on T2-WI, and intense early
    enhancement
  Regional bowel wall thickening, intermediate SI on T1-WI and T2-WI, intense early enhancement
Primary tumor often not detected at imaging
Mesenteric metastases
  Not the primary tumor but regional malignant lymphadenopathy
  Stellate appearance, intermediate SI on T1-WI and T2-WI with intense enhancement
  Calcification: 70% on CT, less accurately detected on MRI
  Associated mesenteric retraction with bowel wall thickening or tethering
Hepatic metastases
  Often hypervascular with early arterial phase enhancement

Carcinoid tumor has a mean age of presentation in the fifth and sixth decades and occurs equally in men and women.[88,91] Appendiceal carcinoids present in a younger patient population than do other gastrointestinal carcinoid tumors, with a peak age at the beginning of the fifth decade of life, occur twice as commonly in women as in men, and are usually incidentally diagnosed at appendectomy.[86,87,89,92,93] However, jejuno-ileal carcinoids usually present at an advanced stage with hepatic metastases and differ from other gastrointestinal tract carcinoid tumors in their presentation.[89]

The symptoms and signs of localized abdominal carcinoid tumor when present are nonspecific.[90] Carcinoid syndrome is a more specific presentation of carcinoid tumor that occurs in approximately 10% of patients whose tumor metabolites have extended beyond the liver. Carcinoid syndrome is caused by a variety of humoral substances, predominantly serotonin, which are produced by tumor cells and secreted into the systemic venous circulation beyond the level of the portal venous circulation.[88] Patients may have watery diarrhea, paroxysmal flushing, asthma-like wheezing, or right-sided heart failure ("carcinoid heart"). Carcinoid heart disease occurs in one to two thirds of those with carcinoid syndrome and has a mortality rate of approximately 50%.[94] Anatomic changes of the heart that result in failure include endocardial fibroelastosis with valvular stenoses or tricuspid regurgitation.[88,91,95]

Metastatic disease is commonly present at initial presentation, approaching 90% in some series, especially with jejuno-ileal and colonic carcinoid tumors.[85,86] The most common sites of carcinoid tumor metastases are the lymph nodes, liver, and lung.[87,88] Secondary mesenteric involvement by carcinoid tumors is common, occurring in approximately two thirds of patients, and is almost always due to metastatic disease from a primary small bowel carcinoid tumor beyond the ligament of Treitz.[89,96] The size of the primary tumor is the most reliable determinant of the risk of metastatic disease. For example, less than 10% of carcinoid tumors smaller than 1 cm are associated with malignant lymphadenopathy or hepatic metastases, whereas more than 80% of carcinoid tumors larger than 2 cm are associated with metastatic disease.[89,97]

On MRI, primary gastrointestinal carcinoid tumors may appear as either well-defined nodular masses or regional relatively uniform areas of bowel wall thickening. The pattern of a well-defined nodular mass tends to have homogeneous intermediate SI on T1-WI, intermediate-high in SI on T2-WI, and intense early enhancement on CE T1-WI (see Fig. 2-22), whereas the pattern of regional bowel wall thickening tends to have intermediate SI on both T1- and T2-WI with intense homogeneous enhancement. Both patterns are difficult to detect, but in both cases delayed fat-suppressed CE T1-WI may reveal moderate enhancement, probably due to a large interstitial space. It is likely more common that an MRI examination will not reveal the primary tumor but only metastatic disease of the mesenteric nodes or liver. In a series of CT examinations of 52 patients with midgut carcinoid tumors, no discrete primary tumors were revealed and only 9 showed nonspecific small bowel thickening.[98]

Mesenteric metastases appear as a stellate soft tissue mass with intermediate SI on T1- and T2-WI and moderate intense enhancement on delayed CE T1-WI.[86] Calcification, present in up to 70% on CT, is often difficult to characterize on MRI, but when revealed appears as foci of very low SI on T1- and T2-WI.[96] Thin linear spicules that extend into the surrounding mesentery in a stellate or spoke-wheel configuration with low SI on T1- and T2-WI and mesenteric retraction are also characteristic (Fig. 6-10).[84,86,96] The soft tissue stranding represents a desmoplastic reaction to the humoral effects of hormonally active substances, particularly serotonin, secreted by the carcinoid tumors.[96] Peritoneal metastases have intermediate SI on T1-WI, intermediate-high SI on T2-WI,

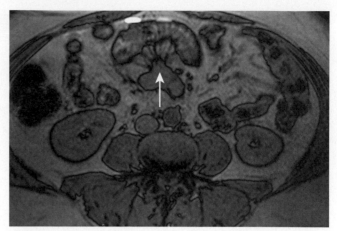

Figure 6-10 ■ Spiculated mesenteric mass of metastatic carcinoid as revealed on MR. Axial T1-WI shows a spiculated mesenteric mass *(arrow)* adjacent to the mesenteric border of a distal small bowel segment. It is not uncommon for cross-sectional imaging to reveal mesenteric masses of malignant carcinoid but fail to reveal the primary distal small bowel tumor.

and moderate-marked enhancement on early CE T1-WI.[86] Hepatic metastases also tend to be hypervascular, often enhancing avidly on the arterial phase of CE T1-WI, and show typical T2-W SI of metastatic disease similar to that of spleen.[85,99] Mesenteric and peritoneal metastases are best depicted on delayed fat-suppressed CE T1-WI.[86]

The treatment of carcinoid tumor is directed at prevention of tumor growth and symptom control.[85,89,93] Surgical resection is the treatment of choice for primary carcinoid tumors and in patients with resectable metastatic disease.[89,100,101] If hepatic metastases are present at the time of diagnosis, the primary tumor is still resected to avoid complications of bowel obstruction, bleeding, and perforation. Hepatic arterial chemoembolization can be used for palliation if there is diffuse liver involvement and severe symptomatology of carcinoid syndrome.[85,89,101] Treatment with octreotide or other somatostatin analogues provides symptomatic relief in carcinoid syndrome, although no associated significant improvement in survival or tumor size has been demonstrated.[93,101,102]

In the absence of metastatic disease, complete resection of localized carcinoid tumors results in 5-year survival rates of greater than 90%.[87,91,92] However, patients with unresectable disease or hepatic metastases at diagnosis have a 30% 5-year survival rate and a 21% 5-year survival rate if carcinoid syndrome is present at diagnosis.[87,92,94] The 5-year survival is excellent for appendiceal (86%) and rectal (72%) carcinoids, since they have lower propensities to metastasize, whereas jejuno-ileal (55%) carcinoids have a less favorable prognosis.[87,89,92]

ABDOMINAL PARAGANGLIOMA

Paragangliomas sometimes called extra-adrenal pheochromocytomas (see Chapter 3 for adrenal pheochromocytomas) are rare neurogenic tumors that arise from specialized neural crest cells called paraganglia which are symmetrically distributed along the aortic axis in close association with the sympathetic chain in the abdomen, pelvis, chest, and neck. The largest collection of paraganglia includes the paired organs of Zuckerkandl that overlie the aorta at the level of the inferior mesenteric artery and have an uncertain physiologic role. Paraganglia are prominent during early infancy and regress after 12 to 18 months.[6,12] Ten percent to 20% of paragangliomas are extra-adrenal in location, and most extra-adrenal paragangliomas arise in the retroperitoneum from the organs of Zuckerkandl, with only a few tumors developing at other locations along the aorta or its branch vessels.[6,12,103,104]

Patients with paragangliomas present in the fourth and fifth decades, with men and women affected equally, although malignant paragangliomas may sometimes arise in younger patients.[12,103,105] Occasionally, paragangliomas may be multicentric, particularly if there is a family history of paraganglioma, or may be associated with other tumors such as gastric malignant gastrointestinal stromal tumors (GIST) and pulmonary chondromas as a component of Carney's syndrome.[104,106] Up to 40% of extra-adrenal paragangliomas are malignant (vs. 10% for pheochromocytoma), as manifested by metastatic spread or locally aggressive behavior, and approximately 10% of patients have with metastatic disease.[12,107] The malignant potential and biological behavior of a paraganglioma cannot be determined from its histologic appearance.[108] Paraganglioma may spread hematogenously or via the lymphatics; the most common sites of metastatic disease are lymph nodes, bone, lung, and liver.[108,109]

Paragangliomas may be considered as functional or nonfunctional, depending on whether catecholamines are secreted. Nonfunctional extra-adrenal abdominal paragangliomas (Box 6-12) present with nonspecific symptoms and signs and are rarely definitively diagnosed prior to surgery. However, functional extra-adrenal paragangliomas cause symptoms and signs similar to pheochromocytomas in 25% to 60% of patients, including chronic or intermittent hypertension, headaches, and palpitations. In affected patients, detection of elevated urinary catecholamines can establish an earlier preoperative diagnosis.[12,103] There is poor correlation between the functional activity of the tumor and the degree of malignancy, however.[12]

On MRI, SI and enhancement characteristics of paragangliomas are similar to those of pheochromocytoma (Fig. 6-11).[6] The masses generally have low-intermediate SI on T1-WI and moderately high SI on T2-WI and are commonly heterogeneous secondary to foci of intratumoral necrosis or hemorrhage, as is revealed at gross pathology.[12,110] Progressive enhancement is present on portal and delayed phases of CE T1-WI; arterial-phase enhancement is variable.[111] Functional paragangliomas are smaller than nonfunctional paragangliomas (mean size of 7 cm vs. 12 cm, respectively).[103,109,112]

6-12 **Features of Abdominal Paraganglioma**

Clinical

10% to 20% of all pheochromocytomas
Common location: organ of Zuckerkandl
Peak age: 4th to 5th decades of life, M:F = 1:1
Gross pathology: heterogeneous solid and/or cystic lesion with necrosis and hemorrhage
Functional tumors (60%) are smaller than nonfunctional lesions (mean size of 7 cm vs. 12 cm, respectively)
Multicentric in 10%
Malignant in 40% (vs. 10% for pheochromocytoma)
Laboratory diagnosis: Elevated urine catecholamines
Treatment: complete surgical resection of primary and localized metastases
5-Year survival = 80%

MRI

SI and enhancement characteristics are similar to those of pheochromocytoma
T1-WI: low SI except for potentially high SI intratumoral hemorrhage
T2-WI: heterogeneous intermediate-high SI, may have low SI foci of coagulative necrosis
Heterogeneous progressive enhancement, intratumoral cysts, and necrosis do not enhance

---

Although malignant paragangliomas tend to be large, necrotic, and poorly marginated, these features also may be present in benign paragangliomas. Furthermore, the SI characteristics and degree of heterogeneity cannot differentiate benign from malignant paragangliomas. As such, the only definitive imaging criterion of malignancy is the presence of metastatic disease.[12,103,110] Complete surgical resection is the treatment of choice for the management of extra-adrenal abdominal paraganglioma, and adjunctive therapies including radiotherapy,[131] I-MIBG, and chemotherapy are considered palliative.[104,108] Surgical resection of localized metastatic disease may also be performed, especially if solitary.[108] If an abdominal paraganglioma is suspected clinically, assessment of the functional activity should be performed prior to surgery. Patients with functional tumors are premedicated with α-blockers to avoid intra-operative hypertensive crises during surgical manipulation of the tumor.[12,113] Overall, the 5-year survival rate may reach 82% for those with abdominal paraganglioma.[107] Extended follow-up is recommended owing to the high propensity for subsequent metastasis, long natural history of the disease, and limitations of histopathologic criteria in predicting malignant behavior.[108] Overall, biological behavior of the tumor is the most important prognostic factor.[12]

RETROPERITONEAL GANGLIONEUROMA

Ganglioneuromas (Box 6-13) are uncommon benign neurogenic tumors that arise from sympathetic ganglia,

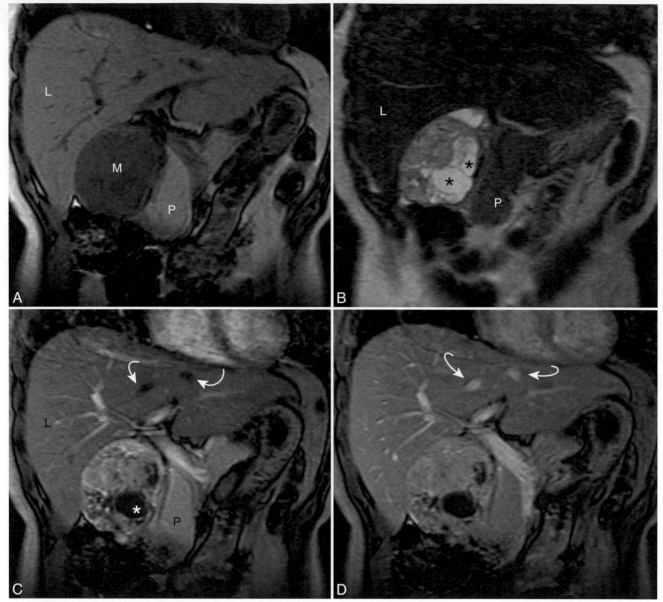

Figure 6-11 ■ MR depiction of a primary retroperitoneal paraganglioma in an asymptomatic 35-year-old woman. A and **B,** Coronal T1-WI (**A**) and T2-WI (**B**) show a well-circumscribed retroperitoneal mass (M) that abuts the right lobe of the liver (L) and the pancreatic head (P) and has heterogeneous low-intermediate T1 and intermediate-to-high T2 SI relative to skeletal muscle. Very T2 hyperintense foci (∗) represent intratumoral cysts or necrosis. **C** and **D,** Coronal arterial (**C**) and portal venous phase (**D**) CE T1-WIs show moderate heterogeneous enhancement of the solid components of the mass. The intratumoral T2 hyperintense foci do not enhance. (∗) The hepatic veins *(curved arrows)* enhance during the portal phase (**D**) but not the arterial phase (**C**) of dynamic imaging.

representing 1% to 2% of all primary retroperitoneal tumors. Ganglioneuromas are three times as common as neuroblastomas.[12,114,115] Ganglioneuromas occur slightly more commonly in women than in men at a ratio of 1.5 to 1, most commonly in the first through fifth decades, with a mean age at diagnosis of 7 years. The posterior mediastinum and retroperitoneum are the two most common locations for ganglioneuroma (80% of lesions).[114-117] Although some ganglioneuromas arise from maturation of neuroblastomas and ganglioneuroblastomas, the majority arise de novo.[12,117]

Most patients with ganglioneuromas are asymptomatic. Otherwise, abdominal pain or a palpable abdominal mass are the most frequent symptoms and signs.[114] Most patients have normal levels of urinary catecholamines.[118] Some hormonally active ganglioneuromas produce catecholamines and patients may have similar signs and symptoms to those of paraganglioma or carcinoid tumor.[116] Secretion of androgenic hormones leading to virilization may also occur with some tumors.[119,120]

Ganglioneuroma are well-circumscribed, encapsulated, benign neoplasms composed of mature Schwann

6-13   Features of Retroperitoneal Ganglioneuroma

Clinical

Rare, benign sympathetic neurogenic tumor
Peak age: 1st decade of life (mean age of 7 years), rare in adults, F:M = 1.5:1
Most arise de novo, some from maturation of neuroblastomas and ganglioneuroblastomas
Weak association with elevated catecholamine or androgenic hormone levels
Treatment: complete surgical resection when symptomatic, conservative approach for some
Prognosis excellent, recurrence rare

MRI

Well-defined retroperitoneal soft tissue mass, infrequently extends into neural foramina
Mean size = 8 cm
Low SI on T1-WI, intermediate-high SI with intratumoral hemorrhage
Intermediate-high SI on T2-WI without intratumoral cysts
Occasionally a whorled appearance on T2-WI
Very low SI punctate calcifications, better detected at CT in 60%
Gradual progressive enhancement
Metastatic disease may be present with ganglioneuroblastoma and neuroblastoma but not with ganglioneuroma

cells, scattered mature ganglion cells, and variable amounts of myxoid stroma and collagen.[12,115,117] On imaging, retroperitoneal ganglioneuromas are well-defined longitudinally oriented masses that are lobulated or oval in shape (Fig. 6-12). Ganglioneuromas that are posterior usually do not result in osseous changes and only infrequently extend into the neural foramina.[114,115,121] Ganglioneuromas have a mean size of 8 cm. Partial or complete encasement of blood vessels without luminal compromise may be present.[119,121]

Ganglioneuromas generally have low SI on T1-WI and intermediate-high SI on T2-WI (see Fig. 6-12).[116,121] Mixed intermediate-high SI on T1-WI may be present if hemorrhagic components are present.[115,119] SI on T2-WI is influenced by the proportion of myxoid stroma to cellular components and collagen fibers.[115] Intermediate T2 SI occurs when there is an abundance of cellular components and collagen fibers relative to myxoid stroma, while high T2 SI is revealed in tumors with a large amount of myxoid stroma with relatively few cellular components and collagen fibers.[115] Occasionally, a whorled appearance may be present on T1- or T2-WI secondary to interlacing bundles of Schwann cells and collagen fibers.[21,115] Unlike in schwannomas, cystic degeneration is not present.[115,122] Calcifications are present in half of tumors at CT, tend to be discrete and punctate as opposed to amorphous and coarse in the neuroblastoma, and may appear as low SI foci on T1- and

T2-WIs when visualized.[116,117,119,123] Ganglioneuromas show gradual progressive enhancement. Since the imaging characteristics of ganglioneuroma overlap with those of ganglioneuroblastoma and neuroblastoma, differentiation on MRI is not possible unless metastatic disease is present.[117]

Generally, management of retroperitoneal ganglioneuromas involves complete surgical resection when possible, particularly if the patient is symptomatic owing to large size or hormonal secretion, although some advocate a more conservative approach.[12,117] The prognosis is excellent, and recurrence after surgical resection is rare, but periodic imaging surveillance is advised following resection.[117,120]

ABDOMINAL SCHWANNOMA

Schwannomas (Box 6-14) are benign tumors of nerve sheaths of peripheral nerves that account for up to 4% of all retroperitoneal tumors and are only rarely located within the omenta or mesentery. Schwannomas are most frequently located within the head and neck region and flexor surfaces of the extremities.[12,124-126] Schwannomas occur most often in the third through sixth decades of life, usually are solitary, and develop twice as commonly in women as in men.[12,122,127] Most individuals with schwannomas are asymptomatic and have a slowly growing, painless soft-tissue mass.[120,122,127] Schwannomas are usually less than 5 cm in diameter, although retroperitoneal schwannomas may be larger at time of presentation.[120]

6-14   Features of Abdominal Schwannoma

Clinical

Up to 4% of retroperitoneal tumors
Rare in omenta or mesentery
Peak age: 3rd to 6th decades of life, M:F = 1:2
Most asymptomatic, malignant transformation rare
Treatment: surgical resection if large or symptomatic

MRI

Solitary, well circumscribed, and fusiform in shape
Eccentric in location to parent nerve if visualized
Generally low-intermediate SI on T1-WI, heterogeneous high SI on T2-WI
Variable low SI capsule on both T1-WI and T2-WI
Heterogeneity of SI more common than with neurofibroma
Hemorrhage revealed as high SI on T1-WI
Cystic degeneration with very high SI on T2-WI without enhancement
Calcification with very low SI on T2-WI, more accurately revealed at CT
"Target sign" is nonspecific, with low SI centrally and high SI peripherally on T2-WI
Solid components reveal late enhancement

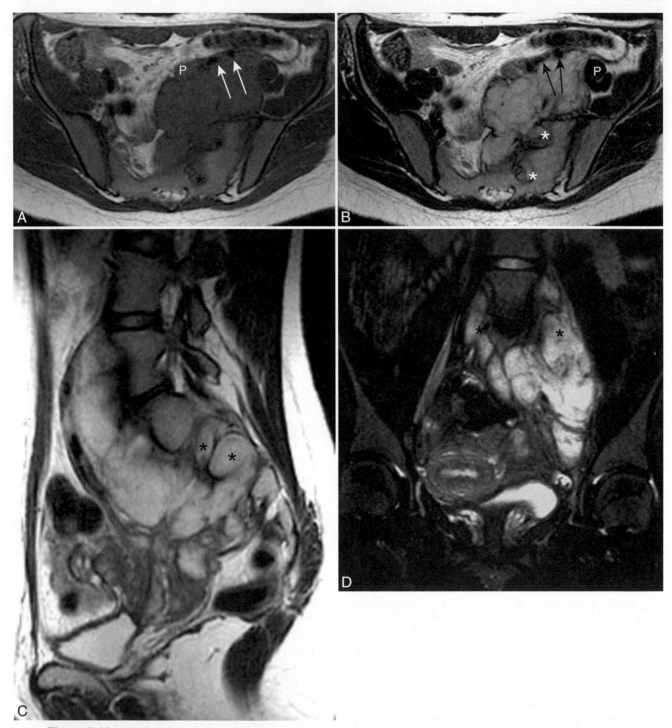

Figure 6-12 ■ **MR illustration of a retroperitoneal ganglioneuroma in a 22-year-old woman with abdominal pain.** **A** and **B**, Axial T1-WI (**A**) and T2-WI (**B**) show an infiltrative lobulated pelvic retroperitoneal mass that has intermediate T1 and heterogeneous high T2 SI relative to skeletal muscle. The mass extends into and expands several left sacral neural foramina (∗), displaces and encases the left external iliac artery and vein *(arrows)* anteriorly, and displaces the left psoas (P) muscle anterolaterally. **C** and **D**, Sagittal T2 (**C**) and coronal fat-suppressed (**D**) T2-WIs show tumoral extension into several left sacral and lower lumbar (∗) neural foramina with associated neural foraminal expansion. Enhanced imaging (not shown) revealed both peripheral and curvilinear internal enhancement. Neural foraminal involvement is usually suggestive of a neoplasm of the nerve or nerve sheath and often is not present in retroperitoneal ganglioneuroma or sarcoma.

Grossly, schwannomas are solitary fusiform masses derived from Schwann cells that are surrounded by a fibrous capsule and are eccentrically located in relation to the parent nerve.[12,127] Histologically, the schwannoma is composed of a highly ordered cellular component of compact spindle cells (Antoni A area) and a less organized and less cellular, loose myxoid component (Antoni B area).[12] Larger retroperitoneal schwannomas are more likely to undergo degenerative changes including cyst formation (up to two thirds) (Fig. 6-13), calcification, hemorrhage, and hyalinization.[12,128]

On MRI, schwannomas are sharply circumscribed fusiform, round, or oval masses that generally have

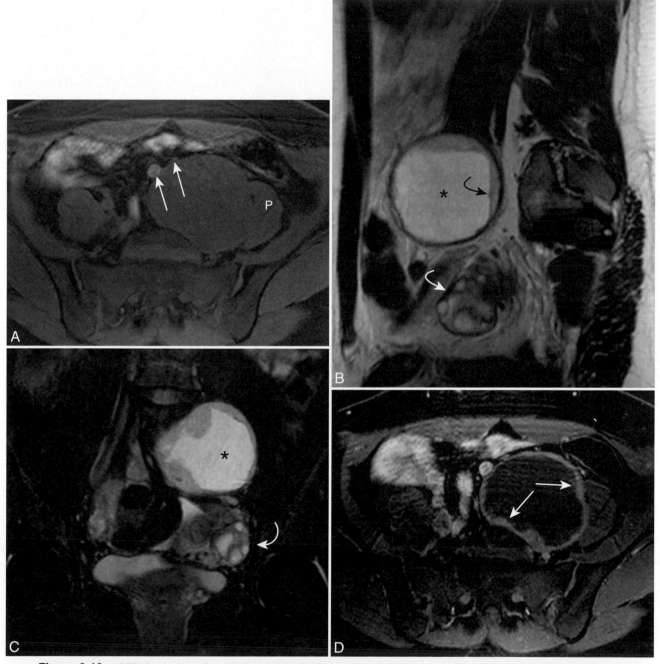

Figure 6-13 ■ **MR depiction of a retroperitoneal schwannoma in a 33-year-old woman who had an adnexal mass revealed on prior sonogram. A,** Axial fat-suppressed T1-WI shows a well-circumscribed left retroperitoneal pelvis mass lesion that is isointense to skeletal muscle and displaces the left psoas (P) muscle to the left and the left common iliac artery and vein *(arrows)* anteriorly. **B** and **C,** Sagittal (**B**) and coronal (**C**) fat-suppressed T2-WIs show central hyperintense cystic degeneration–serous fluid (*) and a fluid-fluid level *(curved black arrow)* with dependent hypointense proteinaceous fluid. The mass is separate from the normal inferiorly located left ovary *(curved white arrow)*. **D,** Axial fat-suppressed CE T1-WI shows enhancement of the solid peripheral components *(arrows)* of the surgically proved benign schwannoma.

nonspecific low-intermediate SI on T1-WI, high SI on T2-WI, and solid enhancing components (see Fig. 6-13). A low SI capsule may be revealed on T1- and T2-WIs.[6,115,122] Heterogeneous SI is much more common in schwannomas than in neurofibromas and may be due to the mixture of Antoni A and B areas along with hemorrhage (usually with increased SI on T1-WI), cystic degeneration (with very high SI on T2-WI without enhancement), or calcification (with very low SI on T2-WI that is often difficult to characterize prospectively).[122,127] Myxoid components have high SI on T2-WI and show variable enhancement.[125] The target sign may be present in both schwannomas and neurofibromas on T2-WI and consists of a central area of low-intermediate SI fibrous tissue surrounded by peripheral high SI myxoid tissue.[21,127] If the parent nerve of a schwannoma can be identified, the schwannoma tends to have an eccentric position in relation to the nerve.[122,127] Schwannomas are treated by surgical excision or enucleation, particularly if large or symptomatic, and surgical excision can usually spare the adjacent nerve as the schwannoma is generally separable from underlying nerve fibers.[127]

ABDOMINAL NEUROFIBROMA

Neurofibromas (Box 6-15) are benign tumors of nerve sheaths of peripheral nerves that represent 5% of all benign soft-tissue neoplasms.[127] They occur sporadically in the third through fifth decades of life and are more common in men. Ten percent of patients with neurofibromatosis (NF)-1 develop neurofibromas.[20,121,127] Approximately one third of patients with solitary neurofibroma have NF-1, and almost all patients with multiple or plexiform neurofibromas have NF-1.[120] Neurofibromas commonly occur in deep anatomic locations in patients with NF-1 (especially in the retroperitoneum and paraspinal locations) that are commonly associated with neurologic symptoms but very rarely may involve the mesentery.[12,127,129] Other symptoms and signs of abdominal neurofibroma are nonspecific. Sporadic neurofibromas are usually smaller than 5 cm,[130] while neurofibromas in those with NF-1 tend to be larger and multiple.[127] Neurofibromas may occur as localized, plexiform, or diffuse types (with the last type typically found in the subcutaneous tissues of patients with NF-1) and rarely undergo malignant transformation (see below).[12,127] Histologically, neurofibromas have variable composition of nerve sheath cells, thick collagenous bundles, and varying amounts of myxoid degeneration. In the most characteristic form, interlacing bundles of elongated cells with wavy dark-staining nuclei are present.[12] Often, longitudinal bundles of residual nerve fibers are centrally situated in neurofibromas.[131]

On MRI, neurofibromas generally have low SI on T1-WI and high SI on T2-WI and enhance on CE T1-WI (Fig. 6-14).[127] The SI on T2-WI may be homogeneous or may be heterogeneous with either a characteristic

---

6-15 Features of Abdominal Neurofibroma

Clinical

5% of all benign soft-tissue neoplasms
Usually develop sporadically
Peak age: 3rd to 5th decades of life, M : F > 1 : 1
Most often asymptomatic
Malignant transformation is rare in sporadic lesions
Treatment: surgical excision, particularly if large, symptomatic, or suspicious for malignant degeneration

Neurofibromatosis Type 1 (NF-1)

10% of patients with NF-1 develop one or more neurofibromas
One third of those with a single neurofibroma have NF-1
99% of those with multiple or plexiform neurofibromas have NF-1
Neurofibromas are larger and in deeper anatomic locations compared with sporadic lesions
Neurofibromas present at a younger age than those with sporadic lesions
Malignant transformation occurs in 2% to 5% of patients with NF-1

MRI

Solitary or multiple, fusiform shape
Centered on parent nerve
Usually in retroperitoneal or paravertebral locations
Dumbbell configuration: neural foraminal expansion when involving a spinal nerve
T1-WI: usually low SI; T2-WI: usually high SI
Homogenous or heterogeneous
Target sign may be present as with schwannoma
Whorled appearance with linear-curvilinear low SI internal foci that correspond to Schwann cell bundles and collagen
"Bag of worms" appearance: multiple diffusely thickened nerve branches as part of a plexiform neurofibroma

---

target sign, as described in the previous section for schwannomas, or with a whorled appearance consisting of linear or curvilinear low SI Schwann cell bundles and collagen fibers in a background of high SI.[21,127] Most neurofibromas have a fusiform shape that are oriented longitudinally in a particular nerve distribution, with tapered ends that are centered on and contiguous with the parent nerve.[127] When they are multiple or of the plexiform type (which is pathognomonic of NF-1), large, conglomerate infiltrative masses of innumerable neurofibromata diffusely thickening a parent nerve and extending into multiple nerve branches may be present, resulting in a characteristic "bag of worms" appearance.[127] Plexiform neurofibromas that infiltrate the mesentery may be associated with vascular encasement and narrowing. Other findings of NF-1 such as scoliosis, dural ectasia, or meningoceles may be present.[132] Surgical treatment

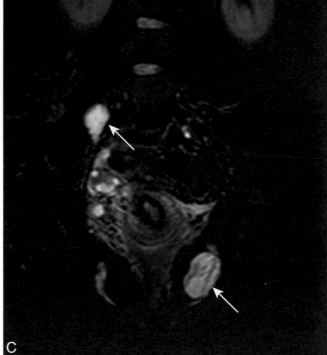

Figure 6-14 ■ **MR illustration of multiple neurofibromas in a 33-year-old woman with neurofibromatosis type 1 with back and right lower extremity pain. A** and **B,** Axial T1-WI (**A**) and T2-WI (**B**) show homogeneous hypointense T1, heterogeneous hyperintense T2 well-circumscribed masses in the left ischiorectal fossa *(arrow)* and the right inguinal region *(curved arrow)* lateral to the common femoral vessels. **C,** Coronal short tau inversion recovery (STIR) image (TE = 68 sec) demonstrates hyperintense neurofibromas *(arrows)* with curvilinear areas of internal low SI, resulting in a whorled appearance.

may be performed for neurofibromas, especially for those which are plexiform, symptomatic, or suspicious for malignant degeneration. Since the neurofibroma is intimately associated with its underlying parent nerve, surgical resection requires removal of the nerve of origin.[127]

MALIGNANT PERIPHERAL NERVE SHEATH TUMOR (MPNST)

Malignant peripheral nerve sheath tumors (MPNSTs; Box 6-16) are malignant tumors arising from or differentiating toward cells of the nerve sheaths of peripheral nerves, representing 5% to 10% of soft-tissue sarcomas. They occur in 2% to 5% of patients with NF-1, usually after a latent period of at least 10 years.[12,127,131,133-135] Conversely, about 50% of patients with MPNST have NF-1.[12,127,131,135]

Ten percent to 20% of MPNSTs arise secondary to irradiation exposure after a latent period of more than 15 years. Most MPNSTs occur during the third through sixth decades of life, which is earlier in onset than other retroperitoneal sarcomas. MPNSTs in those with NF-1 tend to present within the third decade.[12,135,136] MPNSTs that develop in association with NF-1 tend to be of higher histologic grade, larger in size, and more aggressive than those which arise sporadically, and they have a very poor prognosis.[137,138]

As for other abdominal sarcomas, MPNSTs present with nonspecific symptoms and signs of an abdominal mass.[12,127] MPNSTs that arise from major nerves such as the sciatic nerve or sacral plexus may give rise to sensory and motor symptoms including radiated pain, paresthesias, and weakness.[12,127,135] Unexpected growth of a preexisting neurofibroma, especially a plexiform neurofibroma, or associated

**6-16   Features of Malignant Peripheral Nerve
Sheath Tumor (MPNST)**

Clinical

5% to 10% of soft-tissue sarcomas
2% to 5% of patients with NF-1 develop an MPNST
50% of patients with MPNST have NF-1
Compared with sporadic tumors, MPNSTs associated
   with NF-1 are higher grade, larger, and more
   aggressive
Most arise from preexisting neurofibromas after 10
   years of latency
10% to 20% arise following radiation exposure
Peak age: 4th decade of life when sporadic, 3rd decade
   of life when associated with NF-1
M:F slightly <1:1
Pain or rapid growth should raise suspicion of MPNST
Treatment: surgical resection
5-Year survival: 40% if sporadic, 15% if associated
   with NF-1

MRI

Usually solitary, >5 cm ill-defined mass with fusiform,
   round, or ovoid shape in retroperitoneum
Heterogeneous SI on T1-WI and T2-WI with variable
   enhancement
Intratumoral hemorrhage and necrosis common
No imaging findings can reliably differentiate MPNST
   from benign neural tumors
Other findings of NF-1 may be present

pain, particularly if spontaneous and unremitting, should raise clinical suspicion for a MPNST, although benign neurofibromas may also grow and be painful.[127,133,134] Overall, pain associated with a mass in patients with NF-1 is the greatest risk factor for MPNST development, with a relative risk of approximately 30-fold.[136]

On MRI, benign and malignant neural tumors cannot be differentiated reliably, since SI and enhancement characteristics overlap. MPNSTs tend to be larger than 5 cm, may exhibit ill-defined margins suggesting infiltration of surrounding tissues and associated edema, and may expand neural foramina, but these features may also be shown with benign neural tumors (Fig. 6-15). Heterogeneity with central necrosis is common in MPNST, but benign tumors with cystic degeneration may also appear heterogeneous. The most important imaging finding of MPNST is rapid enlargement in size of a tumor mass, particularly if associated with pain.[127,133] Complete surgical resection is the mainstay of treatment of abdominal MPNST as for other abdominal sarcomas.[127] Also as for other abdominal sarcomas, the most important factor influencing patient survival is performance of complete surgical resection.[137] Local recurrence and distant metastatic disease are common complications of MPNST.[127,135] The overall 5-year survival rate for patients with MPNST is approximately 40%, and the 5-year survival rate in patients with NF-1 is 15%.[135,137]

ABDOMINAL WALL AND INTRA-ABDOMINAL FIBROMATOSIS (DESMOID TUMOR)

The fibromatoses are classified as superficial (fascial) or deep (desmoid tumor), and the deep group is divided into extra-abdominal, abdominal wall, and intra-abdominal (mesenteric, mesocolic, omental, retroperitoneal) subgroups.[12,139,140] Abdominal wall and intra-abdominal subgroups of desmoid tumors are discussed here (Box 6-17).

Desmoid tumors are uncommon neoplastic lesions, comprising 0.1% of all tumors and 3.5% of fibrous tumors, occurring either sporadically or in association with familial adenomatous polyposis (FAP).[140] FAP is inherited in autosomal dominant fashion, and patients with a phenotypic variant of FAP known as Gardner's syndrome may develop desmoid tumors in addition to polyposis coli and colon carcinoma.[141,142] The incidence of desmoid tumor in FAP ranges from 3.6% to 34%, and patients with FAP are at an approximately 1,000-fold increased risk compared with the general population.[140] Sporadic desmoid tumor occurs with a female to male ratio of 2 to 5:1, whereas FAP-associated desmoid tumor occurs with equal gender frequency.[140] Both types of desmoid tumor have a peak incidence in the fourth decade of life.[140,143] Sporadic desmoid tumors are solitary in more than 90% of cases; are often present in the retroperitoneum, pelvis, and anterior abdominal wall; and tend to be larger in size (with a mean diameter of 14 cm). In contrast, FAP-associated desmoid tumors are multiple in 40%, are more likely to involve the mesentery (most commonly) and abdominal wall, and tend to be smaller (with a mean diameter 5 cm).[144-147] Even though uncommon, desmoid tumors are the most common primary tumors of the mesentery.[144,148]

Clinically, intra-abdominal desmoid tumors most often present as asymptomatic abdominal masses, although some may cause mild abdominal pain.[12] Less commonly, symptoms and signs are related to local invasion of small bowel or mesenteric vessels or to ureteral obstruction.[149] Minor osseous malformations such as exostoses, enostoses, and incomplete spinal segmentation are present in 80% of sporadic desmoid tumor patients as compared with 5% in the general population.[140]

Abdominal wall fibromatosis tends to occur in young pregnant women or, more frequently, during the first year following childbirth.[12] Most of these tumors are solitary, measure 3 to 10 cm, and arise from and infiltrate the abdominal wall musculoaponeurotic structures, most commonly the rectus abdominis and internal oblique muscles and fascia.[12,148] Rectus and fascial desmoids usually do not cross the abdominal midline but may be associated with intra-abdominal extension.[12,144,148,150] Retroperitoneal desmoid

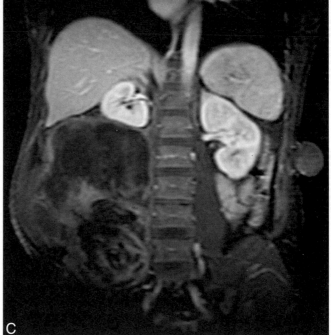

Figure 6-15 ▪ **MR findings of a malignant retroperitoneal nerve sheath tumor (MPNST) and multiple neurofibromas in a 31-year-old man with neurofibromatosis type 1 and a palpable, painful abdominal mass. A**, Coronal T2-WI shows a large, heterogeneous, infiltrative, right retroperitoneal mass (M) with very high SI components (*) relative to skeletal muscle due to cystic degeneration and central necrosis. There is superior displacement of the right kidney (K). A homogeneous, hyperintense, pedunculated cutaneous neurofibroma *(curved arrow)* is present along the left lateral abdominal wall. Multiple other cutaneous neurofibromas were revealed on other images and physical examination. **B** and **C**, Coronal fat-suppressed T1-WIs obtained before (**B**) and after (**C**) contrast show hyperintense intratumoral hemorrhage *(arrows)* in (**B**) and mild heterogeneous central and peripheral enhancement. The IVC was extrinsically compressed without invasion or occlusion (not shown). MPNST should be considered in any patient with neurofibromatosis who has a large or ill-defined abdominal mass, a soft-tissue mass that demonstrates rapid growth, or a mass associated with pain.

tumors are uncommon, occur in less than 20% of patients, may commonly cause ureteral obstruction with a variable clinical presentation, and are rarely completely resectable.[143,151] Mesenteric desmoid tumors usually have an ill-defined whorled configuration but may sometimes appear as a small, discrete mass that later grows into such a whorled soft-tissue lesion with pockets of mesenteric fat.[149,152]

Histologically, desmoids are composed of uniform elongated spindle-shaped fibroblasts surrounded by abundant collagen.[12,140,153] Cellularity is variable, with some portions of tumor showing complete replacement

by dense fibrous tissue and other areas revealing stromal myxoid change.[12] When large, desmoid tumors may rarely reveal cystic degeneration or necrosis.[140] Desmoid tumors are nonencapsulated and have an infiltrative margins.[140] No correlation has been found between the clinical behavior and the histologic appearance.[148]

The exact cause of the desmoid tumor is not known. While most cases are idiopathic, genetic abnormalities, trauma (including surgical trauma), and estrogenic hormones are potential etiologic factors.[12,140] Approximately 20% of sporadic abdominal

6-17 Features of Abdominal Wall and Intra-abdominal Fibromatosis (Desmoid Tumor)

Clinical

Subtype of the deep group of fibromatoses
Uncommon, 0.1% of all tumors, yet most common primary tumor of the small bowel mesentery
Sporadic or associated with familial adenomatous polyposis (FAP)
Patients with FAP have 1,000-fold risk
Peak age: 4th decade of life
Treatment: surgical resection (mainstay of therapy)

Sporadic Desmoid Tumors FAP-associated Desmoid Tumors

Sporadic	FAP-associated
M:F = 1:2-5	M:F = 1:1
Solitary in >90%	Multiple in 40%
Larger, median size = 14 cm	Smaller, median size = 5 cm
Pelvis and retroperitoneum	Small bowel mesentery, several years after colectomy
40% recurrence rate	90% recurrence rate

MRI

Low-intermediate SI on T1-WI and T2-WI
Infiltrative margins: aggressive imaging features even though not malignant
High SI on T2-WI in immature cellular lesions suggests future tumor growth
Enhancement is variable
Decrease in size and SI on T2-WI indicates maturation and/or response to therapy
Poor prognostic findings
  Mesenteric mass >10 cm
  Multiple mesenteric masses
  Extensive SB involvement
  Bilateral hydronephrosis

wall desmoid tumors occur following surgical procedures, with half occurring within 4 years after surgery.[140,154] In addition, approximately 75% of FAP-associated intra-abdominal desmoid tumors develop after abdominal colectomy, at an average of 2 to 3 years following surgery.[140] Abdominal wall desmoid tumors grow the fastest in young women, have a tendency to develop in postpartum women and women who take oral contraceptive medicines, and spontaneously regress after menopause or oophorectomy.[140,147]

Since desmoid tumors may have a variable degree of cellularity, fibrosis, vascularity, and infiltration, they may be well or poorly defined and show variable SI and enhancement on MRI (Fig. 6-16).[155] In general, however, desmoids are infiltrative, are most often low-intermediate in SI on T1- and T2-WI, and tend to appear aggressive on MRI although they are not malignant.[21,147,149,156] Occasionally, a low SI fibrous capsule may be partially or completely visualized on T1-WI, and low SI bands of collagen may be present on T1- and T2-WI.[141,147] The presence of high SI on T2-WI does not exclude a diagnosis of a desmoid

tumor, as immature lesions with higher cellularity and less mature fibrosis can be of higher SI than muscle on T2-WI. These immature, high SI desmoid tumors are associated with rapid growth on follow-up imaging.[147,149] Both mature and immature desmoid tumors tend to enhance.[147,149]

After surgery, recurrent desmoid tumor will have MRI characteristics similar to those of the original lesion, and the site of recurrence is frequently at margins of the original lesion.[147] MRI is also useful in evaluating the effectiveness of nonsurgical therapy, since effective therapy is generally indicated by a size reduction and an increase in the amount of low SI on T2-WI, reflecting increased intratumoral collagen in response to therapy.[147]

Several imaging features of desmoid tumor that suggest a poor prognosis with increased morbidity and mortality include a mesenteric mass greater than 10 cm, multiple mesenteric masses, extensive small bowel involvement, and bilateral hydronephrosis.[152] Overall, the mean survival rate of patients with intra-abdominal desmoid tumors 5 years.[140] The outcome for patients with FAP-associated intra-abdominal desmoid tumors is significantly worse than for those without them.[146,153] For patients with abdominal wall desmoid tumors, a cure rate of up to 20% and a disease-free survival ranging from 5 to 15 years have been reported after surgical treatment.[140]

Surgical removal remains the cornerstone of treatment of desmoid tumors despite frequent local recurrence.[140] Optimally, wide-field surgical resection is performed for abdominal wall or small intra-abdominal tumors in patients who are able to tolerate surgery, so that tumor-free margins may be achieved.[140,153] Large intra-abdominal desmoid tumors cannot be completely removed without sacrificing vital structures such as the mesenteric vessels, have a perioperative mortality rate and major morbidity rate of up to 60%, and recur in up to 90% of cases.[140,157,158] Thus, surgical removal of large intra-abdominal desmoid tumors generally is not recommended unless there is gastrointestinal or genitourinary tract obstruction, fistula formation, or abscess formation.[140,159] Postsurgical radiation therapy may help reduce the risk of recurrent disease.[140,151]

Noncytotoxic drugs, cytotoxic drugs, and observation are nonsurgical treatment options for desmoid tumors, although no single approach has consistently proved effective.[140,153] Noncytotoxic medications including nonsteroidal anti-inflammatory drugs (NSAIDs) and anti-estrogens such as tamoxifen are considered by some as the first line of treatment for desmoid tumors, particularly if small, asymptomatic, and unlikely to cause bowel obstruction.[140,160] Sometimes, though, a trial of watchful waiting may be implemented, especially in patients with FAP or with lesions that are intimately associated with the mesenteric vessels, since spontaneous regression may occur in 5% to 15% of cases.[140,157,158] Infrequently, cytotoxic medications have been used to induce variable degrees of remission for symptomatic,

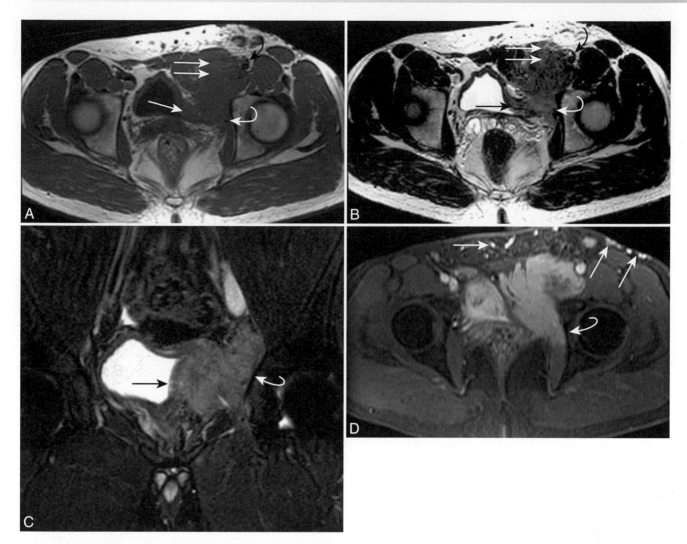

Figure 6-16 ■ **MR depiction of deep pelvic fibromatosis in a 24-year-old man with a palpable inguinal mass.** **A** and **B**, Axial T1-WI (**A**) and T2-WI (**B**) show an infiltrative left pelvic mass that is T1 isointense and T2 intermediate to hyperintense relative to skeletal muscle. The mass infiltrates the bladder wall *(single arrow)*, the left obturator internus muscle *(curved white arrow)*, the left rectus abdominis muscle *(double arrow)*, and the proximal left thigh muscles, with partial encasement of the left common femoral artery and compression of the left common femoral vein *(curved black arrows)*. **C**, Coronal fat-suppressed T2-WI shows desmoid infiltration of the left pelvic sidewall *(curved arrow)* and urinary bladder *(arrow)*. **D**, Axial fat-suppressed CE T1-WI reveals marked homogeneous tumoral enhancement. Anterior collateral vessels *(arrows)* are secondary to obstruction of the left-sided deep pelvic veins. Enhancement of the anterior aspect of the obturator internus muscle indicates invasion *(curved arrow)*.

clinically aggressive, recurrent, nonresectable, or unresponsive desmoid tumors, and may achieve a good initial response for inoperable desmoid tumors that have caused progressive bowel or ureteral obstruction.[140,158,160]

BENIGN NONPARENCHYMAL ABDOMINOPELVIC FAT-CONTAINING LESIONS

Abdominal Lipoma

The lipoma (Box 6-18) is a benign mesenchymal tumor composed of mature fat and represents the most common mesenchymal neoplasm and the most common benign tumor of the retroperitoneum.[5,12]

Lipomatous tumors account for half of all soft-tissue tumors in surgical series.[30] Solitary lipomas usually appear during periods of weight gain most often in the fifth through seventh decades of life, a significantly younger peak age range than for well-differentiated liposarcomas.[12,30] Lipomas occur more commonly in obese men. No treatment is generally implemented, although surgical removal may be performed for large or symptomatic abdominal lipomas.[161] Similar to fat, lipomas are composed of mature adipocytes, although the cells are slightly larger and slightly more variable in size and shape. Admixed mesenchymal elements can be present, most commonly fibrous connective tissue. Lipomas have not been shown to undergo malignant transformation into liposarcomas.[12]

6-18 Features of Abdominal Lipoma

Clinical

Most common mesenchymal neoplasm
Most common benign tumor of the retroperitoneum
May occur in the mesentery, omentum, or
retroperitoneum
Peak age: 5th to 7th decades of life, M:F > 1:1
Increased incidence in obesity
Most asymptomatic and stable in size after
initial growth
No malignant potential
Treatment: surgery for symptoms or cosmesis

MRI

Smaller than well-differentiated liposarcomas
Homogeneous SI similar to fat on all pulse sequences

6-19 Features of Primary Retroperitoneal Teratoma

Clinical

Rare retroperitoneal tumor
Peak age: 1st decade of life, 20% in
adults >30 years old; F:M = 3:1
25% malignant, more frequently malignant in adults
Treatment: surgical removal whether benign or
malignant
Prognosis: excellent if benign

MRI

Usually heterogeneous well-defined solid and
multiloculated cystic lesion
Most common retroperitoneal location is near the
kidneys
Fatty components follow SI of fat on all pulse
sequences
Calcifications, ossifications, or teeth usually have low
SI on T1-WI and T2-WI when recognized

On MRI, lipomas typically have homogeneous SI identical to that of fat on all pulse sequences, in contrast to well-differentiated liposarcomas, and this is the most reliable feature of lipomas at imaging.[1,30] However, a significant number of lipomas have prominent nonadipose areas with an imaging appearance that may overlap with that of well-differentiated liposarcomas. These nonadipose components may be revealed in one third of lipomas and are typically due to fat necrosis and associated calcification, fibrosis, inflammation, and areas of myxoid change. Well-defined thin capsules border the margins of lipomas. Lipomas tend to be smaller than well-differentiated liposarcomas and most often remain stable in size.[12,30]

PRIMARY RETROPERITONEAL TERATOMA

Primary retroperitoneal teratomas (Box 6-19) are rare lesions that represent 5% to 10% of primary retroperitoneal tumors.[162-164] The majority occur in children and less than 20% in adults.[162,164-166] Teratomas in adults have a greater chance of being malignant than those in children (20% vs. 6%, respectively), and primary retroperitoneal teratomas occur 2 to 4 times more frequently in women than in men.[162,165,167] Overall, teratomas are found more commonly in the ovaries, testes, and anterior mediastinum.[162,163] Most patients with primary retroperitoneal teratomas are asymptomatic, but some larger tumors may cause nonspecific symptoms. Alpha-fetoprotein levels are normal in patients with benign teratomas and may be elevated with malignant teratomas.[164]

Primary retroperitoneal teratomas develop from totipotential germ cells that have failed to migrate to their normal gonadal locations.[162] Grossly, teratomas may either be cystic or solid and frequently contain mature tissues including skin and dermal appendages, cartilage, bone, teeth, or fat.[168] Cystic teratomas are generally benign well-defined lesions that contain multiple solid and cystic areas along with mature tissues, sebaceous material, or mucoid fluid.[162,165,168,169] However, solid teratomas are frequently malignant and contain immature embryonic tissue in addition to the mature components.[162,165] Retroperitoneal teratomas tend to be located near the upper poles of the kidneys.[164]

On MRI, teratomas are usually heterogeneous, well-defined solid or multiloculated cystic lesions that may contain fatty components with SI isointense to subcutaneous fat on all pulse sequences. Examples of ovarian teratomas are illustrated in Chapter 7 (see Figs. 7-41 and 7-43) and a case of a metastatic teratoma to the liver is shown in Chapter 1 (see Fig. 1-18). Calcifications, ossifications, and teeth reveal very low SI on T1- and T2-WI when visualized. Other tumoral components have less specific MRI features. Retroperitoneal teratomas are surgically removed if possible, regardless of whether benign or malignant, as even histologically benign lesions may result in significant morbidity from continued growth.[164]

Pelvic Lipomatosis

Pelvic lipomatosis (Box 6-20) is a rare condition characterized by nonencapsulated fatty tissue overgrowth in the perirectal and perivesical regions of the pelvis, resulting in compression of the lower urinary tract and rectosigmoid colon.[170] African American men are affected in approximately two thirds of cases, with a peak age during the third and fourth decades.[170,171] Associated proliferative cystitis, in particular cystitis glandularis (a premalignant bladder condition), is present in 75% of patients.[172-174]

Pelvic lipomatosis is characterized by massive benign hyperplastic overgrowth of pelvic retroperitoneal fat in the perivesical and perirectal locations.

6-20 Pelvic Lipomatosis

Clinical

Uncommon; hyperplastic overgrowth of pelvic retroperitoneal fatty tissue
M:F >> 1:1, two thirds in African Americans
Proliferative cystitis in 80%
Secondary to lymphatic and venous stasis of bladder wall from surrounding fat
Increased risk of bladder adenocarcinoma; requires surveillance
Early irritative voiding symptoms and pain
Late symptoms and signs of ureteral, venous, or bowel obstruction
Treatment: no definitive primary treatment
40% Require urinary diversion

MRI

Homogeneous, nonencapsulated, perivesical and perirectal fatty proliferation
Surrounds pelvic organs symmetrically
SI follows that of fat on all pulse sequences
Pelvic organ changes
   Superior displacement of bladder base
   Pear shape or inverted teardrop shape of bladder
   Smooth narrowing of rectosigmoid colon

The fatty growth is diffuse and composed entirely of mature fat indistinguishable grossly and histologically from fatty tissue elsewhere in the body.[12] The etiology of pelvic lipomatosis is unknown, but a genetic cause is possible.[170] Pelvic lipomatosis is usually asymptomatic. Progressive disease can be complicated by proliferative cystitis, which is hypothesized to be secondary to lymphatic and venous stasis secondary to fatty tissue compressing the urinary bladder.[170,174] Late complications of obstructive renal failure and bladder adenocarcinoma have been reported.[170,175]

On MRI, pelvic lipomatosis appears as homogeneous, nonencapsulated perivesical and perirectal fatty tissue that surrounds the pelvic organs and shows SI similar to mature fat on all pulse sequences (Fig. 6-17). Scattered intratumoral linear foci of fibrosis of low T1- and T2-W SI may also be present.[176,177] Superior displacement of the bladder base, a pear-shaped bladder, elongation of the bladder neck and posterior urethra, elevation of the prostate gland, and superomedial displacement of the seminal vesicles may be revealed.[170,178] Smooth extrinsic narrowing of the rectosigmoid by hypertrophied extramural fat may also be present as well as dilatation and displacement of one or both ureters with or without hydronephrosis.[170,176,177]

No definitive treatment for pelvic lipomatosis has been established.[173,179] Complete surgical removal of the fatty tissue is generally difficult or impossible because of indistinct surgical margins between the fat and adjacent normal structures, and it does not always help improve clinical symptoms or signs.[174]

Other therapeutic measures including weight loss, antimicrobial medication, corticosteroid administration, radiation therapy, and chemotherapy are ineffective.[173,174,179] Although the natural history of pelvic lipomatosis is not entirely clear, approximately 40% of patients will require urinary diversion at a mean of 5 years after diagnosis to prevent renal failure due to obstructive uropathy.[170,179] Since patients with pelvic lipomatosis and proliferative cystitis have a higher incidence of bladder adenocarcinoma, periodic bladder cancer screening should be performed.[174]

Sclerosing Mesenteritis

Sclerosing mesenteritis (Box 6-21) is a rare idiopathic inflammatory fibrosclerotic condition. The three subtypes of sclerosing mesenteritis are termed mesenteric panniculitis, mesenteric lipodystrophy, or retractile mesenteritis, depending on the relative amounts of inflammation, fat necrosis, or fibrosis present.[180-183] Mesenteric panniculitis and mesenteric lipodystrophy are the acute/subacute forms of sclerosing mesenteritis, whereas retractile mesenteritis is the chronic form.[181] The pathogenesis of sclerosing mesenteritis follows the general sequence of nonspecific inflammation and thickening of the mesenteric fat and mesentery, subsequent fat necrosis, and resultant fibrosis with progressive scarring and retraction.[184,185]

Sclerosing mesenteritis occurs most commonly in the fifth or sixth decades of life and is twice as common in men than in women.[181,184-188] Its prevalence is 0.6%, and its etiology is unknown, although an autoimmune response and mesenteric ischemia are possible pathogenetic mechanisms.[185] Sclerosing mesenteritis can coexist with retroperitoneal fibrosis or sclerosing cholangitis.[182] However, in most patients, sclerosing mesenteritis is incidentally identified during imaging for an unrelated condition. There is an association between sclerosing mesenteritis and malignancy (mainly lymphoma but also genitourinary or gastrointestinal adenocarcinoma).[185] As many as 15% of patients with sclerosing mesenteritis may subsequently develop malignant lymphoma.[189]

Symptoms and signs of sclerosing mesenteritis may be related to inflammation or to mass effect on adjacent organs, and may be absent, intermittent, or rapidly progressive.[181,185] One third of patients are asymptomatic.[188] When symptomatic, abdominal pain is the most frequent presenting symptom.[181,184] Laboratory findings are absent or nonspecific.[185] For most symptomatic patients, sclerosing mesenteritis has a benign course, and the most common outcome is spontaneous symptomatic relief although the time course is variable.[184,190,191] Major complications of sclerosing mesenteritis are related to progressive fibrosis, mesenteric shortening, and mesenteric vessel compression with resultant mesenteric venous thrombosis, intestinal obstruction, or intestinal ischemia.[181,184]

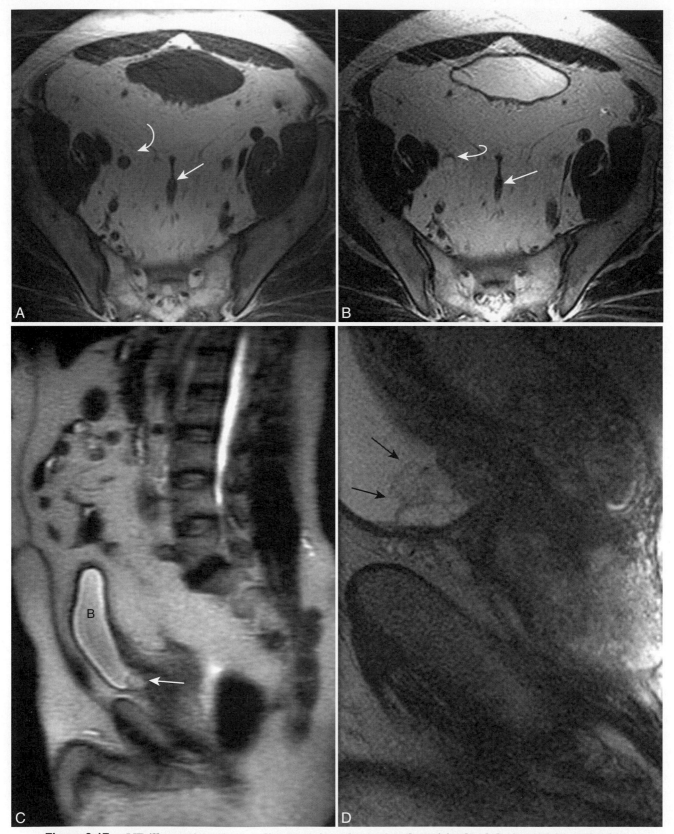

Figure 6-17 ▪ **MR illustration of pelvic lipomatosis and associated cystitis glandularis/cystitis cystica in a 54-year-old man.** The patient required urinary diversion secondary to functional ureteral obstruction. **A** and **B**, Axial T1-WI (**A**) and T2-WI (**B**) show increased pelvic fat that extrinsically compresses the rectosigmoid colon *(arrow)*. The right pelvic ureter is dilated *(curved arrow)* secondary to extrinsic compression. **C**, Sagittal T2-WI shows a bladder (B) that is displaced anteriorly by fat and a hyperintense mucosal lesion of the bladder base *(arrow)*. **D**, Small field-of-view sagittal T2-WI shows a lobulated lesion *(arrows)* of the posteroinferior bladder that is isointense to urine, in keeping with cystitis cystica and cystitis glandularis.

6-21 Features of Sclerosing Mesenteritis

Clinical

Rare, inflammatory-fibrotic process of the mesentery
Acute and subacute forms
  Mesenteric panniculitis (inflammation dominant)
  Mesenteric lipodystrophy (fat necrosis dominant)
Chronic form
  Retractile mesenteritis: mature fibrosis with little
    inflammation or necrosis
Location: small bowel mesentery most common site,
  less commonly mesocolon
Peak age: 5th to 6th decades of life, M:F = 2:1
Usually asymptomatic and incidentally revealed
  on imaging
May be associated with coexistent malignancy:
  10% to 15% of patients may develop lymphoma
Majority of patients have a benign course with
  spontaneous resolution
Potential complications: intestinal obstruction or
  ischemia, mesenteric venous thrombosis
Treatment: most often watchful waiting
Surgery reserved for intestinal obstruction or
  coexistent malignancy
Medical therapy if advanced or progressive

MRI

Diffuse lesion > solitary mass > multiple fatty masses
Intermediate-high SI on T1-WI
Variable SI on T2-WI
Low SI due to fibrosis and calcification (as in retractile
  mesenteritis)
High SI on T2-WI due to inflammation and residual
  fat (equivalent of "misty mesentery" on CT)
Occasional high SI multilocular cystic dilated
  lymphatics on T2-WI
Acute and subacute forms more heterogeneous than
  chronic form
Associated small bowel separation or kinking more
  common in chronic form
"Fat ring" sign: preserved fat about mesenteric vessels
  present in 75% of cases of acute form
Left-sided orientation of maximal diameter in 98%
Scattered, well-defined, <5 mm soft tissue nodules
  often revealed

On MRI, one or more fatty mesenteric masses are typically present with intermediate-high SI on T1-WI and variable SI on T2-WI. If fibrosis and calcifications are dominant (as in retractile mesenteritis), then relatively homogeneous, low T2-W SI components are present. Heterogeneous high T2-W SI occurs within acute/subacute mesenteric panniculitis and mesenteric lipodystrophy that is composed of predominantly inflammatory tissue and fat with a paucity of calcification and mature fibrosis (the MRI equivalent of the "misty mesentery" as described on CT).[180,184,192,193] Occasionally, multilocular cystic foci with very high T2-W SI may be present, representing dilated lymphatics as a result of mesenteric lymphatic obstruction.[186] Separation, tethering, or kinking of

adjacent small bowel segments may be present owing to mesenteric retraction and is more marked in retractile mesenteritis than in mesenteric panniculitis or mesenteric lipodystrophy.[180,181]

The "fat ring" sign, which appears as preservation of the fat immediately surrounding mesenteric vessels, is a useful imaging feature of mesenteric panniculitis, characteristically occurring in up to 75% of cases, although it is not entirely specific.[181,183,194] A tumoral pseudocapsule, appearing as a peripheral band of soft-tissue SI limiting the normal mesentery from the inflammatory process, may be present in mesenteric panniculitis. However, these two findings are not present when mesenteric panniculitis evolves into retractile mesenteritis.[181] A left-sided orientation of the maximum transverse diameter of the lesion (present in up to 98%) and scattered, well-defined soft-tissue nodules smaller than 5 mm are other characteristic imaging features of sclerosing mesenteritis that generally are not present in other mesenteric diseases. The leftward orientation is in keeping with the orientation of the jejunal mesentery, which tends to be involved most often by sclerosing mesenteritis.[185]

No treatment is generally implemented, as surgical resection is technically difficult and of no benefit.[182,185] Treatment for patients with persistent or progressive symptomatology is not well established. Surgical exploration with biopsy and bypass procedures can be performed for intestinal obstruction, with surgical resection reserved for cases highly suggestive of malignancy.[181,184] Occasionally, corticosteroids and immunosuppressants such as azathioprine or cyclophosphamide are given to treat advanced or progressive disease.[181,189,190]

NONPARENCHYMAL ABDOMINAL CYSTS

Mesenteric, omental, mesocolic, and retroperitoneal nonparenchymal abdominal cysts (Boxes 6-22 and 6-23) are rare, with an incidence of 1 in 100,000 in adults and 1 in 20,000 children. Although controversy regarding the etiology and classification of most of these cysts exists, these lesions generally fall into one of several categories: (1) lesions of lymphatic origin (simple lymphatic cyst, lymphangioma), (2) lesions of mesothelial origin (simple mesothelial cyst, multicystic peritoneal mesothelioma[195]), (3) lesions of enteric origin (enteric cyst, enteric duplication cyst), (4) bronchogenic cysts, (5) mature cystic teratoma (dermoid cysts), and (6) nonpancreatic pseudocysts (traumatic or infectious).[168] Mature cystic teratomas and peritoneal inclusion cysts are discussed in Chapter 7 and pancreatic pseudocysts in Chapter 2, respectively.

In general, the first step in the evaluation of a cystic abdominal mass is determination of its organ of origin. If an abdominal cystic mass does not arise from a solid organ but from the mesentery, omentum, or retroperitoneum, the differential diagnosis includes primary mesenteric, omental, mesocolic, or retroperitoneal cysts, as well as benign and malignant

---

6-22 Differential Diagnosis for Nonparenchymal Abdominal Cystic Lesions

Lymphatic Origin
Simple lymphatic cyst
Lymphangioma (see Box 6-24)
Lymphocele

Mesothelial Origin
Simple mesothelial cyst
Multicystic peritoneal mesothelioma

Enteric Origin
Enteric cyst
Enteric duplication cyst

Bronchogenic Origin
Bronchogenic cyst

Miscellaneous
Nonpancreatic pseudocyst/peritoneal inclusion cyst
Loculated fluid collections (see Box 6-34)
  Ascites, hematoma, biloma, urinoma, abscess
Cystic or necrotic neoplasms
  Sarcoma, carcinoma
  Hemangioma (see Box 6-25)
  Schwannoma, paraganglioma

6-23 Features of Nonparenchymal Abdominal Cysts

Clinical
Rare lesions of the mesentery, omentum, mesocolon, and retroperitoneum
Most are incidental
Most common presentation if symptomatic: pain and/or palpable mass
Potential complications: growth, hemorrhage, superinfection, torsion, rupture, and small bowel obstruction
Treatment
  Surgical resection to prevent potential complications, particularly if large or symptomatic
  Imaging follow-up for stable, small, asymptomatic, nonaggressive cystic lesions

Checklist of MRI Features to Assess for a Cystic Abdominal Mass
Site of origin
Purely cystic vs. cyst with solid components
Local extent and involvement of adjacent structures
  Vessels
  Bowel
  Adjacent organs, especially blood vessels and small bowel
SI and enhancement characteristics: evaluate for
  Malignant imaging features
  Malignant ascites
  Suspect lymphadenopathy
  Enhancing solid intracystic components

---

cystic neoplasms and congenital anomalies, among other possibilities.[169] On MRI, the thickness of the cyst wall, the presence of internal septations, calcifications, fat, and the SI and enhancement characteristics of the cyst contents may be useful imaging features to help differentiate among the variety of abdominal cysts.[168] Delineation of the extent and involvement of adjacent structures by the cysts, along with evaluation for features of malignancy such as lymphadenopathy, peritoneal implants, or distant metastatic disease may be performed on MRI.[169] However, often there is overlap in the imaging features of the different kinds of abdominal cysts in addition to overlap with the imaging features of other cystic lesions, and histologic analysis is usually required to establish a definitive diagnosis.

The most common type of nonparenchymal abdominal "cyst" is the lymphangioma, followed by a nonpancreatic pseudocyst, an enteric duplication cyst, a simple mesothelial cyst, and an enteric cyst.[169] All types of nonparenchymal abdominal cysts usually manifest as a large painful abdominal mass when symptomatic, although many are revealed in asymptomatic individuals.[196] Large nonparenchymal abdominal cysts are generally treated with surgical removal to prevent complications such as rupture, hemorrhage, torsion, superinfection, or interval growth and to exclude a cystic malignancy[168,195] Small, asymptomatic, nonparenchymal abdominal cysts, however, may sometimes be followed with imaging if no growth or aggressive imaging features are present.

LYMPHATIC CYSTS

Simple lymphatic cysts are congenital in origin, are usually small (1 to 5 cm) and unilocular, and tend to remain stable and asymptomatic over time.[168,197] Histologically, they are lined by flat endothelial cells with a wall containing smooth muscle fibers, lymphoid tissue, lymphatic space, and/or occasional foam cells containing lipoid material.[198] On MRI, they generally have low SI on T1-WI, high SI on T2-WI, and minimal if any wall enhancement.

Lymphangiomas

Lymphangiomas (Box 6-24) are uncommon cystic lesions that most often occur in the neck (75%) and axillary regions (20%), while the remaining 5% may occur elsewhere, most commonly in the abdomen.[66,197,199,200] The most common location of an abdominal lymphangioma is in the mesentery, followed by the omentum, mesocolon, and retroperitoneum.[12,196,199] Rare multisystemic involvement and extensive intra-abdominal cystic lymphangiomatosis may occur and has a poor prognosis.[197] Forty percent of retroperitoneal and other abdominal lymphangiomas are revealed in older children or adults (the remaining 60% occurring in children), whereas lymphangiomas of the neck and axillary regions more frequently present in infants and children less than 2 years of age.[12,197,201,202]

6-24 Features of Lymphangioma

Clinical

Most common mesenteric or omental "cyst"
40% in adults, 60% in newborns and young children (neck and axilla), M:F > 1:1
5% in abdomen (mesentery > omentum > mesocolon > retroperitoneum), very rare in pelvis
Mesenteric location: usually symptomatic children
Retroperitoneal location: less symptomatic or asymptomatic adults
Prognosis: good unless extensive or multisystemic
May recur if incompletely resected

MRI

Large and infiltrative, affecting a localized portion of the abdomen
Multilocular and thin-walled > unilocular
If serous, low SI on T1-WI and high SI on T2-WI
If chylous, proteinaceous, or hemorrhagic, higher SI on T1-WI
Fat in septa on T1-WI is a suggestive imaging feature
No or minimal wall or septal enhancement
Imaging features to help distinguish lymphangioma from ascites
   Separation of bowel loops
   Absence of fluid in the perihepatic space and cul-de-sac
   Focal septations

The etiology and pathogenesis of lymphangiomas are not entirely clear; some consider them to be acquired malformations secondary to obstruction of lymphatic vessels, and others consider them to be congenital malformations of lymphangiectasia related to failure of communication with the lymphatic system.[197]

Pathologically, lymphangiomas are large, thin-walled, usually multiloculated cystic masses lined by attenuated endothelium resembling that of normal lymphatics. Lymphangiomas are classified as capillary (simple), cavernous, and cystic (hygroma) types depending on the size of the lymphatic spaces. Capillary lymphangiomas are composed of small, thin-walled lymphatics, cavernous lymphangiomas of larger lymphatic channels, and cystic lymphangiomas of large macroscopic lymphatic spaces with intervening collagen and smooth muscle.[12,169,197] The fluid contents are predominantly chylous but may be serous or hemorrhagic.[12,169]

Lymphangiomas of the mesentery, omentum, or mesocolon tend to be symptomatic, particularly in children, reflecting their aggressive behavior.[168] They often present with a palpable abdominal mass and abdominal pain and can be complicated by small bowel obstruction, volvulus, and infarction.[12,168,196,199] In contrast, retroperitoneal lymphangiomas are usually asymptomatic and are diagnosed in older children or adults either by incidental detection on cross-sectional imaging or surgery for unrelated conditions, or by a palpable abnormality.[168,196,197]

On MRI, lymphangiomas usually appear as large, cystic, unilocular or multilocular thin-walled lesions, with multiple cystic components of various sizes (Fig. 6-18) and may be associated with bowel dilatation due to obstruction.[168,169,199] Serous fluid contents have low SI on T1-WI and high SI on T2-WI. Sometimes, the fluid contents may be chylous, proteinaceous, or hemorrhagic, with higher SI on T1-WI and high SI on T2-WI.[169] With complications of infection or hemorrhage, the outer wall and internal septations tend to be thicker.[200] Mild septal or wall enhancement may be present. Separation of bowel loops, absence of fluid in the perihepatic space and cul-de-sac, and focal septations allow for differentiation of an abdominal lymphangioma from ascites.[200]

Complete surgical excision of lymphangioma is performed whenever possible to prevent complications such as progressive growth, superinfection, rupture, hemorrhage, or torsion.[66,197] However, in contrast to simple lymphatic and mesothelial cysts, which are generally easily enucleated, lymphangiomas may be adherent to vital intra-abdominal structures such as small bowel, which may make complete excision difficult or impossible.[168,169]

MESOTHELIAL CYSTS

Simple mesothelial cysts are congenital lesions due to incomplete fusion of the mesothelial-lined peritoneal surfaces.[169,196,197] Most occur in young and middle-aged women and are usually located within the mesentery, although they also occur in the omentum. Mesothelial cysts do not show interval growth and are usually asymptomatic.[168,196] Pathologically, they are thin-walled unilocular cysts lined by flat, cuboidal, or columnar mesothelial cells, usually containing serous fluid, with a fibrous wall without any lymphatic structures.[168,169] Unlike lymphangiomas, mesothelial cysts have no internal septations and have internal content that follows the SI of simple fluid (Fig. 6-19). No T1-shortening is present as can be revealed in some lymphangiomas.[169] Minimal or no wall enhancement may be present.

ENTERIC DUPLICATION CYSTS

Enteric duplication cysts are true diverticula of the bowel that form during gestation and contain an enteric mucosa, a muscle layer, and a nervous plexus. With enteric duplication, the cyst wall "reduplicates" the normal enteric wall.[169] Enteric duplications are usually attached to normal bowel but occasionally migrate into the mesentery.[169] Characteristically, they occur along the mesenteric side of the bowel.[196] Pathologically, they are thick-walled, unilocular cysts with predominantly serous contents, but sometimes chylous or hemorrhagic content is present.[169,196] The wall contains all normal enteric layers including

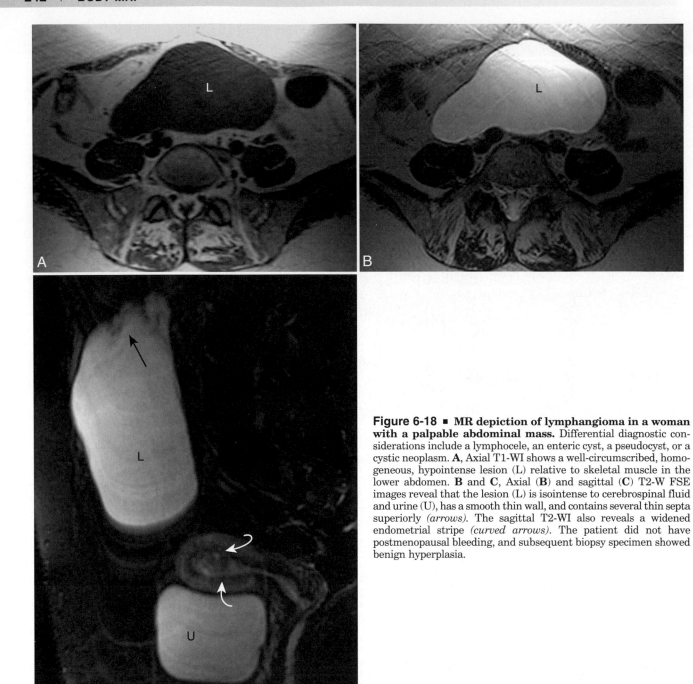

Figure 6-18 ■ MR depiction of lymphangioma in a woman with a palpable abdominal mass. Differential diagnostic considerations include a lymphocele, an enteric cyst, a pseudocyst, or a cystic neoplasm. **A,** Axial T1-WI shows a well-circumscribed, homogeneous, hypointense lesion (L) relative to skeletal muscle in the lower abdomen. **B** and **C,** Axial (**B**) and sagittal (**C**) T2-W FSE images reveal that the lesion (L) is isointense to cerebrospinal fluid and urine (U), has a smooth thin wall, and contains several thin septa superiorly *(arrows).* The sagittal T2-WI also reveals a widened endometrial stripe *(curved arrows).* The patient did not have postmenopausal bleeding, and subsequent biopsy specimen showed benign hyperplasia.

mucosa (usually gastric or pancreatic small bowel epithelium), circular and longitudinal muscle layers, and the mesenteric plexus.[168,169] On MRI, a thick enhancing wall is usually visualized and the contents are usually serous, with low SI on T1-WI and high SI on T2-WI.[169]

Enteric Cysts

Enteric cysts, in contrast, originate from the migration of acquired bowel diverticula into the mesentery and are lined by enteric mucosa only, without reduplication of the bowel wall. Pathologically, they are thin smooth-walled cysts, usually unilocular, with serous contents.[169] They are lined with enteric epithelium and a thin outer fibrous wall without muscle layers or a nervous plexus.[168,169] On MRI, serous fluid contents are present, occasionally with septations but usually without a discernible wall.[169]

Bronchogenic Cysts

Bronchogenic cysts comprise a rare congenital subtype of foregut cysts and usually are located in the

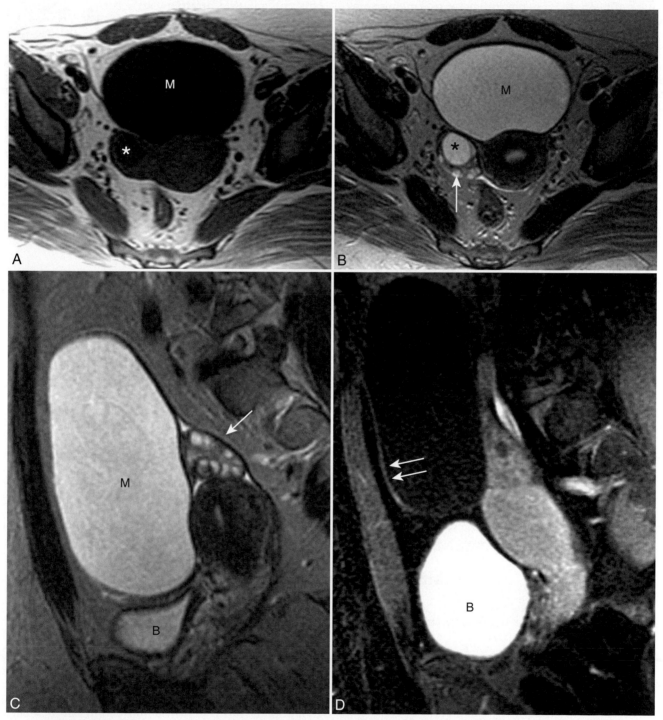

Figure 6-19 ■ **MR illustration of a mesothelial cyst in an asymptomatic 27-year-old woman with a palpable pelvic mass.** **A** and **B**, Axial T1-WI (**A**) and T2-WI (**B**) reveal an 11-cm homogeneous, well-circumscribed, T1 hypointense, T2-hyperintense cyst (M) anterior to the uterus and right ovary *(arrow)*. A 2-cm right ovarian cyst (∗) is present. **C**, Sagittal T2-W FSE image shows that the lesion is separate from the uterus and left ovary *(arrow)* and is located superior to the urinary bladder (B). **D**, Sagittal fat-suppressed CE T1-WI shows smooth peripheral rim enhancement *(arrows)* of the mass without internal enhancement. Excreted hyperintense gadolinium-contrast is present in the bladder (B).

pulmonary parenchyma or mediastinum but can rarely occur in the retroperitoneum. A retroperitoneal bronchogenic cyst is formed when an abnormal bud of the tracheobronchial tree develops during fusion of the pleuroperitoneal membranes with subsequent migration into the abdominal cavity.[203] Pathologically, bronchogenic cysts are thin-walled, usually unilocular cystic masses of nonfunctional pulmonary tissue composed of smooth muscle, cartilage, and glands, with a lining of ciliated columnar epithelium.[203,204] Usually, they are asymptomatic unless large in size, secondarily infected, or ruptured.[203] On MRI, low SI on T1-WI and high SI on T2-WI are usually present due to simple fluid, although high SI on T1-WI may be present if there is hemorrhage, protein, mucus, or debris sometimes with fluid-fluid levels.[203-205] Enhancement is generally absent or may be minimally present peripherally.[204] Most retroperitoneal bronchogenic cysts are found within the upper retroperitoneum adjacent to the diaphragmatic crura.[203,204]

Abdominal Hemangioma

The hemangioma (Box 6-25) is one of the most common soft tissue tumors, accounting for approximately 7% of all benign tumors, and closely resembles normal blood vessels.[12,206] Most hemangiomas occur superficially, with a predilection for the head and neck region, but may also occur commonly deep in parenchymal organs such as the liver and spleen or very rarely within the mesentery, omenta, or retroperitoneum. They may arise in men and women of all ages.[12,206-208]

Mesenteric and omental hemangiomas can present with abdominal pain, gastrointestinal bleeding,

hemoperitoneum, and a palpable abdominal mass.[209-211] Retroperitoneal hemangiomas tend to be asymptomatic, especially in early stages of development, and symptoms, when present, are nonspecific due to mass effect on adjacent anatomic structures.[212] Treatment is conservative, with surgical removal reserved for persistent or severe symptom relief or for the rare occurrence of lesion rupture.[213]

On MRI, a mesenteric or omental hemangioma is generally well defined with round or lobular margins and with low SI on T1-WI and high SI on both T2-WI and heavily T2-WI relative to skeletal muscle.[169,214] Occasional heterogeneity in SI may be present owing to the presence of adipocytes (with loss of SI on T1-WI out-of-phase gradient-echo images relative to in-phase images), hemorrhage (with intermediate-high SI on T1-WI), fibrosis, or thrombosis. Calcified phleboliths, when visualized, have very low SI on both T1- and T2-WI, are better visualized on CT and plain film radiography, and are suggestive of the diagnosis.[206,208,215-217]

ABDOMINOPELVIC LYMPHADENOPATHY

There are approximately 400 to 500 lymph nodes in the human body, with approximately half located in the abdomen and pelvis.[218] Both normal and malignant lymph nodes have intermediate SI on T1-WI, have intermediate-high SI on T2-WI relative to skeletal muscle, and enhance. Fatty hila with SI similar to that of subcutaneous fat may also be present. SI characteristics of lymph nodes on conventional imaging sequences are not accurate in differentiating between benign and malignant lymph nodes.[6,219] Necrotic nodes suggest malignant lymphadenopathy such as from metastatic squamous cell carcinoma or less commonly lymphoma, but may also be encountered in benign infectious diseases including tuberculosis and atypical mycobacterial infection.[220-227]

Short axis size estimation is the most often used imaging criterion to differentiate benign from malignant lymph nodes (Box 6-26).[6] As a general rule, lymph nodes less than or equal to 10 mm in short axis dimension are likely benign, whereas those larger than 10 mm are likely pathologically enlarged.[218,228] However, overlap exists, as malignant lymph nodes can sometimes be smaller than 10 mm and benign reactive or hyperplastic lymph nodes can sometimes be larger than 10 mm.[6,229,230]

Lymphoma

Lymphoma (Box 6-27) is the most common retroperitoneal malignancy, and accounts for one third of retroperitoneal malignant neoplasms.[5] Patients of all ages may be affected although the incidence of non-Hodgkin's lymphoma increases with age, whereas Hodgkin's lymphoma has a bimodal age distribution in young adults and the elderly, and the clinical course may range from indolent to highly aggressive, depending partly on the histology of the tumor.[231,232] While intra-abdominal Hodgkin's lymphoma tends

---

6-25 Features of Abdominal Hemangioma

Clinical

One of the most common soft tissue tumors
Approximately 7% of all benign tumors
Closely resembles normal blood vessels
Most occur superficially, but may commonly occur within parenchymal organs
Mesenteric, omental, or retroperitoneal involvement is extremely rare
Treatment: usually conservative, surgery for symptomatic lesions

MRI

Well-defined, round or lobular in shape
Low SI on T1-WI, high SI on T2-WI and heavily T2-WI similar to lymphangioma
Occasionally heterogeneous in SI due to adipocytes, hemorrhage, fibrosis, or thrombosis
Calcified phleboliths: intralesional foci of very low SI on T1-WI and T2-WI suggestive of diagnosis
Enhancement: progressive (vs. septal for lymphangioma)

6-26　Differential Diagnosis of Abdominopelvic Lymphadenopathy

Neoplasm (Most Common)
Lymphoma, leukemia
Metastatic neoplasm

Infection (Less Common)
Tuberculosis, atypical mycobacterial infection
Bacterial (e.g., cat-scratch disease, Whipple's disease)
Viral (e.g., HIV), fungal (e.g., histoplasmosis)

Inflammation/Miscellaneous (Uncommon)
Mesenteric lymphadenitis
Idiopathic RPF
Sarcoidosis
Amyloidosis
Castleman's disease
　Celiac sprue

MRI
Morphologic Guidelines
Short axis ≤10 mm = suggests benign
Size >10 mm = suggests malignant
Spherical shape more suspect than cylindrically
　shaped nodes
Normal retrocrural and porta hepatis nodes ≤6 mm
Normal gastrohepatic ligament nodes ≤8 mm
Normal pelvic lymph nodes ≤10–15 mm

Evaluation of SI
Most benign and malignant nodes
　Low-intermediate SI on T1-WI
　Intermediate-high SI on T2-WI
　Enhance with gadolinium
　SI alone not accurate in differentiating benign from
　　malignant nodes
Necrotic nodes: high SI on T2-WI with absent central
　enhancement
　Suggests malignancy in patients with squamous cell
　　carcinoma or lymphoma
　Can be present in granulomatous disease
High SI on T1-WI present with hemorrhagic
　metastasis (e.g., melanoma) is uncommon
Foci of very low SI on T1-WI and T2-WI suggests
　calcification
　Uncommon and better revealed with CT
　Differential diagnosis
　　Healed granulomatous disease
　　Treated lymphoma
　　Castleman's disease

6-27　Features of Abdominal Lymphoma

Clinical
One third of retroperitoneal malignancies; peritoneal
　or omental involvement is rare
Hodgkin's Disease (HD)
　Bimodal age distribution in young adults and elderly
　Confined to the spleen and retroperitoneum with
　　spread to contiguous lymph nodes
Non-Hodgkin's Lymphoma (NHL)
　Incidence of NHL increases with age
　Involves multiple lymph nodes and extranodal sites
　　with lymphatic and hematogenous spread
　50% with NHL present with mesenteric
　　lymphadenopathy
　Confluent mesenteric nodes are suggestive
Other conditions tend to have discrete mesenteric
　lymph nodes
Ann Arbor Staging System may be used for both HD
　and NHL (see Box 6-28)

MRI
Lymphadenopathy
　Low-intermediate SI on T1-WI, high SI on T2-WI,
　　with enhancement
　Occasional central necrosis, particularly after
　　treatment
　Low SI on T2-WI after treatment may represent
　　nonviable tumor/fibrosis
　Most experience involves mediastinal nodes in
　　patients with HD
Associated findings: gastrointestinal, bone marrow,
　or parenchymal organ involvement

In contrast, enlarged lymph nodes due to other conditions tend to remain discrete, rarely forming a conglomerate mass.[1] Abdominal pain or a palpable abdominal mass may be present along with constitutional symptoms and signs. The Ann Arbor Staging System for lymphoma (Box 6-28) is used for both Hodgkin's and non-Hodgkin's lymphoma to help predict the prognosis and survival of patients, but it is less useful for non-Hodgkin's lymphoma, since it more frequently disseminates hematogenously.[231,232,235] The management approach to patients with lymphoma is dependent on multiple factors and either may be conservative or involve chemotherapy, radiation therapy, immunotherapy, bone marrow transplantation, or surgical resection.[231,232]

On MRI, lymphoma is typically intermediate-slightly high in SI on T1-WI and high SI on T2-WI relative to muscle (Fig. 6-20).[236] Associated involvement of the bone marrow, gastrointestinal and genitourinary tract, and other parenchymal organs such as the liver or spleen may be present (see Figs. 2-23, 4-15, 5-14, and 7-11). Uncommonly, findings of peritoneal lymphomatosis may also be present. Assessment of the SI of lymphomatous nodal masses after therapy on T2-WI may be useful because low SI

to be confined to the spleen and retroperitoneum, with spread of disease to contiguous lymph nodes, non-Hodgkin's lymphoma more commonly involves a variety of nodal groups and extranodal sites.[231-234] Approximately 50% of patients with non-Hodgkin's lymphoma have mesenteric lymphadenopathy at presentation, which may become confluent, with characteristic encasement of the mesenteric vessels.

6-28 Ann Arbor Staging System for Lymphoma*

Stage I

Involvement of a single lymph node region (stage I), or
Tumor involvement of a single extralymphatic organ or site (stage IE)

Stage II

Involvement of ≥2 lymph node regions on the same side of the diaphragm (stage II), or
Localized involvement of an extralymphatic organ or site (stage IIE)

Stage III

Involvement of lymph nodes on both sides of the diaphragm (stage III), or
Localized involvement of an extralymphatic organ or site (stage IIIE) or spleen (stage IIIS) or both (stage IIIES)

Stage IV

Diffuse or disseminated involvement of ≥1 extralymphatic organ with or without associated lymph node involvement

*The presence or absence of systemic symptoms should be noted with each stage designation: A = asymptomatic, B = presence of fever, sweats, or weight loss >10% of body weight

6-29 Features of Abdominal Tuberculosis (TB)

Clinical

Lymphadenopathy

The most common manifestation of abdominal TB, isolated in 55%
Mesenteric, omental, peripancreatic, periportal, pericaval, and upper para-aortic lymph nodal stations commonly involved

Peritoneal Tuberculosis

Rare (<4% of cases); associated with active disease in 20%
6th most common site of extrapulmonary TB in the USA
Increased incidence in patients with AIDS and in some immigrants
Diagnosis is usually by paracentesis or peritoneal biopsy
Mortality if untreated approaches 50%
Treatment: antituberculous drugs

MRI

Lymphadenopathy

Low-intermediate SI on T1-WI and central high SI on T2-WI in active disease
Degree of high SI on T2-WI parallels amount of central necrosis and severity of symptoms
Central low SI on T1-WI and T2-WI due to fibrosis or calcification
Homogeneous or mildly inhomogeneous enhancement present if minimal/no central necrosis
Peripheral enhancement and lack of central enhancement present with central necrosis in 40%

Peritoneal and Omental Disease

Coexistent abnormal chest radiograph present in 50%
Nonspecific nodular thickening and enhancement of peritoneum
Complex ascites

on T2-WI within treated lymph node masses suggests nonviable tumor or fibrosis. However, most of the published experience of using T2-W SI to document response to treatment has focused on patients with mediastinal Hodgkin's lymphoma.[237]

Abdominal Tuberculosis

Lymphadenopathy is the most common manifestation of abdominal tuberculosis (Box 6-29) and is the only abdominal finding in half of patients.[225,226] The mesenteric, omental, peripancreatic, periportal, pericaval, and upper para-aortic lymph nodes are commonly involved, related to lymphatic drainage from the small bowel and right colon. On MRI, the lymph nodes are usually multiple and large (with a mean size of 2 to 3 cm in diameter) with low-intermediate SI on T1-WI and central high SI on T2-WI relative to skeletal muscle in active disease, without associated urinary, biliary, or gastrointestinal tract obstruction.[224-226,238] The degree of high SI on T2-WI within lymph nodes generally parallels the amount of central necrosis, and the degree of nodal necrosis correlates with clinical signs and symptoms. Less commonly, central low SI on T1-WI and T2-WI relative to skeletal muscle may be present owing to inactive or fibrotic tissue in later stages of disease or to calcification.[224,226] The imaging findings of tuberculosis may mimic other diseases[239]; one should have a low threshold for considering a diagnosis of active tubercular infection in patients at risk.

Whipple's Disease

Whipple's disease is an unusual chronic disorder characterized by lipogranulomatous inflammation of the small bowel with systemic extension to virtually any organ system caused by infection with *Tropheryma whippelii*.[240] The peak age is in the fifth decade of life, Caucasians are most often affected, and men are affected eight times more commonly than women.[241] It is difficult to diagnose, since it may have variable clinical features, but most often presents with arthropathy, weight loss, diarrhea, and abdominal pain, and less commonly with fever, lymphadenopathy, or hepatosplenomegaly.[240,241] The diagnosis is made via biopsy of involved tissues such as the small bowel or peripheral lymph nodes, and reveals PAS-positive granular foamy macrophages on histologic analysis.[241] On MRI, findings may resemble a malignancy such as lymphoma, since hepatosplenomegaly or abdominopelvic

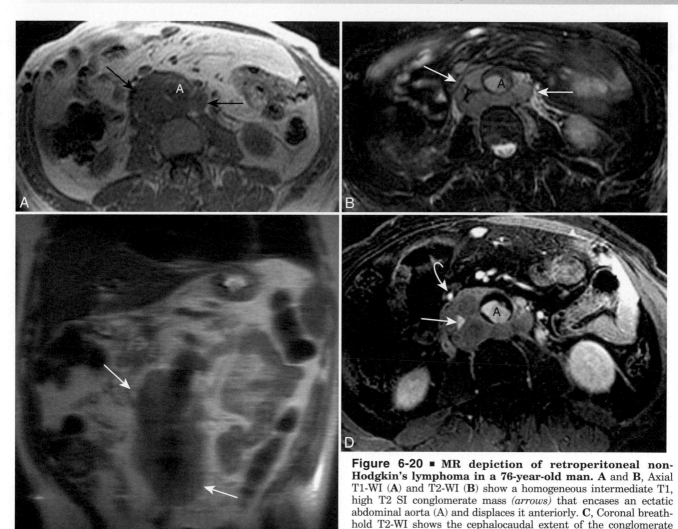

Figure 6-20 ▪ MR depiction of retroperitoneal non-Hodgkin's lymphoma in a 76-year-old man. A and **B**, Axial T1-WI (**A**) and T2-WI (**B**) show a homogeneous intermediate T1, high T2 SI conglomerate mass *(arrows)* that encases an ectatic abdominal aorta (A) and displaces it anteriorly. **C**, Coronal breath-hold T2-WI shows the cephalocaudal extent of the conglomerate lymphadenopathy *(arrows)*. **D**, Axial fat-suppressed CE T1-WI shows homogeneous mild enhancement of the conglomerate mass, with encasement of the abdominal aorta (A) and encasement and narrowing of the inferior vena cava *(arrow)* without occlusion. Malignant lymphadenopathy displaces the right ureter anteriorly *(curved arrow)*. Irregular aortic mural thrombus is present.

lymphadenopathy may be present.[240] Furthermore, lack of central enhancement of lymph nodes due to necrosis may be present.[227] Other findings may include ascites, small bowel mural and fold thickening, and sacroiliitis.[241] In general, treatment is with prolonged antibiotic therapy.[240]

Castleman's Disease

Castleman's disease (Box 6-30), also known as angio-follicular lymph node hyperplasia or benign giant lymph node hyperplasia, is a hyperplastic-dysplastic-neoplastic lymphoproliferative process of uncertain etiology that is a rare cause of abdominopelvic lymph node enlargement.[6,242,243] It tends to present clinically with either unicentric or localized disease confined to a single anatomic lymph node–bearing region

that remains relatively stable, or with multicentric or disseminated disease characterized by generalized lymphadenopathy, constitutional symptoms, organomegaly, and a more aggressive clinical course, with 30% of patients developing malignant transformation.[243-245] Unicentric disease presents at a significantly younger age (peak age in the third decade of life) than does multicentric disease (peak age in the sixth decade of life).[242,243] Patients with unicentric disease usually have intrathoracic disease, whereas in patients with multicentric disease, various anatomic sites including the mesentery, retroperitoneum, and pelvis may be involved (in 7% to 12% of cases).[243,245,246]

On MRI, the lesions of Castleman's disease generally have low-intermediate SI on T1-WI and high SI on T2-WI relative to the liver parenchyma, with

6-30 Features of Castleman's Disease

Clinical

Idiopathic hyperplastic-dysplastic-neoplastic lymphoproliferative process
Rare cause of abdominopelvic lymphadenopathy
Clinical presentation
Unicentric/localized disease
  Peak age: 3rd decade of life, M:F = 1:1
  Rarely associated with malignant transformation
  Prognosis: very good
  Mediastinal or hilar nodal stations most common sites
  Rarely involves the abdomen or pelvis
  Treatment: surgical resection
Multicentric/disseminated disease
  Peak age: 6th decade of life, M:F = 2:1
  Associated with malignant transformation (lymphoma, Kaposi's sarcoma) in 30%
  Prognosis: very poor, median survival of 2-3 years
  Treatment: combination chemotherapy and corticosteroids

MRI

Well-defined, homogeneous, single, large intra-abdominal mass or single dominant mass with satellite nodules in unicentric disease (mean size = 6 cm)
Variably sized, well-defined lymph nodes sometimes with hepatosplenomegaly, ascites, and retroperitoneal fascial thickening in multicentric disease
Low intermediate SI on T1-WI, intermediate to high SI on T2-WI
Occasional central low SI on T1-WI and T2-WI due to fibrosis or calcification
Calcification in one third on CT may have an arborizing linear radial pattern
Enhancement is variable

mild-marked enhancement.[245,247] Calcification may be present in approximately one third of cases of abdominal Castleman's disease and is better revealed on CT.[245,246] Unicentric disease tends to show a well-defined, homogeneous, single, large intra-abdominal mass or a single dominant mass with satellite nodules (with a mean size 6 cm and range of 3 to 10 cm), whereas multicentric disease tends to show variably sized well-defined lymph nodes in multiple locations, sometimes also with associated findings of hepatosplenomegaly, ascites, and retroperitoneal fascial thickening.[245]

Surgical resection generally is standard treatment for unicentric Castleman's disease, usually with resolution of systemic symptoms and laboratory abnormalities within a few months, with a cure rate approaching 100%.[243,244] Combination chemotherapy and corticosteroids are the mainstay of treatment for multicentric Castleman's disease, although interferon may be used alternatively.[243,248] Despite these treatment measures, multicentric Castleman's disease

has a poor prognosis, with a median survival of 24 to 33 months, with death most commonly due to sepsis and lymphoma.[242,244,246]

RETROPERITONEAL FIBROSIS (RPF)

Retroperitoneal fibrosis (RPF; Box 6-31) is a rare fibrotic reactive process with a prevalence of about 1 per 200,000 population.[249] Idiopathic RPF (Ormond's disease) occurs more commonly in men by a ratio of 2:1, which has been attributed to the higher incidence of symptomatic atherosclerotic disease in men.[249,250] Patients of any age may develop RPF, but most are in the fifth or sixth decade of life.[250,251]

Most patients with RPF have vague, nonspecific abdominal symptoms, including dull back, flank, and abdominal pain.[250,251] Symptoms and signs may be related to entrapment and compression of retroperitoneal structures including the ureters, IVC, aorta and its branches, and gonadal vessels.[249] The ureters are the most frequently compressed structures, and pain probably is due to inflammation, ureteral obstruction, or abnormal ureteral peristalsis.[249,251] Oliguria, anuria, and eventual renal failure may occur.

6-31 Features of Retroperitoneal Fibrosis (RPF)

Clinical

Rare fibrotic retroperitoneal process
Peak age: 5th to 6th decades of life
M:F = 2:1 if idiopathic
15% associated with fibrotic processes elsewhere in the body
Etiology
  66% idiopathic, 33% other
  Ergot derivatives
  Retroperitoneal metastatic disease
  Abdominal infection or inflammation
  Retroperitoneal hemorrhage or urine
  Abdominal surgery or irradiation
Treatment
  Corticosteroids
  Ureterolysis, percutaneous nephrostomy, or ureteral stent placement for ureteral obstruction
Prognosis
  Poor if malignant in etiology (mean survival of 3–6 months)
  Excellent if idiopathic
  10-year survival = 70% because of atherosclerotic complications

MRI

Low SI on T1-WI whether benign or malignant
Low SI on T2-WI if mature benign RPF
High SI on T2-WI if immature or malignant RPF
Variable enhancement

Compression of the IVC can result in lower extremity edema, scrotal edema, or deep thrombophlebitis of the lower extremities. In approximately 15% of individuals with RPF, associated fibrotic processes outside the retroperitoneum may be present, including fibrosing mediastinitis, sclerosing mesenteritis, orbital pseudotumor, primary sclerosing cholangitis, and Reidel's thyroiditis.[251,252] Laboratory abnormalities are present in those with obstructive uropathy.[250]

Approximately two thirds of all cases of RPF are considered idiopathic, and approximately one third of cases develop in response to various medications, malignancies, or other causes.[249] Up to 25% of patients with abdominal aortic aneurysms (called inflammatory abdominal aortic aneurysms) may have an association with perianeurysmal fibrosis and are considered by some to be an early or mild form of RPF.[249,251] Inflammatory abdominal aortic aneurysms are discussed separately below.

Approximately 1% of patients who take methysergide, an ergot derivative used to treat migraine headaches, develop RPF, with symptomatic relief commonly occurring after drug withdrawal.[249,251,253] Because of this known side effect of methysergide (as well as pleural and valvular fibrosis), there has been decreased use of this drug and fewer drug-related cases of RPF.[254] Other ergot derivatives such as bromocriptine, used to treat parkinsonism, may also be associated with RPF.

Malignant RPF is an unusual subtype of RPF and is clinically difficult to distinguish from RPF due to benign or idiopathic causes. Malignant RPF occurs when small metastatic foci to the retroperitoneum (usually a lymphoma) elicit an exuberant desmoplastic response.[249] Malignant RPF is distinct from malignant retroperitoneal lymphadenopathy, with the latter typically associated with lateral ureteral displacement.[251] Infections due to tuberculosis, syphilis, actinomycosis, or fungi; nonspecific gastrointestinal inflammation including appendicitis, Crohn's disease, or diverticulitis; retroperitoneal hemorrhage; urine extravasation; or prior irradiation or surgery are all rare reportable causes of RPF.[249,251]

The exact cause of idiopathic RPF is unclear, although some believe that chronic fibrosing periaortitis, possibly due to an immune reaction to a component of ruptured atherosclerotic plaque such as ceroid (an insoluble complex of proteins and oxidized low-density lipoprotein), may play a role.[250,251] The observation that RPF tends to occur in areas where an arterial wall (usually of the aorta) has severe atherosclerotic plaque and attenuation of the media supports this theory.[249] Gross pathologic findings of RPF include a dense, grayish-white, plaque-like mass that surrounds the inferior aspect of the abdominal aorta, often with encasement or compression of the ureters, the aorta, and other retroperitoneal structures.[12] Histologically there is a zonal change in tissue characterization within RPF from central to lateral; the lateral edges of RPF tend to be inflammatory, whereas the central portion tends to be fibrotic.[249,250]

RPF typically originates below the aortic bifurcation at the level of the sacral promontory or lower lumbar vertebrae, and then extends superiorly along the anterior spinal surface in a periaortic and pericaval distribution toward the renal hila, where rarely it may surround the renal pelves.[249] Typically, one or both ureters, usually in the middle third, may be encased, often with resultant hydronephrosis. The anterior margin of RPF respects the posterior peritoneal boundary and is sharply marginated, whereas the posterior margin tends to be less well defined but infiltrative of adjacent structures.[249] The fibrotic plaque may be midline or eccentric, well-circumscribed or ill-defined, and localized or extensive.[249,255] RPF is of low-intermediate SI on T1-WI.[255] On T2-WI, mature fibrotic plaque in benign RPF has low SI (Figs. 6-21 and 6-22), whereas immature fibrotic plaque in early benign RPF and malignant RPF has high SI due to either a high free water content with inflammatory edema or hypercellularity.[249,252,255,256] After corticosteroid therapy and with maturation, there is a decrease in inflammatory reaction with a subsequent in decrease in SI on T2-WI and decreased enhancement on dynamic CE T1-WI.[257,258]

Imaging findings that are more suggestive of a malignant etiology for RPF are the presence of other lymphadenopathy or metastatic disease, subjacent osseous destruction, an ill-defined margin, or inhomogeneity of the plaque or associated high SI changes of the adjacent psoas muscles on T2-WI.[6,255] Malignant retroperitoneal lymphadenopathy is a differential diagnostic consideration for RPF, since it can occasionally become confluent and encase the great vessels and thus mimic the appearance of RPF, particularly with lymphoma (see Fig. 6-20). Generally, however, retroperitoneal metastatic disease most commonly appears as lobulated para-aortic and paracaval masses due to enlarged lymph nodes.[249] Lymphoma and other tumors that result in malignant lymphadenopathy displace the aorta anteriorly and the ureters laterally, whereas benign RPF usually does not cause significant anterior aortic displacement or lateral ureteral displacement (see Fig. 6-22).[249,251]

While rare spontaneous regression of RPF has been reported, most patients require some form of medical or surgical treatment.[12] Patients with methysergide- or bromocriptine-related RPF are treated with drug discontinuation, after which there is often prompt regression of both symptoms and fibrosis.[251] In other patients with RPF, deep biopsies are routinely obtained to exclude a malignant or infectious cause before potential corticosteroid therapy is instituted[250,251] The use of corticosteroids to decrease inflammation in early idiopathic disease typically results in improvement in signs and symptoms and shrinkage/maturation of the RPF on imaging, along with relief of ureteral obstruction within 7 to 10 days.[249,259] If medical therapies alone are not effective, intervention with open or laparoscopic ureterolysis (ureteral dissection from the surrounding fibrotic

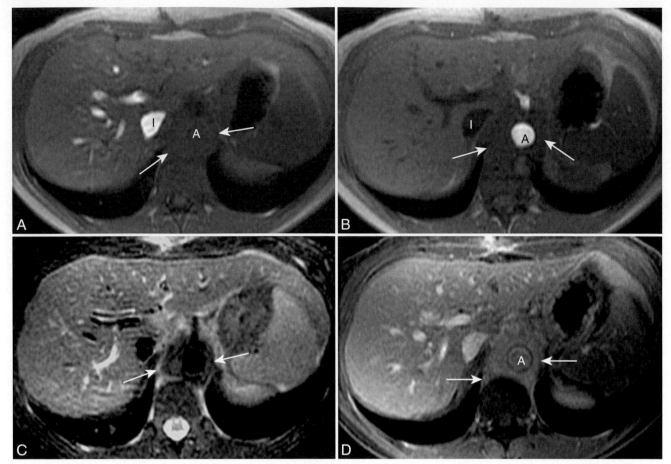

Figure 6-21 ■ MR depiction of periaortic retroperitoneal fibrosis in a 30-year-old woman with abdominal pain and weight loss. A and **B,** Axial T1-WIs show a subtle rim of low SI soft tissue *(arrows)* relative to skeletal muscle around the aorta (A) at the level of the celiac trunk. The hepatic and portal veins and the IVC (I) are hyperintense in **A.** Image **A** was the most inferior of an axial set of gradient echo (GRE) images that did not use inferior or superior saturation bands. Thus, the high SI is secondary to flow-related enhancement. The abdominal aorta and celiac artery are hyperintense in **B** because of flow-related enhancement; the image was acquired as the most superior slice of a second set of GRE images. This "feature" of GRE images obtained without saturation bands provides information regarding vessel patency and direction of flow. **C,** Axial fat-suppressed T2-WI shows low to intermediate SI periaortic soft tissue *(arrows),* suggestive of mature fibrosis. **D,** Axial fat-suppressed CE T1-WI shows mild homogeneous enhancement of the periaortic tissue. The aorta is not displaced anteriorly (see Figure 6-20).

plaque) often is successful in alleviating ureteral obstruction.[260] Although ureterolysis successfully relieves ureteral obstruction in approximately 90% of cases, recurrent obstruction occurs in up to 22% of those treated with ureterolysis alone. Therefore, corticosteroid therapy often is used concomitantly to arrest the inflammatory process, and it is most effective during earlier stages of disease.[251,260]

The prognosis for patients with malignant RPF is exceedingly poor, with a mean survival of 3 to 6 months after diagnosis.[251,252] Conversely, the prognosis for those with idiopathic RPF is generally favorable.[251] In fact, with effective ureterolysis and without renal compromise, a long-term success rate in terms of prevention of recurrent obstructive symptomatology and maintenance of renal function exceeding 90% may be achieved.[252] However, these patients usually have

significant atherosclerotic disease, resulting in future morbidity and mortality secondary to myocardial infarctions and cerebrovascular accidents, and consequently the 10-year survival rate of patients with RPF is usually reported at less than 70%.[250]

INFLAMMATORY ABDOMINAL AORTIC ANEURYSM (IAAA)

Approximately 5% to 15% of patients with abdominal aortic aneurysms (AAAs) have associated asymptomatic perianeurysmal fibrosis, which is similar morphologically and histologically to RPF.[250,261] Perianeurysmal fibrosis is not protective against aneurysm rupture but often renders operative repair of such aneurysms difficult and hazardous.[261-263]

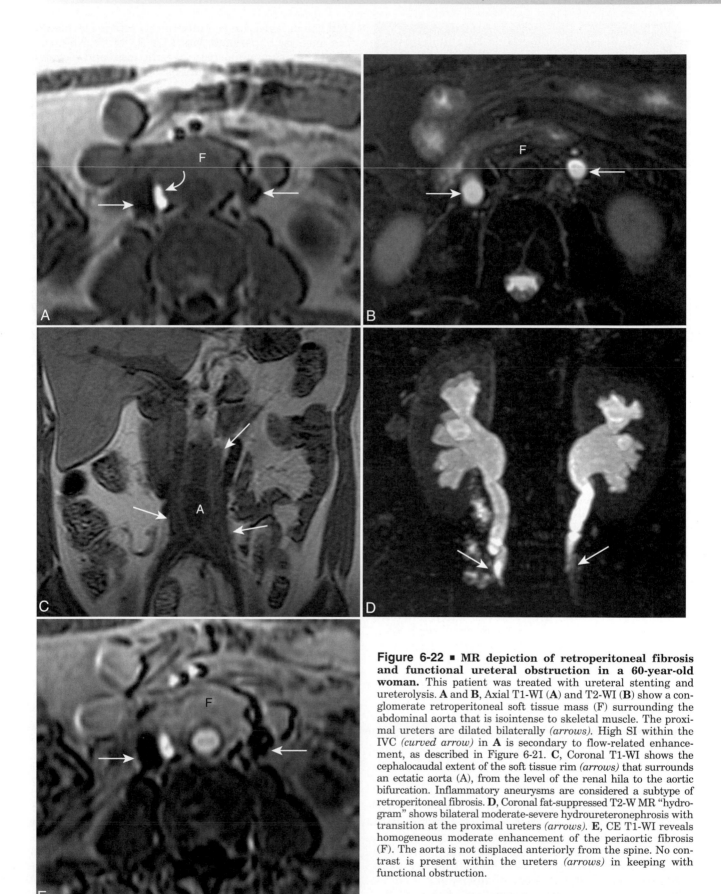

Figure 6-22 ▪ MR depiction of retroperitoneal fibrosis and functional ureteral obstruction in a 60-year-old woman. This patient was treated with ureteral stenting and ureterolysis. **A** and **B**, Axial T1-WI (**A**) and T2-WI (**B**) show a conglomerate retroperitoneal soft tissue mass (F) surrounding the abdominal aorta that is isointense to skeletal muscle. The proximal ureters are dilated bilaterally *(arrows)*. High SI within the IVC *(curved arrow)* in **A** is secondary to flow-related enhancement, as described in Figure 6-21. **C**, Coronal T1-WI shows the cephalocaudal extent of the soft tissue rim *(arrows)* that surrounds an ectatic aorta (A), from the level of the renal hila to the aortic bifurcation. Inflammatory aneurysms are considered a subtype of retroperitoneal fibrosis. **D**, Coronal fat-suppressed T2-W MR "hydrogram" shows bilateral moderate-severe hydroureteronephrosis with transition at the proximal ureters *(arrows)*. **E**, CE T1-WI reveals homogeneous moderate enhancement of the periaortic fibrosis (F). The aorta is not displaced anteriorly from the spine. No contrast is present within the ureters *(arrows)* in keeping with functional obstruction.

6-32 Features of Inflammatory Abdominal Aortic Aneurysm (IAAA)

Clinical

5% to 15% of all AAA
Peak age: 7th decade of life, M : F >> 1 : 1
More likely symptomatic and larger than noninflammatory AAA at presentation
Mean size larger compared with noninflammatory AAA
Most often associated with elevated erythrocyte sedimentation rate (ESR)
Overall survival similar to that of noninflammatory AAA
Treatment: pre-operative corticosteroids, particularly if other retroperitoneal structures are encased

MRI

Aneurysmal dilatation of the abdominal aorta
Perianeurysmal cuff of soft tissue
Intermediate SI on T1-WI
Intermediate-high SI on T2-WI, with concentric rings of high SI alternating with intermediate SI
Homogeneous cuff enhancement
Associated encasement or obstruction of adjacent retroperitoneal structures

The pathogenesis of inflammatory abdominal aortic aneurysm (IAAA) (Box 6-32) is thought to be similar to that of idiopathic RPF, with the perianeurysmal inflammatory response representing an immune reaction to antigens such as ceroid that leak from the aortic wall.[264] Grossly, the anterior and lateral walls of IAAAs are covered with a thick white layer of fibrous tissue that can adhere the duodenum and other adjacent structures to the aneurysm sac. In severe cases, this inflammatory/fibrous tissue may extend to involve the ureters, IVC, left renal vein, small bowel mesentery, or transverse mesocolon with potential obstruction. The periaortic inflammatory tissue partially explains why operative treatment of an IAAA has a higher mortality rate than that of a noninflammatory AAA, and thus pre-operative recognition is important.[261]

Both atherosclerotic AAAs and IAAAs occur more commonly in men than in women, and in patients with IAAA, the mean age at presentation is in the seventh decade (similarly to atherosclerotic AAA), with an age range in the sixth through ninth decades. However, most patients (75%) with IAAAs have abdominal or back pain, compared with only 13.5% of those with noninflammatory AAA.[265] Patients with IAAAs tend to be significantly more symptomatic (most commonly with back and abdominal pain) than those with noninflammatory AAAs (93% vs. 9%), are more likely to have a family history of aneurysms (17% vs. 1.5%), and tend to be current smokers (45% vs. 24%). IAAAs tend to be larger than noninflammatory AAAs at presentation (with a mean size of 8.0 cm vs. 6.4 cm),

and the erythrocyte sedimentation rate is elevated in the majority of patients with IAAAs.[263,265-267] The triad of chronic abdominal pain, weight loss, and elevated sedimentation rate in a patient with an AAA is highly suggestive of an IAAA.[268]

On MRI, the typical imaging appearance of an IAAA consists of a complex layered wall of a dilated aorta with concentric rings of high SI that are most prominent on T2-WI but are also present on T1-WI. These mural concentric rings represent alternating layers of fibrosis and inflammation. IAAAs have three or more concentric layers of high SI, whereas noninflammatory AAAs show at most two rings of high SI.[261] On T1-WI, the surrounding rim of inflammatory tissue shows intermediate SI with poor differentiation from intraluminal thrombus and surrounding structures. On CE T1-WI, the inflammatory cuff enhances homogeneously with distinct definition of intraluminal thrombus and with better definition of adjacent involved structures.[264] Furthermore, on CE T1-WI, the rim of tissue surrounding the aorta may be similar in appearance to retroperitoneal fibrosis, with the exception of aneurysmal dilatation of the abdominal aorta.[249] In patients presenting with a suspected IAAA, MRI-MRA is recommended by some as the diagnostic test of choice as opposed to CE CT, sinxw MRI a has high sensitivity in detecting perianeurysmal inflammatory change and is appropriate in those patients who have renal impairment.[264]

Preoperative treatment of individuals with IAAA with corticosteroids may be useful to control the inflammatory process and facilitate surgical repair, particularly when the inflammatory process is severe or there is associated involvement of adjacent retroperitoneal structures.[269] Aneurysm resection is the treatment of choice for the IAAA, since the risk of aortic rupture does exist and more than 75% of patients undergo spontaneous remission of perianeurysmal fibrosis following surgical repair. Treated patients with IAAAs need to be followed by imaging, as they are at risk of developing perianastomotic aneurysms.[270] The 5-year and 10-year survival rates in surgically treated patients with IAAAs and noninflammatory AAAs are similar.[263,265,270]

RETROPERITONEAL AND PERITONEAL FLUID COLLECTIONS

Fluid collections (Box 6-33) are by far the most common pathologic peritoneal process imaged, and both peritoneal and retroperitoneal fluid collections may result from neoplastic, infectious, inflammatory, and traumatic causes.[1,271] Peritoneal fluid collections, or ascites, may be classified as either transudative or exudative based on biochemical parameters such as the serum-ascites albumin gradient or total protein content. Cirrhosis, nephrotic syndrome, congestive heart failure, and low protein states are some usual causes of transudative ascites, whereas malignancy, infectious peritonitis, and pancreatitis are the common causes of exudative ascites.[1] Peritoneal and retroperitoneal fluid collections may also be classified as simple, proteinaceous, hemorrhagic, bilious, chylous, uriniferous, enteric, infectious, inflammatory, or malignant, based on the composition of the fluid and the underlying etiology (Box 6-34).[1,272]

In most cases, retroperitoneal fluid collections remain confined to their compartment of origin by fascial planes or adhesions.[271,273] However, large, rapidly developing fluid volumes may decompress along laminated, variably fused, potentially expansile retroperitoneal fascial planes.[271] With severe inflammation, infection, or hemorrhage, transfascial spread between compartments as well as extension into the psoas muscle and abdominal wall musculature may occur, frequently with obliteration or displacement of adjacent structures or thickening of surrounding soft tissue planes.[273]

Inflammatory fluid collections are most prominent near the site of origin. Most inflammatory fluid collections originate in the anterior pararenal space of the retroperitoneum from extraperitoneal portions of the gastrointestinal tract including the pancreas, ascending and descending colon, duodenum, and retroperitoneal appendix. Acute pancreatitis is one of the most common causes of an anterior pararenal fluid collection (see Fig. 2-34), and peripancreatic fluid often extends into the lesser peritoneal sac and subperitoneal spaces of the small bowel mesentery and transverse mesocolon.[271,273] Inflammatory fluid collections confined to the posterior pararenal space of the

6-33 Features of Retroperitoneal and Peritoneal Fluid Collections

Common; usually confined by fascial planes or adhesions
May decompress along fascial planes or spread
 transfascially
Etiology
 Transudative fluid
  Causes: cirrhosis, nephrotic syndrome, congestive
   heart failure, hypoproteinemia
 MRI
  Follows the SI of simple fluid on T1-WI and T2-WI
  Nonloculated
 Peritoneal fluid: greater sac > lesser sac favors
  transudate
  Exudative fluid
   Causes: malignancy, infection, inflammation
    (e.g., pancreatitis)

MRI

Varying degrees of T1-shortening, high SI on T2-WI
Loculation common
Peritoneal enhancement may be present
Peritoneal fluid
Greater sac = lesser sac favors malignant ascites
Greater sac < lesser sac favors inflammatory
 pancreatic ascites

6-34 Subtypes of Localized Retroperitoneal and Peritoneal Fluid Collections

Hematoma

Clinical

Risk factors: recent surgery, trauma, coagulopathy
Pain and a drop in hematocrit are typical

MRI

Concentric ring sign is specific for subacute hematoma
Inner rim of high SI methemoglobin on T1-WI
Variable low SI outer rim on T1-WI and T2-WI
 secondary to hemosiderin
No solid enhancing components
Should decrease in size with time

Biloma

Clinical

70% have right upper quadrant pain
Most have history of bile duct surgery or trauma
Can be complicated by peritonitis
Treatment: catheter drainage and repair of site
 of leakage

MRI

Localized fluid in a peribiliary/perihepatic location
Biloma has similar T1-W and T2-W SI to simple fluid
MRI contrast agents with biliary excretion may be
 helpful for characterizing the fluid as bile and
 identifying site of active bile leak

Chylous fluid

Clinical

Chylous ascites is rare, chyloretroperitoneum is very rare
Abdominal malignancy and trauma are two
 leading causes
Morbidity due to metabolic disturbance and
 lymphocytopenia
Treatment: nutritional support, surgical repair
 if necessary

MRI

Fat or lipid containing ascites is specific if identified

Urinoma

Clinical

Risk factors: urinary obstruction, trauma, surgery,
 or instrumentation

MRI

Follows SI of urine in urinary bladder: low SI on
 T1-WI, high SI on T2-WI
May see delayed enhancement from
 gadolinium-excreted contrast in urine

Abscess

Clinical

Risk factors: surgery, inflammatory disease or perforation
 of the gastrointestinal or genitourinary tract, another
 primary site of infection (e.g., spinal osteomyelitis)
Due to bacteria, tuberculosis, or parasitic disease

MRI

Low in SI on T1-WI, intermediate-high in SI on T2-WI,
 sometimes with T2 hypointense lower SI layering
 debris
Up to 50% have very low SI gas on T1-WI and T2-WI
Thick peripheral rim enhancement

retroperitoneum are rare, since no organs are present within this space, but most inflammatory fluid collections involving the posterior pararenal space tend to be secondary to severe infection in another space, such as osteomyelitis of the spine, ribs, or pelvis.[6,273]

Nonloculated fluid collections are shaped by the surrounding structures, do not deform the shapes of the normal organs, and flow to a dependent position.[272] The distribution of a peritoneal fluid collection between the lesser and greater peritoneal sacs may help suggest its etiology. For example, transudative ascites tends to have a smaller lesser sac component, carcinomatosis tends to have similar-sized lesser and greater sac components, and pancreatitis tends to have a larger lesser sac component.[1] On MRI, simple fluid collections and transudative ascites have low SI on T1-WI and very high SI on T2-WI, whereas proteinaceous fluid collections and exudative ascites tend to have similar T2-W SI but variable higher SI on T1-WI.[1,272]

Hemorrhage/Hematoma

Retroperitoneal and intraperitoneal hemorrhage-hematoma (Box 6-35) may be secondary to rupture or leak of an aneurysm or vascular malformation, anticoagulant therapy, a bleeding diathesis, trauma, arterial catheterization, or underlying parenchymal organ pathology with rupture, or it may be spontaneous.[1,6,271,273] Spontaneous retroperitoneal hemorrhage usually originates in the posterior pararenal space and may extend into the properitoneal fat, pelvis, psoas muscle, or abdominal wall musculature.[273] However, most AAAs tend to bleed posteriorly with either confinement by the psoas space or extension into the posterior interfascial plane behind the left kidney, and the IVC often bleeds directly into the right posterior interfascial plane. In such cases, hemorrhage is often present in the perirenal spaces as well, and the anterior interfascial planes are less commonly involved.[271]

On MRI, the appearance of hemorrhage is dependent on on its age.[6,274,275] It is uncommon to perform an abdominal or pelvic MRI examination to evaluate for a hyperacute or acute hematoma. Thus, most hematomas revealed on abdominal MRI examinations are either subacute or chronic. A subacute hematoma may show two outer characteristic layers of SI: a thin peripheral rim with low SI on all pulse sequences corresponding to hemosiderin and an inner peripheral high SI zone that is most distinctive on T1-WI due to methemoglobin (Figs. 6-23 to 6-25; see Fig. 5-15). The central component of the hematoma has variable SI based on the amounts of seroma, deoxyhemoglobin, and methemoglobin present.[6,276] This appearance of the periphery of a fluid collection on T1-WI is known as the concentric ring sign and is pathognomonic for a subacute hematoma.[276] Maturing hematomas decrease in size and the SI of the core diminishes while the outer rim becomes very hypointense on both T1- and T2-WI secondary to hemosiderin deposition.[6] Active hemorrhage may sometimes be present as a focus or jet of extraluminal high SI on T1-WI owing to extravasation of intravenous gadolinium contrast material, and it generally indicates a need for immediate surgical or angiographic therapy.[1,277] Occasionally, a hemorrhagic tumor may be difficult to differentiate from spontaneous nonneoplastic hemorrhage, but hemorrhagic neoplasms typically have conspicuous, solid, enhancing soft tissue components, whereas hemorrhagic lesions with a large component of very high T1-WI SI are usually benign hematomas.[6]

Bile/Biloma

Intraperitoneal bilious fluid collections (bilomas) may be caused by iatrogenic, traumatic, or spontaneous rupture of the biliary tree and are usually located in the upper abdomen, with 70% in the right upper quadrant and 30% in the left upper quadrant.[278] Often, they are asymptomatic, but sometimes bile peritonitis can result. Bilious fluid demonstrates

---

6-35 MRI of Hemorrhage

Age	Time Range	Principal Component	SI on T1-WI	SI on T2-WI
Hyperacute	Minutes–hours	Intracellular oxyhemoglobin	Low-intermediate	High
Acute	Hours–3 days	Intracellular deoxyhemoglobin	Low	Low
Early subacute	3 to 7 days	Intracellular methemoglobin	High	Low
Late subacute	1 Week–months	Extracellular methemoglobin	High	High
Chronic	Months–years	Hemosiderin and ferritin	Very low	Very low

Take-home Points of Chart

1. Methemoglobin results in marked T1-shortening (and thus very high SI) within subacute hematomas
2. Hemosiderin and ferritin within chronic hematomas result in marked T2-shortening (and thus very low SI on both T1-WI and T2-WI)
3. Acute hematomas may be of low SI on both T1-WI and T2-WI secondary to deoxyhemoglobin and the absence of methemoglobin

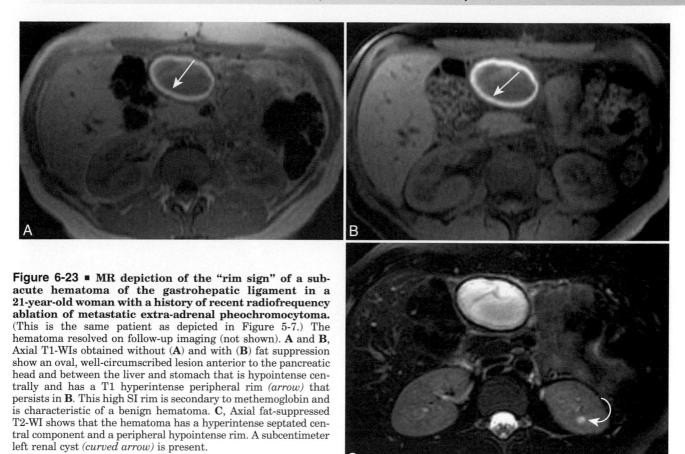

Figure 6-23 ▪ MR depiction of the "rim sign" of a subacute hematoma of the gastrohepatic ligament in a 21-year-old woman with a history of recent radiofrequency ablation of metastatic extra-adrenal pheochromocytoma. (This is the same patient as depicted in Figure 5-7.) The hematoma resolved on follow-up imaging (not shown). **A** and **B**, Axial T1-WIs obtained without (**A**) and with (**B**) fat suppression show an oval, well-circumscribed lesion anterior to the pancreatic head and between the liver and stomach that is hypointense centrally and has a T1 hyperintense peripheral rim *(arrow)* that persists in **B**. This high SI rim is secondary to methemoglobin and is characteristic of a benign hematoma. **C**, Axial fat-suppressed T2-WI shows that the hematoma has a hyperintense septated central component and a peripheral hypointense rim. A subcentimeter left renal cyst *(curved arrow)* is present.

variable SI on T1-WI and high SI on T2-WI, similar to the SI of the gallbladder.[272,278] Both gadolinium- and manganese-based MRI contrast agents are available that are excreted through the biliary system. A delayed enhanced MRI examination using one of these agents could confirm that a localized fluid collection was bile and identify the site of bile leak.[279] Most bilomas are treated successfully with percutaneous catheter drainage and treatment of the underlying site of bile leak.[278]

Chylous Ascites

The rare chyloperitoneum (chylous ascites) and the very rare chyloretroperitoneum are due to collections of lymphatic fluid or chyle in the peritoneal cavity and retroperitoneum, respectively.[1,280-282] The most common cause of chylous ascites in adults is abdominal malignancy, with lymphoma accounting for up to 50% of cases, although any type of cancer and lymph node involvement may lead to chyloperitoneum.[282,283] Iatrogenic and nonsurgical trauma are the second most common cause of chyloperitoneum, which may be present in up to 8% of patients who undergo complex abdominal surgical procedures.[283,284] Primary chylous

disorders may also lead to chylous ascites.[281] The principal mechanisms of chylous ascites formation are leakage from retroperitoneal megalymphatics, usually through a lymphoperitoneal fistula, and leakage from dilated subserosal small bowel and mesenteric lymphatics, usually caused by obstruction of the cisterna chyli or thoracic duct.[282,285]

On MRI, a fat-fluid level may be identified within a chyloperitoneum as a result of its high fat content, which is nearly pathognomonic.[286,287] Chemical shift imaging may reveal the lipid within chylous ascites, but this has not been reported to date. In the absence of detectable fat within the ascites, a diagnosis is established by the clinical history and chemical evaluation of the fluid. The differential diagnosis includes intraperitoneal rupture of a teratoma, which is rare.

Urine/Urinoma

Uriniferous fluid collections are usually found in the retroperitoneum, most commonly within the perinephric spaces, and are most often due to obstructive uropathy and less frequently to abdominopelvic trauma, surgery, or diagnostic

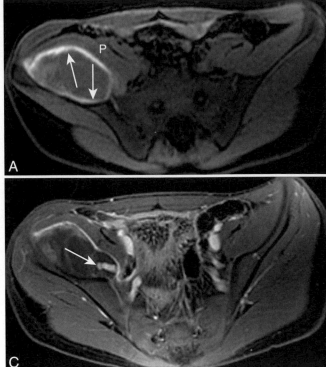

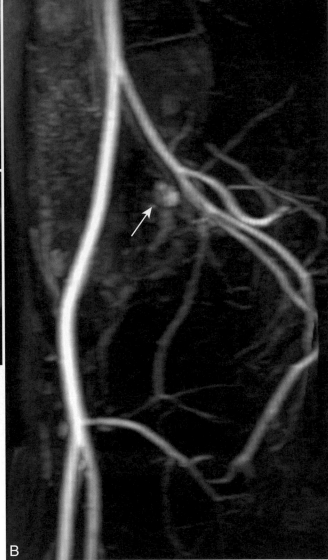

Figure 6-24 ▪ **MR illustration of an internal iliac pseudoaneurysm and retroperitoneal hematoma in a man with lower extremity numbness 2 weeks following trauma.** **A,** Axial fat-suppressed T1-WI shows a well-defined retroperitoneal mass anterior to the right iliac bone that has central intermediate SI and a peripheral high SI rim *(arrows)* relative to skeletal muscle. The mass displaces the right iliopsoas muscle (P) anteriorly. The peripheral hyperintense rim represents methemoglobin in a subacute hematoma. **B,** Oblique sagittal maximum intensity projection (MIP) image obtained during an arterial phase CE MRA shows an enhancing pseudoaneurysm *(arrow)* of the anterior division of the right internal iliac artery. **C,** Axial fat-suppressed CE T1-WI reveals a focal enhancement *(arrow)* within the medial portion of the pseudoaneurysm.

instrumentation.[271,273] Occasionally, intraperitoneal uriniferous ascites may occur if the anatomic boundaries of the retroperitoneal space have been disrupted by trauma or prior surgery, such as in the case of traumatic intraperitoneal bladder rupture.[288] As urine extravasates into the retroperitoneum, it causes lipolysis of the perirenal fat with encapsulation, forming a urinoma.[271,273] On MRI an urinoma or uriniferous ascites tends to have low SI on T1-WI and very high SI on T2-WI, similarly to simple fluid elsewhere in the body. In some cases, urine leakage can be directly demonstrated on CE T1-WI during the excretory phase of enhancement as delayed enhancement of fluid secondary to gadolinium-contrast extravasation from the genitourinary system.[1,272] Management of urinomas generally consists of treatment of the underlying cause of urine leakage, and sometimes percutaneous drainage of the urinomas themselves.[289]

Infectious Fluid Collections/Abscess

Infectious fluid collections in the retroperitoneum are typically subacute, with nonspecific symptoms and signs of nausea, vomiting, weight loss, fever, chills, night sweats, anorexia, flank pain, or hip pain.[6,273] As a result, the diagnosis of retroperitoneal infection may be overlooked in 25% to 50% of patients, with a subsequent increase in morbidity and mortality.[273]

Infectious fluid collections of the peritoneal cavity may either be localized with peritoneal abscess formation or generalized with diffuse peritonitis.[1] An abscess, by definition, is a cavity filled with pus that, when mature, consists of central necrosis-containing cellular debris and peripheral hypervascular connective tissue.[272] The most common site for peritoneal abscess formation is the pouch of Douglas, which is the most dependent site in the peritoneal cavity, although infectious fluid also preferentially ascends in the right paracolic gutter into the right subphrenic and subhepatic peritoneal spaces, which are also common sites of peritoneal abscesses.[1] Peritoneal abscesses form most frequently after surgery, particularly of the gastrointestinal tract, but also form secondary to bowel perforation in the setting of complicated Crohn's disease, appendicitis, or diverticulitis.[1,272] Percutaneous abscess drainage is commonly used to treat both peritoneal and retroperitoneal abscesses along with concomitant antibiotic therapy, since failure to drain an abscess may result in a mortality rate of up to 100%.[273]

On MRI, abscesses appear as localized, complex fluid collections that usually demonstrate low SI on T1-WI, sometimes intermediate-high SI on T1-WI if there is increased protein content, intermediate-high SI on T2-WI, and thick peripheral rim enhancement (Fig. 6-26; see Fig. 7-58).[6,290] Layering debris may be present with low SI on T1- and T2-WI and gas in the form of bubbles, or a gas-fluid level may also be present in 40% to 50% of imaged cases with very low SI on T1- and T2-WI, which may increase the specificity for the diagnosis of a lesion as an abscess.[6,290,291] Most abscesses are round or oval, but those adjacent to solid organs may have a lenticular or crescentic configuration instead.[1]

Retroperitoneal fluid collections related to the psoas muscle, in the absence of pancreatitis, are uncommon. Spread of infection from gastrointestinal disease (e.g., secondary to appendicitis, diverticulitis,

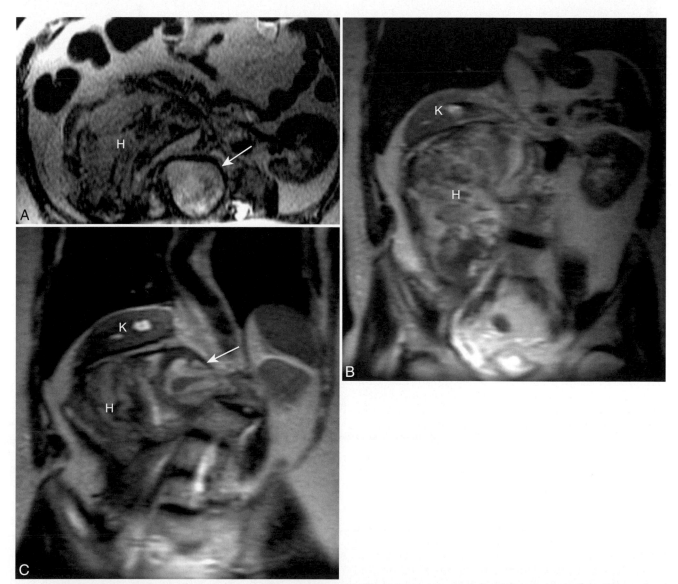

Figure 6-25 ▪ **MR illustration of a lumbar artery pseudoaneurysm in a 53-year-old man with pain, fever, anemia, and a history of prior facet joint injections. A–C,** Axial (**A**) and coronal (**B** and **C**) T2-WIs show a large, heterogeneous, intermediate-to-high SI right retroperitoneal hematoma (H) that displaces and rotates the right kidney (K). A focal hyperintense right lumbar artery pseudoaneurysm *(arrow)* is present. *(Continued)*

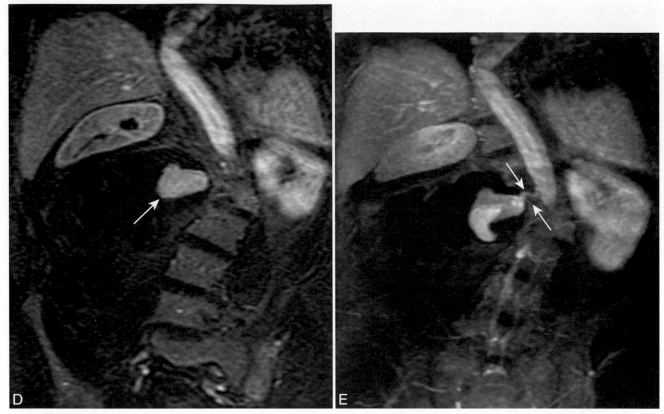

Figure 6-25 ■ Cont'd D and **E**, Coronal fat-suppressed arterial-phase CE T1-W source image (**D**) and MIP image (**E**) depict the enhancing pseudoaneurysm (*arrow* in **D**) and the feeding lumbar artery (*arrows* in **E**). The pseudoaneurysm was successfully treated by coil embolization.

Crohn's disease, or perforated colon carcinoma) is the most common source of a secondary psoas muscle fluid collection, and renal disease (e.g., secondary to a perinephric abscess) is the second most common source. Extension from osteomyelitis of the spine is not uncommon. Primary psoas muscle abscesses are generally rare and idiopathic, although they may have an incidence as high as 20% in some parts of the world, particularly in immunocompromised patients, with up to 90% due to *Staphylococcus aureus* infection. Tuberculosis should be considered in the differential diagnosis of a psoas muscle collection, since tuberculosis is an important cause of retroperitoneal abscess worldwide.[292,293] Five percent of patients with spinal tuberculosis (Pott's disease) develop a tuberculous psoas abscess, although large tuberculous psoas abscesses may occur without concomitant signs of bone involvement.[6,292,294]

On MRI, an abscess of the psoas muscle has findings similar to those of an abscess elsewhere in the body (as described above), sometimes with secondary findings of psoas muscle enlargement, high SI on T2-WI due to muscle edema, bone destruction, and infiltration and loss of surrounding fat planes best visualized on T1-WI.[292,295] Psoas muscle hematomas often have a peripheral rim of high SI on T1-WI secondary to methemoglobin. This finding coupled with a history of trauma or anticoagulation therapy is often diagnostic, and a patient with this combination can be followed clinically. Malignancies with cystic components that involve the psoas muscle are usually large and aggressive and have solid enhancing tissue, so that the distinction between abscess, hematoma, and tumor is not difficult to establish with MRI.

The management of psoas muscle abscesses may include percutaneous drainage, surgical drainage, and/or antibiotic or antituberculous therapy. Successful treatment depends on differentiating primary from secondary psoas collections, as those associated with renal or gastrointestinal disease may additionally require early surgery to correct the underlying disease process. However, percutaneous abscess drainage prior to definitive surgery may be useful to reduce morbidity.[292]

PERITONITIS

Peritonitis (Box 6-36) is inflammation of the peritoneum and is most often due to bacterial infection.[272,296] Bacterial peritonitis may be classified as either primary or secondary. Primary, or spontaneous, bacterial peritonitis (SBP) occurs without an evident

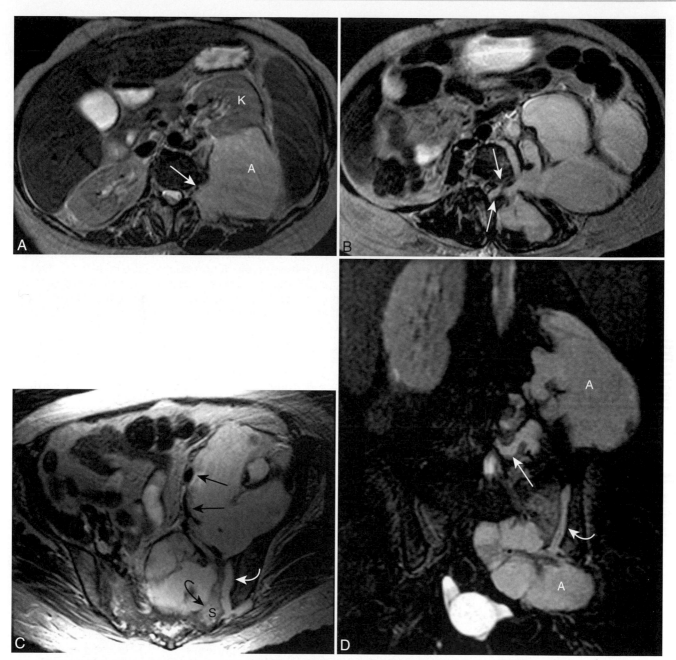

Figure 6-26 ▪ MR depiction of a retroperitoneal abscess secondary to *S. aureus* infection in a 46-year-old immunosuppressed woman. The abscess was subsequently drained percutaneously. **A–C,** Axial T2-WIs show a high SI collection of the left posterior pararenal space (A) that along its superior portion displaces the left kidney (K) anteriorly and partially enters a left thoracic neural foramen *(arrow).* Centrally (**B**), the abscess infiltrates the prevertebral space, paravertebral muscles, and left psoas muscle and extends into the epidural space *(arrows),* with rightward displacement of the thecal sac. The route of extension of fluid from the posterior pararenal space to the paraspinal muscular compartment is identical to the process that results in flank ecchymoses, or Grey Turner's sign, in acute pancreatitis. At the level of the pelvis (**C**), infection extends into the left sacroiliac joint *(curved arrow)* and the left gluteal muscular space. Hyperintense left sacral *(curved arrow, S)* marrow represents osteomyelitis. Medial displacement of the flow voids of left external iliac artery and vein *(black arrows)* confirms the retroperitoneal origin of the infection. **D,** Coronal T2-W STIR image redemonstrates extension of the retroperitoneal abscess (A) into the epidural space through multiple left neural foramina *(long arrow)* and into the left sacroiliac joint *(curved arrow).*

intra-abdominal source of infection and represents colonization of low-protein ascites during a bacteremic episode.[272,296] SBP most often arises in patients with cirrhosis and ascites in whom the incidence of SBP is approximately 12%.[296-298] SBP occurs in 25% of hospitalized cirrhotic patients with ascites and in up to 50% of patients with variceal hemorrhage. For patients who survive an initial episode of SBP, recurrent SBP develops in more than half.[298]

6-36 Features of Peritonitis

Clinical

Subtypes
Infectious (most common cause, most commonly
  bacterial)
Granulomatous (due to foreign materials)
Chemical (due to irritant materials)
Sclerosing peritonitis
Bacterial peritonitis
  Primary or spontaneous (SBP)
    Cirrhotic patients with ascites, 10% annual risk in
      this patient population
    Usually monobacterial, *E. coli* most common
  Diagnosis: paracentesis and ascitic fluid analysis
  Treatment: empiric antibiotic therapy
  Prognosis: poor, mortality approaching 50%
  Secondary
    Due to intra-abdominal disorders involving loss of
      integrity of the gastrointestinal or genitourinary
      tract
    Usually polymicrobial in etiology
    Treatment: antimicrobial therapy, surgical
      correction of the underlying anatomic
      abnormality

MRI

Thickening and enhancement of peritoneal surfaces
Simple or loculated ascites
Findings of cirrhosis or portal hypertension in SBP

---

a diagnosis.[296] SBP has a mortality rate of 15% to 50%, in part due to severe underlying chronic liver disease, and has a very poor long-term prognosis, as 70% to 80% of patients who survive an episode of SBP die of liver disease within the following 2 years.[297,298] Factors associated with a worse prognosis include hepatic encephalopathy, renal insufficiency, hyperbilirubinemia, hypoalbuminemia, and hypothermia. The mainstay of treatment is empiric antibiotic therapy.[296]

Secondary bacterial peritonitis may be due to one of many intra-abdominal disorders including peptic ulcer disease, acute cholecystitis, acute appendicitis, acute diverticulitis, pancreatitis, or penetrating trauma that involve loss of integrity of the gastrointestinal or genitourinary tract with subsequent leak of intraluminal contents into the peritoneal space. At paracentesis, a polymicrobial Gram stain strongly suggests secondary peritonitis, and the treatment of secondary peritonitis entails surgical correction of the underlying cause, along with antimicrobial medications.

On MRI, imaging findings of bacterial peritonitis include thickening and enhancement of peritoneal surfaces, simple or loculated ascites, and septations, sometimes with associated findings of cirrhosis in cases of SBP or findings of other intra-abdominal processes in cases of secondary bacterial peritonitis (Fig. 6-27).[1,272,296] Delayed enhancement of ascites may also be present in SBP but is not specific, since it may occur with other causes of exudative ascites.[299,300]

SCLEROSING ENCAPSULATING PERITONITIS

Sclerosing encapsulating peritonitis is a severe, rare condition characterized by progressive peritoneal sclerosis, inflammation, calcification, and vascular alterations, with partial or total encasement of the small bowel.[301,302] Sclerosing encapsulating peritonitis is multifactorial in etiology but is most commonly associated with chronic ambulatory peritoneal dialysis (in <1% of patients).[301-306] Affected patients tend to have had a long duration of dialysis with bioincompatible substances in the peritoneal dialysis solutions and concomitant bacterial peritonitis, leading to peritoneal cavity fibrin production and organization.[302,307]

Symptoms and signs that may occur include anorexia, nausea, abdominal pain, distension, and loss of peritoneal ultrafiltration.[301,302,307] Onset often is insidious, and in most patients the correct diagnosis frequently is not suspected, resulting in delayed treatment.[301]

At gross pathology, the peritoneal surface appears as a rough, thickened membrane that causes rigidity, thickening, and decreased mobility of small bowel loops. Histopathologically, peritoneal sclerosis with compact layered fibrotic tissue and dystrophic calcifications are present.[302] Often, one area of the

---

SBP in patients with cirrhosis tends to be monobacterial, predominantly involving gram-negative bacilli, most often *Escherichia coli*.[296] Overall, *E. coli*, *Klebsiella*, and *Streptococcus* are responsible for 75% of all cases of SBP.[298] Portosystemic shunting, impairment of phagocytic and metabolic activity of hepatic Kupffer cells, and hypocomplementemia contribute to decreased clearance of bacteremia and increased risk of SBP. A hematogenous route for spread of infection to the peritoneal cavity has been postulated, although bacterial translocation across an intact intestinal mucosa is an alternative route.[296]

Patients with SBP may have classic findings of acute peritonitis such as marked abdominal pain and rebound tenderness, fever, leukocytosis, and hypotension.[298] More commonly, however, patients have more subtle signs and symptoms.[296-298] Approximately one third of patients are asymptomatic. Any medical deterioration in a cirrhotic patient should raise clinical suspicion for SBP, since early diagnostic paracentesis and empiric antibiotic therapy are beneficial.[298] Although SBP can definitively be differentiated from secondary bacterial peritonitis only by laparotomy or laparoscopy, clinical features and laboratory analysis of ascitic fluid are usually sufficient to establish

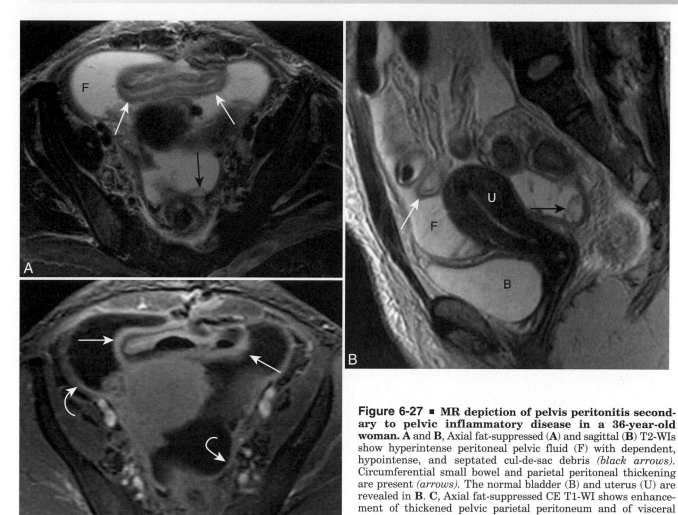

Figure 6-27 ■ MR depiction of pelvis peritonitis secondary to pelvic inflammatory disease in a 36-year-old woman. A and B, Axial fat-suppressed (A) and sagittal (B) T2-WIs show hyperintense peritoneal pelvic fluid (F) with dependent, hypointense, and septated cul-de-sac debris *(black arrows)*. Circumferential small bowel and parietal peritoneal thickening are present *(arrows)*. The normal bladder (B) and uterus (U) are revealed in B. C, Axial fat-suppressed CE T1-WI shows enhancement of thickened pelvic parietal peritoneum and of visceral peritoneum that lines several pelvic small bowel segments *(curved arrows)*, and circumferentially thickened mural portions of small bowel *(arrows)*.

abdomen is more affected than others, forming a mass or an "abdominal cocoon," usually containing segments of small bowel and ascites.[301,306]

On MRI, features suggestive of sclerosing peritonitis include adherent, dilated small bowel loops with gas-fluid levels and mural thickening; very low SI calcification/ossification of the visceral or parietal peritoneum on all pulse sequences, which generally is better visualized on CT; diffuse smooth peritoneal thickening, sometimes with marked enhancement; and loculated ascites (Fig. 6-28).[301,302,305,308]

Surgical treatment generally is performed when there is bowel obstruction and involves lysis of adhesions/membranes and release of obstructed small bowel.[301,302,306] Medical treatment may include corticosteroids, immunosuppressants, or total parenteral nutrition. Antibiotics may be administered if peritoneal infection is suspected.[302] In patients who are undergoing chronic ambulatory peritoneal dialysis, switching from peritoneal dialysis to hemodialysis can result in improvement in both symptoms and signs.

Overall, sclerosing encapsulating peritonitis has a high mortality rate of 25% to 90%, with a mortality rate of 60% at 4 months in one series, due to bowel obstruction, malnutrition, septicemia, or postoperative complications.[302,306,307,309] As such, prevention, when possible, is very important and may include the use of more biocompatible peritoneal dialysis solutions, avoidance of intraperitoneal drugs except antibiotics, prompt management of peritonitis, and peritoneal biopsies when a peritoneal dialysis catheter is placed or removed to assess for peritoneal sclerosis.[302]

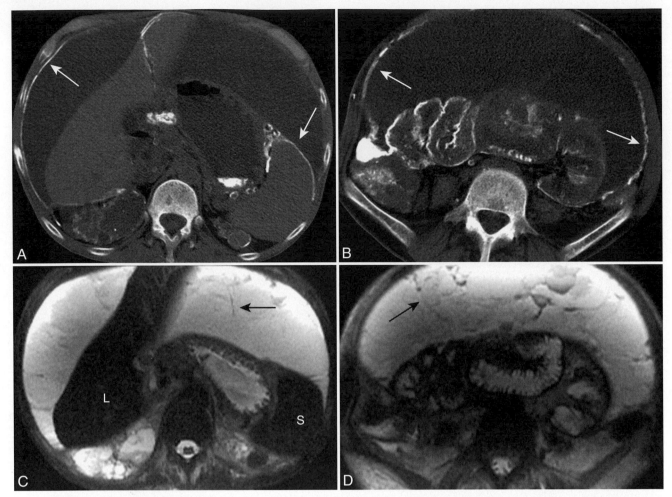

Figure 6-28 ▪ **MR illustration of sclerosing peritonitis in a 47-year-old man with a history of peritoneal dialysis and small bowel obstruction.** CT better detects and characterizes calcification than MRI does. **A** and **B**, Axial unenhanced CT images obtained within the abdomen (**A**) and at the level of the iliac crests (**B**) show curvilinear calcifications *(arrows)* of the visceral peritoneal surfaces of the liver and spleen, falciform ligament, gastrohepatic ligament, gastrosplenic ligament, and parietal peritoneum. Low attenuation complex peritoneal fluid deforms the liver contour. Cystic renal disease of dialysis is present. Inferiorly, small bowel segments are centrally distributed but "tethered" posteriorly, resulting in functional small bowel obstruction. Septated complex ascites is present. **C** and **D**, Axial fat-suppressed T2-WIs at the same anatomic levels as **A** (**C**) and **B** (**D**) demonstrate hypointense liver (L) and spleen (S) from prior transfusions. While hypointense septa *(arrows)* and fluid-fluid levels within the complex ascites are well revealed, the peritoneal calcifications are poorly visualized. Tethering of multiple small bowel segments is present.

REFERENCES

1. Healy JC, Reznek RH. The peritoneum, mesenteries and omenta: normal anatomy and pathological processes. Eur Radiol 1998;8:886-900.
2. Coakley FV, Hricak H. Imaging of peritoneal and mesenteric disease: key concepts for the clinical radiologist. Clin Radiol 1999;54:563-574.
3. Chou CK, Liu GC, Chen LT, Jaw TS. MRI demonstration of peritoneal ligaments and mesenteries. Abdom Imaging 1993;18:126-130.
4. Oliphant M, Berne AS, Meyers MA. Direct spread of subperitoneal disease into solid organs: radiologic diagnosis. Abdom Imaging 1995;20:141-147; discussion 148.
5. Barker CD, Brown JJ. MR imaging of the retroperitoneum. Top Magn Reson Imaging 1995;7:102-111.
6. Engelken JD, Ros PR. Retroperitoneal MR imaging. Magn Reson Imaging Clin North Am 1997;5:165-178.
7. Cyran KM, Kenney PJ. Leiomyosarcoma of abdominal veins: value of MRI with gadolinium DTPA. Abdom Imaging 1994;19:335-338.
8. Low RN, Semelka RC, Worawattanakul S, Alzate GD. Extrahepatic abdominal imaging in patients with malignancy: comparison of MR imaging and helical CT in 164 patients. J Magn Reson Imaging 2000;12:269-277.
9. Low RN, Semelka RC, Worawattanakul S, Alzate GD, Sigeti JS. Extrahepatic abdominal imaging in patients with malignancy: comparison of MR imaging and helical CT, with subsequent surgical correlation. Radiology 1999;210:625-632.
10. Low RN, Sigeti JS. MR imaging of peritoneal disease: comparison of contrast-enhanced fast multiplanar spoiled gradient-recalled and spin-echo imaging. AJR Am J Roentgenol 1994;163:1131-1140.
11. Shibata D, Lewis JJ, Leung DH, Brennan MF. Is there a role for incomplete resection in the management of retroperitoneal liposarcomas? J Am Coll Surg 2001;193:373-379.
12. Weiss SW, Goldblum JR. Enzinger and Weiss's Soft Tissue Tumors. St. Louis: Mosby, 2001.
13. Herman K, Kusy T. Retroperitoneal sarcoma—the continued challenge for surgery and oncology. Surg Oncol 1998;7:77-81.
14. Lewis JJ, Leung D, Woodruff JM, Brennan MF. Retroperitoneal soft-tissue sarcoma: analysis of 500 patients treated and followed at a single institution. Ann Surg 1998;228:355-365.

15. Stoeckle E, Coindre JM, Bonvalot S, et al. Prognostic factors in retroperitoneal sarcoma: a multivariate analysis of a series of 165 patients of the French Cancer Center Federation Sarcoma Group. Cancer 2001;92:359-368.

16. Pirayesh A, Chee Y, Helliwell TR, et al. The management of retroperitoneal soft tissue sarcoma: a single institution experience with a review of the literature. Eur J Surg Oncol 2001;27:491-497.

17. Bautista N, Su W, O'Connell TX. Retroperitoneal soft-tissue sarcomas: prognosis and treatment of primary and recurrent disease. Am Surg 2000;66:832-836.

18. McGinn CJ. The role of radiation therapy in resectable retroperitoneal sarcomas. Surg Oncol 2000;9:61-65.

19. Makela J, Kiviniemi H, Laitinen S. Prognostic factors predicting survival in the treatment of retroperitoneal sarcoma. Eur J Surg Oncol 2000;26:552-555.

20. Nishino M, Hayakawa K, Minami M, Yamamoto A, Ueda H, Takasu K. Primary Retroperitoneal Neoplasms: CT and MR Imaging Findings with Anatomic and Pathologic Diagnostic Clues. Radiographics 2003;23:45-57.

21. Nishimura H, Zhang Y, Ohkuma K, Uchida M, Hayabuchi N, Sun S. MR imaging of soft-tissue masses of the extraperitoneal spaces. Radiographics 2001;21:1141-1154.

22. Hartman DS, Hayes WS, Choyke PL, Tibbetts GP. From the archives of the AFIP. Leiomyosarcoma of the retroperitoneum and inferior vena cava: radiologic-pathologic correlation. Radiographics 1992;12:1203-1220.

23. Alektiar KM, Hu K, Anderson L, Brennan MF, Harrison LB. High-dose-rate intraoperative radiation therapy (HDR-IORT) for retroperitoneal sarcomas. Int J Radiat Oncol Biol Phys 2000;47:157-163.

24. van Geel AN, Pastorino U, Jauch KW, et al. Surgical treatment of lung metastases: The European Organization for Research and Treatment of Cancer-Soft Tissue and Bone Sarcoma Group study of 255 patients. Cancer 1996;77:675-682.

25. Kim T, Murakami T, Oi H, et al. CT and MR imaging of abdominal liposarcoma. AJR Am J Roentgenol 1996;166:829-833.

26. Sung MS, Kang HS, Suh JS, et al. Myxoid liposarcoma: appearance at MR imaging with histologic correlation. Radiographics 2000;20:1007-1019.

27. Lane RH, Stephens DH, Reiman HM. Primary retroperitoneal neoplasms: CT findings in 90 cases with clinical and pathologic correlation. AJR Am J Roentgenol 1989;152:83-89.

28. Jelinek JS, Kransdorf MJ, Shmookler BM, Aboulafia AJ, Malawer MM. Liposarcoma of the extremities: MR and CT findings in the histologic subtypes. Radiology 1993;186:455-459.

29. Arkun R, Memis A, Akalin T, Ustun EE, Sabah D, Kandiloglu G. Liposarcoma of soft tissue: MRI findings with pathologic correlation. Skeletal Radiol 1997;26:167-172.

30. Kransdorf MJ, Bancroft LW, Peterson JJ, Murphey MD, Foster WC, Temple HT. Imaging of Fatty Tumors: Distinction of Lipoma and Well-differentiated Liposarcoma. Radiology 2002;224:99-104.

31. Israel GM, Bosniak MA, Slywotzky CM, Rosen RJ. CT differentiation of large exophytic renal angiomyolipomas and perirenal liposarcomas. Am J Roentgenol 2002;179:769-773.

32. Weiss SW, Rao VK. Well-differentiated liposarcoma (atypical lipoma) of deep soft tissue of the extremities, retroperitoneum, and miscellaneous sites. A follow-up study of 92 cases with analysis of the incidence of "dedifferentiation." Am J Surg Pathol 1992;16:1051-1058.

33. Henricks WH, Chu YC, Goldblum JR, Weiss SW. Dedifferentiated liposarcoma: a clinicopathological analysis of 155 cases with a proposal for an expanded definition of dedifferentiation. Am J Surg Pathol 1997;21:271-281.

34. Kransdorf MJ, Meis JM, Jelinek JS. Dedifferentiated liposarcoma of the extremities: imaging findings in four patients. AJR Am J Roentgenol 1993;161:127-130.

35. Tateishi U, Hasegawa T, Beppu Y, Satake M, Moriyama N. Primary dedifferentiated liposarcoma of the retroperitoneum. Prognostic significance of computed tomography and magnetic resonance imaging features. J Comput Assist Tomogr 2003;27:799-804.

36. Munk PL, Lee MJ, Janzen DL, et al. Lipoma and liposarcoma: evaluation using CT and MR imaging. AJR Am J Roentgenol 1997;169:589-594.

37. Kransdorf MJ. Malignant soft-tissue tumors in a large referral population: distribution of diagnoses by age, sex, and location. AJR Am J Roentgenol 1995;164:129-134.

38. Griffin AS, Sterchi JM. Primary leiomyosarcoma of the inferior vena cava: a case report and review of the literature. J Surg Oncol 1987;34(Suppl):53-60.

39. La Fianza A, Alberici E, Meloni G, Preda L, Campani R. Extraperitoneal pelvic leiomyosarcoma. MR findings in a case. Clin Imaging 2000;24:224-226.

40. Mizoe A, Takebe K, Kanematsu T. Primary leiomyosarcoma of the jejunal mesentery: report of a case. Surg Today 1998;28:87-90.

41. Mahon DE, Carp NZ, Goldhahn RT, Jr., Schmutzler RC 3rd. Primary leiomyosarcoma of the greater omentum: case report and review of the literature. Am Surg 1993;59:160-163.

42. Mingoli A, Cavallaro A, Sapienza P, Di Marzo L, Feldhaus RJ, Cavallari N. International registry of inferior vena cava leiomyosarcoma: analysis of a world series on 218 patients. Anticancer Research 1996;16:3201-3205.

43. Hines OJ, Nelson S, Quinones-Baldrich WJ, Eilber FR. Leiomyosarcoma of the inferior vena cava: prognosis and comparison with leiomyosarcoma of other anatomic sites. Cancer 1999;85:1077-1083.

44. Ko SF, Wan YL, Lee TY, Ng SH, Lin JW, Chen WJ. CT features of calcifications in abdominal malignant fibrous histiocytoma. Clin Imaging 1998;22:408-413.

45. Sebbag G, Yan H, Shmookler BM, Chang D, Sugarbaker PH. Results of treatment of 33 patients with peritoneal mesothelioma. Br J Surg 2000;87:1587-1593.

46. Raptopoulos V. Peritoneal mesothelioma. Crit Rev Diag Imaging 1985;24:293-328.

47. Averbach AM, Sugarbaker PH. Peritoneal mesothelioma: treatment approach based on natural history. Cancer Treat Res 1996;81:193-211.

48. Haliloglu M, Hoffer FA, Fletcher BD. Malignant peritoneal mesothelioma in two pediatric patients: MR imaging findings. Pediatr Radiol 2000;30:251-255.

49. Tandar A, Abraham G, Gurka J, Wendel M, Stolbach L. Recurrent peritoneal mesothelioma with long-delayed recurrence. J Clin Gastroenterol 2001;33:247-250.

50. Sugarbaker PH. Review of a personal experience in the management of carcinomatosis and sarcomatosis. Jpn J Clin Oncol 2001;31:573-583.

51. Begossi G, Gonzalez-Moreno S, Ortega-Perez G, Fon LJ, Sugarbaker PH. Cytoreduction and intraperitoneal chemotherapy for the management of peritoneal carcinomatosis, sarcomatosis and mesothelioma. Eur J Surg Oncol 2002;28:80-87.

52. Stafford-Johnson DB, Bree RL, Francis IR, Korobkin M. CT appearance of primary papillary serous carcinoma of the peritoneum. AJR Am J Roentgenol 1998;171:687-689.

53. Chopra S, Laurie LR, Chintapalli KN, Valente PT, Dodd GD, 3rd. Primary papillary serous carcinoma of the peritoneum: CT-pathologic correlation. J Comput Assist Tomogr 2000;24:395-399.

54. Chu CS, Menzin AW, Leonard DG, Rubin SC, Wheeler JE. Primary peritoneal carcinoma: a review of the literature. Obstet Gynecol Survey 1999;54:323-335.

55. Eltabbakh GH, Piver MS. Extraovarian primary peritoneal carcinoma. Oncology (Huntington) 1998;12:813-819; discussion 820, 825-826.

56. Lauchlan SC. The secondary Mullerian system. Obstet Gynecol Survey. 1972;27:133-146.

57. Kannerstein M, Churg J, McCaughey WT, Hill DP. Papillary tumors of the peritoneum in women: mesothelioma or papillary carcinoma. Am J Obstet Gynecol 1977;127:306-314.

58. Furukawa T, Ueda J, Takahashi S, et al. Peritoneal serous papillary carcinoma: radiological appearance. Abdom Imaging 1999;24:78-81.

59. Sugarbaker PH, Ronnett BM, Archer A, et al. Pseudomyxoma peritonei syndrome. Adv Surg 1996;30:233-280.

60. Ronnett BM, Yan H, Kurman RJ, Shmookler BM, Wu L, Sugarbaker PH. Patients with pseudomyxoma peritonei associated with disseminated peritoneal adenomucinosis have a significantly more favorable prognosis than patients with peritoneal mucinous carcinomatosis. Cancer 2001;92:85-91.

61. Esquivel J, Sugarbaker PH. Clinical presentation of the Pseudomyxoma peritonei syndrome. Br J Surg 2000;87:1414-1418.

62. Sherer DM, Abulafia O, Eliakim R. Pseudomyxoma peritonei: a review of current literature. Gynecol Obstet Invest 2001;51:73-80.

63. Hinson FL, Ambrose NS. Pseudomyxoma peritonei. Br J Surg 1998;85:1332-1339.

64. Sugarbaker PH, Chang D. Results of treatment of 385 patients with peritoneal surface spread of appendiceal malignancy. Ann Surg Oncol 1999;6:727-731.

65. Gupta S, Gupta RK, Gujral RB, Agarwal D, Saxena R, Tandon P. Peritoneal mesothelioma simulating pseudomyxoma peritonei on CT and sonography. Gastrointestinal Radiol 1992;17:129-131.

66. Ozgen A, Akata D, Akhan O, Tez M, Gedikoglu G, Ozmen MN. Giant benign cystic peritoneal mesothelioma: US, CT, and MRI findings. Abdom Imaging 1998;23:502-504.

67. Deans GT, Spence RA. Neoplastic lesions of the appendix. Br J Surg 1995;82:299-306.

68. Sugarbaker PH. Management of peritoneal-surface malignancy: the surgeon's role. Langenbecks Archives of Surgery 1999;384:576-587.

69. Pestieau SR, Jelinek JS, Chang D, Jacquet P, Sugarbaker PH. CT in the selection of patients with abdominal or pelvic sarcoma for reoperative surgery. J Am Coll Surg 2000;190:700-710.

70. Outwater E, Schiebler ML, Brooks JJ. Intraabdominal desmoplastic small cell tumor: CT and MR findings. J Comput Assist Tomogr 1992;16:429-432.

71. Quaglia MP, Brennan MF. The clinical approach to desmoplastic small round cell tumor. Surg Oncol 2000;9:77-81.

72. Goodman KA, Wolden SL, La Quaglia MP, Kushner BH. Whole abdominopelvic radiotherapy for desmoplastic small round-cell tumor. Int J Radiat Oncol Biol Phys 2002;54:170-176.

73. Gerald WL, Miller HK, Battifora H, Miettinen M, Silva EG, Rosai J. Intra-abdominal desmoplastic small round-cell tumor. Report of 19. Am J Surg Pathol 1991;15:499-513.

74. Pickhardt PJ, Fisher AJ, Balfe DM, Dehner LP, Huettner PC. Desmoplastic small round cell tumor of the abdomen: radiologic-histopathologic correlation. Radiology 1999;210:633-638.

75. Wolf AN, Ladanyi M, Paull G, Blaugrund JE, Westra WH. The expanding clinical spectrum of desmoplastic small round-cell tumor: a report of two cases with molecular confirmation. Human Pathol 1999;30:430-435.

76. Tateishi U, Hasegawa T, Kusumoto M, Oyama T, Ishikawa H, Moriyama N. Desmoplastic small round cell tumor: imaging findings associated with clinicopathologic features. J Comput Assist Tomogr 2002;26:579-583.

77. Sabate JM, Torrubia S, Roson N, Matias-Guiu X, Gomez A. Intra-abdominal desmoplastic small round-cell tumor: a rare cause of peritoneal malignancy in young people. Eur Radiol 2000;10:817-819.

78. Choyke PL, Hayes WS, Sesterhenn IA. Primary extragonadal germ cell tumors of the retroperitoneum: differentiation of primary and secondary tumors. Radiographics 1993;13:1365-1375; quiz 1377-1368.

79. Bokemeyer C, Droz JP, Horwich A, et al. Extragonadal seminoma: an international multicenter analysis of prognostic factors and long term treatment outcome. Cancer 2001;91:1394-1401.

80. Comiter CV, Renshaw AA, Benson CB, Loughlin KR. Burned-out primary testicular cancer: sonographic and pathological characteristics. J Urol 1996;156:85-88.

81. Hayashi T, Mine M, Kojima S, Sekine H. Extragonadal germ cell tumor followed by metachronous testicular tumor. A case report. Urol Int 1996;57:194-196.

82. Johnson J, Mattrey R, Phillipson J. Differentiation of seminomatous from nonseminomatous testicular tumors with MR imaging. Am J Roentgenol 1990;154:539-543.

83. Gutierrez Delgado F, Tjulandin SA, Garin AM. Long term results of treatment in patients with extragonadal germ cell tumours. Eur J Cancer. 1993;29A:1002-1005.

84. Wallace S, Ajani JA, Charnsangavej C, et al. Carcinoid tumors: imaging procedures and interventional radiology. World J Surg 1996;20:147-156.

85. Pelage JP, Soyer P, Boudiaf M, et al. Carcinoid tumors of the abdomen: CT features. Abdom Imaging 1999;24:240-245.

86. Bader TR, Semelka RC, Chiu VC, Armao DM, Woosley JT. MRI of carcinoid tumors: spectrum of appearances in the gastrointestinal tract and liver. J Magn Reson Imaging 2001;14:261-269.

87. Modlin IM, Sandor A. An analysis of 8305 cases of carcinoid tumors. Cancer 1997;79:813-829.

88. Soga J, Yakuwa Y, Osaka M. Carcinoid syndrome: a statistical evaluation of 748 reported cases. J Experimental Clin Cancer Research 1999;18:133-141.

89. Lauffer JM, Zhang T, Modlin IM. Review article: current status of gastrointestinal carcinoids. Aliment Pharmacol Ther 1999;13:271-287.

90. Talamonti MS, Goetz LH, Rao S, Joehl RJ. Primary cancers of the small bowel: analysis of prognostic factors and results of surgical management. Arch Surg 2002;137:564-570; discussion 570-561.

91. Shebani KO, Souba WW, Finkelstein DM, et al. Prognosis and survival in patients with gastrointestinal tract carcinoid tumors. Ann Surg 1999;229:815-821; discussion 822-813.

92. Sandor A, Modlin IM. A retrospective analysis of 1570 appendiceal carcinoids. Am J Gastroenterol 1998;93:422-428.

93. Pathirana AA, Vinjamuri S, Byrne C, Ghaneh P, Vora J, Poston GJ. 131I-MIBG radionuclide therapy is safe and cost-effective in the control of symptoms of the carcinoid syndrome. Eur J Surg Oncol 2001;27:404-408.

94. Skogseid B. Nonsurgical treatment of advanced malignant neuroendocrine pancreatic tumors and midgut carcinoids. World J Surg 2001;25:700-703.

95. Kvols LK. Metastatic carcinoid tumors and the malignant carcinoid syndrome. Ann NY Acad Sci 1994;733:464-470.

96. Pantongrag-Brown L, Buetow PC, Carr NJ, Lichtenstein JE, Buck JL. Calcification and fibrosis in mesenteric carcinoid tumor: CT findings and pathologic correlation. AJR Am J Roentgenol 1995;164:387-391.

97. Burke AP, Thomas RM, Elsayed AM, Sobin LH. Carcinoids of the jejunum and ileum: an immunohistochemical and clinicopathologic study of 167 cases. Cancer 1997;79:1086-1093.

98. Woodard PK, Feldman JM, Paine SS, Baker ME. Midgut carcinoid tumors: CT findings and biochemical profiles. J Comput Assist Tomogr 1995;19:400-405.

99. Dromain C, de Baere T, Baudin E, et al. MR imaging of hepatic metastases caused by neuroendocrine tumors: comparing four techniques. AJR Am J Roentgenol 2003;180:121-128.

100. Nilsson O. Gastrointestinal carcinoids—aspects of diagnosis and classification. Apmis. 1996;104:481-492.

101. Halford S, Waxman J. The management of carcinoid tumours. QJM 1998;91:795-798.

102. Taal BG, Hoefnagel CA, Valdes Olmos RA, Boot H, Beijnen JH. Palliative effect of metaiodobenzylguanidine in metastatic carcinoid tumors. J Clin Oncol 1996;14:1829-1838.

103. Hayes WS, Davidson AJ, Grimley PM, Hartman DS. Extraadrenal retroperitoneal paraganglioma: clinical, pathologic, and CT findings. AJR Am J Roentgenol 1990;155:1247-1250.

104. Somasundar P, Krouse R, Hostetter R, Vaughan R, Covey T. Paragangliomas—a decade of clinical experience. J Surg Oncol 2000;74(Suppl):286-290.

105. Clarke MR, Weyant RJ, Watson CG, Carty SE. Prognostic markers in pheochromocytoma. Human Pathol 1998;29:522-526.

106. de Jong E, Mulder W, Nooitgedacht E, Taat CW, Bras J. Carney's triad. Eur J Surg Oncol 1998;24:147-149.

107. Pommier RF, Vetto JT, Billingsly K, Woltering EA, Brennan MF. Comparison of adrenal and extraadrenal pheochromocytomas. Surgery 1993;114:1160-1165; discussion 1165-1166.

108. Hruby G, Lehman M, Barton M, Peduto T. Malignant retroperitoneal paraganglioma: case report and review of treatment options. Australasian Radiol 2000;44:478-482.

109. O'Riordain DS, Young WF, Jr., Grant CS, Carney JA, van Heerden JA. Clinical spectrum and outcome of functional extraadrenal paraganglioma. World J Surg 1996;20:916-921; discussion 922.

110. Maurea S, Cuocolo A, Reynolds JC, et al. [Role of magnetic resonance in the study of benign and malignant pheochromocy-tomas. Quantitative analysis of the intensity of the resonance signal]. Radiologia Medica. 1993;85:803-808.

111. Ichikawa T, Ohtomo K, Uchiyama G, Fujimoto H, Nasu K. Contrast-enhanced dynamic MRI of adrenal masses: classification of characteristic enhancement patterns. Clin Radiol 1995;50: 295-300.

112. Glodny B, Winde G, Herwig R, et al. Clinical differences between benign and malignant pheochromocytomas. Endocr J 2001;48: 151-159.

113. Favia G, Lumachi F, Polistina F, D'Amico DF. Pheochromocytoma, a rare cause of hypertension: long-term follow-up of 55 surgically treated patients. World J Surg 1998;22:689-693; discussion 694.

114. Otal P, Mezghani S, Hassissene S, et al. Imaging of retroperitoneal ganglioneuroma. Eur Radiol 2001;11:940-945.

115. Zhang Y, Nishimura H, Kato S, et al. MRI of ganglioneuroma: histologic correlation study. J Comput Assist Tomogr 2001;25:617-623.

116. Ichikawa T, Ohtomo K, Araki T, et al. Ganglioneuroma: computed tomography and magnetic resonance features. Br J Radiol 1996;69:114-121.

117. Lonergan GJ, Schwab CM, Suarez ES, Carlson CL. Neuroblastoma, ganglioneuroblastoma, and ganglioneuroma: radiologic-pathologic correlation. Radiographics 2002;22:911-934.

118. Lucas K, Gula MJ, Knisely AS, Virgi MA, Wollman M, Blatt J. Catecholamine metabolites in ganglioneuroma. Med Pediatr Oncol 1994;22:240-243.

119. Radin R, David CL, Goldfarb H, Francis IR. Adrenal and extra-adrenal retroperitoneal ganglioneuroma: imaging findings in 13 adults. Radiology 1997;202:703-707.

120. Rha SE, Byun JY, Jung SE, Chun HJ, Lee HG, Lee JM. Neurogenic Tumors in the Abdomen: Tumor Types and Imaging Characteristics. Radiographics 2003;23:29-43.

121. Wang YM, Li YW, Sheih CP, Hsu JC. Magnetic resonance imaging of neuroblastoma, ganglioneuroblastoma, and ganglioneuroma. Chung-Hua Min Kuo Hsiao Erh Ko i Hsueh Hui Tsa Chih. 1995;36:420-424.

122. Hayasaka K, Tanaka Y, Soeda S, Huppert P, Claussen CD. MR findings in primary retroperitoneal schwannoma. Acta Radiologica 1999;40:78-82.

123. Johnson GL, Hruban RH, Marshall FF, Fishman EK. Primary adrenal ganglioneuroma: CT findings in four patients. AJR Am J Roentgenol 1997;169:169-171.

124. Bankier AA, Stanek J, Hubsch P. Case report: benign solitary schwannoma of the greater omentum: a rare cause of acute intraperi-toneal bleeding—diagnosis by CT. Clin Radiol 1996;51:517-518.

125. Murakami R, Tajima H, Kobayashi Y, et al. Mesenteric schwan-noma. Eur Radiol 1998;8:277-279.

126. Nasu K, Arima K, Yoshimatsu J, Miyakawa I. CT and MRI findings in a case of pelvic schwannoma. Gynecol Obstet Invest 1998;46:142-144.

127. Lin J, Martel W. Cross-sectional imaging of peripheral nerve sheath tumors: characteristic signs on CT, MR imaging, and sonography. AJR Am J Roentgenol 2001;176:75-82.

128. Takatera H, Takiuchi H, Namiki M, Takaha M, Ohnishi S, Sonoda T. Retroperitoneal schwannoma. Urology 1986;28:529-531.

129. Yano K, Okamura T, Yoshida Y, Osaki T, Ichiyoshi Y, Yasumoto K. Mesenteric neurofibroma with von Recklinghausen's disease: a case report. Hepatogastroenterology 1998;45:456-458.

130. Murphey MD, Smith WS, Smith SE, Kransdorf MJ, Temple HT. From the archives of the AFIP. Imaging of musculoskeletal neurogenic tumors: radiologic-pathologic correlation. Radiographics 1999;19:1253-1280.

131. Woodruff JM. Pathology of tumors of the peripheral nerve sheath in type 1 neurofibromatosis. Am J Med Genet 1999;89:23-30.

132. Fortman BJ, Kuszyk BS, Urban BA, Fishman EK. Neurofibromatosis type 1: a diagnostic mimicker at CT. Radiographics 2001;21:601-612.

133. Korf BR. Plexiform neurofibromas. Am J Med Genet 1999;89:31-37.

134. Korf BR. Malignancy in neurofibromatosis type 1. Oncologist 2000;5:477-485.

135. Leroy K, Dumas V, Martin-Garcia N, et al. Malignant peripheral nerve sheath tumors associated with neurofibromatosis type 1: a clinicopathologic and molecular study of 17 patients. Arch Dermatol 2001;137:908-913.

136. King AA, Debaun MR, Riccardi VM, Gutmann DH. Malignant peripheral nerve sheath tumors in neurofibromatosis 1. Am J Med Genet 2000;93:388-392.

137. Wong WW, Hirose T, Scheithauer BW, Schild SE, Gunderson LL. Malignant peripheral nerve sheath tumor: analysis of treatment outcome. Int J Radiat Oncol Biol Phys 1998;42:351-360.

138. Ramanathan RC, Thomas JM. Malignant peripheral nerve sheath tumours associated with von Recklinghausen's neurofibromatosis. Eur J Surg Oncol 1999;25:190-193.

139. Lai FM, Allen PW, Chan LW, Chan PS, Cooper JE, Mackenzie TM. Aggressive fibromatosis of the spermatic cord. A typical lesion in a "new" location. Am J Clin Pathol 1995;104:403-407.

140. Kulaylat MN, Karakousis CP, Keaney CM, McCorvey D, Bem J, Ambrus JL Sr. Desmoid tumour: a pleomorphic lesion. Eur J Surg Oncol 1999;25:487-497.

141. Kobayashi H, Kotoura Y, Hosono M, et al. MRI and scintigraphic features of extraabdominal desmoid tumors. Clin Imaging 1997;21:35-39.

142. Richard HM, Thall EH, Mitty H, Gribetz ME, Gelernt I. Desmoid tumor-ureteral fistula in Gardner's syndrome. Urology 1997;49:135-138.

143. Mariani A, Nascimento AG, Webb MJ, Sim FH, Podratz KC. Surgical management of desmoid tumors of the female pelvis. J Am Coll Surg 2000;191:175-183.

144. Kawashima A, Goldman SM, Fishman EK, et al. CT of intra-abdominal desmoid tumors: is the tumor different in patients with Gardner's disease? AJR Am J Roentgenol 1994;162:339-342.

145. Lynch HT, Fitzgibbons R. Surgery, desmoid tumors, and familial adenomatous polyposis: case report and literature review. Am J Gastroenterol 1996;91:2598-2601.

146. Clark SK, Neale KF, Landgrebe JC, Phillips RK. Desmoid tumours complicating familial adenomatous polyposis. Br J Surg 1999;86:1185-1189.

147. Robbin MR, Murphey MD, Temple HT, Kransdorf MJ, Choi JJ. Imaging of musculoskeletal fibromatosis. Radiographics 2001;21:585-600.

148. Casillas J, Sais GJ, Greve JL, Iparraguirre MC, Morillo G. Imaging of intra- and extraabdominal desmoid tumors. Radiographics 1991;11:959-968.

149. Healy JC, Reznek RH, Clark SK, Phillips RK, Armstrong P. MR appearances of desmoid tumors in familial adenomatous polyposis. AJR Am J Roentgenol 1997;169:465-472.

150. Ichikawa T, Koyama A, Fujimoto H, et al. Abdominal wall desmoid mimicking intra-abdominal mass: MR features. Magn Reson Imaging 1994;12:541-544.

151. Ooi BS, Lee CN, Ti TK, Chachlani N, Chua ET. Retroperitoneal fibromatosis presenting as acute duodenal obstruction. ANZ J Surg 2001;71:74-76.

152. Brooks AP, Reznek RH, Nugent K, Farmer KC, Thomson JP, Phillips RK. CT appearances of desmoid tumours in familial adenomatous polyposis: further observations. Clin Radiol 1994;49:601-607.

153. Suit H, Spiro I. Radiation in the multidisciplinary management of desmoid tumors. Front Radiat Ther Oncol 2001;35:107-119.

154. Goy BW, Lee SP, Eilber F, et al. The role of adjuvant radiotherapy in the treatment of resectable desmoid tumors. Int J Radiat Oncol Biol Phys 1997;39:659-665.

155. Ciftci E, Erden I, Koral K, Akyar S. MR imaging in a desmoid tumor of the posterior mediastinum with extension into the abdominal cavity. A case report. Acta Radiologica 1998;39:301-303.

156. Vandevenne JE, De Schepper AM, De Beuckeleer L, et al. New concepts in understanding evolution of desmoid tumors: MR imaging of 30 lesions. Eur Radiol 1997;7:1013-1019.

157. Smith AJ, Lewis JJ, Merchant NB, Leung DH, Woodruff JM, Brennan MF. Surgical management of intra-abdominal desmoid tumours. Br J Surg 2000;87:608-613.

158. Poritz LS, Blackstein M, Berk T, Gallinger S, McLeod RS, Cohen Z. Extended follow-up of patients treated with cytotoxic chemotherapy for intra-abdominal desmoid tumors. Dis Colon Rectum 2001;44:1268-1273.

159. Middleton SB, Phillips RK. Surgery for large intra-abdominal desmoid tumors: report of four cases. Dis Colon Rectum 2000;43:1759-1762; discussion 1762-1753.

160. Samuels BL. Management of recurrent desmoid tumor after surgery and radiation: role of cytotoxic and non-cytotoxic therapies. Surg Oncol 1999;8:191-196.

161. Ilhan H, Tokar B, Isiksoy S, Koku N, Pasaoglu O. Giant mesenteric lipoma. J Pediatr Surg 1999;34:639-640.

162. Panageas E. General diagnosis case of the day. Primary retroperitoneal teratoma. AJR Am J Roentgenol 1991;156:1292-1294.

163. Tezel E, Sare M, Edali N, Oguz M, Uluoglu O, Gokok NH. Retroperitoneal malignant teratoma. A case report. Materia Medica Polona 1995;27:123-125.

164. Wang RM, Chen CA. Primary retroperitoneal teratoma. Acta Obstet Gynecol Scand 2000;79:707-708.

165. Davidson AJ, Hartman DS, Goldman SM. Mature teratoma of the retroperitoneum: radiologic, pathologic, and clinical correlation. Radiology 1989;172:421-425.

166. Ferrero A, Cespedes M, Cantarero JM, Arenas A, Pamplona M. Peritonitis due to rupture of retroperitoneal teratoma: computed tomography diagnosis. Gastrointestinal Radiol 1990;15:251-252.

167. Koroku M, Takagi Y, Suzuki N, Wakabayashi J. Primary retroperitoneal teratoma in an adult: a case report. Int J Urology 1997;4:219-221.

168. de Perrot M, Brundler M, Totsch M, Mentha G, Morel P. Mesenteric cysts. Toward less confusion? Dig Surg 2000;17:323-328.

169. Stoupis C, Ros PR, Abbitt PL, Burton SS, Gauger J. Bubbles in the belly: imaging of cystic mesenteric or omental masses. Radiographics 1994;14:729-737.

170. Tong RS, Larner T, Finlay M, Agarwal D, Costello AJ. Pelvic lipomatosis associated with proliferative cystitis occurring in two brothers. Urology 2002;59:602.

171. Honecke K, Butz M. Pelvic lipomatosis in a female: diagnosis and initial therapy. Urologia Int 1991;46:93-95.

172. Gordon NS, Sinclair RA, Snow RM. Pelvic lipomatosis with cystitis cystica, cystitis glandularis and adenocarcinoma of the bladder: first reported case. Aust New Zealand J Surg 1990;60:229-232.

173. Heyns CF, De Kock ML, Kirsten PH, van Velden DJ. Pelvic lipomatosis associated with cystitis glandularis and adenocarcinoma of the bladder. J Urol 1991;145:364-366.

174. Masumori N, Tsukamoto T. Pelvic lipomatosis associated with proliferative cystitis: case report and review of the Japanese literature. Int J Urol 1999;6:44-49.

175. Sharma S, Nabi G, Seth A, Thulkar S, Ghai S. Pelvic lipomatosis presenting as uraemic encephalopathy. Int J Clin Pract 2001;55:149-150.

176. Baath L, Nyman U, Aspelin P, Wadstrom L. Computed tomography of pelvic lipomatosis. Report of a case. Acta Radiol Diagn (Stockh) 1986;27:311-314.

177. Allen FJ, De Kock ML. Pelvic lipomatosis: the nuclear magnetic resonance appearance and associated vesicoureteral reflux. J Urology. 1987;138:1228-1230.

178. Demas BE, Avallone A, Hricak H. Pelvic lipomatosis: diagnosis and characterization by magnetic resonance imaging. Urol Radiol 1988;10:198-202.

179. Klein FA, Smith MJ, Kasenetz I. Pelvic lipomatosis: 35-year experience. J Urol 1988;139:998-1001.

180. Fujiyoshi F, Ichinari N, Kajiya Y, et al. Retractile mesenteritis: small-bowel radiography, CT, and MR imaging. AJR Am J Roentgenol 1997;169:791-793.

181. Sabate JM, Torrubia S, Maideu J, Franquet T, Monill JM, Perez C. Sclerosing mesenteritis: imaging findings in 17 patients. AJR Am J Roentgenol 1999;172:625-629.

182. Lawler LP, McCarthy DM, Fishman EK, Hruban R. Sclerosing Mesenteritis: Depiction by Multidetector CT and Three-Dimensional Volume Rendering. Am J Roentgenol 2002;178:97-99.

183. Horton KM, Lawler LP, Fishman EK. CT Findings in Sclerosing Mesenteritis (Panniculitis): Spectrum of Disease. Radiographics 2003;23:1561-1567.

184. Kronthal AJ, Kang YS, Fishman EK, Jones B, Kuhlman JE, Tempany CM. MR imaging in sclerosing mesenteritis. AJR Am J Roentgenol 1991;156:517-519.

185. Daskalogiannaki M, Voloudaki A, Prassopoulos P, et al. CT evaluation of mesenteric panniculitis: prevalence and associated diseases. AJR Am J Roentgenol 2000;174:427-431.

186. Kawashima A, Fishman EK, Hruban RH, Kuhlman JE, Lee RP. Mesenteric panniculitis presenting as a multilocular cystic mesenteric mass: CT and MR evaluation. Clin Imaging 1993;17:112-116.

187. Mysorekar VV, Dandekar CP, Rao SG. Mesenteric panniculitis presenting as a huge retroperitoneal mass—a case report. Ind J Med Sci 2000;54:95-97.

188. Bala A, Coderre SP, Johnson DR, Nayak V. Treatment of sclerosing mesenteritis with corticosteroids and azathioprine. Can J Gastroenterol 2001;15:533-535.

189. Mazure R, Fernandez Marty P, Niveloni S, et al. Successful treatment of retractile mesenteritis with oral progesterone. Gastroenterology 1998;114:1313-1317.

190. Kakitsubata Y, Umemura Y, Kakitsubata S, et al. CT and MRI manifestations of intraabdominal panniculitis. Clin Imaging 1993;17:186-188.

191. Parra-Davila E, McKenney MG, Sleeman D, et al. Mesenteric panniculitis: case report and literature review. Am Surg 1998;64:768-771.

192. Mindelzun RE, Jeffrey RB, Jr., Lane MJ, Silverman PM. The misty mesentery on CT: differential diagnosis. AJR Am J Roentgenol 1996;167:61-65.

193. Badiola-Varela CM, Sussman SK, Glickstein MF. Mesenteric panniculitis: findings on CT, MRI, and angiography. Case report. Clin Imaging 1991;15:265-267.

194. Valls C. Fat-ring sign in sclerosing mesenteritis. AJR Am J Roentgenol 2000;174:259-260.

195. Wong WL, Johns TA, Herlihy WG, Martin HL. Best cases from the AFIP: multicystic mesothelioma. Radiographics 2004;24:247-250.

196. Ros PR, Olmsted WW, Moser RP, Jr., Dachman AH, Hjermstad BH, Sobin LH. Mesenteric and omental cysts: histologic classification with imaging correlation. Radiology 1987;164:327-332.

197. Bonhomme A, Broeders A, Oyen RH, Stas M, De Wever I, Baert AL. Cystic lymphangioma of the retroperitoneum. Clin Radiol 2001;56:156-158.

198. de Perrot M, Rostan O, Morel P, Le Coultre C. Abdominal lymphangioma in adults and children. Br J Surg 1998;85:395-397.

199. Ko SF, Ng SH, Shieh CS, Lin JW, Huang CC, Lee TY. Mesenteric cystic lymphangioma with myxoid degeneration: unusual CT and MR manifestations. Pediatr Radiol 1995;25:525-527.

200. Vargas-Serrano B, Alegre-Bernal N, Cortina-Moreno B, Rodriguez-Romero R, Sanchez-Ortega F. Abdominal cystic lymphangiomas: US and CT findings. Eur J Radiol 1995;19:183-187.

201. Hovanessian LJ, Larsen DW, Raval JK, Colletti PM. Retroperitoneal cystic lymphangioma: MR findings. Magn Reson Imaging 1990;8:91-93.

202. Chung JH, Suh YL, Park IA, et al. A pathologic study of abdominal lymphangiomas. J Korean Med Sci 1999;14:257-262.

203. Murakami R, Machida M, Kobayashi Y, Ogura J, Ichikawa T, Kumazaki T. Retroperitoneal bronchogenic cyst: CT and MR imaging. Abdom Imaging 2000;25:444-447.

204. Buckley JA, Siegelman ES, Birnbaum BA, Rosato EF. Bronchogenic cyst appearing as a retroperitoneal mass. AJR Am J Roentgenol 1998;171:527-528.

205. Nakata H, Egashira K, Watanabe H, et al. MRI of bronchogenic cysts. J Comput Assist Tomogr 1993;17:267-270.

206. Chung J, Kim M, Lee JT, Yoo HS. Cavernous hemangioma arising from the lesser omentum: MR findings. Abdom Imaging 2000;25:542-544.

207. Igarashi J, Hanazaki K. Retroperitoneal venous hemangioma. Am J Gastroenterol 1998;93:2292-2293.

208. Takamura M, Murakami T, Kurachi H, et al. MR imaging of mesenteric hemangioma: a case report. Radiat Med 2000;18:67-69.

209. Komi N, Takahashi K, Suzuki S. Klippel-Trenaunay syndrome, omental hemangioma with hemorrhage. Bull Tokyo Med Dent Univ 1970;17:1-7.

210. Hanatate F, Mizuno Y, Murakami T. Venous hemangioma of the mesoappendix: report of a case and a brief review of the Japanese literature. Surg Today 1995;25:962-964.

211. Ruiz AR, Jr., Ginsberg AL. Giant mesenteric hemangioma with small intestinal involvement: an unusual cause of recurrent gastrointestinal bleed and review of gastrointestinal hemangiomas. Dig Dis Sci 1999;44:2545-2551.

212. Adam YG, Alberts W. Retroperitoneal hemangioma. Am Surg 1990;56:374-376.

213. Cappellani A, Zanghi A, Di Vita M, Zanghi G, Tomarchio G, Petrillo G. Spontaneous rupture of a giant hemangioma of the liver. Ann Ital Chir 2000;71:379-383.

214. Lombardo DM, Baker ME, Spritzer CE, Blinder R, Meyers W, Herfkens RJ. Hepatic hemangiomas vs metastases: MR differentiation at 1.5 T. AJR Am J Roentgenol 1990;155:55-59.

215. Ros PR, Lubbers PR, Olmsted WW, Morillo G. Hemangioma of the liver: heterogeneous appearance on T2-weighted images. AJR Am J Roentgenol 1987;149:1167-1170.

216. Dachman AH, Ros PR, Shekitka KM, Buck JL, Olmsted WW, Hinton CB. Colorectal hemangioma: radiologic findings. Radiology 1988;167:31-34.

217. Meyer JS, Hoffer FA, Barnes PD, Mulliken JB. Biological classification of soft-tissue vascular anomalies: MR correlation. AJR Am J Roentgenol 1991;157:559-564.

218. Einstein DM, Singer AA, Chilcote WA, Desai RK. Abdominal lymphadenopathy: spectrum of CT findings. Radiographics 1991;11:457-472.

219. Dooms GC, Hricak H, Moseley ME, Bottles K, Fisher M, Higgins CB. Characterization of lymphadenopathy by magnetic resonance relaxation times: preliminary results. Radiology 1985;155:691-697.

220. van den Brekel MW, Castelijns JA, Stel HV, et al. Detection and characterization of metastatic cervical adenopathy by MR imaging: comparison of different MR techniques. J Comput Assist Tomogr 1990;14:581-589.

221. Radin DR. Disseminated histoplasmosis: abdominal CT findings in 16 patients. AJR Am J Roentgenol 1991;157:955-958.

222. Radin DR. Intraabdominal Mycobacterium tuberculosis vs Mycobacterium avium-intracellulare infections in patients with AIDS: distinction based on CT findings. AJR Am J Roentgenol 1991;156:487-491.

223. Ha HK, Jung JI, Lee MS, et al. CT differentiation of tuberculous peritonitis and peritoneal carcinomatosis. AJR Am J Roentgenol 1996;167:743-748.

224. Moon WK, Im JG, Yu IK, Lee SK, Yeon KM, Han MC. Mediastinal tuberculous lymphadenitis: MR imaging appearance with clinicopathologic correlation. AJR Am J Roentgenol 1996;166:21-25.

225. Harisinghani MG, McLoud TC, Shepard JA, Ko JP, Shroff MM, Mueller PR. Tuberculosis from head to toe. Radiographics 2000;20:449-470; quiz 528-449, 532.

226. Kim SY, Kim MJ, Chung JJ, Lee JT, Yoo HS. Abdominal tuberculous lymphadenopathy: MR imaging findings. Abdom Imaging 2000;25:627-632.

227. Yang WT, Lam WW, Yu MY, Cheung TH, Metreweli C. Comparison of dynamic helical CT and dynamic MR imaging in the evaluation of pelvic lymph nodes in cervical carcinoma. AJR Am J Roentgenol 2000;175:759-766.

228. Vinnicombe SJ, Norman AR, Nicolson V, Husband JE. Normal pelvic lymph nodes: evaluation with CT after bipedal lymphangiography. Radiology 1995;194:349-355.

229. Harisinghani MG, Barentsz J, Hahn PF, et al. Noninvasive detection of clinically occult lymph-node metastases in prostate cancer. N Engl J Med 2003;348:2491-2499.

230. De Gaetano AM, Vecchioli A, Minordi LM, et al. Role of diagnostic imaging in abdominal lymphadenopathy. Rays 2000;25:463-484.

231. Weinshel EL, Peterson BA. Hodgkin's disease. CA Cancer J Clin 1993;43:327-346.

232. Skarin AT, Dorfman DM. Non-Hodgkin's lymphomas: current classification and management. CA Cancer J Clin 1997;47:351-372.

233. Blackledge G, Best JJ, Crowther D, Isherwood I. Computed tomography (CT) in the staging of patients with Hodgkin's Disease: a report on 136 patients. Clin Radiol 1980;31:143-147.

234. Neumann CH, Robert NJ, Canellos G, Rosenthal D. Computed tomography of the abdomen and pelvis in non-Hodgkin lymphoma. J Comput Assist Tomogr 1983;7:846-850.

235. Moormeier JA, Williams SF, Golomb HM. The staging of non-Hodgkin's lymphomas. Semin Oncol 1990;17:43-50.

236. Negendank WG, al-Katib AM, Karanes C, Smith MR. Lymphomas: MR imaging contrast characteristics with clinical-pathologic correlations. Radiology 1990;177:209-216.

237. Rahmouni A, Tempany C, Jones R, Mann R, Yang A, Zerhouni E. Lymphoma: monitoring tumor size and signal intensity with MR imaging. Radiology 1993;188:445-451.

238. Engin G, Acunas B, Acunas G, Tunaci M. Imaging of extrapulmonary tuberculosis. Radiographics 2000;20:471-488; quiz 529-430, 532.

239. Jadvar H, Mindelzun RE, Olcott EW, Levitt DB. Still the great mimicker: abdominal tuberculosis. AJR Am J Roentgenol 1997;168:1455-1460.

240. Friedman HD, Hadfield TL, Lamy Y, Fritzinger D, Bonaventura M, Cynamon MT. Whipple's disease presenting as chronic wastage and abdominal lymphadenopathy. Diagn Microbiol Infect Dis 1995;23:111-113.

241. Marth T, Raoult D. Whipple's disease. Lancet 2003;361:239-246.

242. Shahidi H, Myers JL, Kvale PA. Castleman's disease. Mayo Clinic Proceedings 1995;70:969-977.

243. Chronowski GM, Ha CS, Wilder RB, Cabanillas F, Manning J, Cox JD. Treatment of unicentric and multicentric Castleman disease and the role of radiotherapy. Cancer 2001;92:670-676.

244. McCarty MJ, Vukelja SJ, Banks PM, Weiss RB. Angiofollicular lymph node hyperplasia (Castleman's disease). Cancer Treatment Reviews 1995;21:291-310.
245. Kim TJ, Han JK, Kim YH, Kim TK, Choi BI. Castleman disease of the abdomen: imaging spectrum and clinicopathologic correlations. J Comput Assist Tomogr 2001;25:207-214.
246. Teh HS, Lin MB, Tan AS, Tan TY, Chin CM. Retroperitoneal Castleman's disease in the perinephric space—imaging appearance: a case report and a review of the literature. Ann Acad Med Singapore 2000;29:773-776.
247. Johnson WK, Ros PR, Powers C, Stoupis C, Segel KH. Castleman disease mimicking an aggressive retroperitoneal neoplasm. Abdom Imaging 1994;19:342-344.
248. Andres E, Maloisel F. Interferon-alpha as first-line therapy for treatment of multicentric Castleman's disease. Ann Oncol 2000;11:1613-1614.
249. Amis ES, Jr. Retroperitoneal fibrosis. AJR Am J Roentgenol 1991;157:321-329.
250. Gilkeson GS, Allen NB. Retroperitoneal fibrosis. A true connective tissue disease. Rheumatic Dis Clin North Am 1996;22:23-38.
251. Kottra JJ, Dunnick NR. Retroperitoneal fibrosis. Radiologic Clin North Am 1996;34:1259-1275.
252. Vivas I, Nicolas AI, Velazquez P, Elduayen B, Fernandez-Villa T, Martinez-Cuesta A. Retroperitoneal fibrosis: typical and atypical manifestations. Br J Radiol 2000;73:214-222.
253. Elkind AH, Friedman AP, Bachman A, Siegelman SS, Sacks OW. Silent retroperitoneal fibrosis associated with methysergide therapy. JAMA 1968;206:1041-1044.
254. Silberstein SD. Methysergide. Cephalalgia 1998;18:421-435.
255. Arrive L, Hricak H, Tavares NJ, Miller TR. Malignant versus nonmalignant retroperitoneal fibrosis. Radiology 1989;172:139-143.
256. Lee JK, Glazer HS. Controversy in the MR imaging appearance of fibrosis. Radiology 1990;177:21-22.
257. Burn PR, Singh S, Barbar S, Boustead G, King CM. Role of gadolinium-enhanced magnetic resonance imaging in retroperitoneal fibrosis. Can Assoc Radiol J 2002;53:168-170.
258. Yuh WT, Barloon TJ, Sickels WJ, Kramolowsky EV, Williams RD. Magnetic resonance imaging in the diagnosis and followup of idiopathic retroperitoneal fibrosis. J Urology. 1989;141:602-605.
259. van Bommel EF. Retroperitoneal fibrosis. Neth J Med 2002;60:231-242.
260. Fugita OE, Jarrett TW, Kavoussi P, Kavoussi LR. Laparoscopic treatment of retroperitoneal fibrosis. J Endourol 2002;16:571-574.
261. Tennant WG, Hartnell GG, Baird RN, Horrocks M. Inflammatory aortic aneurysms: characteristic appearance on magnetic resonance imaging. Eur J Vasc Surg 1992;6:399-402.
262. Leseche G, Schaetz A, Arrive L, Nussaume O, Andreassian B. Diagnosis and management of 17 consecutive patients with inflammatory abdominal aortic aneurysm. Am J Surg 1992;164:39-44.
263. Bonamigo TP, Bianco C, Becker M, Puricelli Faccini F. Inflammatory aneurysms of infra-renal abdominal aorta. A case-control study. Minerva Cardioangiol 2002;50:253-258.
264. Wallis F, Roditi GH, Redpath TW, Weir J, Cross KS, Smith FW. Inflammatory abdominal aortic aneurysms: diagnosis with gadolinium enhanced T1-weighted imaging. Clin Radiol 2000;55:136-139.
265. Sasaki S, Yasuda K, Takigami K, Yamauchi H, Shiiya N, Sakuma M. Inflammatory abdominal aortic aneurysms and atherosclerotic abdominal aortic aneurysms—comparisons of clinical features and long-term results. Jpn Circ J 1997;61:231-235.
266. Nitecki SS, Hallett JW, Jr., Stanson AW, et al. Inflammatory abdominal aortic aneurysms: a case-control study. J Vasc Surg 1996;23:860-868; discussion 868-869.
267. Sumino H, Kanda T, Nakamura T, et al. Steroid therapy is effective in a young patient with an inflammatory abdominal aortic aneurysm. J Med 1999;30:67-74.
268. Pennell RC, Hollier LH, Lie JT, et al. Inflammatory abdominal aortic aneurysms: a thirty-year review. J Vasc Surg 1985;2:859-869.
269. Testart J, Plissonnier D, Peillon C, Watelet J. [Inflammatory abdominal aortic aneurysm. Role of corticosteroid therapy]. J Mal Vasc 2000;25:201-207.
270. Bonati L, Rubini P, Japichino GG, et al. Long-term outcome after inflammatory abdominal aortic aneurysm repair: case-matched study. World J Surg 2003;27:539-544.
271. Gore RM, Balfe DM, Aizenstein RI, Silverman PM. The great escape: interfascial decompression planes of the retroperitoneum. AJR Am J Roentgenol 2000;175:363-370.
272. Bennett HF, Balfe DM. MR imaging of the peritoneum and abdominal wall. Magn Reson Imaging Clin North Am. 1995;3:99-120.
273. Alexander ES, Colley DP, Clark RA. Computed tomography of retroperitoneal fluid collections. Semin Roentgenol 1981;16:268-276.
274. Bradley WG, Jr. MR appearance of hemorrhage in the brain. Radiology 1993;189:15-26.
275. Bradley WG, Jr. Hemorrhage and hemorrhagic infections in the brain. Neuroimaging Clin N Am 1994;4:707-732.
276. Hahn PF, Saini S, Stark DD, Papanicolaou N, Ferrucci JT Jr. Intraabdominal hematoma: the concentric-ring sign in MR imaging. AJR Am J Roentgenol 1987;148:115-119.
277. Lane MJ, Katz DS, Shah RA, Rubin GD, Jeffrey RB Jr. Active arterial contrast extravasation on helical CT of the abdomen, pelvis, and chest. AJR Am J Roentgenol 1998;171:679-685.
278. Vazquez JL, Thorsen MK, Dodds WJ, et al. Evaluation and treatment of intraabdominal bilomas. AJR Am J Roentgenol 1985;144:933-938.
279. Vitellas KM, El-Dieb A, Vaswani KK, et al. Using contrast-enhanced MR cholangiography with IV mangafodipir trisodium (Teslascan) to evaluate bile duct leaks after cholecystectomy: a prospective study of 11 patients. AJR Am J Roentgenol 2002;179:409-416.
280. DeHart MM, Lauerman WC, Conely AH, Roettger RH, West JL, Cain JE. Management of retroperitoneal chylous leakage. Spine 1994;19:716-718.
281. Noel AA, Gloviczki P, Bender CE, Whitley D, Stanson AW, Deschamps C. Treatment of symptomatic primary chylous disorders. J Vasc Surg 2001;34:785-791.
282. Amin R. Chylous ascites from prostatic adenocarcinoma. Urology 2002;59:773.
283. Laterre PF, Dugernier T, Reynaert MS. Chylous ascites: diagnosis, causes and treatment. Acta Gastroenterol Belg 2000;63:260-263.
284. Kaas R, Rustman LD, Zoetmulder FA. Chylous ascites after oncological abdominal surgery: incidence and treatment. Eur J Surg Oncol 2001;27:187-189.
285. Browse NL, Wilson NM, Russo F, al-Hassan H, Allen DR. Aetiology and treatment of chylous ascites. Br J Surg 1992;79:1145-1150.
286. Hibbeln JF, Wehmueller MD, Wilbur AC. Chylous ascites: CT and ultrasound appearance. Abdom Imaging 1995;20:138-140.
287. Prasad S, Patankar T. Computed tomography demonstration of a fat-fluid level in tuberculous chylous ascites. Australas Radiol 1999;43:542-543.
288. Healy ME, Teng SS, Moss AA. Uriniferous pseudocyst: computed tomographic findings. Radiology 1984;153:757-762.
289. Lang EK, Glorioso L, 3rd. Management of urinomas by percutaneous drainage procedures. Radiol Clin N Am 1986;24:551-559.
290. Noone TC, Semelka RC, Worawattanakul S, Marcos HB. Intraperitoneal abscesses: diagnostic accuracy of and appearances at MR imaging. Radiology 1998;208:525-528.
291. Gazelle GS, Mueller PR. Abdominal abscess. Imaging and intervention. Radiologic Clin North Am. 1994;32:913-932.
292. Paley M, Sidhu PS, Evans RA, Karani JB. Retroperitoneal collections—aetiology and radiological implications. Clin Radiol 1997;52:290-294.
293. Muttarak M, Peh WC. CT of unusual iliopsoas compartment lesions. Radiographics 2000;20:S53-66.
294. Lindahl S, Nyman RS, Brismar J, Hugosson C, Lundstedt C. Imaging of tuberculosis. IV. Spinal manifestations in 63 patients. Acta Radiol 1996;37:506-511.
295. Kim JY, Park YH, Choi KH, Park SH, Lee HY. MRI of tuberculous pyomyositis. J Comput Assist Tomogr 1999;23:454-457.
296. Laroche M, Harding G. Primary and secondary peritonitis: an update. Eur J Clin Microbiol Infect Dis 1998;17:542-550.
297. Pinzello G, Simonetti RG, Craxi A, Di Piazza S, Spano C, Pagliaro L. Spontaneous bacterial peritonitis: a prospective investigation in predominantly nonalcoholic cirrhotic patients. Hepatology 1983;3:545-549.
298. Hillebrand DJ, Runyon BA. Spontaneous bacterial peritonitis: keys to management. Hospital Practice (Office Edition) 2000;35:87-90, 96-88.
299. Arai K, Makino H, Morioka T, et al. Enhancement of ascites on MRI following intravenous administration of Gd-DTPA. J Comput Assist Tomogr 1993;17:617-622.
300. Kanematsu M, Hoshi H, Murakami T, Tsuda K, Yokoyama R, Nakamura H. Spontaneous bacterial peritonitis in cirrhosis: enhancement of ascites on delayed MR imaging. Radiat Med 1997;15:185-187.
301. Deeb LS, Mourad FH, El-Zein YR, Uthman SM. Abdom cocoon in a man: preoperative diagnosis and literature review. J Clin Gastroenterol 1998;26:148-150.
302. Garosi G, Di Paolo N. Peritoneal sclerosis—an overview. Adv Peritoneal Dialysis 1999;15:185-192.
303. Kaklamanis P, Vayopoulos G, Stamatelos G, Dadinas G, Tsokos GC. Chronic lupus peritonitis with ascites. Ann the Rheumatic Dis 1991;50:176-177.
304. Ngo Y, Messing B, Marteau P, et al. Peritoneal sarcoidosis. An unrecognized cause of sclerosing peritonitis. Dig Dis Sci 1992;37:1776-1780.

305. Reginella RF, Sumkin JH. Sclerosing peritonitis associated with luteinized thecomas. AJR Am J Roentgenol 1996;167:512-513.

306. Garosi G, Di Paolo N. Peritoneal sclerosis: one or two nosological entities? Semin Dialysis 2000;13:297-308.

307. Afthentopoulos IE, Passadakis P, Oreopoulos DG, Bargman J. Sclerosing peritonitis in continuous ambulatory peritoneal dialysis patients: one center's experience and review of the literature. Adv Renal Replacement Therapy 1998;5:157-167.

308. Stafford-Johnson DB, Wilson TE, Francis IR, Swartz R. CT appearance of sclerosing peritonitis in patients on chronic ambulatory peritoneal dialysis. J Comput Assist Tomogr 1998;22:295-299.

309. Rigby RJ, Hawley CM. Sclerosing peritonitis: the experience in Australia. [comment]. Nephrology Dialysis Transplantation. 1998;13:154-159.

7

MRI of the Female Pelvis

Evan S. Siegelman, MD

UTERUS

Normal Uterine Anatomy

The uterus has a zonal anatomy that is well revealed on T2-WI (Box 7-1 and Fig. 7-1; see Figs. 7-3, 7-15, 7-20, 7-30, 7-36, and 7-37). There is a central high SI endometrium, a low SI inner myometrium, and a low-to-intermediate SI outer myometrium. On T1-WI there is poor distinction among the components of the endometrium and myometrium.

Endometrium

The normal uterine endometrium is revealed as homogeneous low SI on T1-WI and high SI on T2-WI. The endometrium may have high SI approaching that of fluid on T2-WIs. However, unlike fluid, the SI decreases on heavily T2-WI and the endometrial glands and stroma do enhance after contrast.[1] The sonographic and MR appearance of the endometrial stripe in premenopausal women during the secretory phase is wider compared with the follicular phase[2-5] secondary to growth of endometrial glands, stroma, and vessels.[6] An endometrial width of less than 10 mm is considered normal in premenopausal women; those women who take oral contraceptives should

have a thin endometrial width of less than 4 mm.[1] Postmenopausal women who do not take hormone replacement therapy should have an endometrial width of less than 5 mm.[7]

INNER MYOMETRIUM (JUNCTIONAL ZONE)

The junctional zone has both structural and functional differences from the outer myometrium.[8] On T2-WI the junctional zone is hypointense relative to the outer myometrium. The histologic features of the inner myometrium that result in lower SI compared with the outer myometrium include increased size and number of nuclei,[9] decreased free water content, and increased density and organization of smooth muscle cells.[10-13] The normal junctional zone thickness on T2-WI is usually less than 10 mm. ROC (receiver operating characteristic) analysis of MR studies in women with and without adenomyosis (described below) showed that a junctional zone thickness of less than 12 mm should be considered as normal.[14]

Functionally, the junctional zone is the site of origin of uterine contractions. Two different types of uterine contractions have been depicted by sonography and MR. Focal sustained, myometrial contractions (FMCs) originate in the junctional zone. FMCs often

269

7-1 Normal Zonal Anatomy of the Uterus on T2-Weighted Images

Layer	Thickness	Signal Intensity Relative to Muscle
Endometrium	<10 mm	Homogeneous ↑ SI
Inner myometrium junctional zone	<12 mm	↓↓ SI
Outer myometrium	Variable	Heterogeneous ↑↓ SI

distort the endometrium but not the outer uterine margin.[15-18] These sustained contractions are most often revealed in pregnant women but can be present in a nongravid uterus. Showing resolution of a questionable myometrial "mass" on a different imaging sequence establishes the diagnosis of FMC (Fig. 7-2).

A second type of uterine contraction is present in menstruating women and has been referred to as uterine peristalsis. Uterine peristalsis is isolated to the junctional zone and occurs with a frequency of one to three times per minute. The direction of the peristaltic wave varies with the phase of the menstrual cycle, being retrograde (towards the fundus) during the follicular and periovulatory phases and antegrade (towards the cervix) during the luteal phase.[19]

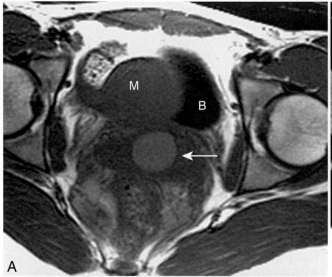

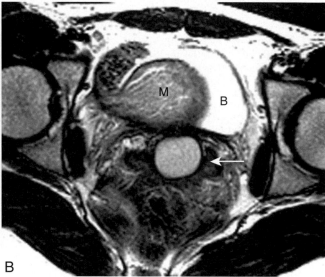

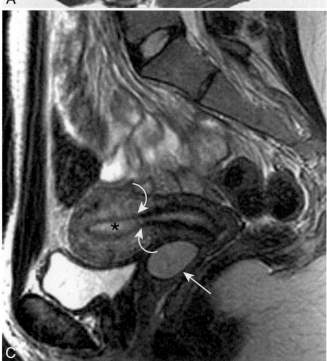

Figure 7-1 ■ **MR findings of normal zonal anatomy of the uterus and cervix in a 22-year-old woman with a palpable midline mucin-containing müllerian cyst. A**, Axial T1-WI shows a well-circumscribed unilocular mass *(arrow)* of the proximal vagina that has higher SI than adjacent myometrium (M) and urine within the bladder (B). **B**, T2-WI shows that the mass *(arrow)* has homogeneous SI that is almost isointense to urine (B). **C**, Sagittal T2-WI reveals that the center of the mass *(arrow)* is located in the midline of the proximal vagina. Mild T2-shortening secondary intracystic mucin is present. Normal zonal anatomy of the uterus and cervix is well depicted. The high SI endometrium (*) is continuous with the endocervical glands. The lower SI junctional zone of the uterus *(curved arrows)* is continuous with the inner fibrous cervical stroma. The outer myometrium has heterogeneous SI and is hyperintense to the adjacent junctional zone and continuous with the outer cervical stroma.

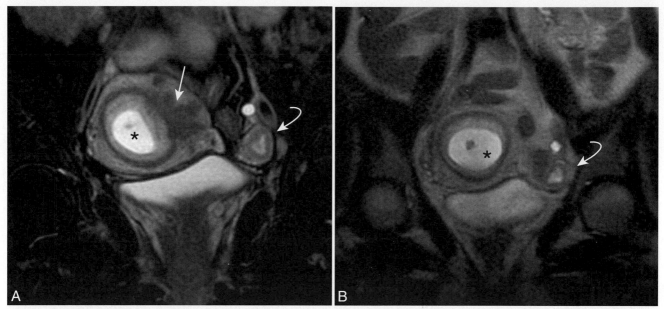

Figure 7-2 ■ MR illustration of a focal myometrium contraction in a pregnant woman. **A,** Coronal fat-suppressed T2-WI shows lobulated low SI within the left-sided myometrium *(arrow).* The widened endometrial cavity (*) represents an early intrauterine gestation. A left-sided corpus luteum cyst is present *(curved arrow).* **B,** Repeat coronal T2-WI shows that the "mass" has resolved, indicating that is was a focal myometrial contraction.

Uterine peristalsis is hypothesized to promote sperm transport to the fallopian tube during ovulation and assist in antegrade menstruation during the luteal phase. MR depiction of uterine peristalsis has been performed using fast sagittal T2-WI[11,20-22] and can be viewed at the following web address: http://www.interscience.wiley.com/jpages/1053-1807/suppmat/index.html (accessed on December 1, 2003).

Outer Myometrium

The outer myometrium has slightly different structure and function than the junctional zone. The higher T2 SI of the outer myometrium compared with the junctional zone is secondary to increased free water and decreased density of smooth muscle cells within the former.[15] Slow flow within myometrial vessels can often be depicted as tubular high SI structures. Leiomyomas (see below) are the most commonly encountered masses of the outer myometrium.

Benign Lesions of the Uterine Myometrium

Uterine Leiomyoma

Leiomyomas (fibroids) are benign neoplasms that are derived from the smooth muscle myoma cells of the uterine myometrium. Leiomyomas are the most common uterine neoplasm and are present in greater than 20% of women older than age 30 years.[23] Most women with leiomyomas are asymptomatic although some may have various signs and symptoms including pelvic mass, pain, abnormal bleeding, and infertility.

Leiomyomas are categorized by location and are termed intramural, subserosal, or submucosal. Most fibroids have an intramural location. Leiomyomas that are centered external to the uterus are termed subserosal. Subserosal leiomyomas can mimic solid adnexal lesions on sonography and physical examination.[24,25] Leiomyomas that have some component extending into the endometrial canal (even if covered by a layer of endometrium) are termed submucosal. Submucosal fibroids that are almost entirely located within the endometrial canal are termed intracavitary. Submucosal and intracavitary fibroids are the most common symptomatic fibroids and are associated with pain, abnormal bleeding, and infertility.[26]

MR findings of uterine leiomyoma. Leiomyomas are composed of compact, smooth muscle myoma cells and a paucity of intercellular matrix that results in characteristic low SI on T2-WI (Figs. 7-3 to 7-5; see Figs. 7-10, 7-40, 7-41, and 7-47).[15,27] Leiomyomas are well circumscribed with well-defined margins. Approximately one third of uterine fibroids are surrounded by a high SI rim on T2-WI that correlates with peritumoral lymphatics, veins, and edema (see Figs. 7-4 and 7-47).[28] MR has shown very high accuracy in the detection and characterization of leiomyomas and the distinction between fibroids and adenomyosis (see Fig. 7-4 and below).[29] MR can also show a distinction between an exophytic subserosal leiomyoma and a solid ovarian neoplasm based on the direct communication of the former with the uterus and the typical low T2-SI.[24] Another MRI feature of exophytic leiomyomas is the "bridging vessel sign,"[30] which refers to the presence of flow voids on T1- and T2-WI from branches of the uterine artery that are localized between the mass and the uterus; this indicates that the tumor is supplied by branches of the uterine artery (see Fig. 7-3).

MR can characterize a submucosal-intracavitary leiomyoma as the cause of an endometrial mass.[2,31]

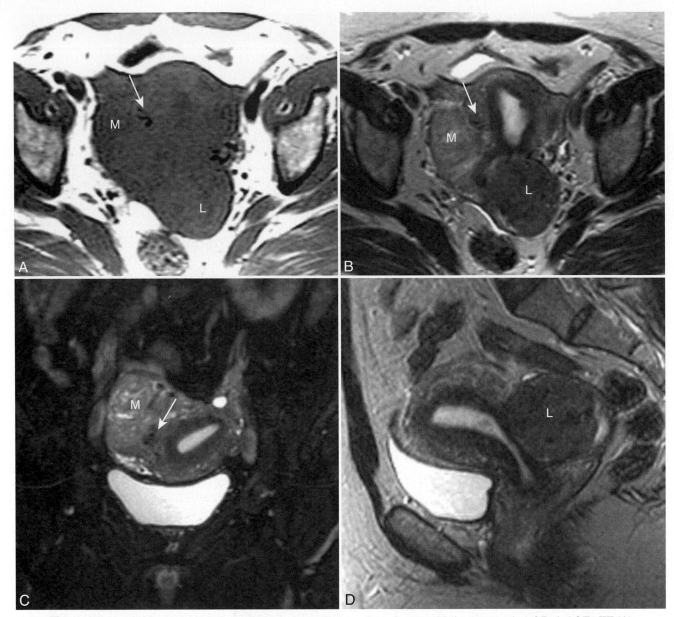

Figure 7-3 ▪ **MR depiction of the "bridging vessel" sign of a subserosal leiomyoma. A** and **B**, Axial T1-WI (**A**) and T2-WI (**B**) show a right-sided pelvic mass (M) located adjacent to the uterus. The mass reveals heterogeneous T2 SI. The presence of low SI flow voids *(arrows)* between the uterus and the mass establishes the uterine origin of the mass. A second exophytic posterior myoma (L) is present. **C**, and **D**, Fat suppressed coronal (**C**) and sagittal (**D**) T2-WIs shows normal uterine zonal anatomy and an additional intramural-subserosal leiomyoma (L).

Neither endometrial polyps nor hyperplasia (see below) are well circumscribed and reveal diffuse low T2-W SI, as do intracavitary myomas. MR can also reveal the presence of a stalk of an intracavitary leiomyoma, which can suggest a myometrial origin of the mass (see Fig. 7-5).[15]

When leiomyomas enlarge, it is common for them to degenerate. The various types of degeneration (the most common subtype being hyaline degeneration) result in heterogeneous SI on T2-WI and decreased enhancement.[32,33] Most of the subtypes of degeneration have little clinical import. As discussed below

under leiomyosarcoma, malignant degeneration of a leiomyoma is rare and is difficult to accurately diagnose on MR in the absence of metastatic disease. Calcium within degenerated fibroids is more accurately detected by radiography than by MR. The characterization of intratumoral calcium is not necessary to establish an MR diagnosis of myoma.

Hemorrhagic, cystic, and fatty degeneration are the three subtypes of myoma degeneration that have suggestive MRI features. Hemorrhagic degeneration of fibroids is uncommon and is associated with leiomyomas during pregnancy. Leiomyomas with

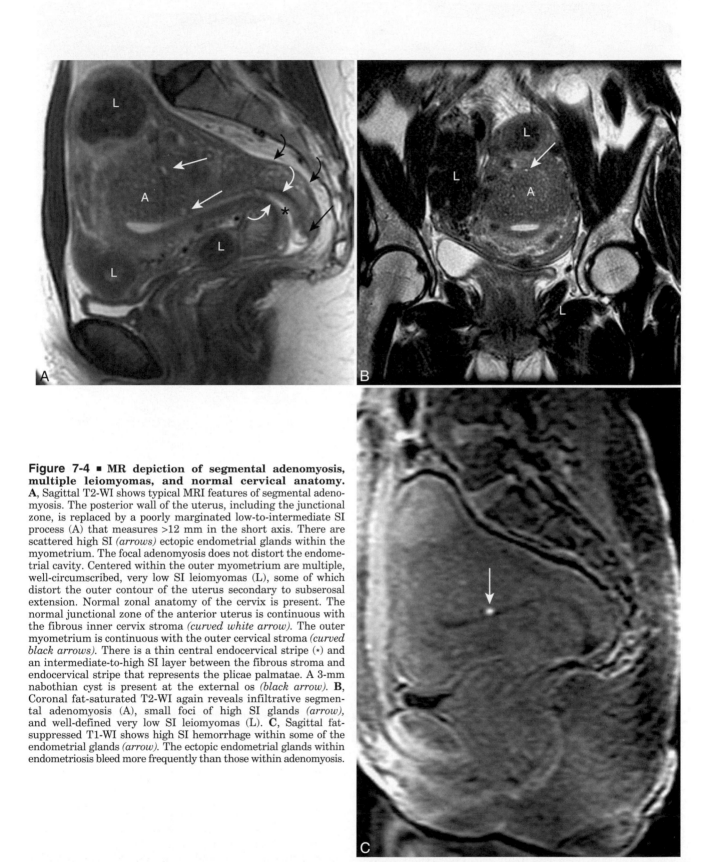

Figure 7-4 ▪ MR depiction of segmental adenomyosis, multiple leiomyomas, and normal cervical anatomy. A, Sagittal T2-WI shows typical MRI features of segmental adenomyosis. The posterior wall of the uterus, including the junctional zone, is replaced by a poorly marginated low-to-intermediate SI process (A) that measures >12 mm in the short axis. There are scattered high SI *(arrows)* ectopic endometrial glands within the myometrium. The focal adenomyosis does not distort the endometrial cavity. Centered within the outer myometrium are multiple, well-circumscribed, very low SI leiomyomas (L), some of which distort the outer contour of the uterus secondary to subserosal extension. Normal zonal anatomy of the cervix is present. The normal junctional zone of the anterior uterus is continuous with the fibrous inner cervix stroma *(curved white arrow)*. The outer myometrium is continuous with the outer cervical stroma *(curved black arrows)*. There is a thin central endocervical stripe (*) and an intermediate-to-high SI layer between the fibrous stroma and endocervical stripe that represents the plicae palmatae. A 3-mm nabothian cyst is present at the external os *(black arrow)*. **B,** Coronal fat-saturated T2-WI again reveals infiltrative segmental adenomyosis (A), small foci of high SI glands *(arrow)*, and well-defined very low SI leiomyomas (L). **C,** Sagittal fat-suppressed T1-WI shows high SI hemorrhage within some of the endometrial glands *(arrow)*. The ectopic endometrial glands within endometriosis bleed more frequently than those within adenomyosis.

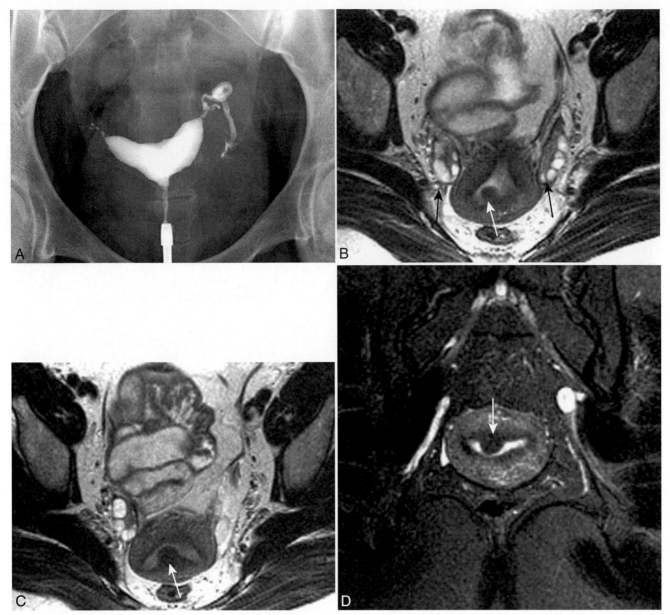

Figure 7-5 ■ **MR illustration of an intracavitary leiomyoma. A,** Radiograph from a hysterosalpingogram reveals contrast within both left- and right-sided endometrial cavities. MR was performed to evaluate a potential developmental uterine anomaly. **B–D,** Two consecutive axial (**B** and **C**) and coronal (**D**) T2-WIs show a well-circumscribed submucosal-intracavitary fundal leiomyoma *(arrow)* with a broad-based stalk that originates from the posterior myometrium. The myoma splays the endometrial cavity; no septate or bicornuate uterus is revealed. Normal ovaries are present *(black arrows)*.

hemorrhagic "red degeneration" often reveal peripheral or central high SI on T1-WI secondary to methemoglobin and show minimal if any enhancement.[34] The approximately 5% of fibroids that have foci of cystic degeneration reveal very high SI on T2-WI and do not enhance after contrast.[32] Fatty degeneration of a leiomyoma into a lipoleiomyoma is rare and has an incidence of less than 0.5%.[35,36] The metamorphosis of smooth muscle cells into adipocytes is the hypothesized etiology.[37] The fat tissue within the myoma can be detected and characterized using fat suppression techniques.[38] MR should be able to distinguish an exophytic lipoleiomyoma from a fat-containing ovarian dermoid by documenting the uterine origin of the former.

Treatment of uterine leiomyoma. Most leiomyomas are asymptomatic and therefore do not require therapy. Women with symptomatic fibroids have multiple treatment options.[39] Surgical options include hysterectomy, myomectomy (via laparotomy, laparoscopy, or hysteroscopy), and myolysis. Nonsurgical treatments include uterine artery embolization (UAE) and medical therapy. To date, no well-designed and -analyzed randomized multicenter trials comparing the various treatment options have been published.[39]

Hysterectomy is still an effective treatment for symptomatic fibroids. Hysterectomy is the second most frequent operation (>600,000/yr) performed in the U. S. Most hysterectomies are performed to treat pain or abnormal bleeding from symptomatic fibroids.[40] Less than 15% of hysterectomies are performed for cancer.[41] Women with abnormal uterine bleeding or infertility secondary to submucosal or intracavitary leiomyomas can be effectively treated with hysteroscopic resection; cessation of excess bleeding occurs in 75%[42] and restoration of fertility may result in up to 50% of treated women.[26,43,44] Imaging could help select those women who might benefit from hysteroscopic resection; the ideal candidate has a uterus that is not enlarged and contains one or two dominant submucosal-intracavitary myomas.[42]

UAE has become an alternative noninvasive treatment of symptomatic uterine fibroids.[45,46] UAE is a viable alternative treatment for many women with symptomatic fibroids who are unwilling to undergo surgical treatment.[47] The cost of UAE is equivalent to or less expensive than that of hysterectomy,[48,49] and it is effective in treating fibroids that are complicated by menorrhagia[50-52] and pain.[53,54] When compared with myomectomy, UAE is a better treatment for fibroid-related menorrhagia and an equivalent method for reducing pain.[52]

MRI-MRA provides data to determine which patients are potential candidates for UAE therapy. MR can document the size, number, location, and vascularity of uterine leiomyomas. MR also can evaluate for other processes that could be the cause or could contribute to the patient's signs and symptoms such as adenomyosis or endometrial carcinoma (see below). A single dominant intracavitary fibroid may be better treated with hysteroscopic resection (see above). Women with very large (>10 cm), dominant leiomyomas have equally good results after UAE as those with smaller myomas.[55] Leiomyomas with high SI on T1-WI and minimal or no enhancement are the one subtype that has shown poor response to UAE.[56] This is likely because the high SI myomas have already undergone ischemia/hemorrhagic necrosis and thus would not lose additional vascularity or volume with additional embolization.[57] Conversely, those myomas that show marked enhancement after contrast appear to have the best response to UAE therapy.[58]

Contrast-enhanced MR arteriography (CE MRA; see Chapter 10) can reveal the presence of normal uterine arteries (Fig. 7-6). If CE MRA shows a separate gonadal arterial supply to the uterus (Fig. 7-6), which is revealed on conventional arteriography in approximately 5% of women,[59,60] then one would consider also performing a gonadal artery embolization at the time of UAE. Not embolizing a gonadal artery that directly supplies the uterus is a cause of UAE failure.[61] Conventional arteriography reveals anastomoses between the uterine and ovarian arteries in 20% of women.[59] Embolic material has been documented in the ovarian arteries after UAE.[62] Inadvertent embolization of ovarian arterioles may explain why 10% to 15% of women experience ovarian failure or premature menopause after UAE.[63] Thus, the desire for future pregnancy is a relative

contraindication to UAE.[15] However, successful term pregnancies after UAE have been reported.[15,64,65]

After UAE, MR can document a decrease in size and enhancement of the fibroids (which reveal varying types of necrosis histologically[66]), preserved enhancement of the remainder of the uterus, and lack of visualization of the uterine arteries on the MRA portion of the examination.[67] Decreased enhancement of the fibroids on MRI immediately after UAE correlates with subsequent successful clinical response.[68] MR has documented a decrease in volume of fibroids by 40% to 60% and decreased enhancement of fibroids, in keeping with successful necrosis.[56,58]

UTERINE ADENOMYOSIS

Adenomyosis is the presence of ectopic endometrial glands and stroma within the uterine myometrium, with surrounding smooth muscle hyperplasia.[69,70] Adenomyosis typically presents in women aged 40 to 50 years. It is hypothesized that multiparous women are at risk for developing adenomyosis because of pregnancy-induced disruption of the endometrial-myometrial complex, especially in women who have had therapeutic abortions with sharp curettage.[71] Two thirds of women with adenomyosis have menorrhagia (excessive menstrual bleeding) or dysmenorrhea (painful menses), symptoms that can also be secondary to leiomyomas or endometriosis.[72] The amount and depth of adenomyosis correlate with symptoms of dysmenorrhea, while the depth of adenomyosis correlates with menorrhagia.[73]

MR can detect and characterize uterine adenomyosis by showing both the ectopic endometrial glands within the junctional zone and the surrounding smooth muscle hyperplasia (Fig. 7-7; see Fig. 7-4). The MR diagnosis of adenomyosis is made when the short axis measurement of the junctional zone is equal to or greater than 12 mm.[14,74] If the junctional zone measures 8 mm or less, then adenomyosis can be excluded with high specificity. Junctional zone thickness that measures between 8 and 12 mm is considered indeterminate.[14,15] Hyperintense 2- to 4-mm foci on T2-WI within the thickened junctional zone represent embedded endometrial glands and add specificity to the MR diagnosis.[75] The endometrial glands of adenomyosis are less hormonally responsive than those present in endometriosis (see next section), and thus the presence of high T1-SI hemorrhage within the glands of adenomyosis is less commonly revealed. MR can more accurately diagnose adenomyosis than can transvaginal sonography,[76,77] especially in women with coexistent leiomyomas.[78] In some patients, the thickened junctional zone can mimic a thickened endometrium on transvaginal sonography.[79]

Adenomyosis can be present in both focal and diffuse forms. The diffuse form is more common and often is distributed asymmetrically within the uterus (see Fig. 7-4).[80] Focal adenomyosis can be present within any segment of inner myometrium (see Figs. 7-4 and 7-7). MRI can distinguish between adenomyosis and uterine leiomyomas (Box 7-2).[29] Adenomyosis reveals poorly defined margins, is often oriented parallel to the endometrial stripe, and has minimal mass effect on the endometrial canal, whereas leiomyomas are well defined and do show mass effect (see Fig. 7-4).[15]

The symptoms of adenomyosis are often resistant to medical therapy, and thus surgery has been advocated for women with refractory symptoms. While MR has documented a decrease in junctional zone width in women with adenomyosis after GnRH analog therapy, no studies correlate the MR changes with improvement in symptoms. The frequent

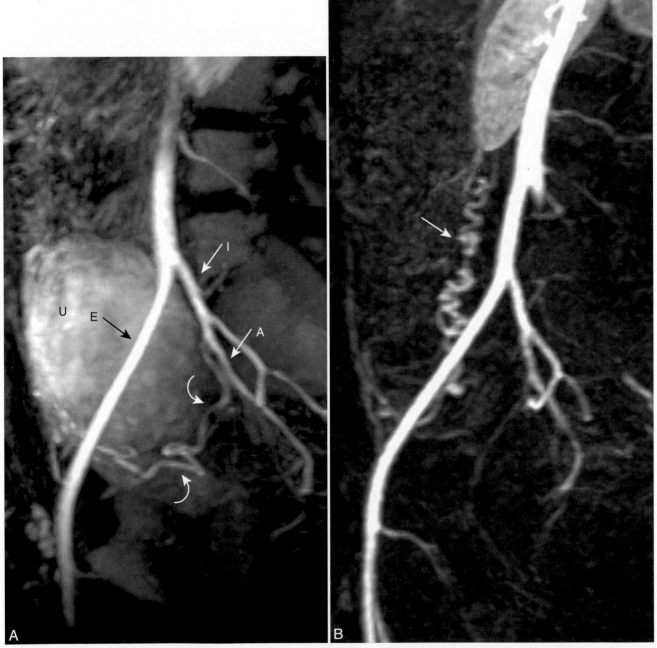

Figure 7-6 ▪ MR demonstration of recruitment of a gonadal artery after uterine artery embolization. **A,** Sagittal maximum intensity projection (MIP) image of the right pelvis from a 3D CE MRA shows the normal external iliac artery (E), internal iliac artery (I), anterior division of the internal iliac artery (A), and right uterine artery *(curved arrows).* Portions of the enhancing uterus are present (U). **B,** Postprocedural MIP image shows nonvisualization of the right uterine artery in keeping with interval embolization. A serpiginous vessel anterior to the aorta and the right common iliac artery is now shown *(arrow).* *(Continued)*

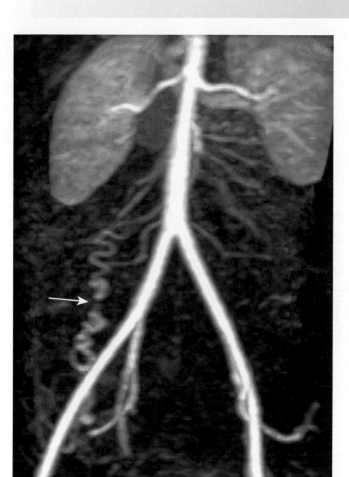

Figure 7-6 ■ Cont'd C, Coronal MIP image shows the vessel to be in the expected location of the right gonadal artery *(arrow)*. Neither uterine artery is identified, in keeping with prior embolization.

Endometrial Carcinoma

Endometrial carcinoma is the fourth most common cancer in women (with breast, lung, and colon cancer being the three most common) and the most common gynecologic malignancy. In 2004, approximately 40,320 women in the U. S. will develop endometrial carcinoma and an anticipated 7,090 women will die of the disease.[83] Endometrial carcinoma accounts for 6% of new tumors in women in the U. S. and results in 3% of cancer-related deaths.[83] Of the 10 most common cancers in women, endometrial carcinoma is the most curable.[84] Approximately 75% of women with endometrial carcinoma are postmenopausal at diagnosis.[85] The peak age range of women with endometrial cancer is 55 to 65 years, with a mean age at presentation of 59 years.[1,86] Excessive estrogen stimulation of the endometrium is a common association with endometrial carcinoma. In the 1960s and 1970s, unopposed estrogen supplements for the treatment of perimenopausal symptoms resulted in a marked increase in endometrial cancer, with an increased risk ratio of between 6 and 8.[84,87] With the subsequent implementation of estrogen-progesterone supplementation, the incidence of endometrial carcinoma has decreased in the last two decades. Tamoxifen has antiestrogenic activity in the breast but estrogen-enhancing effects on the uterine endometrium and is associated with an increased risk of endometrial carcinoma (see below).[2,88] Pregnancy is protective against the development of endometrial carcinoma because it results in a prolonged absence of estrogen stimulation of the endometrium.

The most common symptom of endometrial carcinoma is postmenopausal bleeding. The probability that postmenopausal bleeding is secondary to endometrial carcinoma is approximately 5%.[89,90] The Society of Radiologists in Ultrasound recommends that either transvaginal sonography or endometrial biopsy be performed as the initial procedure of choice in the evaluation of postmenopausal bleeding.[91] Hysteroscopic biopsy has a high diagnostic accuracy for establishing a diagnosis of endometrial carcinoma, especially in postmenopausal women.[92] Cost analysis studies suggest that if the incidence of carcinoma is greater than 31% in a given population, then initial biopsy is the least expensive procedure, while transvaginal sonography is recommended in populations with a lower estimated incidence of cancer.[93] The use of an endometrial

coexistence of endometriosis and lack of controlled studies make the efficacy of drug therapy difficult to evaluate.[81] Conservative surgical therapies are aimed at ablating the endometrium, endometrial-myometrial interface, or both.[81] Many women still resort to hysterectomy to alleviate symptoms that persist after conservative treatment. Results suggest that UAE can effectively treat menorrhagia associated with adenomyosis.[82] MR performed both before and after UAE can document the decrease in width of the junctional zone.[80,82]

7-2	**Uterine Leiomyoma vs. Adenomyosis**	
	Leiomyoma	*Adenomyosis*
Margins	Well circumscribed	Poorly defined
Mass effect on endometrium	+If intracavitary or submucosal	Minimal or none
T2 SI	↓ If not degenerated Variable ↑ SI when degenerated	↓ SI, 2- to 4-mm foci of ↑ SI endometrial glands
Center	Any layer of uterus, although originates in myometrium	Junctional zone

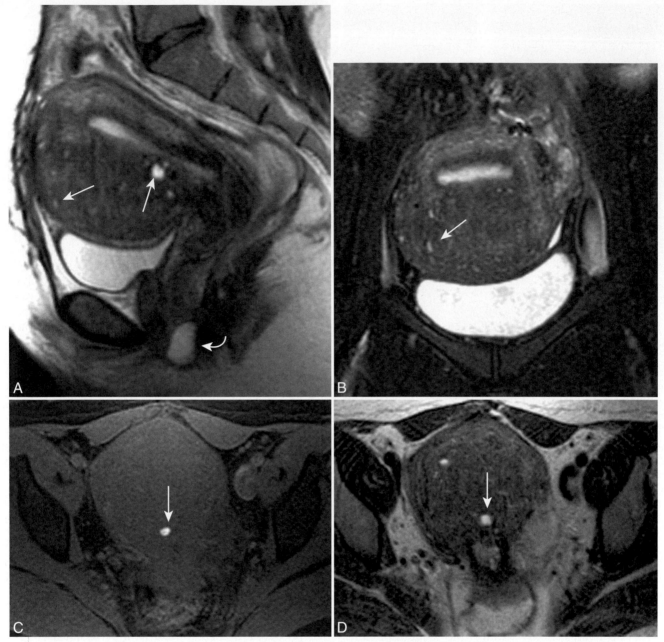

Figure 7-7 ■ **MR illustration of segmental adenomyosis and a Bartholin gland cyst in a woman with dysmenorrhea. A**, Sagittal T2-WI shows marked thickening of the anterior uterine myometrium, whereas the posterior junctional zone is of normal thickness. The anterior junctional zone contains multiple, <5-mm hyperintense foci *(arrows)* that represent ectopic endometrial glands within the myometrium. The adenomyosis does not displace the endometrial stripe. A Bartholin cyst *(curved arrow)* is present in the distal vagina. **B**, Oblique short axis T2-WI through the uterus again shows segmental adenomyosis with high SI glands *(arrow)*. **C** and **D**, Axial fat–saturated T1- (**C**) and T2 (**D**)-WIs show high T1-S1 hemorrhage *(arrow)* within one of the ectopic intramyometrial glands.

suction curette is sufficient for endometrial sampling.[94] Unlike dilation and curettage (D & C), suction curettage can be performed without general anesthesia.

Once a histologic diagnosis of endometrial carcinoma is established, the cancer is staged surgically (Box 7-3). Because many women with endometrial carcinoma have early abnormal uterine bleeding, 75% are diagnosed with stage I disease.[95] The role of

surgical lymphadenectomy at the time of hysterectomy is unclear. Some recommend that women with invasive cancers (stage 1C) have pelvic and para-aortic lymphadenectomy,[96-98] while others suggest that women at risk can be treated with irradiation and that lymphadenectomy is not necessary and only increases morbidity.[99-101] Further experience in laparoscopic lymphadenectomy[102] and sentinel node

7-3 FIGO Classification and MR Findings of Endometrial Carcinoma

FIGO Stage	Clinical Findings	MR Findings on T2-WI and CE T1-WI
Stage 0	Carcinoma in situ	Normal endometrial stripe
Stage I	Tumor confined to corpus	
Stage IA	No myometrial invasion	Variable endometrial abnormalities but intact junctional zone with normal endometrial-myometrial border
Stage IB	<50% Myometrial invasion	Signal intensity of tumor into but not through 50% of myometrium Abnormal endometrial-myometrial border
Stage IC	>50% Myometrial invasion	Signal intensity of tumor through 50% of myometrium Abnormal endometrial-myometrial border Normal contour and signal intensity of outer myometrium
Stage II	Cervical invasion, otherwise confined to uterus	
Stage IIA	Endocervical invasion	Signal intensity of tumor into endocervix with intact low SI cervical stroma
Stage IIB	Invasion on cervical stroma	Signal intensity of tumor into endocervix with disruption of low SI fibrous stroma
Stage III	Tumor beyond uterus but within true pelvis	
Stage IIIA	Invades serosa, invades adnexa, or positive peritoneal cytologic studies	Irregular contour of outer myometrium
Stage IIIB	Vaginal invasion	Disruption of low SI wall of vagina by tumor
Stage IIIC	Regional pelvic adenopathy	Regional lymph nodes with short axis >1 cm
Stage IV	Tumor outside true pelvis, or invasion of rectal mucosa or bladder	
Stage IVA	Invasion of rectal mucosa or bladder	Disruption of low SI detrusor muscle of bladder or low SI muscle of the rectum
Stage IVB	Distant metastasis	Tumor in extrapelvic organs or lymph nodes

evaluation[103] may decrease procedural morbidity and potentially improve patient survival.

MR is not recommended as a screening procedure in the diagnosis of endometrial carcinoma but has been promoted as a method of staging a known cancer. MR can distinguish between superficial and deep muscle invasive tumors by using a combination of T2-WI and dynamic CE MR (Figs. 7-8 and 7-9)[104-107]; MR has a higher staging accuracy than do sonography and CT.[108-112] CE MR is the most accurate technique for evaluating the presence and the depth of myometrial invasion of endometrial carcinoma,[113-115] especially in postmenopausal women or in women with adenomyosis.[116,117] T2-WI has higher diagnostic accuracy for myometrial invasion in premenopausal women. Similar techniques are also used to determine whether a cancer has invaded the cervix (see Fig. 7-9).[118-120]

On T2-WI, endometrial carcinoma can have a variable appearance but typically appears as a heterogenous endometrial mass that is hyperintense to adjacent myometrium and can have hypointense, isointense, and hyperintense components relative to normal endometrium. Hyperintense tissue that extends into more than half the width of the myometrium is the criterion for establishing muscle invasive tumor. On dynamic CE MR, endometrial carcinoma is revealed as hypovascular, hypointense tissue relative to the normal enhancing hyperintense myometrium.

A staging MR may predict the presence or absence of malignant adenopathy based on the presence or absence of muscle invasion of the primary tumor. The prevalence of positive para-aortic lymph nodes without deep myometrial invasion is less than 5% but is greater than 40% in tumors with deep myometrial invasion.[121] MR may be cost effective by indicating women in whom intraoperative lymph node dissection can be avoided.[122] MRI is limited to evaluating the size of nodes that could be involved by endometrial carcinoma. Unfortunately, malignant nodes may be of normal size; more than 50% of para-aortic nodes involved by endometrial carcinoma were enlarged.[123]

Opinions vary concerning the utility of performing a staging MR image in a patient with pathologically proved endometrial carcinoma. The accuracy of MR in determining muscle and cervical invasion is similar to what a surgeon establishes with gross visual inspection at the time of hysterectomy.[122,124] If a surgeon feels comfortable in determining whether to perform a lymphadenectomy at the time of gross visual inspection, then preprocedural staging MRI may not be indicated. However, if knowledge of the presence of myometrial invasion or pelvic adenopathy is desired prior to surgery (e.g., to better inform the patient about

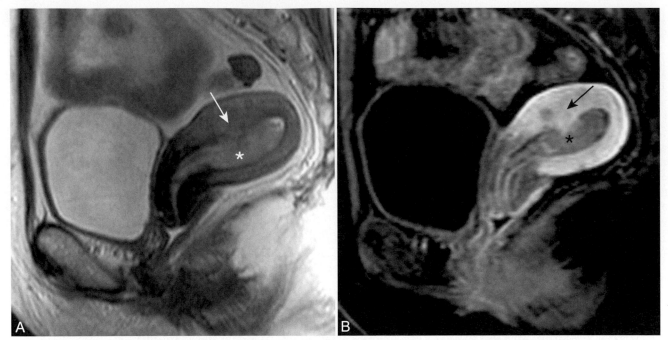

Figure 7-8 ■ MR depiction of a muscle invasive endometrial cancer. **A** and **B**, Sagittal T2-WI (**A**) and fat-suppressed CE T1-WI (**B**) shows an endometrial cavity that is distended by intermediate T2 SI, hypoenhancing tumor (*). The normal T2 hypointense junctional zone is segmentally disrupted in **A**, and hypoenhancing tumor *(arrow)* is well contrasted with the normally enhancing uninvolved myometrium in **B**.

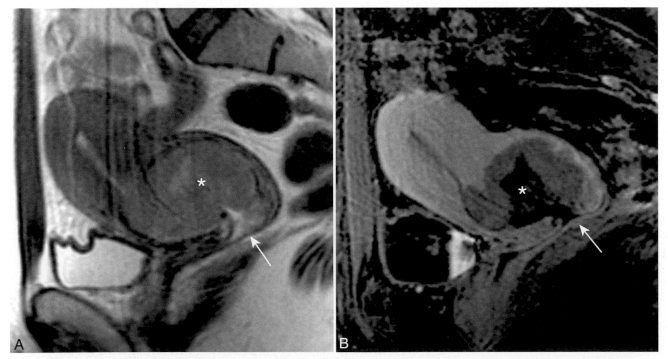

Figure 7-9 ■ MR depiction of deep myometrial and cervical invasion of an endometrial adenocarcinoma of the lower uterine segment. **A** and **B**, Sagittal T2-WI (**A**) and CE T1-WI (**B**) reveals an infiltrative mass (*) of the lower uterine segment that invades the posterior myometrium, endocervix, and stroma of the proximal cervix. The exocervix *(arrow)* is not involved. At surgery, tumor invaded 16 mm into a 20-mm-thick posterior myometrium. Lymphadenectomy revealed no malignant nodes. It is difficult to determine whether this lesion is a cervical cancer with endometrial extension or an endometrial cancer with cervical extension.

the proposed procedure and to effectively estimate operating room times), then obtaining a preoperative MR image could be considered.

Two other situations exist in which pretreatment MRI may be of use. Approximately 5% of women with endometrial carcinoma are poor operative candidates. MR demonstration of advanced disease may influence the patient and surgeon to avoid hysterectomy and to treat with radiation therapy alone.[125] Some centers are utilizing progesterone therapy without hysterectomy to treat some women with stage 1A endometrial carcinoma who want to preserve fertility.[126] MR demonstration of a normal junctional zone may be an appropriate noninvasive screening procedure to ensure the presence of noninvasive disease.

MRI is sometimes performed before a diagnosis of endometrial carcinoma has been established.

The presence of myometrial invasion should suggest a diagnosis of endometrial carcinoma or some other uterine malignancy,[7] as does the presence of necrosis on enhanced imaging.[127] The lack of invasion, the presence of a fibrous core, or the presence of endometrial cysts favor a benign diagnosis such as endometrial polyp–hyperplasia (see below).[127]

SECONDARY UTERINE CANCER

The ovary and vagina are the two most common locations for spread of tumor within the genital tract of women; secondary uterine and cervical cancers are uncommon.[128] Most secondary uterine neoplasms result from direct extension from either bladder and colonic tumors or extension of ovarian tumors via the fallopian tube (Fig. 7-10).[129,130] Less commonly, tumor can reach the uterus through hematogenous

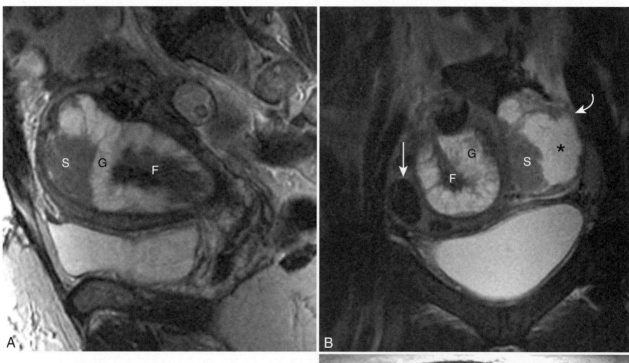

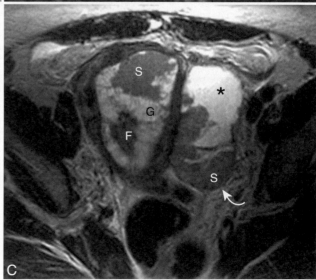

Figure 7-10 ■ **MR illustration of a benign endometrial polyp, benign leiomyomas, and left-sided primary ovarian carcinoma with direct extension to the endometrium.** The route of spread was presumably through the fallopian tube. **A–C.** Sagittal (**A**), coronal (**B**), and axial (**C**) T2-WIs show an aggressive left ovarian, serous papillary cystadenocarcinoma (*curved arrows*; the most common type of ovarian cancer) with both solid (S) and cystic (∗) components. Soft tissue of similar SI is present within the fundal segment of the endometrial canal (S) that was shown to represent local invasion by ovarian cancer. The remainder of the endometrial canal is distended by a mass with two different types of tissue. A benign endometrial polyp with a low SI central core (F) and peripheral, higher SI glands (G) was also present. The coronal image reveals multiple benign intramural leiomyoma.

or lymphatic spread. Secondary uterine cancer should be considered in the differential diagnosis in women who have documented metastatic disease or an infiltrative tumor that preserves the shape of the uterus (Fig. 7-11).[129]

UTERINE SARCOMA

Of all uterine cancers 97% are derived from the endometrial glands of the uterus and are classified as endometrial carcinoma. Only 3% of uterine cancers are sarcomas.[84] In decreasing frequency, the three most common sarcomas are malignant mixed müllerian tumor (MMMT), leiomyosarcoma, and endometrial stromal sarcoma.[131] MMMT has both sarcomatous and carcinomatous elements. Up to one third of women with MMMT have had prior irradiation for other pelvic tumors.[132]

Leiomyosarcomas comprise approximately 30% of uterine sarcomas.[131] They can arise either de novo or from malignant degeneration of a leiomyoma. Less than 1% of leiomyomas undergo malignant degeneration. It has been suggested that a diagnosis of leiomyosarcoma should be suspected when a myoma reveals irregular margins.[133] In my experience, atypical degenerated leiomyomas are more commonly encountered than leiomyosarcomas.

The third most common uterine sarcoma, the endometrial stromal sarcoma (ESS), accounts for approximately 20% of uterine sarcomas. Less aggressive, low-grade ESS occurs in younger women, while high-grade ESS develops in older women. Suggestive MRI findings of ESS include a large aggressive endometrial mass with nodular extension into the myometrium.[134,135] An insensitive but specific MR

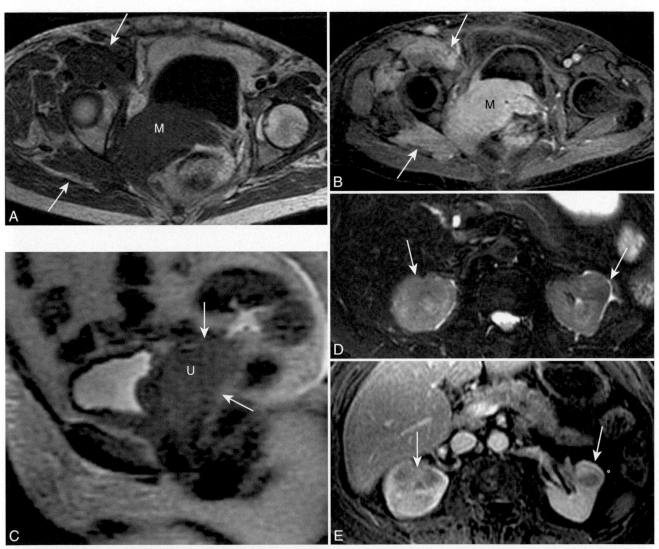

Figure 7-11 ■ MR findings of diffuse pelvic lymphoma with bladder, cervical, and uterine invasion. One year after treatment, the patient developed recurrent disease of the kidneys. **A** and **B**, Axial T1-WIs obtained before (**A**) and after (**B**) contrast show an infiltrative right-sided pelvic mass (M) that invades the cervix, bladder base and muscles of the proximal thigh and buttock *(arrows)*. **C**, Sagittal breath-hold T2-WI reveals lymphomatous extension into the uterus (U, *arrows*). Follow-up imaging after therapy showed resolved pelvic tumor (not shown). **D** and **E**, Axial T2-WI (**D**) and CE T1-WI (**E**) reveal bilateral hypoenhancing renal masses *(arrows)* representing hematogenous spread of recurrent lymphoma.

finding of invasive ESS is that of preserved low SI myometrial bands interspersed by invasive tumor.[74,136] However, the MR findings of most MMMTs, leiomyosarcomas, and high-grade endometrial stromal sarcomas are not specific. The most common MRI finding is that of an aggressive hemorrhagic and necrotic uterine mass with myometrial invasion or metastatic disease (Fig. 7-12).[137] Some uterine sarcomas can appear similar to endometrial carcinoma[137]; thus, tissue sampling is usually required to establish a specific tissue diagnosis.

Tamoxifen, Endometrial Polyps, and Endometrial Hyperplasia

Tamoxifen is a widely used medication that modulates estrogen receptors. Tamoxifen exerts antiestrogenic properties in breast tissue and is used to treat known breast cancer and to prevent the development of breast cancer in women who are at high risk.[138,139] Tamoxifen also has estrogenic effects on the uterus.[140] Women who take tamoxifen are at increased risk of developing both benign (hyperplasia, polyps) and malignant (endometrial carcinoma and sarcoma) lesions of the endometrium[1,88,141] as well as adenomyosis and leiomyomas.[79,142] Long-term users of tamoxifen are at (seven times) greater risk of developing endometrial carcinoma and tend to have higher stage cancers with less favorable histologic features.[143-145] However, the benefit of tamoxifen on survival in women with breast cancer far outweighs the potential development of endometrial carcinoma.[144]

Women who are taking tamoxifen and have abnormal vaginal bleeding require tissue sampling.[1,146] It is unclear whether asymptomatic women who take tamoxifen should be screened with either endometrial sampling or imaging.[147,148] Transvaginal sonography alone may not be an appropriate screening method because of a high percentage of false-positive findings.[149-151] Therefore, women who

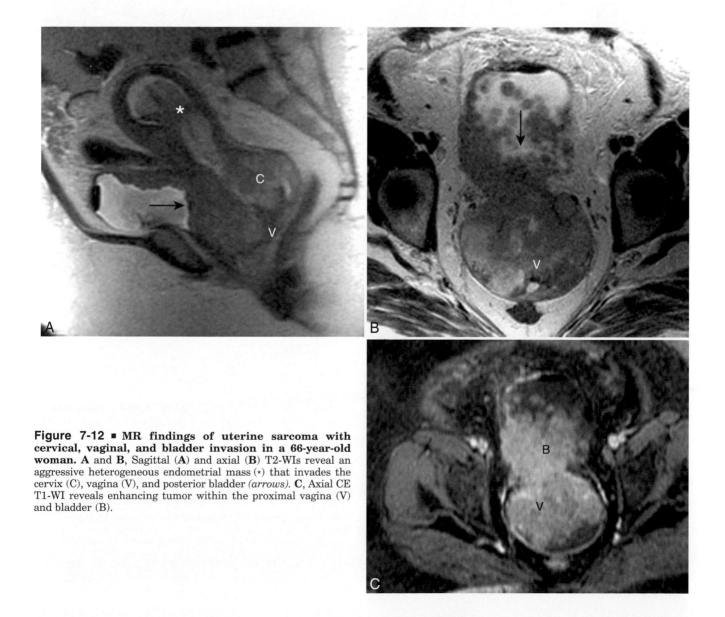

Figure 7-12 ▪ **MR findings of uterine sarcoma with cervical, vaginal, and bladder invasion in a 66-year-old woman. A** and **B,** Sagittal (**A**) and axial (**B**) T2-WIs reveal an aggressive heterogeneous endometrial mass (∗) that invades the cervix (C), vagina (V), and posterior bladder *(arrows).* **C,** Axial CE T1-WI reveals enhancing tumor within the proximal vagina (V) and bladder (B).

are taking tamoxifen and who have an "abnormal" endometrial thickness on a transvaginal ultrasound scan (TVUS; optimally defined using ROC analysis as >6 mm) could be further evaluated with hysterosonography to increase diagnostic specificity. The population of women who might benefit from MR would be those symptomatic women who are being evaluated at centers that do not offer hysterosonography or those women who cannot have the examination for technical reasons, such as cervical stenosis.[88,152]

Two different MR appearances of the endometrium have been described in women who take tamoxifen.[152] In approximately half the women, MR revealed a homogeneous, relatively thin high SI endometrial stripe that did not enhance after contrast. Endometrial atrophy without focal endometrial pathology is revealed in these women at subsequent tissue sampling (Fig. 7-13).[153]

The other half showed a widened heterogeneous endometrium on T2-WI (median width of 18 mm) (Fig. 7-14) that revealed a lattice type of enhancement on postcontrast imaging. Most women with this MRI pattern have endometrial polyps and hyperplasia.[152,154] It can be difficult on MR to distinguish between early, noninvasive endometrial carcinoma and endometrial polyp–hyperplasia (see Figs. 6-18, 7-10, 7-47, and 7-49).[1] While a central fibrous core and intralesional cyst formation are more common in endometrial polyps, tissue sampling usually is needed to exclude endometrial carcinoma.[127] If endometrial hyperplasia is present, histologic distinction between low- and high-risk subtypes can be performed to determine whether conservative follow-up or hysterectomy should be considered.[155]

The MR appearance of leiomyomas and adenomyosis is described above. Postmenopausal women

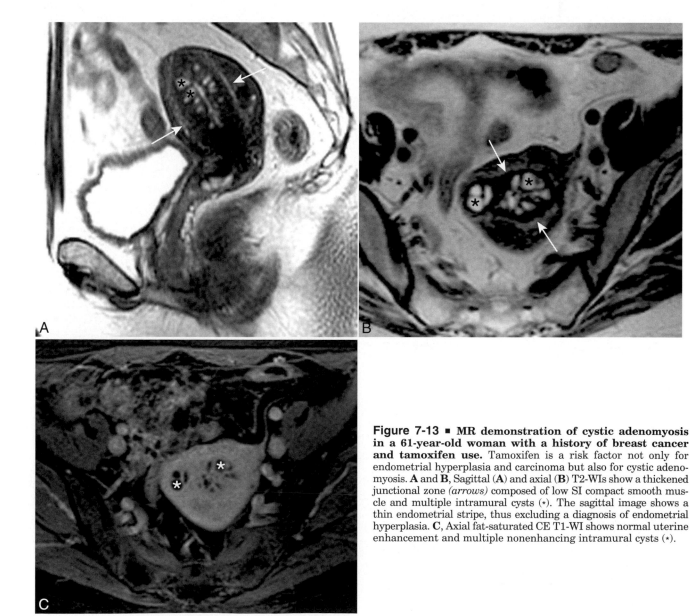

Figure 7-13 ■ MR demonstration of cystic adenomyosis in a 61-year-old woman with a history of breast cancer and tamoxifen use. Tamoxifen is a risk factor not only for endometrial hyperplasia and carcinoma but also for cystic adenomyosis. **A** and **B**, Sagittal (**A**) and axial (**B**) T2-WIs show a thickened junctional zone *(arrows)* composed of low SI compact smooth muscle and multiple intramural cysts (∗). The sagittal image shows a thin endometrial stripe, thus excluding a diagnosis of endometrial hyperplasia. **C**, Axial fat-saturated CE T1-WI shows normal uterine enhancement and multiple nonenhancing intramural cysts (∗).

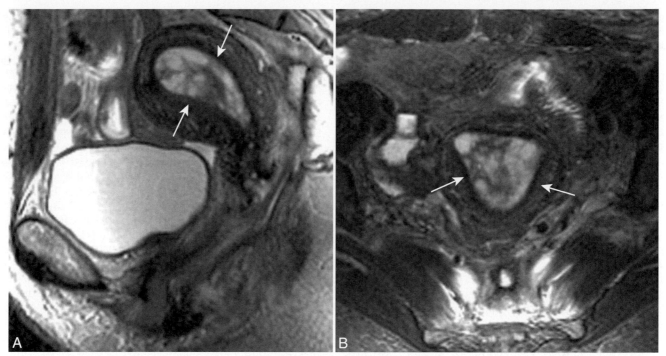

Figure 7-14 ■ **MR findings of tamoxifen-induced proliferative endometrium in a 71-year-old woman with a history of breast cancer. A** and **B**, Axial (**A**) and sagittal (**B**) T2-WIs show a widened endometrial complex *(arrows)* with both cystic and reticular solid soft tissue. This appearance is consistent with endometrial hyperplasia or polyps. Tissue sampling of this endometrium was performed because noninvasive endometrial cancer may have similar imaging features.

who take tamoxifen are also at risk for developing adenomyosis. Tamoxifen-associated adenomyosis often contains an increased number of subendometrial cysts (see Fig. 7-13).[79,152,156]

CERVIX

Normal Cervical Anatomy

Like the uterus, the cervix has a zonal anatomy that is well revealed on T2-WI (Box 7-4; see Figs. 7-4, 7-15, 7-20, 7-22, 7-30, and 7-36).[157] The central endocervical mucosa, secretions, and plicae palmatae (mucosal folds that have a palm-like configuration) have moderate to high SI on T2-WI similarly to the endometrial complex of the uterus. The middle layer of the cervix is revealed as low SI and corresponds to the inner layer of fibromuscular cervical stroma. In many women this cervical layer is contiguous with the junctional zone of the uterus. The outer layer of the cervix reveals low-to-intermediate T2-SI and corresponds to the outer fibromuscular stroma of the cervix. MR-pathology correlation suggests that the lower SI of the inner cervical stroma reflects increased fibroblasts and smooth muscle cells and less vascularized connective tissue when compared with the outer cervical stroma.[158] The outer cervical stroma is often contiguous with the outer myometrium.

Nabothian Cyst

Nabothian cysts are benign retention cysts that develop secondary to obstruction of the mucin-secreting endocervical glands by overgrowth by squamous epithelium.[159] Almost all nabothian cysts are asymptomatic and do not require treatment; they are more common in multiparous women and women with prior cervicitis. When present, nabothian cysts are usually multiple and measure less than 2 cm.[160]

On MR nabothian cysts reveal variable SI on T1-WI that reflects the viscosity of the mucin cyst content. On T2-WI, most nabothian cysts reveal high SI (see Fig. 7-4). They do not enhance after contrast.[161] Nabothian cysts become clinically relevant

7-4	Normal Zonal Anatomy of the Cervix on T2-Weighted Images	
Layer	**Thickness**	**Signal Intensity Relative to Muscle**
Endocervix	<10 mm	↑↑ SI with plicae palmatae
Inner stroma	Variable	↓↓ SI
Outer stroma	Variable	↑ SI

when they are mistakenly characterized as mucinous adenocarcinoma of the cervix (adenoma malignum; see next section).

Cervical Cancer

Cervical cancer is the third most common gynecologic malignancy in women in the U. S. (after endometrial and ovarian cancer, respectively). In 2004 it is estimated that 10,520 new cases of cervical carcinoma will be diagnosed in American women and that 3,900 women will die of the disease.[162] Screening for cervical cancer is done by annual Papanicolaou (Pap) smear[163] beginning at age 18 or the onset of sexual activity, whichever comes first.[164,165] Low-risk women with three prior consecutive negative Pap smears can be screened less frequently.[166] Cervical screening with Pap smears has decreased cervical cancer mortality by 70% in last 50 years[165]; in part because Pap smears are not available to women everywhere, cervical cancer is the second leading cause of cancer mortality worldwide.[167]

Risk factors for the development of cervical carcinoma include low socioeconomic status, cigarette smoking, infection with human papillomavirus (HPV), especially subtypes 16 and 18,[168] and sexual activity with multiple partners.[164,167,169,170] HPV infection is considered to be contributory to almost all cervical cancers; >90% of squamous cell carcinomas of the cervix contain HPV DNA.[86,171] One population that benefits from HPV testing is women who have a PAP smear that shows atypical squamous cells. Only those women who are shown to have HPV infection would require a follow-up colposcopy.[171,172] Vaccines that target the human papillomavirus are being developed.[173]

In the future widespread immunization again HPV may prevent the development of a significant proportion of cervical cancers.[174]

The mean age of women with cervical cancer is 50 years. Symptomatic women have bleeding or a vaginal discharge,[167] while asymptomatic women are diagnosed by a positive PAP smear or by detection of an occult lesion on speculum examination.[167] Of cervical carcinomas 85% are squamous cell cancers.[169] The remaining 15% are mostly adenocarcinomas. Cervical cancer is staged according to the International Federation of Gynecology and Obstetrics (FIGO) clinical classification (Box 7-5).[169,175] Accurate staging of cervical carcinoma is important because it directly influences patient treatment. Women with greater than stage IIB disease are not candidates for hysterectomy and are treated with irradiation. Women with less than stage IIB tumors are candidates for hysterectomy. Women with stage IB tumors (localized but >4 cm) benefit from preoperative irradiation and chemotherapy prior to hysterectomy.[85,176] Women with localized tumors that do not invade the internal os or the uterus and who would like to preserve fertility are candidates for trachelectomy.[177,178]

The FIGO staging system has some limitations. It does not incorporate lymph node status, primary tumor size (with the exception of subdividing stage IB lesions), or tumor histologic grade. The FIGO system can overstage up to 25% of women with stage I disease and understage up to 75% of women with stage III disease.[167,169] MR imaging can accurately stage women with cervical cancer. MR outperforms both examination under anesthesia (EUA) and transrectal sonography in the evaluation of primary tumor size and nodal status.[179] MR is also more accurate

---

7-5   FIGO Classification and MR Findings of Cervical Carcinoma

FIGO Stage	Clinical Findings	MR Findings on T2-WI and CE T1-WI
Stage 0	Carcinoma in situ	Normal endocervix
Stage I	Tumor confined to cervix	
Stage IA	Occult microscopic tumor	Normal endocervix or small tumor
Stage 1B	Visible invasive tumor >5 mm	SI of tumor partially disrupts the low-SI inner cervical stroma
Stage II	Tumor invades beyond uterus but without invasion of lower vagina or pelvic sidewall	
Stage IIA	Vaginal invasion	SI of tumor disrupts the low SI of the proximal wall of the vagina
Stage IIB	Parametrial invasion	SI of tumor extends through both low-SI inner stroma and intermediate-SI outer stroma and into parametrium
Stage III	Tumor extends to lower vagina or pelvic side wall or results in hydronephrosis	
Stage IIIA	Tumor invades lower vagina	SI of tumor disrupts the low SI of the distal vagina
Stage IIIB	Tumor invades pelvic sidewall or results in hydronephrosis	SI of tumor invades normal pelvic sidewall muscles
Stage IV	Tumor outside true pelvis, or invasion of rectal mucosa or bladder	
Stage IVA	Invasion of rectal mucosa or bladder	Disruption of low-SI detrusor muscle of the bladder or the low-SI muscle of the rectum
Stage IVB	Distant metastasis	Tumor in extrapelvic organs

than CT in staging cervical cancer.[180-183] An initial staging MR can reduce costs by obviating the need to obtain other tests such as barium enema and cystoscopy.[184] MR can also help identify those women who may be candidates for trachelectomy.[185]

MR FINDINGS OF CERVICAL CANCER

MR usually is not initially used to diagnose cervical cancer but to stage disease in women who have had a diagnosis established by Pap smear or biopsy. T2-WIs obtained in the sagittal plane and in a plane along the short axis of the cervix (Figs. 7-15 to 7-17)[186] are the most useful for local staging.[159,167,187-191] Most studies have not found that dynamic CE imaging provides significant improvement in local staging.[189,191-193]

On T2-WI, cervical cancer appears as a mass of higher SI than the adjacent fibrous cervical stroma but of lower SI compared with the endometrial and

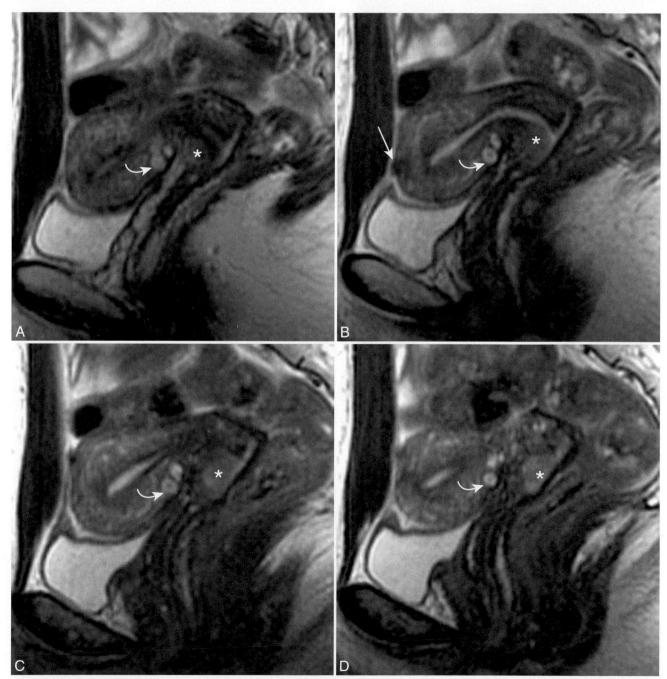

Figure 7-15 ■ **MR illustration of a stage IB cervical carcinoma in a 30-year-old woman.** This patient was treated with trachelectomy to preserve fertility. **A–D,** Four consecutive sagittal T2-WIs reveal normal zonal anatomy of the uterus and cervix. An intermediate SI mass is revealed within the endocervical canal (∗). A subcentimeter intramural-subserosal leiomyoma is present *(arrows)*. The tubular, high SI structures *(curved arrows)* present within the outer myometrium reflect slow flow within veins.

(Continued)

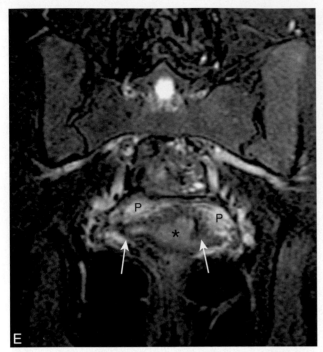

Figure 7-15 ■ Cont'd E, Coronal fat-suppressed T2-WI shows localized hyperintense tumor (*) and adjacent uninvolved fibrous cervical stroma *(arrows)*. The high SI within the parametria (P) is from vascularized connective tissue.

endocervical glands.[167] If an uninterrupted low SI rim of inner cervical stroma is preserved, then one can establish the absence of stage IIB or greater disease negative predictive values between 94% and 100% (see Fig. 7-15).[167,169,191,194] Disruption of the low SI, fibrous cervical stroma does not necessarily indicate parametrial invasion, since the intermediate SI outer cervical stroma may still be preserved. In selected women without parametrial invasion, resection of the cervix with preservation of the uterus (trachelectomy) can be considered.[195] Early results suggest that the rate of tumor recurrence is similar to that for women who are treated by hysterectomy.[196] Successful pregnancy can occur after trachelectomy, but there is an increased incidence of premature rupture of membranes.[197]

Macroscopic extension of tumor into the parametrial fat establishes a diagnosis of stage IIB disease (see Figs. 7-16 and 7-17). MR has an accuracy range of 75% to 95% in evaluating for parametrial invasion.[167,169,187] In women who are not candidates for hysterectomy, MR can more accurately determine the cancer diameter and volume and document the size and number of potentially malignant nodes; all these findings can help predict prognosis.[198,199]

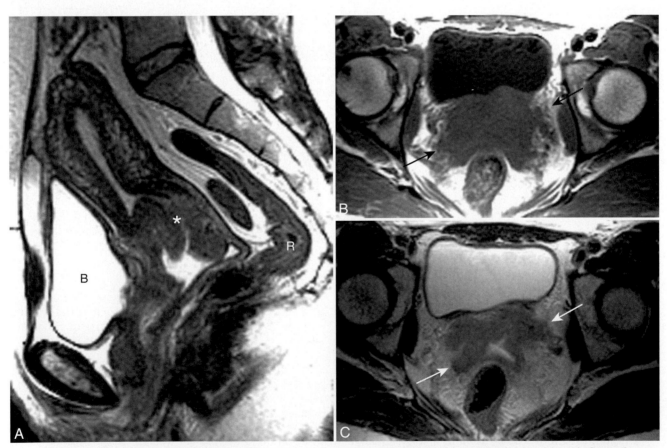

Figure 7-16 ■ MR findings of stage IIB cervical carcinoma with bilateral parametrial invasion. A, Sagittal T2-WI shows an endocervical (*) mass. Urine-filled bladder (B) is present anteriorly and rectum (R) posteriorly. The endometrial stripe is not widened. **B** and **C**, Axial T1-WI (**A**) and T2-WI (**B**) show nonvisualization of the normal low T2 SI cervical stroma. There is tumor infiltration into both the left and right parametria *(arrows)*.

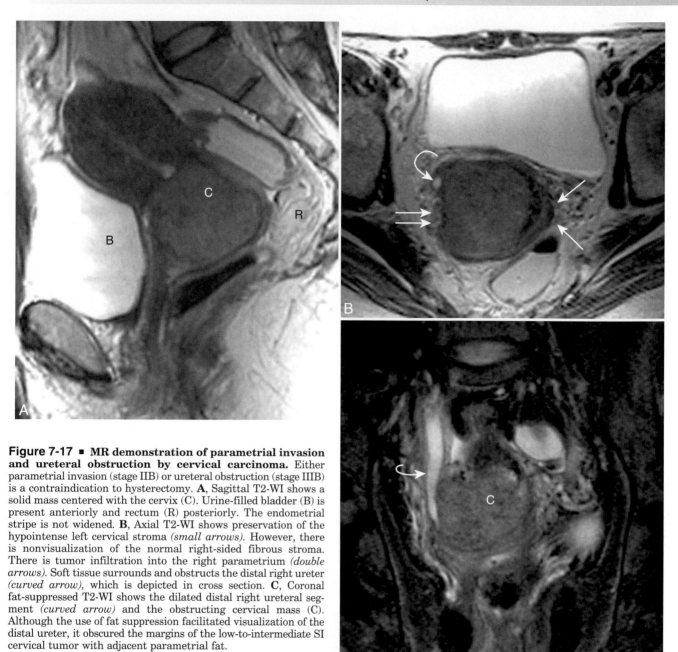

Figure 7-17 ▪ **MR demonstration of parametrial invasion and ureteral obstruction by cervical carcinoma.** Either parametrial invasion (stage IIB) or ureteral obstruction (stage IIIB) is a contraindication to hysterectomy. **A,** Sagittal T2-WI shows a solid mass centered with the cervix (C). Urine-filled bladder (B) is present anteriorly and rectum (R) posteriorly. The endometrial stripe is not widened. **B,** Axial T2-WI shows preservation of the hypointense left cervical stroma *(small arrows)*. However, there is nonvisualization of the normal right-sided fibrous stroma. There is tumor infiltration into the right parametrium *(double arrows)*. Soft tissue surrounds and obstructs the distal right ureter *(curved arrow)*, which is depicted in cross section. **C,** Coronal fat-suppressed T2-WI shows the dilated distal right ureteral segment *(curved arrow)* and the obstructing cervical mass (C). Although the use of fat suppression facilitated visualization of the distal ureter, it obscured the margins of the low-to-intermediate SI cervical tumor with adjacent parametrial fat.

Stage III tumors invade the pelvic sidewall, obstruct the distal ureter, or invade the distal vagina. Distal vaginal invasion is usually evident on clinical examination. MR can accurately evaluate for both pelvic sidewall invasion and obstruction of the distal ureter. Ureteral obstruction can be revealed by the use of heavily T2-WI (MR "urography," a subtype of MR "hydrography"; see Fig. 7-17)[159] or by delayed CE MR with T1-WI (CE MR urography). Women with stage III disease are not candidates for surgery. Localization of tumor and determining the presence or absence of ureteral obstruction provides a road map for radiation therapy and determines whether ureteral stenting is needed. Invasion of the bladder or rectum establishes stage IV disease. The presence of intermediate to high T2 SI tumor extending through the lower SI rectal muscularis or detrusor muscle of the bladder establishes stage IV disease.

MR Evaluation of Lymphadenopathy

While not a direct component of the FIGO classification, the presence and extent of lymphadenopathy is a most important indicator of patient outcome.[169,200] Women with para-aortic adenopathy usually do not undergo hysterectomy.[167] There is no consensus concerning whether women with stage IB or IIA cervical carcinoma and malignant pelvic adenopathy should have hysterectomy. If the patient and her surgical oncologist decide against hysterectomy if there is nodal disease, then sentinel node mapping and laparoscopic lymphadenectomy could be considered for presurgical evaluation.[201,202]

MR is approximately 75% to 90% accurate in characterizing adenopathy in women with cervical cancer (a positive node has a diameter of >1 cm by definition).[169,203,204] The presence of central necrosis is a very specific finding of malignant adenopathy in women with squamous cell carcinoma of the cervix. Thus, the use of contrast can improve the ability of CT and MR to characterize indeterminate lymph nodes. Unfortunately, central necrosis is not often revealed in nodes involved by adenocarcinoma. Thus, current nodal evaluation of adenocarcinoma of the cervix (and adenocarcinoma in other parts of the body) is based on measurements of both the long axis and short axis nodal dimensions. Different classes of contrast agents are in development that may improve the ability of MRI to characterize nodes as benign or malignant.[205,206]

Adenoma Malignum

Adenoma malignum is a rare subtype of mucinous adenocarcinoma that comprises less than 5% of adenocarcinomas of the cervix. Women with Peutz-Jeghers syndrome are increased risk of developing adenoma malignum.[207] Adenoma malignum can be a difficult diagnosis to establish on Pap smear or biopsy because of the well-differentiated appearance of the glands and the similarity to nabothian cysts and other benign glandular elements of the cervix.[208-210] A suggestive presenting symptom in affected women is a watery discharge.[159] Suggestive MRI findings that favor adenoma malignum include thick septa, enhancing solid components,[211,212] and the presence of high T2-WI mucin within the vaginal canal.[213]

Metastatic Disease of the Cervix

Similarly to the uterus, metastatic disease to the cervix is rare and usually secondary to direct extension by adjacent tumors of the uterus, bladder or rectum (Fig. 7-18).[129] Hematogenous metastasis to the cervix is rare. Occasionally a Pap smear will reveal malignant cells and help stage disease in a patient with a known extracervical malignancy.[214]

VAGINA

Normal Vaginal Anatomy

The vagina is a 7- to 9-cm long, fibromuscular tube that is line by stratified squamous epithelium. Three normal zones of the vaginal and paravaginal tissues are often depicted on T2-weighted MR images (Fig. 7-19).[215]

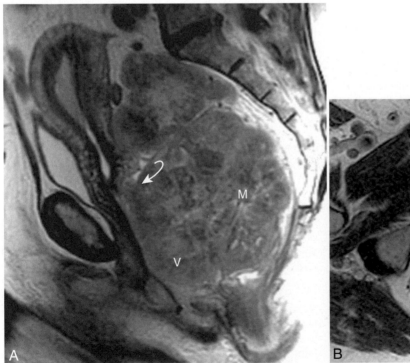
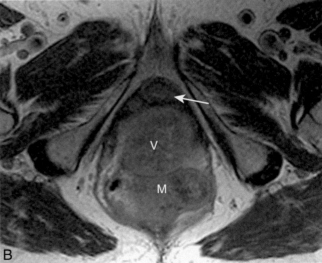

Figure 7-18 ■ MR illustration of recurrent colon cancer that invades the cervix and proximal vagina in a 62-year-old woman. A and **B**, Sagittal (**A**) and axial (**B**) T2-WIs shows an infiltrating soft tissue mass (M) of the presacral space that invades the posterior cervix and the proximal vagina (V). There is disruption of the low SI fibrous cervical stroma *(curved arrow)* The urethra *(arrow)* is not invaded in (**B**).

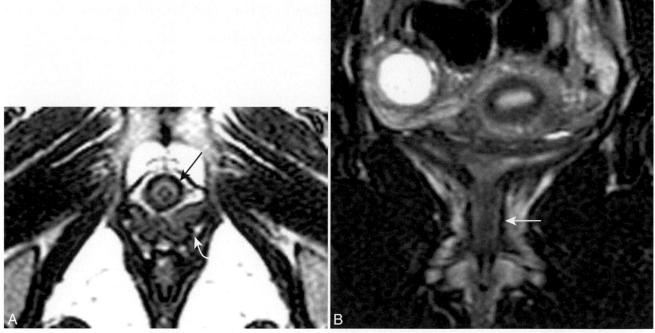

Figure 7-19 ■ **Normal axial vaginal and urethral zonal anatomy as revealed on T2-WIs in a 40-year-old woman. A** and **B,** The four zones of the urethra (from central to peripheral) are (1) inner high SI urine, (2) low SI mucosa, (3) high SI submucosa, and (4) low SI outer muscularis *(arrows).* The vagina has central high SI secretions and outer low SI mucosa and muscularis *(curved arrow).*

The vaginal muscles and collagen-rich submucosal layer appear as a low T1, low T2 SI band. Intraluminally, the vaginal mucosa and any endoluminal secretions have low T1, high T2 SI. A tampon will appear as a homogenous low T1, low T2 SI tubular structure within the vaginal lumen. When depicted along its long axis, a tampon has a characteristic appearance. However, if imaged in cross-section, a tampon can mimic an intracavitary leiomyoma. Surrounding the vaginal muscularis is a rich venous plexus that is revealed as a network of serpentine high SI structures on T2-WIs. The prolonged T2 signal within the veins is secondary to slow flow.[216]

Vaginal Cysts

Most vaginal cysts are asymptomatic and are discovered incidentally on physical examination or on pelvic imaging.[217] The less common symptomatic cysts are usually due to infection. Larger vaginal cysts can present as a palpable mass, urinary symptoms, dyspareunia, or dystocia.[218] At MR imaging, vaginal cysts have variable T1-SI depending on the presence of any intracystic protein or hemorrhage, have high SI on T2-WIs, and do not enhance after contrast.[161] The three most common types of vaginal cysts detected at MR imaging are Gartner duct cysts, Bartholin gland cysts, and müllerian cysts. Distinguishing among these three on MR is likely of little clinical import. Accurately documenting the size, location, and cystic nature of a vaginal mass is usually sufficient.

GARTNER DUCT CYST

Gartner duct cysts are located in the anterolateral aspect of the proximal vagina and are derived from vaginal remnants of the mesonephric (wolffian) ducts (Fig. 7-20). Children with Gartner duct cysts can be symptomatic secondary to communication with an ectopic ureter of the cervix.[219] Since some Gartner duct cysts are associated with developmental anomalies of the genitourinary system,[220,221] imaging the kidneys should be considered when a symptomatic Gartner cyst is revealed on pelvic MR examination.

BARTHOLIN GLAND CYST

Bartholin gland cysts develop as a complication of infection of the vestibular glands of the vagina, which are the female equivalent of the Cowper glands in men.[161] While Gartner cysts are located in the proximal vagina, Bartholin cysts are located in the posterolateral aspect of the distal vagina (Fig. 7-21; see Fig. 7-7) and can often be visualized and palpated on physical examination. Malignant tumors of the Bartholin glands are rare and include squamous cell carcinoma[222] and adenoid cystic carcinoma.[215,223] Both of these unusual tumors should show solid enhancing components at MR and should not be confused with uncomplicated or infected Bartholin cysts.

MÜLLERIAN CYST

The most common vaginal cyst described in the surgery and pathology literature is a müllerian cyst.[224,225]

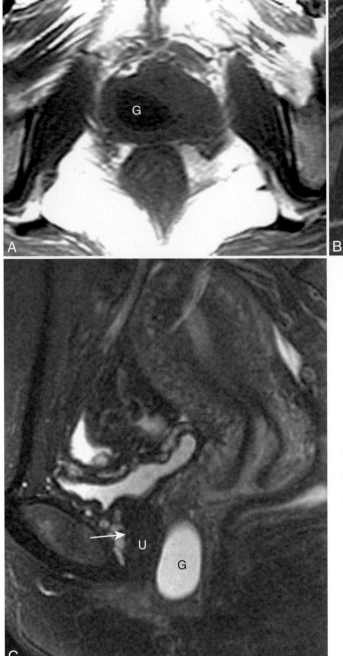

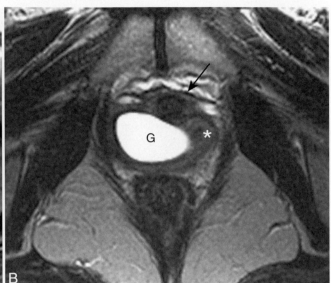

Figure 7-20 ▪ MR imaging features of a Gartner cyst of the proximal vagina in an asymptomatic woman. A–C, Axial T1 (**A**), axial T2 (**B**), and fat-suppressed sagittal T2 (**C**) WIs show an uncomplicated cyst (G) of the anterior lateral aspect of the proximal vagina (*). The normal urethra (*arrows*, U) is located anteriorly. Normal zonal anatomy of the uterus and cervix is present in **C**.

It is characterized on histologic studies by a mucin-producing epithelial lining similar to endocervix, and macroscopic intracystic mucin is sometimes noted on gross inspection. Unlike Gartner or Bartholin cysts, müllerian cysts occur along all vaginal segments (see Fig. 7-1).

Vaginal Fistulas

Fistulas can form between the vagina and adjacent urethra, bladder, bowel, or ureter. The most common etiology of vaginal fistula is prior gynecologic surgery (Fig. 7-22),[226] with radiation therapy, pelvic malignancy (Fig. 7-23), and inflammatory bowel disease being less common causes (Fig. 7-24). Although conventional contrast vaginography detects 80% of fistulae, the technique is suboptimal for evaluation of the extraluminal soft tissues, which may determine what type of repair to perform.[227] For example, in cases of radiated pelvic malignancy, MR might distinguish between sterile radiation fibrosis vs. viable paravaginal tumor. And in instances of rectovaginal fistula, MRI (or endorectal sonography) could evaluate for coexistent defects of the anal sphincter[228,229]

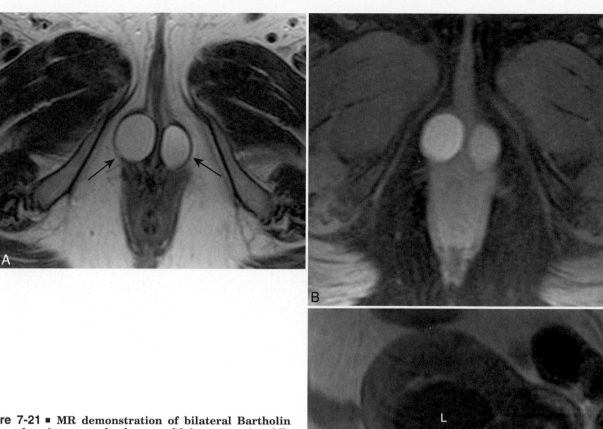

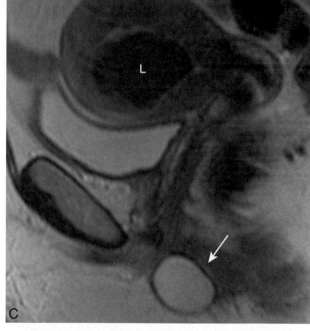

Figure 7-21 ■ **MR demonstration of bilateral Bartholin cysts and an intramural submucosal leiomyoma. A and B,** Axial T2-WI (**A**) and fat-suppressed T1-WI (**B**) show bilateral cysts *(arrows)* of the posterior lateral aspect of the distal vagina. T1 hyperintensity represents intracystic protein or hemorrhage, which is not uncommon in vaginal cysts. **C,** Sagittal T2-WI confirms localization of the cyst *(arrow)* to the distal vagina. A well-circumscribed hypointense leiomyoma (L) exhibits mass effect on the endometrial canal. Segmental adenomyosis would have less well-defined borders and exhibit little or no mass effect.

that could be treated at the time of fistula closure to prevent incontinence. On T2-WI, fistula tracks should appear as high SI material that extends from the vagina to either bowel, bladder, or urethra[230,231] (Figs. 7-22 to 7-25) or as a nonenhancing communication with enhancing walls.[232] To evaluate vesicovaginal or ureterovaginal fistula, delayed CE MR may show the presence of dilute contrast within the vagina (Fig. 7-25).

Vaginal Prolapse

Approximately one third of adult women have signs and symptoms of pelvic floor dysfunction that includes pelvic floor prolapse.[233] Fast T2-weighted

sequences obtained with and without straining can evaluate for abnormal descent of bladder, rectum, and vagina (Fig. 7-26).[234] The normal anatomy, physiology, and pathophysiology of pelvic floor weakness is beyond the purview of this chapter but available elsewhere.[235-239] MRI can provide both anatomic and functional information for the surgeon that may influence whether an abdominal or vaginal approach for potential surgical repair is needed.[240,241]

Vaginal and Vulvar Neoplasms

VAGINAL LEIOMYOMA

Leiomyomas located in the vagina are most often primary pedunculated submucosal uterine leiomyomas

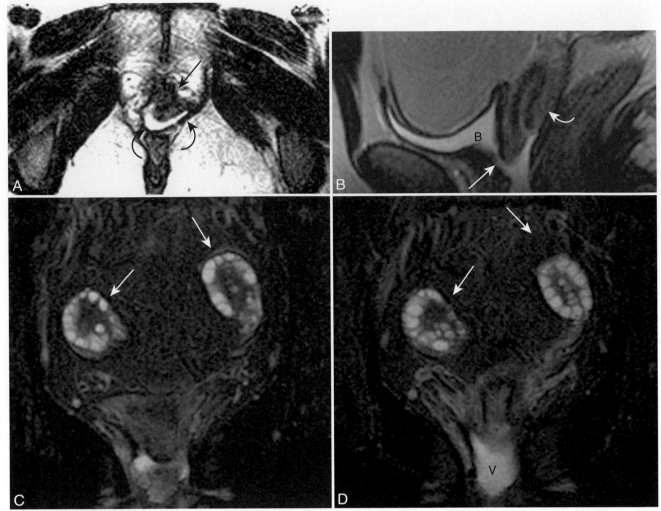

Figure 7-22 ▪ **MR illustration of a vesicovaginal fistula and polycystic ovaries in a 23-year-old woman with incontinence following repair of a vaginal septum. A**, Axial T2-WI shows normal urethral zonal anatomy *(arrow)* and curvilinear fluid within the proximal vagina that communicates with the right posterior urethra *(curved arrows)*. **B**, Sagittal fat-saturated T2-WI reveals the fistulous communication *(arrow)* even with an undistended bladder (B). Normal cervical zonal anatomy is present *(curved arrow)*. **C** and **D**, Two consecutive coronal T2-WIs reveal fluid in the vagina (V). Both ovaries are enlarged *(arrows)* and show peripherally located follicles of similar size and increased hypointense ovarian stroma.

that extend into the vaginal canal.[242] Much less common are primary vaginal leiomyomas that originate within the smooth muscle layer of the anterior vaginal wall.[243] Whether they originate within the uterus or vagina, MR can localize and often characterize such masses as smooth muscle in origin based on the relative low SI on T2-WIs.[244,245]

PRIMARY VAGINAL CANCER

The most common vaginal cancers are not primary but rather direct invasion of the vagina by adjacent tumors of the cervix, uterus, or rectosigmoid colon (see Figs. 7-12 and 7-18).[246,247] Both cervical and endometrial cancer are discussed elsewhere in this chapter. Primary vaginal cancers are not common and account for less than 3% of gynecologic malignancies.[248] It is estimated that 2,160 vaginal cancers and 790 deaths from vaginal cancer will

occur in 2004.[83] Seventy-five percent to 90% of primary vaginal cancer is squamous cell carcinoma.[248,249] The majority of vaginal cancers occur in elderly women. The two most common presenting symptoms are vaginal bleeding (60% to 70%) and vaginal discharge (30%).[248] As for squamous cell carcinoma of the vulva and cervix, women who have been infected with human papillomavirus are at increased risk of developing vaginal cancer. The treatment of choice for stage I and II cancers (Box 7-6) is surgical excision with postoperative radiotherapy.[250] Combination external beam with interstitial brachytherapy is the treatment of choice for advanced cancers.[251] Lymph node extension of cancer that originates within the proximal two thirds of the vagina is to the pelvic lymph nodes. Distal vaginal cancers, like vulvar cancers, tend to spread to inguinal lymph nodes.[252]

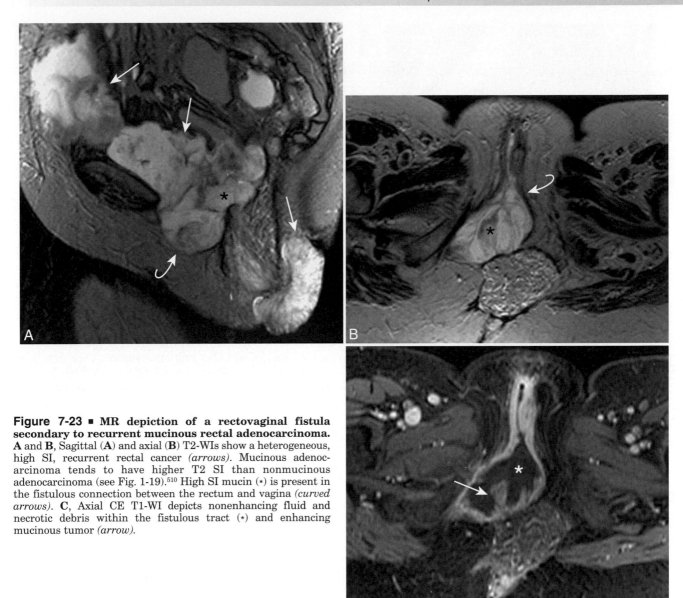

Figure 7-23 ▪ MR depiction of a rectovaginal fistula secondary to recurrent mucinous rectal adenocarcinoma. **A** and **B**, Sagittal (**A**) and axial (**B**) T2-WIs show a heterogeneous, high SI, recurrent rectal cancer *(arrows)*. Mucinous adenocarcinoma tends to have higher T2 SI than nonmucinous adenocarcinoma (see Fig. 1-19).[510] High SI mucin (*) is present in the fistulous connection between the rectum and vagina *(curved arrows)*. **C**, Axial CE T1-WI depicts nonenhancing fluid and necrotic debris within the fistulous tract (*) and enhancing mucinous tumor *(arrow)*.

Primary adenocarcinoma of the vagina is uncommon and comprises less than 5% of primary vaginal cancers.[253] The clear cell variant of vaginal adenocarcinoma develops in approximately 0.1% of women who were exposed to diethylstilbestrol (DES) in utero.[254] Vaginal smears are performed with annual Pap smears in DES-exposed women.[255] MR findings of vaginal clear cell adenocarcinoma have been reported.[256] Suggestive findings include location in the anterior portion of the proximal vagina (the most common location) or relatively high SI on T2-WI (Fig. 7-27). The diagnosis is often known before imaging (based on clinical history of DES exposure or a prior positive vaginal cytologic test) and imaging is used to stage a known cancer. The MRI findings of unusual vaginal neoplasms have been described.[257] However, these tumors are rare and do not have specific MRI findings.

VULVAR CANCER

Vulvar cancer is almost twice as common as primary vaginal cancer. It is the fourth most common gynecologic malignancy after uterine, ovarian, and cervical cancer. An estimated 3,970 cases of vulvar cancer will occur in the U. S. in 2004, and 850 women will die of the disease.[83] Squamous cell carcinoma accounts for more than 85% of vulvar cancers.[258] Vulvar carcinomas are increasing in frequency in young women and are likely secondary to the increase in prevalence of human papillomavirus infection.[258,259] Signs and symptoms of vulvar cancer include pain, bleeding, ulceration, vaginal discharge, or a visible or palpable mass. Unfortunately, many women delay seeking treatment, and up to 40% of women with vulvar cancer have stage III or IV disease at presentation (Box 7-7).[258,260]

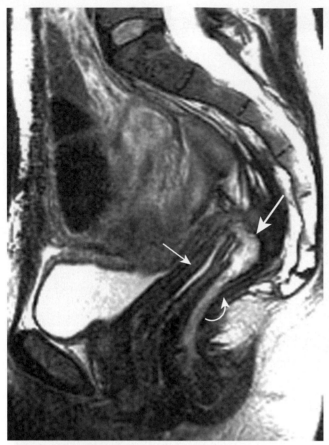

Figure 7-24 ▪ MR illustration of an enterovaginal fistula in a symptomatic 36-year-old woman with Crohn's disease and prior hysterectomy and subtotal colectomy. Sagittal T2-WI shows intermediate-to-high SI within the vagina *(arrow)* and the Hartmann pouch *(curved arrow)*. The fistulous connection at the level of the vaginal fornix *(large arrow)* was surgically confirmed and repaired.

The lymphatic drainage of the vulva is initially to the superficial inguinal lymph nodes and then to the deep inguinal and femoral lymph nodes. Initial studies have evaluated the utility of performing sentinel node sampling in the management of vulvar carcinoma. These studies use nuclear medicine isotopes and not MRI. In an MR-pathology correlation study

7-6	Summary of Staging of Vaginal Cancer[252]		
Clinical/Imaging Findings		**TNM**	**FIGO**
Confined to vagina		T1	I
Extension to paravaginal tissue		T2	II
Extension to pelvic sidewall		T3	III
Invasion of bladder or rectal mucosa, or extension of tumor outside of true pelvis		T4	IVA
Regional adenopathy		N1	III
Distant metastatic disease		M1	IVB

7-7	Summary of Staging of Vulvar Cancer[252,258]		
Clinical/Imaging Findings		**TNM**	**FIGO**
Confined to vulva and <2 cm		T1	I
Confined to vulva and >2 cm		T2	II
Extension to urethra, vagina, or anus		T3	III
Invasion of bladder, proximal urethra, or rectal mucosa, or extension of tumor to pelvic bone		T4	IVA
Unilateral inguinal adenopathy		N1	III
Bilateral inguinal adenopathy		N2	IVA
Distant metastatic disease		M1	IVB

of 22 women with vulvar cancer, superficial lymph nodes with a short axis of greater than 10 mm and deep inguinal nodes with a short axis of greater than 8 mm had respective specificities of 97% and 100% and more modest sensitivities of 40% and 50%.[261] In this same series, the primary tumor was detected only in half the women. Small primary vulvar lesions can easily be missed on MR. However, invasion of the pelvic sidewall or adjacent rectum and urethra can often be revealed (Fig. 7-28). The presence of central necrosis within nodes on CE MR in women with squamous cell cancer of the cervix has 100% positive predictive value for malignancy and may have similar utility in women with vulvar and vaginal cancers.[203]

Developmental Anomalies of the Müllerian Ducts

Developmental uterine anomalies occur in approximately 1% of all women and 3% of women with recurrent pregnancy loss or other poor reproductive outcomes.[262,263] Factors that contribute to an increased rate of pregnancy loss include cervical incompetence, decreased uterine volume, and decreased blood supply to the developing embryo and placenta.[264] Embryologically, the müllerian ducts form the fallopian tubes, uterus, and proximal two thirds of the vagina, while the urogenital sinus forms the urethra and distal third of the vagina. Developmental anomalies can result from one of three categories of abnormality of the müllerian ducts[265]: complete absence of the müllerian ducts, anomalous vertical fusion of the müllerian duct with the ascending urogenital sinus, or abnormalities of lateral fusion of the ducts. The American Fertility Society has a separate classification of uterine anomalies (Box 7-8).[266] MR is useful in the evaluation of developmental anomalies of the müllerian ducts.[262,267-271]

Patients with developmental müllerian duct anomalies may present at puberty with primary amenorrhea, pelvic mass, or pain. In patients with primary amenorrhea, MR can determine the presence or absence of the vagina, cervix, and uterus. In females that have relative or complete obstruction of antegrade menstruation, MR can determine the level

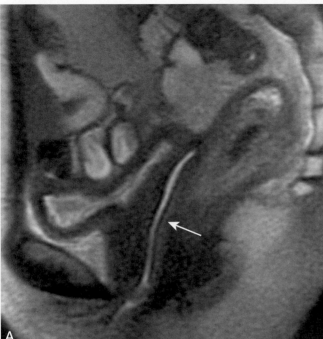

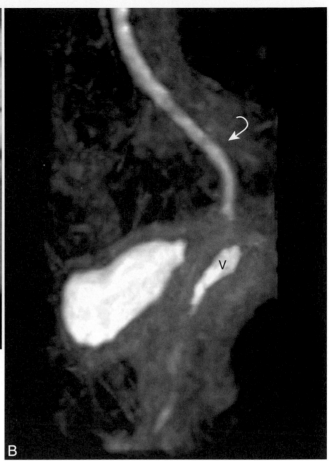

Figure 7-25 ▪ **MR depiction of an ureterovaginal fistula in an incontinent woman with a history of cervical cancer treated by hysterectomy and radiation therapy. A,** Sagittal T2-WI reveals the presence of fluid within the vagina *(arrow).* **B,** Delayed fat-suppressed CE T1-WI shows contrast within the right ureter *(curved arrow)* and proximal vagina (V).

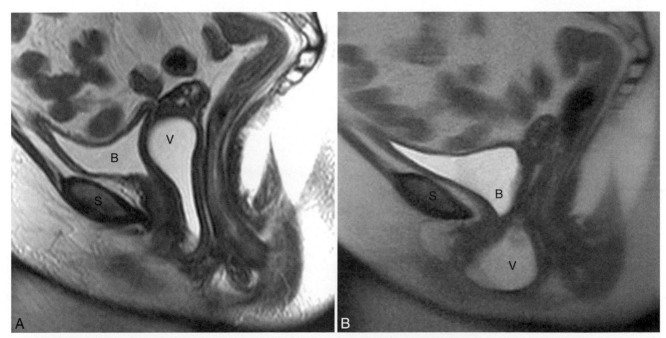

Figure 7-26 ▪ **MR depiction of cystocele and vaginal prolapse in a symptomatic woman. A,** Sagittal T2-WI shows normal position of the bladder (B) and a longitudinally oriented anterior vaginal wall cyst (V). **B,** Sagittal T2-WI obtained during the Valsalva maneuver reveals abnormal descent of both bladder (B) and vagina (V).

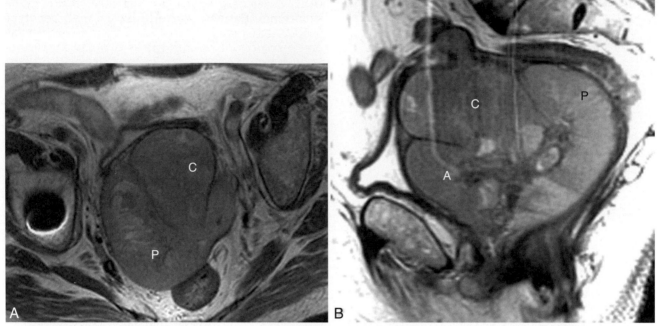

Figure 7-27 ■ MR illustration of clear cell adenocarcinoma of the vagina in a 77-year-old woman with a history of supracervical hysterectomy. A and **B,** Axial (**A**) and sagittal (**B**) T2-WIs show a heterogeneous infiltrative mass of the vagina that expands both the anterior (A) and the posterior (P) vaginal fornices and extends into the cervical canal (C). The MR findings are not specific for clear cell adenocarcinoma, and tissue sampling was required to establish a specific histologic diagnosis.

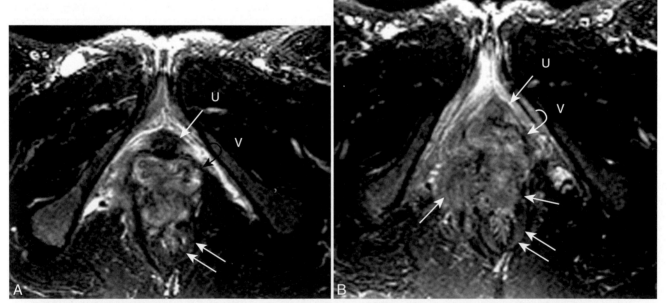

Figure 7-28 ■ MR findings of invasive squamous cell carcinoma of the vulva in a 37-year-old woman with a history of vaginal bleeding and human papillomavirus infection. A and **B,** Two consecutive axial T2-WIs through the superior aspect of the mass show a normal distal urethra (U, *arrow*), anterior portion of the distal vagina (V, *curved arrow*), and posterior rectum *(double arrows)*. A heterogeneous vulvar mass *(arrows* in **B)** invades the low SI posterior vaginal wall and anterior rectal wall. A right-sided inguinal lymph node is indeterminate for malignancy. The presence of central necrosis on enhanced imaging would increase the specificity of metastatic nodal involvement by squamous cell carcinoma. The patient was treated with vulvectomy and radiation therapy without lymphadenectomy and has been disease-free for 7 years.

7-8 American Fertility Society (AFS) Classification of Uterine Anomalies[262,266]

Class	Anomaly	% of Anomalies
Class I	Aplastic hypoplastic uterus	10%
Class II	Unicornuate uterus	15% to 20%
Class III	Uterus didelphys	5% to 7%
Class IV	Bicornuate uterus	10%
Class V	Septate uterus	55%
Class VI	Arcuate uterus (considered a normal variant)	
Class VII	Uterine anomalies associated with DES exposure	1%

of any obstruction and reveal whether retrograde menstruation has resulted in hematosalpinx or endometriosis. The kidneys are partially derived from the mesonephros, which is both spatially and temporally related to the müllerian ducts.[272] Therefore, in individuals with suspected müllerian duct anomalies, the kidneys should be evaluated as well. Women of reproductive age with müllerian duct anomalies may present with a history of infertility, prior miscarriage, or premature delivery. As described below, MR can define the anomaly and suggest if the condition is treatable.

ABSENCE OF THE MÜLLERIAN DUCTS (CLASS I)

Mayer-Rokitansky-Küster-Hauser syndrome (MRKH). The lack of müllerian duct development is part of the spectrum of Mayer-Rokitansky-Küster-Hauser (MRKH) syndrome. MRKH syndrome has an incidence of approximately one in 5,000 and is the most common cause of amenorrhea in women with breast development.[273] This syndrome, which is secondary to müllerian agenesis, results in failure of development of the proximal vagina, cervix, and uterus. Rudimentary functioning endometrial tissue may be present and result in pain secondary to endometriosis. MRI is an ideal modality for evaluating for MRKH syndrome (Fig. 7-29) to confirm the absence of the uterus, cervix, and proximal vagina and the presence of normal ovaries.[265] MR can also reveal persistent endometrial tissue, secondary endometriosis, and associated renal and collecting system anomalies, the latter of which may be present in up to 40% of affected individuals.[265,270,274-276] Treatment includes supportive psychotherapy and creation of a neo-vagina.[277] Rudimentary endometrial tissue should be removed laparoscopically to prevent retrograde menstruation and endometriosis.[278] Because women with MRKH syndrome have normal ovaries, they can become genetic mothers via egg donation.[279]

The differential diagnosis of a phenotypic woman who presents with primary amenorrhea and an absent uterus is androgen insensitivity syndrome (AIS, previously known as testicular feminization syndrome). Patients with AIS have a male genotype (46,XY) but female phenotype. MR can confirm the presence of rudimentary testes and the absence of both uterus and ovaries in patients with AIS.[276] Rudimentary testes in patients with AIS can be located intra-abdominally or inguinally[280]; they are removed laparoscopically after puberty because they are at risk of developing malignant transformation.[281] Many other uncommon disorders result in ambiguous genitalia at birth. MR can help evaluate such infants to determine the presence or absence of a cervix, uterus, and ovaries.[282]

UNICORNUATE UTERUS (CLASS II)

Incomplete or absent development of one of the müllerian ducts results in a unicornuate uterus. The contralateral uterine horn is completely absent in approximately one third of affected women, while a rudimentary horn is present in the remaining two thirds.[283] Approximately half of the rudimentary horns contain a cavity with endometrial tissue and half a noncavitary horn that lacks endometrium.[262] If a rudimentary horn communicates with the normal opposite side, then an ectopic or ruptured pregnancy may result.[283-285] Women with a noncommunicating horn are at risk of endometriosis. Thus, a rudimentary horn should be removed to prevent these complications.[286] Renal agenesis or other anomalies may occur and when present are located ipsilateral to the hypoplastic-aplastic horn. MRI can show the "banana-shaped" unicornuate uterus, evaluate for the presence or absence of a rudimentary uterine horn, and reveal associated findings such as endometriosis, ectopic pregnancy, and renal agenesis (Fig. 7-30).[267,283]

DISORDERS OF VERTICAL FUSION

Anomalies of fusion of the müllerian ducts with the urogenital sinus can result in a variety of disorders. The most common is a transverse vaginal septum (Fig. 7-31). Transverse vaginal septa can occur anywhere along the vagina but are most commonly present in the proximal third. When complete, a transverse vaginal septum results in amenorrhea and proximal hematocolpos. Treatment consists of surgical resection of the septum. More complete lack of fusion can result in proximal vaginal hypoplasia/aplasia and or aplasia of the cervix. If the cervix is present, a vaginal septum can be resected and the vagina reconstructed. In the past, women with cervical aplasia were treated with hysterectomy. However, recent surgical techniques have allowed creation of a uterovaginal anastomosis that allows the resumption of normal antegrade menstruation and restoration of potential fertility.[287]

DISORDERS OF LATERAL FUSION

Disorders of lateral fusion of the müllerian ducts can result in varying degrees of duplication of the uterus and cervix. Possible uterine configurations include uterus didelphys (class III, Fig. 7-32) and bicornuate

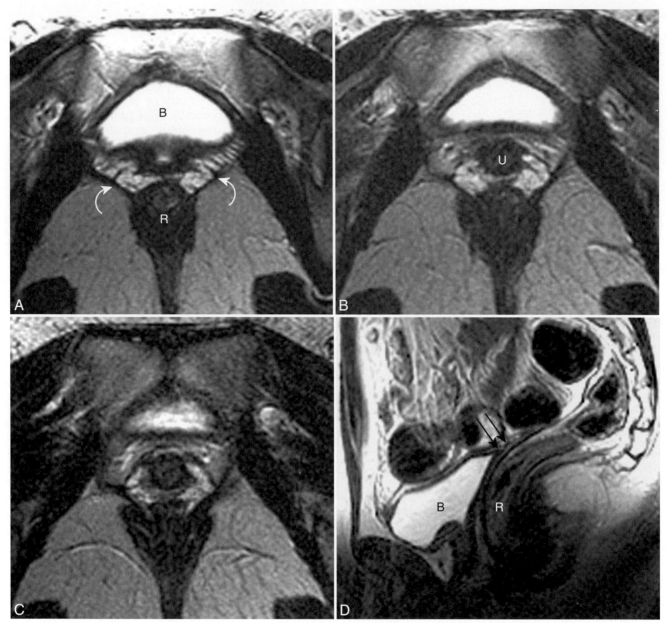

Figure 7-29 ■ **MR findings of Mayer-Rokitansky-Küster-Hauser (MRKH) syndrome in a 17-year-old woman. A–D,** Three consecutive axial (**A–C**) T2-WI and a sagittal (**D**) T2-WI show a normal bladder (B), rectum (R), urethra (U), and paravaginal-paraurethral venous plexus *(curved arrows)*. The vagina, cervix, and uterus are not present. The high SI within the venous plexus is secondary to slow flow. Black arrows indicate fibrous tissue in the expected location of the cervix.

uterus (class IV). After the müllerian ducts fuse, a fibromuscular midline septum can persist. Incomplete resorption of the fibromuscular central septum results in a septate uterus (class V, Fig. 7-33).[269] An arcuate configuration of the uterus (class VI, Fig. 7-34) is considered a normal variant and is not associated with an increased risk of infertility or pregnancy loss.[269,288] The MR appearance of these uterine configurations is described later.

In uterine didelphys there is complete separation of two distinct left and right uteri. The cervix usually is duplicated as well.[262,267,269] MR can readily show two distinct uterine and cervical segments that do not connect. Women with uterus didelphys have normal[289] or minimally impaired fertility. The latter has been hypothesized to be secondary to decreased uterine volumes or decreased vascularity of each uterine horn because of the lack of potential collateral blood supply from the contralateral uterine artery.[262]

Bicornuate and septate uteri are the two most common subtypes of müllerian duct anomaly and comprise approximately two-thirds of all subtypes.[290,291] Differentiating between a bicornuate uterus and a septate uterus is clinically important because of their

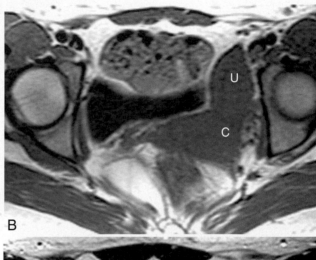

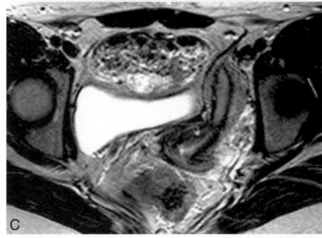

Figure 7-30 ▪ **MR depiction of a left-sided unicornuate uterus and right-sided pelvic kidney in an asymptomatic 30-year-old woman**. **A**, Coronal T1-WI shows a normal left kidney *(arrow)* and absent orthotopic right kidney. **B** and **C**, Axial T1-WI (**B**) and T2-WI (**C**) show a leftward deviation of the cervix (C) and a mildly hypoplastic left-sided uterus (U). Normal uterine and cervical zonal anatomy are present in **C**.

different complications and different treatments. Women with septate uteri may have first trimester miscarriages. It is estimated that the live birth rate of women with untreated septate uterus can be as low as 5%.[291] This has been attributed to implantation of the embryo onto the septum. Women with septate uterus who have had prior pregnancy loss are treated by hysteroscopic resection of the septum; reported live birth rates in treated women are as high as 85%.[262,291,292]

Women with bicornuate uteri do not have early miscarriages. However, some women may have premature labor that is hypothesized to be secondary to a decreased capacity of the endometrial canal. Some advocate the use of hysteroscopic metroplasty (removing some of the midline myometrium that is shared by both the left and right uterine canals) in order to create a single, more capacious endometrial cavity.[293] Women with bicornuate uteri also have an increased prevalence of incompetent cervix, which

can be evaluated with serial sonography during pregnancy.[263] Some advocate that women with bicornuate uterus receive prophylactic cervical cerclage.[294]

Evaluation of the external fundal contour is the key to differentiating between bicornuate and septate uteri.[295] The best imaging plane to evaluate the fundal contour is one that passes through the long axis of the uterus. This plane can be readily identified on sagittal T2-WI. The outer contour of a septate uterus should be convex or flat or at most show less than 10 mm of concavity (see Fig. 7-33). By comparison, the outer fundal contour of a bicornuate uterus or uterus didelphys should have a greater than 10 mm concavity between the left and right horns (see Fig. 7-32).[262,295,296] In indeterminate cases, two other measurements can be obtained.[267,295] The intercornual distance (measured between the distal segments of the left and right horns) is less than 4 cm in septate and more than 4 cm in bicornuate uteri. The intercornual angle (defined as the angle between the

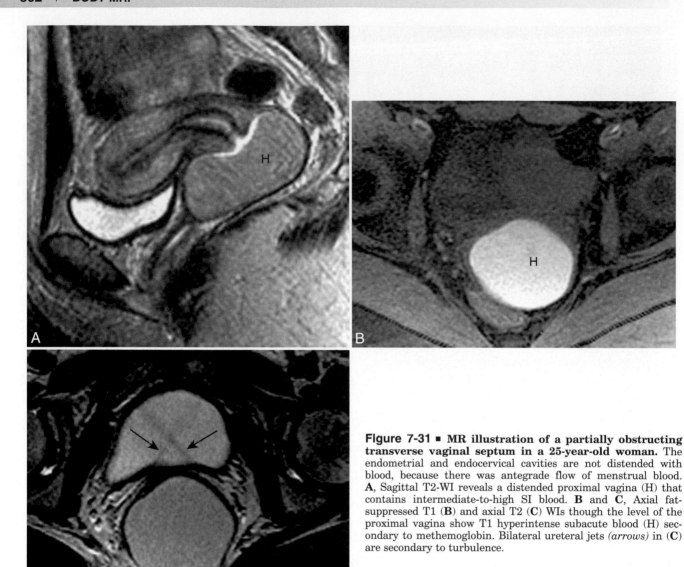

Figure 7-31 ■ MR illustration of a partially obstructing transverse vaginal septum in a 25-year-old woman. The endometrial and endocervical cavities are not distended with blood, because there was antegrade flow of menstrual blood. **A,** Sagittal T2-WI reveals a distended proximal vagina (H) that contains intermediate-to-high SI blood. **B** and **C,** Axial fat-suppressed T1 (**B**) and axial T2 (**C**) WIs though the level of the proximal vagina show T1 hyperintense subacute blood (H) secondary to methemoglobin. Bilateral ureteral jets *(arrows)* in (**C**) are secondary to turbulence.

medial most aspect of the left and right uterine cavities) is less than 60° in both normal and septate uteri and greater than 60° in bicornuate uteri.

Lack of lateral fusion of the müllerian ducts may also result in varying degrees of duplication of the vagina. Vertical vaginal septa are present in 75% of women with uterus didelphys, 25% of women with bicornuate uterus, and 5% of women with septate uterus.[262] Women with nonobstructing vaginal septa may be asymptomatic. Resection of a septum can be performed for dyspareunia. In some women, one of the vaginas forms a blind ending pouch secondary to lateral closure of a longitudinal septum. These women often have ipsilateral hematometrocolpos and/or ipsilateral renal agenesis. They do not have amenorrhea because the contralateral vagina remains patent.[297]

MRI can identify the level of the vaginal obstruction, the type of uterine anomaly, and the presence or absence of an ipsilateral kidney (Fig. 7-35).[272,297] Once again, the treatment of choice is removal of the septum and/or laparoscopic resection of any hematosalpinx.

OVARY AND ADNEXAE

Normal Ovary and Functional Cysts

The appearance of the normal ovary and physiologic functioning ovarian cysts at MRI have been described.[298-300] Like the uterus and cervix, the ovaries in premenopausal women often reveal a zonal anatomy on T2-WI with a lower SI ovarian cortex

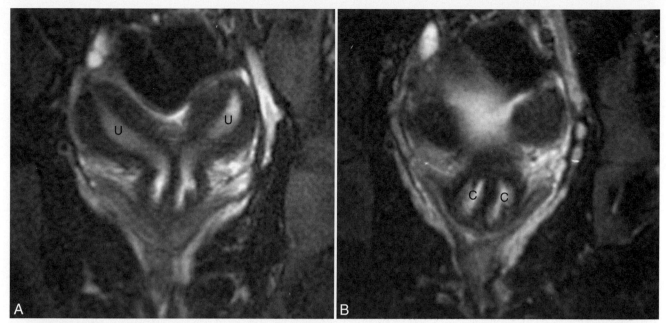

Figure 7-32 ■ MR illustration of uterine didelphys. A and **B**, Two consecutive coronal T2-WIs reveal two separate endometrial (U) and endocervical (C) cavities.

and a low-to-intermediate SI ovarian medulla and high SI ovarian cysts and follicles (see Figs. 7-5, 7-36, 7-41, and 7-56).[25,298,299,301] The higher relative SI of the medulla compared with the cortex is secondary to more vascular, looser connective tissue.

The majority of small cysts revealed within the ovary at MRI represent follicles in various stages of maturation. Normal follicles are less than 3 cm, reveal low T1 and high T2 SI, and have a thin enhancing wall.[25] Another normal cystic ovarian structure that may be present within the ovary is the corpus luteum cyst.[300] Normal corpus luteum cysts may have a thickened low-to-intermediate SI wall on T2-WI (see Fig. 7-2) that enhances after contrast.[25] Proteinaceous corpus luteum cyst content can reveal high SI on T1-WI. However, it is unusual for corpus luteum cysts to show low SI ("shading") on T2-WI as is depicted within most endometriomas.[298,299] In postmenopausal women there is decreased T2-SI within the ovarian medulla secondary to a paucity of follicles and decreased free vascular connective tissue.[25,299]

Ovarian Neoplasms

Ovarian neoplasms can be divided into four categories based on the cell of origin (Box 7-9).[302] The most common subtype of ovarian neoplasm is derived from the epithelial lining cells of the ovary. Ovarian epithelial ovarian neoplasms comprise approximately 60% of all ovarian tumors and more than 85% to 90% of ovarian malignancies.[303-305] Germ cell neoplasms are derived from the primary ovarian germ cells and account for 15% to 30% of ovarian tumors. Tumors derived from cells derived from ovarian sex cord and stromal elements constitute a third type of ovarian neoplasm and comprise 5% to 10% of ovarian tumors.

Metastatic tumors to the ovary are the final category of ovarian tumor and account for 5% to 15% of ovarian tumors.[306]

EPITHELIAL OVARIAN NEOPLASMS AND OVARIAN CANCER

Epithelial ovarian cancer. Ovarian cancer is the second most common gynecologic malignancy in women in the U. S. and the most common cause of death of all gynecologic malignancies. In 2004 it is estimated that 25,580 American women will develop ovarian cancer and that 16,090 will die of the disease. The lifetime risk of developing breast cancer in American women is 1 in 70.[307] Eighty-five percent to 90% of all ovarian cancers are epithelial ovarian cancers.[304,308,309] Nulliparous women have an increased risk of developing ovarian cancer, while parous women and women who use oral contraceptives are at increased risk.[305] Ovarian cancer is more common in older women. In one series, less than 15% of ovarian neoplasms in premenopausal women were malignant compared with a 45% chance of malignancy in postmenopausal women.[304]

Screening for ovarian cancer, either by tumor markers (e.g., CA-125)[310] or transvaginal sonographys[311] not been shown to decrease morbidity or mortality.[312,313] Only 50% of women with stage I ovarian cancer have elevated CA-125 levels, and up to 20% of women with benign adnexal disease have false-positive elevation of CA-125.[305] The one subgroup of women who are screened with sonography and CA-125 are those who are carriers of a BRCA gene.[314] Some of these women choose to have prophylactic oophorectomy in order to eliminate the risk of developing ovarian cancer and to decreased their risk of developing breast cancer.[315]

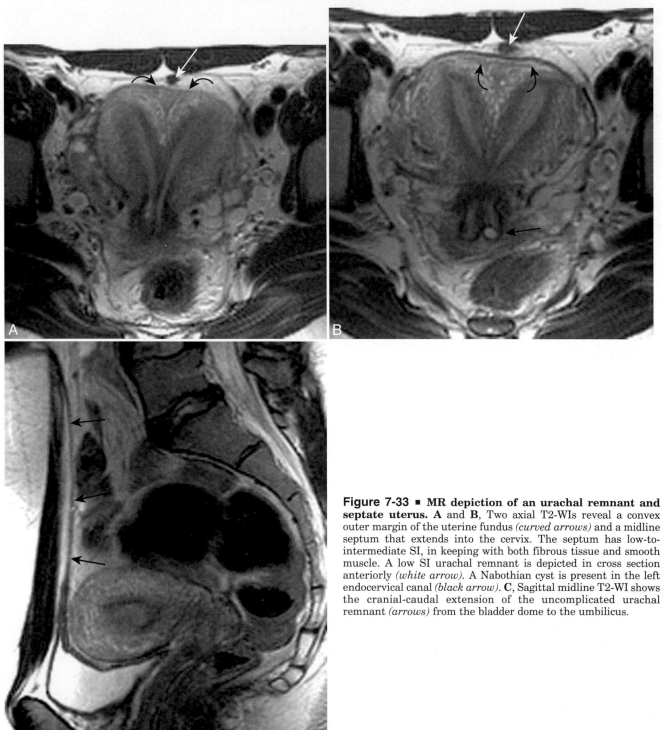

Figure 7-33 ■ MR depiction of an urachal remnant and septate uterus. A and **B**, Two axial T2-WIs reveal a convex outer margin of the uterine fundus *(curved arrows)* and a midline septum that extends into the cervix. The septum has low-to-intermediate SI, in keeping with both fibrous tissue and smooth muscle. A low SI urachal remnant is depicted in cross section anteriorly *(white arrow)*. A Nabothian cyst is present in the left endocervical canal *(black arrow)*. **C**, Sagittal midline T2-WI shows the cranial-caudal extension of the uncomplicated urachal remnant *(arrows)* from the bladder dome to the umbilicus.

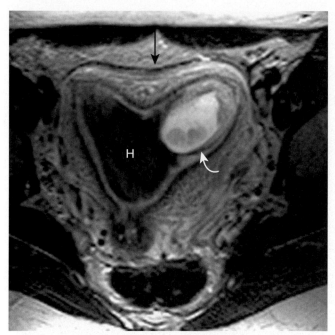

Figure 7-34 ▪ MR depiction of an arcuate configuration of the uterus. A prior sonogram confirmed embryonic demise but could not exclude a cornual ectopic pregnancy. Axial T2-WI shows a mild indentation of the uterine fundus *(black arrow)*. However, no midline fibrous or smooth muscle septum is present in the uterine cavity. An embryo with surrounding amniotic fluid is located in the left fundus *(curved arrow)*. This image unambiguously depicts the intrauterine location of the gestation and was able to exclude an interstitial-cornual ectopic pregnancy. Low SI hemorrhage (H) distends the remainder of the endometrial cavity.

7-9   Classification of Primary Ovarian Tumors

Epithelial Neoplasms (60% to 70%)
Serous cystadenomas and cystadenocarinomas
Mucinous cystadenomas and cystadenocarcinomas
Endometrioid tumor
Clear cell tumor
Brenner tumor

Germ Cell Neoplasms (15% to 20%)
Teratomas
Mature cystic teratoma (dermoid cyst)
Immature teratoma
Monodermal teratomas (e.g., struma ovarii)

Dysgerminoma
Endodermal Sinus Tumor
Embryonal Cell Carcinoma
Choriocarcinoma

Sex Cord–stromal Cell Tumors (5% to 10%)
Granulosa–stromal Cell Tumor
Granulosa cell tumor
Fibroma/fibrothecoma
Sclerosing stromal cell tumor

Sertoli-stromal Cell Tumor
Sertoli-Leydig cell tumor
Sertoli cell tumor
Leydig cell tumor

MRI is not a cost-effective screening modality for ovarian cancer. However, it can be useful to evaluate the female pelvis after an indeterminate sonographic examination. By accurately characterizing benign conditions such as endometriomas and mature cystic teratomas[316] (see below), MR can be cost effective by preventing unnecessary surgery or converting some planned laparotomies to laparoscopic procedures.[317] When compared with CT and sonography, MR was superior in the characterization of malignant ovarian lesions.[318]

The most common subtype of ovarian cancer is the serous cystadenocarcinoma, which comprises half of all epithelial ovarian cancer (see Fig. 7-10).[308] Mucinous cystadenocarcinoma and endometrioid carcinoma each make up 20% of epithelial ovarian cancers. Clear cell carcinoma is the least common subtype of epithelial ovarian cancer. Ovarian cancer is staged surgically

7-10   FIGO Staging of Ovarian Carcinoma

	Five-year Stage	*Survival*
Stage I	Cancer confined to the ovaries	80% to 90%
Stage IA	Unilateral tumor	
Stage IB	Bilateral tumor	
Stage IC	Microscopic peritoneal spread	
Stage II	Extension beyond ovaries; contained within the true pelvis	60% to 70%
Stage IIA	Tumor involves fallopian tube or uterus	
Stage IIB	Tumor involves other pelvic structures	
Stage IIC	Microscopic peritoneal spread	
Stage III	Peritoneal spread outside pelvis, or nodal spread of tumor	20%
Stage IIIA	Microscopic peritoneal implants	
Stage IIIB	Implants <2 cm	
Stage IIIC	Implants >2 cm	
Stage IV	Distant spread of cancer	10%

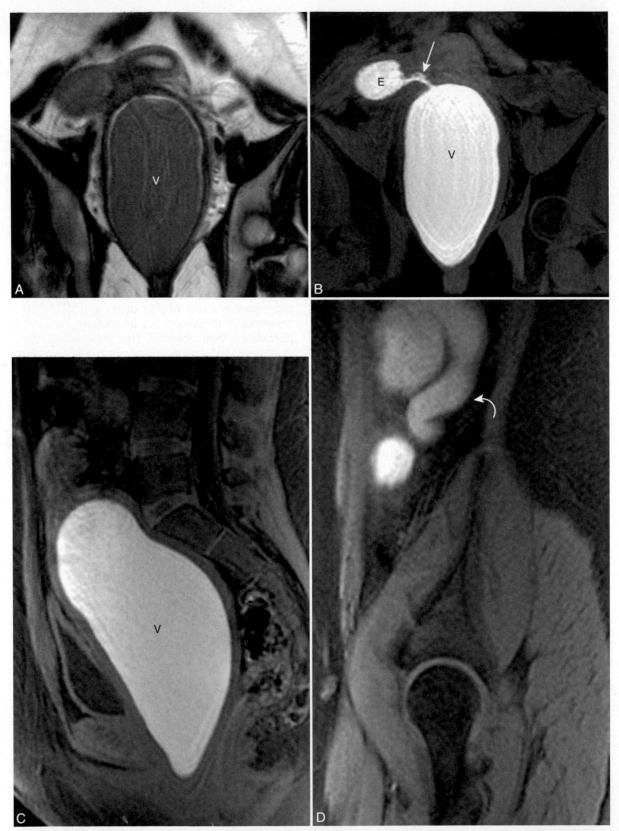

Figure 7-35 ■ MR appearance of uterus didelphys, with an obstructed right-sided system associated with developmental absence of the right kidney and acquired right-sided endometriosis. A and **B,** Oblique coronal T2-WI (**A**) and fat-suppressed T1-WI (**B**) show two widely separate uterine cavities in keeping with uterine didelphys. Normal zonal anatomy is present on the left with a normal endometrial stripe. Antegrade menstruation occurred through patent left-side cervix and vagina. There is obstructive right-sided hematometrocolpos with T1 hyperintense, T2 hypointense blood that distends the right endometrial canal (E), endocervix *(arrow)*, and vagina (V). **C,** Midline fat-suppressed T1-W1 shows the extent of the hematocolpos (V). **D,** Right paramedian fat-suppressed T1-WI shows a hematosalpinx *(curved arrow)* secondary to retrograde menstruation. Abdominal imaging (not shown) revealed normal left kidney and an absent right kidney.

according to the FIGO classification system (Box 7-10). Because of multiple factors including the lack of a cost-effective screening test[319] and the paucity of early specific signs and symptoms,[320] 70% of women have stage III-IV disease at presentation. A pathologist grades removed tissue; 65% of ovarian cancers are poorly differentiated, 25% are moderately differentiated, and the remaining 10% are well differentiated. It is the FIGO stage and histologic grade that determine the prognosis. The subtype of epithelial cancer does not have additional prognostic import.[308]

Most women with suspected ovarian cancer are best treated by total abdominal hysterectomy, bilateral oophorectomy, omentectomy, pelvic and para-aortic lymphadenectomy, peritoneal biopsy, and removal of any implants greater than 1 cm.[308,321] Some gynecologic oncologists will give preoperative chemotherapy to women with advanced ovarian cancer in whom cross-sectional imaging and/or initial direct inspection (via laparoscopy or laparotomy) suggest that cytoreductive surgery (i.e., debulking the abdomen and pelvis of all implants > 1 cm) would be unsuccessful.[322,323] Performing cytoreductive surgery after neoadjuvant chemotherapy improves disease-free survival and decreases the morbidity of surgery.[324] It is estimated that only 35% to 45% of women with advanced ovarian cancer can be optimally debulked without preprocedural chemotherapy.[85,308,325] Either CT or MR[326,327] define the tumor burden within the abdomen and pelvis to determine which women might benefit from preoperative chemotherapy.[308]

After patients are treated with surgery and chemotherapy, cross-sectional imaging can help determine which women have been cured as opposed to those who have residual or recurrent disease. By establishing criteria with high specificity and positive predictive value of residual disease, imaging (including either CT or MR) may prevent many "second look" surgeries to determine which subset of women would benefit from additional treatment.[328-330] Recurrent ovarian cancer is defined as new tumor that develops in women with prior surgery, chemotherapy, and a disease-free interval of longer than 6 months.[331,332] CT, PET (positron emission tomography), and/or MR may be able to point out which subset of these women with recurrent disease may benefit from a second cytoreductive surgery.[332,333] The imaging findings of hydronephrosis or pelvic sidewall tumor suggests unresectable disease that would not be amenable to reoperation.[332]

Subtypes of Epithelial Ovarian Neoplasms

Serous cystadenoma and cystadenocarcinoma. Serous ovarian tumors comprise approximately 25% of benign ovarian neoplasms (Figs. 7-36 and 7-37) and 50% of ovarian cancers (Fig. 7-38; see Fig. 7-10).[309,334] The typical appearance of a serous cystadenoma on MRI is that of a unilocular cyst with cyst content that follows the SI of simple fluid on T1-WI, T2-WI, and enhanced imaging (see Fig. 7-36). In one series of proven ovarian neoplasms, only 1 in 297 unilocular cysts was malignant.[335] Serous neoplasms are bilateral in 20% of tumors but present in 50% of malignant serous neoplasms. Besides bilaterality, other suggestive MRI findings of a serous tumor of low malignant potential (15% of serous tumors) or serous cystadenocarcinoma (25% of serous tumors) include larger size (>6 cm), combined solid and cystic components, and the presence of papillary projections (see Fig. 7-38).[305,336,337] Papillary projections are suggestive but not 100% specific for malignancy (they can be present in serous cystadenomas; see Fig. 7-37), but they are specific for epithelial ovarian neoplasms.[338-340] Outside the ovary, the presence of peritoneal implants[340] and ascites with enhancing peritoneum[341,342] is specific for malignancy and indicates stage III tumor.[337] Intratumoral calcifications (termed psammoma bodies) are present in up to 30% of serous tumors and are poorly depicted on MRI.

Serous epithelial ovarian neoplasms of low malignant potential may look similar to serous cystadenocarcinomas of the ovary on MRI.[343] The best prognostic indicator is determined at subsequent pathologic evaluation of the peritoneum. Peritoneal implants that are classified as invasive behave similarly to serous cystadenocarcinoma, whereas serous ovarian tumors without implants or with noninvasive implants are cured with surgical resection alone.[344]

Mucinous cystadenoma and cystadenocarcinoma. Mucinous ovarian tumors comprise approximately 20% of benign ovarian neoplasms and 10% to 20% of ovarian cancers. Compared with serous epithelial tumors, mucinous ovarian neoplasms are typically larger, multiloculated, and unilateral and do not have papillary projections (Box 7-11). The size of a mucinous tumor does not correlate with malignancy; some of the largest encountered ovarian tumors are benign mucinous adenomas (Fig. 7-39).[345]

A mucinous ovarian neoplasm is often revealed as a multilocular cyst on MR (Fig. 7-40). The SI of the cyst contents varies according to the degree of hydration of the intracellular and extracellular mucin. Hydrated mucin can have an MRI appearance similar to that of simple fluid with low T1 and high T2 SI. Viscous mucin with decreased hydration reveals variable decrease in T2 SI and increase in T1 SI. In the absence of mucinous ascites (see Chapter 6 for a discussion of pseudomyxoma peritonei and malignant mucinous peritoneal implants), differentiating among benign, malignant, and borderline mucinous tumors can be difficult and usually is determined at surgery.

Endometrioid and clear cell adenocarcinomas of the ovary are less common epithelial ovarian neoplasms. Unlike the serous and mucinous subtypes, both the endometrioid and clear cell variants are almost always malignant.[305,309] Although endometrioid ovarian carcinoma does not have specific imaging features, its association with both endometriosis[346] and endometrial hyperplasia/endometrial carcinoma can suggest the diagnosis.

Brenner tumor (transitional cell tumor). Brenner tumor is an uncommon subtype of ovarian neoplasm

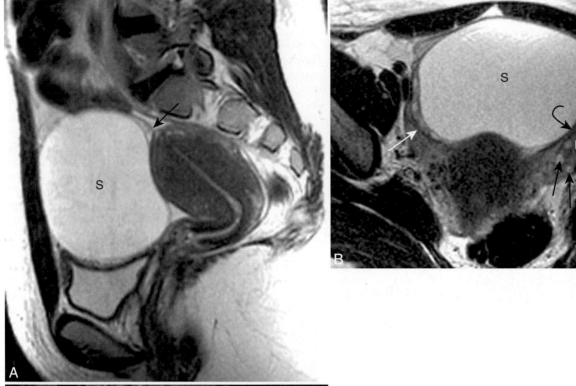

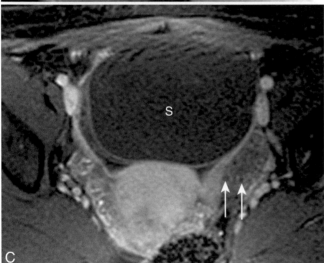

Figure 7-36 ■ **Benign right-sided ovarian serous cystadenoma as revealed on MR. A,** Right parasagittal T2-WI shows a nonaggressive unilocular right adnexal cyst (S). Portions of the normal remaining right ovary are present posteriorly *(arrow).* Normal uterine and cervical zonal anatomy is present. **B** and **C,** Axial T2-WI (**B**) and CE T1-WI (**C**) show no papillary projections or solid components within the lesion (S). A normal left ovary has high SI follicles *(arrows),* low-to-intermediate SI ovarian medulla (M), and very low SI cortex *(curved arrows).* Portions of the adjacent right ovary are also shown *(white arrow).*

composed of ovarian transition cells surrounded by dense fibrous tissue.[347] Most ovarian Brenner tumors are small and detected incidentally in asymptomatic women.[309,348] For unknown reasons, Brenner tumors are associated with other ovarian neoplasms in one third of women.[347,349] It is the predominantly fibrous content of Brenner tumors that results in relatively low SI on T2-WI (see Fig. 7-37).[347,349] The differential diagnosis of a low T2-SI ovarian lesion includes Brenner tumor, ovarian fibroma, and fibrothecoma. The presence of signs or symptoms of estrogen excess would suggest a fibrothecoma, while the presence of a second ovarian neoplasm favors a diagnosis of

Brenner tumor. Otherwise, ovarian fibroma and Brenner tumor may be indistinguishable by imaging.

GERM CELL NEOPLASMS

Germ cell neoplasms (see Box 7-9) comprise approximately 15% to 30% of all ovarian neoplasms.[309] Benign ovarian teratoma is the most common subtype of germ cell tumor and is composed of mature pluripotential germ cells. The other germ cell neoplasms are uncommon and malignant and account for less than 5% of malignant ovarian tumors but comprise two thirds of ovarian malignancies in females below the age of 20 years.[350] Unlike epithelial

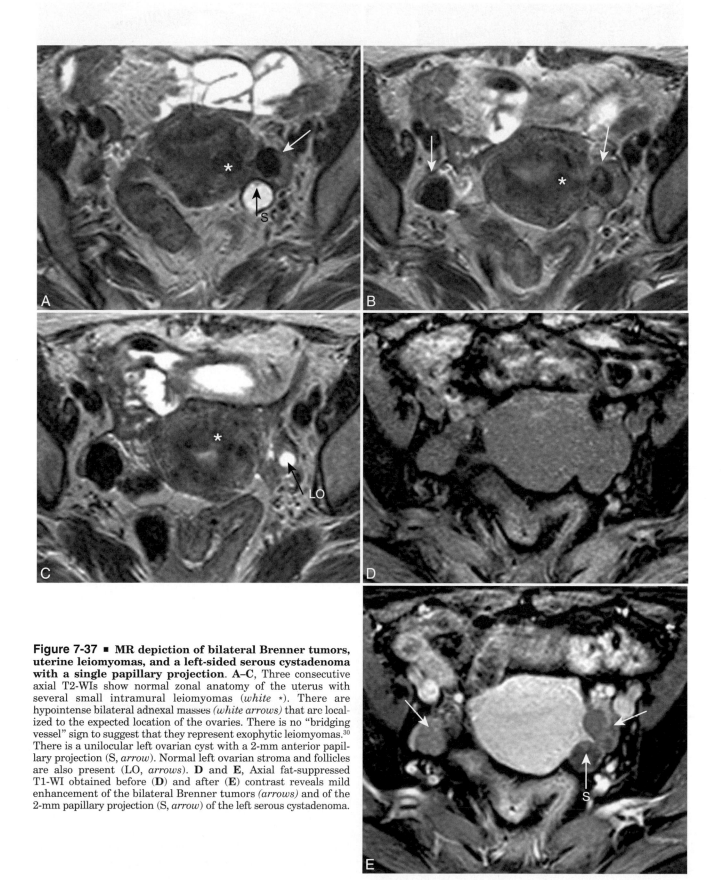

Figure 7-37 ▪ **MR depiction of bilateral Brenner tumors, uterine leiomyomas, and a left-sided serous cystadenoma with a single papillary projection. A–C,** Three consecutive axial T2-WIs show normal zonal anatomy of the uterus with several small intramural leiomyomas *(white ✱)*. There are hypointense bilateral adnexal masses *(white arrows)* that are localized to the expected location of the ovaries. There is no "bridging vessel" sign to suggest that they represent exophytic leiomyomas.[30] There is a unilocular left ovarian cyst with a 2-mm anterior papillary projection (S, *arrow*). Normal left ovarian stroma and follicles are also present (LO, *arrows*). **D** and **E,** Axial fat-suppressed T1-WI obtained before (**D**) and after (**E**) contrast reveals mild enhancement of the bilateral Brenner tumors *(arrows)* and of the 2-mm papillary projection (S, *arrow*) of the left serous cystadenoma.

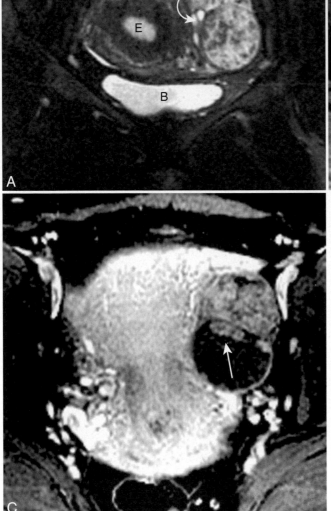

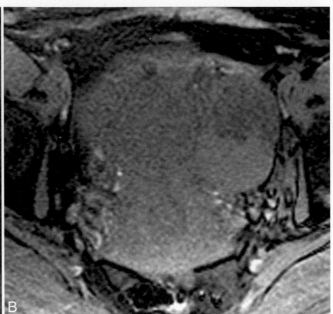

Figure 7-38 ■ MR depiction of multiple papillary projections and solid enhancing tissue within a left-sided serous papillary ovarian neoplasm of low malignant potential. **A**, Coronal fat-suppressed T2-WI reveals a left adnexal mass *(arrow)* with both low and intermediate-high SI components. The low SI foci represent the central fibrous tissue within papillary projections, and the high SI tissue reflects surrounding glandular elements. Portions of the remaining uninvolved left ovary are present medially *(curved arrow)*. Normal zonal anatomy of the uterus is present. (E = endometrium, B = bladder.) **B** and **C**, Axial fat-suppressed T1-WIs obtained before (**B**) and after (**C**) contrast reveals enhancement within the anterior aspect of the mass and within papillary projections *(arrow)* of a cystic posterior component of the mass.

7-11 Classification of Ovarian Cystic Epithelial Neoplasms

	Serous	*Mucinous*
% Benign (B) neoplasms	25%	20%
% Malignant (M) neoplasms	50%	10%
Proportion malignant	63% B, 30% M	73% B, 11% border, 16% M
CA-125	High association	Less reliable (<70% sensitive)
Size	Smaller	Larger
Wall	Thin walled, unilocular	Multilocular
Contour	Irregular/lobular	Smooth
SI	Homogenous	Heterogenous
Papillary projections	Common	Uncommon
Bilateral	Often	Rare
Carcinomatosis	More common	Less common

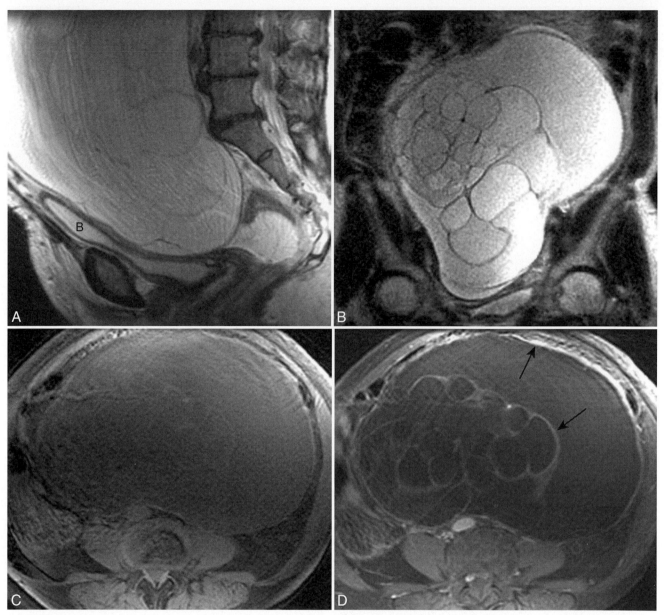

Figure 7-39 ■ **Benign, 22-cm ovarian mucinous cystadenoma as revealed on MR. Size is not an accurate predictor of malignancy of mucinous ovarian tumors.** **A** and **B**, Sagittal (**A**) and coronal (**B**) T2-WIs reveal a multiloculated pelvic mass that displaces the bladder (B) anteriorly and extends into the abdomen. All the cysts do not have the SI of simple fluid. Variable, mild T2-shortening is secondary to variation in mucin content. The uterus is surgically absent. **C** and **D**, Axial fat-suppressed T1-WIs obtained through the superior portion of the mass both before (**C**) and after (**D**) contrast reveals mild enhancement of the cyst wall and of the internal septa *(arrows)*. The large size, lack of papillary projections, and varying T2 SI all suggest a mucinous epithelial ovarian neoplasm.

ovarian neoplasms, which occur in middle-aged to older women, germ cell neoplasms are more common in younger women and are the most common ovarian neoplasm in adolescent girls and pregnant women.[351]

Mature cystic teratoma. Ninety-five percent of ovarian teratomas are benign mature cystic teratomas ("dermoid cysts") that contain a variable combination of mature mesodermal, endodermal, and ectodermal tissues. The median age at presentation is 30 years, the median tumor size is 6 cm, and teratomas are

bilateral in approximately 10%.[352] Most women with mature teratomas are asymptomatic. In symptomatic women, the most common presenting symptom is vague abdominal pain. Torsion is present in 3% to 11% of lesions and is more common is symptomatic, larger lesions.[352-354] The larger size of the tumor may be either or a contributing cause to or a consequence of the torsion. Malignant degeneration is rare and is present in less than 1% of mature cystic teratomas,[353] typically develops in older women, and is

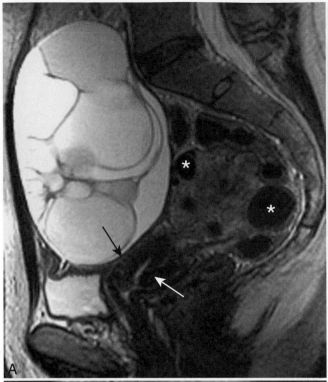

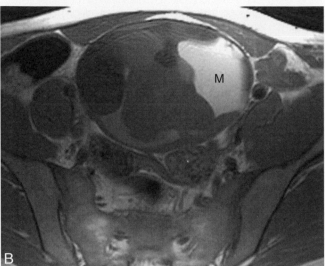

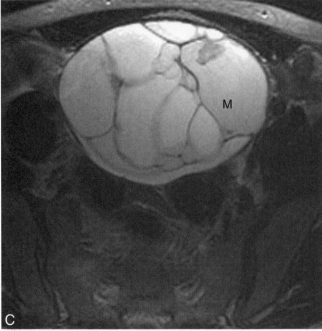

Figure 7-40 ■ **MR illustration of a benign mucinous cystadenoma and uterine leiomyomas. A,** Sagittal T2-WI reveals a multiloculated pelvic mass with cyst contents that vary from intermediate to high SI. Multiple, well-circumscribed, hypointense uterine leiomyomas are present (∗). Prominent hypointense inner fibrous cervical stroma *(arrows)* is considered within normal limits. **B** and **C,** Axial T1-WI (**B**) and T2-WI (**C**) obtained through the central portion of the lesion show variable T1- and T2-shortening of the loculi, which contain viscous mucin (**M**). No papillary projections or enhancing solid components were present on other sequences.

usually secondary to the development of a squamous cell carcinoma.[355,356]

The treatment of choice for mature teratoma is laparoscopic removal.[357-359] Surgical removal prevents the complications of torsion and malignant degeneration. When preserving fertility is desired, cystectomy can be performed and the remainder of the ovary preserved. While some spillage of the cyst contents may occur at the time of surgery, postoperative peritonitis is rarely reported. Some centers manage mature teratomas smaller than 6 cm with serial imaging as opposed to surgery.[360] Mature teratomas show no interval growth in postmenopausal women and average growth of 2 mm/yr in premenopausal women.

The hallmark for establishing the diagnosis of mature cystic teratoma is the presence of intratumoral fat or lipid, which is seen in approximately 95% of lesions.[361-363] In vivo, the cyst contents are in liquid form, so fat-fluid and fat-fat levels may be present. There are three techniques for characterizing the presence of fat or lipid within mature cystic teratomas.[355] Performing a T1-W sequence both with and without fat suppression is the method of choice for establishing the presence of adipose tissue within a mature cystic teratoma and distinguishing a teratoma from other adnexal lesions that have high SI on T1-WIs, namely, endometriosis and hemorrhagic functional cysts (Fig. 7-41).[364-367] Identification of a chemical shift artifact in the frequency encoding direction within an adnexal cyst indicates the presence of a fat-water interface and thus establishes diagnosis of a mature cystic teratoma.[363] This MRI feature of fat is of particular importance on low-field systems where chemically selective fat suppression cannot be performed. While short tau inversion recovery (STIR) sequences do suppress fat on low-field systems, other tissues with similar shortened T1 (such as hemorrhage) may also be hypointense on STIR images, and therefore one cannot rely on STIR images alone to establish a tissue diagnosis of fat (Fig. 7-42).[368]

Some mature cystic teratomas will not contain enough fat that a definitive diagnosis can be established with the use of fat suppression sequences or by detection of a chemical shift artifact. Use of in-phase and opposed-phase chemical shift sequences may allow detection of small amounts of fat that are contained within voxels that also contain nonfatty tissue (Fig. 7-43). The appearance of ovarian torsion is discussed below in a later section.

An uncommon subset of mature teratomas is the monodermal teratoma, which is composed of primarily one tissue subtype. These tumors include ovarian carcinoid and struma ovarii.[355] A suggestive MRI feature of struma ovarii is that of an ovarian mass with cysts of varying T2 SI reflecting the varying

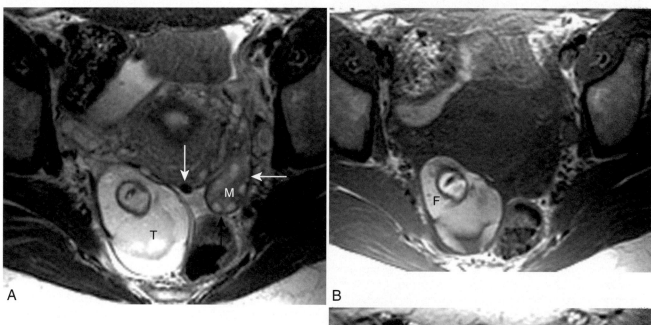

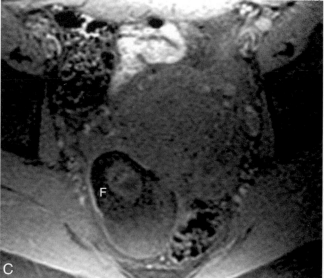

Figure 7-41 ▪ MR findings of a fat-containing mature cystic teratoma of the right ovary, a normal left ovary, and an exophytic leiomyoma. A, Axial T2-WI shows a heterogenous right adnexal mass (T) with low, intermediate, and high SI components. The central lower SI portion of the mass was calcified cartilage on pathologic studies. A normal left ovary is present with high SI follicles, low-to-intermediate SI ovarian medulla (M), and very low SI ovarian cortex *(horizontal arrow).* An exophytic, subserosal, low SI, 6-mm leiomyoma is depicted within the posterior uterus *(vertical arrow).* **B** and **C,** Axial T1-WI **(B)** and fat-suppressed T1-WI **(C)** show intermediate-to-high SI components in **B** that lose SI in **C** and thus establish the presence of macroscopic fat (F).

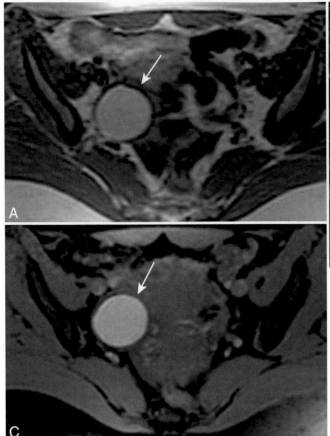

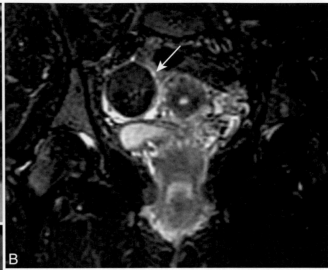

Figure 7-42 ▪ Absence of signal intensity on short tau inversion recovery (STIR) imaging is not specific for fat. MR illustration of a right ovarian endometrioma that shows low SI on STIR imaging. **A**, Axial T1-WI shows a hyperintense right adnexal mass *(arrow)*. **B**, Coronal STIR image shows that the mass is markedly hypointense *(arrow)*. **C**, Axial fat-suppressed T1-WI shows persistent hyperintensity within the lesion *(arrow)*, consistent with protein or hemorrhage. Some proteinaceous or hemorrhagic lesions can also be of very low SI on STIR images if the degree of T1 shortening is similar to that of fat.

concentrations of colloid within the ovarian cystic nodules.[369-372] A preoperative diagnosis can be confirmed with nuclear scintigraphy if necessary.[373]

Immature teratoma. Immature teratomas are uncommon malignant ovarian neoplasms that comprise less than 1% of ovarian germ cell tumors.[309,350,355] Immature and embryonic tissue from all three cell lines may be present within immature teratomas, and primitive neuroectodermal tissue is the most common malignant tissue subtype.[350] Compared with mature teratomas, immature teratomas on average are larger, occur in younger women (in the first three decades of life), and show more solid components on imaging.[355,374] Revealing the presence of small amounts of fat within an aggressive ovarian mass can suggest the diagnosis of malignant immature teratoma (Fig. 7-44).

Dysgerminoma. Dysgerminoma is the female equivalent of a testicular seminoma. While uncommon, dysgerminoma is the most frequently encountered malignant germ cell neoplasm in women below age 20 years.[375] Pure dysgerminomas do not result in elevated levels of human chorionic gonadotrophin (hCG) or α-fetoprotein (AFP). Suggestive imaging findings of dysgerminoma are those of a large, multilobulated solid mass with enhancing internal septa

in a young woman.[376,377] Since two thirds of women with dysgerminomas are found to have stage I disease at surgery, conservative treatment with oophorectomy with or without postsurgical chemotherapy should be considered, especially when preserving fertility is a goal.[378]

Endodermal sinus tumor (yolk sac tumor). Endodermal sinus tumor (yolk sac tumor) is another uncommon, solid, malignant germ cell neoplasm that occurs in young women. Imaging features of endodermal sinus tumor are not specific. Suggestive MRI findings include a large solid mass in a young woman with regions of intratumoral cyst formation and/or intratumoral flow voids secondary to necrosis and prominent tumor vessels, respectively.[379,380] A diagnosis of endodermal sinus tumor can be confirmed prior to surgery by detecting elevated levels of serum AFP. Serial serum AFP measurements can be used to follow treatment.[381] Women with endodermal sinus tumors are treated with surgery and cisplatin-based chemotherapy. Those women who do not respond to chemotherapy have a poor outcome, and none survive beyond 3 years.[382]

Other malignant germ cell tumors. Embryonal cell carcinoma and mixed malignant germ cell tumors are the female counterparts of identically named

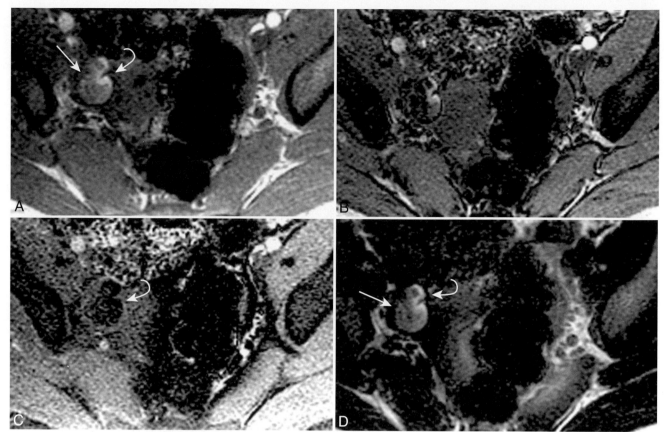

Figure 7-43 ▪ The use of chemical shift imaging to detect the presence of intratumoral lipid within a mature cystic teratoma. A, In-phase T1-WI shows the presence of both intermediate and high SI components within a right adnexal mass *(arrow)*. The high SI region has a C-shaped configuration *(curved arrow)*. **B,** Opposed-phase T1-WI reveals loss of SI within the components of the mass that had intermediate SI in **A**. The tissue within these voxels contained both lipid and water. Some mature teratomas may have a paucity of macroscopic fat; opposed-phase chemical shift imaging is ideal for detecting and characterizing the presence of intratumoral lipid. **C,** Fat-suppressed, opposed-phase T1-WI shows optimal suppression of the C-shaped focus of macroscopic fat *(curved arrow)* and partial suppression of the remainder of the teratoma. **D,** Water-suppressed T1-WI reveals markedly hyperintense macroscopic fat *(curved arrow)* and intermediate SI tissue *(arrow)* that contains both lipid and nonlipid components.

testicular neoplasms. However, they are much less frequently found in women. Primary ovarian choriocarcinoma is extremely rare. Metastatic choriocarcinoma from the uterus and choriocarcinoma derived from an occult ectopic pregnancy are more commonly encountered. Independently of its origin, a diagnosis of choriocarcinoma can be confirmed by elevated serum hCG levels. None of these less common malignant germ cell neoplasms have diagnostic imaging features. However, malignant germ cell tumor should be considered when imaging reveals an aggressive mass in a girl or young woman.[350]

SEX CORD–STROMAL TUMORS

Ovarian tumors that are derived from the gonadal sex cords and mesenchymal cells of the embryonic gonads are terms ovarian sex cord stromal tumors. The five most common cell types in this group of neoplasms are granulosa cells, theca cells, fibroblasts, Sertoli cells, and Leydig cells. The three most common sex cord–stromal tumors are the granulosa cell tumor, ovarian fibrothecoma, and Sertoli-Leydig cell tumor. Unlike the epithelial cell tumors that present in older women and germ cell tumors that present in younger women, sex cord–stromal tumors occur in women of all ages. Sex cord–stromal tumors are the one subtype of ovarian neoplasm that can be hormonally active. Affected women can have with signs or symptoms of hormonal hypersecretion. Finally, women with sex cord–stromal tumors commonly have stage I disease at presentation and are often cured by surgery.

Granulosa Cell Tumor (GCT). Granulosa cell tumors (GCTs) are derived from the cells that surround developing ovarian follicles. GCTs are typically unilateral and solid and secrete estrogen. Pathologists distinguish between two subtypes of GCT based on the cell of origin: 95% are the adult form and 5% the juvenile subtype.[302] The adult GCT typically presents in women in their sixth decade and is the most common estrogen-secreting ovarian neoplasm. Women with GCTs thus commonly have postmenopausal bleeding or irregular bleeding. The excess estrogen

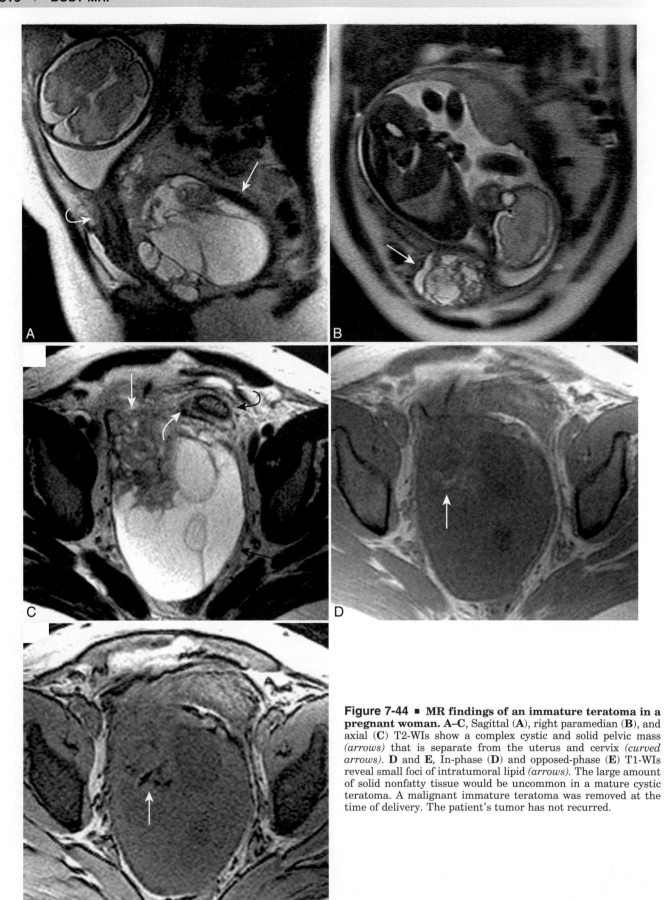

Figure 7-44 ■ **MR findings of an immature teratoma in a pregnant woman. A–C,** Sagittal (**A**), right paramedian (**B**), and axial (**C**) T2-WIs show a complex cystic and solid pelvic mass *(arrows)* that is separate from the uterus and cervix *(curved arrows)*. **D** and **E,** In-phase (**D**) and opposed-phase (**E**) T1-WIs reveal small foci of intratumoral lipid *(arrows)*. The large amount of solid nonfatty tissue would be uncommon in a mature cystic teratoma. A malignant immature teratoma was removed at the time of delivery. The patient's tumor has not recurred.

can also result in endometrial hyperplasia, endometrial polyps, or even endometrial carcinoma, the last of which can develop in up to 25% of women with GCT.[302,383-385] Prepubertal girls with either the juvenile or the adult subtype develop pseudoprecocious puberty ("pseudo" because they still have not ovulated).[386,387] GCTs are treated by surgical removal that is often curative; 90% of women have stage I disease at the time of surgery. However, GCTs can show malignant behavior, and examples of recurrent and metastatic disease have been reported years after "curative" surgeries.[388] Thus, treated women need to be followed clinically to ensure the absence of disease recurrence.

Juvenile and adult types of GCT have similar imaging features and are revealed as solid or cystic unilateral ovarian masses.[309,389,390] An insensitive but suggestive MRI feature of a GCT is the presence of intratumoral hemorrhagic cysts that are revealed as foci of T1-shortening within the mass (Fig. 7-45).[302,339,390,391] One insensitive but specific MRI pattern is that of a "sponge-like" appearance secondary to the interspersed solid and cystic portions of the tumor. Another imaging finding that can suggest a hypersecreting sex cord–stromal tumor is the presence of an abnormally thickened endometrium, reflecting the presence of hyperplasia, polyps, or endometrial carcinoma.

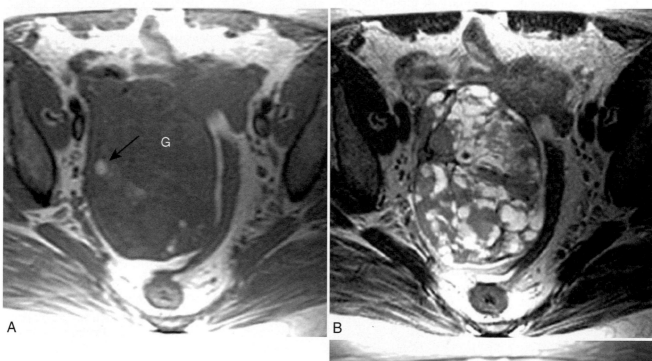

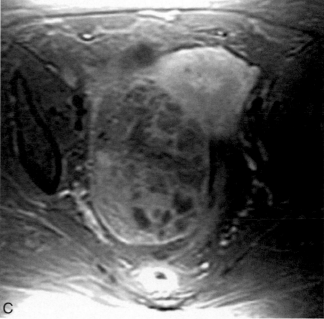

Figure 7-45 ▪ MR findings of a granulosa cell tumor of the right ovary in a 50-year-old woman. A, Axial T1-WI reveals a large right adnexal mass (G) with intratumoral hyperintense foci *(arrow)* that did not lose signal with fat suppression. **B,** Axial T2-WI shows the suggestive "sponge-like" appearance of granulosa tumors with high SI intratumoral cysts and lower SI solid tumoral components. **C,** CE fat-suppressed T1-WI reveals enhancement of the solid components of the tumor and persistent high SI of intratumoral hemorrhage. (Images courtesy of E. K. Outwater, University of Arizona, Tucson.)

Fibrothecoma/Fibroma. Fibrothecomas comprise approximately half of sex cord–stromal ovarian tumors and are composed of variable combinations of fibroblasts and theca cells. When the lesion is composed primarily of fibroblasts with paucity or absence of theca cells, it is termed an ovarian fibroma. Conversely, when theca cells predominate with minimal or absent fibroblasts, the tumor is categorized as a thecoma. Theca cells, like granulosa cells, are hormonally active, and women may have signs or symptoms of estrogen excess. Unlike granulosa cell tumors, fibrothecomas are benign and recurrent and metastatic disease is rare.

MRI can suggest a diagnosis of fibrothecoma. On T2-WI small fibrothecomas usually reveal homogeneous low SI (Fig. 7-46; larger fibrothecomas may have high SI components secondary to intratumoral edema, myxomatous change, or cyst formation.[392,393] A unilateral focal ovarian mass with relative low SI suggests a neoplasm of smooth muscle or fibrous origin[340,347,392] and has a differential diagnosis of fibroma, fibrothecoma, Brenner tumor (see above), and exophytic uterine leiomyoma. MR can readily differentiate an exophytic leiomyoma from an ovarian neoplasm by showing a separate ovary or revealing direct continuity of the mass with the uterus.[24] A thickened endometrium suggests estrogen production by the tumor and favors a diagnosis of fibrothecoma (Fig. 7-47). While it may not be possible to distinguish a fibroma from a Brenner tumor, the distinction is of little clinical import, since both are benign neoplasms that can be similarly cured with simple resection.

Sertoli-Leydig cell tumors. Sertoli-Leydig cell tumors account for approximately 0.5% of ovarian neoplasms and are not as common as fibrothecomas or granulosa cell tumors.[309,394] Sertoli-Leydig cell tumors are usually small and mostly solid and are detected in

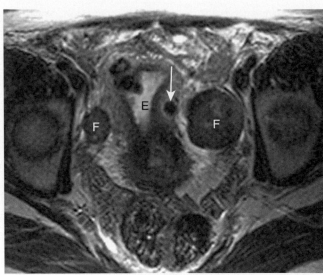

Figure 7-47 ■ MR depiction of bilateral ovarian fibrothecomas and endometrial hyperplasia in a postmenopausal woman who was not taking hormone replacement therapy. Axial T2-WI reveals bilateral low SI adnexal lesions (F) that are separate from the uterus. The uterus shows multiple benign leiomyomas, one of which has a high SI rim *(arrow)*. Thickening of the endometrial stripe (E) suggests that the fibrothecomas are functionally reactive.

younger women. Thirty percent of Sertoli-Leydig cell tumors are hypersecretory; this tumor is the most common ovarian neoplasm associated with virilization. Most lesions present with stage I disease and are cured by surgery. For this uncommon tumor, it is the clinical presentation that is more characteristic than the imaging features.

METASTATIC DISEASE TO THE OVARY

Metastatic disease to the ovary comprised approximately 20% of malignant ovarian masses in the Radiology Diagnostic Oncology Group[306] and in a series of 300 malignant ovarian masses in Japanese women.[395] When the primary tumor involves a signet cell adenocarcinoma of the gastrointestinal tract (typically the stomach), the ovarian metastases are referred to as a Krukenberg tumor.[396] Suggestive imaging features of metastatic disease include the presence of solid bilateral ovarian masses in which the shape of the ovary is preserved or has an ovoid configuration (Fig. 7-48).[396,397] Bilateral ovarian masses that show low SI components on T2-WI are suggestive MRI features.[397,398] The presence of a multilocular mass favors a primary ovarian tumor.[306]

Ovarian Torsion and Massive Ovarian Edema

Adnexal torsion results from the twisting of an ovary or a fallopian tube around its vascular pedicle, resulting in variable ischemia.[399] Untreated torsion can progress to ovarian infarction. Most women with ovarian torsion have an associated benign cystic ovarian neoplasm or enlarged functional cysts (e.g., from ovarian hyperstimulation).[400-403] Ovarian cancer

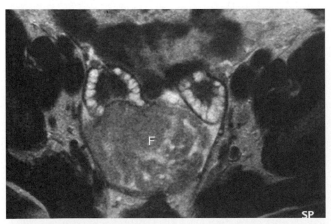

Figure 7-46 ■ MR appearance of polycystic ovaries and right-sided ovarian fibroma. Axial T2-WI shows enlarged ovaries with multiple peripherally located follicles and hypertrophied central stroma, in keeping with the MR findings of classic Stein-Leventhal syndrome. A solid 6-cm mass of the posterior right ovary (F) has intermediate SI between that of smooth muscle and ovarian follicles. The subjacent uterus was normal (not shown).

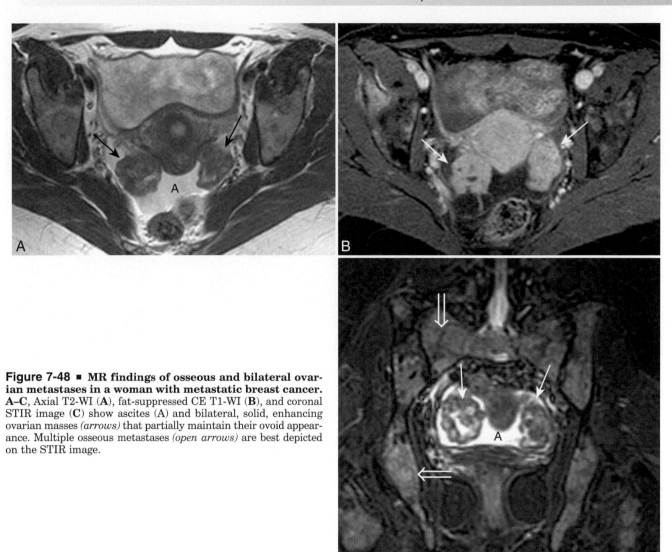

Figure 7-48 ■ MR findings of osseous and bilateral ovarian metastases in a woman with metastatic breast cancer. **A–C**, Axial T2-WI (**A**), fat-suppressed CE T1-WI (**B**), and coronal STIR image (**C**) show ascites (**A**) and bilateral, solid, enhancing ovarian masses *(arrows)* that partially maintain their ovoid appearance. Multiple osseous metastases *(open arrows)* are best depicted on the STIR image.

is rarely (<1%) the cause because associated inflammation and adhesions presumably keep the ovary from twisting.[351,400] The treatment of choice for ovarian torsion is laparoscopic untwisting of the adnexa and resection of any enlarged cysts. Ovaries can remain viable up to 36 hours after twisting, and thus oophorectomy can be avoided in most women.[400,404]

The MR findings of ovarian torsion are variable. A sensitive and specific finding on sonography is that of an enlarged ovary with peripheral 8- to 12-mm follicles.[405] Similar findings have been reported on MR.[406] Additional MRI findings include the presence of acute or subacute hemorrhage within the ovary (as revealed by variable T1 and low T2 SI) (Fig. 7-49), minimal or no contrast enhancement, and deviation of the uterus to the side of torsion.[399,406,407]

When an ovary twists but does not undergo hemorrhagic infarction, massive ovarian edema may result from lymphatic and venous outflow obstruction. Massive ovarian edema is an uncommon entity that typically presents in younger nulliparous women.[351]

Women can be asymptomatic or have pelvic pain and a palpable pelvic mass. On MR the affected ovary is enlarged (the size varies between 5 and 40 cm) with edematous stroma that shows low T1 and high T2 SI (Fig. 7-50).[408,409] Peripherally located ovarian follicles is a characteristic imaging feature and should suggest a diagnosis of either massive ovarian edema or torsion.[351,409,410] However, unlike for ovarian torsion, no high T1-WI hemorrhage should be present and the ovary should enhance after contrast. If massive ovarian edema can be diagnosed preoperatively, then orchiopexy can be performed instead of oophorectomy, since there is no underlying ovarian neoplasm.

Endometriosis

Endometriosis is the presence of endometrial glands and stroma outside the uterus. The etiology of endometriosis is hypothesized to be secondary to retrograde menstruation, which is more pronounced in women with disordered myometrial contractions.[411,412]

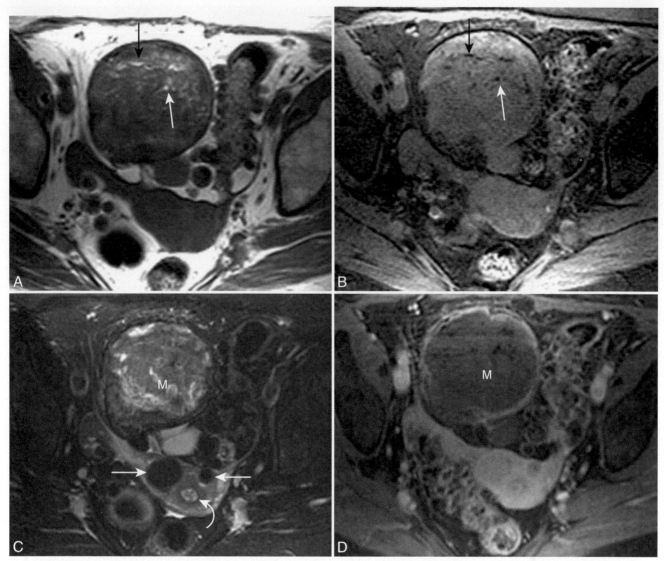

Figure 7-49 ■ **MR findings of chronic infarction of a twisted mature ovarian teratoma, uterine leiomyomas, and a benign endometrial polyp in a 74-year-old woman without acute symptoms. A,** Axial T1-WI shows a 7-cm, low-to-intermediate SI adnexal mass with small foci of high SI *(arrows)*. **B,** Fat-saturated T1-WI shows that the high SI foci in (**A**) lose SI *(arrows)*, thus establishing the presence of intratumoral fat. **C,** Fat-suppressed T2-WI shows low-to-intermediate SI within the mass (M), reflecting fibrosis and old hemorrhage. Two well-circumscribed myomas are present within the myometrium *(arrows)*. The endometrial canal is mildly prominent *(curved arrow)* and has heterogeneous intermediate-to-high SI tissue. It can be difficult to distinguish among endometrial hyperplasia, endometrial polyp, and localized endometrial carcinoma on MR. Tissue sampling established a diagnosis of endometrial polyp with cystic change. **D,** CE fat-suppressed T1-WI shows no enhancement of the infarcted teratoma (M) and mild enhancement of the leiomyomas and endometrial polyp.

Retrograde menstruation alone is not sufficient to result in endometriosis, since only 10% of women with retrograde menstruation develop the disorder.[413] Impaired clearing of endometrial cells from the peritoneal cavity secondary to alterations in the immune system or local peritoneal factors are other risk factors for endometriosis.[414,415] Menstrual factors that place women at risk include dysmenorrhea, early menarche, and short menstrual cycles. Nulliparity can be either a consequence or a contributing cause of endometriosis. Pregnancy lowers the incidence of endometriosis for at least two reasons. The dilation of

the cervix that occurs with labor fosters subsequent antegrade menstruation.[416] With each term pregnancy, a woman stops menstruating for at least 9 months, thus temporarily halting the cycle of retrograde menstruation.

The prevalence of endometriosis in all women is estimated to be 5% to 10%.[417,418] The most common symptoms of endometriosis are dysmenorrhea and pelvic pain. Endometriosis is responsible for 15% to 60% of pelvic pain in women.[419,420] Endometriosis is a common cause of infertility. Approximately 20% of infertile women have endometriosis, and 30% to 50%

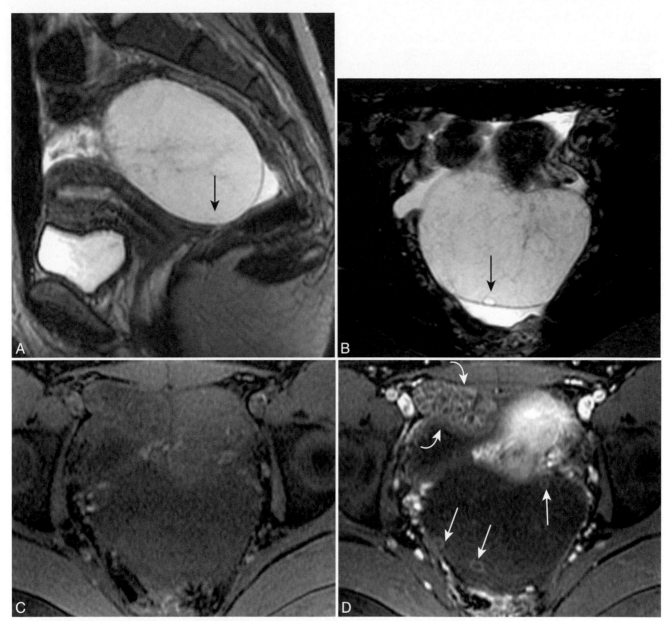

Figure 7-50 ■ **MR findings of massive ovarian edema in a 27-year-old woman. A** and **B**, Sagittal (**A**) and axial (**B**) T2-WIs show a markedly enlarged left ovary that has high SI centrally in keeping with edema. Ovarian follicles *(arrows)* are present along the periphery of the mass, establishing it as ovarian in origin. **C** and **D**, Fat-suppressed T1-WIs obtained before (**C**) and after (**D**) contrast reveal follicular enhancement both within the enlarged left ovary *(arrows)* and within the right ovary *(curved arrows)*.

of women with endometriosis have some degree of infertility.[417,421] The severity of endometriosis does not correlate with degree of pain but does correlate with infertility.

The goals of therapy are to minimize pain and restore fertility. Both medical and surgical therapies are successful in treating the pain associated with endometriosis.[422] No well-performed studies that compare surgical versus medical treatment have been made to date. Some women have a hysterectomy to control pain that is refractory to medical and laparoscopic therapy. Endometriosis is the leading cause for hysterectomy in the U. S.[419] Medical therapy

does not improve fertility in women with endometriosis; however, surgical removal of adhesions and obstructive masses can restore fertility.[422,423]

More than half of women with endometriosis have involvement of the ovaries and the cul-de-sac.[421,424] Approximately one-third of women have involvement of the posterior pelvic wall and the uterosacral ligaments. Less common sites of involvement include the ureter, bladder, sigmoid serosa, and within scars from cesarean sections. The last site is not secondary to retrograde menstruation but from direct implantation of endometrial tissue at the time of surgery.[425,426]

MR Findings of Endometriosis

The MR findings of endometriosis include endometriomas, solid fibrotic masses, and hydrosalpinges.[427] Endometriomas are hemorrhagic/proteinaceous cysts that most commonly occur in the ovary. MR can detect and characterize endometriomas with high accuracy and provide a "road map" for therapeutic laparoscopy.[428] Small endometrial implants and adhesions are two manifestations of endometriosis that are poorly shown by MRI[429] and are more clearly revealed at laparoscopy.[430] MR has only 75% sensitivity for mild endometriosis.[431]

The "chocolate" appearance of an endometrioma on direct inspection is secondary to prior episodes of intracystic bleeding from functional endometrial glands that are present within the cyst wall. The MR findings of ovarian endometriomas are often characteristic. On T1-WIs, endometriomas have increased SI relative to muscle (Figs. 7-51 and 7-52; see Fig. 7-42).

The T1-shortening of the cyst content is secondary to methemoglobin in subacute hemorrhage or the effects of concentrated protein. The capacity to depict the high SI foci within ovarian endometriomas is facilitated by fat suppression. By eliminating the SI present in normal fat, fat-suppressed T1-WI has an improved dynamic range and increased sensitivity for revealing endometriomas[432,433] (see Figs. 7-42, 7-51, and 7-52) and distinguishes endometriomas from fat-containing dermoid cysts of the ovaries (see Figs. 7-41 and 7-43).[434] On T2-WI, endometriomas may reveal lower SI than normal cyst fluid. This process, termed shading, reflects the decrease in free water content of the cyst secondary to hemorrhage or proteinaceous content.[435] Endometriomas that do not decrease in size with hormonal therapy are more likely to reveal shading than do other endometrial cysts.[436]

A single ovarian cyst that reveals high SI on T1 WI (both with and without fat suppression)

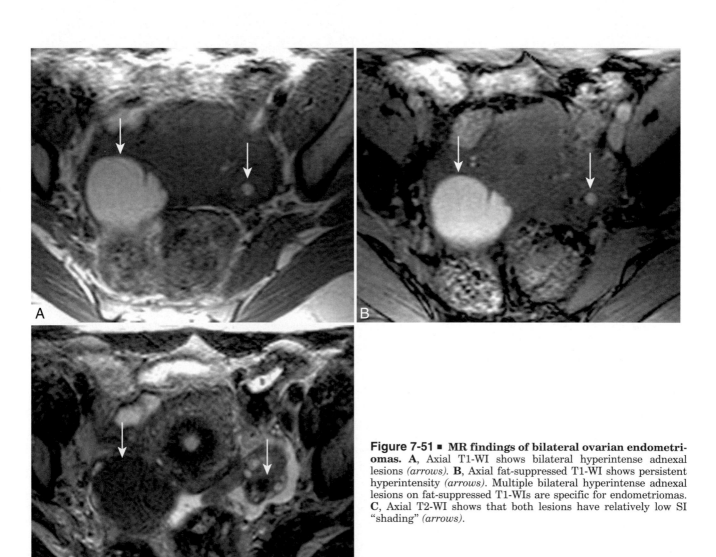

Figure 7-51 ■ **MR findings of bilateral ovarian endometriomas. A,** Axial T1-WI shows bilateral hyperintense adnexal lesions *(arrows)*. **B,** Axial fat-suppressed T1-WI shows persistent hyperintensity *(arrows)*. Multiple bilateral hyperintense adnexal lesions on fat-suppressed T1-WIs are specific for endometriomas. **C,** Axial T2-WI shows that both lesions have relatively low SI "shading" *(arrows)*.

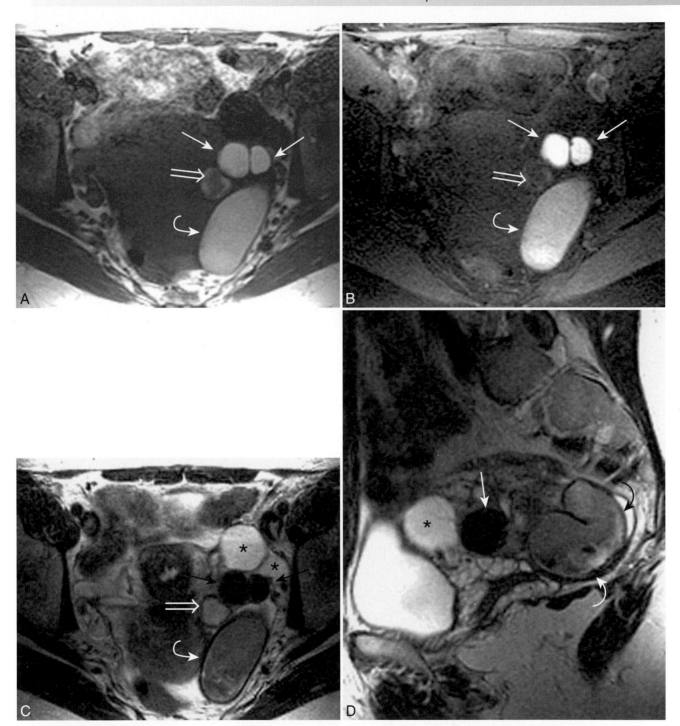

Figure 7-52 ■ MR findings of ovarian endometriomas, functional ovarian cyst, and left-sided hemato-salpinx in a woman with prior right oophorectomy for endometriosis. A, Axial T1-WI shows two hyperintense anterior adnexal lesions *(arrows),* a hyperintense segment of fallopian tube posteriorly *(curved arrow),* and a minimally hyperintense lesion medially *(open arrow)* within the left ovary. **B,** Fat-suppressed T1-WI shows improved dynamic range such that it is easier to appreciate the differences in relative SI among the endometriomas *(arrows),* hematosalpinx *(curved arrow),* and functional cyst *(open arrow).* **C,** T2-WI shows the marked shading of the two endometriomas, moderate shading of the hematosalpinx, and minimal shading of the functional cyst. Two physiologic, simple cysts (*) are now revealed in the anterior portion of the left ovary. **D,** Sagittal T2-WI better depicts the tubular configuration of the hematosalpinx *(curved arrows).* One of the endometriomas *(arrow)* and an ovarian cyst (*) are also shown on this image.

and lower SI than simple fluid on T2-WI is not diagnostic of an endometrioma, since functional ovarian cysts can have similar SI findings.[437] Findings that add specificity for a diagnosis of endometrioma are the presence of multiple and bilateral ovarian lesions with high SI on T1-WI (independent of T2 SI),[438] extraovarian endometriotic cysts (which have similar imaging features to ovarian endometriomas), and other pelvic findings (discussed below).

Endometrial implants can form on both the serosal surface of the fallopian tube and the luminal mucosa. Scarring and adhesions can result in tubal blockage and secondary infertility.[263] MR can detect and characterize an adnexal mass as dilated fallopian tube (see Figs. 7-35 and 7-52).[439] The presence of hyperintensity within the tube on fat-suppressed T1-WIs suggests the presence of hemorrhagic or proteinaceous tubal content and increases the likelihood of endometriosis.[439]

Although MR is insensitive in the detection of small implants, larger, solid fibrotic masses of endometriosis can be revealed on MR.[440] Peritoneum-based solid lesions of endometriosis are composed of endometrial glands and stroma with a large amount of fibrotic tissue and appear as poorly marginated hypointense masses of low SI on both T1- and T2-WIs. The low SI on T2-WIs reflects intralesional mature fibrosis (Figs. 7-53 and 7-54). Some solid masses of endometriosis have small foci of hyperintensity on T2-WIs, reflecting embedded endometrial glands (similar to adenomyosis) (see Fig. 7-54).[427] It is uncommon for these glands to reveal T1 hyperintense hemorrhage that often is present with ovarian endometriomas.

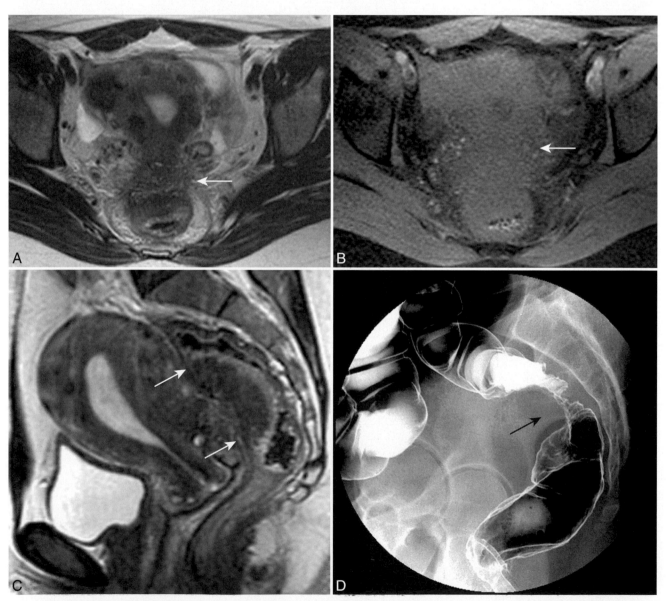

Figure 7-53 ■ **MR illustration of solid endometrial implants within the cul-de-sac that invade the anterior serosa of the sigmoid colon. A** and **B,** Axial T2-WI (**A**) and fat-suppressed T1-WI (**B**) show ill-defined, relatively low SI soft tissue within the cul-de-sac *(arrows)* that invades the anterior wall of the sigmoid. No T1 hyperintense foci of hemorrhagic ectopic endometrial glands are present. **C,** Sagittal T2-WI depicts the cephalocaudal extent of the cul-de-sac endometriosis *(arrows).* **D,** Lateral projection barium enema shows narrowing and tethering of a segment of sigmoid colon *(arrow)* secondary to extrinsic invasion by endometriosis.

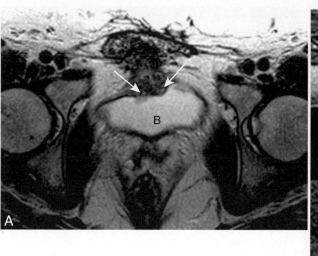

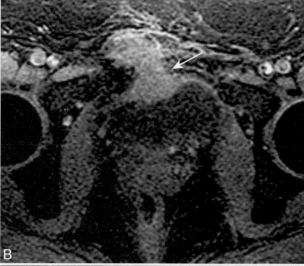

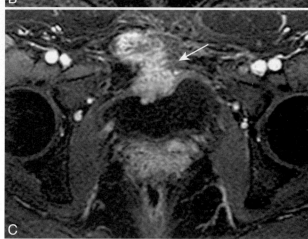

Figure 7-54 ▪ MR findings of solid endometriosis that invades both the rectus muscles and the anterior bladder wall in a woman with prior hysterectomy. A and **B**, Axial T2-WI (**A**) and fat-suppressed T1-WI (**B**) show a poorly marginated low SI mass (*arrow* in **B**). mass that extends from the anterior bladder to the posterior rectus muscles. Small foci of T2 hyperintensity represent intralesional glands (*arrows* in **A**). **C**, Fat-suppressed CE T1-WI shows moderate heterogenous enhancement of the lesion *(arrow)*. Solid endometriosis can have aggressive imaging features but often can be correctly characterized with appropriate clinical history.

Associated imaging findings include other manifestations of endometriosis including endometriomas or dilated fallopian tubes. Solid masses of endometriosis will enhance after contrast. Women with peritoneal spread of ovarian cancer may also have enhancing peritoneum-based lesions. However, these malignant implants usually have higher SI on T2-WIs, are multifocal, and often are associated with malignant ascites and an aggressive ovarian lesion.

Solid masses contained within an abdominal wall incision following cesarean section are a well-described subtype of solid endometriosis (see Fig. 7-54).[425,426] Women may have an abdominal wall mass that may show cyclical change in size or symptoms.[425] This subtype of endometriosis is likely secondary to direct implantation of endometrial glands and stroma at the time of cesarean section, as opposed to retrograde menstruation. Surgical removal is curative.

Another site of solid endometrial implants is the bladder. Endometriosis involves the urinary tract in 1% of affected women. The bladder is affected in 85% of women who have urinary tract involvement.[441] Bladder endometriosis may result from direct invasion of the posterior bladder wall from endometrial implants in the anterior cul-de-sac; women with anteflexed uteri and endometriosis are more likely to develop posterior bladder endometriosis.[442,443] Direct implantation of endometrial glands may occur after cesarean section. Most women with bladder endometriosis do not have catamenial hematuria, because the bladder mucosa is not involved. The MR appearance of bladder endometriosis is similar to that of scar endometriosis and solid masses of endometriosis located elsewhere in the peritoneum (see Fig. 7-54).[440,444] Symptomatic women are treated with surgery.[443]

Women with endometriosis are at risk of developing either the clear cell or endometrioid variants of ovarian carcinoma.[445] Women with endometriosis who develop these subtypes of ovarian cancer tend to have lower grade tumors at an earlier stage at presentation and survive longer than other women with ovarian cancer.[446] Why women with endometriosis are at risk for these two tumors is not understood. One hypothesis is that ovarian endometriosis deactivates a tumor suppression gene that promotes development of the clear cell and endometrioid subtypes of ovarian cancer.[447,448] Fortunately, malignant degeneration of ovarian endometriosis is rare, and the clear cell and endometrioid tumors can be differentiated from endometriosis on MRI by the presence of ascites and solid enhancing mural nodules.[449,450]

Polycystic Ovary Syndrome (PCOS), or Stein-Leventhal Syndrome

Polycystic ovary syndrome (PCOS; Box 7-12) is one of the most common endocrinopathies in women and affects approximately 5% of women of reproductive age.[451] There is no single definition of PCOS, but it is suggested on the basis of clinical, hormonal, and imaging features.[452] The signs and symptoms of obesity, hirsutism, oligomenorrhea/amenorrhea, and infertility clinically characterize PCOS. Women with PCOS show elevated LH/FSH ratios and hyperinsulinemia compared with normal women.[453] Most women with PCOS have insulin resistance; treating these women with insulin sensitizing agents can normalize their reproductive, metabolic, and endocrine function.[451,454,455]

The imaging features of polycystic ovaries include the presence of multiple peripheral ovarian follicles. More than 20% of women have polycystic ovaries on sonography, but only 10% of these women with have typical PCOS.[456] Similar lack of specificity has been shown on MRI.[5,457] In women with PCOS, increased number of peripheral follicles correlates with higher LH/FSH levels.[458] Imaging findings that are more specific for PCOS include the presence of ovarian enlargement and of stromal hypertrophy (see Figs. 7-22 and 7-46).[459] The ratio of ovarian stroma to ovarian area is the best predictor of PCOS by sonography.[460]

Nonovarian Causes of Adnexal Masses

PERITONEAL INCLUSION CYST (PIC)

Peritoneal fluid in premenopausal women is produced by normally functioning ovaries and is reabsorbed by the mesothelial cells of the peritoneal cavity.[461] A peritoneal inclusion cyst (PIC) represents an abnormal accumulation of pelvic peritoneal fluid that is not resorbed secondary to pelvic adhesions (Box 7-13).[462]

7-12　Polycystic Ovary Syndrome

- Epidemiology: 3% to 5% of women of reproductive age
- Etiology: Not known, ? insulin resistance
- Clinical findings: oligo-amenorrhea, infertility, obesity, and hirsutism
- Treatment goals: decrease insulin resistance, restore normal menses and/or fertility, decrease hirsutism, weight loss
- MR imaging findings
  Ovarian enlargement
  Multiple small peripherally based follicles
  Hypertrophied ovarian stroma

7-13　Peritoneal Inclusion Cyst

Etiology
Pelvic adhesions result in inability to reabsorb normal peritoneal fluid
Presents in premenopausal women after surgery

MR Findings
Loculated fluid that abuts or surrounds one or both ovaries
Ill-defined borders that include portions of the peritoneum
Do not confuse with a cystic ovarian tumor—the ovaries are normal

---

Fibrous adhesions and the mesothelial cells of the surrounding peritoneum line the PIC. PICs most commonly develop in premenopausal women who have pain or a palpable mass after pelvic surgery. Untreated PICs can grow secondary to continued cyclic fluid exudation by the ovary that is not resorbed.

On MRI a PIC appears as unilocular or multiloculated pelvic fluid collection that abuts and often surrounds one or both ovaries (Fig. 7-55). The average size range of a PIC is 10 to 12 cm.[463] The fluid content is most often simple but can be complex.[463,464] The borders of a PIC are defined by the pelvic peritoneal cavity, and there is not a well-defined cyst wall.[25] Some adhesions or portions of the vascularized mesothelium-lined wall of a PIC may have a nodular configuration and can enhance. However, the presence of a normal adjacent ovary should exclude a diagnosis of ovarian neoplasm.[463] A loculated cystic collection that surrounds an ovary in a menstruating woman who has had prior pelvic surgery should be considered a PIC. Symptomatic PICs can be treated with hormones to suppress ovarian function so that additional ovarian fluid is not secreted.[462,465] PICs that are resistant to hormonal therapy could be treated with transvaginal sonographic guided aspiration.[466]

PARATUBAL CYST

Paratubal (parovarian) cysts can originate from the paramesonephric ducts, mesonephric (Wolffian) ducts, or mesothelium-derived inclusion cysts.[25] Paratubal cysts can represent up to 10% of adnexal masses revealed on sonography.[25] The most common origin of a paratubal cyst is from the hydatid of Morgagni, a derivative of the paramesonephric ducts that is located in the broad ligament adjacent to the fimbrial end of the fallopian tube.[467] Paratubal cysts are not uncommon and account for 10% to 20% of all cystic adnexal lesions.[25,468] Most paratubal cysts are small and asymptomatic. Larger cysts may become complicated by torsion or internal hemorrhage.[469,470] On MRI, an uncomplicated paratubal cyst is revealed as a unilocular simple hypointense T1, hyperintense T2, nonenhancing lesion located adjacent to an ovary

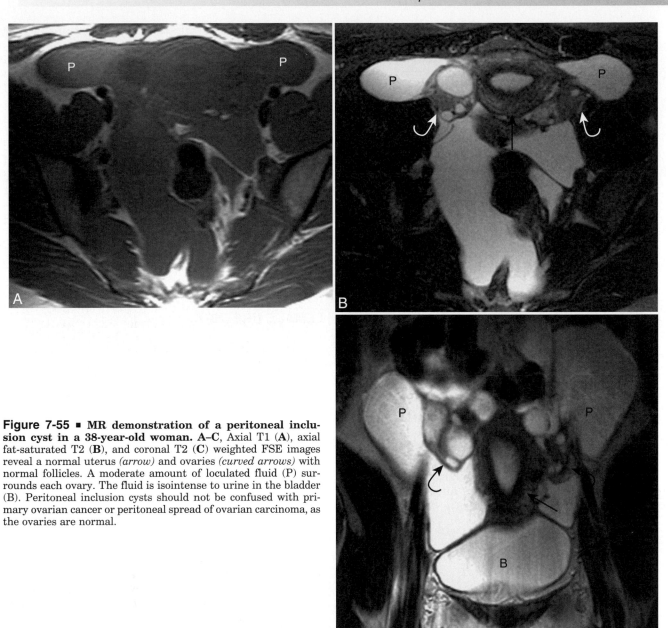

Figure 7-55 ■ **MR demonstration of a peritoneal inclusion cyst in a 38-year-old woman. A–C,** Axial T1 (**A**), axial fat-saturated T2 (**B**), and coronal T2 (**C**) weighted FSE images reveal a normal uterus *(arrow)* and ovaries *(curved arrows)* with normal follicles. A moderate amount of loculated fluid (P) surrounds each ovary. The fluid is isointense to urine in the bladder (B). Peritoneal inclusion cysts should not be confused with primary ovarian cancer or peritoneal spread of ovarian carcinoma, as the ovaries are normal.

within the broad ligament (Fig. 7-56).[471] By showing an adjacent normal ovary, one can exclude a primary ovarian neoplasm.[472] If a separate ipsilateral ovary cannot be revealed, it may be impossible to exclude the presence of a cystic ovarian neoplasm.[473]

TARLOV CYST

Perineural cysts can extend ventrally through the anterior sacral foramina and mimic an ovarian mass or parovarian mass on sonography.[474,475] MRI can readily show the communication of these multilocular cysts with the sacral foramina and thus establish the diagnosis (Fig. 7-57). Although usually asymptomatic, some Tarlov cysts that are larger than 1.5 cm

may result in sacral radiculopathy, which can be treated with cyst aspiration or excision.[476]

DILATED FALLOPIAN TUBE AND PELVIC INFLAMMATORY DISEASE (PID)

Pelvic inflammatory disease (PID) is a common condition in sexually active women. Most cases result from an ascending infection from the vagina and cervix to involve the endometrium,[477] fallopian tube, ovary, and/or remainder of the adnexa.[478,479] The two most common responsible infections are *Neisseria gonorrhoeae* and *Chlamydia trachomatis*. Affected women are given antibiotic therapy for acute disease and also to avoid potential complications of infertility

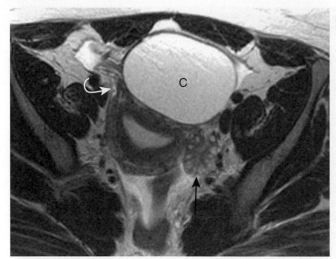

Figure 7-56 ■ **MR illustration of a paratubal cyst.** Axial T2-WI shows a normal uterus and left ovary *(arrow)*. There is a nonaggressive unilocular cyst (C) whose medial border abuts the right broad ligament *(curved arrow)*. Because of chronic pelvic pain, laparoscopy was performed and a right paratubal cyst was removed.

or ectopic pregnancy.[480] Laparoscopy can be performed at the onset of infection to confirm the diagnosis and obtain material for culture.[481] Imaging usually is not needed in women who have typical signs and symptoms. Women who have atypical clinical presentations or who do not respond to initial antibiotic therapy

may be imaged to evaluate for complications of PID or to exclude a neoplasm.

MRI findings of PID include tubo-ovarian abscess and dilated fallopian tube (Fig. 7-58).[5,482] The dilated fallopian tube usually is revealed as a typical C- or S-shaped tubular structure on one or more of the three orthogonal T2-W sequences.[267] When the fallopian tube folds on itself, the walls of the adjacent tubular segments form a false septum.[267] A specific finding for hydrosalpinx is the presence of mucosal folds that extend into the tubular lumen.[25,439] In the setting of acute PID, the presence of wall thickening and hyperemia suggest the presence of pyosalpinx.[25,483] A complicating pelvic abscess due to PID appears similar to abscesses elsewhere in the body. The central contents have high T2-SI (representing pus), and there is a thickened, irregularly enhancing wall.[484]

FEMALE URETHRA

Normal Urethral Anatomy

The normal female urethra is 3 to 4 cm in length. On T1-WI, there is poor distinction among the layers of the urethra. On T2-WI, the urethra reveals a zonal anatomy similar to that of the adjacent vagina (see Figs. 7-19, 7-22, and 7-29). Centrally, intraluminal urine/secretions are hyperintense. The subjacent mucosa shows low SI on T2-WI. The urethral submucosa is prominent and contains richly vascularized connective tissue and smooth muscle that is

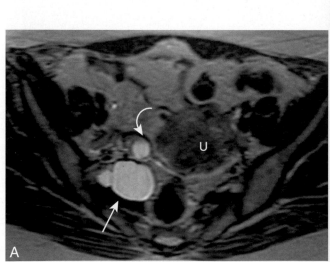

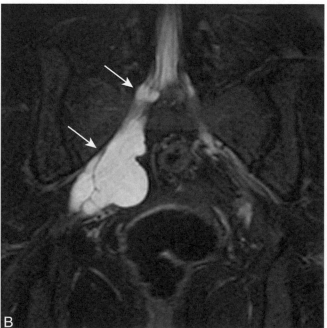

Figure 7-57 ■ **MR appearance of anteriorly located Tarlov cysts that mimicked a cystic ovarian neoplasm on an outside sonogram. A,** Axial T2-WI shows a multiloculated cystic mass of the right posterior pelvis *(arrow)*. The normal ovary is located anterior to the mass *(curved arrow)*. There is volume averaging through the top of the uterus (U). **B,** Coronal fat-saturated T2-WI shows that the cystic mass is continuous with the right S1 nerve root sleeve *(arrows)*.

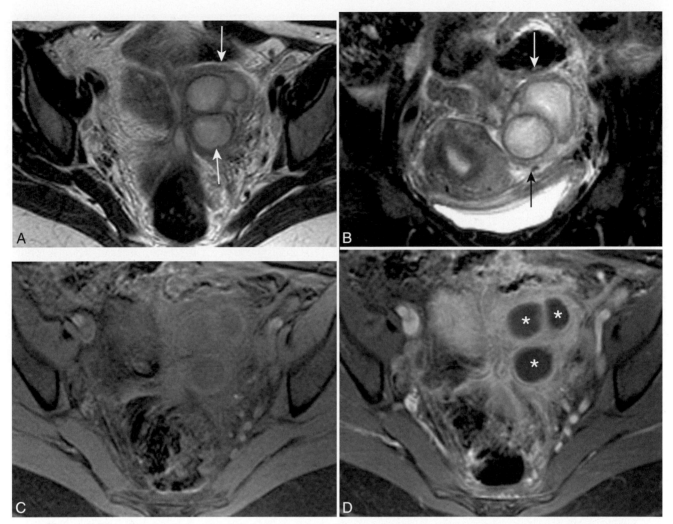

Figure 7-58 ■ **MR findings of pelvic inflammatory disease complicated by a pelvic abscess. A** and **B**, Axial (**A**) and fat-suppressed coronal (**B**) T2-WIs show a complex multiloculated left adnexal mass with thick walls *(arrows)*. Normal uterine zonal anatomy is revealed in **B**. **C** and **D**, CE fat-suppressed T1-WIs obtained before (**C**) and after (**D**) contrast show moderate enhancement of the walls of the abscess but no internal enhancement within three loculi (*) that had higher SI in **A**. Pus was drained from the left side of the pelvis subsequent to this MR.

depicted as high SI.[485] The outer muscle layer, which is composed of striated smooth muscle, shows low T2 SI. It functions to preserve urinary continence. MRI can show thinning of the outer muscularis in women with stress incontinence.[486] Endovaginal or endorectal coil imaging provides high resolution images of the urethra and periurethral soft tissues.[487-490] Endourethral coils have been developed that provide very high resolution urethral images[491]; however, the small field of view of the resultant images limits evaluation of the periurethral soft tissues.

Urethral Diverticula

Urethral diverticula occur more commonly in women than in men. Diverticula result from inflammatory obstruction of or trauma to the periurethral glands that subsequently ruptures into the urethral lumen.[492] The most common symptoms of urethral diverticula are pain, urinary incontinence, and dyspareunia. Because these symptoms are nonspecific, the diagnosis of urethral diverticula may go unrecognized. In a series of 46 consecutive women with symptomatic urethral diverticula, the mean time between onset of symptoms and diagnosis of the diverticulum was more than 5 years.[493] The most common location of a urethral diverticulum is the posterolateral aspect of the mid-urethra.[492] Symptomatic diverticula are best treated by direct excision.[493,494]

Because of its excellent soft tissue contrast and direct multiplanar imaging, high-resolution MR can accurately localize urethral diverticula (Fig. 7-59).[492,495-500] The cephalocaudal extent of a urethral diverticulum (including relationship to the

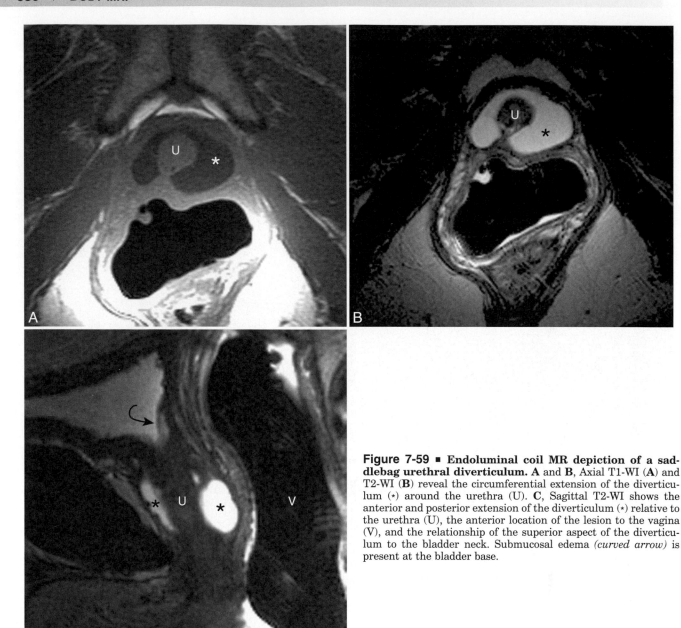

Figure 7-59 ▪ Endoluminal coil MR depiction of a saddlebag urethral diverticulum. A and **B,** Axial T1-WI (**A**) and T2-WI (**B**) reveal the circumferential extension of the diverticulum (*) around the urethra (U). **C,** Sagittal T2-WI shows the anterior and posterior extension of the diverticulum (*) relative to the urethra (U), the anterior location of the lesion to the vagina (V), and the relationship of the superior aspect of the diverticulum to the bladder neck. Submucosal edema *(curved arrow)* is present at the bladder base.

bladder base), degree of circumferential involvement around the urethra, and presence of a diverticular neck should be described to aid in guiding a potential surgical resection. Complications such as infection, calculi, or tumor formation within a diverticulum can also be revealed by MR.[488,501,502]

MRI occasionally is performed in women who have had diverticulectomy in order to evaluate response to therapy and exclude a recurrent diverticulum. The presence of fat within the urethrovaginal space is secondary to a Martius flap (labial fat interposed between urethra and vagina) and is a normal postprocedural finding (Fig. 7-60).[503]

Urethral Cancer

The most commonly encountered cancer of the urethra is direct extension of transitional cell carcinoma of the bladder. In women with bladder cancer who undergo cystectomy, the urethra can be left in situ provided there is no tumor of the bladder neck and that biopsy specimen of the proximal urethra at the time of surgery reveals no tumor.[504] Primary urethral cancers are rare. Squamous cell carcinoma is the most common subtype of the distal female urethra, while transitional cell and adenocarcinomas are more common in the proximal urethra. MR can localize

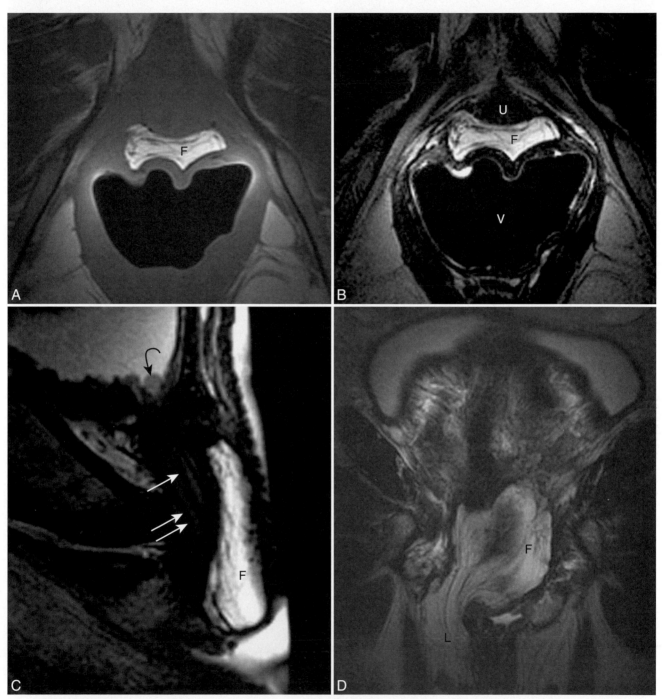

Figure 7-60 ▪ **MR illustration of transposed labial fat between the vagina and urethra in a woman after urethral diverticulectomy and Martius flap reconstruction. A** and **B,** Axial T1-WI (**A**) and T2-WI (**B**) show fatty tissue (F) between the vagina and urethra. No recurrent urethral diverticulum is present. **C,** Sagittal T2-WI shows the longitudinal extent of the interspersed fat (F). Normal urethral zonal anatomy is revealed, with low SI mucosa *(arrow)* and outer muscular layer *(double arrows).* Submucosal bladder edema is present *(curved arrow).* **D,** Coronal T2-WIs reveal the right labial (L) origin of the fat (F).

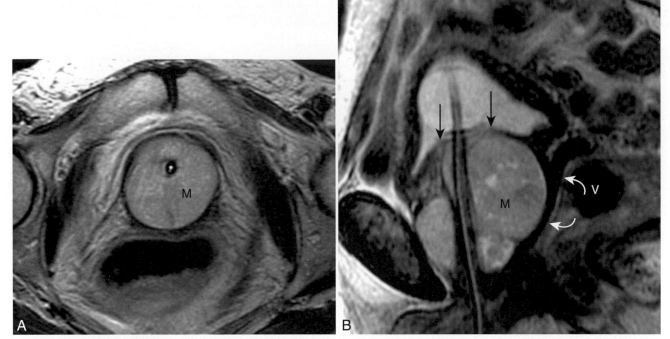

Figure 7-61 ■ **MR depiction of a primary transitional cell carcinoma of the urethra with invasion of the bladder base in a 76-year-old woman with hematuria and urinary retention. A** and **B,** Sagittal T2-WIs show a heterogeneous intermediate-to-high SI mass (M) that surrounds the Foley catheter. The vagina is displaced posteriorly (V, *curved arrows*). The detrusor muscle of the bladder base is attenuated *(arrows)* and poorly defined from below, suggesting secondary bladder invasion, which was confirmed by subsequent cystoscopic study.

a cancer to the urethra and serve to evaluate for adjacent organ invasion, pelvic adenopathy, and metastatic disease (Fig. 7-61). Patients with low-stage disease benefit from complete surgical resection, whereas those with advanced disease are treated with either radiation therapy alone[505] or combined chemotherapy and radiation therapy.[506]

In the differential diagnosis of solid urethral masses is periurethral collagen (Fig. 7-62).[507] Either surgery or periurethral collagen injections are

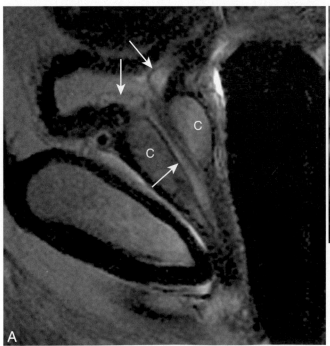

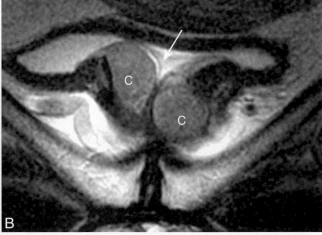

Figure 7-62 ■ **MR illustration of periurethral collagen and submucosal edema in a woman treated for urinary incontinence.** Without a history of prior periurethral injections, an infiltrative neoplasm would be difficult to exclude. **A** and **B,** Sagittal and coronal T2-WIs reveal circumscribed intermediate SI masses (C) that surround the urethra *(lower arrow).* Submucosal bladder edema is revealed as high SI between elevated mucosa *(arrows)* and detrusor muscle.

considered acceptable treatments for stress urinary incontinence.[508] Without an appropriate history, it may be impossible to distinguish periurethral collagen (or other synthetic or biological materials used to treated incontinence) from urethral neoplasm.[509]

REFERENCES

1. Chaudhry S, Reinhold C, Guermazi A, Khalili I, Maheshwari S. Benign and malignant diseases of the endometrium. Top Magn Reson Imaging 2003;14:339-357.
2. Nalaboff KM, Pellerito JS, Ben-Levi E. Imaging the endometrium: disease and normal variants. Radiographics 2001;21:1409-1424.
3. McCarthy S, Tauber C, Gore J. Female pelvic anatomy: MR assessment of variations during the menstrual cycle and with use of oral contraceptives. Radiology 1986;160:119-123.
4. Wiczyk HP, Janus CL, Richards CJ, et al. Comparison of magnetic resonance imaging and ultrasound in evaluating follicular and endometrial development throughout the normal cycle. Fertil Steril 1988;49:969-972.
5. Imaoka I, Wada A, Matsuo M, Yoshida M, Kitagaki H, Sugimura K. MR imaging of disorders associated with female infertility: use in diagnosis, treatment, and management. Radiographics 2003;23:1401-1421.
6. Fleischer AC. Sonographic assessment of endometrial disorders. Semin Ultrasound CT MR 1999;20:259-266.
7. Imaoka I, Sugimura K, Masui T, Takehara Y, Ichijo K, Naito M. Abnormal uterine cavity: differential diagnosis with MR imaging. Magn Reson Imaging 1999;17:1445-1455.
8. Brosens JJ, de Souza NM, Barker FG. Uterine junctional zone: function and disease. Lancet 1995;346:558-560.
9. Scoutt LM, Flynn SD, Luthringer DJ, McCauley TR, McCarthy SM. Junctional zone of the uterus: correlation of MR imaging and histologic examination of hysterectomy specimens. Radiology 1991;179:403-407.
10. Brown HK, Stoll BS, Nicosia SV, et al. Uterine junctional zone: correlation between histologic findings and MR imaging. Radiology 1991;179:409-413.
11. Togashi K, Nakai A, Sugimura K. Anatomy and physiology of the female pelvis: MR imaging revisited. J Magn Reson Imaging 2001;13:842-849.
12. McCarthy S, Scott G, Majumdar S, et al. Uterine junctional zone: MR study of water content and relaxation properties. Radiology 1989;171:241-243.
13. Mitchell DG, Schonholz L, Hilpert PL, Pennell RG, Blum L, Rifkin MD. Zones of the uterus: discrepancy between US and MR images. Radiology 1990;174:827-831.
14. Reinhold C, McCarthy S, Bret PM, et al. Diffuse adenomyosis: comparison of endovaginal US and MR imaging with histopathologic correlation. Radiology 1996;199:151-158.
15. Ascher SM, Jha RC, Reinhold C. Benign myometrial conditions: leiomyomas and adenomyosis. Top Magn Reson Imaging 2003;14:281-304.
16. Ozsarlak O, Schepens E, de Schepper AM, Deckers F, Parizel PM, Campo R. Transient uterine contraction mimicking adenomyosis on MRI. Eur Radiol 1998;8:54-56.
17. Togashi K, Kawakami S, Kimura I, et al. Uterine contractions: possible diagnostic pitfall at MR imaging. J Magn Reson Imaging 1993;3:889-893.
18. Togashi K, Kawakami S, Kimura I, et al. Sustained uterine contractions: a cause of hypointense myometrial bulging. Radiology 1993;187:707-710.
19. Lyons EA, Taylor PJ, Zheng XH, Ballard G, Levi CS, Kredentser JV. Characterization of subendometrial myometrial contractions throughout the menstrual cycle in normal fertile women. Fertil Steril 1991;55:771-774.
20. Masui T, Katayama M, Kobayashi S, et al. Changes in myometrial and junctional zone thickness and signal intensity: demonstration with kinematic T2-weighted MR imaging. Radiology 2001;221:75-85.
21. Masui T, Katayama M, Kobayashi S, Shimizu S, Nozaki A, Sakahara H. Pseudolesions related to uterine contraction: characterization with multiphase-multisection T2-weighted MR imaging. Radiology 2003;4:4.
22. Nakai A, Togashi K, Yamaoka T, et al. Uterine peristalsis shown on cine MR imaging using ultrafast sequence. J Magn Reson Imaging 2003;18:726-733.
23. Schwartz SM. Epidemiology of uterine leiomyomata. Clin Obstet Gynecol 2001;44:316-326.
24. Weinreb JC, Barkoff ND, Megibow A, Demopoulos R. The value of MR imaging in distinguishing leiomyomas from other solid pelvic masses when sonography is indeterminate. AJR Am J Roentgenol 1990;154:295-299.
25. Sala EJ, Atri M. Magnetic resonance imaging of benign adnexal disease. Top Magn Reson Imaging 2003;14:305-327.
26. Pritts EA. Fibroids and infertility: a systematic review of the evidence. Obstet Gynecol Surv 2001;56:483-491.
27. Murase E, Siegelman ES, Outwater EK, Perez-Jaffe LA, Tureck RW. Uterine leiomyomas: histopathologic features, MR imaging findings, differential diagnosis, and treatment. Radiographics 1999;19:1179-1197.
28. Mittl RL, Jr., Yeh IT, Kressel HY. High-signal-intensity rim surrounding uterine leiomyomas on MR images: pathologic correlation. Radiology 1991;180:81-83.
29. Togashi K, Ozasa H, Konishi I, et al. Enlarged uterus: differentiation between adenomyosis and leiomyoma with MR imaging. Radiology 1989;171:531-534.
30. Kim JC, Kim SS, Park JY. "Bridging vascular sign" in the MR diagnosis of exophytic uterine leiomyoma. J Comput Assist Tomogr 2000;24:57-60.
31. Dueholm M, Lundorf E, Hansen ES, Ledertoug S, Olesen F. Evaluation of the uterine cavity with magnetic resonance imaging, transvaginal sonography, hysterosonographic examination, and diagnostic hysteroscopy. Fertil Steril 2001;76:350-357.
32. Ueda H, Togashi K, Konishi I, et al. Unusual appearances of uterine leiomyomas: MR imaging findings and their histopathologic backgrounds. Radiographics 1999;19 Spec No:S131-145.
33. Yamashita Y, Torashima M, Takahashi M, et al. Hyperintense uterine leiomyoma at T2-weighted MR imaging: differentiation with dynamic enhanced MR imaging and clinical implications. Radiology 1993;189:721-725.
34. Kawakami S, Togashi K, Konishi I, et al. Red degeneration of uterine leiomyoma: MR appearance. J Comput Assist Tomogr 1994;18:925-928.
35. Avritscher R, Iyer RB, Ro J, Whitman G. Lipoleiomyoma of the uterus. AJR Am J Roentgenol 2001;177:856.
36. Prieto A, Crespo C, Pardo A, Docal I, Calzada J, Alonso P. Uterine lipoleiomyomas: US and CT findings. Abdom Imaging 2000;25:655-657.
37. Tsushima Y, Kita T, Yamamoto K. Uterine lipoleiomyoma: MRI, CT, and ultrasonographic findings. Br J Radiol 1997;70:1068-1070.
38. Ishigami K, Yoshimitsu K, Honda H, et al. Uterine lipoleiomyoma: MRI appearances. Abdom Imaging 1998;23:214-216.
39. Olive DL. Review of the evidence for treatment of leiomyomata. Environ Health Perspect 2000;108(Suppl 5):841-843.
40. Stewart EA. Uterine fibroids. Lancet 2001;357:293-298.
41. Schaffer JI, Word A. Hysterectomy—still a useful operation. N Engl J Med 2002;347:1360-1362.
42. Emanuel MH, Wamsteker K, Hart AA, Metz G, Lammes FB. Long-term results of hysteroscopic myomectomy for abnormal uterine bleeding. Obstet Gynecol 1999;93:743-748.
43. Fernandez H, Sefrioui O, Virelizier C, Gervaise A, Gomel V, Frydman R. Hysteroscopic resection of submucosal myomas in patients with infertility. Hum Reprod 2001;16:1489-1492.
44. Ubaldi F, Tournaye H, Camus M, Van der Pas H, Gepts E, Devroey P. Fertility after hysteroscopic myomectomy. Hum Reprod Update 1995;1:81-90.
45. Pinto I, Chimeno P, Romo A, et al. Uterine fibroids: uterine artery embolization versus abdominal hysterectomy for treatment: a prospective, randomized, and controlled clinical trial. Radiology 2003;226:425-431.
46. Helmberger TK, Jakobs TF, Reiser MF. Embolization of uterine fibroids. Abdom Imaging 2003;29.
47. Pron G, Cohen M, Soucie J, Garvin G, Vanderburgh L, Bell S. The Ontario Uterine Fibroid Embolization Trial. 1. Baseline patient characteristics, fibroid burden, and impact on life. Fertil Steril 2003;79:112-119.
48. Beinfeld MT, Bosch JL, Isaacson KB, Gazelle GS. Cost-effectiveness of uterine artery embolization and hysterectomy for uterine fibroids. Radiology 2004;230:207-213.
49. Subramanian S, Spies JB. Uterine artery embolization for leiomyomata: resource use and cost estimation. J Vasc Interv Radiol 2001;12:571-574.
50. Pelage JP, Le Dref O, Soyer P, et al. Fibroid-related menorrhagia: treatment with superselective embolization of the uterine arteries and midterm follow-up. Radiology 2000;215:428-431.
51. Pron G, Bennett J, Common A, Wall J, Asch M, Sniderman K. The Ontario Uterine Fibroid Embolization Trial. 2. Uterine fibroid reduction and symptom relief after uterine artery embolization for fibroids. Fertil Steril 2003;79:120-127.
52. Razavi MK, Hwang G, Jahed A, Modanloo S, Chen B. Abdominal myomectomy versus uterine fibroid embolization in the treatment of symptomatic uterine leiomyomas. AJR Am J Roentgenol 2003;180:1571-1575.
53. Spies JB, Benenati JF, Worthington-Kirsch RL, Pelage JP. Initial experience with use of tris-acryl gelatin microspheres for uterine artery embolization for leiomyomata. J Vasc Interv Radiol 2001;12:1059-1063.

54. Katsumori T, Nakajima K, Mihara T, Tokuhiro M. Uterine artery embolization using gelatin sponge particles alone for symptomatic uterine fibroids: midterm results. AJR Am J Roentgenol 2002;178:135-139.

55. Katsumori T, Nakajima K, Mihara T. Is a large fibroid a high-risk factor for uterine artery embolization? AJR Am J Roentgenol 2003;181:1309-1314.

56. Burn PR, McCall JM, Chinn RJ, Vashisht A, Smith JR, Healy JC. Uterine fibroleiomyoma: MR imaging appearances before and after embolization of uterine arteries. Radiology 2000;214:729-734.

57. deSouza NM, Williams AD. Uterine arterial embolization for leiomyomas: perfusion and volume changes at MR imaging and relation to clinical outcome. Radiology 2002;222:367-374.

58. Jha RC, Ascher SM, Imaoka I, Spies JB. Symptomatic fibroleiomyomata: MR imaging of the uterus before and after uterine arterial embolization. Radiology 2000;217:228-235.

59. Razavi MK, Wolanske KA, Hwang GL, Sze DY, Kee ST, Dake MD. Angiographic classification of ovarian artery-to-uterine artery anastomoses: initial observations in oterine fibroid embolization. Radiology 2002;224:707-712.

60. Binkert CA, Andrews RT, Kaufman JA. Utility of nonselective abdominal aortography in demonstrating ovarian artery collaterals in patients undergoing uterine artery embolization for fibroids. J Vasc Interv Radiol 2001;12:841-845.

61. Nikolic B, Spies JB, Abbara S, Goodwin SC. Ovarian artery supply of uterine fibroids as a cause of treatment failure after uterine artery embolization: a case report. J Vasc Interv Radiol 1999;10:1167-1170.

62. Payne JF, Robboy SJ, Haney AF. Embolic microspheres within ovarian arterial vasculature after uterine artery embolization. Obstet Gynecol 2002;100:883-886.

63. Chrisman HB, Saker MB, Ryu RK, et al. The impact of uterine fibroid embolization on resumption of menses and ovarian function. J Vasc Interv Radiol 2000;11:699-703.

64. Ravina JH, Aymard A, Ciraru-Vigneron N, Clerissi J, Merland JJ. [Uterine fibroids embolization: results about 454 cases.] Gynecol Obstet Fertil 2003;31:597-605.

65. Ravina JH, Vigneron NC, Aymard A, Le Dref O, Merland JJ. Pregnancy after embolization of uterine myoma: report of 12 cases. Fertil Steril 2000;73:1241-1243.

66. Colgan TJ, Pron G, Mocarski EJ, Bennett JD, Asch MR, Common A. Pathologic features of uteri and leiomyomas following uterine artery embolization for leiomyomas. Am J Surg Pathol 2003;27:167-177.

67. Banovac F, Ascher SM, Jones DA, Black MD, Smith JC, Spies JB. Magnetic resonance imaging outcome after uterine artery embolization for leiomyomata with use of tris-acryl gelatin microspheres. J Vasc Interv Radiol 2002;13:681-688.

68. deSouza NM, Williams AD. Uterine arterial embolization for leiomyomas: perfusion and volume changes at MR imaging and relation to clinical outcome. Radiology 2002;222:367-374.

69. Azziz R. Adenomyosis: current perspectives. Obstet Gynecol Clin North Am 1989;16:221-235.

70. Reinhold C, Tafazoli F, Mehio A, et al. Uterine adenomyosis: endovaginal US and MR imaging features with histopathologic correlation. Radiographics 1999;19(Spec No.):S147-160.

71. Curtis KM, Hillis SD, Marchbanks PA, Peterson HB. Disruption of the endometrial-myometrial border during pregnancy as a risk factor for adenomyosis. Am J Obstet Gynecol 2002;187:543-544.

72. Ferenczy A. Pathophysiology of adenomyosis. Hum Reprod Update 1998;4:312-322.

73. Levgur M, Abadi MA, Tucker A. Adenomyosis: symptoms, histology, and pregnancy terminations. Obstet Gynecol 2000;95:688-691.

74. Kido A, Togashi K, Koyama T, Yamaoka T, Fujiwara T, Fujii S. Diffusely enlarged uterus: evaluation with MR imaging. Radiographics 2003;23:1423-1439.

75. Outwater EK, Siegelman ES, Van Deerlin V. Adenomyosis: current concepts and imaging considerations. AJR Am J Roentgenol 1998;170:437-441.

76. Ascher SM, Arnold LL, Patt RH, et al. Adenomyosis: prospective comparison of MR imaging and transvaginal sonography. Radiology 1994;190:803-806.

77. Dueholm M, Lundorf E, Hansen ES, Sorensen JS, Ledertoug S, Olesen F. Magnetic resonance imaging and transvaginal ultrasonography for the diagnosis of adenomyosis. Fertil Steril 2001;76:588-594.

78. Bazot M, Cortez A, Darai E, et al. Ultrasonography compared with magnetic resonance imaging for the diagnosis of adenomyosis: correlation with histopathology. Hum Reprod 2001;16:2427-2433.

79. Fong K, Causer P, Atri M, Lytwyn A, Kung R. Transvaginal US and hysterosonography in postmenopausal women with breast cancer receiving tamoxifen: correlation with hysteroscopy and pathologic study. Radiographics 2003;23:137-150; discussion 151-155.

80. Imaoka I, Ascher SM, Sugimura K, et al. MR imaging of diffuse adenomyosis changes after GnRH analog therapy. J Magn Reson Imaging 2002;15:285-290.

81. Wood C. Surgical and medical treatment of adenomyosis. Hum Reprod Update 1998;4:323-336.

82. Siskin GP, Tublin ME, Stainken BF, Dowling K, Dolen EG. Uterine artery embolization for the treatment of adenomyosis: clinical response and evaluation with MR imaging. AJR Am J Roentgenol 2001;177:297-302.

83. Jemal A, Tiwari RC, Murray T, et al. Cancer statistics, 2004. CA Cancer J Clin 2004;54:8-29.

84. Rose PG. Endometrial carcinoma. N Engl J Med 1996;335:640-649.

85. Barakat RR, Hricak H. What do we expect from imaging? Radiol Clin North Am 2002;40:521-526.

86. Szklaruk J, Tamm EP, Choi H, Varavithya V. MR Imaging of common and uncommon large pelvic masses. Radiographics 2003;23:403-424.

87. Gordon J, Reagan JW, Finkle WD, Ziel HK. Estrogen and endometrial carcinoma: an independent pathology review supporting original risk estimate. N Engl J Med 1977;297:570-571.

88. Ascher SM, Imaoka I, Lage JM. Tamoxifen-induced uterine abnormalities: the role of imaging. Radiology 2000;214:29-38.

89. O'Connell LP, Fries MH, Zeringue E, Brehm W. Triage of abnormal postmenopausal bleeding: a comparison of endometrial biopsy and transvaginal sonohysterography versus fractional curettage with hysteroscopy. Am J Obstet Gynecol 1998;178:956-961.

90. Davis PC, O'Neill MJ, Yoder IC, Lee SI, Mueller PR. Sonohysterographic findings of endometrial and subendometrial conditions. Radiographics 2002;22:803-816.

91. Goldstein RB, Bree RL, Benson CB, et al. Evaluation of the woman with postmenopausal bleeding: Society of Radiologists in Ultrasound–Sponsored Consensus Conference statement. J Ultrasound Med 2001;20:1025-1036.

92. Clark TJ, Voit D, Gupta JK, Hyde C, Song F, Khan KS. Accuracy of hysteroscopy in the diagnosis of endometrial cancer and hyperplasia: a systematic quantitative review. JAMA 2002;288:1610-1621.

93. Medverd JR, Dubinsky TJ. Cost analysis model: US versus endometrial biopsy in evaluation of peri- and postmenopausal abnormal vaginal bleeding. Radiology 2002;222:619-627.

94. Dijkhuizen FP, Mol BW, Brolmann HA, Heintz AP. The accuracy of endometrial sampling in the diagnosis of patients with endometrial carcinoma and hyperplasia: a meta-analysis. Cancer 2000;89:1765-1772.

95. Ascher SM, Takahama J, Jha RC. Staging of gynecologic malignancies. Top Magn Reson Imaging 2001;12:105-129.

96. Larson DM, Connor GP, Broste SK, Krawisz BR, Johnson KK. Prognostic significance of gross myometrial invasion with endometrial cancer. Obstet Gynecol 1996;88:394-398.

97. Barnes MN, Kilgore LC. Complete surgical staging of early endometrial adenocarcinoma: optimizing patient outcomes. Semin Radiat Oncol 2000;10:3-7.

98. Mariani A, Webb MJ, Galli L, Podratz KC. Potential therapeutic role of para-aortic lymphadenectomy in node-positive endometrial cancer. Gynecol Oncol 2000;76:348-356.

99. Petereit DG. Complete surgical staging in endometrial cancer provides prognostic information only. Semin Radiat Oncol 2000;10:8-14.

100. Franchi M, Ghezzi F, Riva C, Miglierina M, Buttarelli M, Bolis P. Postoperative complications after pelvic lymphadenectomy for the surgical staging of endometrial cancer. J Surg Oncol 2001;78: 232-237; discussion 237-240.

101. Descamps P, Body G, Calais G, et al. [Stage I and II endometrial cancer: should lymphadenectomy still be done?] J Gynecol Obstet Biol Reprod 1995;24:794-801.

102. Holub Z, Kliment L, Lukac J, Voracek J. Laparoscopically-assisted intraoperative lymphatic mapping in endometrial cancer: preliminary results. Eur J Gynaecol Oncol 2001;22:118-121.

103. Burke TW, Levenback C, Tornos C, Morris M, Wharton JT, Gershenson DM. Intraabdominal lymphatic mapping to direct selective pelvic and paraaortic lymphadenectomy in women with high-risk endometrial cancer: results of a pilot study. Gynecol Oncol 1996;62:169-173.

104. Seki H, Kimura M, Sakai K. Myometrial invasion of endometrial carcinoma: assessment with dynamic MR and contrast-enhanced T1-weighted images. Clin Radiol 1997;52:18-23.

105. Saez F, Urresola A, Larena JA, et al. Endometrial carcinoma: assessment of myometrial invasion with plain and gadolinium-enhanced MR imaging. J Magn Reson Imaging 2000;12:460-466.

106. Minderhoud-Bassie W, Treurniet FE, Koops W, Chadha-Ajwani S, Hage JC, Huikeshoven FJ. Magnetic resonance imaging (MRI) in endometrial carcinoma: preoperative estimation of depth of myometrial invasion. Acta Obstet Gynecol Scand 1995;74:827-831.

107. Hricak H, Rubinstein LV, Gherman GM, Karstaedt N. MR imaging evaluation of endometrial carcinoma: results of an NCI cooperative study. Radiology 1991;179:829-832.

108. Kinkel K, Kaji Y, Yu KK, et al. Radiologic staging in patients with endometrial cancer: a meta-analysis. Radiology 1999;212:711-718.

109. Kim SH, Kim HD, Song YS, Kang SB, Lee HP. Detection of deep myometrial invasion in endometrial carcinoma: comparison of transvaginal ultrasound, CT, and MRI. J Comput Assist Tomogr 1995;19:766-772.

110. Frei KA, Kinkel K. Staging endometrial cancer: role of magnetic resonance imaging. J Magn Reson Imaging 2001;13:850-855.

111. Hardesty LA, Sumkin JH, Hakim C, Johns C, Nath M. The ability of helical CT to preoperatively stage endometrial carcinoma. AJR Am J Roentgenol 2001;176:603-606.

112. Ascher SM, Reinhold C. Imaging of cancer of the endometrium. Radiol Clin North Am 2002;40:563-576.

113. Kinkel K, Tardivon AA, Soyer P, et al. Dynamic contrast-enhanced subtraction versus T2-weighted spin-echo MR imaging in the follow-up of colorectal neoplasm: a prospective study of 41 patients. Radiology 1996;200:453-458.

114. Ito K, Matsumoto T, Nakada T, Nakanishi T, Fujita N, Yamashita H. Assessing myometrial invasion by endometrial carcinoma with dynamic MRI. J Comput Assist Tomogr 1994;18:77-86.

115. Frei KA, Kinkel K, Bonel HM, Lu Y, Zaloudek C, Hricak H. Prediction of deep myometrial invasion in patients with endometrial cancer: clinical utility of contrast-enhanced MR imaging—a meta-analysis and Bayesian analysis. Radiology 2000;216:444-449.

116. Utsunomiya D, Notsute S, Hayashida Y, et al. Endometrial carcinoma in adenomyosis: assessment of myometrial invasion on T2-weighted spin-echo and gadolinium-enhanced T1-weighted images. AJR Am J Roentgenol 2004;182:399-404.

117. Lee EJ, Byun JY, Kim BS, Koong SE, Shinn KS. Staging of early endometrial carcinoma: assessment with T2-weighted and gadolinium-enhanced T1-weighted MR imaging. Radiographics 1999;19:937-945; discussion 946-947.

118. Murakami T, Kurachi H, Nakamura H, et al. Cervical invasion of endometrial carcinoma—evaluation by parasagittal MR imaging. Acta Radiol 1995;36:248-253.

119. Seki H, Takano T, Sakai K. Value of dynamic MR imaging in assessing endometrial carcinoma involvement of the cervix. AJR Am J Roentgenol 2000;175:171-176.

120. Shibutani O, Joja I, Shiraiwa M, et al. Endometrial carcinoma: efficacy of thin-section oblique axial MR images for evaluating cervical invasion. Abdom Imaging 1999;24:520-526.

121. Piver MS, Lele SB, Barlow JJ, Blumenson L. Paraaortic lymph node evaluation in stage I endometrial carcinoma. Obstet Gynecol 1982;59:97-100.

122. Hardesty LA, Sumkin JH, Nath ME, et al. Use of preoperative MR imaging in the management of endometrial carcinoma: cost analysis. Radiology 2000;215:45-49.

123. Morrow CP, Bundy BN, Kurman RJ, et al. Relationship between surgical-pathological risk factors and outcome in clinical stage I and II carcinoma of the endometrium: a Gynecologic Oncology Group study. Gynecol Oncol 1991;40:55-65.

124. Cunha TM, Felix A, Cabral I. Preoperative assessment of deep myometrial and cervical invasion in endometrial carcinoma: comparison of magnetic resonance imaging and gross visual inspection. Int J Gynecol Cancer 2001;11:130-136.

125. Rose PG, Baker S, Kern M, et al. Primary radiation therapy for endometrial carcinoma: a case controlled study. Int J Radiat Oncol Biol Phys 1993;27:585-590.

126. Kaku T, Yoshikawa H, Tsuda H, et al. Conservative therapy for adenocarcinoma and atypical endometrial hyperplasia of the endometrium in young women: central pathologic review and treatment outcome. Cancer Lett 2001;167:39-48.

127. Grasel RP, Outwater EK, Siegelman ES, Capuzzi D, Parker L, Hussain SM. Endometrial polyps: MR imaging features and distinction from endometrial carcinoma. Radiology 2000;214:47-52.

128. Mazur MT, Hsueh S, Gersell DJ. Metastases to the female genital tract: analysis of 325 cases. Cancer 1984;53:1978-1984.

129. Metser U, Haider MA, Khalili K, Boerner S. MR imaging findings and patterns of spread in secondary tumor involvement of the uterine body and cervix. AJR Am J Roentgenol 2003;180:765-769.

130. Lemoine NR, Hall PA. Epithelial tumors metastatic to the uterine cervix: a study of 33 cases and review of the literature. Cancer 1986;57:2002-2005.

131. Rha SE, Byun JY, Jung SE, et al. CT and MRI of uterine sarcomas and their mimickers. AJR Am J Roentgenol 2003;181:1369-1374.

132. Shapeero LG, Hricak H. Mixed mullerian sarcoma of the uterus: MR imaging findings. AJR Am J Roentgenol 1989;153:317-319.

133. Pattani SJ, Kier R, Deal R, Luchansky E. MRI of uterine leiomyosarcoma. Magn Reson Imaging 1995;13:331-333.

134. Gandolfo N, Gandolfo NG, Serafini G, Martinoli C. Endometrial stromal sarcoma of the uterus: MR and US findings. Eur Radiol 2000;10:776-779.

135. Ueda M, Otsuka M, Hatakenaka M, et al. MR imaging findings of uterine endometrial stromal sarcoma: differentiation from endometrial carcinoma. Eur Radiol 2001;11:28-33.

136. Koyama T, Togashi K, Konishi I, et al. MR imaging of endometrial stromal sarcoma: correlation with pathologic findings. AJR Am J Roentgenol 1999;173:767-772.

137. Sahdev A, Sohaib SA, Jacobs I, Shepherd JH, Oram DH, Reznek RH. MR imaging of uterine sarcomas. AJR Am J Roentgenol 2001;177:1307-1311.

138. Neven P, Vergote I. Tamoxifen, screening and new oestrogen receptor modulators. Best Pract Res Clin Obstet Gynaecol 2001;15:365-380.

139. Osborne CK. Tamoxifen in the treatment of breast cancer. N Engl J Med 1998;339:1609-1618.

140. Riggs BL, Hartmann LC. Selective estrogen-receptor modulators—mechanisms of action and application to clinical practice. N Engl J Med 2003;348:618-629.

141. Chourmouzi D, Boulogianni G, Zarampoukas T, Drevelengas A. Sonography and MRI of tamoxifen-associated mullerian adenosarcoma of the uterus. AJR Am J Roentgenol 2003;181:1673-1675.

142. McCluggage WG, Desai V, Manek S. Tamoxifen-associated postmenopausal adenomyosis exhibits stromal fibrosis, glandular dilatation and epithelial metaplasias. Histopathology 2000;37:340-346.

143. Mourits MJ, De Vries EG, Willemse PH, Ten Hoor KA, Hollema H, Van der Zee AG. Tamoxifen treatment and gynecologic side effects: a review. Obstet Gynecol 2001;97:855-866.

144. Bergman L, Beelen ML, Gallee MP, Hollema H, Benraadt J, van Leeuwen FE. Risk and prognosis of endometrial cancer after tamoxifen for breast cancer—Comprehensive Cancer Centres' ALERT Group: assessment of liver and endometrial cancer risk following tamoxifen. Lancet 2000;356:881-887.

145. Deligdisch L, Kalir T, Cohen CJ, de Latour M, Le Bouedec G, Penault-Llorca F. Endometrial histopathology in 700 patients treated with tamoxifen for breast cancer. Gynecol Oncol 2000;78:181-186.

146. American CoOaG, ACOG committee opinion. Tamoxifen and endometrial cancer. Committee on Gynecologic Practice, American College of Obstetricians and Gynecologists. Int J Gynaecol Obstet 1996;53:197-199.

147. Barakat RR. Should women receiving tamoxifen for breast cancer be screened for endometrial cancer? Cancer Invest 2000;18:796-797.

148. Menzin AW, Gal D, Barakat RR. Should women receiving tamoxifen be screened for endometrial cancer? An argument for screening. Cancer Invest 2000;18:793-797.

149. Fong K, Kung R, Lytwyn A, et al. Endometrial evaluation with transvaginal US and hysterosonography in asymptomatic postmenopausal women with breast cancer receiving tamoxifen. Radiology 2001;220:765-773.

150. Gerber B, Krause A, Muller H, et al. Effects of adjuvant tamoxifen on the endometrium in postmenopausal women with breast cancer: a prospective long-term study using transvaginal ultrasound. J Clin Oncol 2000;18:3464-3470.

151. Love CD, Muir BB, Scrimgeour JB, Leonard RC, Dillon P, Dixon JM. Investigation of endometrial abnormalities in asymptomatic women treated with tamoxifen and an evaluation of the role of endometrial screening. J Clin Oncol 1999;17:2050-2054.

152. Ascher SM, Johnson JC, Barnes WA, Bae CJ, Patt RH, Zeman RK. MR imaging appearance of the uterus in postmenopausal women receiving tamoxifen therapy for breast cancer: histopathologic correlation. Radiology 1996;2000:105-110.

153. Marchesoni D, Driul L, Fabiani G, Di Loreto C, Cataldi P, Mozzanega B. Endometrial histologic changes in post-menopausal breast cancer patients using tamoxifen. Int J Gynaecol Obstet 2001;75:257-262.

154. Taieb S, Ceugnart L, Chevalier A, et al. [Value of MRI in symptomatic patients treated with tamoxifen.] J Radiol 2003;84:33-39.

155. Kurman RJ, Kaminski PF, Norris HJ. The behavior of endometrial hyperplasia: a long-term study of "untreated" hyperplasia in 170 patients. Cancer 1985;56:403-412.

156. Hann LE, Gretz EM, Bach AM, Francis SM. Sonohysterography for evaluation of the endometrium in women treated with tamoxifen. AJR Am J Roentgenol 2001;177:337-342.

157. Scoutt LM, McCauley TR, Flynn SD, Luthringer DJ, McCarthy SM. Zonal anatomy of the cervix: correlation of MR imaging and histologic examination of hysterectomy specimens. Radiology 1993;186:159-162.

158. deSouza NM, Hawley IC, Schwieso JE, Gilderdale DJ, Soutter WP. The uterine cervix on in vitro and in vivo MR images: a study of zonal anatomy and vascularity using an enveloping cervical coil. AJR Am J Roentgenol 1994;163:607-612.

159. Okamoto Y, Tanaka YO, Nishida M, Tsunoda H, Yoshikawa H, Itai Y. MR imaging of the uterine cervix: imaging-pathologic correlation. Radiographics 2003;23:425-445.

160. Fogel SR, Slasky BS. Sonography of nabothian cysts. AJR Am J Roentgenol 1982;138:927-930.

161. Kier R. Nonovarian gynecologic cysts: MR imaging findings. AJR Am J Roentgenol 1992;158:1265-1269.

162. Jemal A, Murray T, Saumuels A, Ghafoor A, Ward E, Thun MJ. Cancer statistics, 2003. CA Cancer J Clin 2003;53:5-25.

163. Papanicolaou GN, Traut HF. The diagnostic value of vaginal smears in carcinoma of the uterus. Am J Obstet Gynecol 1941;42:193-205.

164. Sawaya GF, Brown AD, Washington AE, Garber AM. Clinical practice: current approaches to cervical-cancer screening. N Engl J Med 2001;344:1603-1607.

165. Saslow D, Runowicz CD, Solomon D, et al. American Cancer Society guideline for the early detection of cervical neoplasia and cancer. CA Cancer J Clin 2002;52:342-362.

166. Sawaya GF, McConnell KJ, Kulasingam SL, et al. Risk of cervical cancer associated with extending the interval between cervical-cancer screenings. N Engl J Med 2003;349:1501-1509.

167. Scheidler J, Heuck AF. Imaging of cancer of the cervix. Radiol Clin North Am 2002;40:577-590, vii.

168. Munoz N, Bosch FX, de Sanjose S, et al. Epidemiologic classification of human papillomavirus types associated with cervical cancer. N Engl J Med 2003;348:518-527.

169. Kaur H, Silverman PM, Iyer RB, Verschraegen CF, Eifel PJ, Charnsangavej C. Diagnosis, staging, and surveillance of cervical carcinoma. AJR Am J Roentgenol 2003;180:1621-1631.

170. Cannistra SA, Niloff JM. Cancer of the uterine cervix. N Engl J Med 1996;334:1030-1038.

171. Goodman A, Wilbur DC. Case records of the Massachusetts General Hospital, Weekly Clinicopathological Exercises, Case 32-2003: a 37-year-old woman with atypical squamous cells on a Papanicolaou smear. N Engl J Med 2003;349:1555-1564.

172. Results of a randomized trial on the management of cytology interpretations of atypical squamous cells of undetermined significance. Am J Obstet Gynecol 2003;188:1383-1392.

173. Koutsky LA, Ault KA, Wheeler CM, et al. A controlled trial of a human papillomavirus type 16 vaccine. N Engl J Med 2002;347:1645-1651.

174. Crum CP. The beginning of the end for cervical cancer? N Engl J Med 2002;347:1703-1705.

175. Creasman WT. New gynecologic cancer staging. Gynecol Oncol 1995;58:157-158.

176. Keys HM, Bundy BN, Stehman FB, et al. Cisplatin, radiation, and adjuvant hysterectomy compared with radiation and adjuvant hysterectomy for bulky stage IB cervical carcinoma. N Engl J Med 1999;340:1154-1161.

177. Roy M, Plante M. Pregnancies after radical vaginal trachelectomy for early-stage cervical cancer. Am J Obstet Gynecol 1998;179:1491-1496.

178. Dargent D, Martin X, Sacchetoni A, Mathevet P. Laparoscopic vaginal radical trachelectomy: a treatment to preserve the fertility of cervical carcinoma patients. Cancer 2000;88:1877-1882.

179. Hawnaur JM, Johnson RJ, Carrington BM, Hunter RD. Predictive value of clinical examination, transrectal ultrasound and magnetic resonance imaging prior to radiotherapy in carcinoma of the cervix. Br J Radiol 1998;71:819-827.

180. Vorgias G, Katsoulis M, Argyrou K, et al. Preoperative imaging of primary intra-abdominal gynaecological malignancies: diagnostic accuracy of CT-scan and MRI—a Greek cohort study. Eur J Gynaecol Oncol 2002;23:139-144.

181. Bipat S, Glas AS, van der Velden J, Zwinderman AH, Bossuyt PM, Stoker J. Computed tomography and magnetic resonance imaging in staging of uterine cervical cancer: a systematic review. Gynecol Oncol 2003;91:59-66.

182. Oellinger JJ, Blohmer JU, Michniewicz K, et al. Pre-operative staging of cervical cancer: comparison of magnetic resonance imaging (MRI) and computed tomography (CT) with histologic results. Zentralbl Gynakol 2000;122:82-91.

183. Subak LL, Hricak H, Powell CB, Azizi L, Stern JL. Cervical carcinoma: computed tomography and magnetic resonance imaging for preoperative staging. Obstet Gynecol 1995;86:43-50.

184. Hricak H, Powell CB, Yu KK, et al. Invasive cervical carcinoma: role of MR imaging in pretreatment work-up—cost minimization and diagnostic efficacy analysis. Radiology 1996;198:403-409.

185. Peppercorn PD, Jeyarajah AR, Woolas R, et al. Role of MR imaging in the selection of patients with early cervical carcinoma for fertility-preserving surgery: initial experience. Radiology 1999;212:395-399.

186. Shiraiwa M, Joja I, Asakawa T, et al. Cervical carcinoma: efficacy of thin-section oblique axial T2-weighted images for evaluating parametrial invasion. Abdom Imaging 1999;24:514-519.

187. Sheu MH, Chang CY, Wang JH, Yen MS. Preoperative staging of cervical carcinoma with MR imaging: a reappraisal of diagnostic accuracy and pitfalls. Eur Radiol 2001;11:1828-1833.

188. Fujiwara K, Yoden E, Asakawa T, et al. Negative MRI findings with invasive cervical biopsy may indicate stage IA cervical carcinoma. Gynecol Oncol 2000;79:451-456.

189. Lam WW, So NM, Yang WT, Metreweli C. Detection of parametrial invasion in cervical carcinoma: role of short tau inversion recovery sequence. Clin Radiol 2000;55:702-707.

190. Scheidler J, Heuck AF, Steinborn M, Kimmig R, Reiser MF. Parametrial invasion in cervical carcinoma: evaluation of detection at MR imaging with fat suppression. Radiology 1998;206:125-129.

191. Lien HH, Blomlie V, Iversen T, Trope C, Sundfor K, Abeler VM. Clinical stage I carcinoma of the cervix: value of MR imaging in determining invasion into the parametrium. Acta Radiol 1993;34:130-132.

192. Tsuda K, Murakami T, Kurachi H, et al. MR imaging of cervical carcinoma: comparison among T2-weighted, dynamic, and postcontrast T1-weighted images with histopathological correlation. Abdom Imaging 1997;22:103-107.

193. Sironi S, Bellomi M, Villa G, Rossi S, Del Maschio A. Clinical stage I carcinoma of the uterine cervix: value of preoperative magnetic resonance imaging in assessing parametrial invasion. Tumori 2002;88:291-295.

194. Kim SH, Choi BI, Han JK, et al. Preoperative staging of uterine cervical carcinoma: comparison of CT and MRI in 99 patients. J Comput Assist Tomogr 1993;17:633-640.

195. Herzog TJ. New approaches for the management of cervical cancer. Gynecol Oncol 2003;90:S22-27.

196. Burnett AF, Roman LD, O'Meara AT, Morrow CP. Radical vaginal trachelectomy and pelvic lymphadenectomy for preservation of fertility in early cervical carcinoma. Gynecol Oncol 2003;88:419-423.

197. Bernardini M, Barrett J, Seaward G, Covens A. Pregnancy outcomes in patients after radical trachelectomy. Am J Obstet Gynecol 2003;189:1378-1382.

198. Wagenaar HC, Trimbos JB, Postema S, et al. Tumor diameter and volume assessed by magnetic resonance imaging in the prediction of outcome for invasive cervical cancer. Gynecol Oncol 2001;82:474-482.

199. Taylor MB, Carrington BM, Davidson SE, Swindell R, Lawrance JA. Staging of advanced cervical carcinoma using MRI-predictors of outcome after radical radiotherapy. Clin Radiol 2003;58:532-541.

200. Kupets R, Covens A. Is the International Federation of Gynecology and Obstetrics staging system for cervical carcinoma able to predict survival in patients with cervical carcinoma?: An assessment of clinimetric properties. Cancer 2001;92:796-804.

201. Buist MR, Pijpers RJ, van Lingen A, et al. Laparoscopic detection of sentinel lymph nodes followed by lymph node dissection in patients with early stage cervical cancer. Gynecol Oncol 2003;90:290-296.

202. Levenback C, Coleman RL, Burke TW, et al. Lymphatic mapping and sentinel node identification in patients with cervix cancer undergoing radical hysterectomy and pelvic lymphadenectomy. J Clin Oncol 2002;20:688-693.

203. Yang WT, Lam WW, Yu MY, Cheung TH, Metreweli C. Comparison of dynamic helical CT and dynamic MR imaging in the evaluation of pelvic lymph nodes in cervical carcinoma. AJR Am J Roentgenol 2000;175:759-766.

204. Scheidler J, Hricak H, Yu KK, Subak L, Segal MR. Radiological evaluation of lymph node metastases in patients with cervical cancer: a meta-analysis. JAMA 1997;278:1096-1101.

205. Bellin MF, Lebleu L, Meric JB. Evaluation of retroperitoneal and pelvic lymph node metastases with MRI and MR lymphangiography. Abdom Imaging 2003;28:155-163.

206. Koh DM, Cook GJ, Husband JE. New horizons in oncologic imaging. N Engl J Med 2003;348:2487-2488.

207. Tsuruchi N, Tsukamoto N, Kaku T, Kamura T, Nakano H. Adenoma malignum of the uterine cervix detected by imaging methods in a patient with Peutz-Jeghers syndrome. Gynecol Oncol 1994;54:232-236.

208. Tsuda H, Mikami Y, Kaku T, et al. Interobserver variation in the diagnosis of adenoma malignum (minimal deviation adenocarcinoma) of the uterine cervix. Pathol Int 2003;53:440-449.

209. Clement PB, Young RH. Deep nabothian cysts of the uterine cervix: a possible source of confusion with minimal-deviation adenocarcinoma (adenoma malignum). Int J Gynecol Pathol 1989;8:340-348.

210. Yamashita Y, Takahashi M, Katabuchi H, Fukumatsu Y, Miyazaki K, Okamura H. Adenoma malignum: MR appearances mimicking nabothian cysts. AJR Am J Roentgenol 1994;162:649-650.

211. Li H, Sugimura K, Okizuka H, et al. Markedly high signal intensity lesions in the uterine cervix on T2-weighted imaging: differentiation between mucin-producing carcinomas and nabothian cysts. Radiat Med 1999;17:137-143.

212. Doi T, Yamashita Y, Yasunaga T, et al. Adenoma malignum: MR imaging and pathologic study. Radiology 1997;204:39-42.

213. Hricak H, Ascher S, Dodd GD III, Gamsu G, Kucharczyk W, Reiser MF. Image interpretation session: Sunday, December 1, 2002. Radiographics 2002;22:1291-1303.

214. Gupta D, Balsara G. Extrauterine malignancies: role of Pap smears in diagnosis and management. Acta Cytol 1999;43:806-813.

215. Siegelman ES, Outwater EK, Banner MP, Ramchandani P, Anderson TL, Schnall MD. High-resolution MR imaging of the vagina. Radiographics 1997;17:1183-1203.

216. Bluemke DA, Wolf RL, Tani I, Tachiki S, McVeigh ER, Zerhouni EA. Extremity veins: evaluation with fast-spin-echo MR venography. Radiology 1997;204:562-565.

217. Eilber KS, Raz S. Benign cystic lesions of the vagina: a literature review. J Urol 2003;170:717-722.

218. Hagspiel KD. Giant Gartner duct cyst: magnetic resonance imaging findings. Abdom Imaging 1995;20:566-568.

219. Emmons SL, Petty WM. Recurrent giant Gartner's duct cysts: a report of two cases. J Reprod Med 2001;46:773-775.

220. Lee MJ, Yoder IC, Papanicolaou N, Tung GA. Large Gartner duct cyst associated with a solitary crossed ectopic kidney: imaging features. J Comput Assist Tomogr 1991;15:149-151.

221. Rosenfeld DL, Lis E. Gartner's duct cyst with a single vaginal ectopic ureter and associated renal dysplasia or agenesis. J Ultrasound Med 1993;12:775-778.

222. Obermair A, Koller S, Crandon AJ, Perrin L, Nicklin JL. Primary Bartholin gland carcinoma: a report of seven cases. Aust N Z J Obstet Gynaecol 2001;41:78-81.

223. DePasquale SE, McGuinness TB, Mangan CE, Husson M, Woodland MB. Adenoid cystic carcinoma of Bartholin's gland: a review of the literature and report of a patient. Gynecol Oncol 1996;61:122-125.

224. Deppisch LM. Cysts of the vagina: classification and clinical correlations. Obstet Gynecol 1975;45:632-637.

225. Pradhan S, Tobon H. Vaginal cysts: a clinicopathological study of 41 cases. Int J Gynecol Pathol 1986;5:35-46.

226. Filipas D. Vaginal reconstruction/fistulae. Curr Opin Urol 2001;11:267-270.

227. Giordano P, Drew PJ, Taylor D, Duthie G, Lee PW, Monson JR. Vaginography—investigation of choice for clinically suspected vaginal fistulas. Dis Colon Rectum 1996;39:568-572.

228. Stoker J, Rociu E, Schouten WR, Lameris JS. Anovaginal and rectovaginal fistulas: endoluminal sonography versus endoluminal MR imaging. AJR Am J Roentgenol 2002;178:737-741.

229. Yee LF, Birnbaum EH, Read TE, Kodner IJ, Fleshman JW. Use of endoanal ultrasound in patients with rectovaginal fistulas. Dis Colon Rectum 1999;42:1057-1064.

230. Healy JC, Phillips RR, Reznek RH, Crawford RA, Armstrong P, Shepherd JH. The MR appearance of vaginal fistulas. AJR Am J Roentgenol 1996;167:1487-1489.

231. Outwater E, Schiebler ML. Pelvic fistulas: findings on MR images. AJR Am J Roentgenol 1993;160:327-330.

232. Semelka RC, Hricak H, Kim B, et al. Pelvic fistulas: appearances on MR images. Abdom Imaging 1997;22:91-95.

233. Bump RC, Norton PA. Epidemiology and natural history of pelvic floor dysfunction. Obstet Gynecol Clin North Am 1998;25:723-746.

234. Kester RR, Leboeuf L, Amendola MA, Kim SS, Benoit A, Gousse AE. Value of express T2-weighted pelvic MRI in the preoperative evaluation of severe pelvic floor prolapse: a prospective study. Urology 2003;61:1135-1139.

235. Stoker J, Halligan S, Bartram CI. Pelvic floor imaging. Radiology 2001;218:621-641.

236. Fielding JR. Practical MR imaging of female pelvic floor weakness. Radiographics 2002;22:295-304.

237. Maubon A, Aubard Y, Berkane V, Camezind-Vidal MA, Mares P, Rouanet JP. Magnetic resonance imaging of the pelvic floor. Abdom Imaging 2003;28:217-225.

238. Pannu HK. Dynamic MR imaging of female organ prolapse. Radiol Clin North Am 2003;41:409-423.

239. Barbaric ZL, Marumoto AK, Raz S. Magnetic resonance imaging of the perineum and pelvic floor. Top Magn Reson Imaging 2001;12:83-92.

240. Lovatsis D, Drutz HP. Vaginal surgical approach to vaginal vault prolapse: considerations of anatomic correction and safety. Curr Opin Obstet Gynecol 2003;15:435-437.

241. Carey MP, Dwyer PL. Genital prolapse: vaginal versus abdominal route of repair. Curr Opin Obstet Gynecol 2001;13:499-505.

242. Panageas E, Kier R, McCauley TR, McCarthy S. Submucosal uterine leiomyomas: diagnosis of prolapse into the cervix and vagina based on MR imaging. AJR Am J Roentgenol 1992;159:555-558.

243. Shimada K, Ohashi I, Shibuya H, Tanabe F, Akashi T. MR imaging of an atypical vaginal leiomyoma. AJR Am J Roentgenol 2002;178:752-754.

244. Ruggieri AM, Brody JM, Curhan RP. Vaginal leiomyoma. A case report with imaging findings. J Reprod Med 1996;41:875-877.

245. Shadbolt CL, Coakley FV, Qayyum A, Donat SM. MRI of vaginal leiomyomas. J Comput Assist Tomogr 2001;25:355-357.

246. Chagpar A, Kanthan SC. Vaginal metastasis of colon cancer. Am Surg 2001;67:171-172.

247. Heller DS, Kambham N, Smith D, Cracchiolo B. Recurrence of gynecologic malignancy at the vaginal vault after hysterectomy. Int J Gynaecol Obstet 1999;64:159-162.

248. Chang SD. Imaging of the vagina and vulva. Radiol Clin North Am 2002;40:637-658.

249. Goodman A. Primary vaginal cancer. Surg Oncol Clin N Am 1998;7:347-361.

250. Tjalma WA, Monaghan JM, de Barros Lopes A, Naik R, Nordin AJ, Weyler JJ. The role of surgery in invasive squamous carcinoma of the vagina. Gynecol Oncol 2001;81:360-365.

251. Stryker JA. Radiotherapy for vaginal carcinoma: a 23-year review. Br J Radiol 2000;73:1200-1205.

252. Sobin LH, Wittekind C, eds. *TNM Classification of Malignant Tumors.* New York: Wiley, 1997.

253. Merino MJ. Vaginal cancer: the role of infectious and environmental factors. Am J Obstet Gynecol 1991;165:1255-1262.

254. Herbst AL. Diethylstilbestrol and adenocarcinoma of the vagina. Am J Obstet Gynecol 1999;181:1576-1578; discussion 1579.

255. Hanselaar AG, Boss EA, Massuger LF, Bernheim JL. Cytologic examination to detect clear cell adenocarcinoma of the vagina or cervix. Gynecol Oncol 1999;75:338-344.

256. Gilles R, Michel G, Chancelier MD, Vanel D, Masselot J. Case report: clear cell adenocarcinoma of the vagina—MR features. Br J Radiol 1993;66:168-170.

257. Tsuda K, Murakami T, Kurachi H, et al. MR imaging of non-squamous vaginal tumors. Eur Radiol 1999;9:1214-1218.

258. Ghurani GB, Penalver MA. An update on vulvar cancer. Am J Obstet Gynecol 2001;185:294-299.

259. Joura EA, Losch A, Haider-Angeler MG, Breitenecker G, Leodolter S. Trends in vulvar neoplasia: increasing incidence of vulvar intraepithelial neoplasia and squamous cell carcinoma of the vulva in young women. J Reprod Med 2000;45:613-615.

260. Homesley HD, Bundy BN, Sedlis A, et al. Assessment of current International Federation of Gynecology and Obstetrics staging of vulvar carcinoma relative to prognostic factors for survival (a Gynecologic Oncology Group study). Am J Obstet Gynecol 1991;164:997-1003; discussion 1003-1004.

261. Sohaib SA, Richards PS, Ind T, et al. MR imaging of carcinoma of the vulva. AJR Am J Roentgenol 2002;178:373-377.

262. Troiano RN. Magnetic resonance imaging of mullerian duct anomalies of the uterus. Top Magn Reson Imaging 2003;14:269-279.

263. Thurmond AS. Imaging of female infertility. Radiol Clin North Am 2003;41:757-767.

264. Propst AM, Hill JA III. Anatomic factors associated with recurrent pregnancy loss. Semin Reprod Med 2000;18:341-350.

265. Lang IM, Babyn P, Oliver GD. MR imaging of paediatric uterovaginal anomalies. Pediatr Radiol 1999;29:163-170.

266. Buttram VC. The American Fertility Society classifications of adnexal adhesions, distal tubal occlusion, tubal occlusion secondary to tubal ligation, tubal pregnancies, mullerian anomalies and intrauterine adhesions. Fertil Steril 1988;49:944-955.

267. Saleem SN. MR imaging diagnosis of uterovaginal anomalies: current state of the art. Radiographics 2003;23:e13.

268. Minto CL, Hollings N, Hall-Craggs M, Creighton S. Magnetic resonance imaging in the assessment of complex Mullerian anomalies. Bjog 2001;108:791-797.

269. Syed I, Hussain H, Weadock W, Ellis J. Uterus, mullerian duct abnormalities. Emedicine, http://www.emedicine.com/radio/topic738.htm. Last updated August 31, 2002, accessed September 19, 2004.

270. Fielding JR. MR imaging of Mullerian anomalies: impact on therapy. AJR Am J Roentgenol 1996;167:1491-1495.

271. O'Neill MJ, Yoder IC, Connolly SA, Mueller PR. Imaging evaluation and classification of developmental anomalies of the female reproductive system with an emphasis on MR imaging. AJR Am J Roentgenol 1999;173:407-416.

272. Arnold BW, Gilfeather M, Woodward PJ. Mullerian duct anomalies complicated by obstruction: evaluation with pelvic magnetic resonance imaging. J Womens Imaging 2001;3:146-152.

273. Price TM, Bates WG. Adolescent amenorrhea. In: Koehler Carpenter SE, Rock JA (eds). *Pediatric and Adolescent Gynecology,* 2nd ed. Philadelphia: Lippincott Williams and Wilkins, 2000;177-206.

274. Fedele L, Dorta M, Brioschi D, Giudici MN, Candiani GB. Magnetic resonance imaging in Mayer-Rokitansky-Kuster-Hauser syndrome. Obstet Gynecol 1990;76:593-596.

275. Strubbe EH, Cremers CW, Willemsen WN, Rolland R, Thijn CJ. The Mayer-Rokitansky-Kuster-Hauser (MRKH) syndrome without and with associated features: two separate entities? Clin Dysmorphol 1994;3:192-199.

276. Reinhold C, Hricak H, Forstner R, et al. Primary amenorrhea: evaluation with MR imaging. Radiology 1997;203:383-390.

277. Roberts CP, Haber MJ, Rock JA. Vaginal creation for mullerian agenesis. Am J Obstet Gynecol 2001;185:1349-1352; discussion 1352-1353.

278. Sonmezer M, Atabekoglu C, Dokmeci F. Laparoscopic excision of symmetric uterine remnants in a patient with Mayer-Rokitansky-Hauser Kuster syndrome. J Am Assoc Gynecol Laparosc 2003;10:409-411.

279. Ben-Rafael Z, Bar-Hava I, Levy T, Orvieto R. Simplifying ovulation induction for surrogacy in women with Mayer-Rokitansky-Kuster-Hauser syndrome. Hum Reprod 1998;13:1470-1471.

280. Barthold JS, Kumasi-Rivers K, Upadhyay J, Shekarriz B, Imperato-Mcginley J. Testicular position in the androgen insensitivity syndrome: implications for the role of androgens in testicular descent. J Urol 2000;164:497-501.

281. Sills ES, Perloe M, Kaplan CR, Schlegel PN, Palermo GD. Bilateral orchiectomy for the surgical treatment of complete androgen insensitivity syndrome: patient outcome after 1 year of follow-up. J Laparoendosc Adv Surg Tech A 2003;13:193-197.

282. Choi HK, Cho KS, Lee HW, Kim KS. MR imaging of intersexuality. Radiographics 1998;18:83-96.

283. Brody JM, Koelliker SL, Frishman GN. Unicornuate uterus: imaging appearance, associated anomalies, and clinical implications. AJR Am J Roentgenol 1998;171:1341-1347.

284. Ombelet W, Grieten M, Neubourg PD, et al. Undescended ovary and unicornuate uterus: simplified diagnosis by the use of clomiphene citrate ovarian stimulation and magnetic resonance imaging (MRI). Hum Reprod 2003;18:858-862.

285. Smolders D, Deckers F, Pouillon M, Vanderheyden T, Vanderheyden J, De Schepper A. Ectopic pregnancy within a rudimentary horn in a case of unicornuate uterus. Eur Radiol 2002;12:121-124.

286. Heinonen PK. Unicornuate uterus and rudimentary horn. Fertil Steril 1997;68:224-230.

287. Deffarges JV, Haddad B, Musset R, Paniel BJ. Utero-vaginal anastomosis in women with uterine cervix atresia: long-term follow-up and reproductive performance—a study of 18 cases. Hum Reprod 2001;16:1722-1725.

288. Raga F, Bauset C, Remohi J, Bonilla-Musoles F, Simon C, Pellicer A. Reproductive impact of congenital Mullerian anomalies. Hum Reprod 1997;12:2277-2281.

289. Heinonen PK. Clinical implications of the didelphic uterus: long-term follow-up of 49 cases. Eur J Obstet Gynecol Reprod Biol 2000;91:183-190.

290. Nahum GG. Uterine anomalies: how common are they, and what is their distribution among subtypes? J Reprod Med 1998;43:877-887.

291. Grimbizis GF, Camus M, Tarlatzis BC, Bontis JN, Devroey P. Clinical implications of uterine malformations and hysteroscopic treatment results. Hum Reprod Update 2001;7:161-174.

292. Saygili-Yilmaz E, Yildiz S, Erman-Akar M, Akyuz G, Yilmaz Z. Reproductive outcome of septate uterus after hysteroscopic metroplasty. Arch Gynecol Obstet 2003;268:289-292.

293. Maneschi F, Marana R, Muzii L, Mancuso S. Reproductive performance in women with bicornuate uterus. Acta Eur Fertil 1993;24:117-120.

294. Golan A, Langer R, Wexler S, Segev E, Niv D, David MP. Cervical cerclage—its role in the pregnant anomalous uterus. Int J Fertil 1990;35:164-170.

295. Pellerito JS, McCarthy SM, Doyle MB, Glickman MG, DeCherney AH. Diagnosis of uterine anomalies: relative accuracy of MR imaging, endovaginal sonography, and hysterosalpingography. Radiology 1992;183:795-800.

296. Carrington BM, Hricak H, Nuruddin RN, Secaf E, Laros RK, Jr., Hill EC. Mullerian duct anomalies: MR imaging evaluation. Radiology 1990;176:715-720.

297. Li S, Qayyum A, Coakley FV, Hricak H. Association of renal agenesis and mullerian duct anomalies. J Comput Assist Tomogr 2000;24:829-834.

298. Outwater EK, Mitchell DG. Normal ovaries and functional cysts: MR appearance. Radiology 1996;198:397-402.

299. Outwater EK, Talerman A, Dunton C. Normal adnexa uteri specimens: anatomic basis of MR imaging features. Radiology 1996;201:751-755.

300. Outwater EK, Dunton CJ. Imaging of the ovary and adnexa: clinical issues and applications of MR imaging. Radiology 1995;194:1-18.

301. Togashi K. MR imaging of the ovaries: normal appearance and benign disease. Radiol Clin North Am 2003;41:799-811.

302. Outwater EK, Wagner BJ, Mannion C, McLarney JK, Kim B. Sex cord-stromal and steroid cell tumors of the ovary. Radiographics 1998;18:1523-1546.

303. Woodward PJ, Hosseinzadeh K, Saenger JS. From the archives of the AFIP: radiologic staging of ovarian carcinoma with pathologic correlation. Radiographics 2004;24:225-246.

304. Koonings PP, Campbell K, Mishell DR, Jr., Grimes DA. Relative frequency of primary ovarian neoplasms: a 10-year review. Obstet Gynecol 1989;74:921-926.

305. Wagner BJ, Buck JL, Seidman JD, McCabe KM. From the archives of the AFIP: Ovarian epithelial neoplasms—radiologic-pathologic correlation. Radiographics 1994;14:1351-1374; quiz 1375-1376.

306. Brown DL, Zou KH, Tempany CM, et al. Primary versus secondary ovarian malignancy: imaging findings of adnexal masses in the Radiology Diagnostic Oncology Group Study. Radiology 2001;219:213-218.

307. Cannistra SA. Cancer of the ovary. N Engl J Med 1993;329:1550-1559.

308. Coakley FV. Staging ovarian cancer: role of imaging. Radiol Clin North Am 2002;40:609-636.

309. Jung SE, Lee JM, Rha SE, Byun JY, Jung JI, Hahn ST. CT and MR imaging of ovarian tumors with emphasis on differential diagnosis. Radiographics 2002;22:1305-1325.

310. Bast RC, Jr. Status of tumor markers in ovarian cancer screening. J Clin Oncol 2003;21:200-205.

311. DePriest PD, DeSimone CP. Ultrasound screening for the early detection of ovarian cancer. J Clin Oncol 2003;21:194-199.

312. Paley PJ. Ovarian cancer screening: are we making any progress? Curr Opin Oncol 2001;13:399-402.

313. Modugno F. Ovarian cancer and high-risk women-implications for prevention, screening, and early detection. Gynecol Oncol 2003;91:15-31.

314. Levavi H, Sabah G. BRCA susceptibility genes—a review of current conservative management of BRCA mutation carriers. Eur J Gynaecol Oncol 2003;24:463-466.

315. Kauff ND, Satagopan JM, Robson ME, et al. Risk-reducing salpingo-oophorectomy in women with a BRCA1 or BRCA2 mutation. N Engl J Med 2002;346:1609-1615.

316. Rieber A, Nussle K, Stohr I, et al. Preoperative diagnosis of ovarian tumors with MR imaging: comparison with transvaginal sonography, positron emission tomography, and histologic findings. AJR Am J Roentgenol 2001;177:123-129.

317. Schwartz LB, Panageas E, Lange R, Rizzo J, Comite F, McCarthy S. Female pelvis: impact of MR imaging on treatment decisions and net cost analysis. Radiology 1994;192:55-60.

318. Kurtz AB, Tsimikas JV, Tempany CM, et al. Diagnosis and staging of ovarian cancer: comparative values of Doppler and conventional US, CT, and MR imaging correlated with surgery and histopathologic analysis—report of the Radiology Diagnostic Oncology Group. Radiology 1999;212:19-27.

319. Schwartz PE, Taylor KJ. Is early detection of ovarian cancer possible? Ann Med 1995;27:519-528.

320. Olson SH, Mignone L, Nakraseive C, Caputo TA, Barakat RR, Harlap S. Symptoms of ovarian cancer. Obstet Gynecol 2001;98:212-217.

321. Boente MP, Chi DS, Hoskins WJ. The role of surgery in the management of ovarian cancer: primary and interval cytoreductive surgery. Semin Oncol 1998;25:326-334.

322. Meyer JI, Kennedy AW, Friedman R, Ayoub A, Zepp RC. Ovarian carcinoma: value of CT in predicting success of debulking surgery. AJR Am J Roentgenol 1995;165:875-878.

323. Nelson BE, Rosenfield AT, Schwartz PE. Preoperative abdominopelvic computed tomographic prediction of optimal cytoreduction in epithelial ovarian carcinoma. J Clin Oncol 1993;11:166-172.

324. Schwartz PE. Neoadjuvant chemotherapy for the management of ovarian cancer. Best Pract Res Clin Obstet Gynaecol 2002;16:585-596.

325. Chi DS, Venkatraman ES, Masson V, Hoskins WJ. The ability of preoperative serum CA-125 to predict optimal primary tumor cytoreduction in stage III epithelial ovarian carcinoma. Gynecol Oncol 2000;77:227-231.

326. Tempany CM, Zou KH, Silverman SG, Brown DL, Kurtz AB, McNeil BJ. Staging of advanced ovarian cancer: comparison of imaging modalities—report from the Radiological Diagnostic Oncology Group. Radiology 2000;215:761-767.

327. Coakley FV, Choi PH, Gougoutas CA, et al. Peritoneal metastases: detection with spiral CT in patients with ovarian cancer. Radiology 2002;223:495-499.

328. Low RN, Saleh F, Song SY, et al. Treated ovarian cancer: comparison of MR imaging with serum CA-125 level and physical examination—a longitudinal study. Radiology 1999;211:519-528.

329. Park CM, Kim SH, Moon MH, Kim KW, Choi HJ. Recurrent ovarian malignancy: patterns and spectrum of imaging findings. Abdom Imaging 2003;28:404-415.

330. Balestreri L, Bison L, Sorio R, Morra A, Campagnutta E, Morassut S. Abdominal recurrence of ovarian cancer: value of abdominal MR in patients with positive CA125 and negative CT. Radiol Med (Torino) 2002;104:426-436.

331. Bristow RE, Lagasse LD, Karlan BY. Secondary surgical cytoreduction for advanced epithelial ovarian cancer: patient selection and review of the literature. Cancer 1996;78:2049-2062.

332. Funt SA, Hricak H, Abu-Rustum N, Mazumdar M, Felderman H, Chi DS. Role of CT in the management of recurrent ovarian cancer. AJR Am J Roentgenol 2004;182:393-398.

333. Bristow RE, del Carmen MG, Pannu HK, et al. Clinically occult recurrent ovarian cancer: patient selection for secondary cytoreductive surgery using combined PET/CT. Gynecol Oncol 2003;90:519-528.

334. Krigman H, Bentley R, Robboy SJ. Pathology of epithelial ovarian tumors. Clin Obstet Gynecol 1994;37:475-491.

335. Granberg S, Wikland M, Jansson I. Macroscopic characterization of ovarian tumors and the relation to the histological diagnosis: criteria to be used for ultrasound evaluation. Gynecol Oncol 1989;35:139-144.

336. Alcazar JL, Merce LT, Laparte C, Jurado M, Lopez-Garcia G. A new scoring system to differentiate benign from malignant adnexal masses. Am J Obstet Gynecol 2003;188:685-692.

337. Sohaib SA, Sahdev A, Trappen PV, Jacobs IJ, Reznek RH. Characterization of adnexal mass lesions on MR imaging. AJR Am J Roentgenol 2003;180:1297-1304.

338. Outwater EK, Huang AB, Dunton CJ, Talerman A, Capuzzi DM. Papillary projections in ovarian neoplasms: appearance on MRI. J Magn Reson Imaging 1997;7:689-695.

339. Pretorius ES, Outwater EK, Hunt JL, Siegelman ES. Magnetic resonance imaging of the ovary. Top Magn Reson Imaging 2001;12:131-146.

340. Siegelman ES, Outwater EK. Tissue characterization in the female pelvis by means of MR imaging. Radiology 1999;212:5-18.

341. Low RN, Barone RM, Lacey C, Sigeti JS, Alzate GD, Sebrechts CP. Peritoneal tumor: MR imaging with dilute oral barium and intravenous gadolinium-containing contrast agents compared with unenhanced MR imaging and CT. Radiology 1997;204:513-520.

342. Low RN, Carter WD, Saleh F, Sigeti JS. Ovarian cancer: comparison of findings with perfluorocarbon-enhanced MR imaging, in 111-CYT-103 immunoscintigraphy, and CT. Radiology 1995;195:391-400.

343. Takemori M, Nishimura R, Hasegawa K. Clinical evaluation of MRI in the diagnosis of borderline ovarian tumors. Acta Obstet Gynecol Scand 2002;81:157-161.

344. Seidman JD, Kurman RJ. Ovarian serous borderline tumors: a critical review of the literature with emphasis on prognostic indicators. Hum Pathol 2000;31:539-557.

345. Puls LE, Hunter JE, Heidtman EP, Stafford JR, Parker HB. Removal of a 130 pound ovarian neoplasm. J S C Med Assoc 1996;92:216-219.

346. Yoshikawa H, Jimbo H, Okada S, et al. Prevalence of endometriosis in ovarian cancer. Gynecol Obstet Invest 2000;50(Suppl 1):11-17.

347. Outwater EK, Siegelman ES, Kim B, Chiowanich P, Blasbalg R, Kilger A. Ovarian Brenner tumors: MR imaging characteristics. Magn Reson Imaging 1998;16:1147-1153.

348. van der Westhuizen NG, Tiltman AJ. Brenner tumours—a clinico-pathological study. S Afr Med J 1988;73:98-101.

349. Ohara N, Teramoto K. Magnetic resonance imaging of a benign Brenner tumor with an ipsilateral simple cyst. Arch Gynecol Obstet 2001;265:96-99.

350. Brammer HM III, Buck JL, Hayes WS, Sheth S, Tavassoli FA. From the archives of the AFIP—Malignant germ cell tumors of the ovary: radiologic-pathologic correlation. Radiographics 1990;10:715-724.

351. McGee DM, Connolly SA, Young RH. Case records of the Massachusetts General Hospital, Weekly Clinicopathological Exercises, Case 24-2003: A 10-year-old girl with recurrent bouts of abdominal pain. N Engl J Med 2003;349:486-494.

352. Comerci JT, Jr., Licciardi F, Bergh PA, Gregori C, Breen JL. Mature cystic teratoma: a clinicopathologic evaluation of 517 cases and review of the literature. Obstet Gynecol 1994;84:22-28.

353. Wu RT, Torng PL, Chang DY, et al. Mature cystic teratoma of the ovary: a clinicopathologic study of 283 cases. Zhonghua Yi Xue Za Zhi (Taipei) 1996;58:269-274.

354. Benjapibal M, Boriboonhirunsarn D, Suphanit I, Sangkarat S. Benign cystic teratoma of the ovary: a review of 608 patients. J Med Assoc Thai 2000;83:1016-1020.

355. Outwater EK, Siegelman ES, Hunt JL. Ovarian teratomas: tumor types and imaging characteristics. Radiographics 2001;21:475-490.

356. Kido A, Togashi K, Konishi I, et al. Dermoid cysts of the ovary with malignant transformation: MR appearance. AJR Am J Roentgenol 1999;172:445-449.

357. Mecke H, Savvas V. Laparoscopic surgery of dermoid cysts—intraoperative spillage and complications. Eur J Obstet Gynecol Reprod Biol 2001;96:80-84.

358. Zanetta G, Ferrari L, Mignini-Renzini M, Vignali M, Fadini R. Laparoscopic excision of ovarian dermoid cysts with controlled intraoperative spillage: safety and effectiveness. J Reprod Med 1999;44:815-820.

359. Nezhat CR, Kalyoncu S, Nezhat CH, Johnson E, Berlanda N, Nezhat F. Laparoscopic management of ovarian dermoid cysts: ten years' experience. Jsls J Soc Laparoendosc Surg 1999;3:179-184.

360. Caspi B, Appelman Z, Rabinerson D, Zalel Y, Tulandi T, Shoham Z. The growth pattern of ovarian dermoid cysts: a prospective study in premenopausal and postmenopausal women. Fertil Steril 1997;68:501-505.

361. Buy JN, Ghossain MA, Moss AA, et al. Cystic teratoma of the ovary: CT detection. Radiology 1989;171:697-701.

362. Yamashita Y, Hatanaka Y, Torashima M, Takahashi M, Miyazaki K, Okamura H. Mature cystic teratomas of the ovary without fat in the cystic cavity: MR features in 12 cases. AJR Am J Roentgenol 1994;163:613-616.

363. Togashi K, Nishimura K, Itoh K, et al. Ovarian cystic teratomas: MR imaging. Radiology 1987;162:669-673.

364. Stevens SK, Hricak H, Campos Z. Teratomas versus cystic hemorrhagic adnexal lesions: differentiation with proton-selective fat-saturation MR imaging. Radiology 1993;186:481-488.

365. Imaoka I, Sugimura K, Okizuka H, Iwanari O, Kitao M, Ishida T. Ovarian cystic teratomas: value of chemical fat saturation magnetic resonance imaging. Br J Radiol 1993;66:994-997.

366. Guinet C, Buy JN, Ghossain MA, et al. Fat suppression techniques in MR imaging of mature ovarian teratomas: comparison with CT. Eur J Radiol 1993;17:117-121.

367. Bazot M, Boudghene F, Billieres P, Antoine J, Uzan S, Bigot J. Value of fat-suppression gradient-echo MR imaging in the diagnosis of ovarian cystic teratomas. Clin Imaging 2000;24:146-153.

368. Delfaut EM, Beltran J, Johnson G, Rousseau J, Marchandise X, Cotten A. Fat suppression in MR imaging: techniques and pitfalls. Radiographics 1999;19:373-382.

369. Joja I, Asakawa T, Mitsumori A, et al. Struma ovarii: appearance on MR images. Abdom Imaging 1998;23:652-656.

370. Matsuki M, Kaji Y, Matsuo M, Kobashi Y. Struma ovarii: MRI findings. Br J Radiol 2000;73:87-90.

371. Okada S, Ohaki Y, Kawamura T, Hayashi T, Kumazaki T. Cystic struma ovarii: imaging findings. J Comput Assist Tomogr 2000;24:413-415.

372. Kim JC, Kim SS, Park JY. MR findings of struma ovarii. Clin Imaging 2000;24:28-33.

373. Joja I, Asakawa T, Mitsumori A, et al. I-123 uptake in nonfunctional struma ovarii. Clin Nucl Med 1998;23:10-12.

374. Yamaoka T, Togashi K, Koyama T, et al. Immature teratoma of the ovary: correlation of MR imaging and pathologic findings. Eur Radiol 2003;13:313-319.

375. Breen JL, Maxson WS. Ovarian tumors in children and adolescents. Clin Obstet Gynecol 1977;20:607-623.

376. Tanaka YO, Kurosaki Y, Nishida M, et al. Ovarian dysgerminoma: MR and CT appearance. J Comput Assist Tomogr 1994;18:443-448.

377. Kim SH, Kang SB. Ovarian dysgerminoma: color Doppler ultrasonographic findings and comparison with CT and MR imaging findings. J Ultrasound Med 1995;14:843-848.

378. Ayhan A, Bildirici I, Gunalp S, Yuce K. Pure dysgerminoma of the ovary: a review of 45 well staged cases. Eur J Gynaecol Oncol 2000;21:98-101.

379. Levitin A, Haller KD, Cohen HL, Zinn DL, O'Connor MT. Endodermal sinus tumor of the ovary: imaging evaluation. AJR Am J Roentgenol 1996;167:791-793.

380. Yamaoka T, Togashi K, Koyama T, et al. Yolk sac tumor of the ovary: radiologic-pathologic correlation in four cases. J Comput Assist Tomogr 2000;24:605-609.

381. Kurman RJ, Norris HJ. Endodermal sinus tumor of the ovary: a clinical and pathologic analysis of 71 cases. Cancer 1976;38:2404-2419.

382. Nawa A, Obata N, Kikkawa F, et al. Prognostic factors of patients with yolk sac tumors of the ovary. Am J Obstet Gynecol 2001;184:1182-1188.

383. Stenwig JT, Hazekamp JT, Beecham JB. Granulosa cell tumors of the ovary: a clinicopathological study of 118 cases with long-term follow-up. Gynecol Oncol 1979;7:136-152.

384. Segal R, DePetrillo AD, Thomas G. Clinical review of adult granulosa cell tumors of the ovary. Gynecol Oncol 1995;56:338-344.

385. Malmstrom H, Hogberg T, Risberg B, Simonsen E. Granulosa cell tumors of the ovary: prognostic factors and outcome. Gynecol Oncol 1994;52:50-55.

386. Young RH, Dickersin GR, Scully RE. Juvenile granulosa cell tumor of the ovary: a clinicopathological analysis of 125 cases. Am J Surg Pathol 1984;8:575-596.

387. Calaminus G, Wessalowski R, Harms D, Gobel U. Juvenile granulosa cell tumors of the ovary in children and adolescents: results from 33 patients registered in a prospective cooperative study. Gynecol Oncol 1997;65:447-452.

388. Aboud E. A review of granulosa cell tumours and thecomas of the ovary. Arch Gynecol Obstet 1997;259:161-165.

389. Ko SF, Wan YL, Ng SH, et al. Adult ovarian granulosa cell tumors: spectrum of sonographic and CT findings with pathologic correlation. AJR Am J Roentgenol 1999;172:1227-1233.

390. Kim SH. Granulosa cell tumor of the ovary: common findings and unusual appearances on CT and MR. J Comput Assist Tomogr 2002;26:756-761.

391. Morikawa K, Hatabu H, Togashi K, Kataoka ML, Mori T, Konishi J. Granulosa cell tumor of the ovary: MR findings. J Comput Assist Tomogr 1997;21:1001-1004.

392. Troiano RN, Lazzarini KM, Scoutt LM, Lange RC, Flynn SD, McCarthy S. Fibroma and fibrothecoma of the ovary: MR imaging findings. Radiology 1997;204:795-798.

393. Ueda J, Furukawa T, Higashino K, et al. Ovarian fibroma of high signal intensity on T2-weighted MR image. Abdom Imaging 1998;23:657-658.

394. Ayhan A, Tuncer ZS, Hakverdi AU, Yuce K. Sertoli-Leydig cell tumor of the ovary: a clinicopathologic study of 10 cases. Eur J Gynaecol Oncol 1996;17:75-78.

395. Yada-Hashimoto N, Yamamoto T, Kamiura S, et al. Metastatic ovarian tumors: a review of 64 cases. Gynecol Oncol 2003;89:314-317.

396. Holtz F, Hart WR. Krukenberg tumors of the ovary: a clinicopathologic analysis of 27 cases. Cancer 1982;50:2438-2447.

397. Ha HK, Baek SY, Kim SH, Kim HH, Chung EC, Yeon KM. Krukenberg's tumor of the ovary: MR imaging features. AJR Am J Roentgenol 1995;164:1435-1439.

398. Tanaka YO, Nishida M, Yamaguchi M, Kohno K, Saida Y, Itai Y. MRI of gynaecological solid masses. Clin Radiol 2000;55:899-911.

399. Rha SE, Byun JY, Jung SE, et al. CT and MR imaging features of adnexal torsion. Radiographics 2002;22:283-294.

400. Argenta PA, Yeagley TJ, Ott G, Sondheimer SJ. Torsion of the uterine adnexa: pathologic correlations and current management trends. J Reprod Med 2000;45:831-836.

401. Descargues G, Tinlot-Mauger F, Gravier A, Lemoine JP, Marpeau L. Adnexal torsion: a report on forty-five cases. Eur J Obstet Gynecol Reprod Biol 2001;98:91-96.

402. Case records of the Massachusetts General Hospital, Case 3-1996: Severe abdominal pain during early pregnancy in a woman with previous infertility. N Engl J Med 1996;334:255-260.

403. Gorkemli H, Camus M, Clasen K. Adnexal torsion after gonadotrophin ovulation induction for IVF or ICSI and its conservative treatment. Arch Gynecol Obstet 2002;267:4-6.

404. Cohen SB, Oelsner G, Seidman DS, Admon D, Mashiach S, Goldenberg M. Laparoscopic detorsion allows sparing of the twisted ischemic adnexa. J Am Assoc Gynecol Laparosc 1999;6:139-143.

405. Graif M, Itzchak Y. Sonographic evaluation of ovarian torsion in childhood and adolescence. AJR Am J Roentgenol 1988;150:647-649.

406. Bader T, Ranner G, Haberlik A. Torsion of a normal adnexa in a premenarcheal girl: MRI findings. Eur Radiol 1996;6:704-706.

407. Kimura I, Togashi K, Kawakami S, Takakura K, Mori T, Konishi J. Ovarian torsion: CT and MR imaging appearances. Radiology 1994;190:337-341.

408. Hall BP, Printz DA, Roth J. Massive ovarian edema: ultrasound and MR characteristics. J Comput Assist Tomogr 1993;17:477-479.

409. Kramer LA, Lalani T, Kawashima A. Massive edema of the ovary: high resolution MR findings using a phased-array pelvic coil. J Magn Reson Imaging 1997;7:758-760.

410. Umekita Y, Fujiyoshi T, Takasaki T, Kuriwaki K, Yoshida A, Yoshida H. Immunohistochemical studies of S-100 protein expression in myoepithelial cells of benign breast diseases and normal breast tissues. In Vivo 1993;7:415-418.

411. Bulletti C, De Ziegler D, Polli V, Del Ferro E, Palini S, Flamigni C. Characteristics of uterine contractility during menses in women with mild to moderate endometriosis. Fertil Steril 2002;77:1156-1161.

412. Kunz G, Beil D, Huppert P, Leyendecker G. Structural abnormalities of the uterine wall in women with endometriosis and infertility visualized by vaginal sonography and magnetic resonance imaging. Hum Reprod 2000;15:76-82.

413. Taylor RN, Lebovic DI, Mueller MD. Angiogenic factors in endometriosis. Ann N Y Acad Sci 2002;955:89-100; discussion 118, 396-406.

414. Witz CA. Pathogenesis of endometriosis. Gynecol Obstet Invest 2002;53:52-62.

415. Gazvani R, Templeton A. New considerations for the pathogenesis of endometriosis. Int J Gynaecol Obstet 2002;76:117-126.

416. Cramer DW, Missmer SA. The epidemiology of endometriosis. Ann N Y Acad Sci 2002;955:11-22; discussion 34-36, 396-406.

417. Eskenazi B, Warner ML. Epidemiology of endometriosis. Obstet Gynecol Clin North Am 1997;24:235-258.

418. Lu PY, Ory SJ. Endometriosis: current management. Mayo Clin Proc 1995;70:453-463.

419. Murphy AA. Clinical aspects of endometriosis. Ann N Y Acad Sci 2002;955:1-10; discussion 34-36, 396-406.

420. Prentice A. Regular review: Endometriosis. BMJ 2001;323:93-95.

421. Woodward PJ, Sohaey R, Mezzetti TP, Jr. Endometriosis: radiologic-pathologic correlation. Radiographics 2001;21:193-216.

422. Olive DL, Pritts EA. The treatment of endometriosis: a review of the evidence. Ann N Y Acad Sci 2002;955:360-372; discussion 389-393, 396-406.

423. Olive DL, Pritts EA. Treatment of endometriosis. N Engl J Med 2001;345:266-275.

424. Jenkins S, Olive DL, Haney AF. Endometriosis: pathogenetic implications of the anatomic distribution. Obstet Gynecol 1986;67:335-338.

425. Nirula R, Greaney GC. Incisional endometriosis: an underappreciated diagnosis in general surgery. J Am Coll Surg 2000;190:404-407.

426. Dwivedi AJ, Agrawal SN, Silva YJ. Abdominal wall endometriomas. Dig Dis Sci 2002;47:456-461.

427. Gougoutas CA, Siegelman ES, Hunt J, Outwater EK. Pelvic endometriosis: various manifestations and MR imaging findings. AJR Am J Roentgenol 2000;175:353-358.

428. Zanardi R, Del Frate C, Zuiani C, Del Frate G, Bazzocchi M. Staging of pelvic endometriosis using magnetic resonance imaging compared with the laparoscopic classification of the American Fertility Society: a prospective study. Radiol Med (Torino) 2003;105: 326-338.

429. Bis KG, Vrachliotis TG, Agrawal R, Shetty AN, Maximovich A, Hricak H. Pelvic endometriosis: MR imaging spectrum with laparoscopic correlation and diagnostic pitfalls. Radiographics 1997;17:639-655.

430. Porpora MG, Koninckx PR, Piazze J, Natili M, Colagrande S, Cosmi EV. Correlation between endometriosis and pelvic pain. J Am Assoc Gynecol Laparosc 1999;6:429-434.

431. Stratton P, Winkel C, Premkumar A, et al. Diagnostic accuracy of laparoscopy, magnetic resonance imaging, and histopathologic examination for the detection of endometriosis. Fertil Steril 2003;79:1078-1085.

432. Sugimura K, Okizuka H, Imaoka I, et al. Pelvic endometriosis: detection and diagnosis with chemical shift MR imaging. Radiology 1993;188:435-438.

433. Takahashi K, Okada M, Okada S, Kitao M, Imaoka I, Sugimura K. Studies on the detection of small endometrial implants by magnetic resonance imaging using a fat saturation technique. Gynecol Obstet Invest 1996;41:203-206.

434. Kier R, Smith RC, McCarthy SM. Value of lipid- and water-suppression MR images in distinguishing between blood and lipid within ovarian masses. AJR Am J Roentgenol 1992;158:321-325.

435. Glastonbury CM. The shading sign. Radiology 2002;224:199-201.

436. Sugimura K, Okizuka H, Kaji Y, et al. MRI in predicting the response of ovarian endometriomas to hormone therapy. J Comput Assist Tomogr 1996;20:145-150.

437. Outwater E, Schiebler ML, Owen RS, Schnall MD. Characterization of hemorrhagic adnexal lesions with MR imaging: blinded reader study. Radiology 1993;186:489-494.

438. Togashi K, Nishimura K, Kimura I, et al. Endometrial cysts: diagnosis with MR imaging. Radiology 1991;180:73-78.

439. Outwater EK, Siegelman ES, Chiowanich P, Kilger AM, Dunton CJ, Talerman A. Dilated fallopian tubes: MR imaging characteristics. Radiology 1998;208:463-469.

440. Siegelman ES, Outwater E, Wang T, Mitchell DG. Solid pelvic masses caused by endometriosis: MR imaging features. AJR Am J Roentgenol 1994;163:357-361.

441. Shook TE, Nyberg LM. Endometriosis of the urinary tract. Urology 1988;31:1-6.

442. Jenkins S, Olive DL, Haney AF. Endometriosis: pathogenetic implications of the anatomic distribution. Obstet Gynecol 1986;67:335-338.

443. Vercellini P, Frontino G, Pisacreta A, De Giorgi O, Cattaneo M, Crosignani PG. The pathogenesis of bladder detrusor endometriosis. Am J Obstet Gynecol 2002;187:538-542.

444. Umaria N, Olliff JF. MRI appearances of bladder endometriosis. Br J Radiol 2000;73:733-736.

445. Mostoufizadeh M, Scully RE. Malignant tumors arising in endometriosis. Clin Obstet Gynecol 1980;23:951-963.

446. Erzen M, Rakar S, Klancnik B, Syrjanen K, Klancar B. Endometriosis-associated ovarian carcinoma (EAOC): an entity distinct from other ovarian carcinomas as suggested by a nested case-control study. Gynecol Oncol 2001;83:100-108.

447. Sato N, Tsunoda H, Nishida M, et al. Loss of heterozygosity on 10q23.3 and mutation of the tumor suppressor gene PTEN in benign endometrial cyst of the ovary: possible sequence progression from benign endometrial cyst to endometrioid carcinoma and clear cell carcinoma of the ovary. Cancer Res 2000;60:7052-7056.

448. Swiersz LM. Role of endometriosis in cancer and tumor development. Ann N Y Acad Sci 2002;955:281-292; discussion 293-295, 396-406.

449. Tanaka YO, Yoshizako T, Nishida M, Yamaguchi M, Sugimura K, Itai Y. Ovarian carcinoma in patients with endometriosis: MR imaging findings. AJR Am J Roentgenol 2000;175:1423-1430.

450. Matsuoka Y, Ohtomo K, Araki T, Kojima K, Yoshikawa W, Fuwa S. MR imaging of clear cell carcinoma of the ovary. Eur Radiol 2001;11:946-951.

451. Ovalle F, Azziz R. Insulin resistance, polycystic ovary syndrome, and type 2 diabetes mellitus. Fertil Steril 2002;77:1095-1105.

452. Ben-Rafael Z, Orvieto R. Polycystic ovary syndrome: a single gene mutation or an evolving set of symptoms. Curr Opin Obstet Gynecol 2000;12:169-173.

453. Turhan NO, Toppare MF, Seckin NC, Dilmen G. The predictive power of endocrine tests for the diagnosis of polycystic ovaries in women with oligoamenorrhea. Gynecol Obstet Invest 1999;48:183-186.

454. Nardo LG, Rai R. Metformin therapy in the management of polycystic ovary syndrome: endocrine, metabolic and reproductive effects. Gynecol Endocrinol 2001;15:373-380.

455. Smith S, Pfeifer SM, Collins JA. Diagnosis and management of female infertility. JAMA 2003;290:1767-1770.

456. Lakhani K, Seifalian AM, Atiomo WU, Hardiman P. Polycystic ovaries. Br J Radiol 2002;75:9-16.

457. Kimura I, Togashi K, Kawakami S, et al. Polycystic ovaries: implications of diagnosis with MR imaging. Radiology 1996;201:549-552.

458. Battaglia C, Genazzani AD, Salvatori M, et al. Doppler, ultrasonographic and endocrinological environment with regard to the number of small subcapsular follicles in polycystic ovary syndrome. Gynecol Endocrinol 1999;13:123-129.

459. Mitchell DG, Gefter WB, Spritzer CE, et al. Polycystic ovaries: MR imaging. Radiology 1986;160:425-429.

460. Fulghesu AM, Ciampelli M, Belosi C, Apa R, Pavone V, Lanzone A. A new ultrasound criterion for the diagnosis of polycystic ovary syndrome: the ovarian stroma/total area ratio. Fertil Steril 2001;76:326-331.

461. Koninckx PR, Renaer M, Brosens IA. Origin of peritoneal fluid in women: an ovarian exudation product. Br J Obstet Gynaecol 1980;87:177-183.

462. Jain KA. Imaging of peritoneal inclusion cysts. AJR Am J Roentgenol 2000;174:1559-1563.

463. Kim JS, Lee HJ, Woo SK, Lee TS. Peritoneal inclusion cysts and their relationship to the ovaries: evaluation with sonography. Radiology 1997;204:481-484.

464. Kurachi H, Murakami T, Nakamura H, et al. Imaging of peritoneal pseudocysts: value of MR imaging compared with sonography and CT. AJR Am J Roentgenol 1993;161:589-591.

465. Nozawa S, Iwata T, Yamashita H, et al. Gonadotropin-releasing hormone analogue therapy for peritoneal inclusion cysts after gynecological surgery. J Obstet Gynaecol Res 2000;26:389-393.

466. Tsai CC, Shen CC, Changchien CC, et al. Ultrasound-guided transvaginal cyst aspiration for the management of pelvic pseudocyst: a preliminary experience. Chang Gung Med J 2002;25:751-757.

467. Samaha M, Woodruff JD. Paratubal cysts: frequency, histogenesis, and associated clinical features. Obstet Gynecol 1985;65:691-694.

468. Alpern MB, Sandler MA, Madrazo BL. Sonographic features of parovarian cysts and their complications. AJR Am J Roentgenol 1984;143:157-160.

469. Vlahakis-Miliaras E, Miliaras D, Koutsoumis G, Miliaras S, Spyridakis I, Papadopoulos MS. Paratubal cysts in young females as an incidental finding in laparotomies performed for right lower quadrant abdominal pain. Pediatr Surg Int 1998;13:141-142.

470. Wittich AC. Hydatid of morgagni with torsion diagnosed during cesarean delivery: a case report. J Reprod Med 2002;47:680-682.

471. Kishimoto K, Ito K, Awaya H, Matsunaga N, Outwater EK, Siegelman ES. Paraovarian cyst: MR imaging features. Abdom Imaging 2002;27:685-689.

472. Kim JS, Woo SK, Suh SJ, Morettin LB. Sonographic diagnosis of paraovarian cysts: value of detecting a separate ipsilateral ovary. AJR Am J Roentgenol 1995;164:1441-1444.

473. Barloon TJ, Brown BP, Abu-Yousef MM, Warnock NG. Paraovarian and paratubal cysts: preoperative diagnosis using transabdominal and transvaginal sonography. J Clin Ultrasound 1996;24:117-122.

474. Raza S, Klapholz H, Benacerraf BR. Tarlov cysts: a cause of complex bilateral adnexal masses on pelvic sonography. J Ultrasound Med 1994;13:803-805.

475. McClure MJ, Atri M, Haider MA, Murphy J. Perineural cysts presenting as complex adnexal cystic masses on transvaginal sonography. AJR Am J Roentgenol 2001;177:1313-1318.

476. Voyadzis JM, Bhargava P, Henderson FC. Tarlov cysts: a study of 10 cases with review of the literature. J Neurosurg 2001;95:25-32.

477. Eckert LO, Hawes SE, Wolner-Hanssen PK, et al. Endometritis: the clinical-pathologic syndrome. Am J Obstet Gynecol 2002;186:690-695.

478. Sam JW, Jacobs JE, Birnbaum BA. Spectrum of CT findings in acute pyogenic pelvic inflammatory disease. Radiographics 2002;22:1327-1334.

479. Risser WL, Risser JM, Cromwell PF. Pelvic inflammatory disease in adolescents: a review. Tex Med 2002;98:36-40.

480. Padian NS, Washington AE. Pelvic inflammatory disease. A brief overview. Ann Epidemiol 1994;4:128-132.

481. Henry-Suchet J. PID: clinical and laparoscopic aspects. Ann N Y Acad Sci 2000;900:301-308.

482. Tukeva TA, Aronen HJ, Karjalainen PT, Molander P, Paavonen T, Paavonen J. MR imaging in pelvic inflammatory disease: comparison with laparoscopy and US. Radiology 1999;210:209-216.

483. Ha HK, Lim GY, Cha ES, et al. MR imaging of tubo-ovarian abscess. Acta Radiol 1995;36:510-514.

484. Noone TC, Semelka RC, Worawattanakul S, Marcos HB. Intraperitoneal abscesses: diagnostic accuracy of and appearances at MR imaging. Radiology 1998;208:525-528.

485. Strohbehn K, Quint LE, Prince MR, Wojno KJ, Delancey JO. Magnetic resonance imaging anatomy of the female urethra: a direct histologic comparison. Obstet Gynecol 1996;88:750-756.

486. Kim JK, Kim YJ, Choo MS, Cho KS. The urethra and its supporting structures in women with stress urinary incontinence: MR imaging using an endovaginal coil. AJR Am J Roentgenol 2003;180:1037-1044.

487. Aronson MP, Bates SM, Jacoby AF, Chelmow D, Sant GR. Periurethral and paravaginal anatomy: an endovaginal magnetic resonance imaging study. Am J Obstet Gynecol 1995;173:1702-1708; discussion 1708-1710.

488. Siegelman ES, Banner MP, Ramchandani P, Schnall MD. Multicoil MR imaging of symptomatic female urethral and periurethral disease. Radiographics 1997;17:349-365.

489. Soucek M, Carr JJ, Schnall MD, Malkowicz SB, Tomaszewski JE. MR imaging with endorectal surface and multi-array coils in evaluation of lesions of bladder neck, proximal urethra, and posterior bladder wall. Radiology 1994;193(P):167-168.

490. Tan IL, Stoker J, Lameris JS. Magnetic resonance imaging of the female pelvic floor and urethra: body coil versus endovaginal coil. Magma 1997;5:59-63.

491. Quick HH, Serfaty JM, Pannu HK, Genadry R, Yeung CJ, Atalar E. Endourethral MRI. Magn Reson Med 2001;45:138-146.

492. Ryu J, Kim B. MR imaging of the male and female urethra. Radiographics 2001;21:1169-1185.

493. Romanzi LJ, Groutz A, Blaivas JG. Urethral diverticulum in women: diverse presentations resulting in diagnostic delay and mismanagement. J Urol 2000;164:428-433.

494. Fortunato P, Schettini M, Gallucci M. Diagnosis and therapy of the female urethral diverticula. Int Urogynecol J Pelvic Floor Dysfunct 2001;12:51-57.

495. Blander DS, Rovner ES, Schnall MD, et al. Endoluminal magnetic resonance imaging in the evaluation of urethral diverticula in women. Urology 2001;57:660-665.

496. Kim B, Hricak H, Tanagho EA. Diagnosis of urethral diverticula in women: value of MR imaging. AJR Am J Roentgenol 1993;161:809-815.

497. Neitlich JD, Foster HE, Glickman MG, Smith RC. Detection of urethral diverticula in women: comparison of a high resolution fast spin echo technique with double balloon urethrography. J Urol 1998;159:408-410.

498. Daneshgari F, Zimmern PE, Jacomides L. Magnetic resonance imaging detection of symptomatic noncommunicating intraurethral wall diverticula in women. J Urol 1999;161:1259-1261; discussion 1261-1262.

499. Khati NJ, Javitt MC, Schwartz AM, Berger BM. MR imaging diagnosis of a urethral diverticulum. Radiographics 1998;18:517-522.

500. Nurenberg P, Zimmern PE. Role of MR imaging with transrectal coil in the evaluation of complex urethral abnormalities. AJR Am J Roentgenol 1997;169:1335-1338.

501. Hickey N, Murphy J, Herschorn S. Carcinoma in a urethral diverticulum: magnetic resonance imaging and sonographic appearance. Urology 2000;55:588-589.

502. Reuter KL, Young SB, Davidoff A, Colby JM. Magnetic resonance imaging of an infected urethral diverticulum: a case report. Magn Reson Imaging 1991;9:955-957.

503. Rovner ES, Wein AJ. Diagnosis and reconstruction of the dorsal or circumferential urethral diverticulum. J Urol 2003;170:82-86; discussion 86.

504. Bell CR, Gujral S, Collins CM, Sibley GN, Persad RA. Review: the fate of the urethra after definitive treatment of invasive transitional cell carcinoma of the urinary bladder. BJU Int 1999;83:607-612.

505. Milosevic MF, Warde PR, Banerjee D, et al. Urethral carcinoma in women: results of treatment with primary radiotherapy. Radiother Oncol 2000;56:29-35.

506. Eng TY, Naguib M, Galang T, Fuller CD. Retrospective study of the treatment of urethral cancer. Am J Clin Oncol 2003;26:558-562.

507. Maki DD, Banner MP, Ramchandani P, Stolpen A, Rovner ES, Wein AJ. Injected periurethral collagen for postprostatectomy urinary incontinence: MR and CT appearance. Abdom Imaging 2000;25:658-662.

508. Appell RA. Surgery or collagen for the treatment of female stress urinary incontinence: results of a multicenter, randomized trial supports either as first line of treatment. Curr Urol Rep 2001;2:343.

509. Kershen RT, Dmochowski RR, Appell RA. Beyond collagen: injectable therapies for the treatment of female stress urinary incontinence in the new millennium. Urol Clin North Am 2002;29:559-574.

510. Hussain SM, Outwater EK, Siegelman ES. Mucinous versus nonmucinous rectal carcinomas: differentiation with MR imaging. Radiology 1999;213:79-85.

Fetal MRI

Anne M. Hubbard, MD

BACKGROUND

The use of MRI in the evaluation of the developing fetus was revolutionized by the introduction of ultrafast scans developed for adult abdominal MR imaging.[1] Before the development of ultrafast scans, maternal sedation or fetal paralysis was required to eliminate fetal motion and obtain diagnostic images. In the 1990s, faster imaging sequences were developed including half-Fourier acquisition single-shot turbo spin-echo (HASTE) and echo-planar imaging (EPI).[2] These sequences acquire a single slice in less than 400 msec that decrease or eliminate the artifacts caused by fetal motion.

Ultrafast MR imaging is useful for fetal evaluation and reveals detailed and reproducible fetal anatomy.[3-6] MRI is most useful in evaluation of abnormalities of the fetal brain, neck, chest, and abdomen. MR can add additional diagnostic information to sonography in fetuses for which prenatal intervention is being considered.[7] The extremities are not well evaluated with MRI because of motion. Imaging evaluation prior to 18 weeks' gestation is difficult because of the small size of the fetus.

Safety is paramount in evaluating the fetus. To date, no known harmful effects to the developing human fetus have been documented using clinical scanners at field strengths of 1.5 tesla or less.[8] However, safety has not been proved. Animal studies have been performed looking at the effects of radiofrequency (RF) fields on fetal development.[9] Even at high levels, well above maximum permissible human guidelines, consistent morphologic or organ abnormalities have not been identified.[9] Evaluation of health care workers employed in MRI showed no increased incidence of fetal anomalies or spontaneous abortion compared with controls.[10] In utero exposure to echo planar imaging has not been shown to have any effect on fetal growth.[11] One long-term follow-up of children who were imaged in utero showed no demonstrable increase in occurrence of disease.[12]

Heat is a major safety concern. One study evaluated heating affects of MRI with HASTE imaging in a pregnant pig model.[13] Fiberoptic probes showed no heating occurred in the fetal tissues or amniotic fluid during HASTE imaging. Animal models may not be adequate to evaluate human RF deposition and heating, since RF deposition is related to the size, shape, and position of the patient.

As further improvements in MRI technology provide even faster imaging techniques and higher resolution, the applications for fetal imaging will increase. At present, MRI is an adjunct to prenatal US. Fetal MRI provides significant additional information that can affect the accuracy of diagnosis, prenatal counseling, management, prenatal intervention, and delivery planning.

FETAL MRI TECHNIQUE

At the author's institution, MRI is performed in a 1.5 T magnet using a phased array body coil. A phased array surface coil may not accommodate some women who are in the third trimester of pregnancy; body coil imaging may be performed in these patients.[14] The pregnant woman is positioned supine, with the feet placed first into the magnet to minimize claustrophobia. The imaging sequences are obtained are listed in Box 8-1. Similar MRI protocols have been published.[8] The examination takes approximately 40 minutes. Contrast agents are not used in pregnant patients, because gadolinium crosses the placenta. The toxicity of gadolinium to the human fetus is not known. Toxicity has been demonstrated in animal studies, with increased incidence of fetal death and abnormalities.[15]

8-1 Fetal MR Imaging Techniques

T2-weighted Sequence

Subsecond ("ultrafast") technique preferred to minimize artifacts from fetal motion and maternal bowel peristalsis

Suggested parameters: TR = 4400 msec, TE = 64 msec, FA = 150° to 180°, thickness = 4 mm slice

Perform axial, coronal, and sagittal to fetus

Best single sequence for fetal evaluation

Signal Intensity

Very high SI tissues: amniotic fluid, stomach, proximal bowel, gall bladder, urinary bladder, CSF, oropharynx, trachea

Moderate to high SI: lung parenchyma

Intermediate SI: brain, muscles, soft tissues, kidneys, placenta

Low SI: liver

Very low SI: meconium, heart, flowing blood, umbilical cord, calcification

T2-weighted Sequence with Longer TE

Suggested parameters: TR = 400 msec, TE = 95 msec FA = 180°, thickness = 3 mm

Perform sagittal, coronal, and axial to fetal brain

Sequence performed to specifically evaluate the CSF and abnormalities of myelination and migration; poor visualization of remainder of fetus

T1-W GRE Sequence

Suggested parameters: TR = 174 msec, TE = 4.1 msec, FA = 80°, thickness = 4 to 5 mm

Perform sagittal and coronal to fetus

Signal Intensity

High SI: liver and meconium

Will show high SI methemoglobin within hemorrhage

Echo Planar Imaging

Suggested parameters: TR = 800 msec, TE = 56 msec, FA = 90°, thickness = 4 to 5 mm

Perform axial to fetus

Fastest of all sequences, useful for evaluation of moving fetus

Limited by susceptibility artifacts from maternal gas, iron from vitamins, fat

Ideal to use for skeletal anatomy

Signal Intensity

Very low SI: cortical bone, hemorrhage, and calcification

CENTRAL NERVOUS SYSTEM

Ultrasonography (US) is the primary screening modality for evaluation of the fetus. There are pitfalls in the evaluation of the fetal brain and spine with US.[16] The normal and abnormal appearance of the brain on US is based on the ability to obtain specific images of the cerebrum, cerebellum, and spine. Maternal obesity, oligohydramnios, or a suboptimal fetal lie may cause inability to obtain adequate US images. MRI is less affected by these factors. MRI changed the diagnosis and management in up to 40% of fetuses with CNS abnormalities suspected on prior sonography.[17-20]

Normal Brain Maturation

MRI has made a significant impact on the evaluation of the fetal brain, providing more specific information about normal development. Myelination of the fetal brain can be evaluated in vivo. MRI reveals changes in the developing brain due to neuronal migration, gyral formation, and myelination. In vitro MRI shows specific patterns of growth that correlate with known anatomic developments based on pathologic specimens.[21] At 16 to 20 weeks' gestation, the cerebral surface is relatively smooth, with minimal infolding of the sylvian fissures (Fig. 8-1). With brain maturation, increased sulcation is clearly depicted.[22,23] Appearance of specific sulci can be used as an indicator of fetal maturity (Fig 8-2).[24] The in utero MRI visualization of specific sulci lags 2 to 3 weeks behind the visualization in fetal pathologic specimens.[25,26] A multilayered pattern of brain parenchyma corresponding to cellular migration has been shown with in vivo MRI (Fig. 8-3). Normal migration of the parenchymal layers, gray matter, early myelination of the internal capsule, optic radiations, and corona radiata have been shown in the second and third trimesters in vivo. MRI depicts SI changes corresponding to both increased cellularity and maturing myelination.[27] The fast imaging with steady-state free precession technique (TruFISP) is used to evaluate brain maturation. HASTE and TruFISP provide comparable imaging quality in the second trimester when there is little myelination. Myelination in the third trimester is better revealed with TruFISP imaging as hypointense bands. Cortical sulcation is equally shown on both sequences.[28]

MRI has shown normal development of the fetal skull base that correlates with pathologic studies.[29] The width of the posterior cranial fossa increases disproportionately to the length. The growth of

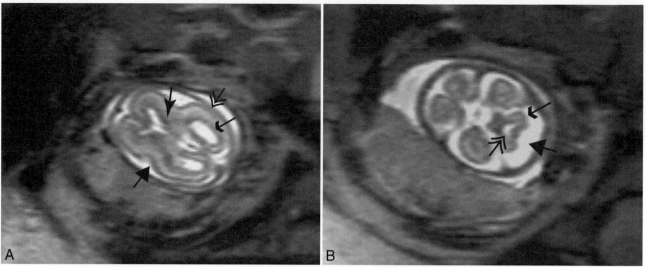

Figure 8-1 ■ **MR findings of a normal 21-week fetal brain. A,** Axial T2-WI of the midventricular level shows the normal appearance of the immature brain. The cortical surface is smooth with minimal infolding of the sylvian fissures *(large arrow)*. The germinal matrix *(curved arrow)* lining the ventricular system is hypointense. There are three discrete parenchymal zones: periventricular *(small arrow)*, cortical *(double arrow)*, and intermediate. **B,** Axial T2-WI through the posterior fossa shows a normal prominent cisterna magna *(large arrow)*, a normal fourth ventricle *(double arrow)*, and normal cerebellar hemispheres *(small arrow)*. (Note: all T2-WIs in this chapter use the half-Fourier acquisition single-shot turbo spin-echo [HASTE] technique.)

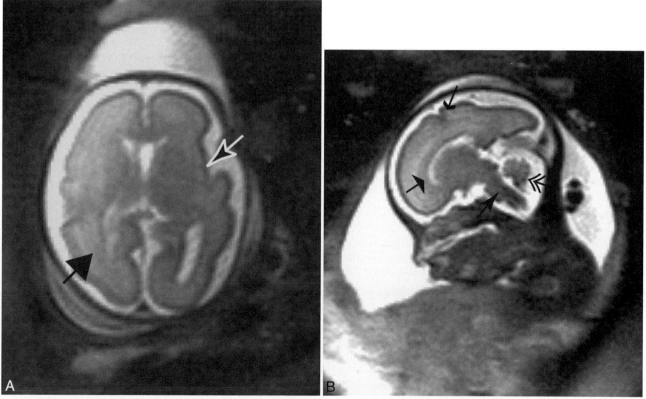

Figure 8-2 ■ **Normal 29-week fetal brain as shown on MRI. A,** Axial T2-WI through the level of the sylvian fissure *(white arrow)* shows increased sulcation of the cortex and increasing complexity of the intermediate zone *(large arrow)*. **B,** Sagittal T2-WI through the midline shows brainstem *(curved arrow)*, cerebellum *(double arrow)*, a well-developed corpus callosum *(broad arrow)*, and increased sulcation of the parietal lobe *(small arrow)*.

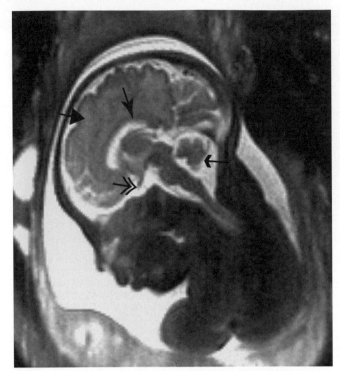

Figure 8-3 ■ MR depiction of a normal 34-week fetal brain. Midline sagittal T2-WI shows increasing size of the cerebellum *(small arrow)* with a well-developed vermis. There is marked infolding of the cortical sulci with increasing complexity of the intermediate zone *(large arrow).* The pituitary stalk is present *(double arrow).* There is a normal corpus callosum *(curved arrow).*

cases of lissencephaly, 73% of polymicrogyria, and 100% of schizencephaly prenatally.[33] Polymicrogyria, the presence of increased number of small gyri, has been documented in utero.[17,32] Polymicrogyria may result from injury to normal cellular interactions at the external limiting membrane, the pial-glial barrier. The most common form of injury is thought to be ischemia.[32] Schizencephaly is a neuronal migration anomaly characterized by gray matter–lined clefts extending from the ventricle to the cortical surface. The lips of the clefts may be fused or separate. Prognosis is related to the amount of cortex involved. The cause may be genetic or ischemic. The defect is better visualized and characterized with MRI.[34] Although in most cases, the abnormality can be documented in the third trimester, it is hoped that abnormalities in neuronal migration will be documented earlier in fetal life.

Ventriculomegaly

Ventriculomegaly is the most common reason for MRI evaluation of the fetal CNS. The criterion for determination of enlargement of the ventricles on US is an atrial measurement greater than 10 mm in width on the transverse image of the brain. Mild-to-moderate enlargement of the ventricles is frequently associated with other anomalies.[35] Outcomes of fetuses born with hydrocephalus reveal normal intelligence in only 50% to 60%. Associated CNS abnormalities have been diagnosed in 84% of fetuses with hydrocephalus. In those cases with severe, rapidly

the anterior skull base is almost twice that of the posterior skull base, and the increases in the width of the posterior cranial fossa exceed the increases in length. MR has shown that the differential growth of the cerebral and cerebellar components of the brain is related to the inferoposterior rotation of the tentorium cerebelli toward the posterior cranial base.[30] This developmental information may result in earlier and more accurate diagnosis of abnormalities. An US study evaluated the clivus to supraocciput angle as a measure of development of the posterior fossa.[31] The angle did not change during gestation in normal fetuses (average value of 79°). All cases of Chiari type II malformations showed a value below the fifth percentile. This may help differentiate ventriculomegaly caused by Chiari malformation from other etiologies. The same measurements can be made on MRI.

Abnormalities of Neuronal Migration

Abnormalities of neuronal migration were previously thought to be rare. However, with MRI they are seen in more than 20% of postnatal diagnoses of CNS anomalies (Fig. 8-4).[32] Abnormalities of neuronal migration may be isolated or be present in association with other cerebral anomalies. MRI visualized areas of heterotopic brain in 54% of third trimester fetuses with a postnatal diagnosis of migrational disorder. Third trimester MRI demonstrated 80% of

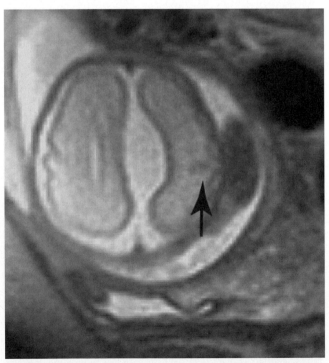

Figure 8-4 ■ MR illustration of gray matter heterotopia in a 25-week fetus. Axial T2-WI through the lateral ventricles shows an area of low SI *(arrow)* in the subcortical area consistent with heterotopic brain with asymmetric infolding of the cortical sulci. There is agenesis of the corpus callosum.

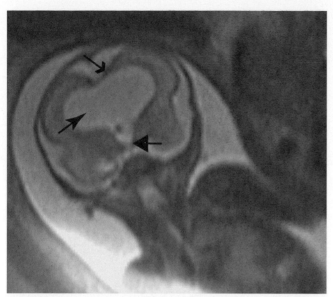

Figure 8-5 ■ **MR demonstration of aqueductal stenosis in a 25-week fetus.** Coronal T2-WI shows dilation of the lateral *(curved arrow)* and the proximal third *(large arrow)* ventricles. There is thinning of the parietal cortex *(small arrow)* that can be present secondary to pressure necrosis or ischemia.

progressing hydrocephalus, there is invariably poor postnatal outcome.[36] MRI is more accurate than US in determining the cause of ventriculomegaly and identifying associated CNS anomalies.[17]

Counseling for mild fetal ventriculomegaly is difficult. No large, long-term follow-up studies document outcome. One study reviewed 26 cases of mild

ventriculomegaly (atria 10 to 15 mm). There was no developmental delay at 2 years of age in fetuses that had regressive ventriculomegaly. Developmental delay occurred in 15% of fetus that developed ventriculomegaly at any time during gestation that did not regress. In fetuses that developed ventriculomegaly in the third trimester, 50% had developmental delay. Late-onset ventriculomegaly has a worse prognosis.[37] The MR findings of congenital aqueductal stenosis are dilation of the lateral and third ventricles and a normal-size fourth ventricle (Fig. 8-5). There is usually obliteration of the subarachnoid space.[17]

Ventriculomegaly may be due to ischemic or infectious events that cause cerebral atrophy (Fig. 8-6). There may be unilateral or bilateral enlargement of the lateral ventricles. There may be associated porencephaly (Fig. 8-7).[38] There is frequently

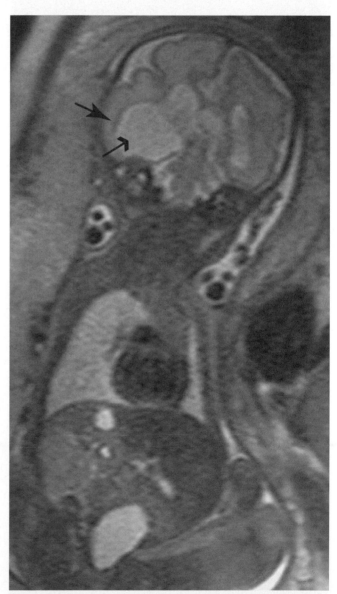

Figure 8-7 ■ **MR demonstration of porencephaly in a 32-week fetus.** Coronal T2-WI through the lateral ventricles shows asymmetry in ventricle size with more focal dilation of the right temporal horn *(small arrow)* and thinning of the cortex *(curved arrow)*.

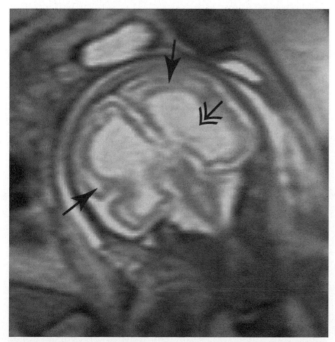

Figure 8-6 ■ **MR findings of cystic encephalomalacia in a 31-week fetus.** Coronal T2-WI through dilated lateral ventricles *(double arrow)* shows thin heterogeneous SI in the thinned intermediate zoned *(curved arrows)*.

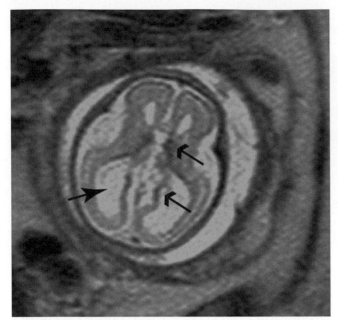

Figure 8-8 ■ MR findings of ischemic hemorrhage following co-twin demise imaged at 25 weeks. Axial T2-WI shows mild ventricular dilation *(curved arrow)* with enlargement of the extra-axial space and mild diffuse cortical thinning. There are areas of low SI *(small arrows)* in the periventricular zone consistent with hemorrhage.

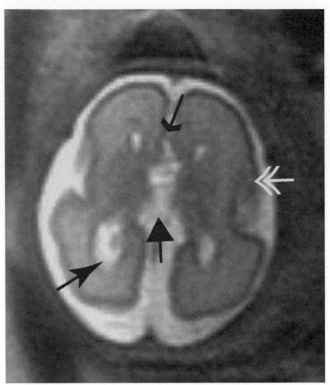

Figure 8-9 ■ MR appearance of agenesis of the corpus callosum in a 28-week fetus. Axial T2-WI shows absence of normal white matter fibers *(small arrow)* crossing the midline. There is widening of the interhemispheric fissure *(large arrow)*, mild colpocephaly with dilation of the occipital horns *(curved arrow)* of the lateral ventricles, and heterotopic gray matter *(double white arrow)*.

enlargement of the extra axial spaces with cerebral atrophy. With postischemic or postinflammatory changes in the brain, there may be irregularity of the ventricular surfaces.

The frequency of in utero cerebral ischemic injuries is not known. Fourteen percent of perinatal deaths in one study were associated with ischemic changes.[39] Ischemic injury to the fetal brain has a variable appearance. The morphology depends on the area affected and the amount of time between the insult and MR imaging.[40] MRI findings include ventricular dilation, microcephaly, hydroencephaly, porencephaly, multicystic encephalomalacia, capsular ischemia, periventricular leukoencephalomalacia with cyst formation, and corpus callosum and cerebral atrophy. MRI is superior to US in demonstrating these changes before birth (Fig. 8-8).

Abnormalities of the Corpus Callosum

Abnormalities of the corpus callosum are often diagnosed on prenatal imaging. There may be complete or partial absence of the corpus callosum. The corpus callosum is normally well developed by 20 weeks, so major abnormalities of the corpus callosum should be present on prenatal MRI (Fig. 8-9). MR reveals associated CNS abnormalities in 60% of patients.[33] MR and US appearance of complete absence of the corpus callosum is similar. There is increased separation of the bodies of the lateral ventricles and upward displacement of the third ventricle, with or without an associated interhemispheric cyst.[33] There is lack of connecting white matter fibers between the cerebral

hemispheres. Partial absence of the corpus callosum may be difficult to diagnose on US. The lack of development of the posterior corpus callosum or thinning is shown with MRI. Arachnoid cysts occur in the midline in the area of the roof of the third ventricle and may be misinterpreted as agenesis of the corpus callosum (Fig. 8-10). MRI can differentiate these two conditions by revealing the wall of the cyst and the presence of a normal corpus callosum.

Holoprosencephaly

Holoprosencephaly is a malformation of the prosencephalon with failure of normal midline cleavage, frequently associated with incomplete midface development. The severe forms, semilobar and alobar holoprosencephaly, are easily diagnosed because of the presence of a monoventricle and obvious fusion of the cerebral hemispheres (Fig. 8-11). MRI is most helpful to distinguish the lobar form of holoprosencephaly from other causes of ventriculomegaly and hydrocephalus.[33,41] In lobar holoprosencephaly there is a falx and some separation of the cerebral hemispheres. In all forms of holoprosencephaly there is some fusion of the thalami and rostral portion of the brain.

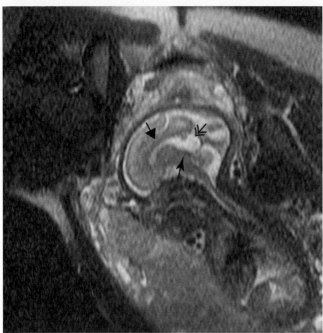

Figure 8-10 ▪ **MR illustration of an arachnoid cyst of the roof of the third ventricle in a 29-week fetus.** Sagittal T2-WI shows a cyst *(double arrow)* in the area of the roof of the third ventricle. The corpus callosum *(large arrow)* and aqueduct *(curved arrow)* are normal.

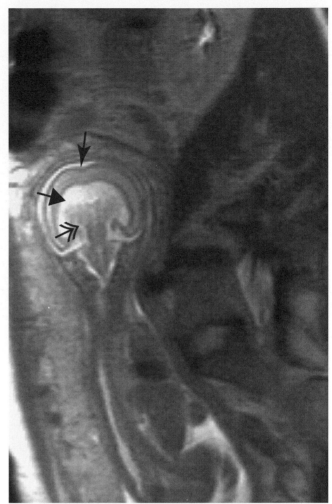

Figure 8-11 ▪ **MR illustration of holoprosencephaly in a 22-week fetus.** Coronal T2-WI shows a large monoventricle *(large arrow)* with no division of the cortex *(curved arrow)* in the midline. The thalami are fused *(double arrow)*.

Vein of Galen Malformation

Vein of Galen malformation is uncommon but is the most common cerebrovascular malformation diagnosed prenatally because the large vein is easy to identify and congestive heart failure is frequently present. A midline mass of low SI is revealed in the region of the dilated straight sinus and vein of Galen on both T1- and T2-WIs secondary to flow within the dilated vascular segments (Fig. 8-12).[42] On US this may be confused with a midline arachnoid cyst or other tumor if Doppler US is not performed. Ventriculomegaly may be present on the basis of obstruction of the third ventricle by the dilated vein, or cerebral atrophy due to a vascular steal phenomenon.

Tuberous Sclerosis (TS)

Tuberous sclerosis (TS) is an autosomal dominant disorder that affects brain, heart, skin, kidneys (see Chapter 4 for a discussion of renal angiomyolipoma), and other organs (Fig. 8-13). Mental retardation and seizures may be mild or severe. Prenatal imaging diagnosis is based on detecting cardiac rhabdomyomas that can be shown in mid–second trimester. The diagnostic accuracy increases with increasing numbers of cardiac rhabdomyomas.[43] Approximately half of patients with postnatal diagnosis of TS have cardiac rhabdomyomas; however, most of these are not present on 20-week gestation US. MRI provides better definition of the periventricular region than does US. Subependymal tubers have been demonstrated in the brain at 21 weeks. The tuber is of low SI on T2-WIs

and high SI on T1-WIs. The lesion may be seen as a defect in the contour of the ventricular wall. Heterotopic brain may be identified in the subcortical region. Hamartomas may not develop in the brain until after birth, which makes screening difficult.[43]

Posterior Fossa Abnormalities

Many abnormalities of the posterior fossa have a poor prognosis.[44] Evaluation of the posterior fossa on US depends on a single-angled axial view through the cerebellar hemispheres and region of the cisterna magna. Dandy-Walker malformation, Dandy-Walker variant, and mega cisterna magna represent a spectrum of developmental abnormalities. Mega cisterna magna demonstrates an intact cerebellar vermis and fourth ventricle with an enlarged posterior fossa cerebrospinal fluid space (Fig. 8-14). Dandy-Walker malformation is agenesis of the inferior vermis, cystic dilation of the fourth ventricle communicating with the cisterna magna, and enlargement of the

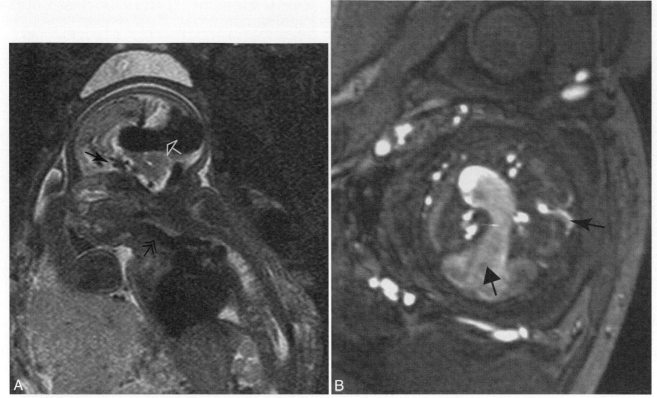

Figure 8-12 ▪ **Vein of Galen malformation in a 34-week fetus revealed by MRI. A,** Sagittal T2-WI shows severe dilation of the straight sinus *(white arrow)* and multiple areas of low SI representing collateral vessels *(curved arrow)*. The heart is enlarged, and there is dilation of the jugular vein *(double arrow)*. **B,** Axial T1-W GRE image shows the enlarged central veins *(large arrow)* and multiple collateral vessels *(curved arrow)*.

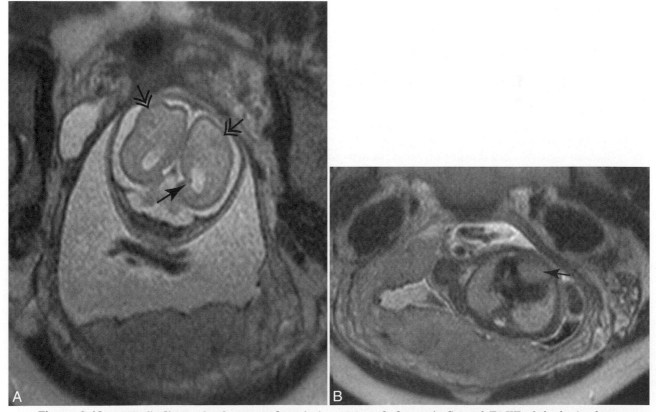

Figure 8-13 ▪ **MR findings of tuberous sclerosis in a 24-week fetus. A,** Coronal T2-WI of the brain shows heterotopic gray matter *(double arrows)* in the subcortical area and a small periventricular nodule *(curved arrow)*. **B,** Axial T2-WI shows a large intermediate SI rhabdomyoma *(arrow)* of the left ventricular wall.

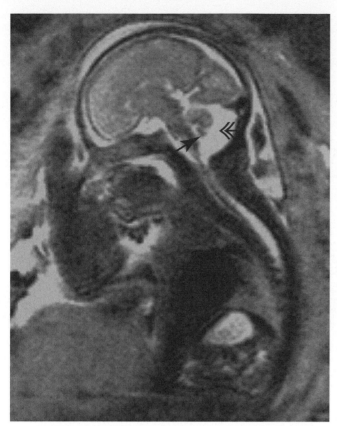

Figure 8-14 ■ **MR illustration of mega cisterna magna in a 28-week fetus.** Sagittal T2-WI though the posterior fossa shows an intact inferior cerebellar vermis *(curved arrow)* and a normal fourth ventricle. The CSF space of the posterior fossa is enlarged *(double arrow).*

posterior fossa with upward displacement of the tentorium (Fig. 8-15).[33] Dandy-Walker variant consists of hypoplasia of the inferior cerebellar vermis, with cystic dilation of the fourth ventricle but without enlargement of the posterior fossa (Fig. 8-16). Isolated mild vermian hypoplasia has a good prognosis. Supratentorial malformations are present in 68% of Dandy-Walker malformations. Hydrocephalus usually develops postnatally. Compared with US, MR better shows the posterior fossa, specifically the vermis, fourth ventricle, and associated abnormalities.[45] MRI differentiates posterior fossa arachnoid cysts from abnormalities of vermian development (Fig. 8-17).

Hematomas have been reported in the tentorium simulating posterior fossa lesions such as Dandy-Walker malformation or arachnoid cysts. Sonography shows a cystic mass with echogenic material and possible thick rim. MRI confirms blood products in the lesion and its position relative to the tentorium and posterior fossa.[46]

Spinal Dysraphism

Various abnormalities of the brain are associated with spinal dysraphism. Ventriculomegaly may be present. The posterior fossa MR findings in Chiari II malformation include a small, cone-shaped posterior fossa, obliteration of the fourth ventricle, and downward herniation of the cerebellar tonsils.[17] Open spina

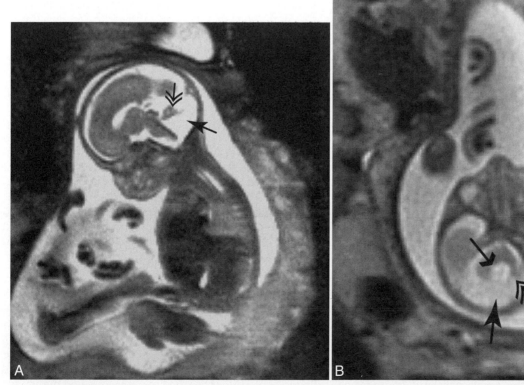

Figure 8-15 ■ **MR illustration of a Dandy-Walker cyst in a 23-week fetus. A,** Sagittal T2-WI shows agenesis of the inferior cerebellar vermis *(double arrow)* and a large cisterna magna *(curved arrow).* **B,** Axial T2-WI shows inferior vermian agenesis *(double arrow).* The dilated fourth ventricle *(small arrow)* communicates with the cisterna magna *(curved arrow).*

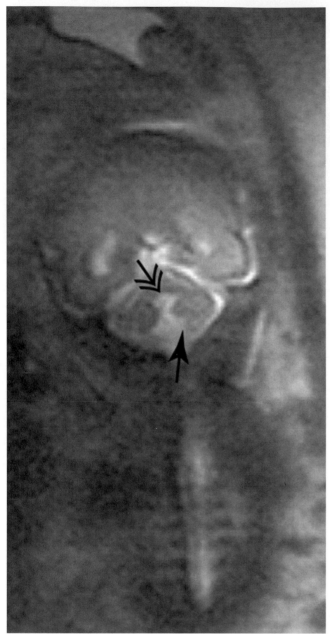

Figure 8-16 ■ MR findings of Dandy-Walker variant in a 30-week fetus. Coronal T2-WI through the posterior fossa demonstrates an intact superior vermis, with mild hypoplasia of the inferior cerebellar vermis *(curved arrow)* and minimal dilation of the fourth ventricle *(double arrow).*

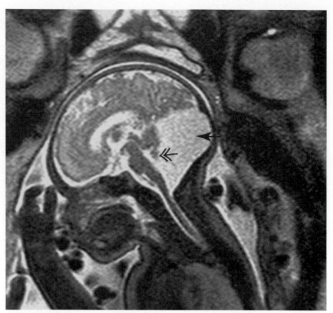

Figure 8-17 ■ MR illustration of a posterior fossa arachnoid cyst in a 34-week fetus. Sagittal T2-WI shows compression of the inferior cerebellar hemisphere *(double arrow)* by a cyst *(curved arrow).* The fourth ventricle is normal.

bifida can be diagnosed with MRI and US. MRI shows a cystic lesion, usually in the lumbosacral spine, with widening of the lamina (Fig. 8-18). There may be a simple meningocele or neural elements within the sac.[47] MRI and US can determine the level of dysraphism. In one study US was more accurate in determining the defect level and evaluating small sacral lesions.[48] MRI has a disadvantage in that spontaneous movement of the lower extremities may be difficult to infer.

In utero fetal surgery can repair meningomyelocele (MMC).[49] Following in utero surgery there is improvement in hindbrain herniation with revisualization of the fourth ventricle and reaccumulation of cerebral spinal fluid within the posterior fossa (Fig. 8-19). Short-term follow-up of patients treated with in utero repair of MMC showed a decreased incidence of postnatal ventricular shunt placement. Only 59% of those treated in utero required shunts, compared to 91% of those who had postnatal MMC closure.[50]

Myelocystoceles represent 5% of skin-covered masses in the lower spine. They may occur in the cervical or sacral region. They are commonly associated with other anomalies, especially midline pelvic and abdominal defects, imperforate anus, caudal regression, and renal anomalies. Myelocystoceles are skin-covered cysts with dilation of the central canal and protrusion of structures through a bony defect. No neural elements are contained within the sac, and the cord ends at a normal level. The posterior fossa structures are usually normal. MRI and US can both differentiate myelocystocele from MMC.[51]

Sacrococcygeal Tumor (SCT)

Sacrococcygeal tumors (SCTs) can be diagnosed in utero. The natural history of prenatal SCT is different from that of neonatal SCT. Prenatal diagnosis has a worse prognosis than do tumors diagnosed in the first year of life.[52] In one series of 17 fetuses with prenatal diagnosis of SCT, three died in utero, one had malignant tumor, one had recurrence of embryonal carcinoma, and

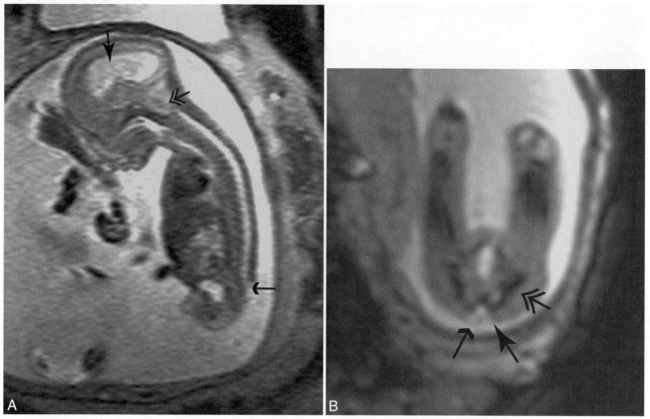

Figure 8-18 ■ **MR findings of a myelomeningocele in a 22-week fetus. A,** Sagittal T2-WI shows mild ventriculomegaly *(curved arrow)* with a small posterior fossa and downward displacement of the cerebellar tonsils *(double arrow)* consistent with Chiari II malformation. In the distal lumbar spine, there are absent posterior spinous processes with a small sac present *(small arrow).* **B,** Axial echo planar T2-WI through L5 shows widening of the lamina *(curved arrow)* with a small thecal sac *(small arrow).* The iliac crests *(double arrow)* are well defined.

two had recurrence with mature histopathology.[53] SCTs arise from the coccyx, are usually benign, and are classified according to the amount of extra or intrapelvic component (Box 8-2 and Fig. 8-20).[54] The classification is important to the surgeon in predicting whether the tumor can be resected. SCT may be cystic, solid, or both (Fig. 8-21). SCT is frequently associated with polyhydramnios. The larger the solid component the more likely the lesion will have increased vascularity. There may be associated hydrops and subsequent fetal demise. Color flow and Doppler US better demonstrate increased flow in the fetal aorta and inferior vena cava (IVC) and increased fetal cardiac output. Poor outcome has been related to the degree of increased vascularity of solid lesions.[55] Size of tumor did not correlate with outcome. MRI correlates well with US in evaluating size of tumor as well as solid versus cystic components. MRI better defines intraspinal and intrapelvic extension of the tumor.[53,56] MRI differentiates predominantly cystic tumors from sacral meningomyelocele. There is rare vascular placental dissemination of SCT with enlargement and inhomogeneity of the placenta.[57]

In fetuses with hydrops, SCT has been successfully removed in utero with resolution of the hydrops. Surgery may also be performed immediately

after delivery.[58] Accurate knowledge of the extension of the tumor into the pelvis, displacement of the urinary bladder, and position of the rectum are important for adequate surgical planning before or at birth.

NECK

Fetal neck masses are uncommon but important to identify, since they may cause life-threatening airway obstruction at birth. The most common neck masses are cystic hygromas, teratomas, and goiters. These lesions can be identified with prenatal US. MRI is used for further characterization of the lesion and delivery planning.[59]

Cystic Hygroma

There are various types of cystic hygromas, a congenital failure of normal cannulation of the lymphatic system.[60] Lesions occurring early in the second trimester in the posterior nuchal region are frequently associated with hydrops and chromosomal abnormalities including trisomy 18, Turner's syndrome, and Down syndrome. Cystic hygromas (also

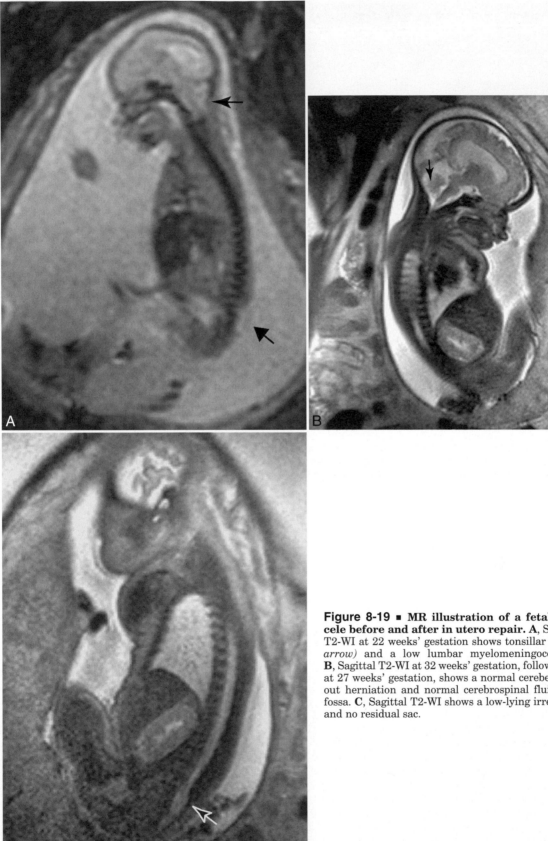

Figure 8-19 ■ **MR illustration of a fetal myelomeningocele before and after in utero repair. A,** Sagittal echo planar T2-WI at 22 weeks' gestation shows tonsillar herniation *(curved arrow)* and a low lumbar myelomeningocele *(large arrow).* **B,** Sagittal T2-WI at 32 weeks' gestation, following in utero repair at 27 weeks' gestation, shows a normal cerebellum *(arrow)* without herniation and normal cerebrospinal fluid in the posterior fossa. **C,** Sagittal T2-WI shows a low-lying irregular cord *(arrow)* and no residual sac.

8-2 Sacrococcygeal Teratoma Staging

Type I	External with small presacral component
Type II	Predominantly external with small intrapelvic component
Type III	Predominantly intrapelvic with small abdominal extension
Type IV	Pelvis and abdomen components, frequently malignant

termed cystic lymphangiomas) of the anterior neck or retropharyngeal area are usually isolated abnormalities. Lymphangiomas may result in morbidity when they infiltrate tissue planes and surround neurovascular structures (Fig. 8-22).[60] Lymphangiomas have a multilocular appearance on MRI with fluid-fluid levels shown on T2-WIs. T1-shortening may be present secondary to intracystic hemorrhage or protein. There may be extension into the anterior mediastinum.[59]

Teratoma

Teratoma of the neck usually occurs in the midline, and 40% contain thyroid tissue.[61] On MRI, these tumors are solid and cystic (Fig. 8-23).[59,62] Occasionally, neck teratomas appear as solitary thick-walled cysts without septations. Calcifications are frequently present in teratomas and are easily identified with US and difficult to show with MRI. Large fetal teratomas often cause hypoplasia of the adjacent facial bones (Fig. 8-24).

CHAOS Syndrome

Congenital high airway obstruction syndrome (CHAOS) is caused by intrinsic complete or partial obstruction of the fetal airway preventing the egress of alveolar fluid from the lungs.[63] The causes include laryngotracheal atresia, laryngeal web, and laryngeal cyst (Fig. 8-25). The prenatal presentation is large, fluid-filled lungs that are echogenic on US with eversion of the diaphragm and dilation of the tracheobronchial tree. The echogenic lungs may be misdiagnosed as bilateral congenital cystic adenomatoid malformation (see next section) although bilateral CCAM is rare. There usually is hydrops with skin and scalp edema and ascites due to compression of the heart and obstruction of venous return. The lungs are large, homogeneous, and very high in SI on T2-WI.[64] The dilated tracheobronchial tree is hyperintense on T2-WI, establishing its fluid content and

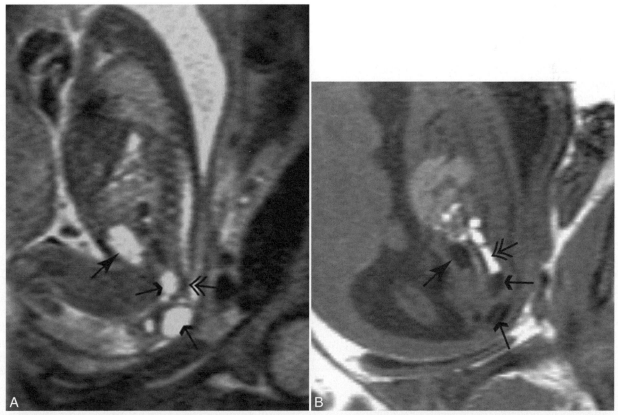

Figure 8-20 ■ MR of a sacrococcygeal teratoma in a 22-week fetus. A, Sagittal T2-WI reveals a multicystic mass *(small arrows)* arising from the distal spine *(double arrow)*. There is intrapelvic extension with superior displacement of the bladder *(curved arrow)*. **B,** Sagittal T1-W GRE image shows a low SI mass *(small arrows)* posterior and inferior to the rectum *(double arrow)* with superior displacement of the bladder *(curved arrow)*.

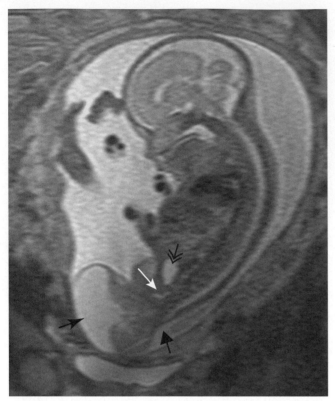

Figure 8-21 ■ MR demonstration of a sacrococcygeal teratoma in a 24-week fetus. Sagittal T2-WI shows a large, mixed solid and cystic lesion *(curved arrow)* arising from the tip of the spine *(large arrow)*. There is intrapelvic extension of the tumor *(white arrow)* with superior displacement of the bladder *(double arrow)*.

the diagnosis. The level of the obstruction can be revealed with MRI.

By means of the EXIT (ex utero intrapartum treatment) procedure, it is now possible to deliver a fetus with a large neck mass or other abnormality associated with ventilation compromise while maintaining umbilical and placental circulation to the fetus.[65] A hysterotomy is performed under deep maternal anesthesia to relax the uterine musculature and delay placental-uterine separation.[66] This allows 40 to 50 minutes of continued perfusion of the fetus to establish an airway, vascular access, and possible removal of the mass. The technique has been successful in maintaining oxygenation of the infant[67] and allows an airway to be established in a controlled fashion. However, deep anesthesia can cause maternal bleeding with the risk of hysterectomy or death. Consequently, as much information as possible about the anatomy of the mass and its relationship to the airway and great vessels is needed to plan delivery and possible immediate surgery.[65,68]

CHEST

The most important determinant of fetal survival after birth is adequate development of the lungs. The bronchi and bronchioles are developed by 16 to 20 weeks' gestational age, with the appearance of a significant number of alveolar ducts and blood vessels by 16 to 24 weeks' gestation. The normal fetal lung on T2-WI is homogeneous, with intermediate-to-high SI relative to muscle. With maturation the SI of the lungs increases with increasing production of alveolar fluid.[64] The best imaging predictor of lung maturity has been comparison of the US-measured circumference of the fetal chest to gestational age and femur length.[69] These measurements, however, will be inaccurate if there is an intrathoracic mass. Normal lung volumes have been documented with echo-planar MR and have been shown to increase exponentially with increasing gestational age.[70] A larger study using fast spin-echo T2-WI showed that the normal fetal lung volume increased with age as a power curve and the spread of values increased with age.[71] The relationship between left and right lung was constant throughout gestation. The MRI lung volumes were 10% less than volumes obtained on pathologic specimens. Fetal lungs have also been shown to have progressive decrease in T1-SI and increase in T2-SI with growth.[72,73] Relaxation time measurements may provide additional information about normal and abnormal development of the lungs in utero. Studies are being done to determine whether lung volumes may be predictive of survival in pulmonary hypoplasia (Fig. 8-26).[74]

Congenital Cystic Adenomatoid Malformation (CCAM)

The most common masses within the fetal chest are congenital cystic adenomatoid malformation (CCAM), bronchopulmonary sequestration, fetal hydrothorax (FHT), and congenital diaphragmatic hernia (see next sections). CCAM is an uncommon lesion characterized by a multicystic mass of pulmonary tissue with an abnormal proliferation of bronchiolar structures that connects to the normal bronchial tree. CCAM differs from normal lung by an increase in cell proliferation and a decrease in apoptosis.[75] The vascular supply is from the pulmonary artery and drains via the pulmonary veins. CCAM may arise from any segment or lobe of the lung and occasionally involves multiple lobes.

On prenatal MRI, the appearance of CCAM is variable and depends on whether they are micro- or macrocystic.[64] Type 1, or microcystic lesions, are hyperintense on T2-WI compared with the normal lung and relatively homogeneous (Fig. 8-27). With increasing numbers of micro- or macrocysts, discrete cysts can be revealed on MRI (Fig. 8-28). MRI demonstrates normal compressed lung tissue better than US does, which is important in determining resectability.[73] The natural history of CCAM is variable. CCAM may decrease in size or involute on prenatal US in 15% to 30% of cases. However, this imaging appearance may be misleading. In a study of infants with prenatal involution of a CCAM, 22 of 23 had postnatal CT scans that showed lung cysts or focal lobar hyperinflation.[76]

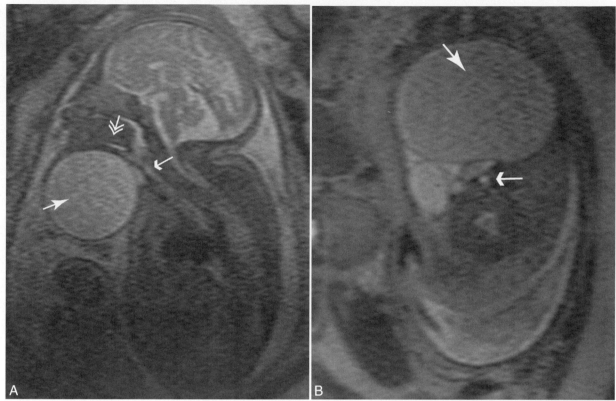

Figure 8-22 ■ **MR illustration of a lymphangioma of the anterior neck in a 36-week fetus. A**, Sagittal T2-WI shows a large multicystic mass *(curved arrow)*. The base of the tongue *(double arrow)* is mildly displaced but not involved. The oropharyngeal airway and trachea *(small arrow)* are patent. **B**, Axial T2-WI through the lower cervical spine reveals a septate cystic mass *(curved arrow)* in the anterior neck with patent, mildly displaced trachea *(small arrow)*.

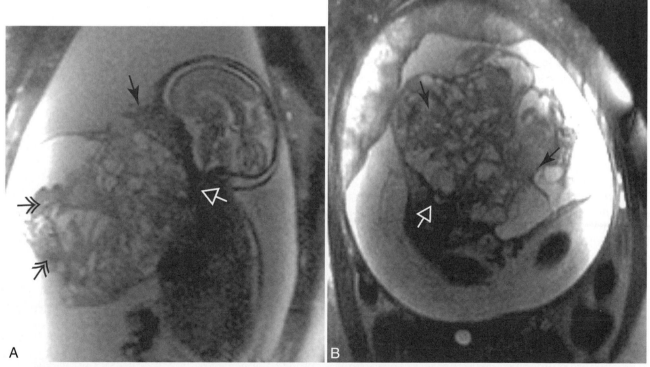

Figure 8-23 ■ **MR depiction of a cervical teratoma in a 30-week fetus. A**, Sagittal T2-WI shows a very large, mixed SI, solid and cystic mass *(double arrows)* in the anterior neck with obliteration of the oropharynx *(white arrow)* and distortion of the facial bones with elevation of the nose and maxilla *(curved arrow)*. There is severe polyhydramnios. **B**, Axial T2-WI reveals severe displacement and compression of the trachea *(white arrow)* at the thoracic inlet by the mass *(curved arrows)*.

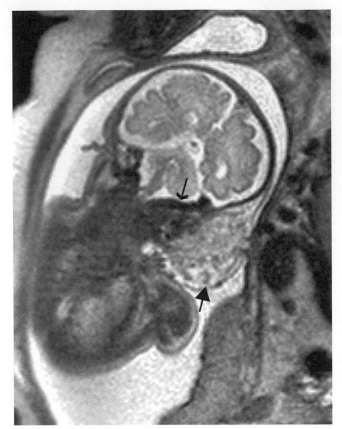

Figure 8-24 ■ **MR illustration of a soft tissue hemangioma of the lateral neck in a 36-week fetus.** Coronal T2-WI shows a large, mixed, heterogeneous solid mass *(large arrow)* in the lateral neck and skull base with multiple enlarged vessels in and around the mass and enlargement of the sigmoid sinus *(small arrow)*.

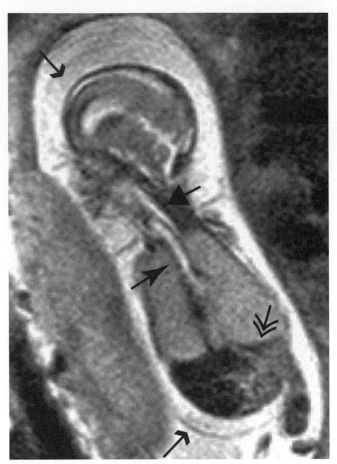

Figure 8-25 ■ **MR of congenital high airway obstruction syndrome (CHAOS) in a 22-week fetus.** Coronal T2-WI shows bilateral, severely enlarged, high SI lungs with eversion of the diaphragm *(double arrow)*. The trachea *(curved arrow)* is dilated below the glottis. The pharynx *(large arrow)* is normal. There is severe skin and scalp edema *(small arrows)*.

Hydrops may be present with large CCAM owing to obstruction of venous return. Hydrops may occur in up to 40% of fetuses with CCAM. A CCAM volume ratio (CVR) normalized for gestational age has been developed to help predict outcome.[77] The tumor volume is divided by the head circumference. A CVR greater than 1.6 at presentation predicts an increased risk of hydrops. A CVR less than 1.6 in the absence of a dominant cyst is associated with less than 3% risk of developing hydrops. Lesions with large cysts have a high incidence of hydrops. Large tumors associated with hydrops and a dominant cyst may be treated with thoracoamniotic shunting. In utero removal of a CCAM with hydrops in a fetus less than 32 weeks' gestation results in a 60% survival rate.[78] After 32 weeks' gestation, the fetus can be delivered and the tumor removed.

Bronchopulmonary Sequestration (BPS)

Bronchopulmonary sequestration (BPS) is a mass of nonfunctioning pulmonary tissue that lacks connection to the tracheobronchial tree. BPS detected prenatally usually is extralobar. Extralobar sequestrations receive

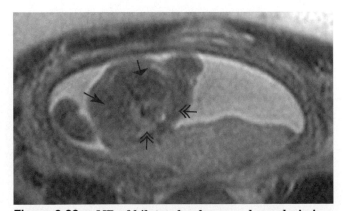

Figure 8-26 ■ **MR of bilateral pulmonary hypoplasia in a 21-week fetus.** Axial T2-WI shows severe hypoplasia of the lungs *(double arrows)* with only minimal low SI tissue in the posterior chest. Normal lung tissue should be of higher SI (see Figs. 8-29 and 8-36). The heart *(broad arrow)* is elevated and rotated posteriorly, and the liver *(curved arrow)* extends into the chest owing to volume loss.

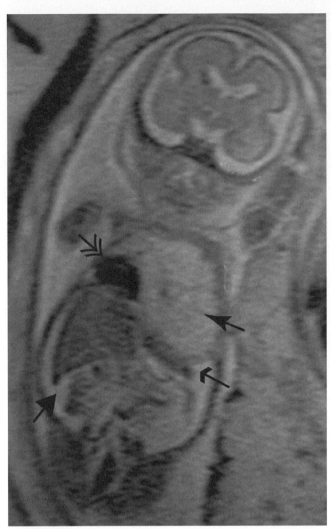

Figure 8-27 ■ MR illustration of congenital cysto-matoid malformation of the lung in a 24-week fetus. Coronal T2-WI shows a large high SI cystic mass *(curved arrow)* that crosses the midline with displacement and compression of the heart *(double arrow)* and eversion of the diaphragm *(small arrow).* There is ascites *(large arrow).*

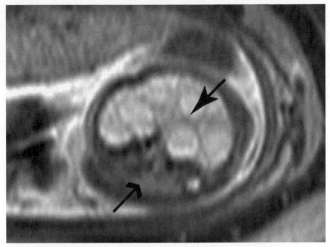

Figure 8-28 ■ MR demonstration of a congenital cystic adenomatoid malformation in a 23-week fetus. Axial T2 SI shows a large high SI mass *(curved arrow)* in the left lower lobe with multiple large cysts that cross the midline. A small amount of compressed contralateral lung *(small arrow)* is present.

because of the ability to perform real time vascular imaging with color flow. Current MR can sometimes show the anomalous vessels on prenatal MRI.[82]

BPS may occur in the upper abdomen and be confused with an adrenal tumor. Although BPS in the chest is usually solid and homogeneous, in the upper abdomen it is usually cystic, is located in the area of the adrenal gland, and may be confused with neuroblastoma.[83]

blood supply from a systemic artery. Although most common in the posterior segment of the left lower lobe, they may occur in any segment or lobe.[79] Half of BPSs are atypical and associated with other anomalies including congenital diaphragmatic hernia (see next section) represents a failure of formation of the diaphragmatic leaflets, occurring most commonly, anomalous pulmonary venous drainage, pulmonary hypoplasia with scimitar syndrome, bronchogenic cyst, bronchial esophageal connection, and horseshoe lung. Pulmonary sequestrations are a subgroup of lung lesion with a favorable prognosis.[80] Hydrops is uncommon unless there is an associated pleural effusion.[81] On T2-WIs, there is a wedge-shaped area of very high, homogeneous SI (Fig. 8-29).[64,82] Prenatal US better demonstrates anomalous systemic vessels

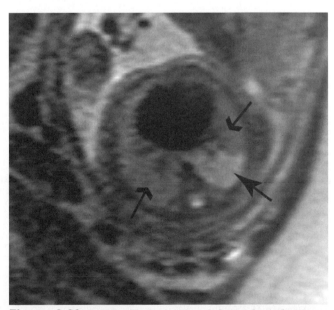

Figure 8-29 ■ MR illustration of bronchopulmonary sequestration in a 26-week fetus. Axial T2-WI shows a focal left lower lobe wedge-shaped mass *(curved arrow)* in the left lower lobe that is of higher SI than the normal lung *(small arrows).*

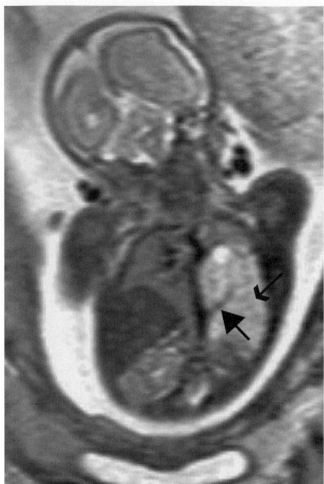

Figure 8-30 ■ **MR illustration of a hybrid lesion (pathologically containing components of congenital cystic adenomatoid malformation, bronchopulmonary sequestration, and/or bronchogenic cyst) in a 23-week fetus.** Coronal T2-WI reveals a mixed high SI mass *(small arrow)* containing cysts in the left lower lobe with a feeding vessel *(large arrow)* that originates from the descending aorta.

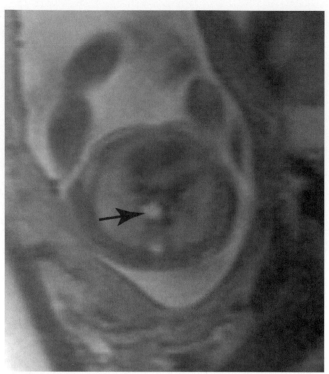

Figure 8-31 ■ **MR illustration of a bronchogenic cyst in a 26-week fetus.** Axial T2-WI through the subcarinal region shows a small, discrete, high SI mass *(arrow)* inferior to the carina tracheae and anterior to the spine.

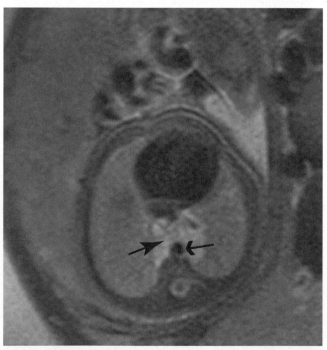

Figure 8-32 ■ **Duplication cyst of the esophagus as revealed on MR in a 29-week fetus.** Axial T2-WI shows a well-defined, high SI mass *(curved arrow)* anterior to the aorta *(small arrow)* and spine.

Multiple chest lesions may be found simultaneously. Although chest lesions such as CCAM, BPS, and bronchogenic cyst used to be thought of as distinct lesions, there is significant overlap in their pathologic occurrence, suggesting similar embryologic development and abnormality (Figs. 8-30 and 8-31). The most common lesion is a hybrid (Fig. 8-32). The cystic lesion has US, MRI, and pathologic characteristics of CCAM and systemic arterial blood supply consistent with BPS.[84] Lesions consisting of BPS, CCAM, and bronchogenic cyst have been described.[85,86]

Congenital Diaphragmatic Hernia (CDH)

Congenital diaphragmatic hernia (CDH) represents a failure of formation of the diaphragmatic leaflets, occurring most commonly in the posterior aspect of the left hemidiaphragm. CDH is present on the left side in 88% and the right side in 10% and is bilateral in 2%. Survival rates in fetuses with CDH range from 40% to 90% with no significant improvement over the last 20 years.[87] Survival is related to the degree of pulmonary hypoplasia associated with the CDH. The best prenatal predictor of outcome remains the lung-to-head (LHR) circumference ratio as revealed by imaging.[88] Fetuses with an LHR greater than 1.4 have a favorable outcome, while those with a ratio of less than 1.0 rarely survive. There is a positive correlation between the lung volume determined on MRI with both fetal outcome and the US-determined LHR in fetuses with isolated left CDH after adjustment for gestational age at delivery and birth weight.[89] In a study at the author's institution it was the percentage of liver that herniated into the chest and not the calculated fetal lung volume that correlated positively with outcome in fetuses with CDH.[90] Herniation of liver into the chest in a patient with CDH has been shown to be associated with a worse outcome and survival of less than 50%. Antenatal branch pulmonary artery (PA) size correlates positively with

postmortem lung weight. In fetuses with CDH, a larger contralateral PA, significant size discrepancy of branch PA, and larger main PA diameter correlated positively with postnatal death andrespiratory morbidity. Progressive ipsilateral PA hypoplasia suggested progressive in utero lung hypoplasia.[91] On US, CDH is diagnosed by demonstrating a shift of the heart away from the midline and an area of increased echogenicity in the base of the chest.[92] Careful evaluation of the position of stomach in the chest is important. Uncertainty in the early diagnosis of CDH that presents as an echogenic chest mass is still described.[93] In a study of patients with postnatal repair of CDH, the diagnosis had not been established on prenatal US in 50% of fetuses.[94] Evaluating the position of the liver on US may be difficult, as the echotexture of liver and lung is similar. US depends on the depiction of the position of the portal and hepatic veins above or below the diaphragm to predict herniation of the liver into the chest, providing indirect information about the hepatic position.[95] With MRI there is direct visualization of the position of the liver (Fig. 8-33).[59] On T1-WIs, the liver is of

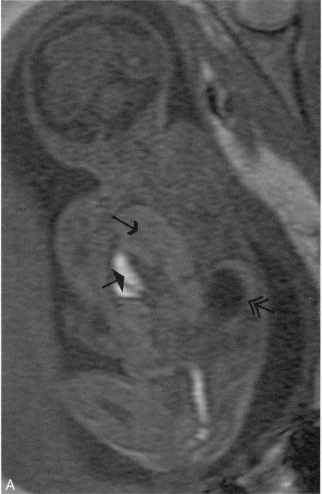

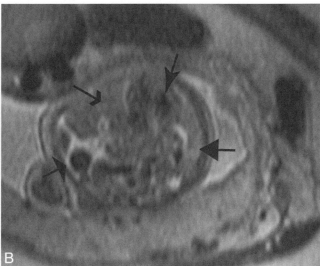

Figure 8-33 ■ **MR illustration of a right congenital diaphragmatic hernia in a 25-week fetus. A,** Coronal T1-W GRE image shows both liver *(small arrow)* and meconium-filled bowel segments *(broad arrow)* in the chest. The stomach *(double arrow)* remains in the left upper quadrant of the abdomen. **B,** Axial T2-WI image reveals displacement of the heart *(curved arrow)* to the left with herniation of bowel *(broad arrow)* and liver *(small arrow)* into the chest. There is a small amount of the left lung tissue present *(large arrow).*

high SI and very conspicuous adjacent to the low SI lungs. Consequently, the position of the liver above or below the diaphragm is easily determined. MRI has been shown to be more sensitive than US in detecting thoracic liver herniation.[59] Meconium-filled bowel is hyperintense on T1-WI, making the position of bowel segments easy to determine. On T2-WI, the liver is of low SI and isointense to muscle (see Fig. 8-33). MRI is most helpful in the evaluation of right-sided CDH, which is more frequently confused with CCAM than left-sided CDH, since the stomach remains in the left upper quadrant.[89] Right-sided CDH usually contains liver and bowel.

The diagnosis of bilateral CDH is easily missed on US.[96] Signs include anterior displacement of the heart with minimal lateral shift.[97] The diagnosis is readily made on MRI by showing liver in the right chest and bowel in the left chest. The prenatal recognition of bilateral CDH is important because of the significant increased incidence of chromosome abnormalities and syndromes compared with unilateral CDH.

Intrauterine therapy has been performed at some institutions using tracheal occlusion to promote lung growth.[98] Criteria for inclusion in this therapy were herniation of liver into the chest and lung volumes that fell into a poor prognostic category. Consequently, accurate knowledge of the position of the liver and the lung volumes was necessary. Tracheal occlusion resulted in significant lung growth in a subset of fetuses with severe CDH, but survival remained poor because of abnormalities in pulmonary function and prematurity.[99]

Eventration of the diaphragm is uncommon but may be confused with CDH. MRI can be helpful in differentiation because of accurate demonstration and localization of the bowel, diaphragm, and lung.[100] The differentiation is important, since the prognosis of eventration is significantly better than that of CDH (Fig. 8-34).

MRI is useful for evaluating atypical chest masses.[64] A foregut cyst on MRI is a fluid-filled cyst with high, homogeneous T2 SI.[101] The cyst may be large, and there is a connection to vertebrae and associated vertebral body anomalies (Fig. 8-35).

Anterior mediastinal masses are uncommon in utero (Fig. 8-36). Fetal mediastinal teratoma has rarely been reported.[102] On US these are complex cystic and solid masses. Because they are unusual lesions they may be misdiagnosed as a CCAM crossing the midline. MRI demonstrates the anatomy of the trachea and great vessels in the thoracic inlet, superior mediastinum, and normal lung. Lymphangiomas may occur anywhere in the body. Lymphangioma is more likely to violate tissue planes. Lymphangiomas appear as complex cystic masses with a variable solid component. Any chest mass may be associated with hydrops if there is obstruction of venous return.

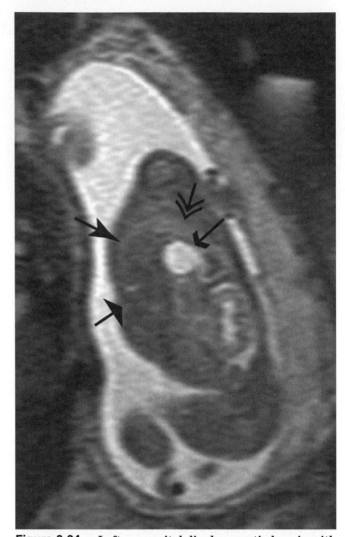

Figure 8-34 ■ **Left congenital diaphragmatic hernia with sac shown by MR in a 22-week fetus.** Sagittal T2-WI reveals stomach *(small arrow)* and liver *(curved arrow)* in the chest above the anterior diaphragmatic leaflet *(broad arrow)*. There is a smooth curved contour to the superior liver and stomach cause by the bowel-containing sac. There is a moderate amount of left lung tissue *(double arrow)*.

ABDOMEN

Liver

The fetal liver is well visualized on prenatal MRI, being very high in SI on T1-WI (see Fig. 8-33) and low to intermediate in SI on T2-WI.[64] Physiologic changes have been demonstrated within the fetal liver using EPI.[103] Iron results in lower SI on EPI and T2-WI owing to susceptibility effects. Early in fetal life, erythropoiesis occurs primarily in the liver; consequently, a large amount of iron is bound to fetal hemoglobin in the liver. Between 20 and 26 weeks' gestation, the site of erythropoiesis changes

Bowel

Fetal bowel is visualized on prenatal MRI as a high-SI meconium-filled tubular structures on T1-WI (see Fig. 8-33).[64,106] Meconium is detectable in the rectum on MRI as early as 14 weeks' gestation. Meconium is seen in the normal mid to distal fetal bowel. If meconium is not revealed, an anomaly of the bowel should be suspected, such as atresia or perforation. On T2-WI, the stomach and proximal bowel are high in SI, similarly to amniotic fluid, and the distal bowel is lower in SI. MRI helps differentiate abnormalities such as bowel obstruction from cystic abdominal masses. MRI can determine the site of bowel atresia.[107]

Adrenal Gland

Neuroblastoma is one of the more common solid childhood tumors, arising from undifferentiated neural tissue in the adrenal medulla or sympathetic ganglia.[108] Neuroblastic nodules are present in the adrenal glands of 100% of second-trimester fetuses

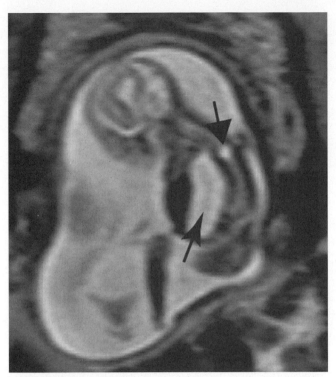

Figure 8-35 ■ MR illustration of a neurenteric cyst in a 19-week fetus. Sagittal T2-WI shows a large cyst *(curved arrow)* in the chest and abdomen connecting to an associated defect in the spine with kyphosis and focal expansion of the dural sac *(broad arrow).*

from the liver to the bone marrow. Changes in liver SI are present throughout fetal development. This has potential use in early noninvasive physiologic assessment of the fetus. Changes in T2* measurements of the fetal liver have been documented following maternal oxygenation based on the blood oxygenation level dependence (BOLD) of the MRI signal.[104] This technique may help in the evaluation of abnormalities such as placental insufficiency and intrauterine growth retardation.

Abdominal masses can be detected with prenatal MRI (Fig. 8-37).[105] Tumors of the liver are rare in the fetus and include hemangioendothelioma, hepatoblastoma, and hamartoma. Hemangioendotheliomas are mixed in intensity depending on the size of the vascular pools and the degree of fibrosis. Hepatomegaly usually is present. Hepatoblastoma is a rare malignant tumor that produces α-fetoprotein. Imaging reveals a solid heterogenous liver mass secondary to intratumoral necrosis and hemorrhage. Hamartomas are typically irregular cystic masses. Calcifications may be present. Hepatomegaly may also be seen with hydrops, infection, anemia, metabolic abnormalities, and Beckwith-Wiedemann syndrome.

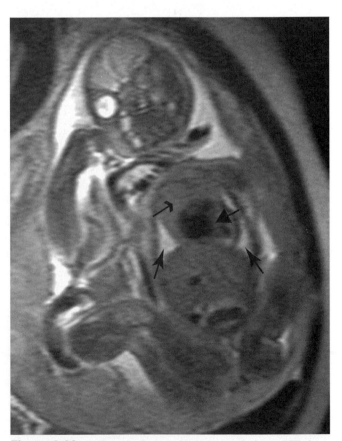

Figure 8-36 ■ Thymic hyperplasia revealed on MR in a 30-week fetus referred for evaluation of a chest tumor. Coronal T2-WI shows an enlarged, intermediate SI, homogeneous thymus *(small arrow)* with normal lungs *(curved arrows)* and heart *(broad arrow).* Thymic hyperplasia can develop secondary to maternal hypothyroidism.

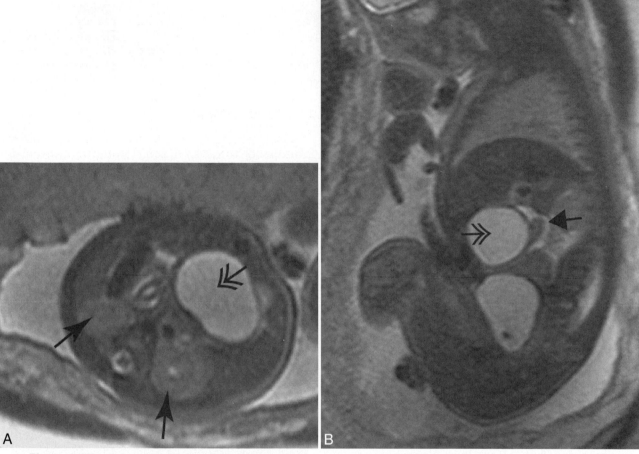

Figure 8-37 ■ **Duodenal duplication cyst revealed on MR in a 32-week fetus referred for evaluation of an anterior chest mass. A,** Axial T2-WI shows a large cyst *(double arrow)* in the anterior upper abdomen. Normal kidneys are present *(curved arrows).* **B,** Sagittal T2-WI shows the cyst *(double arrow)* below the liver without dilation of the biliary tree and anterior to the duodenum *(broad arrow)* intimately related to the duodenal bulb.

and in 2% of neonates and represent a normal embryologic structure that regresses or differentiates with maturation. The incidence of clinical neuroblastoma is 1 in 10,000 to 30,000. Adrenal cysts ar present in fetal neuroblastomas but are uncommon in postnatal neuroblastoma. Cysts may be a variant of the normal development of the fetal adrenal gland.

Kidney and Urinary Tract

Congenital renal masses are rare, but mesoblastic nephroma has been diagnosed in utero.[108] These are predominantly solid masses but may contain cysts. Hemorrhage may be present within areas of

tumor necrosis. This or any abdominal mass may be associated with polyhydramnios secondary to compression of the bowel.

Fetal renal anomalies are often associated with oligohydramnios, a condition that may make the performance of US difficult.[109] MRI is not significantly affected by diminished amniotic fluid. The normal fetal kidney is intermediate in SI on T2-WI and higher than surrounding muscle (see Fig. 8-37). T2 SI of the cortex is slightly lower than of the medulla. The renal pelves and bladder are very high in SI on T2-WI. Normal ureters are not visualized.

Renal anomalies are increasingly detected with US because of significant improvements in

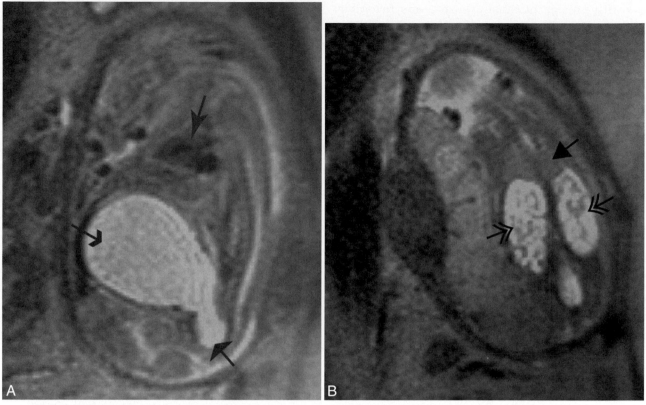

Figure 8-38 ■ **MR demonstration of posterior urethral valves in a 22-week fetus. A,** Sagittal T2-WI shows marked enlargement of the urinary bladder *(small arrow)* with thickening of the bladder wall and dilation of the posterior urethra *(broad arrow).* There is oligohydramnios and a small chest *(curved arrow)* consistent with pulmonary hypoplasia. **B,** Coronal T2-WI reveals severe dysplasia with numerous small renal cortical cysts *(double arrows).* The lungs *(broad arrow)* are hypoplastic and are of decreased SI for this gestational age.

technology. It is estimated that 1 in 1,000 fetuses have a renal anomaly.[110] The mortality after antenatal detection of fetal uropathy ranges from 20% to 50%.[111] Associated anomalies have been found in 50% of fetuses.[110,111]

With uropathy due to lower urinary tract obstruction (LUTO), the urinary bladder is dilated and thick walled (Fig. 8-38). MRI is equal to US in the accuracy of identifying a LUTO but is no better at differentiating the three main causes: posterior urethral valves, urethral atresia, and prune-belly syndrome (Fig. 8-39). With progressive obstruction of the bladder there is dilation of one or both renal collecting systems. Renal dysplastic changes occur with progressive dilation of the renal tubules and progress to cortical and medullary cysts.[112] Renal dysplastic changes are revealed as heterogeneous areas of increased cortical T2 SI and as cysts. In cases of questionable increased echogenicity on US, MRI can help determine whether abnormalities are dysplastic changes or a normal cortical variant. Renal dysplasia associated with a LUTO is a poor prognostic sign and associated with decreased renal function. If dysplastic changes are present prenatally, intervention is usually not indicated. In a

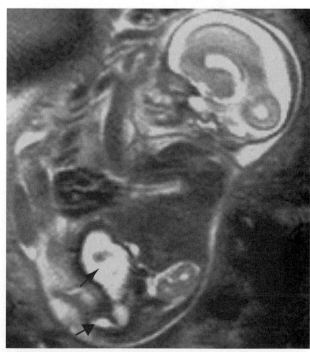

Figure 8-39 ■ **Urethral atresia as revealed on MR in a 25-week fetus.** Sagittal T2-WI shows a dilated thick walled bladder *(curved arrow)* with dilation of the proximal urethra *(broad arrow).*

fetus with no sign of renal dysplasia and favorable levels of urine electrolytes and β-macroglobulins, vesicoamniotic shunting can be offered. Trials of in utero antegrade fetoscopy are being performed to diagnose LUTO and to ablate posterior valves if present.[113]

MRI is accurate in defining urinary tract anatomy (Fig. 8-40).[114] Areas of upper tract obstruction or dilation are revealed, as well as intermittent dilation of the ureter with primary megaureter or reflux. Ureteroceles and duplicated collecting system can be defined (Fig. 8-41).

MRI is most helpful in defining the anatomy of complex renal anomalies, such as bladder extrophy and cloacal anomalies (Fig. 8-42). The ability to define the bowel and the urinary tract helps distinguish these from other forms of LUTO. To date, cloacal anomalies have not been treated successfully in utero.

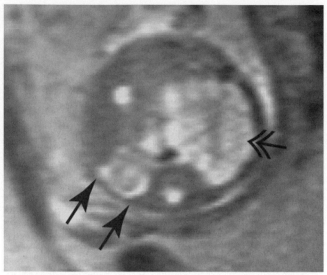

Figure 8-40 ▪ **MR illustration of multicystic dysplastic kidney in a 22-week fetus.** Axial T2-WI shows multiple discrete left renal cysts *(double arrow)* without identifiable renal parenchyma. The right kidney is intermediate in SI with two cysts present *(curved arrows)*, consistent with mild dysplastic changes.

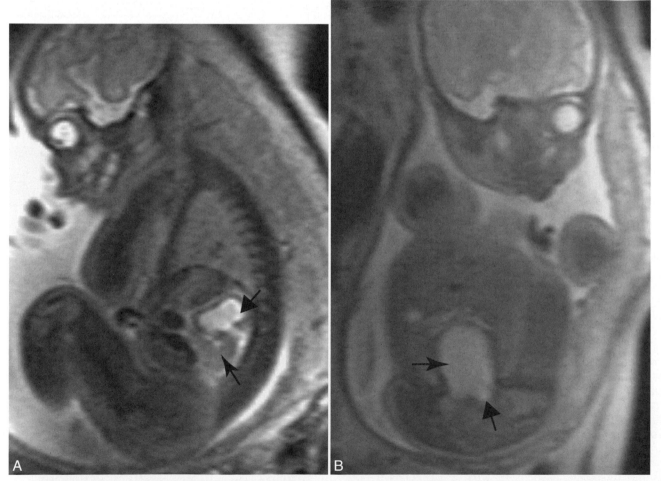

Figure 8-41 ▪ **Duplex renal collecting system with ureterocele as shown on MR in a 30-week fetus.** **A,** Sagittal T2-WI shows dilation of the upper pole *(broad arrow)* renal collecting system with associated cortical thinning. The lower pole is normal *(curved arrow)*. **B,** Coronal T2-WI reveals a distended bladder *(curved arrow)* with a small left ureterocele *(broad arrow)*.

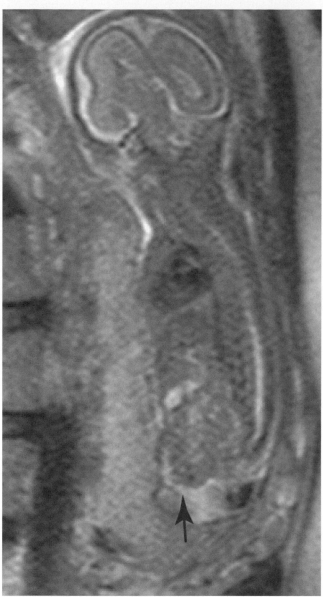

Figure 8-42 ▪ MR illustration of bladder extrophy in a 22-week fetus. Sagittal T2-WI shows absence of fluid in the urinary bladder with a defect *(curved arrow)* in the lower anterior abdominal wall below the umbilicus.

REFERENCES

1. Weinreb JC, Lowe T, Cohen JM, Kutler M. Human fetal anatomy: MR imaging. Radiology 1985;157:715-720.
2. Semelka RC, Kelekis NL, Thomasson D, Brown MA, Laub GA. HASTE MR imaging: description of technique and preliminary results in the abdomen. J Magn Reson Imaging 1996;6:698-699.
3. Johnson IR, Stehling MK, Blamire AM, et al. Study of internal structure of the human fetus in utero by echo-planar magnetic resonance imaging. Am J Obstet Gynecol 1990;163:601-607.
4. Quinn TM, Hubbard AM, Adzick NS. Prenatal magnetic resonance imaging enhances fetal diagnosis. J Pediatr Surg 1998;33:553-558.
5. Levine D, Barnes PD, Sher S, et al. Fetal fast MR imaging: reproducibility, technical quality and conspicuity of anatomy. Radiology 1998;206:549-554.
6. Yamashita Y, Namimoto T, Abe Y, et al. MR imaging of the fetus by a HASTE sequence. AJR Am J Roentgenol 1997;168:513-519.
7. Coakley FV. Role of magnetic resonance imaging in fetal surgery. Top Magn Reson Imaging 2001;12:39-51.
8. Coakley FV, Glenn OA, Qayyum A, Barkovich AJ, Goldstein R, Filly RA. Fetal MRI: a developing technique for the developing patient. AJR Am J Roentgenol 2004;182:243-252.
9. O'Connor ME. Intrauterine effects in animals exposed to radiofrequency and microwave fields. Teratology 1999;59:287-291.
10. Kanal E, Gillen J, Evans JA, Savitz DA, Shellock FG. Survey of reproductive health among female MR workers. Radiology 1993;187:395-399.
11. Myers C, Duncan KR, Gowland PA, Johnson IR, Baker PN. Failure to detect intrauterine growth restriction following in utero exposure to MRI. Br J Radiol 1998;71:549-551.
12. Baker PN, Johnson IR, Harvey PR, Gowland PA, Mansfield P. A three-year follow-up of children imaged in utero with echo-planar magnetic resonance. Am J Obstet Gynecol 1994;170:32-33.
13. Levine D, Zuo C, Faro CB, Chen Q. Potential heating effect in the gravid uterus during MR HASTE imaging. J Magn Reson Imaging 2001;13:856-861.
14. Levine D, Smith AS, McKenzie C. Tips and tricks of fetal MR imaging. Radiol Clin North Am 2003;41:729-745.
15. Okuda Y, Sagami F, Tirone P, Morisetti A, Bussi S, Masters RE. [Reproductive and developmental toxicity study of gadobenate dimeglumine formulation (E7155) (3)—study of embryo-fetal toxicity in rabbits by intravenous administration.] J Toxicol Sci 1999;24(Suppl 1):79-87.
16. Hertzberg BS, Kliewer MA, Bowie JD. Sonographic evaluation of fetal CNS: technical and interpretive pitfalls. AJR Am J Roentgenol 1999;172:523-527.
17. Levine D, Barnes PD, Madsen JR, Abbott J, Mehta T, Edelman RR. Central nervous system abnormalities assessed with prenatal magnetic resonance imaging. Obstet Gynecol 1999;94:1011-1019.
18. Simon EM, Goldstein RB, Coakley FV, et al. Fast MR imaging of fetal CNS anomalies in utero. AJNR Am J Neuroradiol 2000;21:1688-1698.
19. Twickler DM, Magee KP, Caire J, Zaretsky M, Fleckenstein JL, Ramus RM. Second-opinion magnetic resonance imaging for suspected fetal central nervous system abnormalities. Am J Obstet Gynecol 2003;188:492-496.
20. Levine D, Barnes PD, Robertson RR, Wong G, Mehta TS. Fast MR imaging of fetal central nervous system abnormalities. Radiology 2003;229:51-61.
21. Brisse H, Fallet C, Sebag G, Nessmann C, Blot P, Hassan M. Supratentorial parenchyma in the developing fetal brain: in vitro MR study with histologic comparison. AJNR Am J Neuroradiol 1997;18:1491-1497.
22. Garel C, Chantrel E, Brisse H, et al. Fetal cerebral cortex: normal gestational landmarks identified using prenatal MR imaging. AJNR Am J Neuroradiol 2001;22:184-189.
23. Lan LM, Yamashita Y, Tang Y, et al. Normal fetal brain development: MR imaging with a half-Fourier rapid acquisition with relaxation enhancement sequence. Radiology 2000;215:205-210.
24. Naidich TP, Grant JL, Altman N, et al. The developing cerebral surface: preliminary report on the patterns of sulcal and gyral maturation—anatomy, ultrasound, and magnetic resonance imaging. Neuroimaging Clin N Am 1994;4:201-240.
25. Girard N, Raybaud C, Gambarelli D, Figarella-Branger D. Fetal brain MR imaging. Magn Reson Imaging Clin N Am 2001;9:19-56.
26. Girard N, Raybaud C, Poncet M. In vivo MR study of brain maturation in normal fetuses. AJNR Am J Neuroradiol 1995;16:407-413.
27. Levine D, Barnes PD. Cortical maturation in normal and abnormal fetuses as assessed with prenatal MR imaging. Radiology 1999;210:751-758.
28. Chung HW, Chen CY, Zimmerman RA, Lee KW, Lee CC, Chin SC. T2-weighted fast MR imaging with true FISP versus HASTE: comparative efficacy in the evaluation of normal fetal brain maturation. AJR Am J Roentgenol 2000;175:1375-1380.
29. Jeffery N. A high-resolution MRI study of linear growth of the human fetal skull base. Neuroradiology 2002;44:358-366.
30. Jeffery N. Differential regional brain growth and rotation of the prenatal human tentorium cerebelli. J Anat 2002;200:135-144.
31. D'Addario V, Pinto V, Del Bianco A, et al. The clivus-supraocciput angle: a useful measurement to evaluate the shape and size of the fetal posterior fossa and to diagnose Chiari II malformation. Ultrasound Obstet Gynecol 2001;18:146-149.
32. Barkovich AJ, Rowley H, Bollen A. Correlation of prenatal events with the development of polymicrogyria. AJNR Am J Neuroradiol 1995;16:822-827.
33. Sonigo PC, Rypens FF, Carteret M, Delezoide AL, Brunelle FO. MR imaging of fetal cerebral anomalies. Pediatr Radiol 1998;28:212-222.
34. Denis D, Maugey-Laulom B, Carles D, Pedespan JM, Brun M, Chateil JF. Prenatal diagnosis of schizencephaly by fetal magnetic resonance imaging. Fetal Diagn Ther 2001;16:354-359.

35. Nyberg DA, Mack LA, Hirsch J, Pagon RO, Shepard TH. Fetal hydrocephalus: sonographic detection and clinical significance of associated anomalies. Radiology 1987;163:187-191.

36. Oi S, Honda Y, Hidaka M, Sato O, Matsumoto S. Intrauterine high-resolution magnetic resonance imaging in fetal hydrocephalus and prenatal estimation of postnatal outcomes with "perspective classification." J Neurosurg 1998;88:685-694.

37. Mercier A, Eurin D, Mercier PY, Verspyck E, Marpeau L, Marret S. Isolated mild fetal cerebral ventriculomegaly: a retrospective analysis of 26 cases. Prenat Diagn 2001;21:589-595.

38. Toma P, Lucigrai G, Ravegnani M, Cariati M, Magnano G, Lituania M. Hydrocephalus and porencephaly: prenatal diagnosis by ultrasonography and MR imaging. J Comput Assist Tomogr 1990;14:843-845.

39. Low JA, Simpson LL, Ramsey DA. The clinical diagnosis of asphyxia responsible for brain damage in the human fetus. Am J Obstet Gynecol 1992;167:11-15.

40. de Laveaucoupet J, Audibert F, Guis F, et al. Fetal magnetic resonance imaging (MRI) of ischemic brain injury. Prenat Diagn 2001;21:729-736.

41. Toma P, Costa A, Magnano GM, Cariati M, Lituania M. Holoprosencephaly: prenatal diagnosis by sonography and magnetic resonance imaging. Prenat Diagn 1990;10:429-436.

42. Martinez-Lage JF, Garcia Santos JM, Poza M, Garcia Sanchez F. Prenatal magnetic resonance imaging detection of a vein of Galen aneurysm. Childs Nerv Syst 1993;9:377-378.

43. Levine D, Barnes P, Korf B, Edelman R. Tuberous sclerosis in the fetus: second-trimester diagnosis of subependymal tubers with ultrafast MR imaging. AJR Am J Roentgenol 2000;175:1067-1069.

44. Ecker JL, Shipp TD, Bromley B, Benacerraf B. The sonographic diagnosis of Dandy-Walker and Dandy-Walker variant: associated findings and outcomes. Prenat Diagn 2000;20:328-332.

45. Stazzone MM, Hubbard AM, Bilaniuk LT, et al. Ultrafast MR imaging of the normal posterior fossa in fetuses. AJR Am J Roentgenol 2000;175:835-839.

46. Folkerth RD, McLaughlin ME, Levine D. Organizing posterior fossa hematomas simulating developmental cysts on prenatal imaging: report of 3 cases. J Ultrasound Med 2001;20:1233-1240.

47. Nakahara T, Uozumi T, Monden S, et al. Prenatal diagnosis of open spina bifida by MRI and ultrasonography. Brain Dev 1993;15:75-78.

48. Mangels KJ, Tulipan N, Tsao LY, Alarcon J, Bruner JP. Fetal MRI in the evaluation of intrauterine myelomeningocele. Pediatr Neurosurg 2000;32:124-131.

49. Sutton LN, Adzick NS, Bilaniuk LT, Johnson MP, Crombleholme TM, Flake AW. Improvement in hindbrain herniation demonstrated by serial fetal magnetic resonance imaging following fetal surgery for myelomeningocele. JAMA 1999;282:1826-1831.

50. Bruner JP, Tulipan N, Paschall RL, et al. Fetal surgery for myelomeningocele and the incidence of shunt-dependent hydrocephalus. JAMA 1999;282:1819-1825.

51. Kolble N, Huisman TA, Stallmach T, Meuli M, Zen Ruffinen Imahorn F, Zimmermann R. Prenatal diagnosis of a fetus with lumbar myelocystocele. Ultrasound Obstet Gynecol 2001;18:536-539.

52. Kirkinen P, Partanen K, Merikanto J, Ryynanen M, Haring P, Heinonen K. Ultrasonic and magnetic resonance imaging of fetal sacrococcygeal teratoma. Acta Obstet Gynecol Scand 1997;76:917-922.

53. Perrelli L, D'Urzo C, Manzoni C, et al. Sacrococcygeal teratoma. Outcome and management: an analysis of 17 cases. J Perinat Med 2002;30:179-184.

54. Altman RP, Randolph JG, Lilly JR. Sacrococcygeal teratoma: American Academy of Pediatrics Surgical Section Survey—1973. J Pediatr Surg 1974;9:389-398.

55. Westerburg B, Feldstein VA, Sandberg PL, Lopoo JB, Harrison MR, Albanese CT. Sonographic prognostic factors in fetuses with sacrococcygeal teratoma. J Pediatr Surg 2000;35:322-325; discussion 325-326.

56. Avni FE, Guibaud L, Robert Y, et al. MR imaging of fetal sacrococcygeal teratoma: diagnosis and assessment. AJR Am J Roentgenol 2002;178:179-183.

57. Leung JC, Mann S, Salafia C, Brion LP. Sacrococcygeal teratoma with vascular placental dissemination. Obstet Gynecol 1999;93:856.

58. Kitano Y, Flake AW, Crombleholme TM, Johnson MP, Adzick NS. Open fetal surgery for life-threatening fetal malformations. Semin Perinatol 1999;23:448-461.

59. Hubbard AM, Crombleholme TM, Adzick NS, et al. Prenatal MRI evaluation of congenital diaphragmatic hernia. Am J Perinatol 1999;16:407-413.

60. Chervenak FA, Isaacson G, Blakemore KJ, et al. Fetal cystic hygroma: cause and natural history. N Engl J Med 1983;309:822-825.

61. Azizkhan RG, Haase GM, Applebaum H, et al. Diagnosis, management, and outcome of cervicofacial teratomas in neonates: a Childrens Cancer Group study. J Pediatr Surg 1995;30:312-316.

62. Tsuda H, Matsumoto M, Yamamoto K, et al. Usefulness of ultrasonography and magnetic resonance imaging for prenatal diagnosis of fetal teratoma of the neck. J Clin Ultrasound 1996;24:217-219.

63. Kalache KD, Chaoui R, Tennstedt C, Bollmann R. Prenatal diagnosis of laryngeal atresia in two cases of congenital high airway obstruction syndrome (CHAOS). Prenat Diagn 1997;17:577-581.

64. Hubbard AM, Adzick NS, Crombleholme TM, et al. Congenital chest lesions: diagnosis and characterization with prenatal MR imaging. Radiology 1999;212:43-48.

65. Liechty KW, Crombleholme TM, Flake AW, et al. Intrapartum airway management for giant fetal neck masses: the EXIT (ex utero intrapartum treatment) procedure. Am J Obstet Gynecol 1997;177:870-874.

66. Mychaliska GB, Bealer JF, Graf JL, Rosen MA, Adzick NS, Harrison MR. Operating on placental support: the ex utero intrapartum treatment procedure. J Pediatr Surg 1997;32:227-230; discussion 230-221.

67. Bouchard S, Johnson MP, Flake AW, et al. The EXIT procedure: experience and outcome in 31 cases. J Pediatr Surg 2002;37:418-426.

68. Hubbard AM, Crombleholme TM, Adzick NS. Prenatal MRI evaluation of giant neck masses in preparation for the fetal exit procedure. Am J Perinatol 1998;15:253-257.

69. Ohlsson A, Fong K, Rose T, et al. Prenatal ultrasonic prediction of autopsy-proven pulmonary hypoplasia. Am J Perinatol 1992;9:334-337.

70. Duncan KR, Gowland PA, Moore RJ, Baker PN, Johnson IR. Assessment of fetal lung growth in utero with echo-planar MR imaging. Radiology 1999;210:197-200.

71. Rypens F, Metens T, Rocourt N, et al. Fetal lung volume: estimation at MR imaging-initial results. Radiology 2001;219:236-241.

72. Duncan KR, Gowland PA, Freeman A, Moore R, Baker PN, Johnson IR. The changes in magnetic resonance properties of the fetal lungs: a first result and a potential tool for the non-invasive in utero demonstration of fetal lung maturation. Br J Obstet Gynaecol 1999;106:122-125.

73. Levine D, Barnewolt CE, Mehta TS, Trop I, Estroff J, Wong G. Fetal thoracic abnormalities: MR imaging. Radiology 2003;228:379-388.

74. Coakley FV, Lopoo JB, Lu Y, et al. Normal and hypoplastic fetal lungs: volumetric assessment with prenatal single-shot rapid acquisition with relaxation enhancement MR imaging. Radiology 2000;216:107-111.

75. Cass DL, Quinn TM, Yang EY, et al. Increased cell proliferation and decreased apoptosis characterize congenital cystic adenomatoid malformation of the lung. J Pediatr Surg 1998;33:1043-1046; discussion 1047.

76. Blau H, Barak A, Karmazyn B, et al. Postnatal management of resolving fetal lung lesions. Pediatrics 2002;109:105-108.

77. Crombleholme TM, Coleman B, Hedrick H, et al. Cystic adenomatoid malformation volume ratio predicts outcome in prenatally diagnosed cystic adenomatoid malformation of the lung. J Pediatr Surg 2002;37:331-338.

78. Adzick NS, Harrison MR, Crombleholme TM, Flake AW, Howell LJ. Fetal lung lesions: management and outcome. Am J Obstet Gynecol 1998;179:884-889.

79. John PR, Beasley SW, Mayne V. Pulmonary sequestration and related congenital disorders. A clinico-radiological review of 41 cases. Pediatr Radiol 1989;20:4-9.

80. Bratu I, Flageole H, Chen MF, Di Lorenzo M, Yazbeck S, Laberge JM. The multiple facets of pulmonary sequestration. J Pediatr Surg 2001;36:784-790.

81. Lopoo JB, Goldstein RB, Lipshutz GS, Goldberg JD, Harrison MR, Albanese CT. Fetal pulmonary sequestration: a favorable congenital lung lesion. Obstet Gynecol 1999;94:567-571.

82. Dhingsa R, Coakley FV, Albanese CT, Filly RA, Goldstein R. Prenatal sonography and MR imaging of pulmonary sequestration. AJR Am J Roentgenol 2003;180:433-437.

83. Pumberger W, Moroder W, Wiesbauer P. Intraabdominal extralobar pulmonary sequestration exhibiting cystic adenomatoid malformation: prenatal diagnosis and characterization of a left suprarenal mass in the newborn. Abdom Imaging 2001;26:28-31.

84. Cass DL, Crombleholme TM, Howell LJ, Stafford PW, Ruchelli ED, Adzick NS. Cystic lung lesions with systemic arterial blood supply: a hybrid of congenital cystic adenomatoid malformation and bronchopulmonary sequestration. J Pediatr Surg 1997;32:986-990.

85. Kim KW, Kim WS, Cheon JE, et al. Complex bronchopulmonary foregut malformation: extralobar pulmonary sequestration associated with a duplication cyst of mixed bronchogenic and oesophageal type. Pediatr Radiol 2001;31:265-268.

86. MacKenzie TC, Guttenberg ME, Nisenbaum HL, Johnson MP, Adzick NS. A fetal lung lesion consisting of bronchogenic cyst, bronchopulmonary sequestration, and congenital cystic adenomatoid malformation: the missing link? Fetal Diagn Ther 2001;16:193-195.

87. Harrison MR, Adzick NS, Estes JM, Howell LJ. A prospective study of the outcome for fetuses with diaphragmatic hernia. JAMA 1994;271:382-384.
88. Sbragia L, Paek BW, Filly RA, et al. Congenital diaphragmatic hernia without herniation of the liver: does the lung-to-head ratio predict survival? J Ultrasound Med 2000;19:845-848.
89. Paek BW, Coakley FV, Lu Y, et al. Congenital diaphragmatic hernia: prenatal evaluation with MR lung volumetry—preliminary experience. Radiology 2001;220:63-67.
90. Walsh DS, Hubbard AM, Olutoye OO, et al. Assessment of fetal lung volumes and liver herniation with magnetic resonance imaging in congenital diaphragmatic hernia. Am J Obstet Gynecol 2000;183:1067-1069.
91. Sokol J, Bohn D, Lacro RV, et al. Fetal pulmonary artery diameters and their association with lung hypoplasia and postnatal outcome in congenital diaphragmatic hernia. Am J Obstet Gynecol 2002;186:1085-1090.
92. Chinn DH, Filly RA, Callen PW, Nakayama DK, Harrison MR. Congenital diaphragmatic hernia diagnosed prenatally by ultrasound. Radiology 1983;148:119-123.
93. Vettraino IM, Lee W, Comstock CH. The evolving appearance of a congenital diaphragmatic hernia. J Ultrasound Med 2002;21:85-89.
94. Lewis DA, Reickert C, Bowerman R, Hirschl RB. Prenatal ultrasonography frequently fails to diagnose congenital diaphragmatic hernia. J Pediatr Surg 1997;32:352-356.
95. Bootstaylor BS, Filly RA, Harrison MR, Adzick NS. Prenatal sonographic predictors of liver herniation in congenital diaphragmatic hernia. J Ultrasound Med 1995;14:515-520.
96. Paek BW, Danzer E, Machin GA, Coakley F, Albanese CT, Filly RA. Prenatal diagnosis of bilateral diaphragmatic hernia: diagnostic pitfalls. J Ultrasound Med 2000;19:495-500.
97. Song MS, Yoo SJ, Smallhorn JF, Mullen JB, Ryan G, Hornberger LK. Bilateral congenital diaphragmatic hernia: diagnostic clues at fetal sonography. Ultrasound Obstet Gynecol 2001;17:255-258.
98. Hedrick MH, Estes JM, Sullivan KM, et al. Plug the lung until it grows (PLUG): a new method to treat congenital diaphragmatic hernia in utero. J Pediatr Surg 1994;29:612-617.
99. Flake AW, Crombleholme TM, Johnson MP, Howell LJ, Adzick NS. Treatment of severe congenital diaphragmatic hernia by fetal tracheal occlusion: clinical experience with fifteen cases. Am J Obstet Gynecol 2000;183:1059-1066.
100. Tsukahara Y, Ohno Y, Itakura A, Mizutani S. Prenatal diagnosis of congenital diaphragmatic eventration by magnetic resonance imaging. Am J Perinatol 2001;18:241-244.
101. Gulrajani M, David K, Sy W, Braithwaite A. Prenatal diagnosis of a neurenteric cyst by magnetic resonance imaging. Am J Perinatol 1993;10:304-306.
102. Wang RM, Shih JC, Ko TM. Prenatal sonographic depiction of fetal mediastinal immature teratoma. J Ultrasound Med 2000;19:289-292.
103. Duncan KR, Baker PN, Gowland PA, et al. Demonstration of changes in fetal liver erythropoiesis using echo-planar magnetic resonance imaging. Am J Physiol 1997;273:G965-967.
104. Semple SI, Wallis F, Haggarty P, et al. The measurement of fetal liver T*2 in utero before and after maternal oxygen breathing: progress towards a non-invasive measurement of fetal oxygenation and placental function. Magn Reson Imaging 2001;19:921-928.
105. Toma P, Lucigrai G, Dodero P, Lituania M. Prenatal detection of an abdominal mass by MR imaging performed while the fetus is immobilized with pancuronium bromide. AJR Am J Roentgenol 1990;154:1049-1050.
106. Saguintaah M, Couture A, Veyrac C, Baud C, Quere MP. MRI of the fetal gastrointestinal tract. Pediatr Radiol 2002;32:395-404.
107. Benachi A, Sonigo P, Jouannic JM, et al. Determination of the anatomical location of an antenatal intestinal occlusion by magnetic resonance imaging. Ultrasound Obstet Gynecol 2001;18:163-165.
108. Garmel SH, Crombleholme TM, Semple JP, Bhan I. Prenatal diagnosis and management of fetal tumors. Semin Perinatol 1994;18:350-365.
109. Levine D, Goldstein RB, Callen PW, Damato N, Kilpatrick S. The effect of oligohydramnios on detection of fetal anomalies with sonography. AJR Am J Roentgenol 1997;168:1609-1611.
110. Estes JM, Harrison MR. Fetal obstructive uropathy. Semin Pediatr Surg 1993;2:129-135.
111. Cusick EL, Didier F, Droulle P, Schmitt M. Mortality after an antenatal diagnosis of foetal uropathy. J Pediatr Surg 1995; 30:463-466.
112. Lazebnik N, Bellinger MF, Ferguson JE, 2nd, Hogge JS, Hogge WA. Insights into the pathogenesis and natural history of fetuses with multicystic dysplastic kidney disease. Prenat Diagn 1999;19:418-423.
113. Johnson MP, Bukowski TP, Reitleman C, Isada NB, Pryde PG, Evans MI. In utero surgical treatment of fetal obstructive uropathy: a new comprehensive approach to identify appropriate candidates for vesicoamniotic shunt therapy. Am J Obstet Gynecol 1994;170:1770-1776; discussion 1776-1779.
114. Caire JT, Ramus RM, Magee KP, Fullington BK, Ewalt DH, Twickler DM. MRI of fetal genitourinary anomalies. AJR Am J Roentgenol 2003;181:1381-1385.

9

MRI of the Male Pelvis and the Bladder

E. Scott Pretorius, MD
Evan S. Siegelman, MD

MRI OF THE SCROTUM

Sonography remains the primary modality for cross-sectional imaging of the scrotum and penis. However, MRI is an excellent problem-solving tool for situations in which sonography is suboptimal or yields equivocal findings,[1-3] or for patients in whom there is discordance between clinical findings and sonographic results. Selective use of scrotal MR can improve patient care and decrease costs and the frequency of unnecessary surgical procedures.[4]

MR Technique

Appropriate patient positioning facilitates optimal MR of the scrotum and penis. With the patient supine, a folded towel is placed between the patient's legs inferior to the perineum, to elevate the scrotum and penis. For penile imaging, the penis is dorsiflexed against the lower midline abdomen, and taped in position to reduce organ motion during the examination (Box 9-1).

MR protocols depend on the clinical questions to be answered. For imaging of the scrotum and penis, a 3-inch or 5-inch surface coil is placed on the area of interest in order to obtain images with relatively small fields of view (14 to 16 cm), high matrix (256×256), and thin slices (3- to 4-mm skip 1 mm). We acquire axial (short axis) SE T1-WI followed by axial, sagittal, coronal fast spin-echo (FSE) T2-WI, employing fat suppression in one of these planes. Fat-suppression increases the dynamic range so that subtle differences in SI can be distinguished.

For men in whom primary testicular or penile malignancy is known or suspected, body coil or pelvic coil axial T1-WIs are obtained to evaluate for the presence of lymphadenopathy. For penile malignancy, inguinal or obturator nodes are the initial sites of lymphatic spread. For testicular malignancy, images should be acquired superior to the level of the renal hila, as lymphatic drainage of the testicle parallels gonadal blood supply and lymph node metastases can extend to renal hilar nodes.

If contrast injection is required for characterization of a scrotal or penile lesion, the authors obtain either two-dimensional (2D) or three-dimensional (3D) fat-saturated T1-W GRE images. The utility of

---

Sections on the scrotum and penis were primarily authored by E. Scott Pretorius, and those on the prostate and bladder were primarily authored by Evan S. Seigelman.

9-1 Suggested Protocol for MRI of Scrotum and Penis

Positioning
- Towel folded between legs to elevate scrotum
- For penile imaging: tape dorsiflexed penis to lower abdomen, cover with towel

Coil
- For high-resolution images: 5-inch circular coil or similar surface coil
- Pelvic array for larger view of pelvis
  - Evaluate superior extension of disease
  - Establish presence or absence of adenopathy or metastatic disease

Sequences
- Axial T1-WI
- Axial, sagittal, and fat-saturated coronal T2-WIs
- Fat-suppressed T1-WI obtained before and after contrast
- Pelvic or body coil: axial T1/T2 of abdomen/pelvis for tumor staging

Field of View: 14 to 16 cm

Slice Thickness
- 3–4 mm for scrotum and testes
- 6–7 mm for pelvis

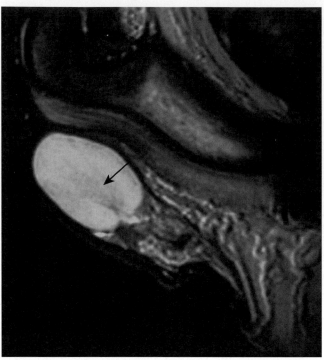

Figure 9-1 ▪ MR illustration of the normal testis. Sagittal T2-WI of a normal testicle shows homogeneous high SI. Thin, hypointense lobular septa *(arrow)* are present that converge on the mediastinum testis and rete testis.

contrast has not been firmly established in MR imaging of the scrotum and penis. In general, contrast is helpful in differentiating testicular cystic lesions from cystic neoplasms, in staging scrotal and penile malignancies, and in establishing the presence of perfusion to an organ, such as in the evaluation of testicular torsion.

For penile imaging, the injection of 10 μg of prostaglandin E_1 (alprostadil) into the proximal third of one of the cavernosal bodies can induce erection[5] and facilitate MR imaging by allowing for easier positioning of the organ and enabling the acquisition of more slices at increased fields of view. Prostaglandin injection is contradicted in patients with predisposition to priapism, including those patients with sickle cell anemia, multiple myeloma, invasive penile malignancy or implanted penile prostheses.

Normal Testes

The normal testes are ovoid structures of homogeneous intermediate T1 SI and high T2 SI relative to skeletal muscle.[6] T2-WIs (Fig. 9-1) are the mainstay of scrotal MR imaging and afford excellent contrast between the testicle and other scrotal structures. T1-WIs are less useful in delineating anatomy but are important for tissue characterization. For example, T1-WIs can reveal high SI secondary to methemoglobin within a subacute hematoma in the setting of trauma or characterize fat within a testicular teratoma or a paratesticular hernia.

Each testicle has approximately 200 to 350 small lobules, which contain the seminiferous tubules. The epithelium of the seminiferous tubules consists of spermatogenic (germ) cells and Sertoli (support) cells. In the interstitium between tubules are the testosterone-secreting Leydig cells.

Individual lobules are separated by septa that coalesce to form the mediastinum testis, which can be identified routinely on MR imaging as a thin, hypointense band on T2-WI relative to the testicular parenchyma (see Fig. 9-1). The mediastinum testis is oriented along the long axis of the testicle, is thickest cranially, and is eccentrically located dorsally within the testicle. The seminiferous tubules converge to form the rete testis, which lies adjacent to the mediastinum testis and which also can be identified on MR.[7] A thick fibrous band of tunica albuginea surrounds each testicle, which is hypointense to the testicle on both T1- and T2-WI.

The epididymis lies posterior to the testicle and consists of a single convoluted tubule that functions as a site for sperm maturation. The epididymis has similar T1 SI and lower T2 SI to the testicle. Sperm cells progress from the rete testis to the epididymal head and course though the epididymal body and tail before entering the vas deferens near the posterior, inferior margin of the testis. The vas deferens proceeds through the inguinal canal as part of the spermatic cord, which also contains the testicular

9-2 Differential Diagnosis of Intratesticular Lesions

Malignant/Potentially Malignant

Germ cell (95% of primary malignancies)
Seminomas: 40% of all primary malignancies
Mixed germ cell types: second most common subtype
Embryonal cell
Teratoma
Choriocarcinoma
Stromal cell (often histologically benign)
   (5% of primary malignancies)
Leydig cell
Sertoli cell
Gonadoblastoma
Lymphoma (most common intratesticular lesion in
   men over age 50 yr)
Metastases

Benign

Epidermoid inclusion cyst
Testicular cyst

artery and veins, lymphatics, nerves, and spermatic cord fascia. The vas deferens receives fluid from the seminal vesicles before forming the ejaculatory duct, which in turn enters the urethra. Superior to the epididymal head lies the tortuous, tubular, pampiniform venous plexus, which receives the venous return from the testicle. Slow flow within these veins is revealed as high SI on T2-WI.

The parietal and visceral layers of the tunica vaginalis, which lie in contiguity with the mesothelial layers lining the peritoneal cavity, surround the testicle and epididymis. A small amount of fluid (1 to 3 mm thick) is normally present between these layers. Larger amounts of fluid are termed hydroceles.

Intratesticular Lesions

MALIGNANT INTRATESTICULAR LESIONS

A primary indication for imaging the scrotum is to exclude the presence of an intratesticular mass (Box 9-2). Solid intratesticular lesions are highly suspicious for malignancy, whereas the vast majority of extratesticular lesions are benign. A major goal of diagnostic imaging, therefore, is to determine whether a palpable scrotal mass lies within the testicle or in an extratesticular location.

In the U. S. in 2004 there will be an estimated 8,980 new cases of testicular malignancy with an estimated 360 deaths.[8] Carcinoma of the testicle presents most commonly as a palpable intrascrotal abnormality, but it may present as a sensation of "heaviness" of the affected testicle or, in a minority of cases, as testicular pain. Carcinoma of the testicle is of germ cell origin in 95% of cases (see Box 9-2).[9] Seminoma is the most common cell type (Figs. 9-2 and 9-3). Nonseminomatous germ cell tumors include embryonal carcinoma (Fig. 9-4), yolk sac tumor teratoma (Fig. 9-5), and choriocarcinoma. A mixed cell type that includes both seminomatous and nonseminomatous elements also is common (Fig. 9-6).

Non–germ cell tumors include Leydig cell and Sertoli cell neoplasms. These are malignant in a minority (5% to 10%) of cases. Gonadoblastoma is a rare tumor arising from both germ cell and stromal elements and is seen primarily in patients with

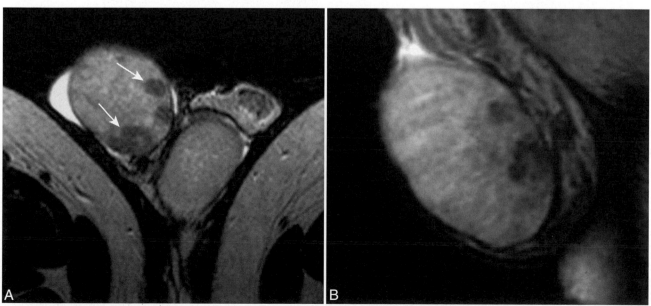

Figure 9-2 ▪ MR demonstration of a seminoma in a 34-year-old man with a palpable mass. A and **B,** Axial (**A**) and sagittal (**B**) T2-WIs show a hypointense, multifocal intratesticular neoplasm *(arrows)*. Seminomas tend to have more homogeneous SI compared with nonseminomatous tumors.

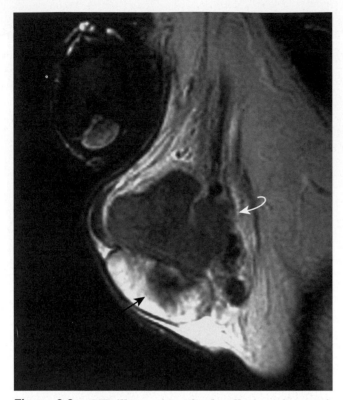

Figure 9-3 ▪ MR illustration of a locally invasive seminoma in a 43-year-old man with palpable mass and scrotal pain. Sagittal T2-WI reveals an intratesticular mass *(arrow)* that extends from the superior aspect of the left testicle and invades the adjacent epididymis and spermatic cord *(curved arrow).*

gonadal dysgenesis; affected individuals often have chromosomal abnormalities.

Lymphoma is the most common intratesticular neoplasm in men over age 50 years, and it may represent primary lymphoma or a manifestation of systemic disease (Fig. 9-7). The testicle is a common site of recurrence for lymphoma, since the blood-testis barrier limits delivery of chemotherapeutic agents.

Most intratesticular tumors are relatively iso-intense to the normal testis on T1-W images and hypointense on T2-W images. Testicular malignancies tend to enhance more heterogeneously than normal testicular parenchyma. MRI cannot reliably differentiate the different subtypes of testicular neoplasms. However, seminomas are generally homogeneous on all pulse sequences and discrete in location, while non-seminomatous tumors tend to be more heterogeneous in MR SI owing to hemorrhage and mixed cell types. Lymphomas tend to be multifocal (Box 9-3) and infiltrative and present in an older age group.

Metastatic disease is present at time of diagnosis in 20% to 25% of seminomas and approximately 40% of nonseminomatous tumors (Box 9-4).[10] Testicular lymphatic drainage parallels blood supply, and the para-aortic lymph nodes near the renal hilum are among the first sites of disease extension. Invasion of the epididymis or spermatic cord, which have different lymphatic drainage from the testes, may lead to early involvement of the internal iliac and external iliac nodes.

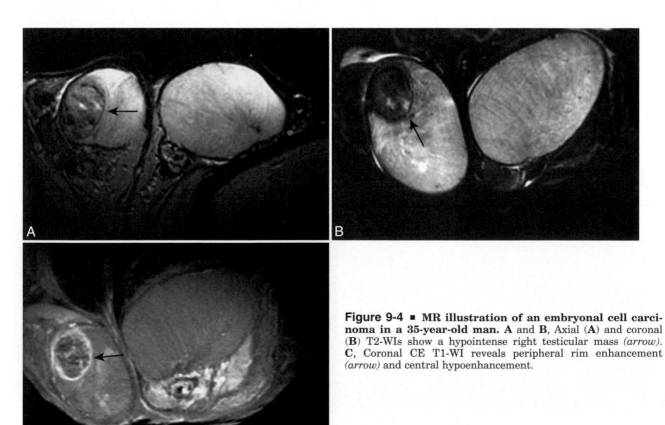

Figure 9-4 ▪ MR illustration of an embryonal cell carcinoma in a 35-year-old man. A and **B**, Axial **(A)** and coronal **(B)** T2-WIs show a hypointense right testicular mass *(arrow).* **C,** Coronal CE T1-WI reveals peripheral rim enhancement *(arrow)* and central hypoenhancement.

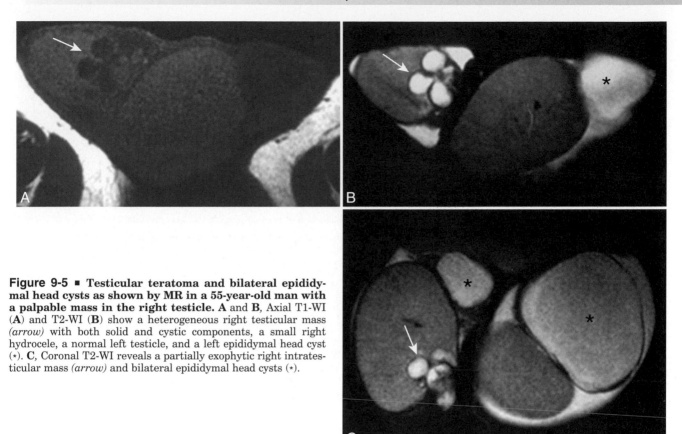

Figure 9-5 ■ **Testicular teratoma and bilateral epididymal head cysts as shown by MR in a 55-year-old man with a palpable mass in the right testicle. A** and **B**, Axial T1-WI (**A**) and T2-WI (**B**) show a heterogeneous right testicular mass *(arrow)* with both solid and cystic components, a small right hydrocele, a normal left testicle, and a left epididymal head cyst (*). **C**, Coronal T2-WI reveals a partially exophytic right intratesticular mass *(arrow)* and bilateral epididymal head cysts (*).

BENIGN INTRATESTICULAR LESIONS

Testicular cyst. Testicular cysts can occur in up to 10% of men[11] and can originate within either the testicle or the tunica albuginea.[12] Intratesticular cysts are sharply demarcated, thin-rimmed, and isointense to fluid on all pulse sequences, and display

no enhancement following gadolinium injection (Fig. 9-8). Contrast-enhanced (CE) images are highly recommended in the evaluation of such lesions, to differentiate simple cysts from cystic components of testicular neoplasms, such as cystic teratomas.[13] Unlike testicular malignancy, most testicular cysts

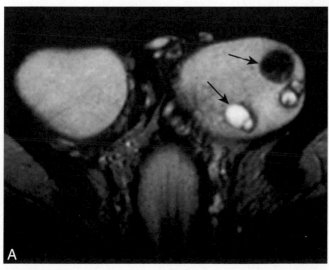

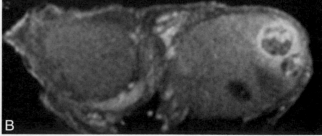

Figure 9-6 ■ MR depiction of a mixed malignant germ cell tumor in a 24-year-old man with palpable abnormality. **A**, Axial T2-WI shows multifocal, heterogeneous solid and cystic intratesticular lesions *(arrows)*. **B**, Axial CE T1-WI reveals heterogeneous tumoral enhancement.

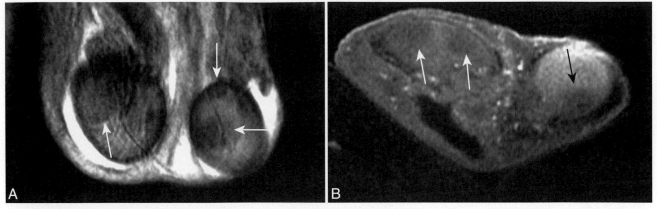

Figure 9-7 ■ **MR illustration of bilateral intratesticular lymphoma in a 40-year-old man with AIDS and non-Hodgkin's lymphoma. A**, Coronal T2-WI shows bilateral hypointense intratesticular lesions *(arrows)*. **B**, Axial CE T1-WI reveals that the lesions enhance less *(arrows)* than the normal testes.

are not palpable. They are usually incidental findings of ultrasound (US) or MRI examination, and are most commonly found near the mediastinum testis and may originate from the rete testis.[12,14]

Epidermoid inclusion cyst. Epidermoid inclusion cysts are the most common benign intratesticular neoplasm (Box 9-5). They are of uncertain origin, and some authors have speculated that they represent monodermal, benign teratomas. They are composed of cystic cavities lined by stratified squamous epithelium, surrounded by multiple lamellated layers of keratin debris.[15] US examination displays concentric rings of alternating hypo- and hyperechogenicity.[16] MRI shows an "onion ring" appearance, with alternating whirled bands of high and low SI (Fig. 9-9).[17] With gadolinium injection, epidermoid inclusion cysts are avascular and usually sharply demarcated against the background of the enhancing testicle. Since preoperative imaging can identify most epidermoid inclusion cysts, they can be treated with enucleation and frozen-section diagnosis rather than with orchiectomy.

DILATION OF THE RETE TESTIS

Dilation of the rete testis can in some cases simulate an intratesticular mass on US, although most cases are depicted on US examination as a region composed of small hypoechoic foci.[18] Dilation of the rete testis may indicate distal partial or complete obstruction, as the condition is associated with prior vasectomy, hernia repair, epididymal head cysts, and spermatoceles.[19]

MR examination demonstrates the characteristic appearance of this benign finding[7,20] (Fig. 9-10). Oriented along the superior portion of the mediastinum testis, cystic dilation or ectasia of the multiple small tubules of the rete testis will be identified. These will be either isointense or hyperintense to the normal testicular parenchyma on T2-WIs. Following gadolinium enhancement, the ectatic, fluid-filled tubules do not enhance.

ADRENAL RESTS

Testicular adrenal rests are of uncertain etiology, but their existence is likely related to the common embryologic origin of the adrenal gland and testes. Bilateral testicular lesions identified in the setting of congenital adrenal hyperplasia and elevated ACTH are almost certainly due to adrenal rests.

On US, affected testes display bilateral homogeneous hypoechoic nodules.[21] On MRI,[22,23] lesions are hypointense to the normal testicular tissue on T2-WIs and enhance following contrast administration (Fig. 9-11). Since these imaging findings are

---

9-3 Types of Multiple Bilateral Intratesticular Lesions

Leukemia/lymphoma
Metastatic disease
Adrenal rests (in congenital adrenal hyperplasia; check ACTH)
Leydig cell hyperplasia (if LH or hCG elevated)

9-4 Testicular Carcinoma Staging*

Stage I	Tumor confined to testis
Stage II	Metastases to subdiaphragmatic lymph nodes
IIA	Retroperitoneal nodes less than 2 cm
IIB	Retroperitoneal nodes 2-5 cm
IIC	Retroperitoneal nodes >5 cm
Stage III	Metastases to nodes above the diaphragm
Stage IV	Extranodal metastases

*Adapted from Testicular tumors and tumor like lesions. In: Hricak H, Hamm B, Kim B (Eds.): Imaging of the Scrotum. New York, Raven Press, 1995, p. 67.

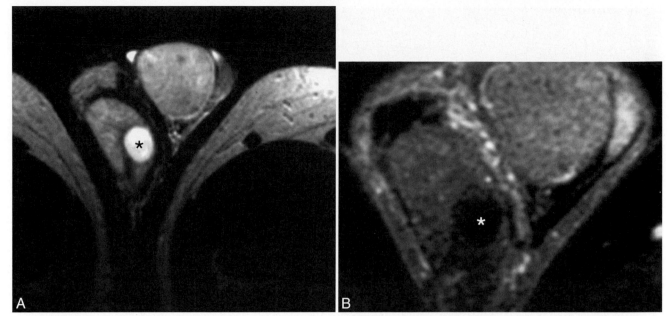

Figure 9-8 ■ **Benign intratesticular cyst as revealed on MR in a 48-year-old man. A**, Axial T2-WI shows a homogeneous hyperintense lesion (*) in the right testicle. **B**, Axial CE T1-WI shows normal testicular enhancement and absent enhancement in the simple testicular cyst (*).

nonspecific, endocrinologic workup is needed to evaluate for elevated ACTH and congenital adrenal hyperplasia. Serial imaging of patients with congenital adrenal hyperplasia and testicular adrenal rests may reveal that the lesions remain stable in size, grow larger or smaller, or resolve.[24]

LEYDIG CELL HYPERPLASIA

Testicular Leydig cell hyperplasia is a rare, benign condition characterized by small (1 to 6 mm), multifocal, bilateral testicular nodules. Adult patients with Leydig cell hyperplasia are usually asymptomatic, although some patients may present with testicular pain, swelling, or infertility. Lesions typically are not palpable, and serum tumor markers usually are normal.

Histologically, Leydig cell hyperplasia is characterized by an increased number of hyperplastic testicular Leydig cells that infiltrate between seminiferous tubules rather than displacing and compressing them, as occurs with Leydig cell tumors.[25] Leydig cell hyperplasia is thought to be due to a faulty hypothalamic-pituitary-testicular axis with resultant chronic Leydig cell stimulation, and patients often have elevated serum luteinizing hormone or human chorionic gonadotropin (hCG).[26] Causes of Leydig cell hyperplasia include cryptorchidism, congenital adrenal hyperplasia, hCG production by germ cell tumors or choriocarcinoma, pituitary abnormalities, Klinefelter's syndrome, exogenous hCG therapy, and anti-androgen therapy for prostate cancer.

On MRI, Leydig cell hyperplasia may be depicted as multiple, bilateral solid lesions that are hypointense on T2-WIs relative to normal testicular parenchyma, display mild contrast-enhancement, and range in size from 1 to 6 mm (Fig. 9-12).[27] Other differential possibilities include lymphoma, leukemia, metastatic disease, and bilateral primary testicular neoplasm. If clinical history and laboratory workup reveal an etiology for Leydig cell hyperplasia, medical treatment may be feasible, thereby obviating the need for operative exploration and possible radical orchiectomy.

POLYORCHIDISM

Polyorchidism is a rare condition in which division of the genital ridge during genital formation (between weeks 6 and 8 of intrauterine development) results in development of one or more supernumerary testicles.[2] This condition is more common on the left (71%) than on the right (20%), although both sides (10%) may be involved.[28] Seventy-five percent of the supernumerary testicles are intrascrotal, 20% are inguinal, and 5% are located within the retroperitoneum.[2] US[29] and MR imaging[30] demonstrate one or more supernumerary testicles, which are often

---

9-5   Features of Epidermoid Inclusion Cysts

Intratesticular and benign
Sonography: concentric rings of alternating hypo- and hyperechogenicity
MRI: alternating high and low SI on T2-WI ("onion ring" appearance)
Relatively avascular
Pathologic: multiple layers of keratin debris

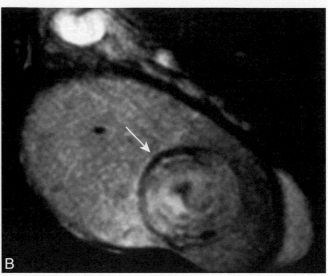

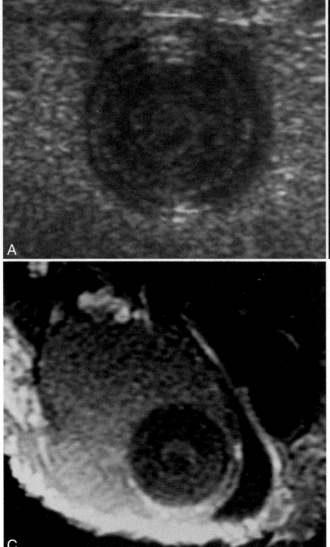

Figure 9-9 ▪ **MR depiction of an intratesticular epidermoid inclusion cyst in a 26-year-old man with a palpable scrotal mass. A,** Sonography shows an intratesticular mass with multiple concentric rings. **B,** Sagittal T2-WI confirms the intratesticular location of the mass *(arrow)* and reveals the "onion skin" appearance that is characteristic of epidermoid inclusion cyst. **C,** Sagittal CE T1-WI shows absent enhancement within the lesion. There is mild internal SI, which was present on precontrast images (not shown). (**A–C** adapted from Langer JE, Ramchadani P, Siegelman ES, Banner MP. Epidermoid cysts of the testicle: sonographic and MR imaging factors. AJR Am J Roentgenol 1999;173:1295–1299, with permission.)

slightly smaller than the normal testes (Fig. 9-13). The supernumerary testicle may share an epididymis and vas with another testicle or may be missing these structures. Torsion of a supernumerary testicle can occur de novo[31] or complicate an inadequate fixation.[32]

TESTICULAR PROSTHESIS

Testicular prostheses are placed for either cosmetic or psychological purposes, following orchiectomy or for a congenitally absent testicle. They are of variable appearance on MR, as they may contain internal fluid silicone or be composed of solid materials.[33] No evidence suggests that silicone testicular prostheses place men at risk for systemic disease (Fig. 9-14).[34] Most testicular prostheses are of homogeneous high T2 SI, similarly to the normal testis, but can easily be differentiated from native testicles by their lack of normal internal testicular architecture.

Extratesticular Processes

HYDROCELE

Hydrocele is fluid (Box 9-6) between the parietal and visceral layers of tunica vaginalis testis.[2] A small amount of physiologic fluid is revealed by sonography in this space in greater than 80% of asymptomatic men.[35] Hydroceles can be either congenital or acquired. Acquired hydroceles can be idiopathic or secondary to torsion or associated with infection or tumor. The cause of these hydroceles is hypothesized to be secondary to increased production of fluid from the mesothelial cell lining, decreased absorption of fluid from the mesothelium, or decreased lymphatic drainage.[2] Hydroceles are generally an asymptomatic finding on MR imaging of the scrotum. High T2 SI fluid surrounds the entire testicle, with the exception of the "bare area" (Fig. 9-15). Symptomatic hydroceles can be treated with sclerotherapy.[36]

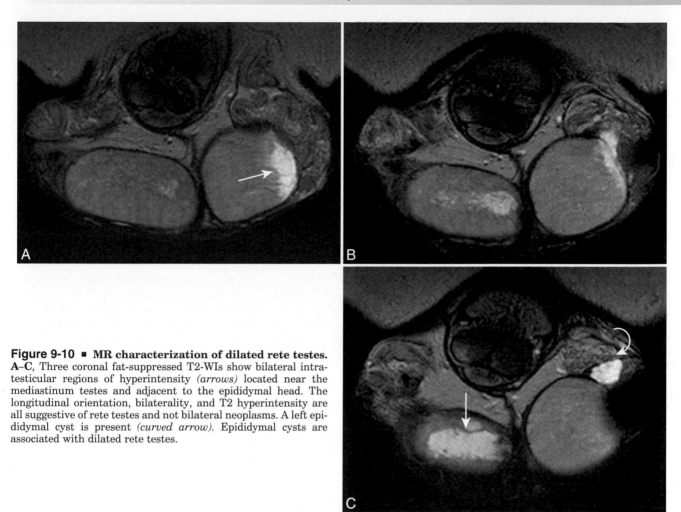

Figure 9-10 ▪ MR characterization of dilated rete testes.
A–C, Three coronal fat-suppressed T2-WIs show bilateral intra-testicular regions of hyperintensity *(arrows)* located near the mediastinum testes and adjacent to the epididymal head. The longitudinal orientation, bilaterality, and T2 hyperintensity are all suggestive of rete testes and not bilateral neoplasms. A left epi-didymal cyst is present *(curved arrow).* Epididymal cysts are associated with dilated rete testes.

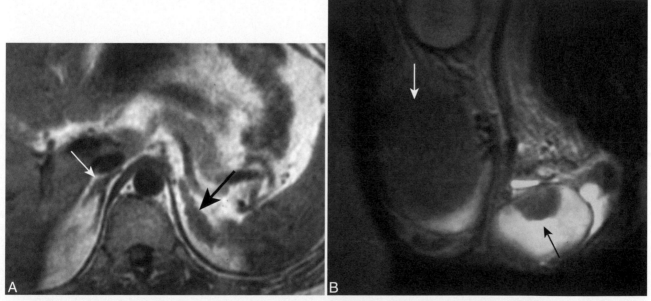

Figure 9-11 ▪ MR depiction of adrenal rests in a young adult man with congenital adrenal hyperplasia.
A, Axial T1-WI shows bilateral adrenal hyperplasia *(arrows).* **B,** Coronal T2-WI reveals bilateral hypointense intratesticular adrenal rests *(arrows).* In patients with known or suspected congenital adrenal hyperplasia, testicular masses that are revealed on physical examination or imaging are more likely to represent benign adrenal rests than testicular cancers.

Hemorrhagic fluid between the layers of the tunica vaginalis testis is termed a hematocele and may be a complication of scrotal trauma.[6] MR SI characteristics depend on the amount and age of the hemorrhage. In general, subacute hemorrhage will have higher T1 SI than will simple fluid. Unlike a simple hydrocele, a hematocele may distort the adjacent testicle.[2] In the pediatric population, scrotal swelling from hematocele may originate from blood in the peritoneum due to splenic trauma.[37] Blood reaches the scrotum through a patent processus vaginalis.

Infected fluid between the layers of the tunica vaginalis is termed pyocele or scrotal abscess. Pyoceles generally have thick walls and multiple septations. Diagnosis is based largely on clinical presentation, although US, and rarely MRI, may play a confirmatory role. Scrotal abscess is most commonly a complication of adjacent epididymo-orchitis.[2] Less commonly, peritoneal infection (e.g., appendicitis) can extend into the scrotum via a patent processus vaginalis.[38]

SPERMATOCELE AND EPIDIDYMAL CYST

Spermatoceles are sperm-filled retention cysts, often located within the epididymal head in close association with the rete testis. They are associated with distal obstruction and are especially common following vasectomy or herniorrhaphy. Spermatoceles most commonly present as palpable scrotal masses, superior and posterior to the testis. Spermatoceles may contain higher T1 SI than does simple fluid owing to their internal content of dead spermatozoa. Torsion of a spermatocele is rare and reportable and can clinically mimic testicular torsion.[39] Epididymal cysts are congenital lesions also located most commonly in the epididymal head. On MRI, epididymal cysts have content similar to simple fluid[6] (see Fig. 9-5). Differentiating between a spermatocele and an epididymal head cyst has little clinical importance. A large epididymal head cyst–spermatocele can be differentiated from a hydrocele at MRI because the latter surrounds the testicle while the former displaces the adjacent testicle.[40] Asymptomatic epididymal cysts and spermatoceles are present in up to

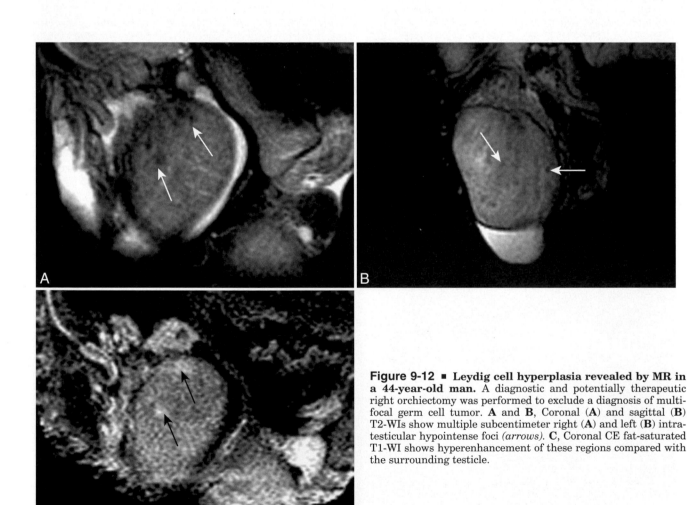

Figure 9-12 ■ Leydig cell hyperplasia revealed by MR in a 44-year-old man. A diagnostic and potentially therapeutic right orchiectomy was performed to exclude a diagnosis of multifocal germ cell tumor. **A** and **B**, Coronal (**A**) and sagittal (**B**) T2-WIs show multiple subcentimeter right (**A**) and left (**B**) intratesticular hypointense foci *(arrows).* **C**, Coronal CE fat-saturated T1-WI shows hyperenhancement of these regions compared with the surrounding testicle.

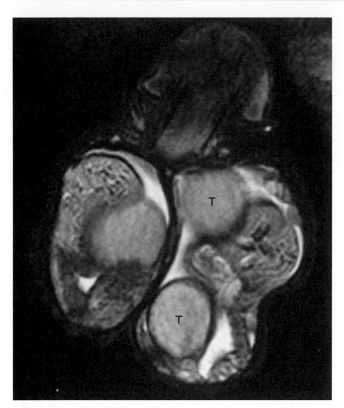

Figure 9-13 ▪ MR depiction of polyorchidism in a 34-year-old man with a left palpable mass. Coronal T2-WI shows the presence of a left supernumerary testicle. The right testicle is normal, but the left hemiscrotum contains two smaller testicles (T) of similar normal SI.

40% of men at sonography and do not require treatment.[35] Symptomatic lesions are successfully treated with aspiration and sclerotherapy.[36,41]

TUNICA ALBUGINEA CYST

Small cysts (generally <5 m) can be found in the tunica albuginea. They may present as a palpable mass and are readily identified by US or MR examination.[42] If US cannot establish the diagnosis of an extratesticular cyst, multiplanar imaging with MRI is helpful in demonstrating the cystic nature and paratesticular location of these lesions, which, being simple fluid, are isointense to fluid on all pulse sequences.

VARICOCELE

A varicocele is dilation of the veins of the pampiniform plexus. Varicoceles are revealed in 15% of all men and 40% of infertile men.[2,43] Although long thought to be a common cause of male infertility, recent meta-analyses have questioned this relationship and the benefits of varicocele treatment.[44,45] Reviews of this topic are available elsewhere.[46,47] MRI is not required for diagnosis, but varicocele may be diagnosed by MR imaging when dilated tubular structures are identified superior to the testicle, in the expected region of the pampiniform plexus. Because of slow flow within these tortuous veins, internal flow voids generally are not present; varicoceles most commonly are depicted as serpiginous structures with high SI on T2-WI (Fig. 9-16).[48]

SCROTAL HERNIA

Inguinal hernias are readily identified by MR examination. The contents of the hernia sac are variable

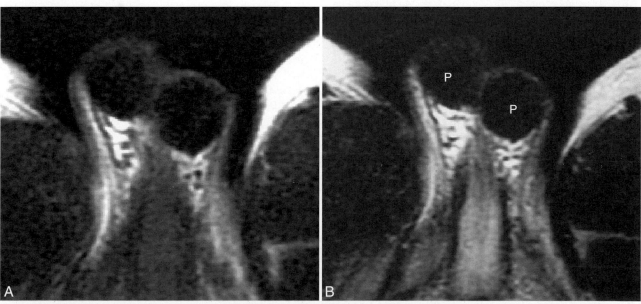

Figure 9-14 ▪ MR illustration of testicular prostheses in a 45-year-old man with a history of prior orchiectomies for seminoma. The prostheses were placed for cosmesis. **A** and **B**, Axial T1-WI (**A**) and T2-WI (**B**) show bilateral, spherical, low T1, low T2 SI structures (P) in the scrotum. The T2-SI of normal testicles is much higher (see Fig. 9-1).

9-6 Scrotal Fluid Collections

Hydrocele
Fluid between visceral and parietal layers of tunica vaginalis
Causes: idiopathic, infection, torsion, tumor

Hematocele
Blood between walls of tunica vaginalis.
Usually posttraumatic.

Pyocele
Infected fluid between walls of tunica vaginalis
Often thick walled with septa

Tunica Albuginea Cyst
SI: simple fluid
Usually small (<5 mm)

Spermatocele
Usually in epididymal head
Retention cyst containing spermatozoa
Often has debris
SI depends on content

Epididymal Cyst
SI: simple fluid
Congenital

Varicocele
Dilation of testicular veins of pampiniform plexus
Usually idiopathic
Can occur secondary to testicular vein compression
Controversial cause of male infertility

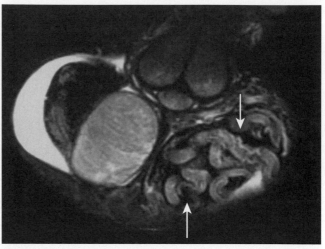

Figure 9-16 ■ MR illustration of a varicocele in a 33-year-old man with a palpable scrotal mass. Coronal T2-WI shows intermediate-to-high SI serpiginous left varicocele *(arrows)*, which correspond to the palpable abnormality. Slow flow within veins often has high SI on T2-WIs. There is a normal right testis. The left testis (not shown) also was normal.

and may consist only of fluid within the processus vaginalis testis or may contain mesenteric fat with mesenteric vessels or fluid- and air-containing loops of bowel. The MR appearance of an inguinal hernia extending into the scrotum is variable and dependent on the nature of the herniated contents. Mesenteric fat within the inguinal canal will appear similar to mesenteric fat in an orthotopic location. Oblique coronal or oblique sagittal images can show contiguity of intrascrotal bowel segment with adjacent bowel in the peritoneal cavity (Figs. 9-17 and 9-18).

Paratesticular Lesions

Most paratesticular lesions are benign (Box 9-7). The three most common neoplasms of paratesticular tissues are spermatic cord lipoma, adenomatoid tumor, and papillary cystadenoma.[3,40,49] Spermatic cord lipomas comprise approximately 45% of paratesticular neoplasms.[49] They are benign, usually are asymptomatic, and follow simple fat on all MR pulse

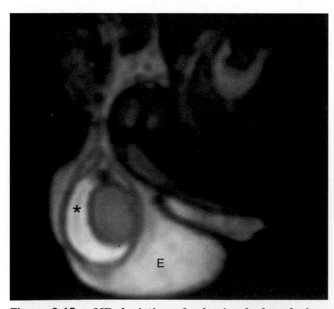

Figure 9-15 ■ MR depiction of a benign hydrocele in a 35-year-old man with signs and symptoms of epididymo-orchitis. Imaging was performed to exclude an underlying mass lesion. Coronal T2-WI reveals a large hydrocele (*) and skin thickening and marked subcutaneous edema (E). No occult testicular neoplasm was present.

9-7 Paratesticular Solid Masses

Adenomatoid Tumor of the Testicle
Benign
Usually in epididymal tail
Solid

Papillary Cystadenoma
Benign epididymal lesion
Common in patients with von Hippel–Lindau disease

Rhabdomyosarcoma
Malignant
Pediatric population

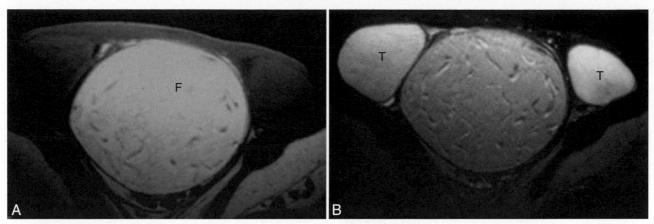

Figure 9-17 ■ **MR characterization of a fat-containing inguinal hernia as the cause of a palpable scrotal mass in a 27-year-old man.** **A** and **B**, Axial T1-WI (**A**) and T2-WI (**B**) show that the "mass" represents herniated mesenteric fat (F) with small mesenteric vessels and is situated between normal testes (T). A testicular or scrotal neoplasm was excluded.

sequences. A spermatic cord lipoma could be considered a normal developmental variant, since dissection reveals them in more than half of individuals examined at autopsy.[50] Adenomatoid tumor is a benign intrascrotal, extratesticular solid lesion that can originate from the epididymis, tunica vaginalis, or spermatic cord.[3] Adenomatoid tumor is most commonly found in or near the epididymal tail and represents the most common neoplasm of the epididymis.[2,49] On MR imaging, adenomatoid tumors are generally of higher SI than epididymis on T2-WI (Figs. 9-19 and 9-20). Papillary cystadenomas are benign epididymal lesions, present in 25% of patients with von Hippel–Lindau (VHL) disease. Two thirds of individuals with a papillary cystadenoma have VHL disease; 40% of men have bilateral papillary cystadenomas, which is more specific for VHL.[2]

Malignant paratesticular lesions are rare. The most common is rhabdomyosarcoma, which is seen almost exclusively in children.[51,52] In adults, the most common malignant neoplasm is liposarcoma.[2] MR imaging can be useful in demonstrating the paratesticular nature of these lesions and excluding the presence of an intratesticular mass.

Scrotal Inflammatory Disease

Epididymitis is the most common cause of scrotal pain in adult men. Imaging is not generally required for diagnosis, which can in most cases be made by clinical history, physical examination, and urinalysis. Epididymitis is usually due to an ascending urethritis from *Neisseria gonorrhoeae* or *Chlamydia trachomatis* in younger men[2] and

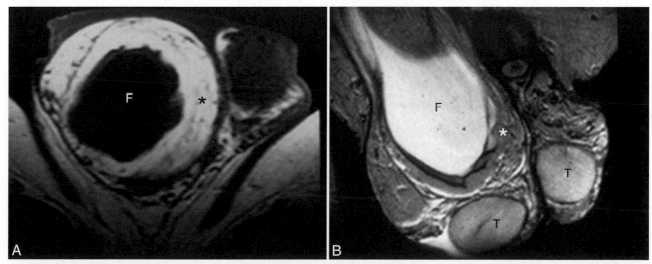

Figure 9-18 ■ **MR illustration of a fat- and fluid-containing hernia sac in a 59-year-old man with a palpable scrotal mass.** **A** and **B**, Axial T1-WI (**A**) and coronal (**B**) T2-WIs reveal an inguinal hernia containing both fluid (F) and fat (∗). No bowel segments were present. Normal testes (T) are revealed in **B**.

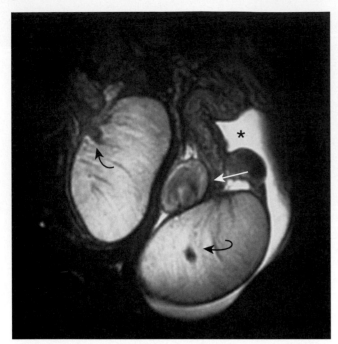

Figure 9-19 ■ **MR findings of an adenomatoid tumor in a 56-year-old man with a palpable mass.** Coronal T2-WIs show a hyperintense extratesticular mass *(arrow)* located adjacent to the epididymis. A small left hydrocele (✳) is present. The bilateral hypointense testicular foci *(curved arrows)* represent segments of the mediastinum testes depicted in cross-section.

Escherichia coli in older men.[40] US or MRI may be performed when clinical findings are equivocal or when there is suspicion of abscess. MRI generally demonstrates a large epididymis which is hypointense on T2-WI compared with the unaffected contralateral epididymis and which enhances avidly following gadolinium administration.[53]

Testicular infection and inflammation, orchitis, is depicted on MRI as heterogeneous regions of low SI on T2-WIs[53] and heterogeneous enhancement following gadolinium administration (Fig. 9-21; see Fig. 9-15). A reactive hydrocele is almost always present.

Orchitis may be difficult to distinguish from testicular malignancy, but in the case of infection normal testicular architecture will remain present, along with ipsilateral epididymitis, hydrocele, and scrotal skin thickening.[6]

Testicular Torsion

Testicle torsion is a surgical emergency and results when the testis abnormally rotates and twists the spermatic cord, compromising testicular perfusion. Absence of or defect in the testicular fixation at the "bare area" predisposes to torsion. Testicular torsion is most common in patients below age 25 years, and 85% of cases occur in patients between the ages of 12 and 18 years. Prompt surgical intervention with orchiopexy is curative and organ saving, provided the testicle has not yet infarcted.

US, or less often, scintigraphy, is used as a confirmatory procedure prior to surgical correction.[54] MRI is a not a primary modality for evaluation of the acutely twisted testicle, largely because of the greater availability of other modalities on an emergent basis. On MRI, the acutely twisted testicle is usually enlarged and hyperintense compared with the normal testicle on both T1- and T2-WI owing to small areas of hemorrhage. Gadolinium enhancement can be used to demonstrate blood flow to the testicle.[55] MR may be more useful in the diagnosis of subacute or chronic torsion, and especially in differentiating these entities from epididymitis. In chronic torsion, the testicle generally becomes hypointense on T2-WIs. The twisted spermatic cord may be directly visualized, and the affected testicle will enhance less than the normal testicle on enhanced images.[53]

Testicular Trauma

Testicular fracture is defined by rupture of the tunica albuginea. As there is exceptionally high contrast between the testicular parenchyma and the tunica albuginea on both T2-WI and gadolinium-enhanced images, MR is an excellent modality for

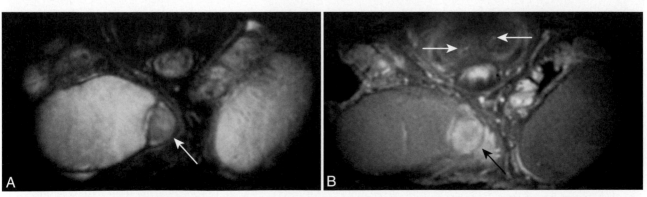

Figure 9-20 ■ **MR depiction of an adenomatoid tumor. A** and **B**, Coronal T2-WI (**A**) and CE T1-WI (**B**) show a T2-hypointense enhancing paratesticular mass *(arrow)*. Enhancing cavernosal arteries *(white arrows)* are revealed in **B**.

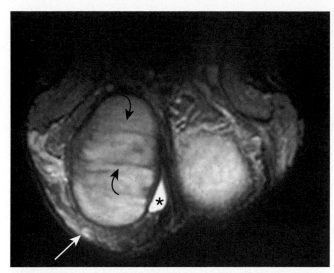

Figure 9-21 ■ MR illustration of orchitis in a 28-year-old man with scrotal pain. Coronal T2-WI shows no intratesticular mass. However, there is scrotal skin thickening *(arrow)* and a small hydrocele (*). There are hypointense bands *(curved arrows)* within the right testicle, an imaging feature characteristic of orchitis.

9-8 **Undescended Testes**
May be intra-abdominal or in inguinal canal Increased risk of malignancy, 38-45 times baseline MRI superior to sonography for identification

diagnosis of testicular fracture. MR can identify tears of the tunica albuginea not revealed by US examination.[56] Acquisition of images in multiple planes is indicated, to evaluate the entire tunica. Associated intratesticular hematoma (Fig. 9-22) or scrotal hematocele (Fig. 9-23) may be present.

Undescended Testis

One or both testes remain undescended in 3% of full-term male births and 30% of premature

infants (Box 9-8). Most undescended testes will spontaneously descend within the first year of life, so surgery is generally deferred until age 1 year, when the incidence of undescended testis is 0.8%. The inguinal canal is the most common location for a cryptorchid testis. The risk of malignancy developing within an undescended testicle is approximately 35 to 48 times baseline,[57] and testicular malignancies associated with cryptorchidism comprise 10% of all testicular carcinomas. After age 32, however, the risk of surgery outweighs the risk of malignancy, and surgery is generally not performed after this age.[58]

A complete imaging evaluation for an undescended testicle extends from the renal hila to the scrotum. MRI is superior to US at identifying undescended testes, largely due to the superiority of MRI at identifying intra-abdominal testes.[59] A cryptorchid testis is depicted on MR imaging (T2-WI) as a high SI, round or oval mass located along the path of testicular descent, parallel to the course of the gonadal vessels (Figs. 9-24 and 9-25). In some patients, enhanced sequences may be helpful in identifying the pampiniform plexus of the undescended, atrophic testis.[60]

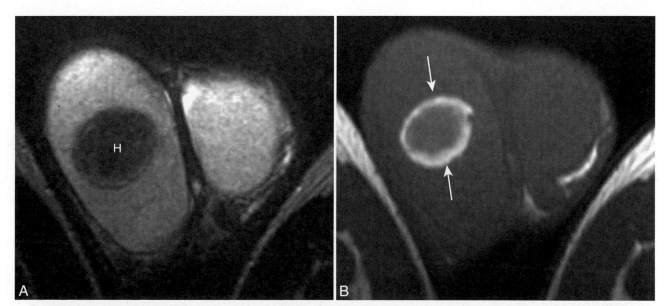

Figure 9-22 ■ MR depiction of an intratesticular hematoma. A, Axial T2-WI shows a low SI mass (H) within the right testicle. A testicular neoplasm could have a similar T2 appearance. **B,** Axial T1-WI reveals a hyperintense rim *(arrows)* in the right testicle that is characteristic of the rim sign of a subacute hematoma. Since testicular neoplasms may sometimes develop intratumoral hemorrhage, the images should be reviewed carefully to ensure that there is no occult tumor.

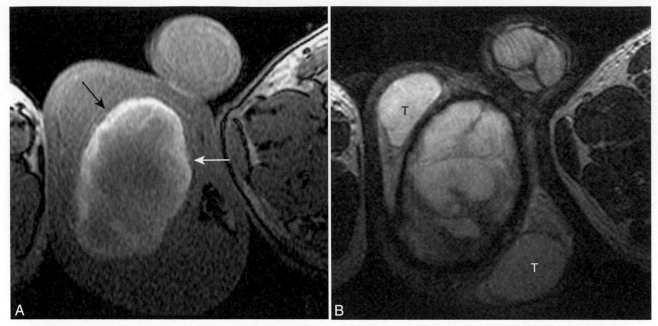

Figure 9-23 ■ Scrotal hematoma revealed on MR in a man after trauma. A and **B**, Axial T1-WI opposed-phase gradient echo image (**A**) and T2-WI (**B**) show a large, T1-hyperintense *(arrows)* scrotal hematoma. The testes (T), which are of normal SI, remain intact. The right testicle is hyperintense compared with the left testicle because the former is closer to the anteriorly placed surface coil.

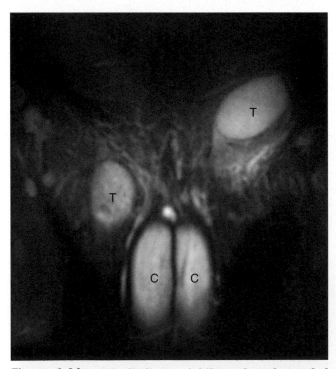

Figure 9-24 ■ MR findings of bilateral undescended testes in a 25-year-old man with an "empty scrotum" on physical examination. Coronal fat-saturated T2-WI shows bilateral undescended inguinal testes (T) that have similar high SI to the paired corpora cavernosa (C).

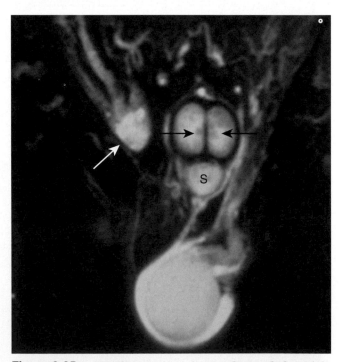

Figure 9-25 ■ MR illustration of an undescended testicle in a 57-year-old man. Coronal T2-WI shows a normal left testicle and small left hydrocele. The right testicle *(white arrow)* is atrophic, maldescended, and located within the inguinal canal. No intratesticular mass lesion is seen. The paired dorsal corpora cavernosa, with their medially located central cavernosal arteries *(black arrows),* are also depicted. The corpus spongiosum (S) is unpaired and is located midline and ventrally.

MRI OF THE PENIS

Normal Penis

MR imaging of the penis[61,62] is performed rarely, as US and physical examination are sufficient to answer most clinical questions. MRI, however, is a useful adjunct to US for imaging a wide range of penile pathology.[63] MR imaging of the penis is best reserved for those men for whom US is equivocal or those in whom there is discordance between clinical and US findings.

The penis consists of three tubular endothelium-lined vascular spaces: the paired, dorsolateral corpora cavernosa and the single, ventral corpus spongiosum (Fig. 9-26). Posteriorly, the corpora cavernosa flare laterally to form the crura and attach to the ischial tuberosities. The bulbar and pendulous portions of the urethra traverse the corpus spongiosum, which forms the penile bulb posteriorly and the glans penis anteriorly.

All three corporal bodies tend to be of intermediate T1 SI and high T2 SI relative to skeletal muscle. The corpora cavernosa are isointense to one another, as their vascular sinuses communicate through fenestrations in the membranous intercavernosal septum. The corpus spongiosum may normally have a different MR SI from that of the corpus cavernosum, since its vascular channels are functionally separate (see Fig. 9-26). The differential SI is related to different rates of flow of sinusoidal blood. Both the corpus spongiosum and the corpora cavernosa are surrounded by a low T1 and T2 SI tunica albuginea. This hypointense band appears thicker around the corpora cavernosa than around the spongiosum, since the corpora cavernosa are also surrounded by Buck's fascia, a separate fibrous layer that is inseparable from the tunica on imaging.

The cavernosal arteries are revealed on short-axis T2-WI as hypointense foci located medially within the corpora cavernosa. The cavernosal arteries are end branches of the common penile artery, which arises on each side from the internal pudendal artery, which in turn originates from the anterior division of the internal iliac artery. Vascular resistance to flow within the flaccid penis is high. Following appropriate psychological or physical stimulation, parasympathetic nerves relax the smooth muscle within the corporal sinusoids, increasing inflow of blood from the cavernosal arteries. The corporal bodies normally drain to veins within the wall of the tunica albuginea, but the expanding sinusoids compress these veins, trapping blood within the corporal bodies and sustaining penile erection.

Penile Malignancies

Squamous Cell Carcinoma of the Penis

Squamous cell carcinoma of the penis (Box 9-9) is rare in the U. S., with an estimated 1,570 cases that will arise in 2004 and result in 270 deaths.[8] In Africa and Asia, it is among the most common malignancies of adult male patients.[64] This difference in incidence is in part related to the practice of circumcision, as the chronic irritative effect of smegma is an important risk factor in the development of penile cancer. Human papillomaviruses 16 and 18, which have been implicated in the development of carcinoma of the female genital tract, are also known risk factors. In the U. S., penile squamous cell carcinoma usually presents in men in the sixth or seventh decade of life. Delays in diagnosis are common because the lesions often are not painful and many men delay in seeking medical attention.

Carcinoma of the penis has traditionally been staged clinically using the Jackson classification (Box 9-10). Carcinoma of the penis most commonly arises in the skin of the glans penis. On MRI,

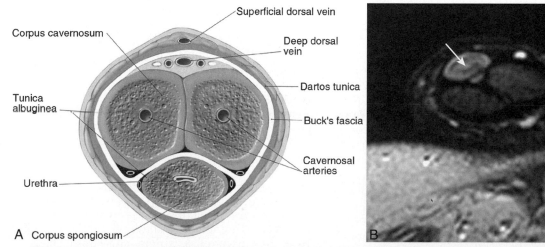

Figure 9-26 ■ Normal penile anatomy. A, Cross-sectional illustration of penile anatomy. (Courtesy of F. M. Corl; reproduced from Pretorius ES, Siegelman ES, Ramchandani P, Banner, MP. MR imaging of the penis. Radiographics 2001;21(Spec No.):S283–S298; discussion S298–S299, with permission.) **B,** Axial T2-WI shows the penis dorsiflexed against the lower abdominal wall. Although the corpora cavernosa are isointense to one another, they are of different SI from the corpus spongiosum. This is a normal finding. The collapsed, low SI urethra *(arrow)* is visible within the corpus spongiosum.

9-9 Features of Squamous Cell Carcinoma (SCC)

Most common in 6th to 7th decades
1,200 cases/yr in U. S.
Much more common in Africa and Asia
Risk factors
    Human papillomavirus, especially subtypes 16 and 18
    Lack of circumcision
MRI
    Most common on the glans
    Hypointense to corpora on T1- and T2-WI
    SCC enhances less than corporal bodies

squamous cell carcinoma of the penis is hypointense to the corpora on both T1- and T2-WI (Fig. 9-27) and enhances less than the normal corpora. Both T2-WI and enhanced images can determine the presence and extent of invasion of the corpora. Although a small surface coil is required for genital imaging, pelvic or body coil images should be obtained of the pelvis to detect regional lymph nodes. Unlike testicular carcinomas, the primary lymphatic drainage of penile malignancies is to pelvic lymph node chains. Treatment of carcinoma of the penis is usually surgical, with radical or partial penectomy.

NONSQUAMOUS PRIMARY PENILE MALIGNANCIES

Squamous cell carcinoma of the penis accounts for 95% of primary penile malignancies. The remaining cases are mostly primary penile melanomas and penile sarcomas, which include epithelioid sarcoma, Kaposi's sarcoma, leiomyosarcoma, and, particularly in children, rhabdomyosarcoma.[65] Penile melanomas present in similar fashion to melanomas at other sites.[66] Imaging rarely is required, although, as with other penile malignancies, MR may be used to determine whether cavernosal invasion has occurred. Primary melanoma is most commonly hyperintense to skin on both T1- and T2-WI. Following gadolinium administration, the tumor enhances avidly.

PRIMARY URETHRAL CARCINOMA

The cell type of normal urothelium changes along the course of the urethra. Transitional cells line the prostatic and membranous urethra, pseudostratified columnar epithelium is present in the bulbar and pendulous segments, and squamous cells line the fossa navicularis and urethral meatus. Primary urethral carcinomas are most common in men with a history of

9-10 Jackson Classification for Staging SCC of Penis

Stage I	Lesions confined to the glans or prepuce
Stage II	Involves the penile shaft
Stage III	Extends to inguinal nodes
Stage IV	Involves deep pelvic nodes or distant metastases

urethritis and urethral strictures, and tumors occur most commonly in the bulbar and membranous portions of the urethra, followed by the fossa navicularis.[6] Squamous cell carcinomas of the urethra are the most common primary urethral malignancy.[67]

On MR imaging, primary urethral carcinomas are most commonly depicted as bulky masses, often in association with proximal urethral dilation. A major goal of imaging is to determine the proximal extent of tumor, as this determines appropriate surgical management.[68] Urethral carcinomas involving the glans or distal penile shaft are treated by partial or radical penectomy. Lesions involving the proximal shaft or posterior urethra are treated by radical penectomy, with or without cystoprostatectomy.

METASTASES TO THE PENIS

Metastases to the penis constitute distant organ spread and therefore connote a very poor prognosis. Genitourinary tumors, particularly prostate and bladder malignancies, are the most common primary tumors of origin.[69] Penile metastases present with single or multiple palpable nodules, superficial ulcer, pain, swelling, hematuria, obstructive urinary symptoms, or even malignant priapism. Metastases to the penis have variable MR appearance.[70] In most cases, one or more discrete enhancing masses are seen in the corpora cavernosa, with or without invasion of the tunica albuginea or corpus spongiosum. Simultaneous imaging of the pelvis is recommended and may reveal the genitourinary or rectosigmoid primary and associated pelvic lymphadenopathy.

Benign Penile Disorders

Several benign conditions of the penis may present as palpable masses. Although history and physical examination are the mainstays of diagnosis, MR imaging can play an important role in equivocal cases or in confirming a clinically suspected diagnosis.

COWPER'S DUCT SYRINGOCELE

The bulbourethral glands are located inferior to the prostatic apex in the urogenital diaphragm and drain into the bulbar urethra. Cystic dilation of the main duct of the bulbourethral (Cowper's) glands is termed Cowper's duct syringocele. Patients with this entity may have postvoid dribbling, urinary frequency, recurrent infection, weak stream, or hematuria. Surgical marsupialization is curative.[71] MRI of the penile bulb most commonly demonstrates a midline high T2 SI structure near the bulbourethral glands (Fig. 9-28).

PARTIAL CAVERNOSAL THROMBOSIS

Segmental thrombosis of a corpus cavernosum may occur as a result of trauma or a hypercoagulable state and most commonly presents as partial priapism or focal hardness of a single cavernosal body. The affected corporal body will appear distended and compress its normal, contralateral mate. The MR signal intensity of the affected segment dependson the age of the thrombus, but in general will be hyperintense

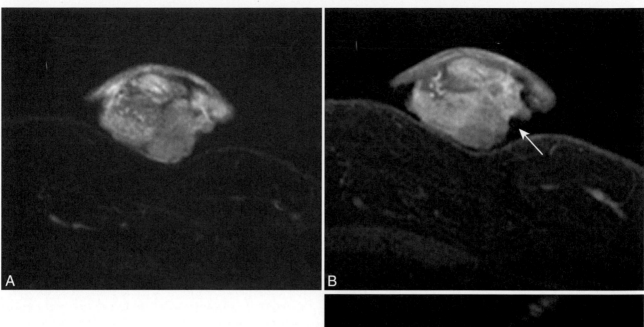

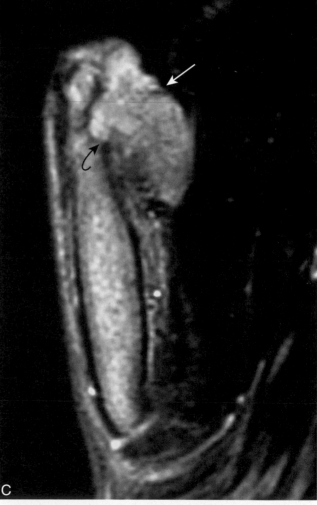

Figure 9-27 ■ MR depiction of a squamous cell carcinoma in a 75-year-old man with a palpable penile mass. **A** and **B**, Axial fat-suppressed T2-WI (**A**) and CE T1-WI (**B**) reveal an infiltrative necrotic mass *(arrow)* of the glans penis. **C**, Sagittal T2-WI shows that the mass *(arrow)* originates from the dorsal glans and invades the distal corpus spongiosum, as revealed by interruption of the low SI tunica albuginea *(curved arrow).*

to the normal corpora on T1-WI and hypointense on T2-WI (Fig. 9-29).[72,73]

PEYRONIE'S DISEASE

Peyronie's disease is an idiopathic chronic disorder in middle-aged men. It begins as an area of vasculitic inflammation subjacent to the tunica albuginea and progresses to focal fibrous thickening of the tunica that may extend into the intercavernosal septum. The resulting fibrous plaques can be single or multiple and may calcify, in which case they will be visible on radiography. Clinical manifestations of Peyronie's

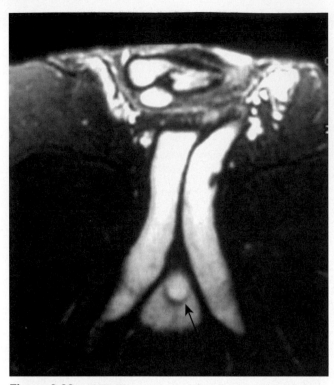

Figure 9-28 ■ **MR illustration of Cowper's syringocele in a 43-year-old man with a palpable mass at the base of the penis.** Axial T2-WI shows a high SI midline structure *(arrow)* near the penile bulb, representing a Cowper syringocele. (Reproduced from Vossough A, Pretorius ES, Siegelman ES, Ramchandani P, Banner MP. Magnetic resonance imaging of the penis. Abdom Imaging 2002;27:640–659, with permission.)

disease include painful erection, penile deviation, poor-quality erection distal to the involved area, and even inability to perform intercourse.

The disease starts with an active inflammatory stage, lasting 12 to 18 months, associated with painful erections. This is followed by a second stage of mature scar formation associated with painless penile deformity. Sonography and MRI are similar in their ability to demonstrate fibrous plaques,[74] although CE MRI may depict active inflammation within or around a fibrous plaque.[75] This may be helpful in guiding therapy, as the early stage of Peyronie's disease is generally treated not with surgery but with anti-inflammatory medications. On MRI, the fibrous plaques of Peyronie's disease appear as thickened and irregular low SI areas on both T1- and T2-WI in and around the tunica albuginea (Fig. 9-30).

Penile Trauma

Fracture of the penis is defined as a tear in the tunica albuginea, and MRI is the most sensitive means of identifying this finding. Penile fracture usually results from blunt trauma to the erect organ, such as might be incurred during vigorous intercourse or masturbation.[76,77] A tear in the tunica albuginea or disruption of the urethra is an indication for surgical repair, whereas other cases of blunt penile trauma, such as isolated corporal or subcutaneous hematoma, may be managed conservatively.

Fracture of the tunica albuginea is depicted on MR imaging as discontinuity of the T2-hypointense tunica albuginea (Fig. 9-31).[78] Associated hematoma may also be present. CE MRI may more easily demonstrate a tunical tear or the extent of hematoma, but

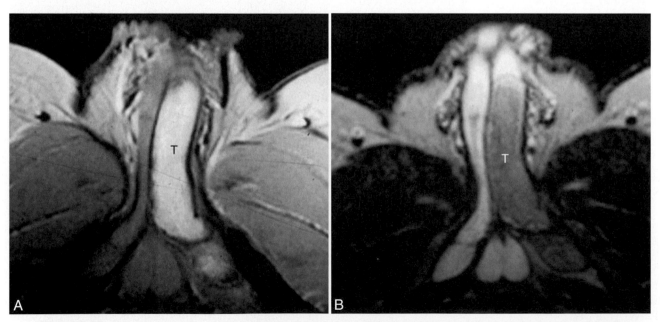

Figure 9-29 ■ **Partial cavernosal thrombosis revealed on MR in an 18-year-old man who presented with a firm mass at the base of his penis. A,** Axial T1-WI shows a hyperintense expanded left corpus cavernosum (T). **B,** Corresponding T2-WI reveals the region to be hypointense to the remainder of the corpus cavernosum. This represented segmental cavernosal thrombosis. (Reproduced from Pretorius ES, Siegelman ES, Ramchandani P, Banner MP. MR imaging of the penis. Radiographics 2001;21(Spec No.):S283–S298; discussion S298–S299, with permission.)

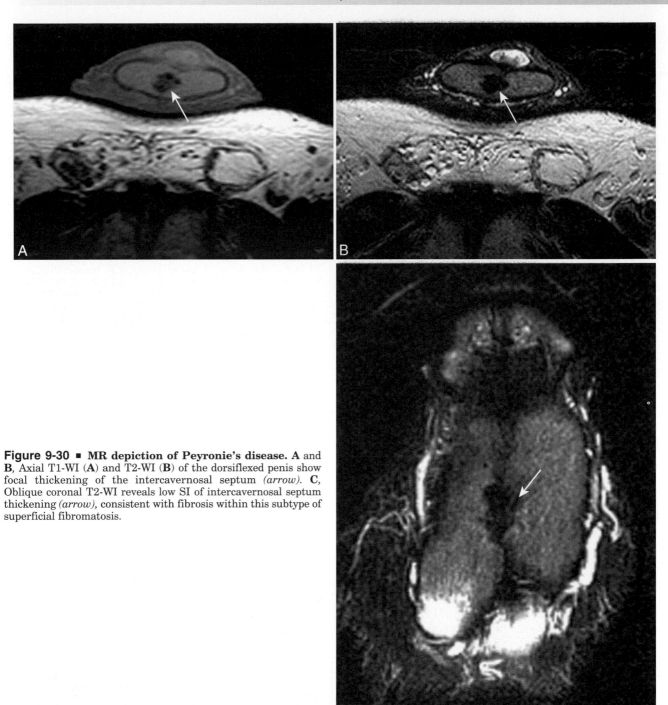

Figure 9-30 ■ **MR depiction of Peyronie's disease. A** and **B**, Axial T1-WI (**A**) and T2-WI (**B**) of the dorsiflexed penis show focal thickening of the intercavernosal septum *(arrow)*. **C**, Oblique coronal T2-WI reveals low SI of intercavernosal septum thickening *(arrow),* consistent with fibrosis within this subtype of superficial fibromatosis.

unenhanced MR images are sufficient for almost all cases. Extravasation of urine from an injured urethra will appear as a high SI collection on T2-WIs. Although complications of urethral injuries can be revealed on MR imaging, they are best evaluated with retrograde urethrography.

Penile Prostheses

Most penile prostheses are MR compatible, but the OmniPhase and Duraphase penile implants (Dacomed, Minneapolis, MN) have test positive for relatively strong ferromagnetic deflection forces when exposed to static 1.5 tesla magnetic fields.[79,80] In theory, any implanted device can result in heat generation in the scanner, and the patient should be removed from the scanner immediately if he complains of pain.

The most common indication for the placement of a penile prosthesis is erectile dysfunction that is not responsive to pharmacologic therapy. There are many kinds of penile prosthesis, but the most common is the inflatable prosthesis, consisting of paired

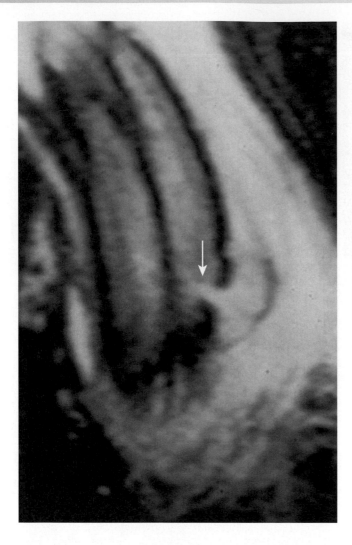

Figure 9-31 ▪ MR illustration of a tunical fracture in a 32-year-old man with pain and palpable abnormality following vigorous sexual intercourse. Coronal T1-WI shows a fracture of the tunica albuginea *(arrow)* with associated hyperintense hematoma in the pericavernosal soft tissues. (Reproduced from Vossough A, Pretorius ES, Siegelman ES, Ramchandani P, Banner MP. Magnetic resonance imaging of the penis. Abdom Imaging 2002;27:640–659, with permission.)

inflatable rubber tubes within the cavernosa, an abdominal fluid reservoir, and a small scrotal pump used to fill the tubes from the reservoir. On MR imaging, the cavernosal cylinders have internal SI isointense to fluid, surrounded by a low T1, low T2 hypointense rim (Fig. 9-32).

Complications of penile prostheses include infection and mechanical failure. Infection may lead to abscess formation and/development of a sinus tract, both of which can be demonstrated by MR imaging. Mechanical failures include fluid leakage, tube kinking, and aneurysmal dilation of the cylinders.[81] Some patients with chronic penile pain following device placement have been demonstrated by MR to have buckling of the penile cylinders.[82]

MRI OF THE PROSTATE

MRI Techniques

Most MR imaging of the prostate is performed for the staging of prostate cancer.[83] The ideal technique includes a combination of a phased-array pelvic coil and an endorectal coil and multiple imaging planes.[84-86] Initially we perform a large-field-of-view sagittal sequence to confirm optimal placement of the endorectal coil and to provide survey images of the lumbar spine and retroperitoneum. If the coil is appropriately positioned, small-field-of-view, high-resolution images of the prostate are obtained that include axial T1-WI and axial, coronal, and sagittal T2-WI. Fast spin-echo T2-WI is preferred to conventional T2-WI because of decreased motion artifact from rectal spasm and patient motion.[85] Finally, larger field-of-view axial imaging is performed of the pelvis to evaluate for adenopathy and osseous metastatic disease. The use of gadolinium contrast does not improve the ability of MRI to stage prostate cancer,[87,88] although some have found dynamic CE MRI useful to detect prostate cancer.[89]

A staging MR examination in a man with biopsy-proved prostate cancer should be confined to the pelvis. CT of the abdomen and pelvis is not cost effective for detecting comorbid disease in men with prostate cancer.[90,91] The pelvis should be evaluated for osseous metastatic disease and adenopathy. It is rare

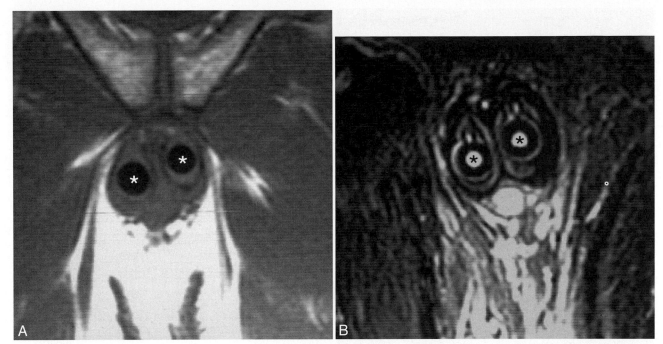

Figure 9-32 ▪ **A 40-year-old man with an uncomplicated penile prosthesis as revealed by MRI. A** and **B**, Coronal T1-WI (**A**) and T2-WI (**B**) show paired, fluid-filled prosthetic tubes (∗) within the corpora cavernosa. The corpus spongiosum retains its normal intermediate T1 and high T2 SI.

for a man with isolated metastatic disease to the abdomen to not also have demonstrable metastatic disease within the pelvis.

Zonal Anatomy of the Prostate

Before the MR appearance of normal prostate tissue and prostate cancer are described, a brief description of the zonal anatomy of the prostate is provided.[92,93] The peripheral zone of the prostate accounts for 70% of the volume of the prostate in young men and contains most of the prostate glandular tissue (Fig. 9-33). Seventy percent of prostate cancers originate in the peripheral zone. The transitional zone makes up only 5% of the prostate volume in young men and comprises the glandular prostatic tissue that surrounds the proximal prostatic urethra. The transition zone is the site of benign prostatic hyperplasia (BPH) and progressively enlarges as men age. The central zone makes up 25% of the prostate volume in young men and surrounds the transition zone at the prostate base. The central zone becomes compressed and is less well visualized in older men. Twenty percent of prostate cancers originate within the transition zone, and the remaining 10% arise from the central zone. The central gland is the term used to describe the region of the prostate composed of the central and transitional zones.

Normal MR Appearance of the Prostate and Periprostatic Soft Tissues

On T1-WI the normal prostate has relatively homogeneous low-to-intermediate SI with poor differentiation between the central gland and the peripheral zone (Fig. 9-34A; see Fig. 9-33A). On T2-WI the normal peripheral zone of the prostate reveals relative high SI secondary to the presence of mucin-rich glandular tissue (Fig. 9-34B; see Fig. 9-33B). Reticular low SI foci within the peripheral zone on T2-WI represent a supporting network of collagenous septa. The true prostate capsule is a 2- to 3-mm fibromuscular layer that has low SI on T2-WI and separates the high SI peripheral zone of the prostate from the periprostatic soft tissues (Box 9-11).

The periprostatic soft tissues are composed of variable amounts of fat and the paired neurovascular bundles. The neurovascular bundles are composed of nerves that innervate the corpora cavernosa and branches of Santorini's venous plexus; these nerves and vessels are present along the posterolateral aspect of the left and right sides of the gland. These bundles have low SI compared with the surrounding periprostatic fat. The SI is variable on T2-WI. While the nerves show low SI relative to fat, the veins may reveal high SI secondary to slow flow.

Most men who have an MR examination to stage established prostate cancer have some degree of BPH. BPH originates from the periurethral transition zone that is part of the central gland. BPH is revealed as multiple nodules of varying SI on T2-WI[94,95] (see Fig. 9-34). Relatively low SI nodules are stroma-rich foci of BPH, while higher SI foci are glandular-rich nodules.[95] The central gland (composed of both central and transitional zones) is separated from the peripheral zone by a low T2-SI band of tissue known as the surgical capsule, which is of little clinical import.

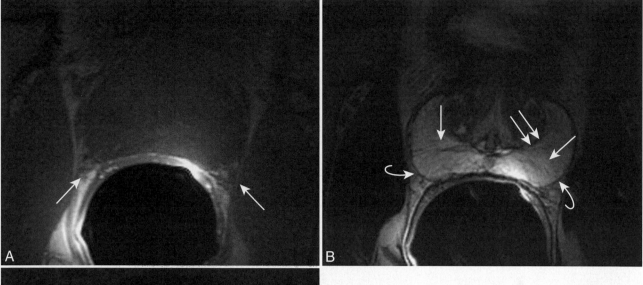

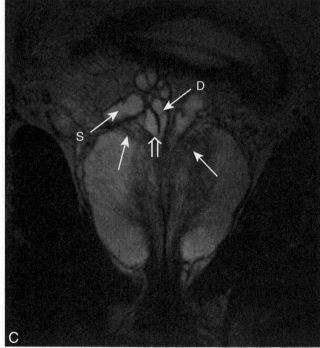

Figure 9-33 ▪ MR depiction of normal prostate gland anatomy in a 45-year-old man with symptoms of prostatitis. In younger men, the central gland comprises a minority of the volume of the prostate. **A,** Axial T1-WI shows poor distinction between the central gland and peripheral zone of the prostate. The periprostatic fat is of high SI. The paired neurovascular bundles are revealed as tubular low SI structures *(arrows)* within the periprostatic fat at the 5 and 7 o'clock positions. **B,** Axial T2-WI shows excellent distinction between the heterogeneous low-to-intermediate SI central gland and the higher SI peripheral zone. The low SI curvilinear structures within the peripheral gland are normal fibrous septa *(arrows)*. The central gland and peripheral zone are separated by a low SI surgical capsule *(double arrows)* that has little clinical import. The true prostatic capsule *(curved arrows)* is revealed as a low SI structure between the peripheral zone and the high SI periprostatic soft tissue. The latter is hyperintense secondary to fat and slow flow within veins. **C,** Coronal T2-WI again shows excellent contrast differentiation between the hyperintense peripheral zone and the heterogeneous lower SI central gland. There is a normal superior extension of hypointense central gland *(arrows)* located immediately subjacent to the seminal vesicles that should not be confused with peripheral zone tumor of the prostate base. The central segments of the right seminal vesicle (S) and vas deferens *(arrow, D)* join to form the ejaculatory duct *(open arrow)*.

The seminal vesicles are paired structures located above the prostate that are responsible for the formation and storage of the ejaculate. Each seminal vesicle is composed of multiple lobules whose contents have SI of relatively simple fluid and whose walls have low SI on both T1- and T2-WI (Fig. 9-35). The ampullae of the vas deferens are paired tubular structures that pass through the medial aspect of the seminal vesicles. The walls of the ampullae can measure up to 3 to 4 mm. The vas deferens joins the outflow of the seminal vesicles to form the ejaculatory ducts, which empty into the prostatic urethra (see Fig. 9-35).

Prostate Cancer

EPIDEMIOLOGY OF PROSTATE CANCER

Prostate cancer is the most commonly diagnosed malignancy and the second leading cause of cancer deaths in American men.[96] In 2004 it is expected that 230,110 men in the U. S. will be newly diagnosed with prostate cancer and that 29,900 men will die of this disease.[8] In 2004 prostate cancer will account for one third of new cancers in American men and 10% of cancer-related deaths.[8] The number of men with newly diagnosed prostate cancer is stabilizing, in part because the number of tumors detectable by

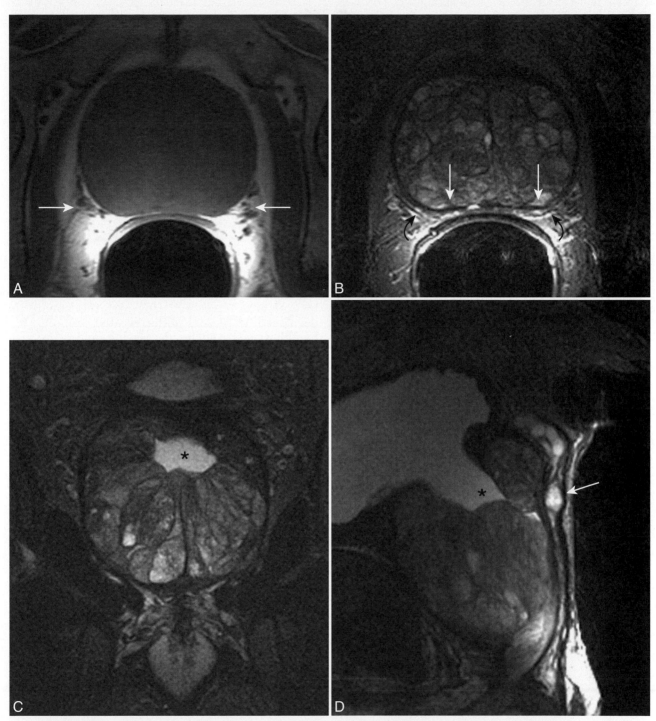

Figure 9-34 ■ MR findings of benign prostatic hyperplasia, a midline prostatic cyst, and a defect due to prior transurethral resection in a 67-year-old man. A, Axial T1-WI shows an enlarged prostate with poor definition of prostate zonal anatomy but good contrast between the peripheral zone and the normal periprostatic fat. The normal neurovascular bundles are revealed in cross-section *(arrows)*. **B,** Axial T2-WI shows a markedly enlarged and heterogeneous central gland secondary to benign prostatic hyperplasia. The hyperintense central gland foci represent glandular-rich BPH nodules, while the lower SI foci represent stromal dominant foci. The peripheral zone is compressed between the inner hypointense surgical capsule *(arrows)* and the less well delineated outer low SI surgical capsule *(curved arrows)*. **C** and **D,** Coronal **(C)** and sagittal **(D)** T2-WIs show segmental dilation of the intraprostatic urethra (*) that is secondary to a prior transurethral resection of the prostate (TURP) performed for symptomatic BPH. Low T2 SI fibrosis can develop around a TURP defect and should not be diagnosed as central gland tumor. With the advent of successful medical therapies for symptomatic BPH, it is expected that fewer TURP procedures will be performed. A midline prostatic cyst is present *(arrow)*.

9-11 MR Appearance of Prostate and Periprostatic Soft Tissues

	T1-Weighted Images	T2-Weighted Images
Prostate		
Peripheral zone	Low SI	High SI with low SI septa
Postbiopsy hemorrhage	High SI	Variable SI
Prostate cancer	Low SI	Low SI
Prostate capsule	Low SI	Low SI
Periprostatic Soft Tissues		
Neurovascular Bundles	Low SI	Low to intermediate SI / Slow flow in veins: higher SI
Periprostatic Fat	High SI	Intermediate to high SI
Seminal Vesicles		
Luminal wall	Low SI	Low SI
Luminal content	Low SI	High SI
Tumor invasion	Low SI	Low SI with adjacent tumor
Hemorrhage	High SI	High SI

current screening methods is diminishing.[97] This is a reversal of the trend that occurred between 1983 and 1992 when the incidence of prostate cancer in the U. S. tripled.[98]

African American men have an increased incidence of prostate cancer and almost twice the mortality of prostate cancer compared with Caucasian men.[99] The reasons are multifactorial and include social, genetic, and environmental factors.[100] Genetic risk factors for prostate cancer are reviewed elsewhere.[101] Finasteride, an inhibitor of 5α-reductase,

reduced the prevalence of prostate cancer in men by 25% after 7 years.[102] However, the tumors that developed were less differentiated tumors. It is hypothesized that by decreasing androgen levels within the prostate finasteride gave a survival advantage to the less differentiated tumors that were less reliant on androgens for growth.[103]

SCREENING FOR PROSTATE CANCER

The American Cancer Society states that the screening for prostate cancer consists of an annual digital

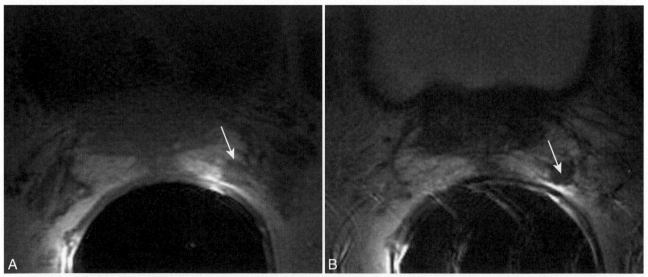

Figure 9-35 ■ **MR illustration of normal seminal vesicles, confined peripheral zone tumor, and postbiopsy peripheral zone hemorrhage. A,** Axial T1-WI obtained at the level of the midgland to base reveals hyperintense peripheral zone from postbiopsy hemorrhage. Areas of T1 hyperintensity within the peripheral zone suggest the absence of infiltrative cancer, especially when imaging is performed more than 2 weeks after biopsy. Infiltrative tumors are resistant to developing intratumoral hemorrhage, whereas normal glandular tissue is not. The hypointense focus of peripheral zone *(arrow)* represents either normal glandular tissue or prostate cancer. **B,** Corresponding axial T2-WI shows that the spared segment of peripheral zone hemorrhage is hypointense and thus is consistent with prostate cancer. Peripheral zone hemorrhage can have variable T2 SI depending on the amounts of extracellular and intracellular methemoglobin.

(Continued)

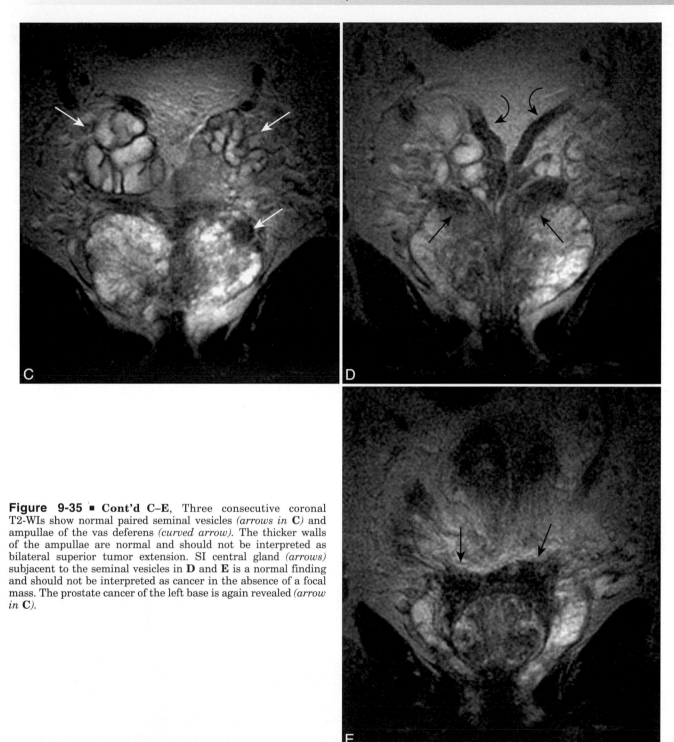

Figure 9-35 ▪ Cont'd C–E, Three consecutive coronal T2-WIs show normal paired seminal vesicles *(arrows in* **C***)* and ampullae of the vas deferens *(curved arrow)*. The thicker walls of the ampullae are normal and should not be interpreted as bilateral superior tumor extension. SI central gland *(arrows)* subjacent to the seminal vesicles in **D** and **E** is a normal finding and should not be interpreted as cancer in the absence of a focal mass. The prostate cancer of the left base is again revealed *(arrow in* **C***)*.

rectal examination (DRE) and a measurement of serum prostatic specific antigen (PSA) for men above age 50 years who have a life expectancy of at least 10 years.[104] This strategy of screening with DRE and PSA can be performed at reasonable cost, and eligible men benefit from screening.[105] If either the DRE or the PSA level is abnormal (>4 ng/mL), then a transrectal sonogram with biopsies is recommended.

In men with borderline elevated PSA values (between 4 and 10 ng/mL) and a normal DRE, it is recommended that a free PSA level be measured to increase specificity without significantly decreasing the sensitivity of prostate cancer detection. Free PSA levels are lower in men with prostate cancer than in men without prostate cancer. Only those men with free PSA values of less than 25% in this indeterminate subgroup would then proceed to US-guided biopsy.[106] Another recommended strategy to improve the specificity of the PSA screening test is to confirm an abnormal value (>4 ng/mL) with a repeat PSA test after several weeks.[107] Up to 40% of men may have a subsequent normal PSA value due to normal fluctuations or resolution of occult prostatitis.

At the time of sonography, biopsy specimens should be taken of any focal abnormalities of the peripheral zone of the prostate gland. Since sonography is not sensitive enough to act as screening test, at least six random biopsy specimens are also tested.[108] US is not accurate for establishing the presence or absence of extracapsular tumor, and so other parameters are used.[109]

A pathologist evaluates for the presence or absence of cancer within each tissue sample, estimates the percentage of each core that was involved by tumor, and assigns a Gleason grade. The Gleason grade can range from 1 through 5. Grade 1 tumors closely resemble the normal prostate and are well-differentiated cancers, while grade 5 tumors are poorly differentiated. The most prevalent type of cancer cell in the sampled tissue is assigned a Gleason grade. The two most prevalent types of cancer cells are added together to form a Gleason sum or Gleason score.[110] The higher the Gleason score, the more likely the tumor is not confined to the prostate.

Once the diagnosis of prostate cancer has been made, accurate staging is important because it influences treatment and prognosis (Box 9-12). Men with localized tumor (stage I and II disease) who have a life expectancy of at least 10 years are candidates for prostatectomy.[96] Prostatectomy decreased cancer-specific mortality and the frequency of metastatic disease by approximately 50% when compared with watchful waiting in a randomized study of Scandinavian men.[111] When experienced surgeons perform a prostatectomy at a high-volume hospital, there is significant reduction in postoperative morbidity and late urinary complications.[112] Men with extracapsular tumor, seminal vesicle invasion,

malignant adenopathy, or bone metastases are not ideal candidates for prostatectomy[113] and would derive greater benefit from radiation therapy, cryotherapy, or hormonal therapy. The presence of extracapsular tumor can be difficult to evaluate. Approximately 60% of men who are diagnosed with prostate cancer are considered to have localized disease.[114] However, approximately 40% to 50% of men who do undergo prostatectomy are shown not to have had organ-confined disease.[110,115-117]

To improve the ability to establish the presence of resectable or unresectable prostate cancer, nomograms that estimate the likelihood of confined disease based on the results of the DRE, PSA test, and Gleason score were created.[118,119] These nomograms have been prospectively evaluated and updated.[120] Those men who have an intermediate-to-high probability of extracapsular tumor would most benefit from MR imaging. Such men would have clinically localized disease, PSA value of greater than 10, and at least 50% positive core tissue specimens.[121,122] Staging MRI of the prostate can be cost effective if selectively performed in this subset of men.[123,124]

Men with nonpalpable tumor, a low PSA value, low tumor volume, and low tumor grade based on the biopsy specimen can be managed expectantly with serial PSA measurements, DREs, and annual biopsies.[125] After 81 such men were followed, 70% were able to avoid treatment, with a median follow-up of 2 years. The prevalence of extracapsular tumor in this subset of men would be so low that MR imaging probably is not warranted.

MRI APPEARANCE OF PROSTATE CANCER AND POSTBIOPSY HEMORRHAGE

Prostate cancer is isointense to surrounding prostatic tissue on T1-WI. Thus, based on T1-WI alone, it is difficult to detect the presence of confined prostate cancer. Postbiopsy hemorrhage results in high T1-SI secondary to the presence of methemoglobin (Fig. 9-36; see Fig. 9-35). Since most cancers are resistant to the development of intratumoral hemorrhage, one can use the presence of high SI on T1-WI to determine where cancer *is not* present (the "MR exclusion sign").

On T2-WI, prostate cancer is of lower SI than the normal peripheral zone of the prostate (see Fig. 9-35). Postbiopsy hemorrhage has variable T2-SI but shows low SI components in approximately 80% of foci secondary to the presence of intracellular methemoglobin.[126] When the T1- and T2-WI are viewed together, one can usually determine whether a low T2-SI focus represents cancer or hemorrhage. Blood has high SI on the T1-WI, whereas cancer does not.[93] If any low T2-SI focus in the peripheral zone is characterized as prostate cancer independently of the T1-SI, then foci of bland hemorrhage will be mischaracterized as tumor.[127]

Small central gland tumors often are not detected on prostate MR imaging. It can be difficult, if not impossible, to distinguish between stromal dominant BPH and central gland adenocarcinoma.

9-12	TNM System of Staging Prostate Cancer
T1	Tumor is occult on basis of digital rectal examination (DRE) and imaging
T2	Tumor is palpable on DRE
T2a	Tumor present on ≤ one side of the gland
T2b	Tumor present on ≥ one side of gland
T2c	Tumor present on both left and right sides of gland
T3	Tumor not confined to the prostate
T3a	Tumor extension beyond the prostate but does not involve seminal vesicles
T3b	Tumor extension to seminal vesicle
T4	Tumor extension to bladder, rectum, or pelvic sidewalk

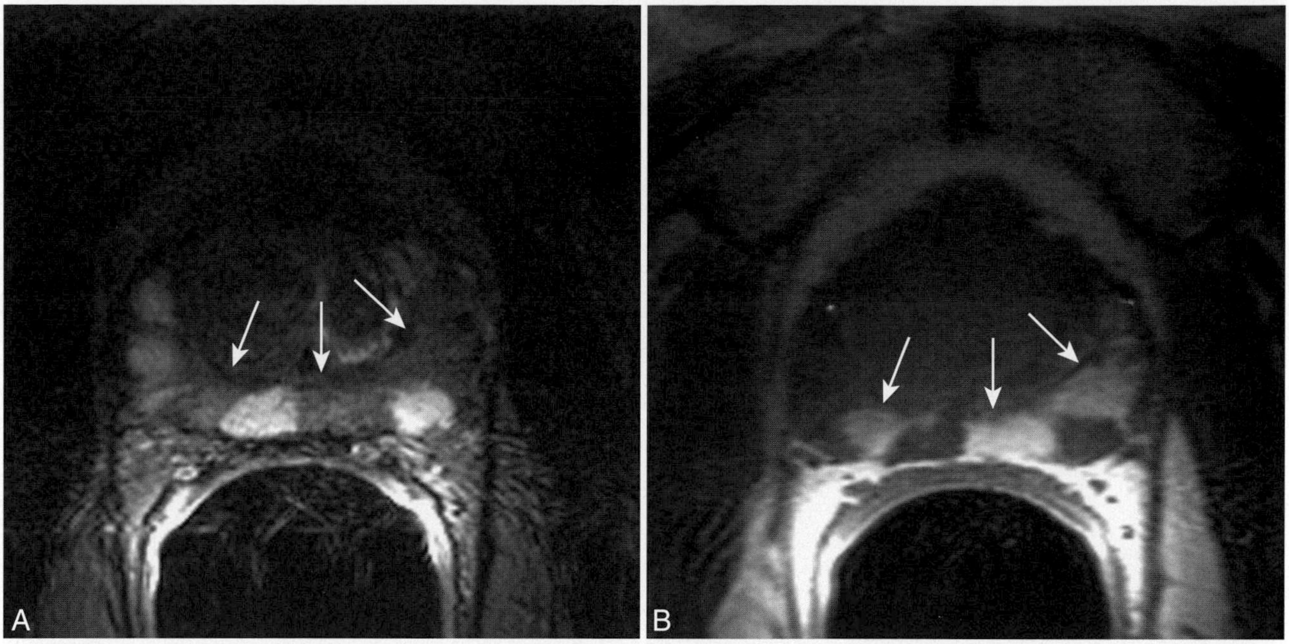

Figure 9-36 ■ **MR illustration of benign postprocedural peripheral zone hemorrhage. A,** Axial T2-WI through the prostate midgland reveals an alternating pattern of low *(arrows)* and high SI. The hypointense foci are potential prostate cancers, while the hyperintense foci represent normal glandular tissue. **B,** T1-WI shows that the hypointense foci in **A** correspond to hyperintense hemorrhage *(arrows)*. No midgland tumor was present on prior biopsy specimen or subsequent prostatectomy.

As stated previously, most central gland cancers are of little clinical import and do not affect the staging or management of a man with biopsy-proved prostate cancer of the peripheral zone. One subpopulation for whom MRI could be considered for primary prostate cancer detection are those men who have elevated PSA values with or without an abnormal DRE and prior prostate tissue samples that did not reveal cancer.[128-130] Some of these men may have infiltrative cancers, especially of the central gland, that can be shown with MRI (Fig. 9-37).[131] If these men do not have MRI, then tissue sampling of the transitional zone should be considered in order to diagnose an occult central gland tumor.[132] Some urologists suggest that the transition zone and anterior aspect of the peripheral gland be sampled along with the peripheral zone at the time of initial biopsy in order to decrease the false-negative rate of initial prostate biopsy, which can be as high as 25%.[133]

MRI FINDINGS OF UNRESECTABLE PROSTATE CANCER

Most MR evaluations of men with prostate cancer are for cancer staging and not detection. Evaluation of the extraprostatic tissues has greater clinical importance than evaluation of the prostate itself. The four extraprostatic regions to evaluate for tumor involvement are the periprostatic fat, seminal vesicles, pelvic lymph nodes, and pelvic bone marrow.

Invasion of periprostatic fat. Tumor extension through the prostatic capsule into the periprostatic fat indicates T3a, stage III disease. Most surgeons will

not operate on men with established extracapsular tumor. By limiting the MR criteria to either the presence of an irregular bulge of the prostate capsule or the presence of tumor in the periprostatic fat (Figs. 9-38 and 9-39),[134] greater than 90% specificity may be achieved for establishing extracapsular tumor with modest sensitivity.[122,135] False-positive diagnoses should be avoided, since they could prevent a potentially curative resection. A false-negative MR for extracapsular tumor, while less than ideal, does not necessarily mean that the patient will have an unsatisfactory postsurgical result. Some of these men are found to have microscopic invasion of the capsule ("focal capsular penetration") and not extensive spread of tumor through the capsule ("established capsular penetration").[136] In a postprostatectomy group of men who had T3a disease without malignant adenopathy or seminal vesicle invasion, almost 50% had focal capsular penetration alone; this subset of men had similar cure rates after prostatectomy to those men with confined disease.[136]

Seminal vesicle invasion. Seminal vesicle invasion is found histologically in approximately 15% of men who undergo prostatectomy for clinically localized disease.[137] The route of spread of tumor to the seminal vesicles is most commonly by direct superior extension by subjacent tumors of the base of the prostate.[138] Thus, if a patient's biopsy specimen does not show tumor of the prostate base, it is unlikely that the patient will have seminal vesicle invasion revealed at MR imaging or prostatectomy.[139]

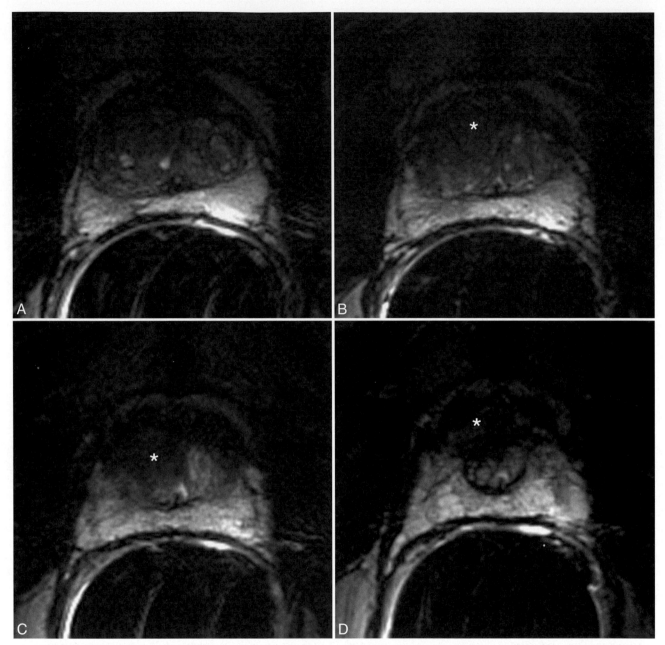

Figure 9-37 ■ **MR depiction of occult central gland tumor in a man with an elevated PSA and prior negative prostate biopsies.** Occult central gland cancer is one of the causes of false-negative prostate biopsy. **A–D,** Four consecutive axial T2-WIs show normal, high SI peripheral zone. The left side of the central gland reveals heterogeneous SI in keeping with BPH. The central to right portions of the central gland show low SI (*). There was no corresponding hyperintensity on the T1-WI (not shown) to suggest bland hemorrhage (the central gland was not sampled on the prior biopsy). This is the typical MRI appearance of an infiltrating central gland tumor.

Conversely, if a man has an abnormal DRE or transrectal ultrasound (TRUS) examination of the prostate base, then sampling of the seminal vesicles at the time of initial biopsy should be considered. In addition, some authors advocate taking biopsy specimens of the seminal vesicles and neurovascular bundles in all men with suspected prostate cancer who come to TRUS examination, independently of the DRE and sonographic findings.[140]

MR has approximately 80% to 90% accuracy in evaluating for seminal vesicle invasion, with greater than 90% specificity and more modest sensitivity.[122,141,142] The MR findings of seminal vesicle invasion are that of low T1 and T2 SI within the lobules of the seminal vesicles and an adjacent cancer of the prostatic base (Figs. 9-40 and 9-41). The corresponding T1-WI should always be evaluated to exclude the presence of seminal vesicle hemorrhage (Fig. 9-42), which may appear similar to tumor on T2-WI. A rare and reportable cause of abnormal, low SI seminal vesicles on T2-WI is secondary to infiltration by amyloidosis.[143,144] Although seminal vesicle

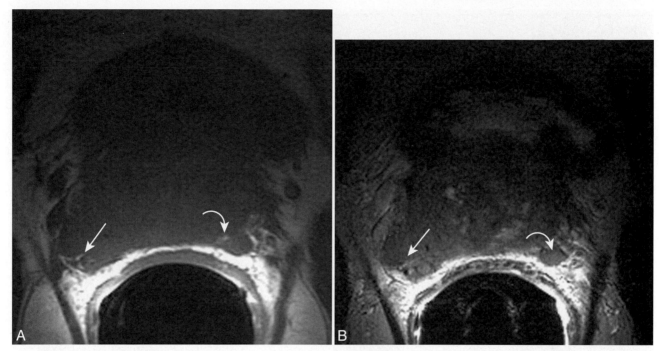

Figure 9-38 ■ **MR depiction of macroscopic extension of prostate cancer into the periprostatic fat. A** and **B,** Axial T1-WI (**A**) and T2-WI (**B**) of the prostate base reveal an infiltrative, low SI peripheral zone tumor that extends into both the right *(arrow)* and left *(curved arrow)* periprostatic fat.

amyloid can mimic tumor, there usually is no adjacent cancer within the prostate base.

Malignant pelvic lymphadenopathy. An MR examination of the prostate should include larger field-of-view images of the pelvis to evaluate for adenopathy. Diagnosing malignant adenopathy is important in men with prostate cancer because these individuals are not candidates for either curative prostatectomy or local radiation therapy. T1- and T2-SI do not distinguish between benign and malignant nodes. However, larger nodes (short axis >6 mm) and nodes that are spherical are more likely to be malignant (Fig. 9-43). As for other primary malignancies, micrometastasis can be present in normal-sized nodes and enlarged pelvic lymph nodes can be reactive.[145] Ultrasmall super paramagnetic iron oxide–enhanced MR can help distinguish between reactive and malignant lymph nodes when imaging men with prostate cancer.[146,147]

The main lymphatic sites of spread of prostate cancer include the obturator lymph nodes and the external, internal, and common iliac lymph node chains.[148] Biopsy specimens can be taken from suspicious lymph nodes under imaging guidance, or the nodes can be removed laparoscopically.[145,149,150] As mentioned above, abdominal imaging is not cost effective in patients with prostate cancer. When enlarged mesenteric lymph nodes are detected on abdominal imaging studies in patients with prostate cancer, the nodes are more likely to be involved by lymphoma than by metastatic prostate cancer.[151] Some urologists do not perform lymphadenectomies

at time of prostatectomy in men at low risk of nodal extension.[152-155] The most conservative reference suggests that men with PSA values of less than 10 with either well or moderately differentiated tumors can forego lymphadenectomy.[148,156]

Osseous metastases. Patients with bone metastases from prostate cancer such as men with malignant adenopathy are not candidates for curative surgery or irradiation (Fig. 9-44). Because the prevalence of bone metastases is so low in men with PSA values below 10 ng/mL, bone scanning is not recommended.[157-159] Only 1% of men with untreated prostate cancer with PSA value below 50 ng/mL, clinical stage T2b or lower, and Gleason score less than 8 had a positive bone scan.[160] Independent of the PSA, it is still prudent to obtain images of the pelvic bone marrow when performing a staging MR examination for patients with prostate cancer. Uncommonly, men with poorly differentiated or undifferentiated cancers have bone metastases on initial presentation with PSA values below 10 ng/mL.[161] MRI can reveal intramedullary metastatic disease in men with normal bone scans when the tumor has not yet involved the cortical bone[162]; MR can also evaluate for complications such as cord compression.[163]

ROLE OF IMAGING AFTER TREATMENT OF PROSTATE CANCER

MRI after prostatectomy. While radical prostatectomy is an effective treatment for men with clinically localized prostate cancer, up to one third of patients will not be cured and will have localized recurrent disease

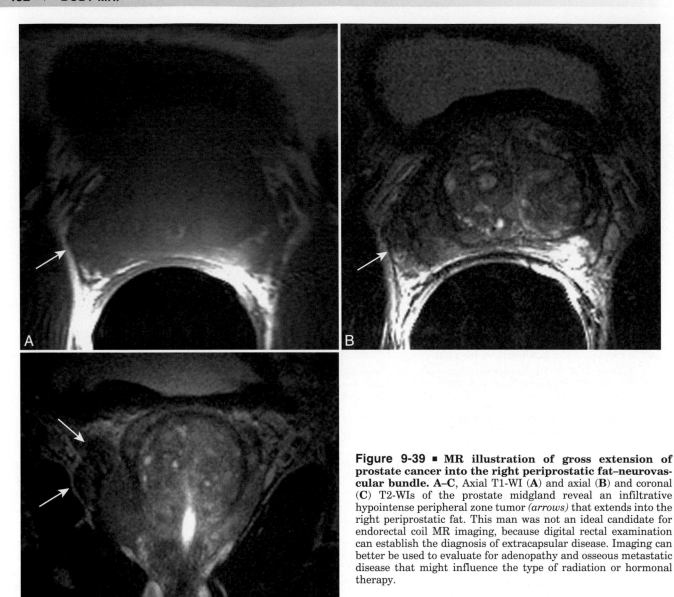

Figure 9-39 ■ MR illustration of gross extension of prostate cancer into the right periprostatic fat–neurovascular bundle. A–C, Axial T1-WI (**A**) and axial (**B**) and coronal (**C**) T2-WIs of the prostate midgland reveal an infiltrative hypointense peripheral zone tumor *(arrows)* that extends into the right periprostatic fat. This man was not an ideal candidate for endorectal coil MR imaging, because digital rectal examination can establish the diagnosis of extracapsular disease. Imaging can better be used to evaluate for adenopathy and osseous metastatic disease that might influence the type of radiation or hormonal therapy.

or metastatic disease (Fig. 9-45).[164] Patients who have isolated recurrent disease within the prostate bed may benefit from localized radiation therapy,[165] while those with metastatic disease are better treated with hormonal therapies. There is no consensus concerning the importance of confirming the presence of localized recurrent disease either by imaging or by biopsy in men with detectable PSA after surgery.[164] The postprostatectomy PSA level and doubling time are the best predictors of which men will benefit from radiation therapy.[166] The subgroup of men who best benefit from radiation to the prostate bed are those who do not develop a detectable PSA level until at least 2 years after

surgery and have a PSA doubling time of greater than one year.[167] Thus, imaging studies that reveal the presence of osseous metastatic disease or tumor outside the prostate bed may better change patient management than will high-resolution imaging of the prostate bed.[168] Some men who become incontinent after prostatectomy are injected with periurethral collagen in order to increase urethral closure and increase resistance of the perisphincteric tissues.[169] On MRI, periurethral collagen is revealed as focal nodules of low SI on T1- and T2-WIs and can mimic recurrent disease (Fig. 9-46).

MRI after radiation seed placement. Radiation seed therapy (brachytherapy) is another treatment

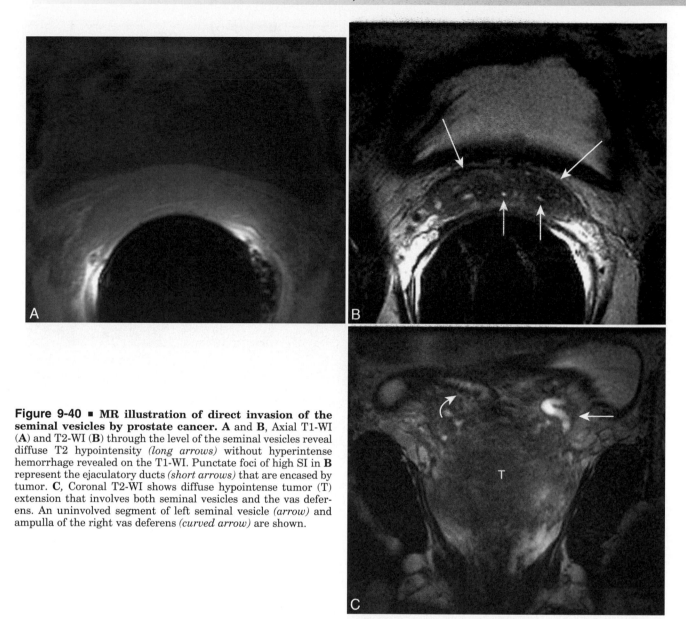

Figure 9-40 ■ MR illustration of direct invasion of the seminal vesicles by prostate cancer. A and **B**, Axial T1-WI (**A**) and T2-WI (**B**) through the level of the seminal vesicles reveal diffuse T2 hypointensity *(long arrows)* without hyperintense hemorrhage revealed on the T1-WI. Punctate foci of high SI in **B** represent the ejaculatory ducts *(short arrows)* that are encased by tumor. **C**, Coronal T2-WI shows diffuse hypointense tumor (T) extension that involves both seminal vesicles and the vas deferens. An uninvolved segment of left seminal vesicle *(arrow)* and ampulla of the right vas deferens *(curved arrow)* are shown.

option for men with prostate cancer. Although no randomized controlled trials comparing radiation seed therapy with either prostatectomy or external beam therapy have been performed, men treated with brachytherapy appear to have equivalent survival to men who have prostatectomy.[170] When MRI was performed prior to planned brachytherapy in a series of 327 men, the number and distribution of seeds was modified in over half based on the MR findings.[171] In some centers the brachytherapy seeds are being placed in an interventional MR system.[172] After brachytherapy, MRI can confirm satisfactory distribution of radiation seeds and evaluate for potential untreated cancer or developing sites of tumor (Fig. 9-47; see Fig. 9-41).[173] After radiation seed therapy or external beam therapy, the normal high SI peripheral zone loses SI because of decreased free water and mucin. It can be extremely

difficult to distinguish sterile radiation fibrosis and granulation tissue from viable prostate cancer. As described below, MR spectroscopy may help in this evaluation.

FUTURE ROLE OF MRI IN THE EVALUATION OF PROSTATE CANCER

MR spectroscopy (MRS) and MR elastography are two potential imaging techniques that may play a larger role in prostate imaging in the future. MRS can detect the presence and amount of hydrogen-containing metabolites such as citrate, creatine, lysine, and choline within a chosen voxel of tissue. The prostate peripheral zone contains abundant citrate and choline, whereas prostate cancer depletes choline and increases citrate concentrations.[174] One can infer the presence of prostate cancer on MRS when the ratio of (choline + creatinine) / citrate > 0.75 which is

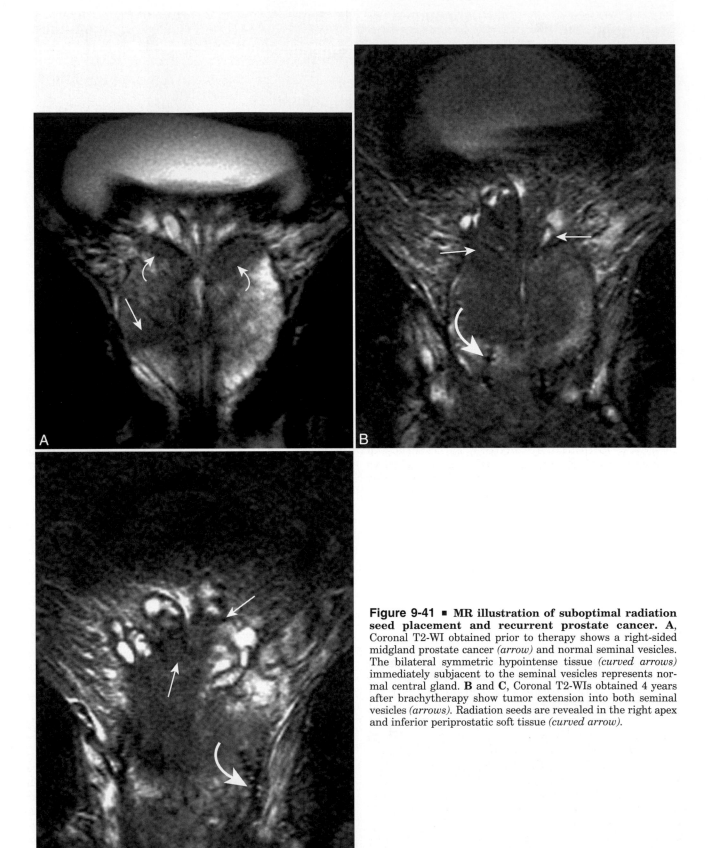

Figure 9-41 ■ MR illustration of suboptimal radiation seed placement and recurrent prostate cancer. A, Coronal T2-WI obtained prior to therapy shows a right-sided midgland prostate cancer *(arrow)* and normal seminal vesicles. The bilateral symmetric hypointense tissue *(curved arrows)* immediately subjacent to the seminal vesicles represents normal central gland. **B** and **C,** Coronal T2-WIs obtained 4 years after brachytherapy show tumor extension into both seminal vesicles *(arrows).* Radiation seeds are revealed in the right apex and inferior periprostatic soft tissue *(curved arrow).*

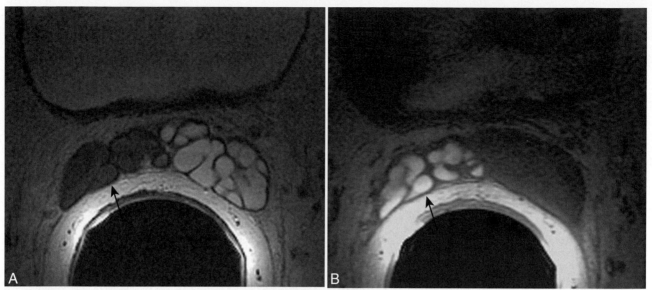

Figure 9-42 ■ MR depiction of right-sided seminal vesicle hemorrhage. Seminal vesicle hemorrhage can be secondary to direct biopsy or retrograde extension of prostatic blood. **A**, Axial T2-WI reveals normal hyperintense fluid of the left seminal vesicle lobules and abnormal, low SI right seminal vesicle content *(arrow)*. However, the right seminal vesicle walls are thin and uniform. **B**, Corresponding T1-WI reveals hyperintense right seminal vesicle blood *(arrow)* that is well contrasted with the normal adjacent walls. No subjacent tumor was present within the right prostate base, and the seminal vesicles were free of tumor at subsequent prostatectomy.

greater than two standard deviations from normal.[135] Thus, in vivo MRS may increase the accuracy of endorectal coil MR imaging in the staging of prostate cancer.[135,175,176] MRS may be able to detect the presence of viable prostate cancer in men who have been treated with hormone or radiation therapy[173,177] and to evaluate the success of future therapies. MRS can complement MRI in the evaluation of men with suspicion of prostate cancer and a prior negative biopsy. MRS shows promise in distinguishing between the benign entities of fibrosis, prostatitis, and hemorrhage and malignant tumor.[130,178]

MR elastography is a phase contrast technique that evaluates the stiffness of tissue.[179] Prostate cancer has decreased elasticity compared with normal prostate tissue. This maturing MR technique may increase the accuracy of prostate cancer detection and staging.

Other Prostate Malignancies

Adenocarcinoma of the prostate accounts for greater than 95% of primary prostate malignancies. The next most common primary tumor of the prostate is transitional cell carcinoma, which arises within the periurethral prostatic ducts and accounts for approximately 3% of primary prostatic cancers.[180] More than half the tumors are associated with bladder carcinoma. Patients have urinary obstruction with or without hematuria.[181]

Prostate sarcomas are rare aggressive lesions.[182] The most common presenting symptom is urinary retention. The two most common subtypes are rhabdomyosarcoma and leiomyosarcoma (Fig. 9-48). The two factors that predict long-term survival are negative margins at time of surgery and absence of metastatic disease at presentation.[182] Tumor size, subtype, and histologic features do not influence patient survival. MR can evaluate for metastatic disease and help determine whether the prostatic sarcoma is resectable.[183]

Figure 9-43 ■ MR depiction of malignant adenopathy from prostate cancer. Subsequent laparoscopic lymph node dissection confirmed the diagnosis of metastatic adenopathy, and prostatectomy was avoided. Axial T1-WI shows multiple bilateral iliac lymph nodes *(arrows)* with short-axis dimensions of >10 mm.

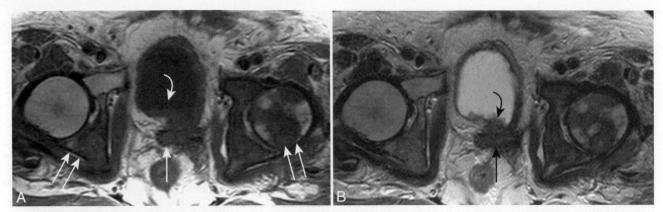

Figure 9-44 ▪ **MR findings of bladder extension of prostate cancer and osseous metastatic disease. A** and **B,** Axial T1-WI (**A**) and T2-WI (**B**) show the superior aspect of an aggressive, infiltrative, low SI prostate cancer *(arrow)* that extends anteriorly to invade the bladder base *(curved arrow)*. Osseous metastatic disease involves both acetabula and the left femoral head *(double arrows)*.

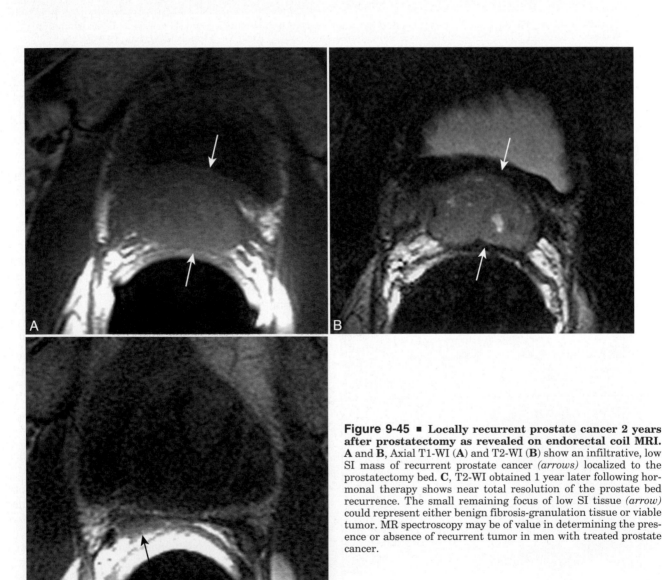

Figure 9-45 ▪ **Locally recurrent prostate cancer 2 years after prostatectomy as revealed on endorectal coil MRI. A** and **B,** Axial T1-WI (**A**) and T2-WI (**B**) show an infiltrative, low SI mass of recurrent prostate cancer *(arrows)* localized to the prostatectomy bed. **C,** T2-WI obtained 1 year later following hormonal therapy shows near total resolution of the prostate bed recurrence. The small remaining focus of low SI tissue *(arrow)* could represent either benign fibrosis-granulation tissue or viable tumor. MR spectroscopy may be of value in determining the presence or absence of recurrent tumor in men with treated prostate cancer.

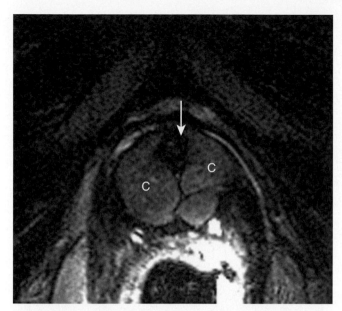

Figure 9-46 ■ **MR findings of periurethral collagen that was used to treat postprostatectomy incontinence.** Without the clinical history of prior collagen injections, recurrent prostate cancer would have to be considered in the differential diagnosis. Axial T2-WI shows low-to-intermediate SI masses (C) in the prostate bed that surround the urethra *(arrow).* No recurrent disease was present based on serial PSA and subsequent stable examinations.

Metastatic disease to the prostate cancer is uncommon and accounts for approximately 2% of solid prostatic tumors. More than half these tumors are direct extensions of either bladder or rectal cancers.[184] Patients usually have hematuria, pelvic

pain, and imaging findings of metastatic disease elsewhere.

Nonneoplastic Disease of the Prostate and Seminal Vesicles

PROSTATITIS

Prostatitis has been termed the "neglected third disease" of the prostate after prostate cancer and BPH.[185] Chronic prostatitis is considered part of the chronic pelvic pain syndrome that affects up to 15% of young and middle-aged men.[186] Only a minority of affected patients have active prostatic bacterial infection requiring antibiotic therapy. Many men with clinical prostatitis have nonprostatic causes of their symptoms, which include pelvic floor muscular dysfunction and functional somatic and myofascial pain syndromes.[187] Imaging is rarely performed in the evaluation of affected men. Occasionally MR imaging is performed to exclude an abscess or an obstructing müllerian duct cyst (see below).[188] Chronic inflammation of the prostate can appear similar to prostate cancer on MR in that both chronic inflammation and cancer can demonstrate low SI on T2-WI.[189,190] Prostatitis can result in relatively diffuse low T2 SI of the peripheral zone without focal mass or capsular irregularity (Fig. 9-49).

PROSTATIC AND EJACULATORY DUCT CYSTS

Approximately 5% to 8% of men will have a prostate cyst depicted on imaging.[191,192] Cysts can be categorized as either midline or paramedian. There are two types of midline prostatic cysts: utricle cysts and müllerian duct cysts.[193,194] Utricle cysts are smaller, usually less

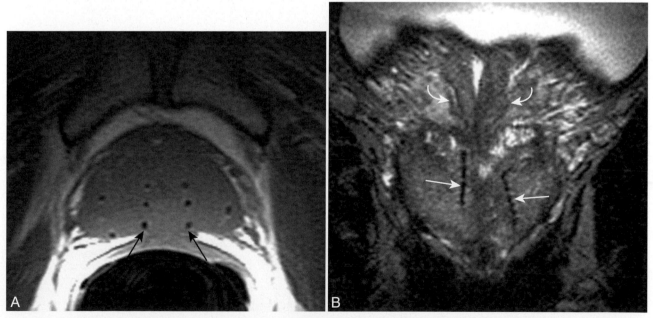

Figure 9-47 ■ **MR depiction of the distribution of brachytherapy seeds. A** and **B**, Axial T1-WI (**A**) and coronal T2-WI (**B**) show linear, low SI peripheral zone foci *(arrows)* that represent susceptibility artifact from brachytherapy seeds. MR spectroscopy may be of value in determining whether viable tumor is present in the low T2 SI peripheral zone or the thick-walled ampullae of the vas deferens *(curved arrows)* in **B**.

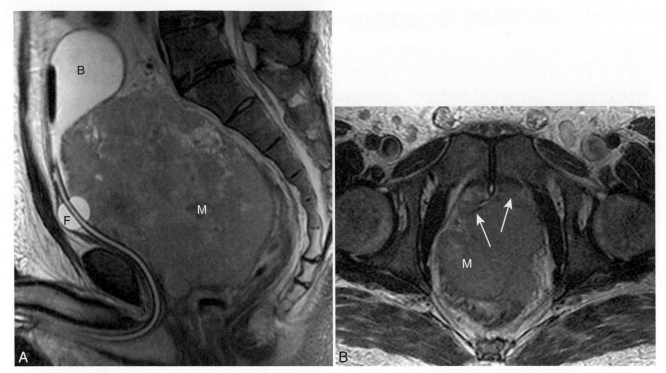

Figure 9-48 ■ **MR depiction of a prostate sarcoma in a 37-year-old man with pain and urinary retention.** **A** and **B**, Sagittal (**A**) and axial (**B**) T2-WIs show an aggressive infiltrative mass (M) of the posterior aspect of the prostate with superior extension. A Foley catheter balloon (F) is present in situ, and an air-fluid level is present in the bladder (B). The axial image shows that the mass originates from the posterior aspect of the prostate *(arrows)*. Prostate adenocarcinoma would be unusual in a man of this age.

than 1 cm, and rarely extend above the prostate gland (Fig. 9-50), while müllerian duct cysts are larger and can extend above the prostate gland (Fig. 9-51).[195] Most of these cysts are smaller than 10 mm and asymptomatic;[192] however, an occasional cyst can cause pain or urinary tract infection. Symptomatic cysts can be treated with either aspiration or resection.[193] Another potential complication of prostatic and periprostatic cysts is obstruction of the ejaculatory ducts with secondary infertility. The obstruction of the ejaculatory ducts can be relieved and fertility restored by transurethral resection of the obstructing cyst.

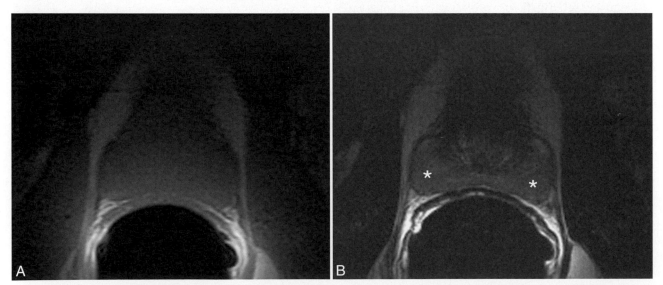

Figure 9-49 ■ **MR findings of diffuse prostatitis in a 22-year-old man with signs and symptoms of prostatitis/chronic pelvic pain syndrome.** **A** and **B**, Axial T1-WI (**A**) and T2-WI (**B**) of the prostate midgland reveal a diffuse, homogeneous, T2 hypointense peripheral zone (*). No focal mass or abscess is present. No BPH is present in this young man, and thus the central gland is not enlarged.

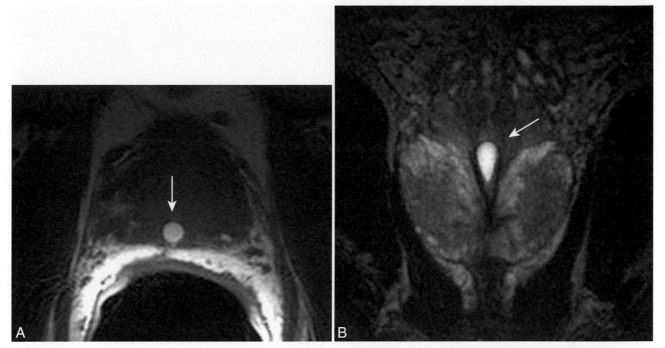

Figure 9-50 ■ **MR illustration of an incidental <10 mm utricle cyst revealed on a staging examination for prostate cancer. A**, Axial T1-WI obtained at the level of the base of the prostate shows a hyperintense midline structure *(arrow)*. Hemorrhagic and proteinaceous content within utricle cysts, müllerian cysts, and seminal vesicles is common after prostate biopsy is performed. **B**, Coronal T2-WI reveals hyperintense fluid *(arrow)* and the cephalocaudal extension of the cyst.

Focal dilation of the prostatic urethra from a prior transurethral resection of the prostate (TURP; see Fig. 9-34) can be misinterpreted as a utricle or müllerian duct cyst. Knowledge of the history of a TURP procedure as treatment for symptomatic BPH is usually sufficient to establish a diagnosis of a TURP defect. The low T2 SI tissue that surrounds a TURP defect is secondary to postprocedural fibrosis/scarring and should not be interpreted as central gland cancer (see Fig. 9-34). Effective treatments are available for symptomatic BPH. Combination therapy with an α-adrenergic-receptor antagonist and 5α-reductase inhibitors has been shown to decrease progression of symptomatic BPH.[196] As mentioned above, it is unclear whether dual therapy should be recommended because of the potential risk of 5α-reductase inhibitors promoting the growth of higher grade tumors.[102,197]

ABSENT SEMINAL VESICLES AND VAS DEFERENS

Another cause of male infertility that can be depicted by MR is absence of the vas deferens or the seminal vesicles.[198] Absence of the vas deferens is responsible for infertility in men with cystic fibrosis.[199] Some asymptomatic or minimally symptomatic men who are infertile secondary to absent vas deferens have a single mutation of the cystic fibrosis gene.[200] This subtype of obstructive azoospermia cannot be directly treated. However, these men can reproduce through the use of intracytoplasmic sperm injection. Men with absent vas deferens who request assisted reproduction should consider seeking genetic counseling.[199]

SEMINAL VESICLE CYSTS

Seminal vesicle cysts are uncommon benign lesions that are occasionally revealed in US or MR images of men with prostate cancer. When this occurs, additional renal imaging should be considered because seminal vesicle cysts are associated with ipsilateral renal agenesis[201,202] and autosomal dominant polycystic kidney disease in 40% of affected individuals.[203] Men with symptomatic seminal vesicle cysts can be treated with endoscopic incision[204] or laparoscopic cystectomy.[201]

MRI OF THE BLADDER

MRI Techniques

The use of a phased-array pelvic coil increases the signal-to-noise ratio of bladder MRI so that smaller field-of-view, higher resolution images can be obtained.[205] When the body coil is used, bladder lesions less than 15 mm may be undetectable.[206] Endorectal coil MR can be used for the specific evaluation of the bladder neck, base, or posterior bladder wall and can provide a further increase in signal-to-noise ratio and spatial resolution compared with a phased-array pelvic coil.[207]

For tumor staging, T1-WIs are useful for showing extension of bladder cancers into the perivesical fat (Figs. 9-52 and 9-53) and for revealing pelvic lymphadenopathy (see Fig. 9-52) and osseous metastatic disease (see above).[208] T2-WIs are performed in three

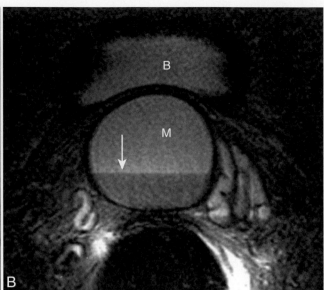

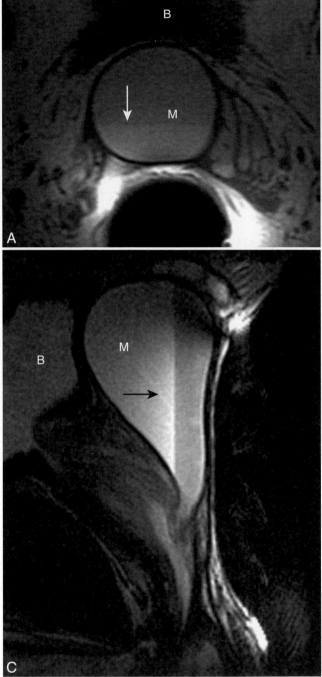

Figure 9-51 ■ **MR findings of a müllerian duct cyst in a 61-year-old man with hematospermia. A** and **B,** Axial T1-WI (**A**) and T2-WI (**B**) of prostate base reveal a 3-cm cystic midline structure (M) with hyperintense T1 components. Fluid-fluid levels *(arrows)* are present on both sequences. The urine-filled bladder (B) shows the SI of relatively simple fluid. **C,** Sagittal T2-WI reveals the cephalocaudal extent of the cyst. Cysts of this size can result in infertility by obstructing antegrade flow of sperm. Sonographically guided cyst aspiration or resection can restore fertility in many of these men.

orthogonal planes to optimize tumor detection and staging. Imaging in a plane that is perpendicular to the tumor-bladder wall interface most accurately shows the presence and extent of tumor invasion of the bladder wall.[209] The patient should void 2 hours prior to scanning. An underdistended bladder has a thickened contracted wall that can obscure some bladder lesions, while an overdistended bladder can limit a patient's ability to tolerate scanning.[210] Dynamic CE-MRI is a useful technique

for determining the presence and depth of bladder carcinoma invasion.

MR Appearance of Normal Bladder

Urine has low SI on T1-WI and high SI on T2-WI (similarly to other relatively simple stagnant fluids). Excreted gadolinium within the bladder can have variable SI that is dependent on the concentration of gadolinium and on the type of T1 sequence used.

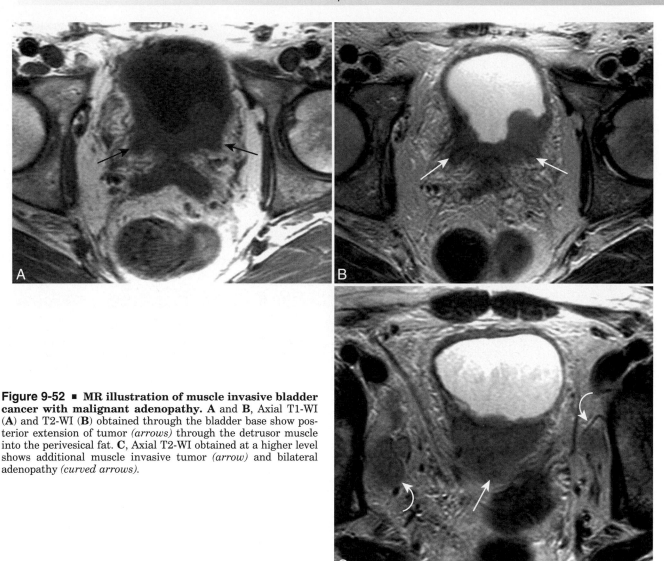

Figure 9-52 ■ **MR illustration of muscle invasive bladder cancer with malignant adenopathy. A** and **B**, Axial T1-WI (**A**) and T2-WI (**B**) obtained through the bladder base show posterior extension of tumor *(arrows)* through the detrusor muscle into the perivesical fat. **C**, Axial T2-WI obtained at a higher level shows additional muscle invasive tumor *(arrow)* and bilateral adenopathy *(curved arrows)*.

Gadolinium is paramagnetic and results in both T1 and T2 shortening (Fig. 9-54). Dilute gadolinium within the bladder is hyperintense on T1-WI, whereas concentrated gadolinium may show lower SI on T1-WI because of T2-shortening effects.[211] Similarly to delayed enhanced CT, excreted intravesical gadolinium can mimic intraluminal soft tissue.[212] Similarly to sonography and CT plus sonography, ureteral jets can be revealed on MRI as curvilinear high SI or low SI on enhanced T1-WI or T2-WI, respectively (see Figs. 7-31C and 9-53).

The bladder wall is composed of four layers. From the bladder lumen outward, they are the mucosa, submucosa, detrusor muscle, and serosa. The normal bladder wall is revealed as homogeneous low-to-intermediate T1 SI and low T2 SI secondary to the dominant detrusor muscle.[213] Normal bladder mucosa, submucosa, and serosa are not normally depicted as distinct layers. Submucosal edema is hyperintense to detrusor muscle and minimally hypointense to urine on T2-WI (see Figs. 7-60 and 7-62). In the presence of submucosal

edema, the bladder mucosa will be revealed as a low SI layer located between high SI urine and edema. Bladder mucosa, submucosa, and transitional cell carcinomas enhance during dynamic CE MRI, whereas the detrusor muscle enhances on delayed imaging.

Bladder Cancer

Transitional cell carcinoma of the bladder is the most common malignancy of the genitourinary tract (Box 9-13). Bladder cancer is more common in men than in women (M:F = 3:1) and the mean age at time of diagnosis is approximately 65 years.[214] More than 70% of patients with bladder cancer have microscopic or gross hematuria. Less than 25% have pain. In the U. S. in 2004 it is estimated that 60,240 people will develop bladder cancer and that 12,710 will die of the disease.[8] Bladder cancer accounts for 6% of developing cancers in American men and 3% of cancer deaths. Greater than 90% of bladder cancers are transitional cell carcinomas.[208] The remainder

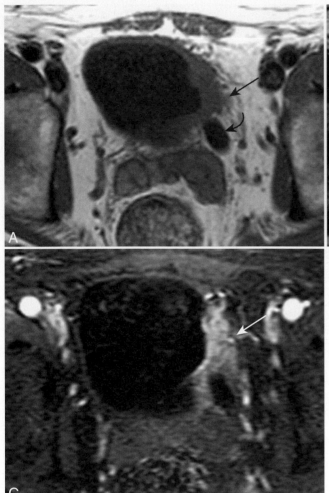

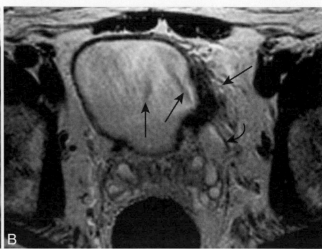

Figure 9-53 ■ MR findings of invasive transitional cell carcinoma of the left ureteropelvic junction and normal ureteral jets. A and **B,** Axial T1-WI (**A**) and T2-WI (**B**) obtained through the bladder base reveal an aggressive infiltrative muscle invasive cancer that extends into the adjacent left perivesicular fat *(arrows)*. The distal left ureter is dilated *(curved arrow)* secondary to obstruction. Low SI ureteral jets *(black arrows in bladder)* are revealed in **B. C,** CE T1-WI shows that bladder cancer enhances *(arrow)* before normal bladder. In this patient, the enhanced images did not provide additional information concerning the extent of tumor invasion.

consist of squamous cell carcinomas (approximately 5%), adenocarcinoma (approximately 2%), and other rare sarcomas.[215] In Egypt and many other parts of Africa, bladder cancer is the most prevalent malignancy. Unlike in the U. S., the most common subtype of cancer is squamous cell carcinoma; chronic infection by schistosomiasis (bilharziasis) contributes to the development of most of these squamous cell bladder cancers.[215]

In the U. S., cigarette smoking is the most prevalent risk factor for the development of bladder cancer, secondary to carcinogens that are excreted by the kidneys. Smokers have a two- to sixfold increased risk of developing bladder cancer compared with nonsmokers; smoking contributes to the development of up to half of bladder cancers.[213,214,216,217] Compared with the urothelium of the renal pelvis and ureter, the bladder urothelium has a larger surface area and a longer exposure to potential toxins in the urine. These factors partially explain why bladder cancer is 40 times more common than cancers of the upper urinary tracts.

Patients with suspected bladder cancer are evaluated with cystoscopy to inspect the bladder mucosa and take tissue samples of any visualized lesions.[218] Bladder cancer is staged by the TNM classification,[219]

which has replaced the older Jewitt-Strong-Marshall[220] scheme (Box 9-14). Initial pathologic evaluation of a bladder biopsy specimen is not necessarily the gold standard for staging bladder cancer. When biopsy specimens are re-evaluated by specialized bladder pathologists, patient stage and management can be affected.[221,222] For example, some T1 tumors will be reinterpreted as T2 lesions that require cystectomy. Conversely, initial overstaging can result in unnecessary cystectomy. When lamina propria is not present in the biopsy specimen, one cannot evaluate for muscle invasion. Cystoscopy and transurethral biopsy cannot be used to evaluate for lymphadenopathy or metastatic disease.

From 60% to 80% of transitional cell carcinomas of the bladder are superficial and of the papillary subtype (Fig. 9-55).[223,224] Ninety-nine percent of bladder tumors that are less than 1 cm in size are superficial[218] (Tis, Ta, and T1 lesions) and are successfully treated with transurethral resection. Depending on factors such as tumor grade and number, patients may receive additional treatment. Intravesical BCG (bacille Calmette-Guérin) therapy is the adjuvant agent of choice[225] and can improve survival, slow progression rate, and decrease the

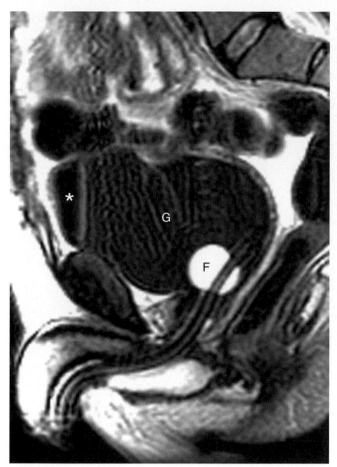

Figure 9-54 ▪ MR illustration of the T2-shortening effects of concentrated gadolinium. Sagittal T2-WI obtained after introduction of gadolinium shows variable low SI urine (G) secondary to the T2-shortening effects of gadolinium. Nondependent air (*) is present anteriorly within the bladder. Simple hyperintense fluid is present within the Foley catheter balloon (F). Excreted gadolinium may mimic a solid bladder mass or an enhancing lesion on T2- or T1-WIs, respectively.

need for future cystectomy in patients with high-risk superficial tumors.

Approximately one third of bladder tumors greater than 1 cm are muscle invasive.[218] The 20% to 40% of bladder cancers that are muscle invasive tumors are most often treated with radical cystectomy with or without neoadjuvant chemotherapy.[226,227] In selected patients, a bladder-sparing approach to surgical resection can be performed.[228] Eligible patients are treated with a wide local excision and close clinical follow-up, since they are at risk of developing locally recurrent disease of a new focus of bladder cancer.[228] For individuals who are not candidates for surgery, attempt at curative radiation can be performed.[229] Radiation therapy after cystectomy can effectively treat residual or locally recurrent disease. Systemic chemotherapy for advanced disease has shown modest survival benefit.[230] For patients with extensive malignant adenopathy or metastatic disease, palliative radiation therapy and chemotherapy are used and cystectomy is not routinely performed.[224]

9-13 Features of Bladder Cancer

Clinical

Most common malignant tumor of the urinary tract
In U. S., >90% of bladder malignancies are transitional cell carcinomas
In Egypt and Africa, squamous cell carcinoma is most common secondary to chronic infection by schistosomiasis or bilharziasis
In U.S., 5% of developing cancers and 2% of cancer deaths
M:F = 3:1, mean age = 65
70% have hematuria

Pathology

60% to 80% of bladder cancers are superficial
20% to 40% of cancers are muscle invasive
Lesion size <1 cm: 99% are superficial
Tumor >1 cm: one third are muscle invasive
Papillary growth pattern: 85% are superficial

MRI

T1-WI

Isointense to bladder wall
Higher SI than urine
Lower SI than perivesical fat

T2-WI

Higher SI than bladder wall
Lower SI than urine
Low SI central stalk within papillary lesion suggests superficial tumor

Dynamic Enhanced MR

Enhances earlier than normal bladder wall
Enhances on average 6 sec before inflammation-granulation tissue in biopsy specimen

Delayed Enhanced MR

Presence of continuous enhancing submucosa subjacent to tumor suggests superficial disease

9-14 Bladder Cancer Staging (Adapted from reference 219)

TNM	Pathology-Imaging
Tis	Carcinoma in situ
Ta	Superficial papillary tumor
T1	Submucosal invasion
T2a	Superficial muscle invasion
T2b	Deep muscle invasion
T3	Tumor invades perivesical fat
T4a	Adjacent organ invasion
T4b	Invades pelvic sidewalk
N1	Single malignant lymph node <2 cm
N2	Single malignant node >2 cm or multiple nodes none >5 cm
N3	Malignant node >5 cm
M1	Distant metastatic disease

	T	N	M
Stage 0	Ta or Tis	N0	M0
Stage I	T1	N0	M0
Stage II	T2a or T2b	N0	M0
Stage III	T3a or T3b or T4a	N0	M0
Stage IV	T4b	N0	M0
	Any T	N1-N3	M0
	Any T	Any N	M1

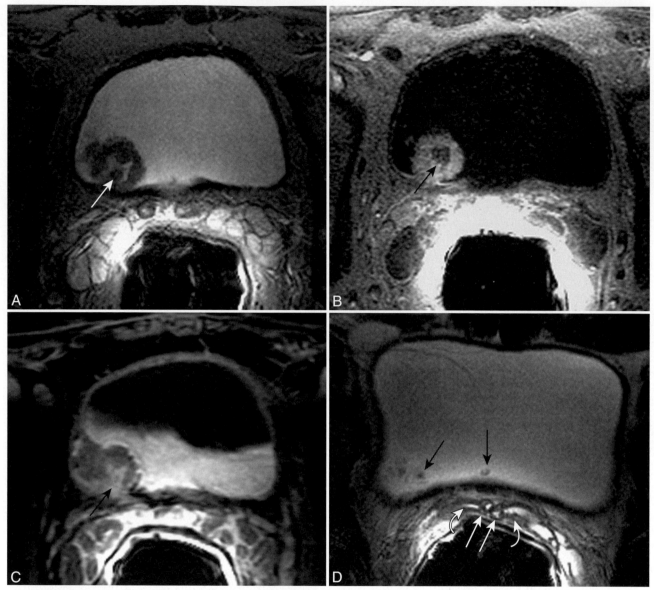

Figure 9-55 ■ **MR demonstration of a superficial papillary transitional cell carcinoma with a fibrous core.**
The patient was successfully treated by transurethral resection. **A,** Axial endorectal coil T2-WI reveals an intraluminal
bladder mass with a low SI central core *(arrow)* and heterogeneous SI outer portion. The subjacent detrusor muscle is
intact. **B,** Dynamic CE T1-WI reveals moderate enhancement of the outer portion of the tumor with a nonenhancing
central core *(arrow)*. No deep muscle invasion is revealed. **C,** Interstitial phase CE T1-WI shows delayed enhancement of
the fibrous core *(arrow)* and relative washout of contrast from the peripheral tumor. **D,** Axial T2-WI in another patient
shows similar-appearing superficial papillary tumors with low SI fibrous cores *(black arrows)*. The ampullae of the vas deferens *(white arrows)* and the ducts of the seminal vesicles *(curved arrows)* are well depicted proximal to the formation of
the ejaculatory ducts.

MRI of Bladder Cancer

MRI of the bladder can help evaluate and
stage patients with biopsy-proved bladder cancer. On
T1-WIs, bladder cancer has similar SI to detrusor
muscle, higher SI than urine, and lower SI than
perivesical fat. Macroscopic extension of low SI
tumor into the perivesical fat is specifically diagnostic of T3b disease and is well depicted on T1-WI (see
Figs. 9-52 and 9-53).[231] On T2-WI, cancer is of lower
SI than urine but of higher SI than adjacent detrusor
muscle. Thus, visualization of an intact low SI detrusor
muscle subjacent to a bladder tumor suggests
absence of muscle invasion (see Fig. 9-55).[208] If either
a T2-W "MR hydrogram" or a delayed-phase CE
T1-W urogram shows a dilated ureter to the level of
an ureteropelvic junction bladder tumor, then a
muscle invasive tumor can be inferred (see Fig. 9-53).
MR techniques of evaluating the ureter ("MR urography") are discussed in Chapter 4. In patients with
bladder cancer who were treated with radiation therapy, the MRI T stage, size of tumor, and presence
of hydronephrosis provided additional prognostic

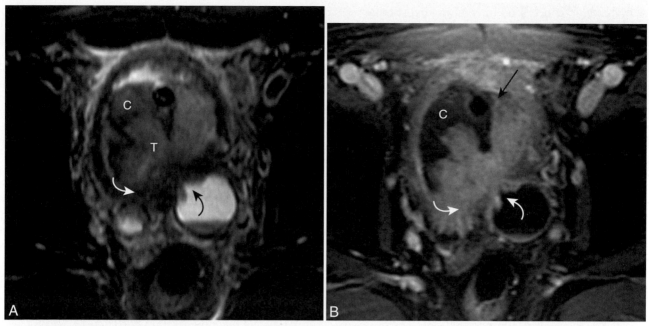

Figure 9-56 ■ MR depiction of muscle invasive transitional cell carcinoma with extension into bilateral periureteral Hutch diverticula. A, Axial fat-suppressed T2-WI reveals bilateral fluid-filled periureteral Hutch diverticula (distal ureters were present on adjacent images that are not shown). Tumor extends through the orifices of both diverticula *(curved arrows),* indicating extramural tumor extension. There are two different types of soft tissue in the bladder lumen: higher SI tumor posteriorly (T) and lower SI clot-debris (C) anteriorly. A fluid-fluid level is present in the left-sided diverticulum. **B,** Axial CE fat-saturated T1-WI shows heterogeneous enhancement of the tumor with extension through the wall of the bladder into both diverticula *(curved arrows).* The anterior clot and necrotic debris do not enhance. A Foley catheter is depicted in cross-section *(arrow).*

information to the clinical T stage and histologic grade; 20% and 30% of these patients were clinically downstaged and upstaged, respectively.[232]

Suspected or indeterminate muscle invasive cancers are most accurately evaluated with dynamic CE MRI (Fig. 9-56).[210,231,233-235] Bladder cancer enhances earlier than both normal detrusor muscle and postbiopsy inflammation and granulation tissue, and so dynamic MR imaging can improve tumor staging.[208,236] Barentsz and colleagues have reported that bladder cancer enhanced 6 to 7 seconds after the arterial phase of enhancement while postbiopsy noncancerous tissue enhanced after 13 to 14 seconds.[237] Another criterion for distinguishing between noninvasive and invasive cancers is the presence or absence of a continuous enhancing layer of submucosa on enhanced imaging obtained after 5 minutes.[238] Thus, both dynamic and delayed enhanced MR provide useful information for determining the T stage of bladder cancer.

The MR evaluation of malignant adenopathy in patients with bladder cancer is challenging because metastatic transitional cell carcinoma can be present in normal-sized nodes.[145,217] Like CT and sonography, MR can measure the dimensions of the node to estimate the probability of malignancy. Some have used 3D T1-WI to facilitate the distinction between spherical and cylindrical shaped nodes; the former are more likely to be malignant.[145] Individuals with T2B

tumors have a 30% prevalence of malignant adenopathy, which increases to 60% in those with T3 lesions. If the presence or absence of tumor within a suspect node influences the decision to perform cystectomy, a laparoscopic or image-guided biopsy of the node can be performed.[145,239] MR evaluation of bone metastases has greater sensitivity and specificity compared with bone scanning,[240] and thus MR could be a "one-stop" imaging modality for the staging of bladder cancer.

Subtypes of Bladder Cancer

SUPERFICIAL PAPILLARY TUMORS

Superficial papillary transitional cell cancers contain a central stalk composed of fibrous connective tissue with variable edema, vascularity, and inflammatory change.[241] From 80% to 90% of papillary (mushroom-like) tumors revealed at cystoscopy are noninvasive.[218] Ninety-five percent of pedunculated bladder tumors that contain a stalk are benign. MR can reveal both the papillary configuration of a bladder tumor and the fibrous tissue within the stalk as low SI on T2-WI (see Fig. 9-55).[213]

TRANSITIONAL CELL CARCINOMA ARISING WITHIN BLADDER DIVERTICULA

There is a 5% to 7% incidence of transitional cell carcinoma within bladder diverticula, and approximately

7% of bladder cancers occur within diverticula.[217,242] Bladder diverticula are at increased risk for developing dysplasia and carcinoma because their urothelial lining has increased exposure to static urine.[243] Because diverticula do not contain detrusor muscle, diverticular tumors often have invaded the perivesical fat at diagnosis[231] (see Fig. 9-56). If a diverticular neck is occluded or not visualized at cystoscopy, diverticular tumors may go undetected for prolonged periods. If diagnosed early, a superficial tumor within a diverticulum can be cured by cystoscopic resection or a bladder sparing diverticulectomy.[244,245] The direct multiplanar capability of MRI facilitates distinguishing between a tumor within an exophytic diverticulum and a solid extravesical mass.[246] Uncommonly, a large bladder diverticulum can mimic an adnexal cyst in a woman.

URACHAL CANCER

The urachus is the remnant of the embryonic segment of the allantois. The involuted urachus forms the median umbilical ligament, which extends from the anterior bladder dome to the umbilicus (see Fig. 7-33). Incomplete regression of the urachus can result in an urachal cyst, sinus, or diverticulum. Urachal remnants can be present in the mucosa or intramural segment of the bladder dome or be located above the bladder. The most common complication of an urachal remnant is infection.

A less common complication of a urachal remnant is the development of urachal carcinoma (Fig. 9-57 and Box 9-15).[247,248] Greater than 80% of urachal cancers are adenocarcinomas that develop from columnar metaplasia of the urachal epithelium.[215] While urachal carcinomas comprise less than 1% of bladder cancers,

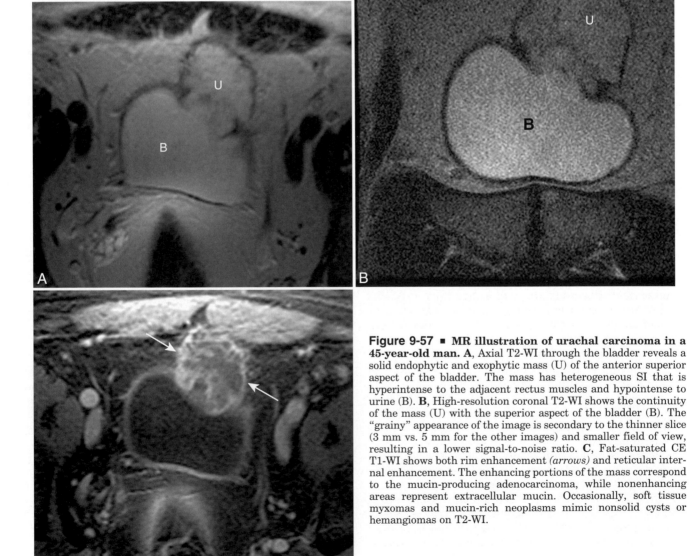

Figure 9-57 ■ MR illustration of urachal carcinoma in a 45-year-old man. A, Axial T2-WI through the bladder reveals a solid endophytic and exophytic mass (U) of the anterior superior aspect of the bladder. The mass has heterogeneous SI that is hyperintense to the adjacent rectus muscles and hypointense to urine (B). **B**, High-resolution coronal T2-WI shows the continuity of the mass (U) with the superior aspect of the bladder (B). The "grainy" appearance of the image is secondary to the thinner slice (3 mm vs. 5 mm for the other images) and smaller field of view, resulting in a lower signal-to-noise ratio. **C**, Fat-saturated CE T1-WI shows both rim enhancement *(arrows)* and reticular internal enhancement. The enhancing portions of the mass correspond to the mucin-producing adenocarcinoma, while nonenhancing areas represent extracellular mucin. Occasionally, soft tissue myxomas and mucin-rich neoplasms mimic nonsolid cysts or hemangiomas on T2-WI.

9-15   Features of Urachal Carcinoma

Clinical

Rare: ≤1% of bladder cancers, 1 case/5 million/yr
90% of cases are adenocarcinoma
Two thirds of patients are male; two thirds are
  between 40 and 70 years of age
Intramural or juxtavesical location
Hematuria in 70%

MRI

Bladder dome or juxtavesical mass

T2-WI

High SI represents intratumoral mucin
Dystrophic calcification better revealed on CT

---

they represent one third of bladder adenocarcinomas. At histology 75% of urachal adenocarcinomas contain intratumoral mucin and 25% of patients have mucinuria.[247] The mucinous components of an urachal adenocarcinoma are revealed as high SI on T2-WI (see Fig. 9-57). MR can differentiate mucinous vs. nonmucinous adenocarcinomas in other organs as well based on the difference in T2 SI.[249,250] MR can differentiate intratumoral cyst formation and liquefactive necrosis from mucinous adenocarcinomas with the use of contrast; the latter enhances, while the former does not. Intratumoral dystrophic calcification within urachal tumors is more readily detected and characterized by CT.[251]

Other Neoplastic Bladder Diseases

METASTATIC DISEASE

Metastatic disease to the bladder is rare. Most reported cases involved adjacent spread of prostate and rectal cancers in men (see Fig. 9-44)[252] and uterine and cervical cancers in women (see Fig. 7-12). When other carcinomas have metastasized to the bladder by hematogenous or lymphatic spread, there is usually widespread metastatic disease present at other sites.[253] An exception is renal carcinoma that may present as an isolated bladder "drop-metastasis" via the ureter.[254]

LYMPHOMA

Lymphoma of the bladder can present in one of three clinical situations. In order of decreasing frequency, they are lymphoma of bladder in the setting of widespread extranodal disease (see Fig. 7-11), recurrent secondary lymphoma, and primary lymphoma of the bladder.[255] Primary bladder lymphoma is often from a low grade B-cell lymphoma and has a good prognosis, whereas the former two diseases involve large cell lymphoma and have a poorer prognosis. Endometriosis of the bladder (see Fig. 7-54) can mimic a bladder neoplasm (see Chapter 7).

Nonneoplastic Bladder Diseases

BLADDER CALCULI

Bladder calculi are uncommon intraluminal masses. Most bladder stones develop in situ within stagnant urine in the setting of bladder outlet obstruction or within bladder diverticula.[256] Less commonly, bladder calculi originate more proximally within the kidney and ureter and migrate distally. Independent of stone composition, MR usually reveals calculi as low SI on T2-WI (Fig. 9-58). To demonstrate that a bladder calculus is not located within the distal ureter or does not originate from the bladder wall, repeat scanning in the prone position can be performed to show bladder stone mobility.[257]

CYSTITIS

Inflammatory and infectious diseases of the bladder do not routinely require imaging. Interstitial cystitis, termed the "great enigma of urology,"[258] is an idiopathic, sterile, inflammatory condition of the bladder. Affected patients may experience suprapubic pain, urinary frequency, and urgency. No specific imaging findings have been reported. Infectious cystitis can usually be diagnosed by clinical symptoms and urine culture. Imaging can help establish the unusual diagnosis of emphysematous cystitis.[259,260] Cystitis glandularis is an uncommon inflammatory condition that is associated with pelvic lipomatosis[261] (see Fig. 6-17). Foci of cystitis glandularis have been reported to mimic bladder neoplasms on both imaging and cystoscopic studies.[262,263]

INFLAMMATORY PSEUDOTUMOR

Included in the differential diagnosis of solid bladder neoplasms is inflammatory pseudotumor.[264-266]

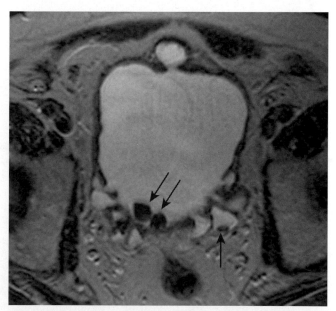

Figure 9-58 ■ **MR depiction of bladder calculi and small diverticula.** Axial T2-WI shows multiple bladder diverticula and dependent hypointense bladder stones *(arrows)*.

Other names for this nonneoplastic lesion include atypical myofibroblastic tumor and pseudosarcomatous fibromyxoid tumor. Inflammatory pseudotumor can mimic other bladder tumors in terms of tumor size, symptomatology, and imaging features. A suggestive MR imaging feature is relative low SI on T2-WI (Fig. 9-59). However, tissue sampling usually is necessary to establish the diagnosis and exclude a neoplasm.[264,266] Patients with inflammatory pseudotumor of the bladder can be treated conservatively. Metastatic disease has not been reported.

CYSTOCELE

Pelvic floor relaxation is characterized by abnormal descent of the bladder, vagina/uterus, and/or rectum. The support of the bladder and other pelvic floor structures is by the urogenital diaphragm. The muscles that contribute the most to the stability of the pelvic floor are the puborectalis and iliococcygeus; both are components of the levator ani. Abnormal descent of the bladder (as well as the vagina, rectum, and other pelvic floor structures) can be evaluated with the use of breath-hold T2-WIs.[267-272] Breath-hold sequences are obtained with and without having the patient perform the Valsalva maneuver. If the bladder descends below a line drawn from the last joint of the coccyx to the most inferior portion of the symphysis during straining, then an MR diagnosis of cystocele is established (see Fig. 7-26).

URETEROCELE

Ureterocele is defined as a congenital dilation of the submucosal segment of the intravesicular portion of a ureter. The incidence of ureterocele on autopsy is up to 1 in 500. Ureteroceles are four to seven times more common in females and are bilateral in 10%. Orthotopic ureteroceles are located at the normal position of the ureterovesicular junction. They are less likely to be asymptomatic and are more commonly discovered in adults incidentally. Children more frequently present with ectopic ureteroceles and are more likely to have secondary symptoms. Ectopic ureteroceles are associated with the upper pole moiety of a duplex collecting system. The most common complication of ectopic ureterocele is urinary tract infection secondary to obstruction. Heavily T2-WIs (MR hydrography; Fig. 9-60) or delayed T1-WIs following administration of furosemide (Lasix) and gadolinium (MR urography) can be used for ureterocele evaluation.[273] MR hydrography can better evaluate dilated and obstructed ureters; CE MR urography can better evaluate normal-caliber functioning ureters. Symptomatic orthotopic ureteroceles and intravesical ectopic ureteroceles may be treatable by endoscopic puncture, whereas extravesical ureteroceles and those associated with a duplex collecting system more often require open surgical repair.[274]

FISTULA

Bladder fistulas are uncommon complications of surgery, inflammatory bowel disease, diverticulitis, and cancer. Most cases of vesicovaginal fistula are secondary to either gynecologic surgery or complications of childbirth in developing countries[275,276] (see Fig. 7-22). Affected women have urinary incontinence. Surgical repair can be performed though a transabdominal or vaginal approach.[277] Enterovesical fistula is less common than vesicovaginal fistula. The three main causes of enterovesical fistula are inflammatory bowel disease, infiltrative cancer, and complications of diverticulitis.[278,279] Patients may have with pneumaturia, fecaluria, or recurrent urinary tract infections. Treatment consists of surgical removal of the affected bowel segment with or without urinary diversion.

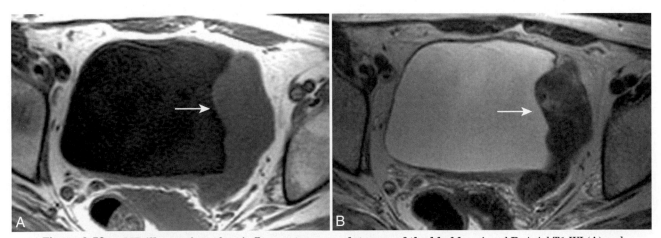

Figure 9-59 ▪ MR illustration of an inflammatory pseudotumor of the bladder. A and **B**, Axial T1-WI (**A**) and T2-WI (**B**) show a lobular solid mass *(arrow)* of the left bladder wall. The hypointense T2 SI suggested a lesion of smooth muscle or fibrous origin. Since this biopsy-proved inflammatory pseudotumor has caused no symptoms, the patient has been treated conservatively. The mass has not grown in 5 years.

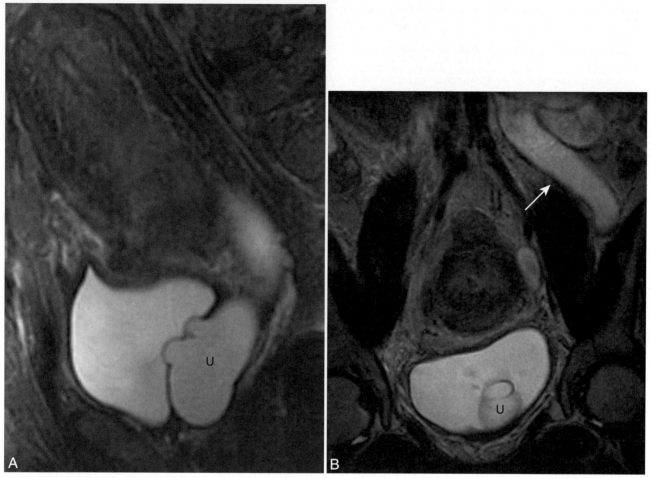

Figure 9-60 ■ **MR findings of an ectopic ureterocele.** A subsequent conventional urogram confirmed a duplicated left collecting system with an obstructed upper tract moiety. **A** and **B,** Sagittal (**A**) and fat-saturated coronal (**B**) T2-WIs show a cystic intramural bladder mass (U) that represents the dilated distal ureteral segment. The obstructed dilated proximal ureter is revealed in **B** *(arrow).*

REFERENCES

1. Muglia V, Tucci S, Jr., Elias J, Jr., Trad CS, Bilbey J, Cooperberg PL. Magnetic resonance imaging of scrotal diseases: when it makes the difference. Urology 2002;59:419-423.
2. Woodward PJ, Schwab CM, Sesterhenn IA. From the archives of the AFIP: extratesticular scrotal masses: radiologic-pathologic correlation. Radiographics 2003;23:215-240.
3. Patel MD, Silva AC. MRI of an adenomatoid tumor of the tunica albuginea. AJR Am J Roentgenol 2004;182:415-417.
4. Serra AD, Hricak H, Coakley FV, et al. Inconclusive clinical and ultrasound evaluation of the scrotum: impact of magnetic resonance imaging on patient management and cost. Urology 1998;51:1018-1021.
5. Shabsigh R, Padma-Nathan H, Gittleman M, McMurray J, Kaufman J, Goldstein I. Intracavernous alprostadil alfadex is more efficacious, better tolerated, and preferred over intraurethral alprostadil plus optional actis: a comparative, randomized, crossover, multicenter study. Urology 2000;55:109-113
6. Sica GT, Teeger S. MR imaging of scrotal, testicular, and penile diseases. Magn Reson Imaging Clin N Am 1996;4:545-563.
7. Monette RJ, Woodward PJ. MR appearance of dilated rete testis. AJR Am J Roentgenol 1994;163:482.
8. Jemal A, Tiwari RC, Murray T, et al. Cancer statistics, 2004. CA Cancer J Clin 2004;54:8-29.
9. Bosl GJ, Motzer RJ. Testicular germ-cell cancer. N Engl J Med 1997;337:242-253.
10. Einhorn LH, Crawford ED, Shipley WU, Loehrer RJ, Williams SD. Cancer of the testes. In De Vita VT, Hellman S, Rosenberg SA (eds). *Cancer: Principles and Practice of Oncology,* 3rd ed. Philadelphia: Lippincott, 1989;1071-1098.
11. Gooding GA, Leonhardt W, Stein R. Testicular cysts: US findings. Radiology 1987;163:537-538.
12. Woodward PJ, Sohaey R, O'Donoghue MJ, Green DE. From the archives of the AFIP: tumors and tumorlike lesions of the testis: radiologic-pathologic correlation. Radiographics 2002;22:189-216.
13. Fritzsche PJ, Wilbur MJ. The male pelvis. Semin Ultrasound CT MR 1989;10:11-28.
14. Hamm B, Fobbe F, Loy V. Testicular cysts: differentiation with US and clinical findings. Radiology 1988;168:19-23.
15. Langer JE, Ramchandani P, Siegelman ES, Banner MP. Epidermoid cysts of the testicle: sonographic and MR imaging features. AJR Am J Roentgenol 1999;173:1295-1299.
16. Dogra VS, Gottlieb RH, Rubens DJ, Oka M, Di Sant Agnese AP. Testicular epidermoid cysts: sonographic features with histopathologic correlation. J Clin Ultrasound 2001;29:192-196.
17. Cho JH, Chang JC, Park BH, Lee JG, Son CH. Sonographic and MR imaging findings of testicular epidermoid cysts. AJR Am J Roentgenol 2002;178:743-748.
18. Brown DL, Benson CB, Doherty FJ, et al. Cystic testicular mass caused by dilated rete testis: sonographic findings in 31 cases. AJR Am J Roentgenol 1992;158:1257-1259.
19. Burrus JK, Lockhart ME, Kenney PJ, Kolettis PN. Cystic ectasia of the rete testis: clinical and radiographic features. J Urol 2002;168:1436-1438.
20. Meyer DR, Huppe T, Lock U, Hodek E, Friedrich M. Pronounced cystic transformation of the rete testis: MRI appearance. Invest Radiol 1999;34:600-603.
21. Proto G, Di Donna A, Grimaldi F, Mazzolini A, Purinan A, Bertolissi F. Bilateral testicular adrenal rest tissue in congenital adrenal hyperplasia: US and MR features. J Endocrinol Invest 2001;24:529-531.

22. Stikkelbroeck NM, Suliman HM, Otten BJ, Hermus AR, Blickman JG, Jager GJ. Testicular adrenal rest tumours in postpubertal males with congenital adrenal hyperplasia: sonographic and MR features. Eur Radiol 2003;13:1597-1603.

23. Avila NA, Premkumar A, Merke DP. Testicular adrenal rest tissue in congenital adrenal hyperplasia: comparison of MR imaging and sonographic findings. AJR Am J Roentgenol 1999;172:1003-1006.

24. Avila NA, Shawker TS, Jones JV, Cutler GB, Jr., Merke DP. Testicular adrenal rest tissue in congenital adrenal hyperplasia: serial sonographic and clinical findings. AJR Am J Roentgenol 1999;172:1235-1238.

25. Leung AC, Kogan SJ. Focal lobular spermatogenesis and pubertal acceleration associated with ipsilateral Leydig cell hyperplasia. Urology 2000;56:508-509.

26. Naughton CK, Nadler RB, Basler JW, Humphrey PA. Leydig cell hyperplasia. Br J Urol 1998;81:282-289.

27. Carucci LR, Tirkes AT, Pretorius ES, Genega EM, Weinstein SP. Testicular Leydig's cell hyperplasia: MR imaging and sonographic findings. AJR Am J Roentgenol 2003;180:501-503.

28. Ozok G, Taneli C, Yazici M, Herek O, Gokdemir A. Polyorchidism: a case report and review of the literature. Eur J Pediatr Surg 1992;2:306-307.

29. Chung TJ, Yao WJ. Sonographic features of polyorchidism. J Clin Ultrasound 2002;30:106-108.

30. Spranger R, Gunst M, Kuhn M. Polyorchidism: a strange anomaly with unsuspected properties. J Urol 2002;168:198.

31. Shah SN, Miller BM, Geisler E. Polyorchidism discovered as testicular torsion. Urology 1992;39:543-544.

32. Hricak H, Hamm B, Kim B. Congenital anomalies of the testis. In: Hricak H, Hamm B, Kim B (Eds.): Imaging of the Scrotum. New York: Raven Press, 1995, p 46.

33. Semelka R, Anderson M, Hricak H. Prosthetic testicle: appearance at MR imaging. Radiology 1989;173:561-562.

34. Pidutti R, Morales A. Silicone gel-filled testicular prosthesis and systemic disease. Urology 1993;42:155-157.

35. Leung ML, Gooding GA, Williams RD. High-resolution sonography of scrotal contents in asymptomatic subjects. AJR Am J Roentgenol 1984;143:161-164.

36. Braslis KG, Moss DI. Long-term experience with sclerotherapy for treatment of epididymal cyst and hydrocele. Aust NZ J Surg 1996;66:222-224.

37. Shirvani AR, Ortenberg J. Communicating hematocele in children following splenic rupture: diagnosis and management. Urology 2000;55:590.

38. Thakur A, Buchmiller T, Hiyama D, Shaw A, Atkinson J. Scrotal abscess following appendectomy. Pediatr Surg Int 2001;17:569-571.

39. Takimoto K, Okamoto K, Wakabayashi Y, Okada Y. Torsion of spermatocele: a rare manifestation. Urol Int 2002;69:164-165.

40. Holden A, List A. Extratesticular lesions: a radiological and pathological correlation. Australas Radiol 1994;38:99-105.

41. Beiko DT, Morales A. Percutaneous aspiration and sclerotherapy for treatment of spermatoceles. J Urol 2001;166:137-139.

42. Martinez-Berganza MT, Sarria L, Cozcolluela R, Cabada T, Escolar F, Ripa L. Cysts of the tunica albuginea: sonographic appearance. AJR Am J Roentgenol 1998;170:183-185.

43. Kim ED, Lipshultz LI. Role of ultrasound in the assessment of male infertility. J Clin Ultrasound 1996;24:437-453.

44. Evers JL, Collins JA, Vandekerckhove P. Surgery or embolisation for varicocele in subfertile men. Cochrane Database Syst Rev 2001;1.

45. Silber SJ. The varicocele dilemma. Hum Reprod Update 2001;7:70-77.

46. Schoor RA, Elhanbly SM, Niederberger C. The pathophysiology of varicocele-associated male infertility. Curr Urol Rep 2001;2:432-436.

47. Redmon JB, Carey P, Pryor JL. Varicocele—the most common cause of male factor infertility? Hum Reprod Update 2002;8:53-58.

48. Bluemke DA, Wolf RL, Tani I, Tachiki S, McVeigh ER, Zerhouni EA. Extremity veins: evaluation with fast-spin-echo MR venography. Radiology 1997;204:562-565.

49. Akbar SA, Sayyed TA, Jafri SZ, Hasteh F, Neill JS. Multimodality imaging of paratesticular neoplasms and their rare mimics. Radiographics 2003;23:1461-1476.

50. Heller CA, Marucci DD, Dunn T, Barr EM, Houang M, Dos Remedios C. Inguinal canal "lipoma." Clin Anat 2002;15:280-285.

51. Mason BJ, Kier R. Sonographic and MR imaging appearances of paratesticular rhabdomyosarcoma. AJR Am J Roentgenol 1998;171:523-524.

52. Sugita Y, Clarnette TD, Cooke-Yarborough C, Chow CW, Waters K, Hutson JM. Testicular and paratesticular tumours in children: 30 years' experience. Aust NZ J Surg 1999;69:505-508.

53. Trambert MA, Mattrey RF, Levine D, Berthoty DP. Subacute scrotal pain: evaluation of torsion versus epididymitis with MR imaging. Radiology 1990;175:53-56.

54. Sidhu PS. Clinical and imaging features of testicular torsion: role of ultrasound. Clin Radiol 1999;54:343-352.

55. Cheng HC, Khan MA, Bogdanov A, Jr., Kwong K, Weissleder R. Relative blood volume measurements by magnetic resonance imaging facilitate detection of testicular torsion. Invest Radiol 1997;32:763-769.

56. Pavlica P, Barozzi L. Imaging of the acute scrotum. Eur Radiol 2001;11:220-228.

57. Rajfer J. Congenital Anomalies of the testis and scrotum. In Campbell MF, Retik AB, Vaugham ED, Walsh PC (Eds.): Campbell's Urology. Philadelphia, WB Saunders, 1998, pp 2172-2183.

58. Friedland GW, Chang P. The role of imaging in the management of the impalpable undescended testis. AJR Am J Roentgenol 1988;151:1107-1111.

59. Yeung CK, Tam YH, Chan YL, Lee KH, Metreweli C. A new management algorithm for impalpable undescended testis with gadolinium enhanced magnetic resonance angiography. J Urol 1999;162:998-1002.

60. Lam WW, Tam PK, Ai VH, Chan KL, Chan FL, Leong L. Using gadolinium-infusion MR venography to show the impalpable testis in pediatric patients. AJR Am J Roentgenol 2001;176:1221-1226.

61. Vossough A, Pretorius ES, Siegelman ES, Ramchandani P, Banner MP. Magnetic resonance imaging of the penis. Abdom Imaging 2002;27:640-659.

62. Pretorius ES, Siegelman ES, Ramchandani P, Banner MP. MR imaging of the penis. Radiographics 2001;21(Spec No.):S283-S298; discussion S298-299.

63. Pavlica P, Menchi I, Barozzi L. New imaging of the anterior male urethra. Abdom Imaging 2003;28:180-186.

64. Jemal A, Thomas A, Murray T, Thun M. Cancer statistics, 2002. CA Cancer J Clin 2002;52:23-47.

65. Burgers JK, Badalament RA, Drago JR. Penile cancer: clinical presentation, diagnosis, and staging. Urol Clin North Am 1992;19:247-256.

66. de Bree E, Sanidas E, Tzardi M, Gaki B, Tsiftsis D. Malignant melanoma of the penis. Eur J Surg Oncol 1997;23:277-279.

67. Pow-Sang MR, Benavente V, Pow-Sang JE, et al. Cancer of the penis. Cancer Control 2002;9:305-314.

68. Ryu J, Kim B. MR imaging of the male and female urethra. Radiographics 2001;21:1169-1185.

69. Robey EL, Schellhammer PF. Four cases of metastases to the penis and a review of the literature. J Urol 1984;132:992-994.

70. Lau TN, Wakeley CJ, Goddard P. Magnetic resonance imaging of penile metastases: a report on five cases. Australas Radiol 1999;43:378-381.

71. Bevers RF, Abbekerk EM, Boon TA. Cowper's syringocele: symptoms, classification and treatment of an unappreciated problem. J Urol 2000;163:782-784.

72. Kimball DA, Yuh WT, Farner RM. MR diagnosis of penile thrombosis. J Comput Assist Tomogr 1988;12:604-607.

73. Ptak T, Larsen CR, Beckmann CF, Boyle DE, Jr. Idiopathic segmental thrombosis of the corpus cavernosum as a cause of partial priapism. Abdom Imaging 1994;19:564-566.

74. Vosshenrich R, Schroeder-Printzen I, Weidner W, Fischer U, Funke M, Ringert RH. Value of magnetic resonance imaging in patients with penile induration (Peyronie's disease). J Urol 1995;153:1122-1125.

75. Andresen R, Wegner HE, Miller K, Banzer D. Imaging modalities in Peyronie's disease: an intrapersonal comparison of ultrasound sonography, X-ray in mammography technique, computerized tomography, and nuclear magnetic resonance in 20 patients. Eur Urol 1998;34:128-134; discussion 135.

76. Uder M, Gohl D, Takahashi M, et al. MRI of penile fracture: diagnosis and therapeutic follow-up. Eur Radiol 2002;12:113-120.

77. Eke N. Fracture of the penis. Br J Surg 2002;89:555-565.

78. Choi MH, Kim B, Ryu JA, Lee SW, Lee KS. MR imaging of acute penile fracture. Radiographics 2000;20:1397-1405.

79. Sawyer-Glover AM, Shellock FG. Pre-MRI procedure screening: recommendations and safety considerations for biomedical implants and devices. J Magn Reson Imaging 2000;12:92-106.

80. Shellock FG, Curtis JS. MR imaging and biomedical implants, materials, and devices: an updated review. Radiology 1991; 180:541-550.

81. Mulcahy JJ. Surgical management of penile prosthesis complications. Int J Impot Res 2000;12 (Suppl 4):S108-S111.

82. Moncada I, Hernandez C, Jara J, et al. Buckling of cylinders may cause prolonged penile pain after prosthesis implantation: a case control study using magnetic resonance imaging of the penis. J Urol 1998;160:67-71.

83. Adusumilli S, Pretorius ES. Magnetic resonance imaging of prostate cancer. Semin Urol Oncol 2002;20:192-210.

84. Schnall MD, Connick T, Hayes CE, Lenkinski RE, Kressel HY. MR imaging of the pelvis with an endorectal-external multicoil array. J Magn Reson Imaging 1992;2:229-232.

85. Engelbrecht MR, Jager GJ, Laheij RJ, Verbeek AL, van Lier HJ, Barentsz JO. Local staging of prostate cancer using magnetic resonance imaging: a meta-analysis. Eur Radiol 2002;12:2294-2302.

86. Hricak H, White S, Vigneron D, et al. Carcinoma of the prostate gland: MR imaging with pelvic phased-array coils versus integrated endorectal-pelvic phased-array coils. Radiology 1994;193:703-709.

87. Jager GJ, Ruijter ET, van de Kaa CA, et al. Dynamic TurboFLASH subtraction technique for contrast-enhanced MR imaging of the prostate: correlation with histopathologic results. Radiology 1997;203:645-652.

88. Siegelman ES, Schnall MD. Contrast enhanced MR of bladder and prostate. MR Clin North Am 1996;4:1-17.

89. Engelbrecht MR, Huisman HJ, Laheij RJ, et al. Discrimination of prostate cancer from normal peripheral zone and central gland tissue by using dynamic contrast-enhanced MR imaging. Radiology 2003;229:248-254.

90. Miller JS, Puckett ML, Johnstone PA. Frequency of coexistent disease at CT in patients with prostate carcinoma selected for definitive radiation therapy: is limited treatment-planning CT adequate? Radiology 2000;215:41-44.

91. Forman HP, Heiken JP, Brink JA, Glazer HS, Fox LA, McClennan BL. CT screening for comorbid disease in patients with prostatic carcinoma: is it cost-effective? AJR Am J Roentgenol 1994;162:1125-1128; discussion 1129-1130.

92. Sickler GK, Chen PC, Dubinsky TJ, Maklad N. Free echogenic pelvic fluid: correlation with hemoperitoneum. J Ultrasound Med 1998;17:431-435.

93. Siegelman ES. Magnetic resonance imaging of the prostate. Semin Roentgenol 1999;34:295-312.

94. Grossfeld GD, Coakley FV. Benign prostatic hyperplasia: clinical overview and value of diagnostic imaging. Radiol Clin North Am 2000;38:31-47.

95. Banner MP. Imaging of benign prostatic hyperplasia. Semin Roentgenol 1999;34:313-324.

96. Walsh PC. Surgery and the reduction of mortality from prostate cancer. N Engl J Med 2002;347:839-840.

97. Haas GP, Sakr WA. Epidemiology of prostate cancer. CA Cancer J Clin 1997;47:273-287.

98. Jacobsen SJ, Katusic SK, Bergstralh EJ, et al. Incidence of prostate cancer diagnosis in the eras before and after serum prostate-specific antigen testing. JAMA 1995;274:1445-1449.

99. Mitka M. Disparity in cancer statistics changing. JAMA 2002;287: 703-704.

100. Farkas A, Marcella S, Rhoads GG. Ethnic and racial differences in prostate cancer incidence and mortality. Ethn Dis 2000;10:69-75.

101. Nelson WG, De Marzo AM, Isaacs WB. Prostate cancer. N Engl J Med 2003;349:366-381.

102. Thompson IM, Goodman PJ, Tangen CM, et al. The influence of finasteride on the development of prostate cancer. N Engl J Med 2003;349:215-224.

103. Scardino PT. The prevention of prostate cancer—the dilemma continues. N Engl J Med 2003;349:297-299.

104. Smith RA, Cokkinides V, von Eschenbach AC, et al. American Cancer Society guidelines for the early detection of cancer. CA Cancer J Clin 2002;52:8-22.

105. Cookson MM. Prostate cancer: screening and early detection. Cancer Control 2001;8:133-140.

106. Catalona WJ, Southwick PC, Slawin KM, et al. Comparison of percent free PSA, PSA density, and age-specific PSA cutoffs for prostate cancer detection and staging. Urology 2000; 56:255-260.

107. Eastham JA, Riedel E, Scardino PT, et al. Variation of serum prostate-specific antigen levels: an evaluation of year-to-year fluctuations. JAMA 2003;289:2695-2700.

108. Kuligowska E, Barish MA, Fenlon HM, Blake M. Predictors of prostate carcinoma: accuracy of gray-scale and color Doppler US and serum markers. Radiology 2001;220:757-764.

109. Rifkin MD, Zerhouni EA, Gatsonis CA, et al. Comparison of magnetic resonance imaging and ultrasonography in staging early prostate cancer: results of a multi-institutional cooperative trial [see comments]. N Engl J Med 1990;323:621-626.

110. Wilkinson BA, Hamdy FC. State-of-the-art staging in prostate cancer. BJU Int 2001;87:423-430.

111. Holmberg L, Bill-Axelson A, Helgesen F, et al. A randomized trial comparing radical prostatectomy with watchful waiting in early prostate cancer. N Engl J Med 2002;347:781-789.

112. Begg CB, Riedel ER, Bach PB, et al. Variations in morbidity after radical prostatectomy. N Engl J Med 2002;346:1138-1144.

113. Engelbrecht MR, Barentsz JO, Jager GJ, et al. Prostate cancer staging using imaging. BJU Int 2000;86 Suppl 1:123-134.

114. Parker SL, Tong T, Bolden S, Wingo PA. Cancer statistics, 1996 [see comments]. CA Cancer J Clin 1996;46:5-27.

115. Yu KK, Hricak H, Alagappan R, Chernoff DM, Bacchetti P, Zaloudek CJ. Detection of extracapsular extension of prostate carcinoma with endorectal and phased-array coil MR imaging: multivariate feature analysis. Radiology 1997;202:697-702.

116. Presti JC, Jr., Hricak H, Narayan PA, Shinohara K, White S, Carroll PR. Local staging of prostatic carcinoma: comparison of transrectal sonography and endorectal MR imaging. AJR Am J Roentgenol 1996;166:103-108.

117. O'Dowd GJ, Veltri RW, Orozco R, Miller MC, Oesterling JE. Update on the appropriate staging evaluation for newly diagnosed prostate cancer. J Urol 1997;158:687-698.

118. Partin AW, Kattan MW, Subong EN, et al. Combination of prostate-specific antigen, clinical stage, and Gleason score to predict pathological stage of localized prostate cancer. A multi-institutional update. JAMA 1997;277:1445-1451.

119. Presti JC, Jr. Prostate cancer: assessment of risk using digital rectal examination, tumor grade, prostate-specific antigen, and systematic biopsy. Radiol Clin North Am 2000;38:49-58.

120. Partin AW, Mangold LA, Lamm DM, Walsh PC, Epstein JI, Pearson JD. Contemporary update of prostate cancer staging nomograms (Partin tables) for the new millennium. Urology 2001;58:843-848.

121. D'Amico AV, Schnall M, Whittington R, et al. Endorectal coil magnetic resonance imaging identifies locally advanced prostate cancer in select patients with clinically localized disease. Urology 1998;51:449-454.

122. Cornud F, Flam T, Chauveinc L, et al. Extraprostatic spread of clinically localized prostate cancer: factors predictive of pT3 tumor and of positive endorectal MR imaging examination results. Radiology 2002;224:203-210.

123. Jager GJ, Severens JL, Thornbury JR, de La Rosette JJ, Ruijs SH, Barentsz JO. Prostate cancer staging: should MR imaging be used? A decision analytic approach. Radiology 2000;215:445-451.

124. Langlotz CP. Benefits and costs of MR imaging of prostate cancer. Magn Reson Imaging Clin N Am 1996;4:533-544.

125. Carter HB, Walsh PC, Landis P, Epstein JI. Expectant management of nonpalpable prostate cancer with curative intent: preliminary results. J Urol 2002;167:1231-1234.

126. Kaji Y, Kurhanewicz J, Hricak H, et al. Localizing prostate cancer in the presence of postbiopsy changes on MR images: role of proton MR spectroscopic imaging. Radiology 1998;206:785-790.

127. White S, Hricak H, Forstner R, et al. Prostate cancer: effect of postbiopsy hemorrhage on interpretation of MR images. Radiology 1995;195:385-390.

128. Perrotti M, Han KR, Epstein RE, et al. Prospective evaluation of endorectal magnetic resonance imaging to detect tumor foci in men with prior negative prostatic biopsy: a pilot study. J Urol 1999;162:1314-1317.

129. Lui PD, Terris MK, McNeal JE, Stamey TA. Indications for ultrasound guided transition zone biopsies in the detection of prostate cancer. J Urol 1995;153:1000-1003.

130. Beyersdorff D, Taupitz M, Winkelmann B, et al. Patients with a history of elevated prostate-specific antigen levels and negative transrectal US-guided quadrant or sextant biopsy results: value of MR imaging. Radiology 2002;224:701-706.

131. Ikonen S, Karkkainen P, Kivisaari L, et al. Magnetic resonance imaging of clinically localized prostatic cancer. J Urol 1998;159: 915-919.

132. Liu IJ, Macy M, Lai YH, Terris MK. Critical evaluation of the current indications for transition zone biopsies. Urology 2001;57:1117-1120.

133. Cookson MS. Update on transrectal ultrasound-guided needle biopsy of the prostate. Mol Urol 2000;4:93-97; discussion 99.

134. Outwater EK, Petersen RO, Siegelman ES, Gomella LG, Chernesky CE, Mitchell DG. Prostate carcinoma: assessment of diagnostic criteria for capsular penetration on endorectal coil MR images. Radiology 1994;193:333-339.

135. Yu KK, Scheidler J, Hricak H, et al. Prostate cancer: prediction of extracapsular extension with endorectal MR imaging and three-dimensional proton MR spectroscopic imaging. Radiology 1999;213:481-488.

136. Epstein JI, Carmichael MJ, Pizov G, Walsh PC. Influence of capsular penetration on progression following radical prostatectomy: a study of 196 cases with long-term followup. J Urol 1993;150:135-141.

137. Linzer DG, Stock RG, Stone NN, Ratnow R, Ianuzzi C, Unger P. Seminal vesicle biopsy: accuracy and implications for staging of prostate cancer. Urology 1996;48:757-761.

138. Chuang YC, Chen KK, Chang KM, et al. The route of seminal vesicle involvement in adenocarcinoma of prostate: lymphaticovascular or local extension? Zhonghua Yi Xue Za Zhi (Taipei) 1997;59:95-98.

139. Guillonneau B, Debras B, Veillon B, Bougaran J, Chambon E, Vallancien G. Indications for preoperative seminal vesicle biopsies in staging of clinically localized prostatic cancer. Eur Urol 1997;32:160-165.

140. Saliken JC, Gray RR, Donnelly BJ, et al. Extraprostatic biopsy improves the staging of localized prostate cancer. Can Assoc Radiol J 2000;51:114-120.

141. Bartolozzi C, Crocetti L, Menchi I, Ortori S, Lencioni R. Endorectal magnetic resonance imaging in local staging of prostate carcinoma. Abdom Imaging 2001;26:111-122.

142. Sanchez-Chapado M, Angulo JC, Ibarburen C, et al. Comparison of digital rectal examination, transrectal ultrasonography, and multicoil magnetic resonance imaging for preoperative evaluation of prostate cancer. Eur Urol 1997;32:140-149.

143. Jager GJ, Ruijter ET, de la Rosette JJ, van de Kaa CA. Amyloidosis of the seminal vesicles simulating tumor invasion of prostatic carcinoma on endorectal MR images. Eur Radiol 1997;7:552-554.

144. Ramchandani P, Schnall MD, LiVolsi VA, Tomaszewski JE, Pollack HM. Senile amyloidosis of the seminal vesicles mimicking metastatic spread of prostatic carcinoma on MR images. AJR Am J Roentgenol 1993;161:99-100.

145. Jager GJ, Barentsz JO, Oosterhof GO, Witjes JA, Ruijs SJ. Pelvic adenopathy in prostatic and urinary bladder carcinoma: MR imaging with a three-dimensional TI-weighted magnetization-prepared-rapid gradient-echo sequence. AJR Am J Roentgenol 1996;167:1503-1507.

146. Harisinghani MG, Saini S, Weissleder R, et al. MR lymphangiography using ultrasmall superparamagnetic iron oxide in patients with primary abdominal and pelvic malignancies: radiographic-pathologic correlation. AJR Am J Roentgenol 1999;172:1347-1351.

147. Harisinghani MG, Barentsz J, Hahn PF, et al. Noninvasive detection of clinically occult lymph-node metastases in prostate cancer. N Engl J Med 2003;348:2491-2499.

148. Heidenreich A, Varga Z, Von Knobloch R. Extended pelvic lymphadenectomy in patients undergoing radical prostatectomy: high incidence of lymph node metastasis. J Urol 2002;167:1681-1686.

149. Van Arsdalen KN, Broderick GA, Malkowicz SB, Wein AJ. Laparoscopic lymphadenectomy based on magnetic resonance imaging: is a unilateral dissection adequate for staging prostate cancer? Tech Urol 1996;2:93-98.

150. Oyen RH, Van Poppel HP, Ameye FE, Van de Voorde WA, Baert AL, Baert LV. Lymph node staging of localized prostatic carcinoma with CT and CT-guided fine-needle aspiration biopsy: prospective study of 285 patients [see comments]. Radiology 1994;190:315-322.

151. Coakley FV, Lin RY, Schwartz LH, Panicek DM. Mesenteric adenopathy in patients with prostate cancer: frequency and etiology. AJR Am J Roentgenol 2002;178:125-127.

152. Ekman P. Predicting pelvic lymph node involvement in patients with localized prostate cancer. Eur Urol 1997;32:60-64.

153. Meng MV, Carroll PR. When is pelvic lymph node dissection necessary before radical prostatectomy? A decision analysis. J Urol 2000;164:1235-1240.

154. Sandblom G, Holmberg L, Damber JE, et al. Prostate-specific antigen for prostate cancer staging in a population-based register. Scand J Urol Nephrol 2002;36:99-105.

155. Fergany A, Kupelian PA, Levin HS, Zippe CD, Reddy C, Klein EA. No difference in biochemical failure rates with or without pelvic lymph node dissection during radical prostatectomy in low-risk patients. Urology 2000;56:92-95.

156. Parkin J, Keeley FX, Jr., Timoney AG. Laparoscopic lymph node sampling in locally advanced prostate cancer. BJU Int 2002;89:14-17; discussion 17-18.

157. Lee CT, Oesterling JE. Using prostate-specific antigen to eliminate the staging radionuclide bone scan. Urol Clin North Am 1997;24:389-394.

158. Ataus S, Citci A, Alici B, et al. The value of serum prostate specific antigen and other parameters in detecting bone metastases in prostate cancer. Int Urol Nephrol 1999;31:481-489.

159. Kosuda S, Yoshimura I, Aizawa T, et al. Can initial prostate specific antigen determinations eliminate the need for bone scans in patients with newly diagnosed prostate carcinoma? A multicenter retrospective study in Japan. Cancer 2002;94:964-972.

160. Lee N, Fawaaz R, Olsson CA, et al. Which patients with newly diagnosed prostate cancer need a radionuclide bone scan? An analysis based on 631 patients. Int J Radiat Oncol Biol Phys 2000;48:1443-1446.

161. Yamamoto S, Ito T, Akiyama A, Aizawa T, Miki M, Tachibana M. M1 prostate cancer with a serum level of prostate-specific antigen less than 10 ng/mL. Int J Urol 2001;8:374-379.

162. Taoka T, Mayr NA, Lee HJ, et al. Factors influencing visualization of vertebral metastases on MR imaging versus bone scintigraphy. AJR Am J Roentgenol 2001;176:1525-1530.

163. Fujii Y, Higashi Y, Owada F, Okuno T, Mizuno H, Mizuno H. Magnetic resonance imaging for the diagnosis of prostate cancer metastatic to bone. Br J Urol 1995;75:54-58.

164. Leventis AK, Shariat SF, Slawin KM. Local recurrence after radical prostatectomy: correlation of US features with prostatic fossa biopsy findings. Radiology 2001;219:432-439.

165. Rogers R, Grossfeld GD, Roach M, 3rd, Shinohara K, Presti JC, Jr., Carroll PR. Radiation therapy for the management of biopsy proved local recurrence after radical prostatectomy. J Urol 1998;160:1748-1753.

166. Leventis AK, Shariat SF, Kattan MW, Butler EB, Wheeler TM, Slawin KM. Prediction of response to salvage radiation therapy in patients with prostate cancer recurrence after radical prostatectomy. J Clin Oncol 2001;19:1030-1039.

167. Ornstein DK, Oh J, Herschman JD, Andriole GL. Evaluation and management of the man who has failed primary curative therapy for prostate cancer. Urol Clin North Am 1998;25:591-601.

168. Silverman JM, Krebs TL. MR imaging evaluation with a transrectal surface coil of local recurrence of prostatic cancer in men who have undergone radical prostatectomy. AJR Am J Roentgenol 1997;168:379-385.

169. Tiguert R, Gheiler EL, Gudziak MR. Collagen injection in the management of post-radical prostatectomy intrinsic sphincteric deficiency. Neurourol Urodyn 1999;18:653-658.

170. Norderhaug I, Dahl O, Hoisaeter PA, et al. Brachytherapy for prostate cancer: a systematic review of clinical and cost effectiveness. Eur Urol 2003;44:40-46.

171. Clarke DH, Banks SJ, Wiederhorn AR, et al. The role of endorectal coil MRI in patient selection and treatment planning for prostate seed implants. Int J Radiat Oncol Biol Phys 2002;52:903-910.

172. D'Amico AV, Cormack RA, Tempany CM. MRI-guided diagnosis and treatment of prostate cancer. N Engl J Med 2001;344:776-777.

173. Coakley FV, Hricak H, Wefer AE, Speight JL, Kurhanewicz J, Roach M. Brachytherapy for prostate cancer: endorectal MR imaging of local treatment-related changes. Radiology 2001;219:817-821.

174. Costello LC, Franklin RB. The intermediary metabolism of the prostate: a key to understanding the pathogenesis and progression of prostate malignancy. Oncology 2000;59:269-282.

175. Wefer AE, Hricak H, Vigneron DB, et al. Sextant localization of prostate cancer: comparison of sextant biopsy, magnetic resonance imaging and magnetic resonance spectroscopic imaging with step section histology. J Urol 2000;164:400-404.

176. Thornbury JR, Ornstein DK, Choyke PL, Langlotz CP, Weinreb JC. Prostate cancer: what is the future role for imaging? AJR Am J Roentgenol 2001;176:17-22.

177. Mueller-Lisse UG, Vigneron DB, Hricak H, et al. Localized prostate cancer: effect of hormone deprivation therapy measured by using combined three-dimensional 1H MR spectroscopy and MR imaging: clinicopathologic case-controlled study. Radiology 2001;221:380-390.

178. Swindle P, McCredie S, Russell P, et al. Pathologic characterization of human prostate tissue with proton MR spectroscopy. Radiology 2003;228:144-151.

179. Manduca A, Oliphant TE, Dresner MA, et al. Magnetic resonance elastography: non-invasive mapping of tissue elasticity. Med Image Anal 2001;5:237-254.

180. Khan A, Ramchandani P. Unusual and uncommon prostatic lesions. Semin Roentgenol 1999;34:350-363.

181. Donat SM, Wei DC, McGuire MS, Herr HW. The efficacy of transurethral biopsy for predicting the long-term clinical impact of prostatic invasive bladder cancer. J Urol 2001;165:1580-1584.

182. Sexton WJ, Lance RE, Reyes AO, Pisters PW, Tu SM, Pisters LL. Adult prostate sarcoma: the M. D. Anderson Cancer Center Experience. J Urol 2001;166:521-525.

183. Russo P, Demas B, Reuter V. Adult prostatic sarcoma. Abdom Imaging 1993;18:399-401.

184. Bates AW, Baithun SI. Secondary solid neoplasms of the prostate: a clinico-pathological series of 51 cases. Virchows Arch 2002;440:392-396.

185. Nickel JC. Prostatitis: the last frontier. World J Surg 2000;24:1197-1199.

186. Schaeffer AJ, Datta NS, Fowler JE, Jr., et al. Overview summary statement: diagnosis and management of chronic prostatitis/chronic pelvic pain syndrome (CP/CPPS). Urology 2002;60:1-4.

187. Potts JM. Chronic pelvic pain syndrome: a non-prostatocentric perspective. World J Urol 2003;21:54-56.

188. Atilla MK, Sargin H, Odabas O, Yilmaz Y, Aydin S. Evaluation of 42 patients with chronic abacterial prostatitis: are there any underlying correctable pathologies? Int Urol Nephrol 1998;30:463-469.

189. Parsons RB, Fisher AM, Bar-Chama N, Mitty HA. MR imaging in male infertility. Radiographics 1997;17:627-637.

190. Ikonen S, Kivisaari L, Tervahartiala P, Vehmas T, Taari K, Rannikko S. Prostatic MR imaging: accuracy in differentiating cancer from other prostatic disorders. Acta Radiol 2001;42:348-354.

191. Kim ED, Onel E, Honig SC, Lipschultz LI. The prevalence of cystic abnormalities of the prostate involving the ejaculatory ducts as detected by transrectal ultrasound. Int Urol Nephrol 1997;29:647-652.

192. Ishikawa M, Okabe H, Oya T, et al. Midline prostatic cysts in healthy men: incidence and transabdominal sonographic findings. AJR Am J Roentgenol 2003;181:1669-1672.

193. Coppens L, Bonnet P, Andrianne R, de Leval J. Adult mullerian duct or utricle cyst: clinical significance and therapeutic management of 65 cases. J Urol 2002;167:1740-1744.

194. McDermott VG, Meakem TJr, Stolpen AH, Schnall MD. Prostatic and periprostatic cysts: findings on MR imaging. AJR Am J Roentgenol 1995;164:123-127.

195. Nghiem HT, Kellman GM, Sandberg SA, Craig BM. Cystic lesions of the prostate. Radiographics 1990;10:635-650.

196. McConnell JD, Roehrborn CG, Bautista OM, et al. The long-term effect of doxazosin, finasteride, and combination therapy on the clinical progression of benign prostatic hyperplasia. N Engl J Med 2003;349:2387-2398.

197. Vaughan ED, Jr. Medical management of benign prostatic hyperplasia—are two drugs better than one? N Engl J Med 2003;349:2449-2451.

198. Engin G, Kadioglu A, Orhan I, Akdol S, Rozanes I. Transrectal US and endorectal MR imaging in partial and complete obstruction of the seminal duct system: a comparative study. Acta Radiol 2000; 41:288-295.

199. Sokol RZ. Infertility in men with cystic fibrosis. Curr Opin Pulm Med 2001;7:421-426.

200. Chillon M, Casals T, Mercier B, et al. Mutations in the cystic fibrosis gene in patients with congenital absence of the vas deferens. N Engl J Med 1995;332:1475-1480.

201. Cherullo EE, Meraney AM, Bernstein LH, Einstein DM, Thomas AJ, Gill IS. Laparoscopic management of congenital seminal vesicle cysts associated with ipsilateral renal agenesis. J Urol 2002;167:1263-1267.

202. Livingston L, Larsen CR. Seminal vesicle cyst with ipsilateral renal agenesis. AJR Am J Roentgenol 2000;175:177-180.

203. Belet U, Danaci M, Sarikaya S, et al. Prevalence of epididymal, seminal vesicle, prostate, and testicular cysts in autosomal dominant polycystic kidney disease. Urology 2002;60:138-141.

204. Gonzalez CM, Dalton DP. Endoscopic incision of a seminal vesicle cyst. Urology 1998;51:831-832.

205. McCauley TR, McCarthy S, Lange R. Pelvic phased array coil: image quality assessment for spin-echo MR imaging. Magn Reson Imaging 1992;10:513-522.

206. Fisher MR, Hricak H, Tanagho EA. Urinary bladder MR imaging. 2. Neoplasm. Radiology 1985;157:471-477.

207. Siegelman ES, Schnall MD. Contrast-enhanced MR imaging of the bladder and prostate. Magn Reson Imaging Clin N Am 1996;4:153-169.

208. Tekes A, Kamel IR, Imam K, Chan TY, Schoenberg MP, Bluemke DA. MR imaging features of transitional cell carcinoma of the urinary bladder. AJR Am J Roentgenol 2003;180:771-777.

209. Narumi Y, Kadota T, Inoue E, et al. Bladder tumors: staging with gadolinium-enhanced oblique MR imaging. Radiology 1993;187:145-150.

210. Barentsz JO, Jager GJ, Witjes JA. MR imaging of the urinary bladder. Magn Reson Imaging Clin N Am 2000;8:853-867.

211. Elster AD, Sobol WT, Hinson WH. Pseudolayering of Gd-DTPA in the urinary bladder. Radiology 1990;174:379-381.

212. Olcott EW, Nino-Murcia M, Rhee JS. Urinary bladder pseudolesions on contrast-enhanced helical CT: frequency and clinical implications. AJR Am J Roentgenol 1998;171:1349-1354.

213. Lawler LP. MR imaging of the bladder. Radiol Clin North Am 2003;41:161-177.

214. Wong-You-Cheong JJ, Wagner BJ, Davis CJ, Jr. Transitional cell carcinoma of the urinary tract: radiologic-pathologic correlation. Radiographics 1998;18:123-142; quiz 148.

215. Tekes A, Kamel IR, Chan TY, Schoenberg MP, Bluemke DA. MR imaging features of non-transitional cell carcinoma of the urinary bladder with pathologic correlation. AJR Am J Roentgenol 2003;180:779-784.

216. Pirastu R, Iavarone I, Comba P. Bladder cancer: a selected review of the epidemiological literature. Ann Ist Super Sanita 1996;32:3-20.

217. MacVicar AD. Bladder cancer staging. BJU Int 2000;86(Suppl 1):111-122.

218. Satoh E, Miyao N, Tachiki H, Fujisawa Y. Prediction of muscle invasion of bladder cancer by cystoscopy. Eur Urol 2002;41:178-181.

219. Sobin LH, Wittekind C (Eds.). TNM Classification of Malignant Tumors. New York, Wiley, 1997.

220. Marshall VF. The relation of the preoperative estimate to the pathologic demonstration of the extent of vesical neoplasms. J Urol 1952;68:714-723.

221. Coblentz TR, Mills SE, Theodorescu D. Impact of second opinion pathology in the definitive management of patients with bladder carcinoma. Cancer 2001;91:1284-1290.

222. Van Der Meijden A, Sylvester R, Collette L, Bono A, Ten Kate F. The role and impact of pathology review on stage and grade assessment of stages Ta and T1 bladder tumors: a combined analysis of 5 European Organization for Research and Treatment of Cancer trials. J Urol 2000;164:1533-1537.

223. Kiemeney LA, Witjes JA, Verbeek AL, Heijbroek RP, Debruyne FM. The clinical epidemiology of superficial bladder cancer. Dutch South-East Cooperative Urological Group. Br J Cancer 1993; 67:806-812.

224. Barentsz JO. Bladder cancer. In: Pollack HM, McClennan BL (Eds.): Clinical Urography, 2nd ed. Philadelphia, WB Saunders, 2000, pp 1642-1668.

225. Bassi P. BCG (bacillus of Calmette-Guérin) therapy of high-risk superficial bladder cancer. Surg Oncol 2002;11:77-83.

226. Grossman HB, Natale RB, Tangen CM, et al. Neoadjuvant chemotherapy plus cystectomy compared with cystectomy alone for locally advanced bladder cancer. N Engl J Med 2003;349:859-866.

227. O'Connor RC, Alsikafi NF, Steinberg GD. Therapeutic options and treatment of muscle invasive bladder cancer. Expert Rev Anticancer Ther 2001;1:511-522.

228. Kaufman DS, Shipley WU, McDougal WS, Young RH. Case records of the Massachusetts General Hospital, Weekly clinicopathological exercise, Case 3-2004: A 57-year-old man with invasive transitional-cell carcinoma of the bladder. N Engl J Med 2004;350:394-402.

229. Santacaterina A, Settineri N, De Renzis C, et al. Muscle-invasive bladder cancer in elderly-unfit patients with concomitant illness: can a curative radiation therapy be delivered? Tumori 2002;88:390-394.

230. Raghavan D, Quinn D, Skinner DG, Stein JP. Surgery and adjunctive chemotherapy for invasive bladder cancer. Surg Oncol 2002;11:55-63.

231. Kundra V, Silverman PM. Imaging in the diagnosis, staging, and follow-up of cancer of the urinary bladder. AJR Am J Roentgenol 2003;180:1045-1054.

232. Robinson P, Collins CD, Ryder WD, et al. Relationship of MRI and clinical staging to outcome in invasive bladder cancer treated by radiotherapy. Clin Radiol 2000;55:301-306.

233. Neuerburg JM, Bohndorf K, Sohn M, Teufl F, Gunther RW. Staging of urinary bladder neoplasms with MR imaging: is Gd-DTPA helpful? J Comput Assist Tomogr 1991;15:780-786.

234. Scattoni V, Da Pozzo LF, Colombo R, et al. Dynamic gadolinium-enhanced magnetic resonance imaging in staging of superficial bladder cancer. J Urol 1996;155:1594-1599.

235. Beyersdorff D, Taupitz M, Giessing M, et al. [The staging of bladder tumors in MRT: the value of the intravesical application of an iron oxide-containing contrast medium in combination with high-resolution T2-weighted imaging]. Rofo Fortschr Geb Rontgenstr Neuen Bildgeb Verfahr 2000;172:504-508.

236. Venz S, Ilg J, Ebert T, et al. [Determining the depth of infiltration in urinary bladder carcinoma with contrast medium enhanced dynamic magnetic resonance tomography: with reference to postoperative findings and inflammation]. Urologe A 1996;35:297-304.

237. Barentsz JO, Jager GJ, van Vierzen PB, et al. Staging urinary bladder cancer after transurethral biopsy: value of fast dynamic contrast-enhanced MR imaging. Radiology 1996;201:185-193.

238. Hayashi N, Tochigi H, Shiraishi T, Takeda K, Kawamura J. A new staging criterion for bladder carcinoma using gadolinium-enhanced magnetic resonance imaging with an endorectal surface coil: a comparison with ultrasonography. BJU Int 2000;85:32-36.

239. Barentsz JO. MR intervention in the pelvis: an overview and first experiences in MR-guided biopsy in nodal metastases in urinary bladder cancer. Abdom Imaging 1997;22:524-530.

240. Ghanem N, Altehoefer C, Hogerle S, et al. Comparative diagnostic value and therapeutic relevance of magnetic resonance imaging and bone marrow scintigraphy in patients with metastatic solid tumors of the axial skeleton. Eur J Radiol 2002;43:256-261.

241. Saito W, Amanuma M, Tanaka J, Heshiki A. Histopathological analysis of a bladder cancer stalk observed on MRI. Magn Reson Imaging 2000;18:411-415.

242. Lawler LP, Fishman EK. Bladder imaging using multidetector row computed tomography, volume rendering, and magnetic resonance imaging. J Comput Assist Tomogr 2003;27:553-563.

243. Dondalski M, White EM, Ghahremani GG, Patel SK. Carcinoma arising in urinary bladder diverticula: imaging findings in six patients. AJR Am J Roentgenol 1993;161:817-820.

244. Sulaiman MN, Buchholz NP, Khan MA. Carcinoma in a bladder diverticulum: the place of diverticulectomy. Arch Ital Urol Androl 1998;70:195-197.

245. Baniel J, Vishna T. Primary transitional cell carcinoma in vesical diverticula. Urology 1997;50:697-699.

246. Durfee SM, Schwartz LH, Panicek DM, Russo P. MR imaging of carcinoma within urinary bladder diverticulum. Clin Imaging 1997;21:290-292.

247. Mangiacapra FJ, Scheraga JL, Jones LA. Mucinous colloid adenocarcinoma of the urachus. Radiographics 2001;21:965-969.

248. Mengiardi B, Wiesner W, Stoffel F, Terracciano L, Freitag P. Case 44: adenocarcinoma of the urachus. Radiology 2002;222:744-747.

249. Hussain SM, Outwater EK, Siegelman ES. MR imaging features of pelvic mucinous carcinomas. Eur Radiol 2000;10:885-891.

250. Kim MJ, Park JS, Park SI, et al. Accuracy in differentiation of mucinous and nonmucinous rectal carcinoma on MR imaging. J Comput Assist Tomogr 2003;27:48-55.

251. Brick SH, Friedman AC, Pollack HM, et al. Urachal carcinoma: CT findings. Radiology 1988;169:377-381.

252. Mai KT, Ford JC, Morash C, Gerridzen R. Primary and secondary prostatic adenocarcinoma of the urinary bladder. Hum Pathol 2001;32:434-440.

253. Feldman PA, Madeb R, Naroditsky I, Halachmi S, Nativ O. Metastatic breast cancer to the bladder: a diagnostic challenge and review of the literature. Urology 2002;59:138.

254. Raviv S, Eggener SE, Williams DH, Garnett JE, Pins MR, Smith ND. Long-term survival after "drop metastases" of renal cell carcinoma to the bladder. Urology 2002;60:697.

255. Kempton CL, Kurtin PJ, Inwards DJ, Wollan P, Bostwick DG. Malignant lymphoma of the bladder: evidence from 36 cases that low-grade lymphoma of the MALT-type is the most common primary bladder lymphoma. Am J Surg Pathol 1997;21:1324-1333.

256. Douenias R, Rich M, Badlani G, Mazor D, Smith A. Predisposing factors in bladder calculi: review of 100 cases. Urology 1991;37:240-243.

257. Levine J, Neitlich J, Smith RC. The value of prone scanning to distinguish ureterovesical junction stones from ureteral stones that have passed into the bladder: leave no stone unturned. AJR Am J Roentgenol 1999;172:977-981.

258. Bouchelouche K, Nordling J. Recent developments in the management of interstitial cystitis. Curr Opin Urol 2003;13:309-313.

259. O'Connor LA, De Guzman J. Emphysematous cystitis: a radiographic diagnosis. Am J Emerg Med 2001;19:211-213.

260. Asada S, Kawasaki T. Images in clinical medicine: emphysematous cystitis. N Engl J Med 2003;349:258.

261. Heyns CF, De Kock ML, Kirsten PH, van Velden DJ. Pelvic lipomatosis associated with cystitis glandularis and adenocarcinoma of the bladder. J Urol 1991;145:364-366.

262. Lin HY, Wu WJ, Jang MY, et al. Cystitis glandularis mimics bladder cancer—three case reports and literature review. Kaohsiung J Med Sci 2001;17:102-106.

263. Young RH, Bostwick DG. Florid cystitis glandularis of intestinal type with mucin extravasation: a mimic of adenocarcinoma. Am J Surg Pathol 1996;20:1462-1468.

264. Iczkowski KA, Shanks JH, Gadaleanu V, et al. Inflammatory pseudotumor and sarcoma of urinary bladder: differential diagnosis and outcome in thirty-eight spindle cell neoplasms. Mod Pathol 2001;14:1043-1051.

265. Poon KS, Moreira O, Jones EC, Treissman S, Gleave ME. Inflammatory pseudotumor of the urinary bladder: a report of five cases and review of the literature. Can J Urol 2001; 8:1409-1415.

266. Heney NM, Young RH. Case records of the Massachusetts General Hospital, Weekly clinicopathological exercises, Case 39-2003: A 33-year-old woman with gross hematuria. N Engl J Med 2003;349:2442-2447.

267. Stoker J, Halligan S, Bartram CI. Pelvic floor imaging. Radiology 2001;218:621-641.

268. Fielding JR. Practical MR imaging of female pelvic floor weakness. Radiographics 2002;22:295-304.

269. Pannu HK. Magnetic resonance imaging of pelvic organ prolapse. Abdom Imaging 2002;27:660-673.

270. Pannu HK. Dynamic MR imaging of female organ prolapse. Radiol Clin North Am 2003;41:409-423.

271. Maubon A, Aubard Y, Berkane V, Camezind-Vidal MA, Mares P, Rouanet JP. Magnetic resonance imaging of the pelvic floor. Abdom Imaging 2003;28:217-225.

272. Barbaric ZL, Marumoto AK, Raz S. Magnetic resonance imaging of the perineum and pelvic floor. Top Magn Reson Imaging 2001;12:83-92.

273. Staatz G, Rohrmann D, Nolte-Ernsting CC, et al. Magnetic resonance urography in children: evaluation of suspected ureteral ectopia in duplex systems. J Urol 2001;166: 2346-2350.

274. Hagg MJ, Mourachov PV, Snyder HM, et al. The modern endoscopic approach to ureterocele. J Urol 2000;163:940-943.

275. Kochakarn W, Ratana-Olarn K, Viseshsindh V, Muangman V, Gojaseni P. Vesico-vaginal fistula: experience of 230 cases. J Med Assoc Thai 2000;83:1129-1132.

276. Hadley HR. Vesicovaginal fistula. Curr Urol Rep 2002;3:401-407.

277. Huang WC, Zinman LN, Bihrle W, 3rd. Surgical repair of vesicovaginal fistulas. Urol Clin North Am 2002;29:709-723.

278. Gruner JS, Sehon JK, Johnson LW. Diagnosis and management of enterovesical fistulas in patients with Crohn's disease. Am Surg 2002;68:714-719.

279. Liu CH, Chuang CK, Chu SH, et al. Enterovesical fistula: experiences with 41 cases in 12 years. Changgeng Yi Xue Za Zhi 1999;22:598-603.

10

MRI of the Breast

Mark A. Rosen, MD

Evan S. Siegelman, MD

INTRODUCTION

Why Perform Breast MRI?

While mammography and sonography are the mainstays of breast imaging for detection of malignancy and evaluation of clinical breast abnormalities, breast MRI is being more commonly used as an adjunctive imaging modality in a variety of clinical situations. MRI is the most accurate modality for evaluation of breast implants and has high sensitivity for detecting invasive cancer. Breast MR is also useful for evaluating the patient after breast conservation therapy or following reconstruction. The use of breast MRI for screening high-risk patients is currently under evaluation.

Breast MRI in Cancer Detection and Lesion Characterization

Both mammography and sonography have shown efficacy as an adjunct to the physical examination in the evaluation of known or suspected breast cancer.[1-3] The efficacy of screening mammography for the detection of unsuspected breast cancer has achieved near universal acceptance.[4] Nevertheless, both mammography and sonography have several shortcomings in the detection of cancer and the characterization of palpable lesions. Estimates of the sensitivity of mammography for cancer detection vary between 50% and 90%.[5,6] In certain patient groups, such as younger women or women who are taking hormone replacement therapy, the sensitivity may be lower.[7] The positive predictive value of mammography ranges between 20% and 60%,[8,9] resulting in a large number of biopsies and surgical procedures for benign disease.

Traditionally, sonography has been used as a means of differentiating solid lesions from cysts. Although sonography may also be able to distinguish between benign and malignant solid masses,[2] the evaluation is operator-dependent. Even with refined criteria, the false-positive rate of solid mass characterization by sonography and mammography combined may be as high as 60%.[10]

Many features of breast MRI make it an attractive modality for breast imaging. The sensitivity of MRI for invasive breast cancer is nearly 100%.[11-16] Its specificity is not nearly so high. However, research is ongoing toward improving specificity through refined interpretation criteria.[17,18]

Several obstacles limit the use of breast MRI in general clinical practice. MRI is unlikely to be a

10-1 Potential Indications for Breast MRI

- Evaluating implants
- Evaluating an indeterminate mammographic or sonographic abnormality (e.g., asymmetric breast density, probably benign solid mass)
- Localizing a mammographic abnormality revealed on only one view
- Evaluating spontaneous nipple discharge
- Detecting an occult primary breast cancer in women with negative mammography/physical exam and axillary nodal metastases
- Determining the extent of local disease in biopsy-proved breast cancer
- Monitoring neoadjuvant therapy for locally advanced breast cancer
- Following up breast conservation or reconstruction
- Screening patients at high risk for breast cancer (e.g., BRCA1/2 mutation carriers)

10-2 Ideal Features of Breast MRI Coil Design

- Patient comfort and ease of positioning
- Adequate coverage of breast and chest wall
- Signal uniformity
- High signal-to-noise ratio
- Easy access to breast for interventional procedures

cost-effective screening modality for the general population. Additionally, there are limited numbers of MR systems capable of performing optimized breast imaging and of radiologists trained in breast MRI interpretation. Furthermore, routine integration of breast MRI in the imaging diagnosis of breast disease is limited by the absence of agreed-upon uniform standards for both breast MR examination protocols and interpretation criteria.[19] Only though continued evaluation of breast MRI in well-controlled clinical trials will its proper role in various clinical circumstances be defined.

Indications for Breast MRI

Breast MRI has potential value as an adjunctive imaging modality for a variety of clinical indications (Box 10-1).[20-30]

The high sensitivity and negative predictive value of contrast-enhanced MRI for detection of invasive tumor make it an attractive modality for patient evaluation when physical, mammographic, and sonographic findings are indeterminate. This is true for the patient with increased breast density but also in patients whose normal breast architecture has been disrupted by surgery, irradiation, or chemotherapy.

TECHNICAL CONSIDERATIONS

Magnetic Field Strength

Breast MRI is ideally performed on high-field (1.0 tesla or greater) clinical imaging systems. Breast MRI obtained on lower field systems is limited by the difficulty in achieving selective fat saturation.[31] Another potential disadvantage of breast MRI at lower fields is that the degree of contrast enhancement may be reduced owing to the dependence of tissue T1 values on magnetic field.[32] As such, enhancing lesions may be less apparent on low-field MRI examinations.

Radiofrequency Coils

As for all MRI examinations, choice of the proper detection coil is critical for obtaining a high-quality study. There is no current uniform standard breast coil or agreed-upon design that combines all the desirable features of an MRI coil (Box 10-2).

The ideal breast coil should have a high degree of patient and technologist acceptance, while maintaining good signal-to-noise ratio and receptive field uniformity throughout the breast. Since many potentially cancerous lesions are detectable only by MRI, access to the breast during MR imaging is important for MR-guided localization procedures and biopsies.

Breast MRI coils may be unilateral or bilateral. They may be of a single loop, solenoid, or phased-array design.[33-35] Breast coils may or may not allow for breast compression or access for interventional procedures. All these factors, which can affect the quality of the MRI examination, must be considered when evaluating the performance of a breast MR imaging system.

A unilateral breast coil with sagittal compression and a four-coil phased array design[36,37] allows for high-resolution imaging of the breast with optimal signal-to-noise characteristics.[35] Four-coil array bilateral breast imaging coils (two coils for each breast) are also available (Fig. 10-1).[38] While these devices

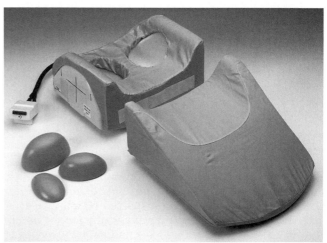

Figure 10-1 ■ Breast coil for 1.5 T MR systems. (Courtesy of MEDRAD, Pittsburgh, PA.)

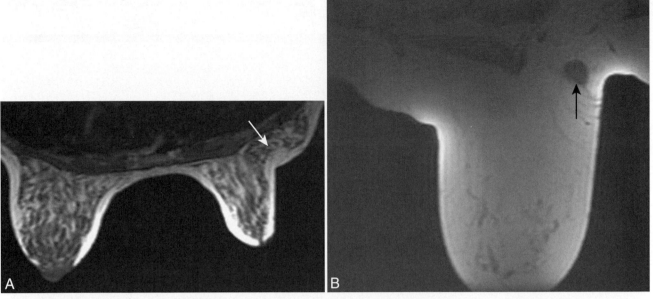

Figure 10-2 ■ Examples of incorrect and correct positioning of the breast within a sagittal compression coil. A, Axial T1-WI shows incorrect positioning of the breast for an MRI examination. Much of the glandular tissue has not been included *(arrow)* between the compression plates. This can lead to inadvertent exclusion of glandular tissue from the imaged volume. **B,** Axial T1-WI in a different patient with proper positioning reveals satisfactory coverage of the breast parenchyma, which includes a primary cancer *(arrow)* of the axillary tail (same patient as depicted in Fig. 10-17).

have a signal-to-noise ratio approximately 30% less than that of the dedicated unilateral coil, they offer the advantage of simultaneous bilateral breast examination.

Patient Positioning

For any breast MRI study, optimized patient positioning is required. Breast MRI is performed with the patient in the prone position, with the breast or breasts positioned dependent in the receiver coil. Prone positioning minimizes excursions of the chest wall and breast during respiration and displaces the breast away from the heart, thus limiting the degree of pulsatility artifact. Dependent positioning also allows for compression of the breast, which facilitates immobilization, more rapid volumetric imaging, and access to the breast for interventional procedures. If a breast coil with a compression array is utilized, care should be taken by the technologist to insure that compression includes all of the breast tissue, as axillary parenchyma may be inadvertently excluded from the field of view (Fig. 10-2).

THE FEMALE BREAST

Anatomy

The female breast develops between the superficial and deep layers of the superficial fascia. It has between 8 and 20 segments, each of which contains a major duct extending from the nipple. Each major duct ramifies into smaller ducts, all of which end in a terminal ductal lobular unit (TDLU). The individual TDLU is composed of a grouping of glandular tissue arranged in separate lobules, each of which feeds into a separate terminal ductule. Most breast cancers originate within the TDLU.

In addition to the lobular and ductal glandular tissue, the breast contains fibrous connective tissue, which lends structural support to the breast. This fibrous tissue is arranged in a regular array of oriented sheets and fibers within which the glandular elements are arrayed. The breast lymphatics are also found within this fibrous supporting framework. In mammography, the fibrous and glandular tissues are often grouped together as the "fibroglandular elements" of the breast. Finally, variable amounts of fat are present in the subcutaneous and retromammary spaces, leading to variation in size and density of the mature female breast.

MRI Features of the Normal Breast

On T1-WI (Fig. 10-3A), the fat within the breast reveals high signal intensity (SI) owing to the short T1 of adipose tissue. The fibroglandular tissue is of lower SI because of its longer T1. In general, fibrous and glandular tissue cannot be distinguished solely on the basis of T1 SI. In a breast with a moderate or large amount of fat, the fibrous septa appear as thin, low SI strands between fatty lobules, whereas glandular tissue has a more mass-like appearance. However, in breasts with a paucity of fat, it is difficult to distinguish fibrous tissue from glandular elements.

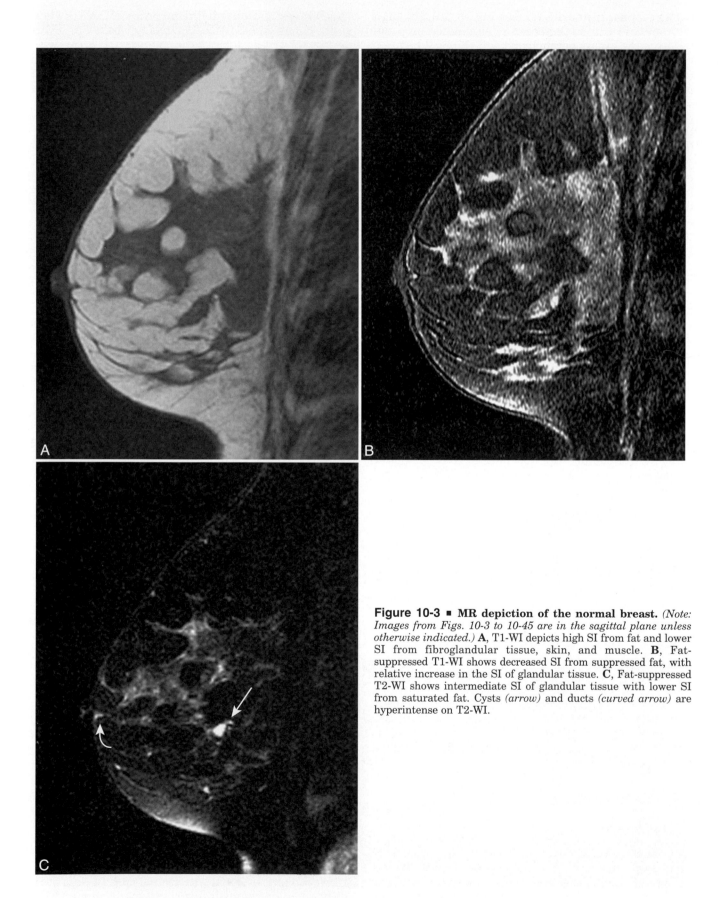

Figure 10-3 ▪ MR depiction of the normal breast. *(Note: Images from Figs. 10-3 to 10-45 are in the sagittal plane unless otherwise indicated.)* **A,** T1-WI depicts high SI from fat and lower SI from fibroglandular tissue, skin, and muscle. **B,** Fat-suppressed T1-WI shows decreased SI from suppressed fat, with relative increase in the SI of glandular tissue. **C,** Fat-suppressed T2-WI shows intermediate SI of glandular tissue with lower SI from saturated fat. Cysts *(arrow)* and ducts *(curved arrow)* are hyperintense on T2-WI.

On fat-saturated T1-WI (see Fig.10-3B), the high SI from lipid will be decreased or eliminated, and signal from the breast parenchyma and skin will be more readily shown secondary to the improved dynamic range. Fat saturation will also improve the conspicuity of enhancing lesion lesions, which, following contrast administration, may achieve SI equal to that of non-suppressed fat. Fat-suppressed T1-WI images are therefore ideal for evaluating enhancing breast lesions.[13,39]

On T2-WI (see Fig. 10-3C), glandular tissue is of intermediate SI, hyperintense to muscle, and hypointense to fluid. In most clinical applications, fast spin echo (FSE) T2-WI is used. Since fat has relatively high SI on FSE sequences, the relative SI of glandular tissue on T2-weighted FSE images will be hypointense to surrounding fat. On fat-saturated T2-WI, glandular tissue is isointense or slightly hyperintense to suppressed fat, and there is greater conspicuity of fluid-containing structures such as cysts and ducts. On lower field systems that do not allow for selective fat suppression, short tau inversion recovery (STIR) imaging may be used to suppress the signal from fat on T2-WI.

Contrast Enhancement of Normal Breast Parenchyma

Given the importance of enhancement for breast lesion detection and characterization, there has been much investigation into the behavior of normal glandular tissue on CE MRI. The biologic behavior of the breast changes during the menstrual cycle with corresponding cyclical fourth weeks of the menstrual cycle, with the least enhancement in the second week.[40-43] Thus, breast MRI in premenopausal women should ideally be performed mid-cycle (second week), when baseline parenchymal enhancement is at its lowest.[44]

In the nonproliferating breast, low-level parenchymal enhancement is common.[45] Typically, there is a generalized mild increase in SI of the glandular tissue after contrast administration but much less than for adjacent peripheral and intrathoracic vessels, axillary lymph nodes, and the cardiac chambers. The skin overlying the breast enhances to a variable degree. Mild to moderately intense nipple enhancement is also common (Fig. 10-4)[46,47] and should not be confused with an enhancing neoplasm. Typically in premenopausal women, glandular tissue will demonstrate low-to-moderate levels of diffuse or regional enhancement. This pattern of enhancement usually is gradual and often will resolve on follow-up imaging (Fig. 10-5).[41,42] In addition, diffuse or regional enhancement patterns featuring a fine stippled appearance (Fig. 10-6) are thought to represent a spectrum of normal parenchymal enhancement.[48]

In the actively proliferating breast, during the early or late phases of the menstrual cycle, there is more variability in the degree and pattern

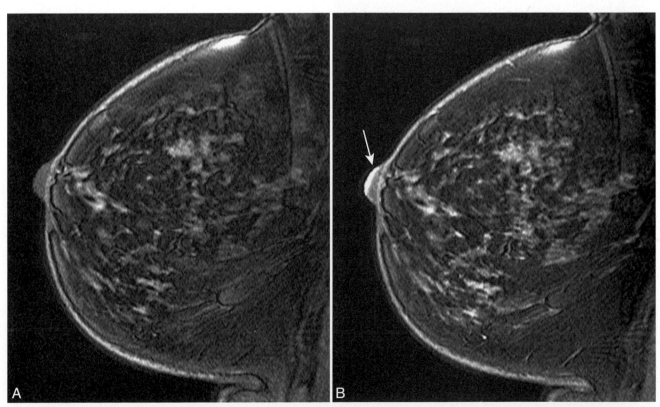

Figure 10-4 ▪ MR illustration of normal nipple enhancement. A and **B**, Fat-suppressed T1-WIs obtained before (**A**) and after (**B**) contrast show intense enhancement of the superficial aspect of the nipple *(arrow)*.

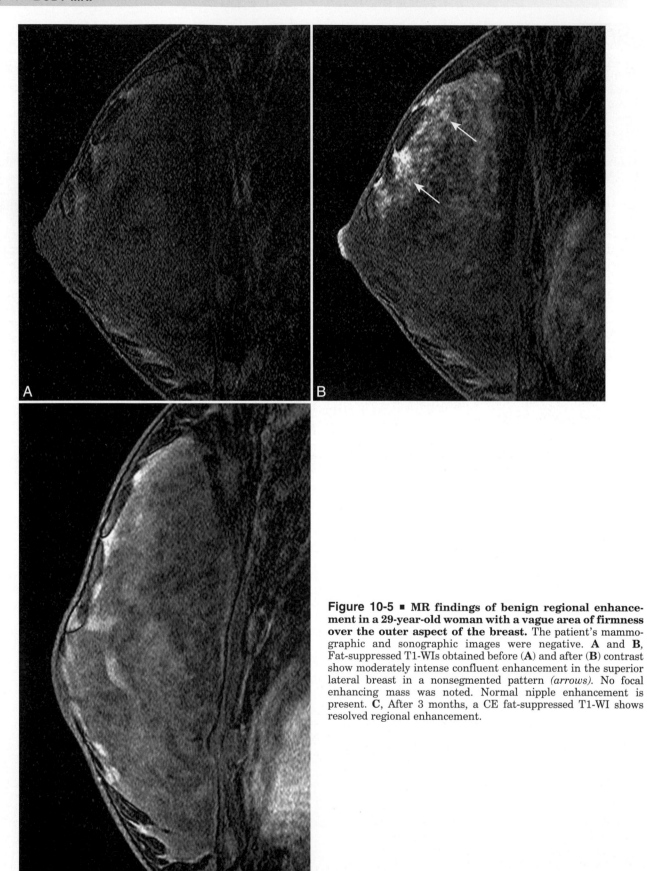

Figure 10-5 ■ MR findings of benign regional enhancement in a 29-year-old woman with a vague area of firmness over the outer aspect of the breast. The patient's mammographic and sonographic images were negative. **A** and **B**, Fat-suppressed T1-WIs obtained before (**A**) and after (**B**) contrast show moderately intense confluent enhancement in the superior lateral breast in a nonsegmented pattern *(arrows)*. No focal enhancing mass was noted. Normal nipple enhancement is present. **C**, After 3 months, a CE fat-suppressed T1-WI shows resolved regional enhancement.

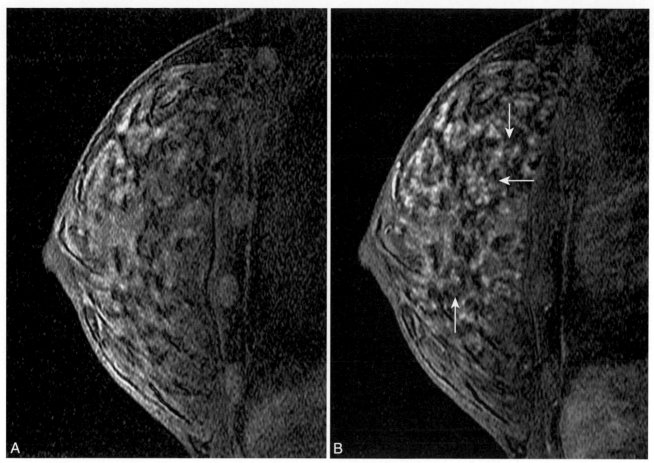

Figure 10-6 ▪ MR depiction of benign diffuse glandular enhancement. A and **B**, Fat-suppressed T1-WI obtained before (**A**) and after (**B**) contrast shows diffusely scattered punctate, or stippled, 1- to 3-mm foci of glandular enhancement *(arrows)*.

of enhancement. Moderate or even intensely enhancing parenchyma may be present, with variable morphologic appearances. While this pattern is generally diffuse, local or regional enhancement has been described,[45] potentially complicating the interpretation of a breast MRI examination. During high-level hormonal activity in the breast, such as pregnancy or lactation, there maybe extensive parenchymal enhancement, making the detection and characterization of a breast malignancy a challenge.[49]

IMAGING PROTOCOLS AND INTERPRETATION

Implant Evaluation

PURPOSE

In 1992, the U. S. FDA issued a moratorium on the use of silicone implants, allowing for their use only under strict criteria and in controlled clinical studies [http://www.fda.gov/cdrh/breastimplants/bichron.html, accessed January 2004]. Currently placed breast implants, whether for cosmetic or reconstructive purposes, are of the saline type. It is estimated that 1 to 2 million women in the U. S. underwent breast implant placement prior to 1992.[50,51] While many of these women have undergone elective explantation, the prevalence of silicone implants in the population remains high.

The purpose of an MRI examination for implant evaluation is to detect disruptions of the external elastomer shell of the implant. MRI is the most reliable imaging technique for evaluation of implant integrity.[52] Furthermore, MRI may reliably demonstrate the presence of silicone in the soft tissues of the breast or chest wall.[53]

TECHNIQUE

Implant evaluation requires examination of the entire external surface of the implant. Imaging is performed in two orthogonal planes—usually sagittal and axial. T1-WI is of less value than T2-WI, since both saline and silicone are hyperintense and differentially depicted on T2-WI.[54] Fat saturation is desirable but is complicated by the location of the up-field silicone resonance near that of the lipid resonance. At 1.5 T, approximately 220 Hz separates the fat and water resonances. At the same field strength, lipid and silicone are separated by approximately 80 Hz (Box 10-3).[55]

10-3 Comparison of Lipid, Water, and Silicone in Breast Implant Evaluation

	Water	Lipid	Silicone
Chemical shift (ppm)	4.7	1.2 to 1.5	~0
Resonance frequency relative to water (1.5 T)	—	−220 Hz	−300 Hz
T1 weighted SI	Low	High	Low
T2 weighted SI (TE = 90 ms)	High	Intermediate-high	High
T2 weighted SI (TE > 180 ms)	High	Low-intermediate	Intermediate
Short tau inversion recovery (STIR) SI	High	Low	High
STIR SI with water suppression	Low	Low	High

Chemical selective fat-suppression techniques may therefore be compromised by inadvertent silicone suppression (Fig. 10-7).[56] Unwanted silicone suppression may be more pronounced on lower strength scanners and scanners with nonuniform magnetic field homogeneity.

To avoid the possibility of artifact arising from chemical selective fat suppression, alternative sequences are available. Heavily T2-WI (with echo time (TE) >180 ms) accentuates the slight differences in T2 relaxation between silicone and saline (Fig. 10-8A).[57] A second type of sequence that is invaluable in evaluating silicone implants is a "silicone-only" sequence (see Fig. 10-8B). To achieve selective silicone imaging, a three-point Dixon technique[58] or a sequence that utilizes a combination of chemical selective water suppression and STIR fat suppression[59] may be used.

Silicone-only sequences are ideally suited for detection of extracapsular silicone in the adjacent breast tissue or lymph nodes (Fig. 10-9). Other strategies utilizing chemical shift artifacts may be used for evaluation of water/silicone interfaces.[60]

NORMAL AND ABNORMAL IMPLANT APPEARANCE

A large variety of breast implant designs are in current and past use. In general, implants are saline-only or silicone-containing types.[61] Silicone implants may have additional saline components (Fig. 10-10A). All breast implants have a thin outer elastomer shell that maintains implant integrity.

Following implant placement, there is a local inflammatory reaction at the site of placement, which results in the formation of a fibrous capsule of varying thickness. This thick layer of fibrous tissue lies immediately adjacent to, and often adheres to, the elastomer shell of the implant. As such, the elastomer shell of an intact implant is not revealed as a separate structure on MRI; instead, a hypointense band of tissue representing the fibrous capsule and the adherent elastomer shell is shown.

Saline-only implants are revealed as a single lumen with uniform hyperintensity on T2-WI. Saline implants are often used as tissue expanders for cosmesis following unilateral mastectomy. An access port is revealed as a low SI structure protruding into the lumen of the implant on T2-WI (see Fig. 10-10B). Silicone-containing implants reveal high SI on silicone-only sequences and are readily distinguishable from the saline-only type.

Intact implants are generally round or oval. Infolding of the elastomer shell is not uncommon and can lead to a confusing appearance on MRI. Imaging in at least two orthogonal planes is needed for complete evaluation of the outer contour of the implant. Small amounts of fluid accumulation may be present within the outer fibrous capsule, but external to the elastomer shell, in areas of incomplete adherence between the implant shell and the fibrous capsule. These regions of "condensation" are particularly common in areas of shell infolding, and MRI will often depict small water droplets that appear to be located within the silicone-containing lumen (Fig. 10-11). This is not a sign of rupture.

For silicone-containing implants, three types of ruptures are described. Extracapsular rupture

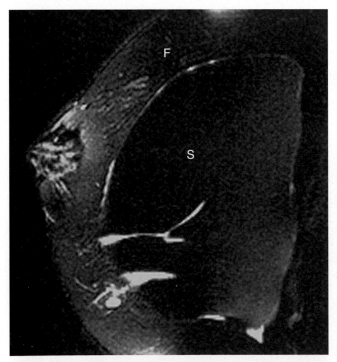

Figure 10-7 ▪ MR illustration of inadvertent silicone suppression during frequency-selective fat saturation. Fat-suppressed T2-WI in a woman with a silicone implant. The SI of the intraluminal silicone has been suppressed (S) along with fatty (F) breast tissue.

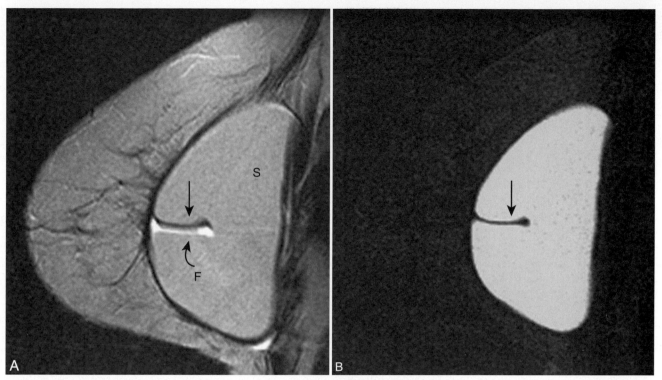

Figure 10-8 ■ **MR techniques of silicone/fluid differentiation as illustrated in an uncomplicated, single-lumen, retropectoral silicone implant. A**, Heavily T2-WI (TE = 180 ms) accentuates the SI differences between silicone (S) and fluid (F). The two parallel bands of low and high SI within the anterior implant represent chemical shift displacement of physiologic fluid (F, *curved arrow*) in the frequency-encoding direction within a normal radial fold *(arrow)*. This phenomenon is explained in Chapter 3. **B**, Short tau inversion recovery (STIR) imaging with frequency-selective water suppression allows for silicone-only imaging, which is useful for excluding extracapsular extension of silicone into adjacent tissues. The physiologic fluid within the radial fold *(arrow)* depicted in **A** has been suppressed.

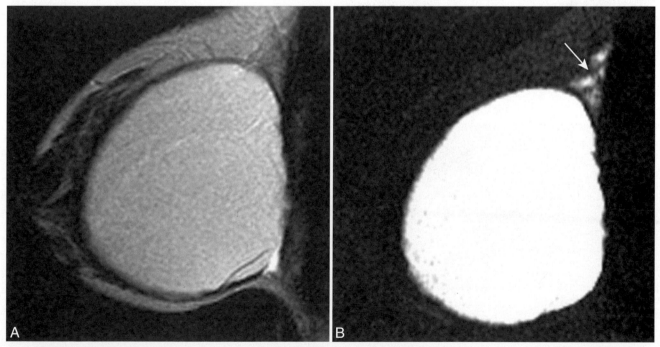

Figure 10-9 ■ **MR findings of extracapsular silicone in a woman with implant rupture. A**, T2-WI shows normal extracapsular tissues and a single-lumen retroglandular implant. On an adjoining slice (not shown), there were findings of implant and capsular rupture. **B**, Silicone-only imaging with STIR and frequency-selective water suppression reveals extracapsular silicone *(arrow)* in the adjacent soft tissues. This silicone leak was not depicted in **A** because of relative isointensity with adjacent fat.

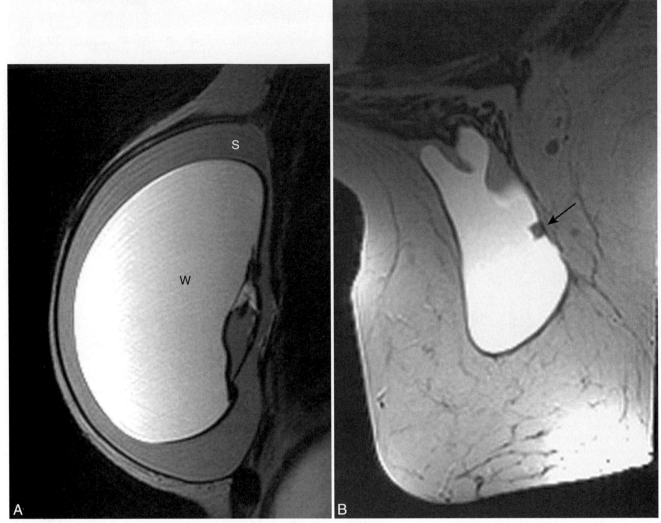

Figure 10-10 ■ **MR depictions of breast implant models. A**, T2-WI of a double-lumen implant with silicone in the outer shell and saline in the inner lumen. The fluid/saline (W) is hyperintense to silicone (S). **B**, Axial T2-WI of a single-lumen saline implant reveals the tissue expander port as a small focus of low SI defect protruding into the lumen (arrow).

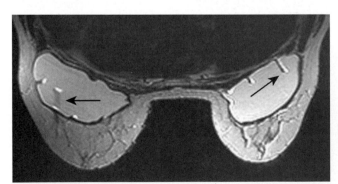

Figure 10-11 ■ **MR illustration of normal radial folds in a silicone implant.** Axial T2-WI shows several low SI folds (arrows) of the elastomer shell projecting into the lumen of the implant. Physiologic fluid present within these radial folds is depicted as higher SI relative to the intermediate SI of the silicone. Displacement of these droplets along the frequency axis (right to left in this image) reflects the difference in chemical shift between silicone and water (see Chapter 3).

represents the presence of silicone beyond the confines of the fibrous capsule. Focal extracapsular silicone can be present in the adjacent breast parenchyma or lymph nodes. A less severe form of silicone leak comes from intracapsular rupture, in which there is collapse of the elastomer shell, but the silicone remains contained by the outer fibrous capsule. In intracapsular rupture, low SI linear structures, representing remnants of the elastomer shell, are revealed interspersed with contained silicone (Fig. 10-12). This finding, termed the "linguine sign"[62] is specific for implant rupture. Finally, a gel bleed can be present in which small amounts of silicone protrude beyond the elastomer shell, without rupture of the surrounding fibrous capsule (Fig. 10-13). This results from of transudation of silicone gel through small tears in an otherwise intact elastomer shell. Small collections of silicone gel accumulate between folds of the elastomer shell and the intact fibrous

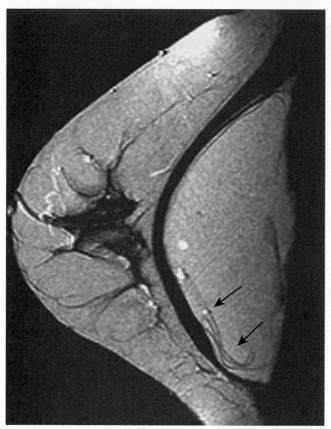

Figure 10-12 ■ MR depiction of intracapsular rupture of a single-lumen retropectoral silicone implant. Sagittal T2-WI depicts fine linear bands *(arrows)* of the elastomer shell freely floating within the fibrous capsule ("linguine" sign). No silicone extension beyond the fibrous capsule is revealed.

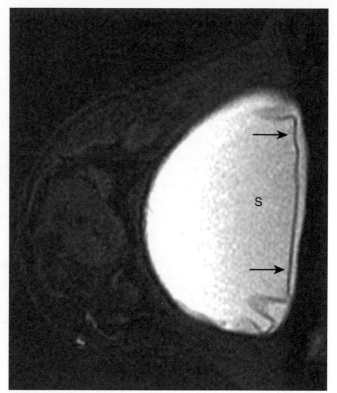

Figure 10-13 ■ MR findings of extensive gel bleed. STIR image with water saturation shows silicone (S) on either side of the elastomer shell *(arrows)* but contained within the outer fibrous capsule. No elastomer shell disruption is present.

capsule; when located solely within a radial fold this has been termed the "noose" or "keyhole" sign.[63]

Breast Cancer

BACKGROUND

It is estimated that in 2004, approximately 215,990 women in the U. S. will develop breast cancer, which will represent nearly one third of all new cancers.[64] Breast cancer mortality rates have fallen in recent years, largely due to a combination of early detection and improved treatment regimens. Nevertheless, in 2004, it is estimated that breast cancer will account for 15% of cancer-related deaths among American women and that 40,110 women will die of their disease.[64]

Early investigations of unenhanced breast MRI for evaluation of breast cancer had low diagnostic accuracy.[65] However, with the use of contrast-enhanced imaging, improved accuracy was obtained.[12,45] CE MRI is now used as a means of detecting and characterizing benign and malignant breast diseases.

TECHNIQUE

Specific protocols and approaches to MR imaging for breast cancer differ among imaging centers. Optimal imaging plane, slice thickness, and in-plane resolution depend on the type of detector coil as well as the performance of the imaging system. Regardless of the exact imaging protocol utilized, a breast MR examination includes both T1-WI and T2-WI, followed by a dynamic CE T1-WI series.

T1-WI before contrast is useful for assessing overall glandular volume and architecture. T1-WI can depict focal masses, which appear hypointense against the background of hyperintense fat and areas of architectural distortion. T1-WI obtained without fat suppression may also be useful for depicting fat within masses, or the fatty hilum of an intramammary lymph node. In addition, fat necrosis and breast hamartomas contain macroscopic lipid SI on T1-WI. Subacute blood in postprocedural seromas or within ducts also is hyperintense on T1-WI. However, hyperintense blood and proteinaceous material are better revealed on fat-suppressed T1-WI.

T2-WI is useful for evaluating dilated ducts, cysts, fibroadenomas, intratumoral cystic necrosis, and postprocedural seromas.[14] With T2-WI, fat suppression often is performed. This may be accomplished by either an inversion-recovery (IR) technique or the use of chemical selective suppression. Fat saturation can be used to minimize the hyperintense SI of adipose tissue commonly present on FSE imaging. The increased dynamic range of fat-suppressed T2-WI is useful for increasing the conspicuity of hyperintense cysts and ducts as well as for revealing fine detail of hyperintense lesions, such as the notched configuration of a lymph node or the presence of hypointense internal septations in a fibroadenoma.

USE OF FAT SATURATION

Regardless of the specific imaging protocol chosen, some form of contrast-enhanced T1-WI sequence is always performed. Adipose tissue will show the highest SI on T1-WI. Following contrast administration, enhancing lesions may achieve SI equal to that of fat, rendering them less conspicuous. For these reasons, the authors recommend the use of fat suppression for breast MRI.

While various fat-suppression techniques are available, current manufactures offer schemes tailored to rapid imaging, including selective water excitation[66] and partial selective lipid inversion.[54] Nonselective inversion recovery techniques are not appropriate for CE T1-WI. Contrast agent accumulation in breast lesions will lower the T1 relaxation rate, thereby decreasing the SI of these lesions on IR imaging.

A fat-saturated T1-W sequence should be obtained prior to contrast administration. This is usually followed by one or several repetitions of the same imaging sequence immediately following contrast administration. In this way, meaningful comparisons between pre- and postcontrast images can be made regarding the pattern and degree of enhancement. Gradient echo (GRE) sequences (two- or three-dimensional) are preferred over spin-echo (SE) sequences for more rapid acquisition.[67] Computer-generated subtraction methods are useful for increasing the conspicuity of enhancing tissue.[20,68] Subtraction image depiction becomes more important when fat saturation cannot be performed, such as on low-field MR systems or MR systems that cannot achieve homogeneous fat suppression. Of note, if an opposed-phase echo time (e.g., ~2 ms at 1.5 T) is used in GR imaging, paradoxic suppression of the SI of small enhancing lesions may occur owing to chemical shift cancellation effects if fat suppression is not used.[69] Thus, if GR T1-WI is used without fat suppression (not recommended), then the shortest in-phase echo time should be chosen.

Dynamics of contrast enhancement. Breast cancers will generally enhance more rapidly than benign lesions or normal parenchyma.[12,45] This observation led to early investigations into the use of kinetic measures of contrast enhancement with MRI as a means of discriminating between benign and malignant breast lesions.[70-72] Measurement of such parameters as the time to peak enhancement or the rate of early enhancement of breast lesions has been used to discriminate between benign and malignant lesions.[20,73-75] Rapid temporal sampling of a specific lesion or region of anatomy following gadolinium administration allows such parameters to be determined with a higher degree of precision. However, since the units of MR signal intensity are arbitrary, the value of such measurements may vary depending on the specific imaging sequence parameters, magnetic field strength, and amount and rate of contrast administration. As such, rigorous comparison among different imaging protocols is problematic. Furthermore, with existing MR gradient technology, rapid temporal sampling (on the order of one image every 2 to 3 seconds) generally restricts the imaging evaluation to only a small portion of the breast.

Sophisticated pharmacokinetic analyses of breast lesion enhancement kinetics, which eliminate the dependence of machine settings, have been performed.[76-78] However, other variables, such as reader definition of the area of enhancement, may complicate quantitative measures,[79-81] and pharmacokinetic modeling does not appear to give added clinical benefit over a more qualitative analysis of the kinetics of lesion enhancement.[82,83] The latter method requires one to obtain fewer sequences after contrast—sometimes as few as two—and generate an enhancement curve that falls into one of three patterns: progressively enhancing, plateau, or washout (Fig. 10-14).[84,85] This strategy is more compatible with high-resolution scanning of the entire breast, allowing simultaneous evaluation of lesion morphology and qualitative lesion enhancement dynamics. Since the lower rate of temporal sampling allows for the acquisition of higher resolution images, internal heterogeneity of dynamic enhancing patterns within a lesion may be shown.[86]

Lesions that reach peak enhancement during the first 1 to 2 minutes following contrast administration are classified as either "plateau" or "washout," based on the relative degree of enhancement on delayed imaging. Lesions that continue to increase in SI for 3 or more minutes following contrast administration are labeled as progressively enhancing. Using either plateau or washout curve types as a sign of malignancy, Kuhl and colleagues demonstrated sensitivity of 91% and specificity of 83% for detection of malignancy.[87] Only nine of 146 lesions that demonstrated type I enhancement curves were malignant, whereas 137 of 165 benign enhancing lesions (83%) demonstrated this type of enhancement profile. Other researchers have confirmed that the presence of contrast washout following initial enhancement is predictive of malignancy.[88-90]

MORPHOLOGY OF FOCALLY ENHANCING BREAST LESIONS

Characterization of enhancing breast lesions requires evaluation of not only the temporal pattern of lesion enhancement, but also lesion shape, borders, and enhancement morphology. The vocabulary for description and categorization of focal enhancing lesions is MRI has been derived in large part from the successful use of such descriptors to categorize focal masses in mammography or sonography, as codified in the Breast Imaging Reporting and Data System (BI-RADS) lexicon.[91] In 1999, the Lesion Diagnosis International Working Group on Breast MRI issued a technical report[92] summarizing the

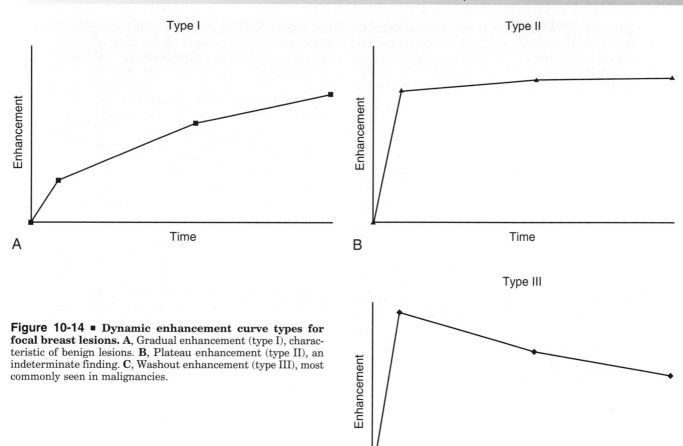

Figure 10-14 ■ **Dynamic enhancement curve types for focal breast lesions. A**, Gradual enhancement (type I), characteristic of benign lesions. **B**, Plateau enhancement (type II), an indeterminate finding. **C**, Washout enhancement (type III), most commonly seen in malignancies.

consensus results regarding the use of descriptors in reporting the characteristics of focally enhancing lesions. These results classified the shape (round, oval, lobulated, irregular, stellate), margin (smooth, scalloped, irregular, spiculated), and enhancement morphology (homogeneous, heterogeneous, rim-enhancing, and enhancing or nonenhancing internal septations) of lesions. This report was issued in the hope of arriving at a standard set of descriptors to be used for classifying lesions present on breast MRI, so that future single- and multisite studies evaluating the performance of breast MRI in various clinical settings would generate reproducible data.[93,94]

Border classification of focally enhancing masses has proved to be the most reliable static descriptor for differentiating benign and malignant enhancing lesions. As is true in mammography, lesions with irregular or spiculated margins (Fig. 10-15) have the highest rate of malignancy, with the positive predictive value (PPV) ranging between 76% and 91%.[15,16,18,95,96] The margins of benign lesions, in comparison, are more likely to be smooth or lobulated, with negative predictive values for malignancy in the range of 90% (see Fig. 10-15).[16,95,96] These results suggest that the morphologic characteristics of invasive breast cancers

(infiltrative growth, desmoplastic reaction) that allow for accurate mammographic characterization can also be identified on MRI.

Beside border characterization, the morphology of lesion enhancement has diagnostic value. Certain enhancement patterns, particularly irregular rim enhancement, are associated with invasive cancer (Fig. 10-16).[97,98] The PPV of rim enhancement for malignancy ranges from 79% to 92%.[16] Heterogeneous enhancement in a mass also is associated with malignancy,[99] and the PPV of heterogeneous enhancement for malignancy was 84% in one study.[100] Homogeneously enhancing lesions are more likely to be benign. Of note, the presence of thin, nonenhancing internal septations within an otherwise uniformly enhancing lesion is not considered to be a form of heterogeneous enhancement, since this pattern of enhancement is commonly present in fibroadenomas (see Fig. 10-15).[16,101]

Regional enhancement. Regional enhancement refers to ill-defined enhancement (usually low-to-moderate in degree but occasionally intensely enhancing) that occupies only a portion of the breast. Unlike a focally enhancing lesion, regional enhancement has borders that fade into the background parenchyma, defying

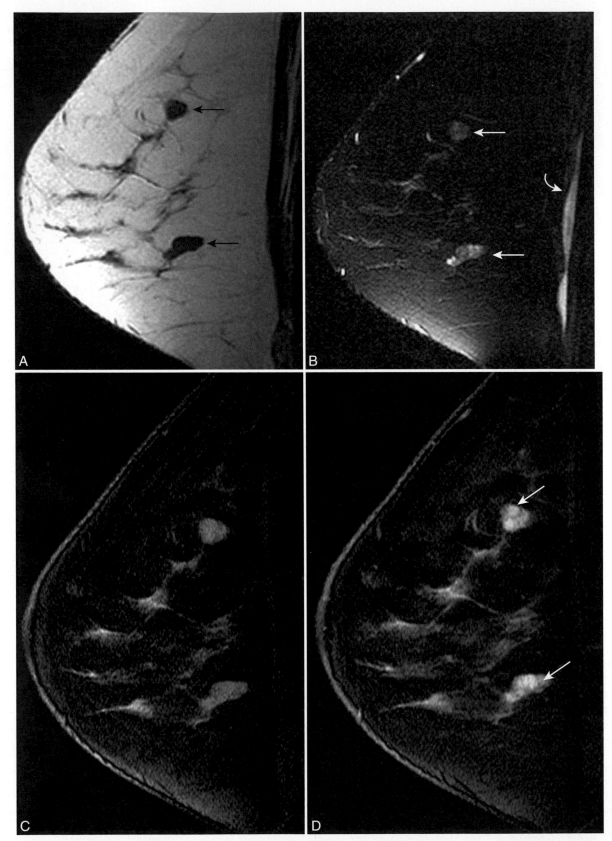

Figure 10-15 ■ **MR findings of fibroadenomas. A** and **B**, T1-WI (**A**) and T2-WI (**B**) depict two smooth lobulated masses *(arrows)* with low T1 and intermediate-to-high T2-SI. In **B**, internal hypointense collagenous septations are well contrasted with hyperintense adenomatous lobules. High, SI-dependent layering pleural fluid *(curved arrow)* is a normal finding. **C** and **D**, Fat-suppressed T1-WIs obtained before (**C**) and after (**D**) contrast reveal low-level enhancement *(arrows)* with internal nonenhancing septa, a characteristic of fibroadenomas.

(Continued)

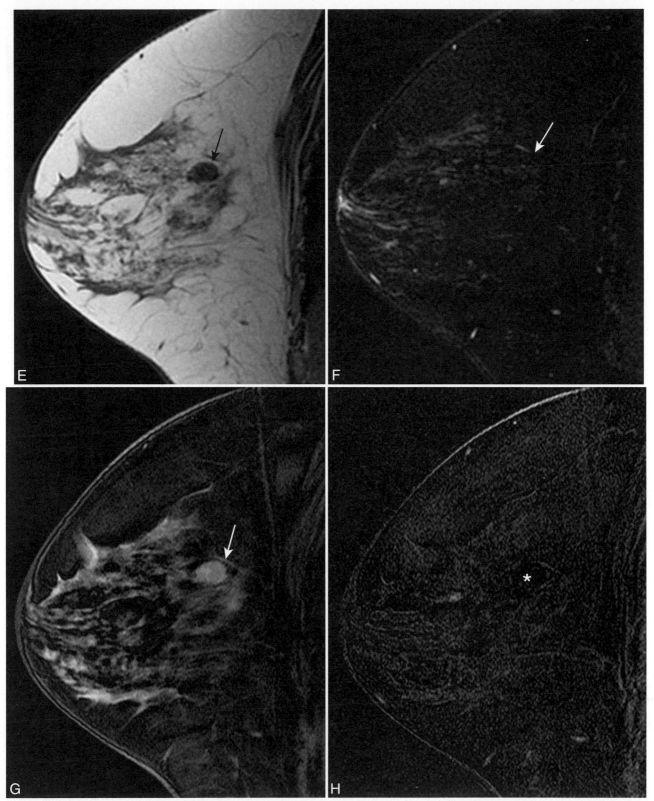

Figure 10-15 ■ Cont'd E–H, MR illustration of a mature fibroadenoma in a different woman. E and **F,** Sagittal T1-WI (**E**) and fat-suppressed T2-WI (**F**) show a well-circumscribed, low SI mass on both images *(arrows)*. The lesion is difficult to depict in **F** because it is relatively isointense to the adjacent suppressed fat. **G,** Fat-suppressed T1-WI obtained before contrast shows improved depiction of the mass *(arrow)* due to improvements in dynamic range. **H,** Subtraction image from the portal phase of enhancement show absent enhancement within the mature fibroadenoma (*). There is minimal low-level enhancement of the surrounding glandular tissue. A 2-mm focus of enhancement present anteriorly corresponds to a T2 hyperintense focus in **F** and likely represents an immature fibroadenoma or focus of glandular tissue.

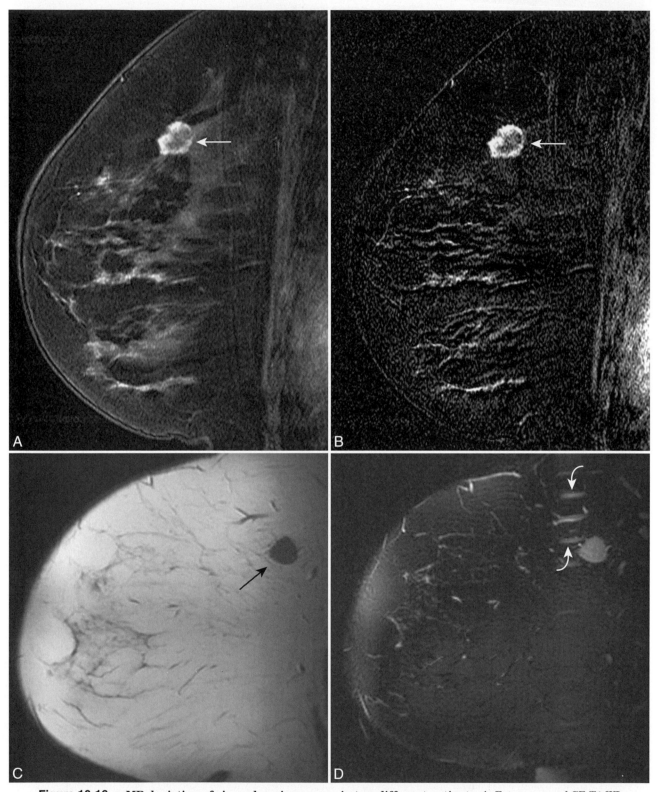

Figure 10-16 ■ **MR depiction of rim-enhancing cancer in two different patients. A**, Fat-suppressed CE T1-WI reveals a small, irregular, enhancing mass *(arrow)*. **B**, Subtraction image better depicts the thick rim enhancement of this lesion *(arrow)*. **C** and **D**, T1-WI **(C)** and T2-WI **(D)** in a second woman show a spiculated mass *(arrow)* of the axillary portion of the upper outer quadrant of the breast (same patient as depicted in Fig. 10-2B). Pulsatility artifact *(curved arrows)* from a blood vessel is present in the phase-encoding direction on the T2-WI **(D)**. *(Continued)*

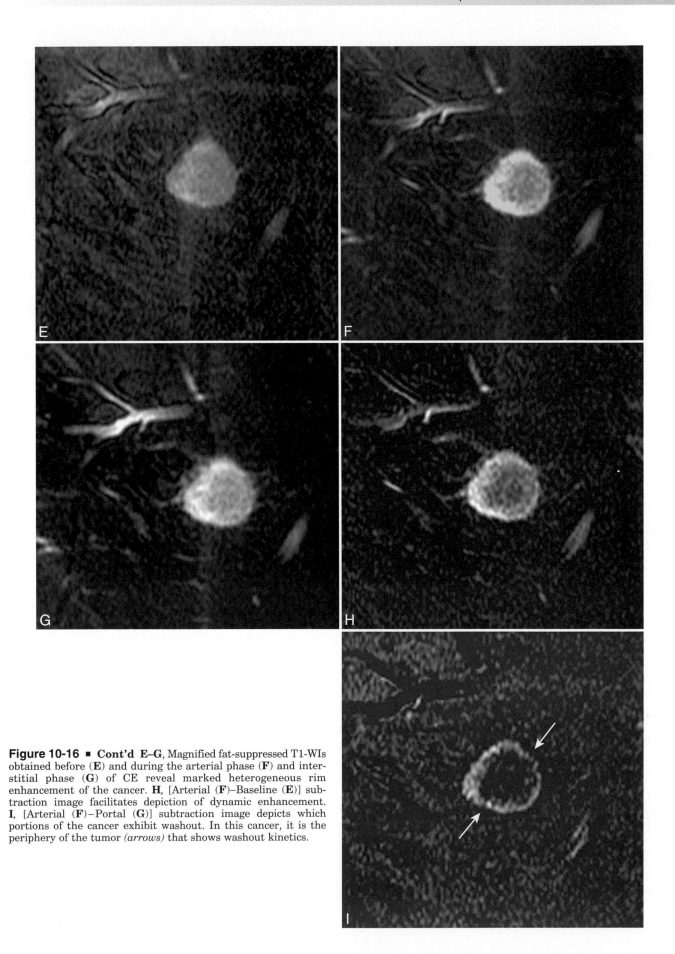

Figure 10-16 ■ **Cont'd** **E–G**, Magnified fat-suppressed T1-WIs obtained before (**E**) and during the arterial phase (**F**) and interstitial phase (**G**) of CE reveal marked heterogeneous rim enhancement of the cancer. **H**, [Arterial (**F**)–Baseline (**E**)] subtraction image facilitates depiction of dynamic enhancement. **I**, [Arterial (**F**)–Portal (**G**)] subtraction image depicts which portions of the cancer exhibit washout. In this cancer, it is the periphery of the tumor *(arrows)* that shows washout kinetics.

border classification schemes. Terms such as clumped, confluent, or stippled are often used to categorize such patterns of enhancement (Fig. 10-17).[92]

Confluent enhancement is enhancement that is continuous within a region of the breast, without intervening nonenhancing areas. *Stippled enhancement*

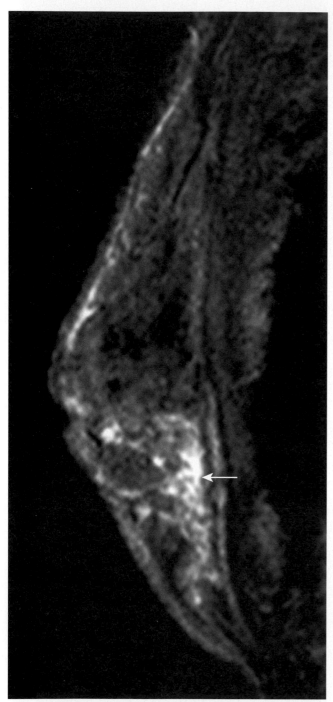

Figure 10-17 ■ **MR illustration of DCIS revealed as segmental enhancement in a 40-year-old woman with a strong family history of breast cancer.** Mammography (not shown) revealed dense breasts with no suspicious abnormality. Fat-suppressed CE T1-WI depicts intense regional enhancement *(arrow)* in the lower breast, in a segmental pattern. MR-guided core biopsy and subsequent lumpectomy showed DCIS without invasive cancer.

is characterized by multiple punctate 1- to 2-mm foci of enhancement that are separated by intervening nonenhancing tissue. Both confluent and stippled enhancement represent a uniform pattern of enhancement and often are associated with benign etiologies. *Clumped enhancement* is more heterogeneous and is characterized by clustering of larger enhancing foci (usually >5 mm in diameter) that can be separated by nonenhancing or minimally enhancing parenchyma. Clumped enhancement has been associated with malignancy, particularly ductal carcinoma in situ (DCIS).[48,102] *Segmental enhancement* is enhancement that is confined to a single ductal distribution,[103] although the enhancement itself may not appear to be confined solely to the ducts themselves.

Regional enhancement is a nonspecific finding. If the degree of enhancement is low (i.e., only slightly greater than that of background parenchymal enhancement), then the probability of malignancy is low (negative predictive value [NPV] for malignancy of 92%).[18] Regional enhancement that is segmental, demonstrates clumped morphology, or is exceedingly more intense than that of the background parenchymal enhancement suggests malignancy, specifically DCIS (Fig. 10-18).[101,104,105] Low-level regional enhancement may resolve on short-term follow-up examination, especially when timed at a different phase of the menstrual cycle.[42] Regional enhancement that is markedly hyperintense to parenchymal tissue after contrast, or persists on follow-up examination, requires histologic sampling to exclude DCIS.

Ductal enhancement. Ductal enhancement is a subtype of regional enhancement. It refers to a linear or branching pattern of enhancement isolated to a portion of the ductal system (Fig. 10-19). When a pattern of ductal enhancement is identified, biopsy to exclude DCIS is recommended.[101,106-108] Architecture-based models of enhancement patterns suggest that the positive-predictive value of ductal-type enhancement is 80% to 85%,[16,18] including both isolated DCIS and DCIS associated with invasive cancer. However, ductal enhancement can be present in benign conditions, including fibrocystic change.[16] A lower PPV for malignancy of 24% has been reported for linear or ductal enhancement in patients without a corresponding mammographic abnormality.[102,109] A clumped pattern of ductal enhancement is more likely to be associated with malignancy than either smooth or irregular linear/branching enhancement.

TEMPORAL VERSUS SPATIAL RESOLUTION

The optimal breast MR imaging protocol would yield high-resolution images in rapid temporal sequence following gadolinium administration. Different breast MR imaging groups advocate protocols that vary the emphasis between morphologic and kinetic information. With high-resolution imaging using optimized surface coils, in-plane resolution of several hundred microns per pixel is achievable although imaging time is proportionately increased. Alternatively, rapid temporal sampling of 2 to 3 seconds per image

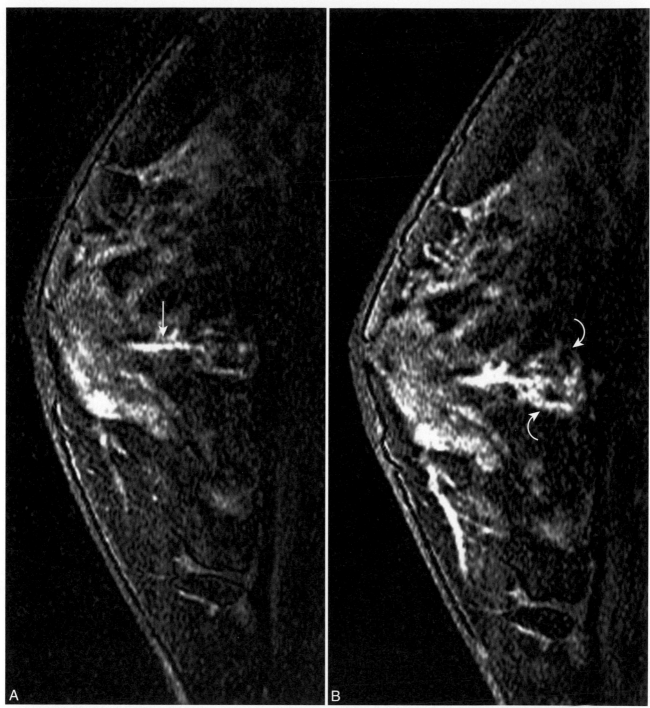

Figure 10-18 ▪ MR findings of ductal enhancement secondary to DCIS in a 48-year-old woman with bloody nipple discharge. A, Fat-suppressed T1-WI shows a central duct with high SI content *(arrow)* extending into the deep central breast tissue. High SI within ducts is usually secondary to hemorrhagic or proteinaceous content. **B**, Fat-suppressed CE T1-WI reveals branching linear enhancement *(curved arrows)* at the termination of the central high T1-SI duct.   *(Continued)*

may be achieved, but only by compromising image resolution or anatomic coverage. The larger anatomic coverage required in simultaneous imaging of both breasts limits the ability to acquire high-resolution imaging with rapid temporal resolution. The authors recommend the use of unilateral breast MR imaging with sagittal compression, to obtain high-resolution

images with a sampling rate of approximately 80 seconds. Exceptions are made for patients for whom bilateral imaging is desirable (e.g., high-risk screening), in which case the authors utilize an imaging protocol with slightly lower spatial resolution, to allow for imaging of both breasts with sufficient temporal resolution.

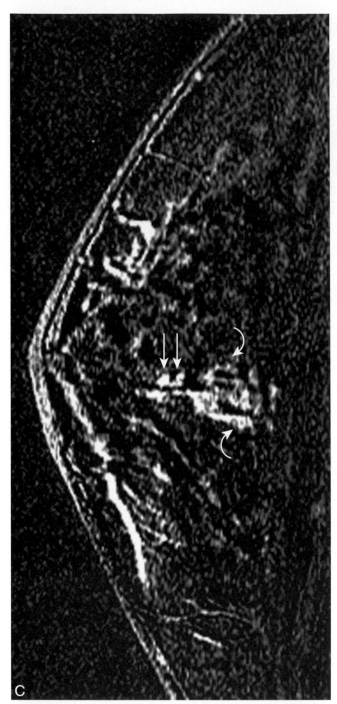

Figure 10-18 ▪ Cont'd C, Subtraction image facilitates depiction both of the ductal morphology of the enhancement and of the enhancement within the proximal duct segment that has T1 hyperintense content *(double arrow).*

MR APPEARANCE OF SPECIFIC BREAST LESIONS

Non-neoplastic Conditions

CYSTS

Breast cysts are commonly revealed on MRI and generally do not pose a diagnostic dilemma. As for sonography, specific MR criteria exist that enable

one to define a simple cyst. Simple cysts are composed of uniformly hyperintense fluid on T2-WI, with corresponding low SI on T1-WI (see Fig. 10-19). Cysts may have internal protein or hemorrhage that can result in relative increase in T1-SI and decrease in T2-SI (Fig. 10-20). Fluid-debris and fluid-fluid levels can also be present in complex cysts.

All cysts should have thin uniform walls. Following gadolinium administration, cyst walls may enhance (Fig. 10-21). However, the wall should remain thin and uniform throughout. A cyst with rim enhancement should not be confused with a rim-enhancing tumor or breast abscess. These latter entities will have thicker and more irregular wall enhancement.

Certain solid lesions, such as fibroadenomas or mucinous tumors, can demonstrate relatively high SI on T2-WI.[110-112] However, both mucinous tumors and mature fibroadenomas will demonstrate internal enhancement not present in cysts.

DUCT ECTASIA

The major subareolar ducts may distend and fill with simple or proteinaceous fluid, a process termed duct ectasia. The patient may be asymptomatic or have tenderness or a palpable abnormality. Spontaneous discharge may be present. Dilated ducts extending from the retroareolar region will generally be hyperintense on T2-WI (Fig. 10-22A) and have variable SI on T1-WI.[113] Ducts filled with simple fluid will demonstrate low T1 SI, whereas proteinaceous or hemorrhagic ductal contents reveal variable T1 shortening. On unenhanced fat-suppressed T1-WI, these ducts may have the highest SI in the image (see Fig. 10-22B). Strict attention to image interpretation is needed, so that subtle ductal enhancement—which may represent DCIS—is not overlooked. Inspection of baseline and subtracted images can detect ductal enhancement. However, artifactual enhancement may be produced on subtracted images if there has been even a small degree of motion between the pre- and post-contrast sequences.[114] Automated motion correction schemes have been proposed that adjust for breast motion between pre- and postcontrast images,[115,116] although such algorithms are not routinely available for clinical use.

PROLIFERATIVE BREAST DISEASE

Proliferative breast disease encompasses a range of histologic abnormalities, from fibrocystic changes to atypical ductal or lobular hyperplasia and lobular carcinoma in situ (LCIS). MRI findings in these cases are variable and nonspecific. In 192 women with palpable or mammographic lesions who underwent breast MRI,[95] 67 were subsequently found to have fibrocystic changes, and an additional 14 women had hyperplastic or other proliferative findings (including lobular carcinoma in situ). Of these 81 women, 32 (40%) had no enhancing lesion; 39 (48%) had focal enhancing masses (Fig. 10-23), the majority of which were smooth or lobulated; and 10 (12%) had regional or ductal enhancement.

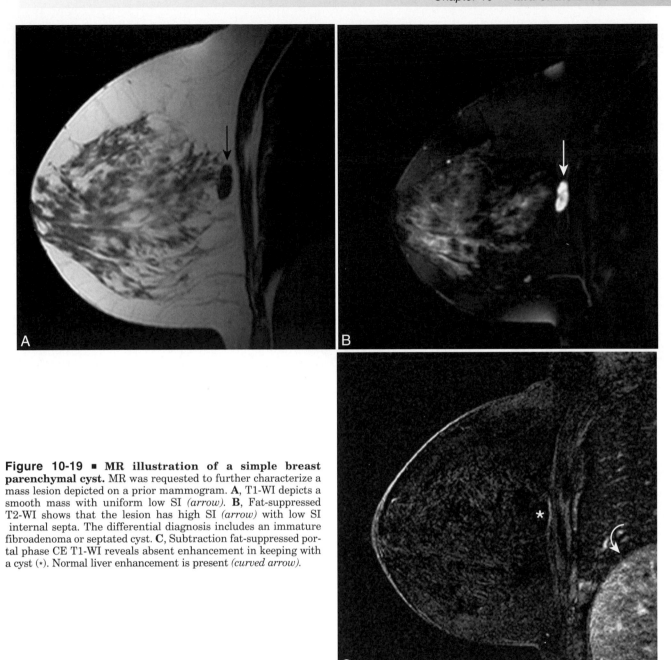

Figure 10-19 ■ **MR illustration of a simple breast parenchymal cyst.** MR was requested to further characterize a mass lesion depicted on a prior mammogram. **A**, T1-WI depicts a smooth mass with uniform low SI *(arrow)*. **B**, Fat-suppressed T2-WI shows that the lesion has high SI *(arrow)* with low SI internal septa. The differential diagnosis includes an immature fibroadenoma or septated cyst. **C**, Subtraction fat-suppressed portal phase CE T1-WI reveals absent enhancement in keeping with a cyst (*). Normal liver enhancement is present *(curved arrow)*.

Proliferative breast disease also demonstrates heterogeneous enhancement dynamics in breast MRI. Kuhl and colleagues[87] studied the dynamic properties of 266 enhancing breast lesions, all with pathologic confirmation. Sixty-two of these lesions were fibrocystic change, accounting for approximately 40% of all benign enhancing lesions. The majority of these lesions demonstrated progressive, low-level enhancement. However, 15 of these lesions demonstrated early enhancement rates of 80% or greater, and 8 lesions demonstrated plateau or washout type enhancement curves.

RADIAL SCAR

A radial scar, or complex sclerosing lesion, is a non-neoplastic breast abnormality characterized by bands of connective tissue radiating outward from a central nidus, often containing fat (Box 10-4).[117]

The mammographic appearance reflects this histologic finding: stellate lesions, often with lucent centers, causing surrounding architectural distortion. However, there is considerable overlap in the mammographic appearance of radial scars and invasive cancers, and excisional biopsy is often required for pathologic confirmation.

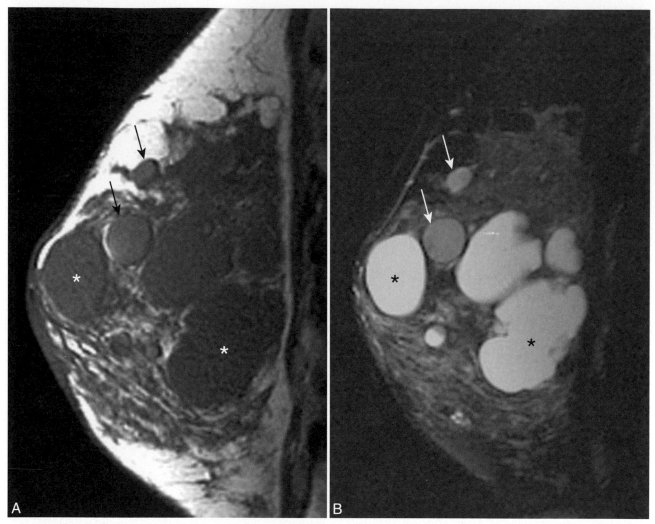

Figure 10-20 ▪ MR illustration of complex and simple breast cysts. A, T1-WI shows multiple low SI simple cysts (∗). Some of the cysts *(arrows)* contain increased SI owing to hemorrhagic or proteinaceous contents. **B,** Fat-suppressed T2-WI shows lower SI in the complicated cysts *(arrows)* and uniform high SI within the simple cysts. None of the cysts revealed internal enhancement or solid components.

On MRI, radial scars may be depicted as irregular or spiculated masses.[95] Enhancement can be variable (Fig. 10-24).[118] While the degree and kinetics of enhancement may suggest benignity, the irregular morphology of radial scars is usually reason enough for diagnostic concern, and excision is ultimately required to exclude an invasive cancer. The presence of intralesional fat, a finding that is not found within breast cancers, may suggest the diagnosis of radial scar.

FAT NECROSIS

Fat necrosis involves traumatic injury to the breast, with hemorrhagic infarction and delayed scarring. It can also follow anticoagulation therapy. Fat necrosis usually occurs in the setting of surgery or radiation therapy to the breast. Lesions representing fat necrosis are generally focal, usually

measuring 2 cm or less. If superficially located fat necrosis may be accompanied by skin thickening or retraction.

Fat necrosis may be difficult to distinguish from carcinoma, both by clinical examination and by imaging. Lipid cysts are commonly present in fat necrosis, and may be represented mammographically as a lucent round or oval mass, occasionally with rim calcification.[119] However, other findings, including spiculated masses indistinguishable from invasive cancer have been reported.[119,120]

The appearance of fat necrosis on MRI has been described. A classic lipid cyst with rim enhancement is one benign MR appearance (Fig. 10-25).[121] Fat necrosis can also be revealed as a focal mass with irregular or rim enhancement.[122-125] This MR appearance of fat necrosis may confound the MR interpretation in women following breast conservation therapy.[122,124]

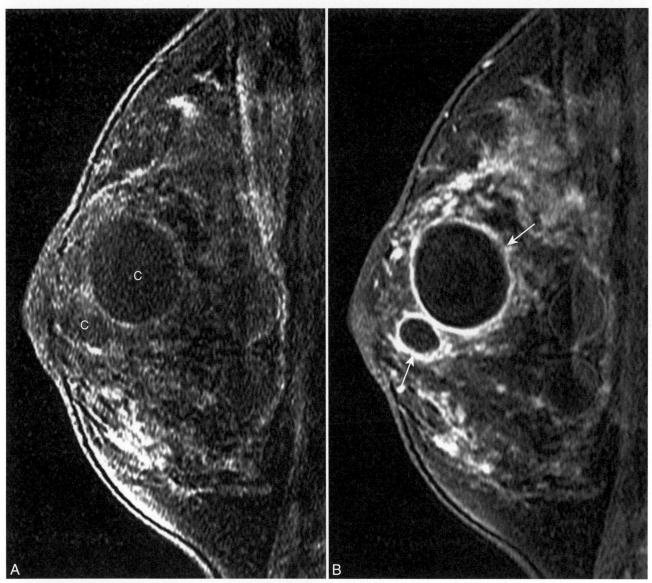

Figure 10-21 ▪ MR depiction of cysts with rim enhancement. A and **B**, Fat-suppressed T1-WIs obtained before (**A**) and after (**B**) contrast shows several cysts (C) with thin uniform rim enhancement *(arrows),* reflecting inflammation.

INTRAMAMMARY LYMPH NODES

Lymph nodes, both axillary and intramammary can often be identified on breast MR examinations. Lymph nodes have well-defined borders and typically demonstrate an oval or notched appearance. They are uniformly of low-to-intermediate SI on T1-WI and intermediate-to-high SI on T2-WI. A central fatty hilum can often be identified on non-fat-suppressed T1-W sequences, a pathognomonic finding. Intramammary lymph nodes are most commonly present in the upper and lower outer quadrants but can be found in any portion of the breast.[126,127] Lymph nodes may enhance following gadolinium administration, sometimes avidly (Fig. 10-26).[128] Nevertheless, their location adjacent and parallel to vessels and their characteristic appearance usually are sufficient for definitive diagnosis. Occasionally, intramammary lymph nodes may present as enlarging enhancing masses, necessitating biopsy to exclude an underlying malignancy.

GYNECOMASTIA

Gynecomastia is unilateral or bilateral breast enlargement secondary to proliferation of the rudimentary glandular tissue of the male breast. Gynecomastia is a common finding, especially during puberty or in the elderly. Causes are various and include androgen-estrogen imbalance, estrogen-secreting tumors (testicular or adrenal), exogenous medication, or

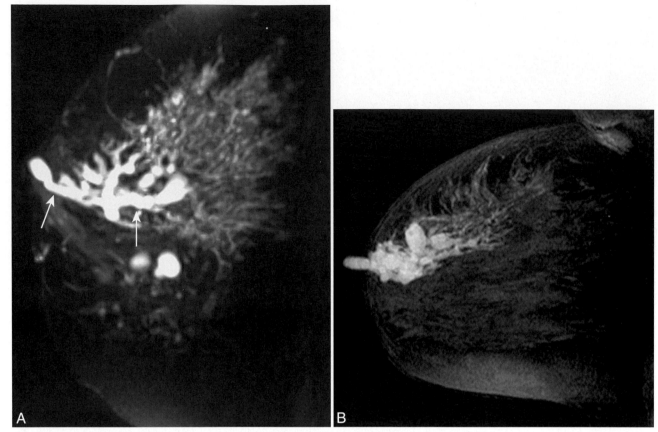

Figure 10-22 ■ MR findings of ductal ectasia. A, Multiplanar thin-slab sagittal maximal intensity projection image from a fat-suppressed T2-W sequence reveals segmental retroareolar ductal distension *(arrows)*. CE T1-WI (not shown) revealed no enhancement. **B,** MR illustration of serosanguineous fluid in the retroareolar ducts after a breast biopsy. The patient did not have a discharge prior to the biopsy but developed serosanguineous drainage after the procedure. Fat-suppressed maximal intensity projection obtained from a fat-suppressed unenhanced T1-WI reveals complex hyper-intense fluid within distended ducts. The ducts did not enhance after contrast (not shown).

underlying liver or renal disease.[129] Sudden enlargement of the breast in the male patient will often lead to concern for breast cancer. Male breast cancer, however, is a relatively rare entity. It is estimated that 1,450 new cases will be diagnosed in 2004 and result in 470 deaths in American men.[64] Male breast cancer presents later in life (mean age at presentation of approximately 60 years) but at an earlier age in men with Klinefelter's syndrome.[130]

Clinically, differentiation between gynecomastia and male breast cancer can be established based on history and physical examination. Unilateral breast enlargement that is focal and firm raises concern for breast cancer. In a man with unilateral or asymmetric breast swelling, mammography is the preferred imaging modality to differentiate between benign gynecomastia and male breast cancer, with sonography used as an adjunctive modality.[131] In selected cases, MRI may be used for evaluation of gynecomastia (Fig. 10-27).[132] Unlike male breast cancer, which will usually enhance avidly following gadolinium administration, gynecomastia will demonstrate no or low-level heterogeneous enhancement, akin to that of normal parenchyma in the female breast.

10-4 Features of Radial Scar

Clinical
Small lesions, usually <1 cm
Rarely palpable
Usually mammographically detected or incidentally noted in biopsy specimens of adjacent abnormalities
Frequency in mastectomy specimens: 4% to 26%
Age range: 30 to 60 years

Pathology
Sclerotic core of obliterated ducts with fibrosis
Ductal proliferation extends peripherally from central core
Entrapped ducts centrally may simulate invasive cancer on core biopsy, especially tubular carcinoma

MRI
Spiculated mass, usually hypointense on T1- and T2-WI
Central nidus may contain high T1-SI of fat
Variable enhancement, often gradual

Differential Diagnosis
Tubular carcinoma
Fat necrosis
Postoperative scarring

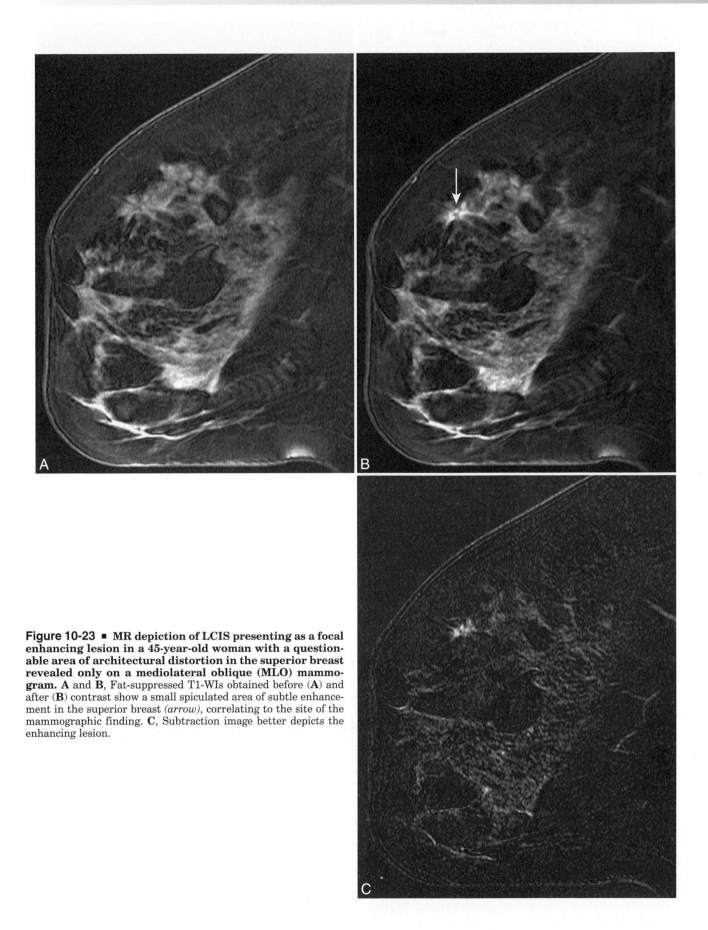

Figure 10-23 ▪ **MR depiction of LCIS presenting as a focal enhancing lesion in a 45-year-old woman with a questionable area of architectural distortion in the superior breast revealed only on a mediolateral oblique (MLO) mammogram. A** and **B**, Fat-suppressed T1-WIs obtained before (**A**) and after (**B**) contrast show a small spiculated area of subtle enhancement in the superior breast *(arrow)*, correlating to the site of the mammographic finding. **C**, Subtraction image better depicts the enhancing lesion.

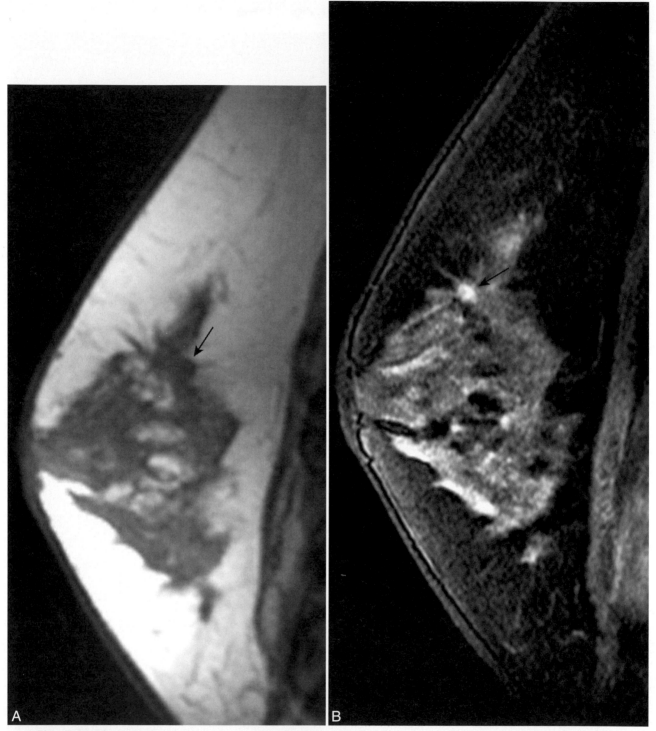

Figure 10-24 ■ **MR illustration of a radial scar in a 48-year-old woman with discomfort at a prior biopsy site in the inferior breast. A**, T1-WI image reveals subtle architectural distortion *(arrow)* superiorly in a region that was remote from the site of focal symptoms. **B**, Fat-suppressed CE T1-WI reveals irregular focus of enhancement *(arrow)* at the site of distortion.

Benign Neoplastic Lesions

FIBROADENOMA

Fibroadenomas are benign neoplasms of the fibrous and glandular elements of the lobule and one of the most common benign entities that present as a focal mass on (Box 10-5).[133]

While certain fibroadenomas demonstrate a pathognomonic appearance on mammography and sonography, many are more variable in appearance

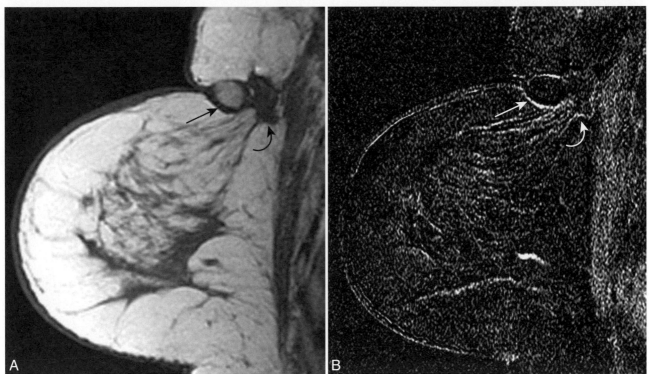

Figure 10-25 ■ **MR depiction of fat necrosis. A,** T1-WI reveals a mass with a central hyperintense interior and hypointense rim *(arrow)*. Postlumpectomy fibrosis and scarring are present posteriorly to this lesion *(curved arrow)*. The fat-suppressed T1-WI obtained prior to contrast confirmed that the hyperintense T1 signal was secondary to fat. **B,** Fat-suppressed CE T1-WI subtraction image reveals thin rim enhancement of the fat necrosis *(arrow)* and no enhancement of the mature postprocedural scar *(curved arrow)*.

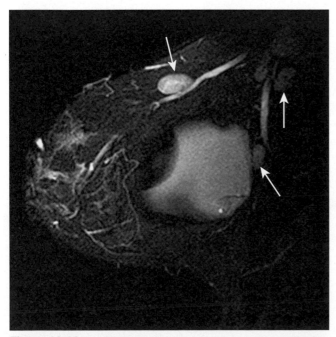

Figure 10-26 ■ **MR illustration of reactive intramammary lymph nodes in a woman with breast implant rupture.** At surgery, the removed nodes showed inflammatory changes without tumor. Fat-suppressed T2-WI shows multiple lymph nodes *(arrows)* of the upper outer quadrant, axillary tail, and axilla.

and may not be reliably differentiated from cancer. On sonography, roughly two thirds of fibroadenomas are prospectively diagnosed correctly.[2,134]

On MRI, fibroadenomas are revealed as round, oval, or lobulated masses with well-defined borders.[101] The appearance of fibroadenomas on T2-WI is variable and correlates with the degree of involution and sclerosis on histologic specimens. A sclerotic fibroadenoma is hypointense on T2-WI and may not be revealed on fat-saturated T2-WI. The more common immature, nondegenerated fibroadenoma is hyperintense on T2-WI (see Fig. 10-15). T2 hyperintensity is a reassuring MR imaging feature when a focally enhancing mass with indeterminate morphologic and enhancing characteristics is revealed, since cancers tend to have more intermediate SI on T2-WI, akin to that of normal breast parenchyma.[135] However, an enhancing mass that is hyperintense on T2-WI is not diagnostic of a benign fibroadenoma, because certain malignancies, such as the mucinous subtype of invasive ductal cancers[136] and phyllodes tumors,[137] can also show high SI on T2-WI.

Most fibroadenomas will enhance following intravenous (IV) gadolinium administration although the degree of enhancement can be variable. Low-level, gradually increasing enhancement is most typical, but higher levels of enhancement, with "plateau" or

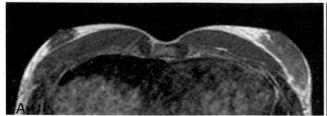

Figure 10-27 ■ **MR depiction of gynecomastia in a 44-year-old man. A**, Axial T1-WI of the entire chest reveals asymmetric breast enlargement. **B**, T1-WI of the left breast shows glandular proliferation *(arrows)* with no focal mass. No enhancement was seen following contrast administration (not shown).

occasionally "washout" enhancement curves, occur in up to 20% of fibroadenomas.[138] In general, enhancement patterns correspond with the degree of stromal cellularity, with immature cellular fibroadenomas demonstrating more rapid and intense enhancement than mature degenerated fibroadenomas.[139]

An MR imaging feature of enhancing breast masses that is highly specific for fibroadenomas is the presence of thin, nonenhancing, internal septations.[101] The nonenhancing septa correlate with collagenous bands on histopathology, while the enhancing tissue represents nodules of glandular and stromal elements. Generally, fibroadenomas enhance in a relatively uniform manner. This may reflect the even distribution of microvessel density within the lobules of the fibroadenoma.[139,140]

INTRADUCTAL PAPILLOMA

Intraductal papillomas are benign neoplasms arising from the epithelial lining of the breast ducts (Box 10-6). Papillomas are often asymptomatic, and may be an incidental finding following a biopsy for an adjacent abnormality. The presence of a papilloma may incite an inflammatory reaction within the duct, and women may have nipple discharge.[141] Papillomas may be shown as filling defects during galactography[142] or as one or several solid masses associated with a dilated duct on sonography.[143]

On MRI, an intraductal papilloma is usually depicted as a well-marginated mass within a duct and associated duct dilation (Fig. 10-28).[113] Frequently, segmental ductal dilatation can be seen both centrally and peripherally to the lesion, and this finding also is

10-5 Features of Fibroadenoma

Clinical

Most common benign neoplasm of the breast
More common in adolescents and young women
Found in 8% to 10% of women at autopsy
Comprises 10% to 20% of mammographically detected masses
Multiple in 10% to 15% of cases

Pathology

Usually several millimeters to 3 to 4 cm in diameter
Lobular proliferation of glandular and stromal elements with intervening collagenous bands
Histologic patterns
    Immature: increased stromal cellularity, myxoid change
    Mature or degenerated: sclerotic stroma, calcification

MRI

Isolated, round or lobular mass
Hypointense on T1-WI
Variable appearance on T2-WI
    Cellular or myxoid stroma: hyperintense on T2-WI
    Sclerotic stroma: hypointense on T2-WI
    Gadolinium enhancement
    Usually low level, gradual
    Uniform enhancement, with internal nonenhancing septa pathognomonic
    Occasional increased enhancement and washout

Differential Diagnosis

Lymph node
Phyllodes tumor
Mucinous carcinoma

10-6 Features of Intraductal Papilloma

Clinical

Most frequently found in postmenopausal women but can occur throughout life
Spontaneous nipple discharge most common presenting symptom
Small lesions (<1 cm) present with discharge
Larger lesions may present as palpable mass or mammographic abnormality

Pathology

Intraductal epithelial tumor of mammary ducts
Often solitary; multiple papillomas occur in younger women
Most frequently seen in central (subareolar) duct (75%)

MRI

Duct dilatations with or without intraductal filling defect on T2-WI
Enhancing lesions, usually round and smooth

Differential Diagnosis

DCIS
IDC

---

noted on sonography.[113,144] Small papillomas (<1 cm) are often incidental findings unless the patient has with spontaneous nipple discharge on presentation. Larger lesions (2 to 3 cm) usually present as a mammographically detected lesion or a palpable mass. Enhancement following contrast administration was frequently noted in one report.[113] In a different series,[145] enhancement beyond a threshold of 100% in the first 3 minutes only occurred for papillomas with associated malignancy.

Malignancy, generally DCIS, can be associated with papillomas, as can invasive papillary cancer. Papillomas that harbor in situ or invasive malignancy are more likely to demonstrate contrast enhancement on MRI.[145] Furthermore, the MR imaging findings of intraductal papillomas overlap with other forms of in situ and invasive malignancy. Regardless of the shape of a lesion, an enhancing abnormality associated with ductal dilatation merits histologic evaluation to exclude associated malignancy.

BREAST HAMARTOMA

A breast hamartoma (fibroadenolipoma) is a rare, benign mass composed of well-encapsulated fatty, fibrous, and adenomatous elements. Breast hamartomas often present as a prominent palpable mass or as gross breast asymmetry; they vary in size from 1 and 20 cm, with a mean size of 6 cm.[146] The mammographic appearance of hamartomas is usually diagnostic, and excision is generally performed for cosmesis. Although MRI is not generally indicated for evaluation of a suspected hamartoma, it can be used to confirm the presence of intratumoral fat (Fig. 10-29).[147] The parenchymal elements of a hamartoma may enhance following IV gadolinium administration, though usually to a much lesser degree than will a malignant lesion.

Malignant Tumors

INVASIVE DUCTAL CARCINOMA (IDC)

Greater than 90% of invasive cancers in women are ductal in origin. Approximately 85% to 90% of invasive ductal cancers (IDCs) are categorized as invasive ductal cancer, not otherwise specified (IDC-NOS). However, invasive ductal cancer also includes several distinct categories of less common histologic types, including medullary, mucinous (colloid), and tubular cancers. Mammographically IDC is most likely to present as either a focal mass or an area of architectural distortion. A spiculated mass is the classic mammographic appearance of IDC; however, it may present as smooth or lobulated solid masses at mammography.

On MRI, IDC generally presents as focally enhancing mass, often with either spiculated or irregular margins (Fig. 10-30).[95] Border evaluation can be more difficult in smaller lesions, and even smooth or lobulated borders in a focally enhancing lesion do not in themselves exclude malignancy.[18,95,102] Certain enhancement patterns, including rim enhancement (see Fig. 10-16), are highly suggestive of malignancy and are commonly present in IDC.[97,148] IDC most commonly demonstrates either washout or plateau enhancement pattern (Fig 10-14).[87] Gradual enhancement does not exclude malignancy, however, and a gradually enhancing lesion with suspicious morphology merits histologic sampling.

MEDULLARY CARCINOMA

Medullary cancers are a subtype of infiltrating ductal carcinoma in which certain macro- and microscopic pathologic features predominate. These include a well-circumscribed tumor, with a syncytial growth pattern and a large peripheral lymphocytic infiltrate. The relative lack of fibrotic stroma in these cancers lends them a soft, "fleshy" appearance, as indicated by their nomenclature. Medullary cancers constitute between 5% and 7% of invasive ductal cancers.[149] They are often unifocal, although they can present as multifocal tumors in 8% to 10% of cases. Bilaterality is also reported with medullary carcinoma. They present at a slightly earlier age than other types of IDC, are associated with BRCA1 mutation carriers, and generally carry a more favorable prognosis (Box 10-7).[150]

At mammography or sonography, medullary cancers are typically unifocal masses with lobulated or smooth, well-defined borders.[151] However, medullary carcinomas are more likely than other types of ductal cancers to be mammographically occult.[152] Medullary cancers are revealed as well-marginated, enhancing lobulated masses,[95] correlating well with their histologic and mammographic features. With their smooth borders, medullary cancers could conceivably be mischaracterized as fibroadenoma on MRI. At high-resolution MR imaging, fibroadenomas usually have nonenhancing internal septations and show progressive enhancement kinetics. Medullary cancers are not hyperintense on T2-WI, do not have internal septations, and are more likely to show heterogeneous enhancement.[97]

TUBULAR CARCINOMA

Tubular carcinomas comprise 1% to 2% of invasive cancers. Tubular cancers are generally slow growing and metastasize less often than other forms of invasive cancer. Histologically, the tumors reveal intratumoral desmoplasia, often with a stellate configuration (Box 10-8). This architectural feature of tubular cancers, combined with the typical slow growth of the tumor, lends itself to mammographic detection before the lesion is clinically evident.[153]

Tubular cancer frequently presents as a spiculated mass on mammography and MRI and is often difficult to differentiate from radial scars.[72,95] The frequent incidence of tubular carcinoma within

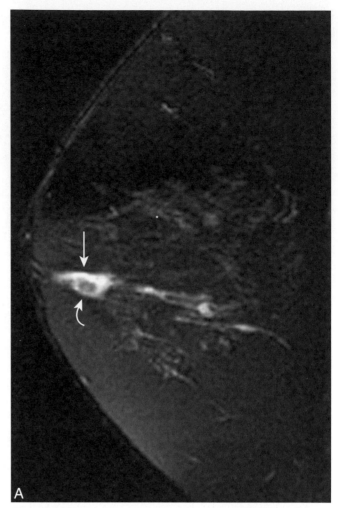

Figure 10-28 ■ MR depiction of an intraductal papilloma in a 58-year-old woman with nipple discharge. A, Fat-suppressed T2-WI reveals a mildly distended hyperintense retroareolar duct *(arrow)* with a focal intraductal low SI lesion *(curved arrow).*   *(Continued)*

radial scar further compounds the diagnostic difficulty. Therefore, a spiculated or stellate enhancing breast lesion, regardless of its dynamic enhancement profile, warrants excision to exclude carcinoma.

MUCINOUS CARCINOMA

Mucinous carcinoma is a subtype of invasive ductal carcinoma characterized by abundant mucin-producing glands. The prognosis of this subtype of invasive cancer is more favorable that that of other invasive ductal carcinomas, and metastatic lymphadenopathy is infrequent. On mammography, mucinous tumors appear as lobulated masses, with borders that may be either well- or ill-defined.[154,155] Mucin-containing breast masses that are ill defined on mammography are more likely to represent mixed mucinous tumors (e.g., invasive ductal cancers with mucinous features).[156]

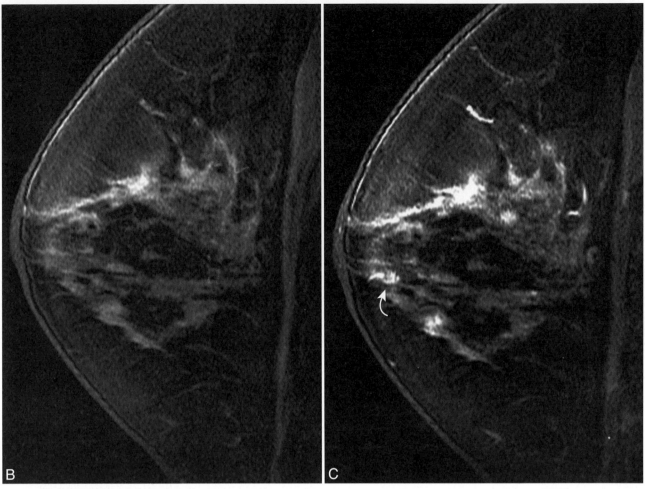

Figure 10-28 ▪ Cont'd B and **C,** Fat-suppressed T1-WI obtained before (**B**) and after (**C**) CE reveals enhancement *(curved arrow)* of the intraductal lesion.

10-7   Features of Medullary Carcinoma

Clinical

More frequent in younger women (<50 yr)
Rapidly growing tumor; median size 2 to 3 cm
Associated with multicentric (8% to 10%) and bilateral (3% to 18%) tumors (contralateral tumor usually is not medullary)

Pathology

Round, well-marginated tumor
Cellular with reactive lymphocytic reaction
Can be associated with reactive (nonmetastatic) axillary lymphadenopathy

MRI

Smooth, round or oval, enhancing lesions
Well-marginated
Heterogeneous enhancement

Differential Diagnosis

Fibroadenoma

10-8   Features of Tubular Carcinoma

Clinical Presentation

Wide range of age at presentation (20 to 90 yr)
Slow-growing tumor; median size 2 to 3 cm
Skin retraction secondary to desmoplastic reaction
Common mammographically detected tumor (architectural distortion)

Pathology

Generally small size (<2 cm)
Stellate lesion with fibrotic reaction
Associated with radial scars

MRI

Spiculated lesion
Variable degree of enhancement, often progressive
Multifocality rare

Differential Diagnosis

Radial scar
Proliferative breast disease (e.g., sclerosing adenosis)

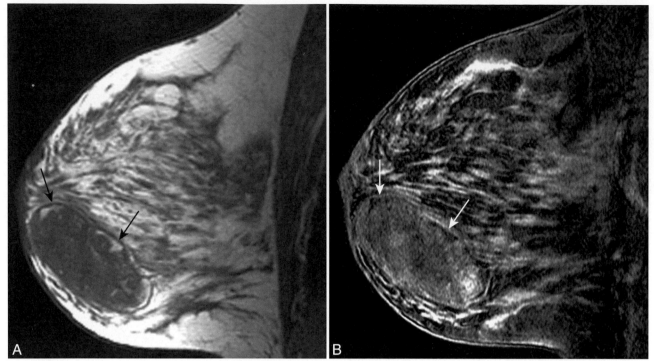

Figure 10-29 ■ **MR findings of a breast hamartoma in a 31-year-old woman with a large, palpable breast mass. A**, T1-WI reveals a large, well-encapsulated breast mass. The mass is largely of low SI, with small foci of higher SI *(arrows)*. **B**, Fat-suppressed T1-WI shows loss of SI *(arrows)* within the hyperintense foci depicted in **A**, thereby establishing the presence of intratumoral fat. The enhanced images (not shown) revealed minimal intralesional enhancement. The characterization of fat within a well-circumscribed breast mass is characteristic of a hamartoma.

Because of their high mucin content, these tumors have a distinctive appearance on MR imaging (Box 10-9). They are hyperintense to glandular tissue on T2-WI (Fig. 10-31) and hypo- or isointense to parenchyma on T1-WI.[136] Thus, mucinous tumors are different from most other breast malignancies, which demonstrate isointensity to normal glandular tissue on T2-WI. This distinctive appearance of mucinous tumors represents a pitfall in breast MRI, as hyperintensity on T2-WI is more commonly associated with benign lesions such as lymph nodes and immature fibroadenomas.

The enhancement pattern of mucinous tumors may also be variable. The intratumoral extracellular mucin shows no enhancement, while the mucin-producing glandular elements do enhance. The kinetic pattern of solid enhancement in these tumors may be variable, and mucinous tumors can demonstrate a delayed or gradual enhancement pattern.[26,97,110,136,157]

INVASIVE LOBULAR CARCINOMA

Invasive lobular carcinoma (ILC) comprises only 10% of all invasive breast cancers but is increasing in frequency.[158,159] ILC is less likely to invoke a desmoplastic reaction in the breast and thus is more insidious in its clinical and imaging presentation.[160] Among mammographically detected cancers, invasive lobular cancers tend to be larger, often with poorer prognostic features at the time of detection.[4,161] Compared with IDC, ILCs are more likely to have positive surgical margins after breast-conserving surgery.[162] This may be due, in part, to the difficulty in recognizing the boundaries of the tumor, either clinically or mammographically.

10-9 Features of Mucinous Carcinoma

Clinical

Slightly older age at presentation (7% of tumors in women >75 yr)
Presents as slow-growing mass
Mammographic calcifications in 40%

Pathology

Well-defined, lobulated mass
Mixed histologic patterns are common
Pure mucinous tumors carry more favorable prognosis

MRI

Solitary lesion
Bright T2-WI secondary to mucin content
Enhancement of solid portions only

Differential Diagnosis

Fibroadenoma
Intramammary lymph node
Complex cyst

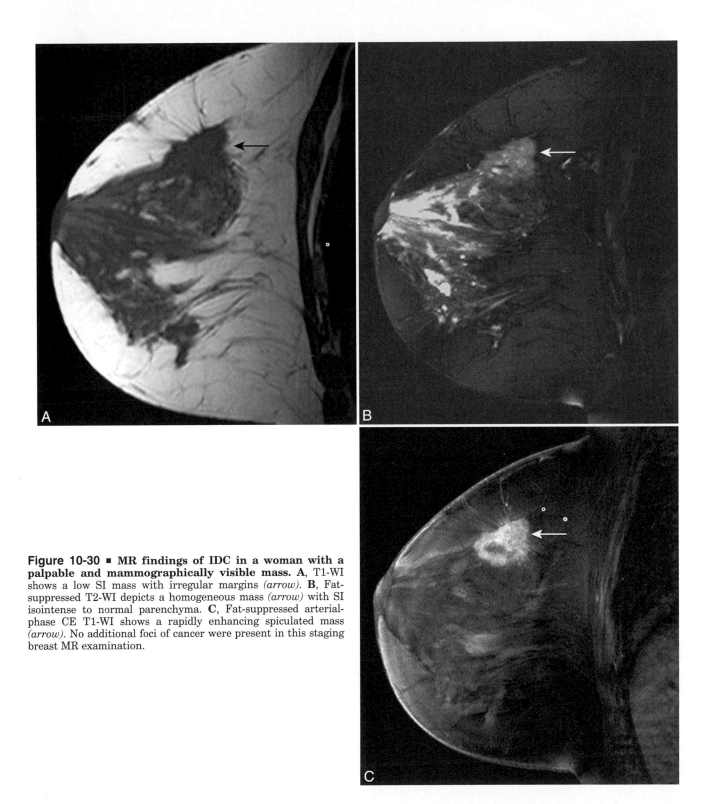

Figure 10-30 ■ **MR findings of IDC in a woman with a palpable and mammographically visible mass. A,** T1-WI shows a low SI mass with irregular margins *(arrow)*. **B,** Fat-suppressed T2-WI depicts a homogeneous mass *(arrow)* with SI isointense to normal parenchyma. **C,** Fat-suppressed arterial-phase CE T1-WI shows a rapidly enhancing spiculated mass *(arrow)*. No additional foci of cancer were present in this staging breast MR examination.

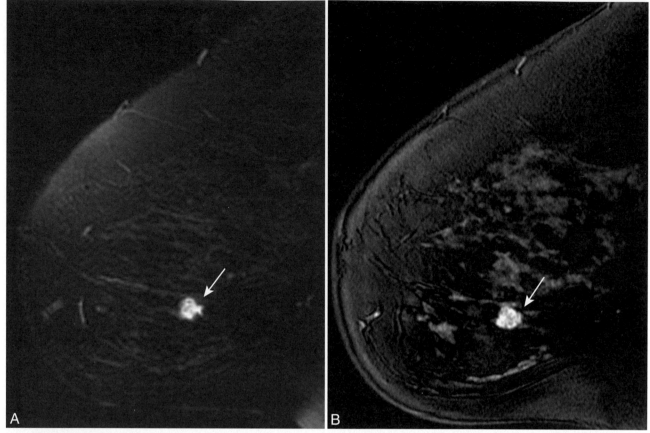

Figure 10-31 ■ MR illustration of a mucinous carcinoma. Mucinous tumors may mimic cysts or fibroadenomas on T2-WI, and thus CE imaging is required for characterization. **A,** Fat-suppressed T2-WI reveals an irregular lesion with uniform high SI *(arrow).* **B,** Fat-suppressed CE T1-WI reveals moderate uniform enhancement *(arrow).* The irregular margins and lack of nonenhancing internal septa distinguish this lesion from a fibroadenoma.

ILC has a high propensity toward bilaterality (6% to 28%),[163,164] and patients with ILC are approximately twice as likely as patients with IDC to harbor or develop contralateral breast cancer (Box 10-10).[165]

ILC can present on MRI as a focal irregular mass, similarly to IDC. However, ILC may also commonly appear as multiple small foci of discontinuous enhancement or as diffuse parenchymal enhancement (Fig. 10-32).[166,167] This type of imaging pattern reflects the propensity of ILC toward infiltrative growth, rendering it difficult to visualize mammographically.

MRI defines the histologic extent of resected invasive lobular cancers more accurately than mammography.[168-171] In a retrospective evaluation of MR in patients with pure ILC,[167] clinical management was altered in 50%[16,32] of patients on the basis of MRI findings. These included identification of mammographically occult multifocal/diffuse tumor or residual tumor following excisional biopsy.

Owing to its propensity for infiltrative growth, MRI findings of ILC can be subtle. ILC is more likely than IDC to present without a focally enhancing mass, and the pattern of ill-defined enhancement may

---

10-10 Invasive Lobular Carcinoma

Clinical

No particular age predilection
  Ill-defined mass or breast enlargement
    Variable mammographic appearance
Focal mass
Asymmetric density
Unilateral breast enlargement

Pathology

Ill-defined or infiltrating mass
Multi-focality and bilaterality
Mixed ductal-lobular tumors not uncommon
Surgical margins more frequently positive following
  lumpectomy

MRI

Isolated mass less commonly seen
Infiltrative or discontinuous enhancement
Variable enhancement kinetics

Differential Diagnosis

Benign glandular enhancement
Proliferative breast disease

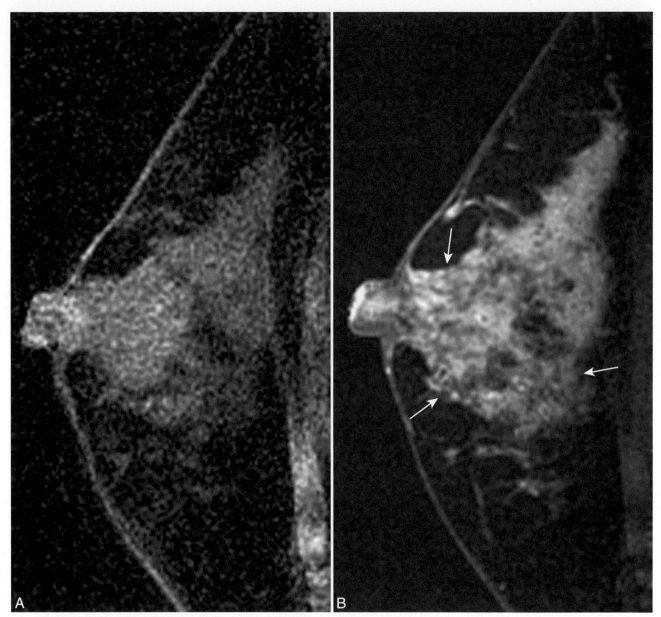

Figure 10-32 ■ **MR depiction of a diffusely infiltrating lobular carcinoma in a 46-year-old woman who presented with painless enlargement of the breast.** On mammography there was asymmetric density but no focal mass. **A** and **B**, Fat-suppressed T1-WIs obtained before (**A**) and after (**B**) contrast reveal diffuse moderate-intense enhancement of the glandular tissue *(arrows)* without a well-defined focal mass.

be misinterpreted as normal enhancing glandular tissue. ILC is commonly represented among patients with false-negative MRI examinations.[172] One third of ILCs may show a more gradual pattern of dynamic enhancement, or they may lack discernible enhancement (Fig. 10-33).[44]

INFLAMMATORY CARCINOMA

Inflammatory breast cancer does not represent a separate histologic subtype of breast cancer but instead is a clinical entity of tumor infiltration to the lymphatics of the skin. Signs and symptoms of diffuse breast swelling, erythema, and skin thickening and axillary adenopathic findings similar to those of mastitis characterize inflammatory breast cancer. When symptoms do not respond to empiric medical therapy, skin biopsy often is used to establish a diagnosis.

Mammographic findings of inflammatory breast cancer include breast enlargement, skin thickening, nipple retraction, and increased density.[173] Focal masses or abnormal calcifications are less commonly present,[174,175] and differentiation from nonmalignant causes of breast enlargement may be difficult.

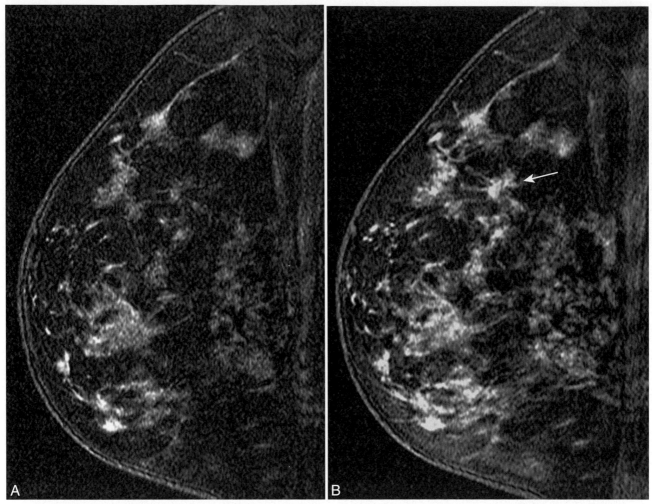

Figure 10-33 ■ MR findings of a subtle ILC with low-level enhancement in a 47-year-old woman with questionable architectural distortion revealed only on the craniocaudal mammogram (not shown). **A** and **B**, Fat-suppressed T1-WIs obtained before (**A**) and after (**B**) contrast reveal a hypoenhancing spiculated lesion (*arrow*). *(Continued)*

The findings of inflammatory cancer in MRI follow those of mammography and physical examination. Diffuse or peritumoral breast edema on T2-WI may be present.[176] Skin thickening and trabecular thickening are also common (Fig. 10-34). Following contrast administration, there is usually diffuse enhancement, similar to or somewhat greater than that revealed with mastitis.[177,178] In women in whom the diagnosis of inflammatory cancer is clinically suspected but cannot be confirmed, MRI may be useful for guiding tissue biopsy of the most focally enhancing region.

DUCTAL CARCINOMA IN SITU (DCIS)

Unlike invasive cancers, ductal carcinoma in situ (DCIS) represents a malignant proliferation of ductal epithelial cells without invasion beyond the basement membrane. The term intraductal carcinoma is often used for DCIS, to avoid confusion with lobular carcinoma in situ (LCIS), a pathologically and clinically distinct entity. DCIS is a precursor of invasive ductal cancer, and surgical resection is the treatment of choice. DCIS may be associated with invasive tumors or may be present without invasive cancer.[179] The fraction of breast cancer representing pure DCIS has increased with the advent of screening mammography.[1] Although DCIS may occasionally present as a mass lesion, it is more often asymptomatic and usually presents as mammographically detected calcifications.[180]

Histologically, DCIS demonstrates two dominant subtypes: comedo and noncomedo. The noncomedo subtypes are further distinguished as solid, cribriform, and papillary. Comedo DCIS is the more aggressive subtype and is more frequently associated with invasive ductal cancers. Like its invasive counterpart, comedo DCIS is more likely to promote tumor angiogenesis.

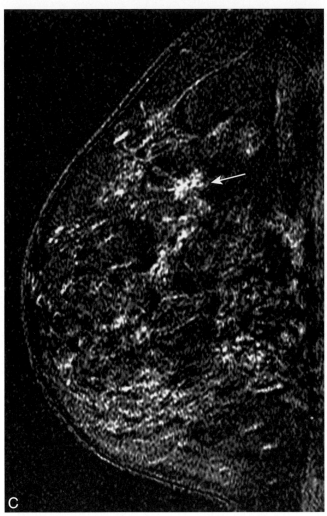

Figure 10-33 ▪ **Cont'd C,** Subtraction image better depicts the tumoral enhancement *(arrow).*

The MR imaging characteristics of DCIS are more variable than those of IDC. DCIS is more likely than IDC to be occult on MR imaging.[106,107,181-184] While the vast majority of invasive cancers will be depicted on a technically adequate breast MRI, a false-negative image may occur in 5% to 60% of cases of DCIS. DCIS lesions that are inapparent on MRI tend to be smaller[171] and lack findings of angiogenesis on histologic specimens.[106]

Given its intraductal distribution, one would expect DCIS to manifest as linear or branching enhancement on MR imaging. This pattern often is present in patients with DCIS with or without associated invasive ductal cancer.[15,44,106] More commonly, however, DCIS presents as regional enhancement on MRI, often with a clumped appearance (Fig. 10-35).[95,107] DCIS may also occasionally present as a focally enhancing mass, especially when associated with invasive tumor.

There is also more variability in the dynamics of contrast enhancement with DCIS.[106,108,183] While higher grade foci of DCIS lesions tend to show contrast dynamics suggestive of malignancy (plateau or washout), many cases of DCIS show progressive enhancement,[108] a pattern more suggestive of benignity.[182] Therefore, regardless of specific enhancement dynamics, certain regional patterns of enhancement, especially those following a ductal or segmental distribution, should be sampled and tested to exclude DCIS.

Paget's Disease

Involvement of the nipple by breast cancer (invasive or in situ) is termed Paget's disease, described first by James Paget in 1874. Women have scaly eczematous or psoriatic changes of the nipple and areola that generally precede the diagnosis of underlying malignancy. The cancer may be limited to the subareolar ducts or may be deeper within the breast parenchyma, with ductal extension toward the nipple.

Mammography in Paget's disease is often normal,[185,186] although a retroareolar tumor can be depicted in some women.[186,187] In women with invasive cancers who underwent mastectomy,[46] MRI was 100% accurate in identifying those with or without nipple involvement. Diffuse enhancement of the nipple and retroareolar complex suggested malignant involvement, whereas the uninvolved or contralateral nipple demonstrated linear superficial enhancement only.

Phyllodes Tumor (PT)

Phyllodes tumors (PTs) are a class of breast neoplasms arising from periductal stromal tissue. The older term cystosarcoma phyllodes was changed because phyllodes tumors have a wide range of neoplastic potential, from benign to borderline to frankly malignant. There are no reliable clinical or imaging indicators to distinguish benign from borderline or malignant PT; classification requires analysis of histologic features such as mitotic index. Phyllodes tumors are related histologically to fibroadenomas but generally present as larger masses. The median size of phyllodes tumors is 4 to 5 cm,[188,189] while the majority of fibroadenomas are less than 3 cm.[190] Phyllodes tumors, even histologically benign lesions, have a propensity toward local recurrence following excision.

On mammography, PTs are revealed as lobulated, well-circumscribed masses.[191,192] Sonography demonstrates mixed tumors with cystic and solid spaces.[193,194] Mammographic and sonographic features are not reliable in distinguishing between phyllodes tumors and fibroadenomas,[191,192] nor between benign and malignant variants of phyllodes tumors.[194] Larger size and more prominent cystic spaces suggest malignancy.[193]

The MR appearance of PTs have been reported.[137,195,196] The tumor is hyperintense relative to glandular tissue on T2-WI, with some tumors having low SI internal septations. The typically "leafy" pattern of solid papillary projection into cystic spaces has been depicted in larger tumors.[196] Rapid enhancement is present for both benign and borderline malignant tumors. Thus, masses with otherwise benign morphologic features should be excised if they are large (>4 cm) or rapidly growing.

SPECIFIC CLINICAL APPLICATIONS OF BREAST MRI

Lesion Identification and Diagnosis

EVALUATION OF THE INDETERMINATE MAMMOGRAPHIC FINDING

Given its high sensitivity for invasive cancer, MR has been increasingly used as a adjunctive imaging modality for problematic mammographic abnormalities.[22,197] These include lesions that are only revealed on one view, or indeterminate lesions that cannot be readily characterized as benign or malignant on mammographic and sonographic evaluation.

Since MRI is nearly 100% sensitive for invasive cancers, it has been suggested that a negative MRI evaluation may obviate the need for biopsy or additional short-term follow-up of mammographic masses or asymmetric density.[198] Absence of enhancement for a palpable or mammographic abnormality has an NPV of 97% to 100%.[15,95] In a study of MR for evaluation of indeterminate mammographic findings,[21] 60/89 cases demonstrated no corresponding enhancing lesion on MRI and all with negative histologic or stable mammographic findings on follow-up.

Despite these findings, false-negative MR results have been reported.[44,172,183] Technical limitations (e.g., lesion not included in imaging volume; misadministration of intravenous contrast) account for some instances of tumor nonvisualization. In other women, the malignancy could not be identified because of either minimal enhancement or unrecognized infiltrative pattern of growth. False-negative studies can occur in patients with pure DCIS or invasive lobular cancers. In the setting of a negative MRI examination, a suspicious mammographic abnormality—particularly indeterminate mammographic calcifications—may still require biopsy to exclude malignancy.

With values ranging between 37% and 97%, the specificity of MR for characterization of focal lesions is not as high as its sensitivity.[12,13,20,45,74,184,199] Improvements in specificity through careful evaluation of architectural features of focal and regional areas of enhancement have been proposed.[15,16,18,95,96] In addition, kinetic enhancement features have been utilized to improve specificity in lesion characterization.[17,72,87]

Despite these advances, it is not clear whether routine use of MR as an adjunct to mammography and sonography will improve the overall accuracy of breast imaging. While a negative MR examination may be reassuring, a positive MR examination may still result in a negative biopsy. Furthermore, additional unsuspected enhancing lesions are frequently identified in MRI, and only a small portion of these findings result in a diagnosis of malignancy.[102,200]

EVALUATION OF NIPPLE DISCHARGE

Spontaneous nipple discharge is a relatively common symptom and may represent a diagnostic dilemma for the breast surgeon. Discharge that is bilateral or involves multiple ducts is more commonly physiologic. Unilateral discharge, especially that which is serosanguineous or frankly bloody, can be a sign of underlying malignancy. Nevertheless, in the majority of women with nipple discharge, the underlying etiology is benign. The most common causes of breast discharge are solitary papilloma or papillomatosis (present in 35% to 50% of women with spontaneous nipple discharge) or ductal ectasia (15% to 35%), with malignancy reported in only 5% to 20%.[201]

MRI can be useful for evaluating women with nipple discharge.[145] In an MRI study in women with spontaneous nipple discharge of uncertain etiology,[23] an enhancing lesion was identified in 11 of 23 patients (48%). Of the 12 patients with normal MR examinations, 4 underwent ductal exploration. Of these 4 women, 2 were found to have papillomas, one had a fibroadenoma, and the fourth had normal tissue. The remaining eight women with normal MRI examinations underwent clinical and mammographic follow-up, and all had complete or partial resolution of discharge.

Of the 11 patients with enhancing abnormalities at MRI, excisional biopsy demonstrated four papillomas, one fibroadenoma, and six malignancies (all DCIS, two with microinvasion). In one patient, a small focus of DCIS not depicted on MRI was detected adjacent to a 15-mm papilloma revealed by MRI. In another MRI study in 48 women with nipple discharge,[145] MRI successfully depicted pathologic enhancement in all 8 women who were ultimately shown to have invasive carcinoma.

DEPICTION OF OCCULT PRIMARY BREAST CANCER

In slightly less than 1% of patients with breast cancer, metastatic adenopathy to the axilla is the only presenting sign.[202] Mammographic examination yields variable results, depicting nonpalpable cancers in from 0% to 56% of these patients.[24,203,204] When breast cancer is suspected in women with malignant axillary adenopathy but no palpable or mammographic abnormality, breast MRI may depict the site of primary malignancy in 36% to 86% of women (Fig. 10-36).[13,24,205-208] This finding may can allow the patient to avoid mastectomy in favor of lumpectomy and local irradiation. MRI may also be useful for confirming or excluding breast cancer in a patient with distant metastatic adenocarcinoma and no known primary cancer.

Breast Cancer Staging

Accurate staging of breast cancer aids in the planning of appropriate therapy (i.e., mastectomy vs. breast

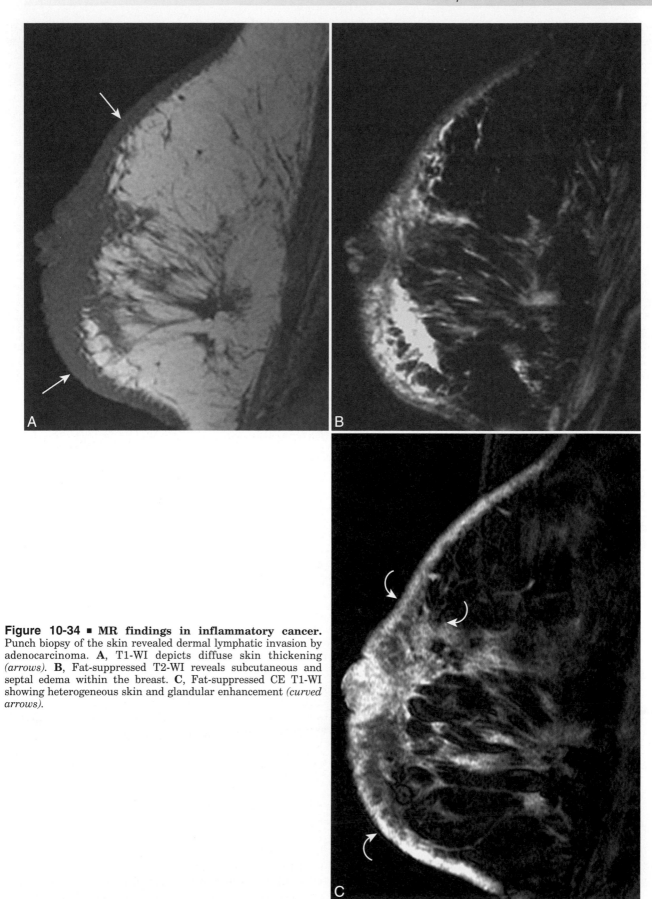

Figure 10-34 ■ **MR findings in inflammatory cancer.** Punch biopsy of the skin revealed dermal lymphatic invasion by adenocarcinoma. **A**, T1-WI depicts diffuse skin thickening *(arrows)*. **B**, Fat-suppressed T2-WI reveals subcutaneous and septal edema within the breast. **C**, Fat-suppressed CE T1-WI showing heterogeneous skin and glandular enhancement *(curved arrows)*.

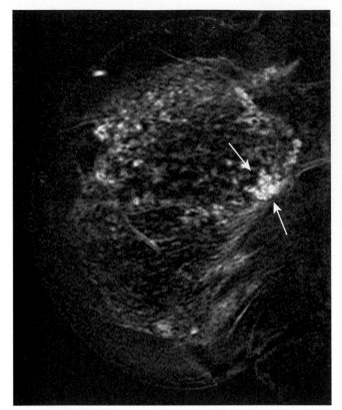

Figure 10-35 ■ **MR illustration of DCIS in a 35-year-old woman.** Fat-suppressed CE T1-WI (subtraction image) shows heterogeneous clumped regional enhancement *(arrows)*.

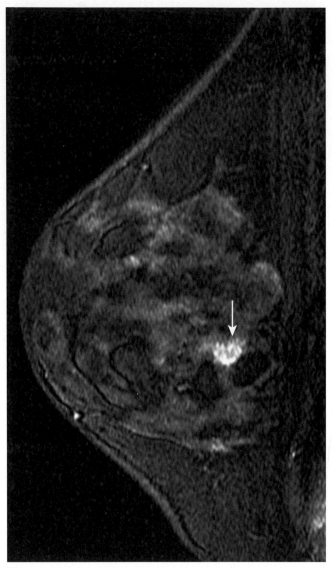

Figure 10-36 ■ **MR depiction of occult IDC in a 29-year-old woman with malignant axillary adenopathy.** The patient did not have a primary breast cancer revealed on physical examination or mammography. Fat-suppressed CE T1-WI reveals a heterogeneously enhancing occult primary cancer *(arrow)*.

conservation). The TMN staging system (Box 10-11) identifies characteristics of the primary tumor, presence and degree of regional nodal tumor spread, and presence of distant metastatic disease. Staging of breast cancer helps determine prognosis and guide decisions regarding local and systemic therapy.

LOCAL STAGING

Local breast cancer staging reflects the size of the primary tumor and associated spread to the adjacent skin or chest wall. Multifocality (two or more distinct foci of cancer within a single quadrant of the breast) or multicentricity (two or more foci in separate breast quadrants) are additional features of local disease extent that, while not formally part of the TMN staging system, may affect the surgical and radiotherapeutic approach.

MRI is superior to traditional clinical staging (physical examination plus mammography) in depicting the size and overall extent of tumor in patients suspected of having confined disease.[171,209,210] MRI is particularly valuable in defining local extent of disease in patients with lobular carcinoma[167,168] and in patients whose cancer includes an extensive intraductal component.[107,170]

Breast MRI can depict unsuspected multifocal or multicentric disease in 10% and 37% of patients, respectively (Fig. 10-37).[13,26,171,211-214] MRI is also the most accurate imaging modality for evaluation of pectoral muscle invasion.[215] In patients whose tumors are more extensive or invasive than initially presumed, MRI can redirect surgical management from local excision to wider excision or mastectomy, thereby avoiding the need for multiple surgical procedures.

AXILLARY NODAL STAGING

In women with invasive breast cancer, accurate nodal staging helps determine patient prognosis and appropriate therapeutic regimens. The use of sentinel mapping has made nodal staging possible without incurring the increased cost and morbidity of extensive axillary nodal dissection. Patients with a positive sentinel lymph node evaluation will typically undergo intensive adjuvant systemic treatment

10-11   TMN Staging System for Breast Cancer*

Definitions

Tumor (T)

T0	No primary tumor
Tis	Intraductal tumor only
T1	Invasive tumor <2 cm in greatest dimension
T2	Invasive tumor 2 to 5 cm in greatest dimension
T3	Invasive tumor >5 cm in greatest dimension
T4	Tumor of any size with chest wall or skin invasion (includes inflammatory cancer)

Lymph Nodes (N)

N0	No regional lymph node metastasis
N1	Metastasis to moveable axillary lymph nodes
N2	Metastasis to fixed axillary lymph nodes
N3	Metastasis to internal mammary lymph nodes

Metastases (M)

M0	No distant metastases
M1	Distant metastases (including ipsilateral supraclavicular lymph nodes)

Staging

Stage	Tumor	Nodes	Metastases
0	Tis	N0	M0
I	T1	N0	M0
IIA	T0-T1	N1	M0
	T2	N0	M0
IIB	T2	N1	M0
	T3	N0	N0
IIIA	T0-T2	N2	M0
	T3	N1-N2	M0
IIIB	T0-T3	N3	M0
	T4	N0-N2	M0
IV	Any T	Any N	M1

*Used with permission of the American Joint Committee on Cancer (AJCC), Chicago, IL. The original source for this material is the *AJCC Cancer Staging Manual*, 6th ed. New York, Springer-Verlag, 2002, www.springer-ny.com

(chemotherapy ± hormonal therapy) following surgery and irradiation. Node-negative patients may be treated with local therapy alone or with less intensive adjuvant therapies.

In the setting of breast cancer, enlarged lymph nodes with loss or distortion of the normal nodal architecture are characteristic of metastatic disease.[216,217] Dynamic enhancement patterns may provide additional diagnostic information concerning nodal characterization.[217-219] In one study,[217] the combination of small lymph node size and lack of intense enhancement had 100% NPV for the presence of axillary metastases. However, the results of conventional MRI of the axilla do not obviate the need for diagnostic sentinel node biopsy.

Ultrasmall superparamagnetic iron oxide particles (USPIOs) as negative contrast agents on T2-WI. USPIOs are phagocytosed up the reticuloendothelial system (RES), including regional lymph nodes. Since metastatic tumor cells within lymph nodes are unable to take up iron particles by phagocytosis, USPIOs have been developed as a subtype of MR contrast agent for differentiating between reactive and metastatic lymph nodes.[220,221] Owing to the pharmacokinetics of these contrast agents, postcontrast imaging must be performed from 24 to 36 hours following IV administration for optimal lymph node characterization.

Enhanced MR imaging of axillary lymph nodes with USPIOs[222,223] shows improved accuracy for defining malignant axillary involvement relative to unenhanced MRI. However, additional studies are required to determine the value of RES-directed MR imaging for assessment of axillary lymph nodes in women with newly diagnosed breast cancer.

MRI and Breast Cancer Treatment

MRI PRIOR TO RE-EXCISION

In patients with breast cancer treated with breast conservation surgery, pathologic assessment of the surgical margins is required. Local recurrence rates are increased when invasive or intraductal tumor is transected by or lies close to the surgical margin.[224,225] Knowing the true extent of residual macroscopic disease prior to surgical re-excision can help guide subsequent treatment options involving the extent of surgery. In patients whose true extent of disease is much greater than initially suspected, mastectomy may ultimately be required for definitive surgical treatment.[226]

MRI following excisional biopsy may be used to determine the extent of residual tumor.[28,29,227,228] The optimal time for imaging is between 28 and 35 days following surgery.[29] If imaging is performed less than 4 weeks after excisional biopsy, enhancing granulation tissue can resemble residual tumor.

Postbiopsy seromas or hematomas are demonstrated as irregular fluid-filled cavities, usually with a thin, uniform rim of enhancement (Fig. 10-38). Thick or nodular foci of enhancement are more suggestive of residual tumor. In a subset of patients imaged prior to re-excision, MRI may depict unsuspected extensive residual or multicentric tumor (Fig. 10-39), necessitating alteration of surgical management from re-excision to mastectomy.[28]

LOCAL RECURRENCE FOLLOWING LUMPECTOMY AND RADIATION THERAPY

Following lumpectomy and radiation therapy, local breast cancer recurrence rates range from 8% to 20%.[229] Recurrence may be at or near the site of original tumor, elsewhere within the same breast, or solely within regional lymph nodes. Most local recurrences at or near the original tumor site occur within the first 5 to 7 years following lumpectomy and radiation therapy, while the recurrence rate for tumors more distantly located from the original surgical site peaks at 8 to 10 years.[230] This latter finding suggests that some of these remote

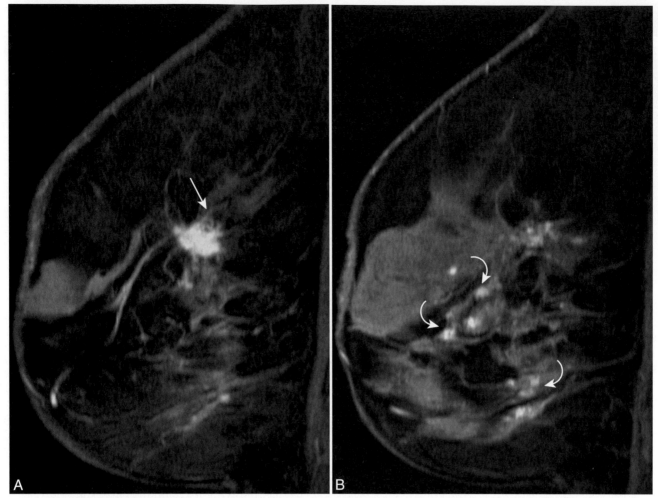

Figure 10-37 ■ **MR findings of a multifocal tumor in a 62-year-old woman with biopsy-proved IDC. A** and **B**, Fat-suppressed CE T1-WIs reveal a dominant enhancing lesion representing the known cancer *(arrow)*. Several additional foci of enhancement *(curved arrows)* are present that were not clinically or mammographically evident. MR-guided needle localization of secondary nodule proved the existence of multifocal tumor.

recurrences may, in fact, represent new primary breast cancers.

Changes due to surgery and radiation therapy can mimic local recurrence on physical examination and mammography, confounding the evaluation of the postlumpectomy breast. In one series, following lumpectomy and irradiation, 28% of patients with suspicious findings on both mammography and physical examination demonstrated benign findings on biopsy.[231] Benign biopsy rates were even greater for patients with suspicious findings on only physical examination or only mammography. In these patients, fibrosis and fat necrosis were the most common benign entities at histology.

MRI is useful in the evaluation of the postoperative breast. In cases of suspected local tumor recurrence due to an evolving palpable or mammographic abnormality, MRI can be used to differentiate recurrent malignancy from benign posttreatment changes. In patients treated with lumpectomy and irradiation, MRI often shows

regional or focal areas of low SI on T1-WI.[232] Secondary findings of architectural distortion or skin thickening are also common following radiation therapy and are not specific for recurrent tumor. Masses with low SI on T2-WI are suggestive of a benign process, such as mature fibrosis,[232] although some authors have not found T2-WI useful in distinguishing benign treatment changes from recurrent tumor.[233]

As is true of primary tumors, recurrent breast cancers tend to enhance rapidly following contrast administration. The sensitivity of dynamic enhanced T1-WI for detecting recurrent tumor is between 90% and 100%,[11,30,83,124,209,233-237] which is significantly greater than that of mammography or physical examination (Fig. 10-40).[209,237] However, the specificity of MRI in the irradiated breast may vary. In the first year following irradiation, foci of immature fibrosis and scar tissue may enhance, mimicking the appearance of locally recurrent tumor.[11,235] However, in the 9 to 18 months following irradiation, fibrosis matures and becomes less vascular. These mature

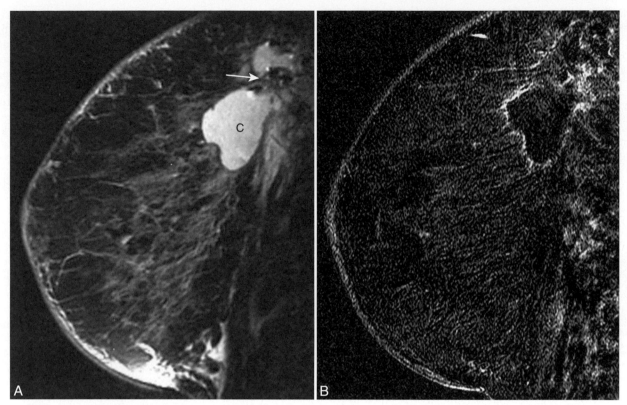

Figure 10-38 ■ **MR findings of a postbiopsy seroma. A**, Fat-suppressed T2-WI reveals an irregular fluid-filled cavity (C) in the deep upper breast. Clip artifact is present *(arrow)*. **B**, Fat-suppressed CE T1-WI subtraction image shows thin rim enhancement only.

areas of fibrosis therefore enhance minimally, with gradual enhancement kinetics.[11,235] Fat necrosis also may demonstrate solid enhancement and can occasionally mimic recurrent tumor.[122,238]

LOCAL RECURRENCE AFTER MASTECTOMY

Local recurrence of breast cancer following mastectomy occurs within the chest wall or beneath the skin of the reconstructed breast (Fig. 10-41). Rates of such recurrence are similar to local recurrence rates in conservatively treated patients. Concurrent distant metastases are present in 50% of patients with local recurrence following mastectomy, with nearly all patients eventually developing metastatic disease.

In patients treated without reconstruction, local recurrence is generally evident on clinical examination. However, for patients with prosthetic or myocutaneous flap reconstruction (e.g., transverse rectus abdominis myocutaneous [TRAM] flap), recurrent disease may be difficult to distinguish from postoperative changes within the reconstructed breast. Scarring along the surgical planes is common and can mimic local tumor recurrence on physical examination or mammography.

The normal and abnormal appearance of implants for breast reconstruction are discussed above. The MR imaging appearance of the TRAM flap–reconstructed breast can vary but is characterized by the replacement of normal glandular tissue with subcutaneous abdominal fat. The rectus abdominis may appear mass-like in the early postoperative period[239,240] and should not be misdiagnosed as a tumor. With time, the rectus abdominis muscle undergoes progressive atrophy and fatty replacement.

On MRI, local tumor recurrence is demonstrated as a rapidly enhancing mass, often with contrast washout on delayed imaging, similarly to local recurrence following lumpectomy. Seroma and fat necrosis are other common complications, which generally may be differentiated by MRI.[240,241]

RESPONSE TO NEOADJUVANT CHEMOTHERAPY

For patients with locally advanced breast cancer (T3 or T4 tumors), preoperative ("neoadjuvant") chemotherapy can be used in an attempt to down-stage the extent of local tumor. While such therapy does not reduce the incidence of local recurrence, neoadjuvant chemotherapy can allow for less radical surgical treatments, such as lumpectomy, rather than full mastectomy.[242] The use of neoadjuvant chemotherapy also provides an opportunity to observe the response of the patient to chemotherapeutic regimens, which then may be

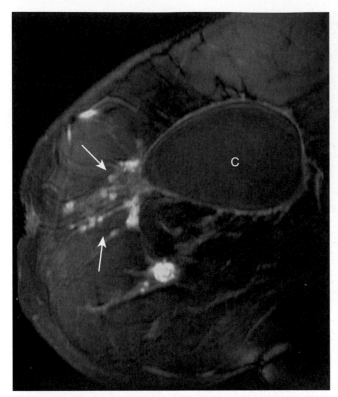

Figure 10-39 ▪ **MR findings of extensive residual carcinoma in a 32-year-old woman following excisional biopsy for IDC, with positive surgical margins.** Fat-suppressed CE T1-WI reveals seroma cavity (C) with extensive confluent enhancement extending anterior to the biopsy site *(arrows)*. Additional foci of confluent enhancement were seen in other quadrants of the breast. Subsequent mastectomy revealed extensive residual invasive and intraductal tumor.

used subsequent to surgery in the hope of preventing distant metastatic disease.

Evaluation of chemotherapeutic response is a critical component in the assessment of these patients and in the determination of appropriate operative therapy. However, both physical examination and mammography may be inadequate in assessing the true extent of residual tumor following neoadjuvant therapy.[243,244] Interestingly, morphologic phenotyping of locally advanced tumors (circumscribed vs. diffuse/infiltrating) has been used successfully to predict response to neoadjuvant therapy.[245] In addition, chemotherapy-induced alterations in the degree of linear/ductal enhancement extending from tumor margins has been shown to increase the likelihood of negative pathologic margins following lumpectomy.[246]

MRI is more accurate than either physical examination or mammography in defining the extent of viable tumor following chemotherapy (Fig. 10-42).[247-251] However, chemotherapy may diminish the dynamic enhancement pattern of tumor.[76,246] Conversely, granulation tissue in response to tumor regression may enhance avidly. Thus, MRI

can over- or underestimate the true extent of residual disease.[25,252,253] Since microscopic foci of tumor cannot be excluded in the setting of a complete imaging response,[254] surgery (mastectomy or lumpectomy) is required following completion of chemotherapy. However, the physical findings in the patient undergoing neoadjuvant therapy can be confusing. Therefore, preoperative MRI may allow for more definitive surgical planning. In addition, MRI can document lack of clinical response to ongoing chemotherapy, allowing the oncologist the option of changing chemotherapy regimens.

Breast Cancer Screening with MRI

SCREENING OF WOMEN AT HIGH RISK

The overall lifetime risk for the development of breast cancer in women is estimated as high as 13% (American Cancer Society, Cancer Facts and Figures 2004, http://www.cancer.org/docroot/STT/stt_0.asp, accessed September 2004). However, certain groups of women are at higher than average risk for breast cancer development. Most prominently, women with a mutation in one of two breast cancer (BRCA) susceptibility genes, termed BRCA1 and BRCA2, have a lifetime breast cancer risk of between 50% and 85%.[255] These women also experience breast cancer at an earlier age than the general population does.[256] Other risk categories include women with a history of "high-risk" non-malignant conditions, such as atypical ductal hyperplasia (ADH) and lobular carcinoma in situ (LCIS), and women with a strong family history of breast cancer.

In high-risk women, such as those known or suspected to be carriers of BRCA mutations, management options include prophylactic mastectomy and chemoprevention. Aggressive screening programs that include frequent clinical examinations and early mammography have also been recommended.[257] The results of such a screening regimen have been disappointing, as mammographic sensitivity in these women appears to be low.[258,259] This may be due to the changing nature of the breast examination in premenopausal patients as well as the higher percentage of women with dense breasts in this population. Early mammographic examination also carries a potential added morbidity by exposing patients to increased irradiation at an age when the breast parenchymal tissue is potentially more sensitive to irradiation.

Several studies have evaluated the role of breast MRI as a screening tool in selected high-risk populations.[260-265] MRI has been shown to detect mammographically occult cancer in these women at rates between 1% and 4%. However, false-positive results are also commonly reported, leading to additional follow-up examinations and biopsies. Additional larger scale studies are needed to determine which populations, if any, would truly benefit from MR screening. Other issues such as examination protocol (high temporal vs. high spatial resolution) and optimal screening intervals need to

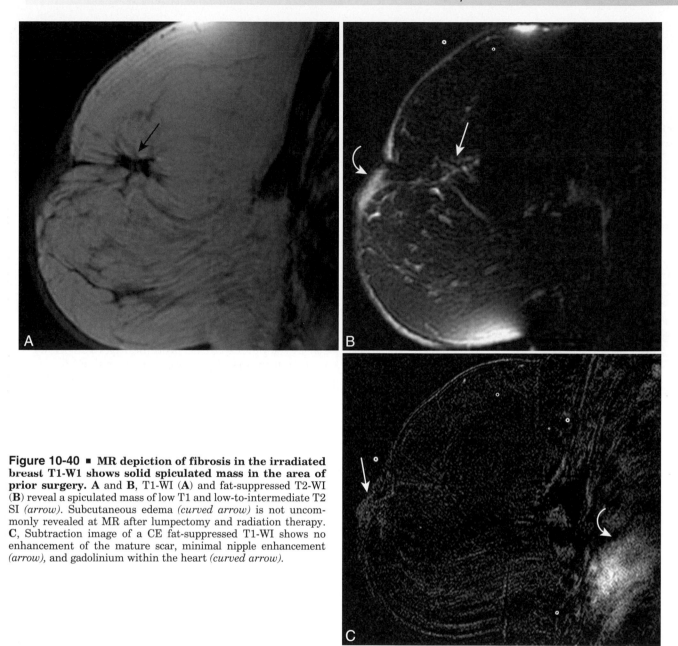

Figure 10-40 ▪ MR depiction of fibrosis in the irradiated breast T1-W1 shows solid spiculated mass in the area of prior surgery. A and **B,** T1-WI (**A**) and fat-suppressed T2-WI (**B**) reveal a spiculated mass of low T1 and low-to-intermediate T2 SI *(arrow)*. Subcutaneous edema *(curved arrow)* is not uncommonly revealed at MR after lumpectomy and radiation therapy. **C,** Subtraction image of a CE fat-suppressed T1-WI shows no enhancement of the mature scar, minimal nipple enhancement *(arrow),* and gadolinium within the heart *(curved arrow).*

be addressed in carefully constructed clinical trials to maximize the potential benefit of MR screening in high-risk populations.

CONTRALATERAL BREAST CANCER
SCREENING

There is a 1% to 3% incidence of clinically or mammographically detected synchronous bilateral breast cancer.[266-268] However, the frequency of pathologically identified cancers in patients undergoing elective contralateral mastectomy is higher,[269] as is the frequency of metachronous bilateral cancers,[266,267,270] suggesting that a number of patients may have clinically and mammographically occult

contralateral malignancies at the time of initial presentation.

MRI also has been investigated as a means of screening for contralateral breast cancer in patients with recently diagnosed unilateral tumors. In patients with cancers initially detected by mammography or physical examination, MR can demonstrate occult contralateral malignancy in 4% to 9% of patients (Fig. 10-43).[26,176,271,272] The variability in the reported detection rates likely reflects the small number of patients in some series. False-positive MRI findings in the contralateral breast in these series range between 3% and 6%, with positive predictive values between 45% and 80%.

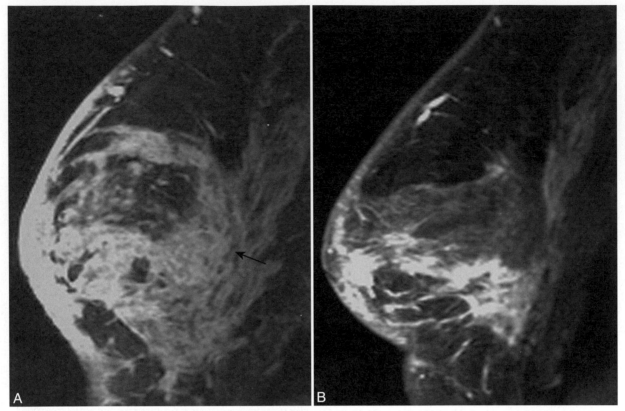

Figure 10-41 ▪ MR documentation of the response to neoadjuvant chemotherapy in a 44-year-old woman with inflammatory breast cancer. A, Fat-suppressed CE T1-WI prior to therapy shows extensive confluent enhancement throughout a large portion of the breast. Enhancement of the subjacent pectoral muscle suggests chest wall invasion *(arrow)*. **B**, Corresponding fat-suppressed CE T1-WI obtained after four cycles of chemotherapy shows a marked reduction in the amount of enhancing glandular tissue. At surgery, there was no evidence of pectoral muscle invasion.

Given the usefulness of MRI for local staging of breast cancer, it has been suggested that a bilateral breast MRI examination be performed following a new cancer diagnosis, allowing for simultaneous ipsilateral staging and contralateral screening. However, given the potential costs associated with routine use of MRI following cancer detection, additional controlled studies are required to examine the true clinical benefit of this approach. Ongoing studies are examining the clinical and economic outcomes of routine implementation of bilateral breast MRI in all patients with newly diagnosed breast cancer.

INTERVENTIONAL BREAST MRI

Lesion Localization and MRI-guided Biopsy

The usefulness of breast MRI is limited if MRI-detected lesions cannot be sampled. Some MR-detectable breast lesions will have a preexisting mammographic, sonographic, or palpable correlate that can serve as the guiding modality for interventional procedures. In other cases, directed sonography toward a particular portion of the breast can lead to depiction of a previously undetected abnormality.[206,273] However, in many women, a suspicious enhancing lesion can be shown only by MRI,[274] and MRI-guided localization procedures are therefore required for histologic evaluation.[275]

Image-guided options for tissue diagnosis of suspicious nonpalpable breast lesions include fine needle aspiration (FNA), core biopsy, vacuum-assisted large-core biopsy, and excisional biopsy following wire localization. MRI-compatible needles are designed with nondeflecting metallic components, so that patients may be safely reimaged within the MRI scanner following placement of a localization device. The use of nonmagnetic components lessens the degree of metallic artifact, so that image distortion and lesion obscuration are minimized following placement of the device.

Although freehand localization under MR guidance has been reported,[276-278] most MR-guided localization has been performed with targeted access to the immobilized breast.[279-282] Immobilization facilitates needle placement and allows one to

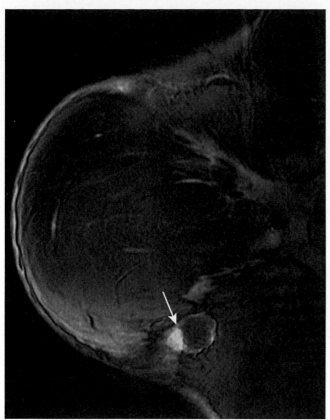

Figure 10-42 ■ MR findings of local tumor recurrence in a 31-year-old woman 1 year after mastectomy and TRAM flap reconstruction for IDC. The new abnormality was palpated at the inframammary crease of the neo-breast. Fat-suppressed CE T1-WI image identifies enhancing recurrent cancer *(arrow)* at the site of palpable abnormality.

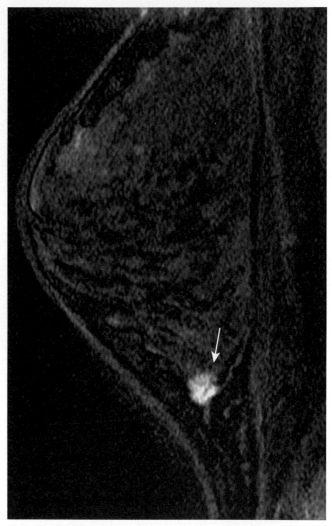

Figure 10-43 ■ MR depiction of occult contralateral breast cancer in a 43-year-old woman with DCIS identified in the left breast on screening mammography. Right breast mammogram showed no suspicious findings. Fat-suppressed CE T1-WI of the right breast performed at the time of initial diagnosis shows an 8-mm enhancing lesion *(arrow)* in the lower breast. Core biopsy revealed IDC with tubular features.

localize lesions that, owing to the washout phenomenon, are only transiently revealed during the early phase of contrast enhancement. Overcompression of the breast during these procedures can impede contrast flow to the breast and thus lesion visualization.[283] Therefore, short-term follow-up may be required if a suspicious lesion does not enhance at the time of anticipated MR-guided biopsy.

Histologic evaluation of solid lesions via FNA may be performed.[284-286] However, the diagnostic accuracy of FNA of solid breast masses varies widely[287] and requires an experienced cytopathologist to determine whether adequate cellular material has been obtained. Percutaneous MR-guided core biopsy has also been reported.[288,289] Vacuum-assisted biopsy with MR guidance allows for complete removal of small lesions (Fig. 10-44).[290,291] The failure rate of these MR-guided procedures is low and often secondary to far medial lesions not easily accessed from the lateral approach required by many biopsy systems.[289]

For women who require an excisional biopsy, MR-guided wire localization can be performed.[280,282,292-294] An MR-compatible needle is inserted into the lesion (Fig. 10-45). Following verification of its position,

the needle is exchanged for a hook wire device. Complications, including wire breakage or migration, have been reported.[294]

An alternative strategy is MR guidance for coil or clip placement at the site of an MR-visible lesion without sampling.[295] Traditional mammographic-based localization can be performed subsequently. This allows MR localization at a tertiary center, with subsequent surgery at a different site where access to breast MRI is limited.

Monitoring of Minimally Invasive Therapy of Breast Lesions

Minimally invasive therapy of breast lesions involves the use of interstitial laser therapy, focused ultrasound, or cryotherapy for tissue ablation. These therapies

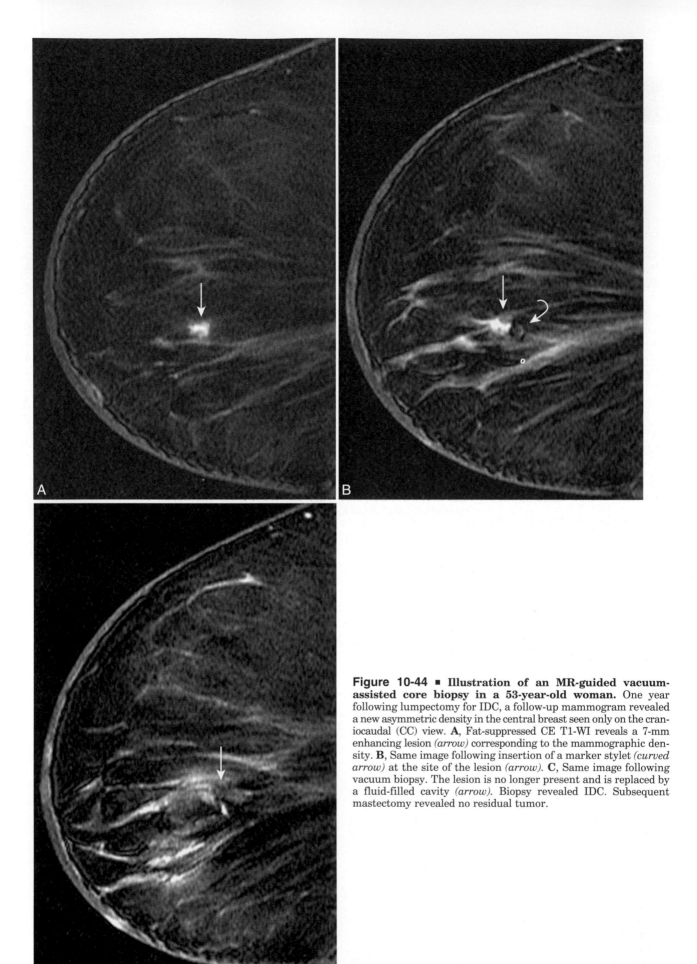

Figure 10-44 ▪ Illustration of an MR-guided vacuum-assisted core biopsy in a 53-year-old woman. One year following lumpectomy for IDC, a follow-up mammogram revealed a new asymmetric density in the central breast seen only on the craniocaudal (CC) view. **A**, Fat-suppressed CE T1-WI reveals a 7-mm enhancing lesion *(arrow)* corresponding to the mammographic density. **B**, Same image following insertion of a marker stylet *(curved arrow)* at the site of the lesion *(arrow)*. **C**, Same image following vacuum biopsy. The lesion is no longer present and is replaced by a fluid-filled cavity *(arrow)*. Biopsy revealed IDC. Subsequent mastectomy revealed no residual tumor.

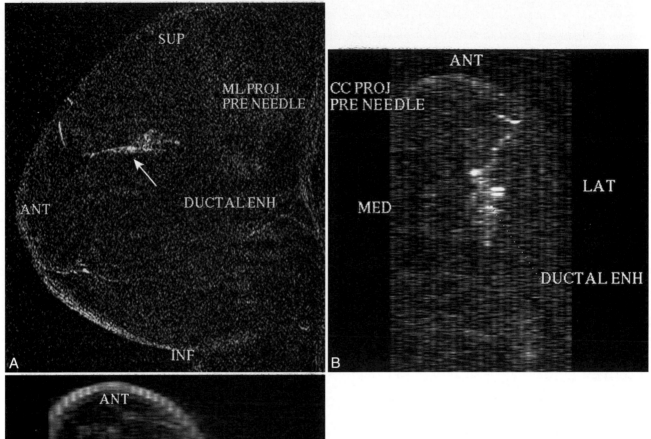

Figure 10-45 ■ **Illustration of MR-guided needle localization in a 48-year-old woman with linear and segmental enhancement identified on bilateral breast MRI.** MRI was performed for the evaluation of a contralateral abnormality. Surgical excision revealed DCIS with a 4-mm invasive tumor. **A**, Fat-suppressed CE T1-WI subtraction image reveals linear and branching enhancement *(arrow)*. **B**, Reformatted CC projection of **A** depicts location of enhancement in the medial-lateral plane. **C**, Reformatted CC projection of sagittal fat-suppressed CE T1-WI following needle placement under MR guidance. The needle tip is shown to end in the vicinity of the lesion.

are now routinely utilized to treat a variety of malignancies of the liver, kidney, and other organs.[296-298] However, since breast cancer is often amenable to curative surgery, the use of minimally invasive therapy for breast cancer treatment is controversial. Such therapies are more often utilized for ablation of benign breast lesions (e.g., fibroadenomas) in symptomatic patients who wish to avoid surgery.[299]

MRI also has a potential role in monitoring the performance and results of minimally invasive therapies in the breast.[300] Real-time monitoring of tissue changes can be performed.[301,302] Since MRI often is the optimal modality for delineating the exact location and extent of disease, it would be a logical choice for image-guided delivery of therapy[299] as well as for post-therapeutic follow-up.

REFERENCES

1. Tabard L, Fagerberg CJ, Gad A, et al. Reduction in mortality from breast cancer after mass screening with mammography: randomised trial from the Breast Cancer Screening Working Group of the Swedish National Board of Health and Welfare. Lancet 1985;1:829-832.
2. Stavros AT, Thickman D, Rapp CL, Dennis MA, Parker SH, Sisney GA. Solid breast nodules: use of sonography to distinguish between benign and malignant lesions. Radiology 1995;196:123-134.
3. Feig SA. Breast masses: mammographic and sonographic evaluation. Radiol Clin North Am 1992;30:67-92.

4. Tabar L, Vitak B, Chen HH, et al. The Swedish Two-County Trial twenty years later: Updated mortality results and new insights from long-term follow-up. Radiol Clin North Am 2000;38:625-651.
5. Flobbe K, Nelemans PJ, Kessels AG, Beets GL, von Meyenfeldt MF, van Engelshoven JM. The role of ultrasonography as an adjunct to mammography in the detection of breast cancer. A systematic review. Eur J Cancer 2002;38:1044-1050.
6. Rosenberg RD, Hunt WC, Williamson MR, et al. Effects of age, breast density, ethnicity, and estrogen replacement therapy on screening mammographic sensitivity and cancer stage at diagnosis: review of 183,134 screening mammograms in Albuquerque, New Mexico. Radiology 1998;209:511-518.
7. Peer PG, Verbeek AL, Straatman H, Hendriks JH, Holland R. Age-specific sensitivities of mammographic screening for breast cancer. Breast Cancer Res Treat 1996;38:153-160.
8. Mushlin AI, Kouides RW, Shapiro DE. Estimating the accuracy of screening mammography: a meta-analysis. Am J Prev Med 1998;14:143-153.
9. Fletcher SW, Black W, Harris R, Rimer BK, Shapiro S. Report of the International Workshop on Screening for Breast Cancer. [Comment.] J Natl Cancer Inst 1993;85:1644-1656.
10. Rahbar G, Sie AC, Hansen GC, et al. Benign versus malignant solid breast masses: US differentiation. Radiology 1999;213:889-894.
11. Heywang-Kobrunner SH, Schlegel A, Beck R, et al. Contrast-enhanced MRI of the breast after limited surgery and radiation therapy. J Comput Assist Tomogr 1993;17:891-900.
12. Kaiser WA, Zeitler E. MR imaging of the breast: fast imaging sequences with and without Gd-DTPA: preliminary observations. Radiology 1989;170:681-686.
13. Harms SE, Flamig DP, Hesley KL, et al. MR imaging of the breast with rotating delivery of excitation off resonance: clinical experience with pathologic correlation. Radiology 1993;187:493-501.
14. Orel SG, Schnall MD, LiVolsi VA, Troupin RH. Suspicious breast lesions: MR imaging with radiologic-pathologic correlation. Radiology 1994;190:485-493.
15. Nunes LW, Schnall MD, Siegelman ES, et al. Diagnostic performance characteristics of architectural features revealed by high spatial-resolution MR imaging of the breast. AJR Am J Roentgenol 1997;169:409-415.
16. Nunes LW, Schnall MD, Orel SG, et al. Breast MR imaging: interpretation model. Radiology 1997;202:833-841.
17. Schnall MD, Rosten S, Englander S, Orel SG, Nunes LW. A combined architectural and kinetic interpretation model for breast MR images. Acad Radiol 2001;8:591-597.
18. Nunes LW. Architectural-based interpretations of breast MR imaging. Magn Reson Imaging Clin North Am 2001;9:303-320.
19. Ikeda DM. Progress report from the American College of Radiology Breast MR Imaging Lexicon Committee. Magn Reson Imaging Clin North Am 2001;9:295-302.
20. Boetes C, Barentsz JO, Mus RD, et al. MR characterization of suspicious breast lesions with a gadolinium-enhanced TurboFLASH subtraction technique. Radiology 1994;193:777-781.
21. Lee CH, Smith RC, Levine JA, Troiano RN, Tocino I. Clinical useful-ness of MR imaging of the breast in the evaluation of the problematic mammogram. AJR Am J Roentgenol 1999;173:1323-1329.
22. Orel SG. High-resolution MR imaging for the detection, diagnosis, and staging of breast cancer. Radiographics 1998;18:903-912.
23. Orel SG, Dougherty CS, Reynolds C, Czerniecki BJ, Siegelman ES, Schnall MD. MR imaging in patients with nipple discharge: initial experience. Radiology 2000;216:248-254.
24. Orel SG, Weinstein SP, Schnall MD, et al. Breast MR imaging in patients with axillary node metastases and unknown primary malignancy. Radiology 1999;212:543-549.
25. Gilles R, Guinebretiere JM, Toussaint C, et al. Locally advanced breast cancer: contrast-enhanced subtraction MR imaging of response to preoperative chemotherapy. Radiology 1994;191:633-638.
26. Fischer U, Kopka L, Grabbe E. Breast carcinoma: effect of preoperative contrast-enhanced MR imaging on the therapeutic approach. Radiology 1999;213:881-888.
27. Harms SE, Flamig DP, Hesley KL, et al. Fat-suppressed three-dimensional MR imaging of the breast. Radiographics 1993;13:247-267.
28. Orel SG, Reynolds C, Schnall MD, Solin LJ, Fraker DL, Sullivan DC. Breast carcinoma: MR imaging before re-excisional biopsy. Radiology 1997;205:429-436.
29. Frei KA, Kinkel K, Bonel HM, Lu Y, Esserman LJ, Hylton NM. MR imaging of the breast in patients with positive margins after lumpectomy: influence of the time interval between lumpectomy and MR imaging. AJR Am J Roentgenol 2000;175:1577-1584.
30. Viehweg P, Heinig A, Lampe D, Buchmann J, Heywang-Kobrunner SH. Retrospective analysis for evaluation of the value of contrast-enhanced MRI in patients treated with breast conservative therapy. Magma 1998;7:141-152.
31. Daniel BL, Butts K, Glover GH, Cooper C, Herfkens RJ. Breast cancer: gadolinium-enhanced MR imaging with a 0.5-T open imager and three-point Dixon technique. Radiology 1998;207:183-190.
32. Hittmair K, Turetschek K, Gomiscek G, Stiglbauer R, Schurawitzki H. Field strength dependence of MRI contrast enhancement: phantom measurements and application to dynamic breast imaging. Br J Radiol 1996;69:215-220.
33. Sinha S, Gorczyca DP, DeBruhl ND, Shellock FG, Gausche VR, Bassett LW. MR imaging of silicone breast implants: comparison of different coil arrays. Radiology 1993;187:284-286.
34. Sun L, Olsen JO, Robitaille PM. Design and optimization of a breast coil for magnetic resonance imaging. Magn Reson Imaging 1993;11:73-80.
35. Konyer NB, Ramsay EA, Bronskill MJ, Plewes DB. Comparison of MR imaging breast coils. Radiology 2002;222:830-834.
36. Insko EK, Connick TJ, Schnall MD, Orel SG. Multicoil array for high resolution imaging of the breast. Magn Reson Med 1997;37:778-784.
37. Greenman RL, Lenkinski RE, Schnall MD. Bilateral imaging using separate interleaved 3D volumes and dynamically switched multiple receive coil arrays. Magn Reson Med 1998;39:108-115.
38. Stelling CB, Wang PC, Lieber A, Mattingly SS, Griffen WO, Powell DE. Prototype coil for magnetic resonance imaging of the female breast: work in progress. Radiology 1985;154:457-462.
39. Hylton NM, Frankel SD. Imaging techniques for breast MR imaging. Magn Reson Imaging Clin North Am 1994;2:511-525.
40. Sambrook M, Bamber JC, Minasian H, Hill CR. Ultrasonic Doppler study of the hormonal response of blood flow in the normal human breast. Ultrasound Med Biol 1987;13:121-129.
41. Muller-Schimpfle M, Ohmenhauser K, Stoll P, Dietz K, Claussen CD. Menstrual cycle and age: influence on parenchymal contrast medium enhancement in MR imaging of the breast. Radiology 1997;203:145-149.
42. Kuhl CK, Bieling HB, Gieseke J, et al. Healthy premenopausal breast parenchyma in dynamic contrast-enhanced MR imaging of the breast: normal contrast medium enhancement and cyclical-phase dependency. Radiology 1997;203:137-144.
43. Rieber A, Nussle K, Merkle E, Kreienberg R, Tomczak R, Brambs HJ. MR mammography: influence of menstrual cycle on the dynamic contrast enhancement of fibrocystic disease. Eur Radiol 1999;9:1107-1112.
44. Kinkel K, Hylton NM. Challenges to interpretation of breast MRI. J Magn Reson Imaging 2001;13:821-829.
45. Heywang SH, Wolf A, Pruss E, Hilbertz T, Eiermann W, Permanetter W. MR imaging of the breast with Gd-DTPA: use and limitations. Radiology 1989;171:95-103.
46. Friedman EP, Hall-Craggs MA, Mumtaz H, Schneidau A. Breast MR and the appearance of the normal and abnormal nipple. Clin Radiol 1997;52:854-861.
47. Adusumilli S, Siegelman ES, Schnall MD. MR Findings of nipple adenoma. AJR Am J Roentgenol 2002;179:803-804.
48. Nakahara H, Namba K, Fukami A, et al. Three-dimensional MR imaging of mammographically detected suspicious microcalcifications. Breast Cancer 2001;8:116-124.
49. Talele AC, Slanetz PJ, Edmister WB, Yeh ED, Kopans DB. The lactating breast: MRI findings and literature review. Breast J 2003;9:237-240.
50. Bright RA, Moore RM, Jr. Estimating the prevalence of women with breast implants. [Comment.] Am J Public Health 1996;86:891-892.
51. Cook RR, Perkins LL. The prevalence of breast implants among women in the United States. Curr Top Microbiol Immunol 1996;210:419-425.
52. Berg WA, Caskey CI, Hamper UM, et al. Single- and double-lumen silicone breast implant integrity: prospective evaluation of MR and US criteria. Radiology 1995;197:45-52.
53. Berg WA, Nguyen TK, Middleton MS, Soo MS, Pennello G, Brown SL. MR imaging of extracapsular silicone from breast implants: diagnostic pitfalls. AJR Am J Roentgenol 2002;178:465-472.
54. Gorczyca DP, Schneider E, DeBruhl ND, et al. Silicone breast implant rupture: comparison between three-point Dixon and fast spin-echo MR imaging. AJR Am J Roentgenol 1994;162:305-310.
55. Gorczyca DP, Sinha S, Ahn CY, et al. Silicone breast implants in vivo: MR imaging. Radiology 1992;185:407-410.
56. Gorczyca DP. MR imaging of breast implants. Magn Reson Imaging Clin N Am 1994;2:659-672.
57. Berg WA, Caskey CI, Hamper UM, et al. Single- and double-lumen silicone breast implant integrity: prospective evaluation of MR and US criteria. Radiology 1995;197:45-52.
58. Schneider E, Chan TW. Selective MR imaging of silicone with the three-point Dixon technique. Radiology 1993;187:89-93.
59. Monticciolo DL, Nelson RC, Dixon WT, Bostwick J III, Mukundan S, Hester TR. MR detection of leakage from silicone breast implants: value of a silicone-selective pulse sequence. AJR Am J Roentgenol 1994;163:51-56.
60. Murphy TJ, Piccoli CW, Mitchell DG. Correlation of single-lumen silicone implant integrity with chemical shift artifact on T2-weighted magnetic resonance images. J Magn Reson Imaging 2002;15:159-164.
61. Middleton MS. Magnetic resonance evaluation of breast implants and soft-tissue silicone. Top Magn Reson Imaging 1998;9:92-137.

62. Gorczyca DP. MR imaging of breast implants. Magn Reson Imaging Clin North Am 1994;2:659-672.

63. Berg WA, Anderson ND, Zerhouni EA, Chang BW, Kuhlman JE. MR imaging of the breast in patients with silicone breast implants: normal postoperative variants and diagnostic pitfalls. AJR Am J Roentgenol 1994;163:575-578.

64. Jemal A, Tiwari RC, Murray T, et al. Cancer Statistics, 2004. CA Cancer J Clin 2004;54:8-29.

65. Turner DA, Alcorn FS, Shorey WD, et al. Carcinoma of the breast: detection with MR imaging versus xeromammography. Radiology 1988;168:49-58.

66. Harms SE, Flamig DP. MR imaging of the breast: technical approach and clinical experience. Radiographics 1993;13:905-912.

67. Hylton NM, Kinkel K. Technical aspects of breast magnetic resonance imaging. Top Magn Reson Imaging 1998;9:3-16.

68. Flanagan FL, Murray JG, Gilligan P, Stack JP, Ennis JT. Digital subtraction in Gd-DTPA enhanced imaging of the breast. Clin Radiol 1995;50:848-854.

69. Heywang-Kobrunner SH, Wolf HD, Deimling M, Kosling S, Hofer H, Spielmann RP. Misleading changes of the signal intensity on opposed-phase MRI after injection of contrast medium. J Comput Assist Tomogr 1996;20:173-178.

70. Stack JP, Redmond OM, Codd MB, Dervan PA, Ennis JT. Breast disease: tissue characterization with Gd-DTPA enhancement profiles. Radiology 1990;174:491-494.

71. Flickinger FW, Allison JD, Sherry RM, Wright JC. Differentiation of benign from malignant breast masses by time-intensity evaluation of contrast enhanced MRI. Magn Reson Imaging 1993;11:617-620.

72. Gilles R, Guinebretiere JM, Lucidarme O, et al. Nonpalpable breast tumors: diagnosis with contrast-enhanced subtraction dynamic MR imaging. Radiology 1994;191:625-631.

73. Hulka CA, Edmister WB, Smith BL, et al. Dynamic echo-planar imaging of the breast: experience in diagnosing breast carcinoma and correlation with tumor angiogenesis. Radiology 1997;205: 837-842.

74. Hulka CA, Smith BL, Sgroi DC, et al. Benign and malignant breast lesions: differentiation with echo-planar MR imaging. Radiology 1995;197:33-38.

75. Kelcz F, Santyr GE, Cron GO, Mongin SJ. Application of a quantitative model to differentiate benign from malignant breast lesions detected by dynamic, gadolinium-enhanced MRI. J Magn Reson Imaging 1996;6:743-752.

76. Knopp MV, Brix G, Junkermann HJ, Sinn HP. MR mammography with pharmacokinetic mapping for monitoring of breast cancer treatment during neoadjuvant therapy. Magn Reson Imaging Clin North Am 1994;2:633-658.

77. Tofts PS, Berkowitz B, Schnall MD. Quantitative analysis of dynamic Gd-DTPA enhancement in breast tumors using a permeability model. Magn Reson Med 1995;33:564-568.

78. Port RE, Knopp MV, Hoffmann U, Milker-Zabel S, Brix G. Multicompartment analysis of gadolinium chelate kinetics: blood-tissue exchange in mammary tumors as monitored by dynamic MR imaging. J Magn Reson Imaging 1999;10:233-241.

79. Mussurakis S, Buckley DL, Horsman A. Dynamic MRI of invasive breast cancer: assessment of three region-of-interest analysis methods. J Comput Assist Tomogr 1997;21:431-438.

80. Gribbestad IS, Nilsen G, Fjosne HE, Kvinnsland S, Haugen OA, Rinck PA. Comparative signal intensity measurements in dynamic gadolinium-enhanced MR mammography. J Magn Reson Imaging 1994;4:477-480.

81. Liney GP, Gibbs P, Hayes C, Leach MO, Turnbull LW. Dynamic contrast-enhanced MRI in the differentiation of breast tumors: user-defined versus semi-automated region-of-interest analysis. J Magn Reson Imaging 1999;10:945-949.

82. Muller-Schimpfle M, Ohmenhauser K, Sand J, Stoll P, Claussen CD. Dynamic 3D-MR mammography: is there a benefit of sophisticated evaluation of enhancement curves for clinical routine? J Magn Reson Imaging 1997;7:236-240.

83. Buckley DL, Mussurakis S, Horsman A. Effect of temporal resolution on the diagnostic efficacy of contrast-enhanced MRI in the conservatively treated breast. J Comput Assist Tomogr 1998;22:47-51.

84. Degani H, Gusis V, Weinstein D, Fields S, Strano S. Mapping pathophysiological features of breast tumors by MRI at high spatial resolution. Nature Med 1997;3:780-782.

85. Kinkel K, Helbich TH, Esserman LJ, et al. Dynamic high-spatial-resolution MR imaging of suspicious breast lesions: diagnostic criteria and interobserver variability. AJR Am J Roentgenol 2000;175:35-43.

86. Furman-Haran E, Grobgeld D, Kelcz F, Degani H. Critical role of spatial resolution in dynamic contrast-enhanced breast MRI. J Magn Reson Imaging 2001;13:862-867.

87. Kuhl CK, Mielcareck P, Klaschik S, et al. Dynamic breast MR imaging: are signal intensity time course data useful for differential diagnosis of enhancing lesions? [Comments.] Radiology 1999;211:101-110.

88. Sherif H, Mahfouz AE, Oellinger H, et al. Peripheral washout sign on contrast-enhanced MR images of the breast. Radiology 1997;205:209-213.

89. Siegmann KC, Muller-Schimpfle M, Schick F, et al. MR imaging-detected breast lesions: histopathologic correlation of lesion characteristics and signal intensity data. AJR Am J Roentgenol 2002;178:1403-1409.

90. Ikeda O, Yamashita Y, Morishita S, et al. Characterization of breast masses by dynamic enhanced MR imaging: a logistic regression analysis. Acta Radiol 1999;40:585-592.

91. Bassett LW. Imaging of breast masses. Radiol Clin North Am 2000;38:669-691.

92. Schnall MD, Ikeda DM. Lesion Diagnosis Working Group report. J Magn Reson Imaging 1999;10:982-990.

93. Ikeda DM, Baker DR, Daniel BL. Magnetic resonance imaging of breast cancer: clinical indications and breast MRI reporting system. J Magn Reson Imaging 2000;12:975-983.

94. Ikeda DM, Birdwell RL, Daniel BL. Potential role of magnetic resonance imaging and other modalities in ductal carcinoma in situ detection. Magn Reson Imaging Clin North Am 2001;9:345-356.

95. Nunes LW, Schnall MD, Orel SG, et al. Correlation of lesion appearance and histologic findings for the nodes of a breast MR imaging interpretation model. Radiographics 1999;19:79-92.

96. Nunes LW, Schnall MD, Orel SG. Update of breast MR imaging architectural interpretation model. Radiology 2001;219:484-494.

97. Matsubayashi R, Matsuo Y, Edakuni G, Satoh T, Tokunaga O, Kudo S. Breast masses with peripheral rim enhancement on dynamic contrast-enhanced MR images: correlation of MR findings with histologic features and expression of growth factors. Radiology 2000;217:841-848.

98. Mussurakis S, Gibbs P, Horsman A. Peripheral enhancement and spatial contrast uptake heterogeneity of primary breast tumours: quantitative assessment with dynamic MRI. J Comput Assist Tomogr 1998;22:35-46.

99. Issa B, Buckley DL, Turnbull LW. Heterogeneity analysis of Gd-DTPA uptake: improvement in breast lesion differentiation. J Comput Assist Tomogr 1999;23:615-621.

100. Buadu LD, Murakami J, Murayama S, et al. Breast lesions: correlation of contrast medium enhancement patterns on MR images with histopathologic findings and tumor angiogenesis. Radiology 1996;200:639-649.

101. Hochman MG, Orel SG, Powell CM, Schnall MD, Reynolds CA, White LN. Fibroadenomas: MR imaging appearances with radiologic-histopathologic correlation. Radiology 1997;204: 123-129.

102. Liberman L, Morris EA, Lee MJ, et al. Breast lesions detected on MR imaging: features and positive predictive value. AJR Am J Roentgenol 2002;179:171-178.

103. Kuhl CK. MRI of breast tumors. Eur Radiol 2000;10:46-58.

104. Kuhl CK, Schild HH. Dynamic image interpretation of MRI of the breast. J Magn Reson Imaging 2000;12:965-974.

105. Satake H, Shimamoto K, Sawaki A, et al. Role of ultrasonography in the detection of intraductal spread of breast cancer: correlation with pathologic findings, mammography and MR imaging. Eur Radiol 2000;10:1726-1732.

106. Gilles R, Zafrani B, Guinebretiere JM, et al. Ductal carcinoma in situ: MR imaging-histopathologic correlation. Radiology 1995; 196:415-419.

107. Soderstrom CE, Harms SE, Copit DS, et al. Three-dimensional RODEO breast MR imaging of lesions containing ductal carcinoma in situ. Radiology 1996;201:427-432.

108. Viehweg P, Lampe D, Buchmann J, Heywang-Kobrunner SH. In situ and minimally invasive breast cancer: morphologic and kinetic features on contrast-enhanced MR imaging. Magma 2000;11:129-137.

109. Liberman L, Morris EA, Dershaw DD, Abramson AF, Tan LK. Ductal enhancement on MR imaging of the breast. AJR Am J Roentgenol 2003;181:519-525.

110. Fischer U, Kopka L, Grabbe E. Invasive mucinous carcinoma of the breast missed by contrast-enhancing MR imaging of the breast. Eur Radiol 1996;6:929-931.

111. Miller RW, Harms S, Alvarez A. Mucinous carcinoma of the breast: potential false-negative MR imaging interpretation. AJR Am J Roentgenol 1996;167:539-540.

112. Kawashima M, Tamaki Y, Nonaka T, et al. MR imaging of mucinous carcinoma of the breast. AJR Am J Roentgenol 2002;179:179-183.

113. Rovno HD, Siegelman ES, Reynolds C, Orel SG, Schnall MD. Solitary intraductal papilloma: findings at MR imaging and MR galactography. AJR Am J Roentgenol 1999;172:151-155.

114. Yu JS, Rofsky NM. Dynamic subtraction MR imaging of the liver: advantages and pitfalls. AJR Am J Roentgenol 2003;180: 1351-1357.

115. Denton ER, Sonoda LI, Rueckert D, et al. Comparison and evaluation of rigid, affine, and nonrigid registration of breast MR images. J Comput Assist Tomogr 1999;23:800-805.

116. Zuo CS, Jiang A, Buff BL, Mahon TG, Wong TZ. Automatic motion correction for breast MR imaging. Radiology 1996; 198:903-906.

117. Alleva DQ, Smetherman DH, Farr GH, Jr., Cederbom GJ. Radial scar of the breast: radiologic-pathologic correlation in 22 cases. Radiographics 1999;19:S27-35; discussion S36-27.

118. Baum F, Fischer U, Fuzesi L, Obenauer S, Vosshenrich R, Grabbe E. [The radial scar in contrast media-enhanced MR mammography.] Rofo Fortschr Geb Rontgenstr Neuen Bildgeb Verfahr 2000;172:817-823.

119. Bilgen IG, Ustun EE, Memis A. Fat necrosis of the breast: clinical, mammographic and sonographic features. Eur J Radiol 2001;39:92-99.

120. Bassett LW, Gold RH, Cove HC. Mammographic spectrum of traumatic fat necrosis: the fallibility of "pathognomonic" signs of carcinoma. AJR Am J Roentgenol 1978;130:119-122.

121. Coady AM, Mussurakis S, Owen AW, Turnbull LW. Case report: MR imaging of fat necrosis of the breast associated with lipid cyst for-mation following conservative treatment for breast carcinoma. Clin Radiol 1996;51:815-817.

122. Solomon B, Orel S, Reynolds C, Schnall M. Delayed development of enhancement in fat necrosis after breast conservation therapy: a potential pitfall of MR imaging of the breast. AJR Am J Roentgenol 1998;170:966-968.

123. Kinoshita T, Yashiro N, Yoshigi J, Ihara N, Narita M. Fat necrosis of breast: a potential pitfall in breast MRI. Clin Imaging 2002;26: 250-253.

124. Gilles R, Guinebretiere JM, Shapeero LG, et al. Assessment of breast cancer recurrence with contrast-enhanced subtraction MR imaging: preliminary results in 26 patients. Radiology 1993;188:473-478.

125. Villeirs G, Van Damme S, Heydanus R, Serreyn R, Kunnen M, Mortier M. Heparin-induced thrombocytopenia and fat necrosis of the breast. Eur Radiol 2000;10:527-530.

126. Svane G, Franzen S. Radiologic appearance of nonpalpable intramammary lymph nodes. Acta Radiol 1993;34:577-580.

127. McSweeney MB, Egan RL. Prognosis of breast cancer related to intramammary lymph nodes. Recent Results Cancer Res 1984;90:166-172.

128. Gallardo X, Sentis M, Castaner E, Andreu X, Darnell A, Canalias J. Enhancement of intramammary lymph nodes with lymphoid hyperplasia: a potential pitfall in breast MRI. Eur Radiol 1998;8:1662-1665.

129. Braunstein GD. Gynecomastia. [Comment.] N Engl J Med 1993;328:490-495.

130. Evans DB, Crichlow RW. Carcinoma of the male breast and Klinefelter's syndrome: is there an association? CA Cancer J Clin 1987;37:246-251.

131. Jackson VP, Gilmor RL. Male breast carcinoma and gynecomastia: comparison of mammography with sonography. Radiology 1983; 149:533-536.

132. Tochika N, Takano A, Yoshimoto T, et al. Intracystic carcinoma of the male breast: report of a case. Surg Today 2001;31:806-809.

133. Hunter TB, Roberts CC, Hunt KR, Fajardo LL. Occurrence of fibroadenomas in postmenopausal women referred for breast biopsy. J Am Geriatr Soc 1996;44:61-64.

134. Jackson VP, Rothschild PA, Kreipke DL, Mail JT, Holden RW. The spectrum of sonographic findings of fibroadenoma of the breast. Invest Radiol 1986;21:34-40.

135. Kuhl CK, Klaschik S, Mielcarek P, Gieseke J, Wardelmann E, Schild HH. Do T2-weighted pulse sequences help with the differential diagnosis of enhancing lesions in dynamic breast MRI? J Magn Reson Imaging 1999;9:187-196.

136. Kawashima M, Tamaki Y, Nonaka T, et al. MR imaging of mucinous carcinoma of the breast. AJR Am J Roentgenol 2002;179: 179-183.

137. Farria DM, Gorczyca DP, Barsky SH, Sinha S, Bassett LW. Benign phyllodes tumor of the breast: MR imaging features. AJR Am J Roentgenol 1996;167:187-189.

138. Brinck U, Fischer U, Korabiowska M, Jutrowski M, Schauer A, Grabbe E. The variability of fibroadenoma in contrast-enhanced dynamic MR mammography. AJR Am J Roentgenol 1997; 168:1331-1334.

139. Weinstein D, Strano S, Cohen P, Fields S, Gomori JM, Degani H. Breast fibroadenoma: mapping of pathophysiologic features with three-time-point, contrast-enhanced MR imaging—pilot study. Radiology 1999;210:233-240.

140. Weind KL, Maier CF, Rutt BK, Moussa M. Invasive carcinomas and fibroadenomas of the breast: comparison of microvessel distributions—implications for imaging modalities. Radiology 1998;208:477-483.

141. Woods ER, Helvie MA, Ikeda DM, Mandell SH, Chapel KL, Adler DD. Solitary breast papilloma: comparison of mammographic, galactographic, and pathologic findings. AJR Am J Roentgenol 1992;159:487-491.

142. Cardenosa G, Eklund GW. Benign papillary neoplasms of the breast: mammographic findings. Radiology 1991;181:751-755.

143. Yang WT, Suen M, Metreweli C. Sonographic features of benign papillary neoplasms of the breast: review of 22 patients. J Ultrasound Med 1997;16:161-168.

144. March DE, Coughlin BF, Polino JR, Goulart RA, Makari-Judson G. Single dilated lactiferous duct due to papilloma: ultrasonographically guided percutaneous biopsy with a vacuum-assisted device. J Ultrasound Med 2002;21:107-111.

145. Kramer SC, Rieber A, Gorich J, et al. Diagnosis of papillomas of the breast: value of magnetic resonance mammography in comparison with galactography. Eur Radiol 2000;10:1733-1736.

146. Weinzweig N, Botts J, Marcus E. Giant hamartoma of the breast. Plast Reconstr Surg 2001;107:1216-1220.

147. Kievit HC, Sikkenk AC, Thelissen GR, Merchant TE. Magnetic resonance image appearance of hamartoma of the breast. Magn Reson Imaging 1993;11:293-298.

148. Nunes LW. Architectural-based interpretations of breast MR imaging. Magn Reson Imaging Clin N Am 2001;9:303-320, vi.

149. Rapin V, Contesso G, Mouriesse H, et al. Medullary breast carcinoma. A reevaluation of 95 cases of breast cancer with inflammatory stroma. Cancer 1988;61:2503-2510.

150. Ridolfi RL, Rosen PP, Port A, Kinne D, Mike V. Medullary carcinoma of the breast: a clinicopathologic study with 10 year follow-up. Cancer 1977;40:1365-1385.

151. Meyer JE, Amin E, Lindfors KK, Lipman JC, Stomper PC, Genest D. Medullary carcinoma of the breast: mammographic and US appearance. Radiology 1989;170:79-82.

152. Newcomer LM, Newcomb PA, Trentham-Dietz A, et al. Detection method and breast carcinoma histology. Cancer 2002;95:470-477.

153. Holland DW, Boucher LD, Mortimer JE. Tubular breast cancer experience at Washington University: a review of the literature. Clin Breast Cancer 2001;2:210-214.

154. Chopra S, Evans AJ, Pinder SE, et al. Pure mucinous breast cancer—mammographic and ultrasound findings. Clin Radiol 1996;51:421-424.

155. Goodman DN, Boutross-Tadross O, Jong RA. Mammographic features of pure mucinous carcinoma of the breast with pathological correlation. Can Assoc Radiol J 1995;46:296-301.

156. Wilson TE, Helvie MA, Oberman HA, Joynt LK. Pure and mixed mucinous carcinoma of the breast: pathologic basis for differences in mammographic appearance. AJR Am J Roentgenol 1995;165:285-289.

157. Isomoto I, Koshiishi T, Okimoto T, Okada H, Uetani M, Hayashi K. Gradually enhancing breast cancer on dynamic MRI. Nippon Igaku Hoshasen Gakkai Zasshi—Nippon Acta Radiol 2000;60:514-519.

158. Li CI, Anderson BO, Daling JR, Moe RE. Trends in incidence rates of invasive lobular and ductal breast carcinoma. JAMA 2003;289:1421-1424.

159. Li CI, Anderson BO, Porter P, Holt SK, Daling JR, Moe RE. Changing incidence rate of invasive lobular breast carcinoma among older women. [Comment.] Cancer 2000;88:2561-2569.

160. Sickles EA. The subtle and atypical mammographic features of invasive lobular carcinoma. [Comment.] Radiology 1991;178:25-26.

161. Krecke KN, Gisvold JJ. Invasive lobular carcinoma of the breast: mammographic findings and extent of disease at diagnosis in 184 patients. AJR Am J Roentgenol 1993;161:957-960.

162. Moore MM, Borossa G, Imbrie JZ, et al. Association of infiltrating lobular carcinoma with positive surgical margins after breast-conservation therapy. Ann Surg 2000;231:877-882.

163. Lesser ML, Rosen PP, Kinne DW. Multicentricity and bilaterality in invasive breast carcinoma. Surgery 1982;91:234-240.

164. Slanetz PJ, Edmister WB, Yeh ED, Talele AC, Kopans DB. Occult contralateral breast carcinoma incidentally detected by breast magnetic resonance imaging. Breast J 2002;8:145-148.

165. Broet P, de la Rochefordiere A, Scholl SM, et al. Contralateral breast cancer: annual incidence and risk parameters. J Clin Oncol 1995;13:1578-1583.

166. Qayyum A, Birdwell RL, Daniel BL, et al. MR imaging features of infiltrating lobular carcinoma of the breast: histopathologic correlation. AJR Am J Roentgenol 2002;178:1227-1232.

167. Weinstein SP, Orel SG, Heller R, et al. MR imaging of the breast in patients with invasive lobular carcinoma. AJR Am J Roentgenol 2001;176:399-406.

168. Rodenko GN, Harms SE, Pruneda JM, et al. MR imaging in the management before surgery of lobular carcinoma of the breast: correlation with pathology. AJR Am J Roentgenol 1996;167:1415-1419.

169. Munot K, Dall B, Achuthan R, Parkin G, Lane S, Horgan K. Role of magnetic resonance imaging in the diagnosis and single-stage surgical resection of invasive lobular carcinoma of the breast. Br J Surg 2002;89:1296-1301.

170. Mumtaz H, Hall-Craggs MA, Davidson T, et al. Staging of symptomatic primary breast cancer with MR imaging. AJR Am J Roentgenol 1997;169:417-424.

171. Boetes C, Mus RD, Holland R, et al. Breast tumors: comparative accuracy of MR imaging relative to mammography and US for demonstrating extent. Radiology 1995;197:743-747.

172. Teifke A, Hlawatsch A, Beier T, et al. Undetected malignancies of the breast: dynamic contrast-enhanced MR imaging at 1.0 T. Radiology 2002;224:881-888.

173. Dershaw DD, Moore MP, Liberman L, Deutch BM. Inflammatory breast carcinoma: mammographic findings. Radiology 1994;190:831-834.

174. Gunhan-Bilgen I, Ustun EE, Memi A. Inflammatory breast carcinoma: mammographic, ultrasonographic, clinical, and pathologic findings in 142 cases. Radiology 2002;223:829-838.

175. Kushwaha AC, Whitman GJ, Stelling CB, Cristofanilli M, Buzdar AU. Primary inflammatory carcinoma of the breast: retrospective review of mammographic findings. AJR Am J Roentgenol 2000;174:535-538.

176. Rieber A, Merkle E, Bohm W, Brambs HJ, Tomczak R. MRI of histologically confirmed mammary carcinoma: clinical relevance of diagnostic procedures for detection of multifocal or contralateral secondary carcinoma. J Comput Assist Tomogr 1997;21:773-779.

177. Fischer U, Vosshenrich R, von Heyden D, Knipper H, Oestmann JW, Grabbe E. [Inflammatory lesions of the breast: indication for MR-mammography?]. Rofo Fortschr Geb Rontgenstr Neuen Bildgeb Verfahr 1994;161:307-311.

178. Rieber A, Tomczak RJ, Mergo PJ, Wenzel V, Zeitler H, Brambs HJ. MRI of the breast in the differential diagnosis of mastitis versus inflammatory carcinoma and follow-up. J Comput Assist Tomogr 1997;21:128-132.

179. Dershaw DD, Abramson A, Kinne DW. Ductal carcinoma in situ: mammographic findings and clinical implications. Radiology 1989;170:411-415.

180. Ikeda DM, Andersson I. Ductal carcinoma in situ: atypical mammographic appearances. [Comment.] Radiology 1989;172:661-666.

181. Orel SG, Mendonca MH, Reynolds C, Schnall MD, Solin LJ, Sullivan DC. MR imaging of ductal carcinoma in situ. Radiology 1997;202:413-420.

182. Daniel BL, Yen YF, Glover GH, et al. Breast disease: dynamic spiral MR imaging. Radiology 1998;209:499-509.

183. Boetes C, Strijk SP, Holland R, Barentsz JO, Van Der Sluis RF, Ruijs JH. False-negative MR imaging of malignant breast tumors. Eur Radiol 1997;7:1231-1234.

184. Fobben ES, Rubin CZ, Kalisher L, Dembner AG, Seltzer MH, Santoro EJ. Breast MR imaging with commercially available techniques: radiologic-pathologic correlation. Radiology 1995;196:143-152.

185. Ceccherini AF, Evans AJ, Pinder SE, Wilson AR, Ellis IO, Yeoman LJ. Is ipsilateral mammography worthwhile in Paget's disease of the breast? Clin Radiol 1996;51:35-38.

186. Burke ET, Braeuning MP, McLelland R, Pisano ED, Cooper LL. Paget disease of the breast: a pictorial essay. Radiographics 1998;18:1459-1464.

187. Sawyer RH, Asbury DL. Mammographic appearances in Paget's disease of the breast. Clin Radiol 1994;49:185-188.

188. Reinfuss M, Mitu SJ, Smolak K, Stelmach A. Malignant phyllodes tumours of the breast: a clinical and pathological analysis of 55 cases. Eur J Cancer 1993;29A:1252-1256.

189. Cohn-Cedermark G, Rutqvist LE, Rosendahl I, Silfversward C. Prognostic factors in cystosarcoma phyllodes: a clinicopathologic study of 77 patients. Cancer 1991;68:2017-2022.

190. Foster ME, Garrahan N, Williams S. Fibroadenoma of the breast: a clinical and pathological study. J R Coll Surg Edinb 1988;33:16-19.

191. Cosmacini P, Zurrida S, Veronesi P, Bartoli C, Coopmans de Yoldi GF. Phyllode tumor of the breast: mammographic experience in 99 cases. Eur J Radiol 1992;15:11-14.

192. Page JE, Williams JE. The radiological features of phylloides tumour of the breast with clinico-pathological correlation. Clin Radiol 1991;44:8-12.

193. Liberman L, Bonaccio E, Hamele-Bena D, Abramson AF, Cohen MA, Dershaw DD. Benign and malignant phyllodes tumors: mammographic and sonographic findings. Radiology 1996;198:121-124.

194. Jorge Blanco A, Vargas Serrano B, Rodriguez Romero R, Martinez Cendejas E. Phyllodes tumors of the breast. Eur Radiol 1999;9:356-360.

195. Ogawa Y, Nishioka A, Tsuboi N, et al. Dynamic MR appearance of benign phyllodes tumor of the breast in a 20-year-old woman. Radiat Med 1997;15:247-250.

196. Cheung HS, Tse GM, Ma TK. "Leafy" pattern in phyllodes tumour of the breast: MRI-pathologic correlation. Clin Radiol 2002;57:230-231.

197. Orel SG, Schnall MD. MR imaging of the breast for the detection, diagnosis, and staging of breast cancer. Radiology 2001;220:13-30.

198. Kelcz F, Santyr G. Gadolinium-enhanced breast MRI. Crit Rev Diagn Imaging 1995;36:287-338.

199. Stomper PC, Herman S, Klippenstein DL, et al. Suspect breast lesions: findings at dynamic gadolinium-enhanced MR imaging correlated with mammographic and pathologic features. Radiology 1995;197:387-395.

200. Brown J, Smith RC, Lee CH. Incidental enhancing lesions found on MR imaging of the breast. AJR Am J Roentgenol 2001;176:1249-1254.

201. Winchester D. Nipple discharge. In: Harris JR, Lippman ME, Morrow M, Hellman S (Eds.). Diseases of the Breast. Philadelphia: Lippincott-Raven, 1996, pp 106-109.

202. Forurquet A, De La Rochefordiere A, Campana, F. Occult primary cancer with axillary metastases. In: Harris JR, Lippman ME, Morrow M, Hellman S (Eds.). Diseases of the Breast. Philadelphia: Lippincott-Raven, 1996, pp 892-896.

203. Knapper WH. Management of occult breast cancer presenting as an axillary metastasis. Semin Surg Oncol 1991;7:311-313.

204. Baron PL, Moore MP, Kinne DW, Candela FC, Osborne MP, Petrek JA. Occult breast cancer presenting with axillary metastases: updated management. Arch Surg 1990;125:210-214.

205. Brenner RJ, Rothman BJ. Detection of primary breast cancer in women with known adenocarcinoma metastatic to the axilla: use of MRI after negative clinical and mammographic examination. J Magn Reson Imaging 1997;7:1153-1158.

206. Obdeijn IM, Brouwers-Kuyper EM, Tilanus-Linthorst MM, Wiggers T, Oudkerk M. MR imaging-guided sonography followed by fine-needle aspiration cytology in occult carcinoma of the breast. AJR Am J Roentgenol 2000;174:1079-1084.

207. Morris EA, Schwartz LH, Dershaw DD, van Zee KJ, Abramson AF, Liberman L. MR imaging of the breast in patients with occult primary breast carcinoma. Radiology 1997;205:437-440.

208. Schorn C, Fischer U, Luftner-Nagel S, Westerhof JP, Grabbe E. MRI of the breast in patients with metastatic disease of unknown primary. Eur Radiol 1999;9:470-473.

209. Mumtaz H, Davidson T, Hall-Craggs MA, et al. Comparison of magnetic resonance imaging and conventional triple assessment in locally recurrent breast cancer. Br J Surg 1997;84:1147-1151.

210. Esserman L, Hylton N, Yassa L, Barclay J, Frankel S, Sickles E. Utility of magnetic resonance imaging in the management of breast cancer: evidence for improved preoperative staging. J Clin Oncol 1999;17:110-119.

211. Drew PJ, Chatterjee S, Turnbull LW, et al. Dynamic contrast enhanced magnetic resonance imaging of the breast is superior to triple assessment for the preoperative detection of multifocal breast cancer. Ann Surg Oncol 1999;6:599-603.

212. Drew PJ, Turnbull LW, Chatterjee S, et al. Prospective comparison of standard triple assessment and dynamic magnetic resonance imaging of the breast for the evaluation of symptomatic breast lesions. Ann Surg 1999;230:680-685.

213. Orel SG, Schnall MD, Powell CM, et al. Staging of suspected breast cancer: effect of MR imaging and MR-guided biopsy. Radiology 1995;196:115-122.

214. Liberman L, Morris EA, Dershaw DD, Abramson AF, Tan LK. MR imaging of the ipsilateral breast in women with percutaneously proven breast cancer. AJR Am J Roentgenol 2003;180:901-910.

215. Morris EA, Schwartz LH, Drotman MB, et al. Evaluation of pectoralis major muscle in patients with posterior breast tumors on breast MR images: early experience. Radiology 2000;214:67-72.

216. Yoshimura G, Sakurai T, Oura S, et al. Evaluation of axillary lymph node status in breast cancer with MRI. Breast Cancer 1999;6:249-258.

217. Murray AD, Staff RT, Redpath TW, et al. Dynamic contrast enhanced MRI of the axilla in women with breast cancer: comparison with pathology of excised nodes. Br J Radiol 2002;75:220-228.

218. Mussurakis S, Buckley DL, Horsman A. Dynamic MR imaging of invasive breast cancer: correlation with tumour grade and other histological factors. Br J Radiol 1997;70:446-451.

219. Kvistad KA, Rydland J, Smethurst HB, Lundgren S, Fjosne HE, Haraldseth O. Axillary lymph node metastases in breast cancer: preoperative detection with dynamic contrast-enhanced MRI. Eur Radiol 2000;10:1464-1471.

220. Harisinghani MG, Barentsz J, Hahn PF, et al. Noninvasive detection of clinically occult lymph-node metastases in prostate cancer. N Engl J Med 2003;348:2491-2499.

221. Koh DM, Cook GJ, Husband JE. New horizons in oncologic imaging. N Engl J Med 2003;348:2487-2488.

222. Michel SC, Keller TM, Frohlich JM, et al. Preoperative breast cancer staging: MR imaging of the axilla with ultrasmall superparamagnetic iron oxide enhancement. Radiology 2002;225:527-536.

223. Stets C, Brandt S, Wallis F, Buchmann J, Gilbert FJ, Heywang-Kobrunner SH. Axillary lymph node metastases: a statistical analysis of various parameters in MRI with USPIO. J Magn Reson Imaging 2002;16:60-68.

224. Pittinger TP, Maronian NC, Poulter CA, Peacock JL. Importance of margin status in outcome of breast-conserving surgery for carcinoma. Surgery 1994;116:605-608; discussion 608-609.

225. Park CC, Mitsumori M, Nixon A, et al. Outcome at 8 years after breast-conserving surgery and radiation therapy for invasive breast cancer: influence of margin status and systemic therapy on local recurrence. J Clin Oncol 2000;18:1668-1675.

226. Jardines L, Fowble B, Schultz D, et al. Factors associated with a positive reexcision after excisional biopsy for invasive breast cancer. Surgery 1995;118:803-809.

227. Soderstrom CE, Harms SE, Farrell RS, Jr., Pruneda JM, Flamig DP. Detection with MR imaging of residual tumor in the breast soon after surgery. AJR Am J Roentgenol 1997;168:485-488.

228. Kawashima H, Tawara M, Suzuki M, Matsui O, Kadoya M. Effectiveness of dynamic MRI for diagnosing pericicatricial minimal residual breast cancer following excisional biopsy. Eur J Radiol 2001;40:2-9.

229. Harris J, Morrow M. Treatment of early stage breast cancer. In: Harris JR, Lippman ME, Morrow M, Hellman S (Eds.). Diseases of the Breast. Philadelphia, Lippincott-Raven, 1996, pp 487-547.

230. Gage I, Recht A, Gelman R, et al. Long-term outcome following breast-conserving surgery and radiation therapy. [Comment.] Int J Radiat Oncol Biol Phys 1995;33:245-251.

231. Solin LJ, Fowble BL, Schultz DJ, Rubenstein JR, Goodman RL. The detection of local recurrence after definitive irradiation for early stage carcinoma of the breast: an analysis of the results of breast biopsies performed in previously irradiated breasts. Cancer 1990;65:2497-2502.

232. Lewis-Jones HG, Whitehouse GH, Leinster SJ. The role of magnetic resonance imaging in the assessment of local recurrent breast carcinoma. Clin Radiol 1991;43:197-204.

233. Dao TH, Rahmouni A, Campana F, Laurent M, Asselain B, Fourquet A. Tumor recurrence versus fibrosis in the irradiated breast: differentiation with dynamic gadolinium-enhanced MR imaging. Radiology 1993;187:751-755.

234. Murray AD, Redpath TW, Needham G, Gilbert FJ, Brookes JA, Eremin O. Dynamic magnetic resonance mammography of both breasts following local excision and radiotherapy for breast carcinoma. Br J Radiol 1996;69:594-600.

235. Muuller RD, Barkhausen J, Sauerwein W, Langer R. Assessment of local recurrence after breast-conserving therapy with MRI. J Comput Assist Tomogr 1998;22:408-412.

236. Rieber A, Merkle E, Zeitler H, et al. Value of MR mammography in the detection and exclusion of recurrent breast carcinoma. J Comput Assist Tomogr 1997;21:780-784.

237. Kramer S, Schulz-Wendtland R, Hagedorn K, Bautz W, Lang N. Magnetic resonance imaging in the diagnosis of local recurrences in breast cancer. Anticancer Res 1998;18:2159-2161.

238. Cohen EK, Leonhardt CM, Shumak RS, et al. Magnetic resonance imaging in potential postsurgical recurrence of breast cancer: pitfalls and limitations. Can Assoc Radiol J 1996;47:171-176.

239. LePage MA, Kazerooni EA, Helvie MA, Wilkins EG. Breast reconstruction with TRAM flaps: normal and abnormal appearances at CT. Radiographics 1999;19:1593-1603.

240. Devon-Karpati R. Transverse rectus abdominim myocutaneous flap breast reconstruction: spectum of normal and abnormal MRI findings. Radiographics; in press.

241. Rieber A, Schramm K, Helms G, et al. Breast-conserving surgery and autogenous tissue reconstruction in patients with breast cancer: efficacy of MRI of the breast in the detection of recurrent disease. Eur Radiol 2003;13:780-787.

242. Hortobagyi GN. Multidisciplinary management of advanced primary and metastatic breast cancer. Cancer 1994;74:416-423.

243. Cocconi G, Di Blasio B, Alberti G, Bisagni G, Botti E, Peracchia G. Problems in evaluating response of primary breast cancer to systemic therapy. Breast Cancer Res Treat 1984;4:309-313.

244. Segel MC, Paulus DD, Hortobagyi GN. Advanced primary breast cancer: assessment at mammography of response to induction chemotherapy. Radiology 1988;169:49-54.

245. Esserman L, Kaplan E, Partridge S, et al. MRI phenotype is associated with response to doxorubicin and cyclophosphamide neoadjuvant chemotherapy in stage III breast cancer. Ann Surg Oncol 2001;8:549-559.

246. Tsuboi N, Ogawa Y, Inomata T, et al. Changes in the findings of dynamic MRI by preoperative CAF chemotherapy for patients with breast cancer of stage II and III: pathologic correlation. Oncol Rep 1999;6:727-732.

247. Abraham DC, Jones RC, Jones SE, et al. Evaluation of neoadjuvant chemotherapeutic response of locally advanced breast cancer by magnetic resonance imaging. Cancer 1996;78:91-100.

248. Drew PJ, Kerin MJ, Mahapatra T, et al. Evaluation of response to neoadjuvant chemoradiotherapy for locally advanced breast cancer with dynamic contrast-enhanced MRI of the breast. Eur J Surg Oncol 2001;27:617-620.

249. Nakamura S, Kenjo H, Nishio T, Kazama T, Do O, Suzuki K. 3D-MR mammography-guided breast conserving surgery after neoadjuvant chemotherapy: clinical results and future perspectives with reference to FDG-PET. Breast Cancer 2001; 8:351-354.

250. Weatherall PT, Evans GF, Metzger GJ, Saborrian MH, Leitch AM. MRI vs. histologic measurement of breast cancer following chemotherapy: comparison with x-ray mammography and palpation. J Magn Reson Imaging 2001;13:868-875.

251. Rosen E, Blackwell KL, Baker JA, et al. Accuracy of MRI in the detection of residual breast cancer after neoadjuvant chemotherapy. AJR Am J Roentgenol 2003;181:1275-1282.

252. Rieber A, Zeitler H, Rosenthal H, et al. MRI of breast cancer: influence of chemotherapy on sensitivity. Br J Radiol 1997;70: 452-458.

253. Wasser K, Sinn HP, Fink C, et al. Accuracy of tumor size measurement in breast cancer using MRI is influenced by histological regression induced by neoadjuvant chemotherapy. Eur Radiol 2003;13:1213-1223.

254. Mumtaz H, Davidson T, Spittle M, et al. Breast surgery after neoadjuvant treatment: is it necessary? Eur J Surg Oncol 1996;22:335-341.

255. Brody LC, Biesecker BB. Breast cancer susceptibility genes: BRCA1 and BRCA2. Medicine 1998;77:208-226.

256. Claus EB, Schildkraut JM, Thompson WD, Risch NJ. The genetic attributable risk of breast and ovarian cancer. Cancer 1996;77: 2318-2324.

257. Garber J, Smith BL. Management of the high-risk and the concerned patient. In: Harris JR, Lippman ME, Morrow M, Hellman S (Eds.). Diseases of the Breast. Philadelphia, Lippincott-Raven, 1996, pp 323-334.

258. Tilanus-Linthorst M, Verhoog L, Obdeijn IM, et al. A BRCA1/2 mutation, high breast density and prominent pushing margins of a tumor independently contribute to a frequent false-negative mammography. [Erratum in Int J Cancer 2002;102:665.] Int J Cancer 2002;102:91-95.

259. Brekelmans CT, Seynaeve C, Bartels CC, et al. Effectiveness of breast cancer surveillance in BRCA1/2 gene mutation carriers and women with high familial risk. [Comment.] J Clin Oncol 2001;19:924-930.

260. Kuhl CK, Schmutzler RK, Leutner CC, et al. Breast MR imaging screening in 192 women proved or suspected to be carriers of a breast cancer susceptibility gene: preliminary results. Radiology 2000;215:267-279.

261. Warner E, Plewes DB, Shumak RS, et al. Comparison of breast magnetic resonance imaging, mammography, and ultrasound for surveillance of women at high risk for hereditary breast cancer. J Clin Oncol 2001;19:3524-3531.

262. Stoutjesdijk MJ, Boetes C, Jager GJ, et al. Magnetic resonance imaging and mammography in women with a hereditary risk of breast cancer. J Natl Cancer Inst 2001;93:1095-1102.

263. Tilanus-Linthorst MM, Obdeijn IM, Bartels KC, de Koning HJ, Oudkerk M. First experiences in screening women at high risk for breast cancer with MR imaging. Breast Cancer Res Treat 2000;63:53-60.

264. Tilanus-Linthorst MM, Bartels CC, Obdeijn AI, Oudkerk M. Earlier detection of breast cancer by surveillance of women at familial risk. Eur J Cancer 2000;36:514-519.

265. Morris EA, Liberman L, Ballon DJ, et al. MRI of occult breast carcinoma in a high-risk population. AJR Am J Roentgenol 2003;181:619-626.

266. Carmichael AR, Bendall S, Lockerbie L, Prescott R, Bates T. The long-term outcome of synchronous bilateral breast cancer is worse than metachronous or unilateral tumours. Eur J Surg Oncol 2002;28:388-391.

267. Heron DE, Komarnicky LT, Hyslop T, Schwartz GF, Mansfield CM. Bilateral breast carcinoma: risk factors and outcomes for patients with synchronous and metachronous disease. Cancer 2000;88:2739-2750.

268. Hungness ES, Safa M, Shaughnessy EA, et al. Bilateral synchronous breast cancer: mode of detection and comparison of histologic features between the 2 breasts. Surgery 2000; 128:702-707.

269. Gershenwald JE, Hunt KK, Kroll SS, et al. Synchronous elective contralateral mastectomy and immediate bilateral breast reconstruction in women with early-stage breast cancer. Ann Surg Oncol 1998;5:529-538.

270. Kollias J, Ellis IO, Elston CW, Blamey RW. Prognostic significance of synchronous and metachronous bilateral breast cancer. World J Surg 2001;25:1117-1124.

271. Lee SG, Orel SG, Woo IJ, et al. MR imaging screening of the contralateral breast in patients with newly diagnosed breast cancer: preliminary results. Radiology 2003;226:773-778.

272. Liberman L, Morris EA, Kim CM, et al. MR imaging findings in the contralateral breast of women with recently diagnosed breast cancer. AJR Am J Roentgenol 2003;180:333-341.

273. LaTrenta LR, Menell JH, Morris EA, Abramson AF, Dershaw DD, Liberman L. Breast lesions detected with MR imaging: utility and histopathologic importance of identification with US. Radiology 2003;227:856-861.

274. Warren RM, Hayes C. Localization of breast lesions shown only on MRI: a review for the UK Study of MRI Screening for Breast Cancer. Advisory Group of MARIBS. Br J Radiol 2000;73:123-132.

275. Helbich TH. Localization and biopsy of breast lesions by magnetic resonance imaging guidance. J Magn Reson Imaging 2001;13:903-911.

276. Brenner RJ, Shellock FG, Rothman BJ, Giuliano A. Technical note: magnetic resonance imaging-guided preoperative breast localization using "freehand technique." Br J Radiol 1995;68:1095-1098.

277. Daniel BL, Birdwell RL, Ikeda DM, et al. Breast lesion localization: a freehand, interactive MR imaging-guided technique. Radiology 1998;207:455-463.

278. Daniel BL, Birdwell RL, Butts K, et al. Freehand iMRI-guided large-gauge core needle biopsy: a new minimally invasive technique for diagnosis of enhancing breast lesions. J Magn Reson Imaging 2001;13:896-902.

279. Heywang-Kobrunner SH, Heinig A, Pickuth D, Alberich T, Spielmann RP. Interventional MRI of the breast: lesion localisation and biopsy. Eur Radiol 2000;10:36-45.

280. Heywang-Kobrunner SH, Huynh AT, Viehweg P, Hanke W, Requardt H, Paprosch I. Prototype breast coil for MR-guided needle localization. J Comput Assist Tomogr 1994;18:876-881.

281. Lo LD, Orel SG, Schnall MD. MR imaging-guided interventions in the breast. Magn Reson Imaging Clin North Am 2001;9:373-380.

282. Orel SG, Schnall MD, Newman RW, Powell CM, Torosian MH, Rosato EF. MR imaging-guided localization and biopsy of breast lesions: initial experience. Radiology 1994;193:97-102.

283. Hefler L, Casselman J, Amaya B, et al. Follow-up of breast lesions detected by MRI not biopsied due to absent enhancement of contrast medium. Eur Radiol 2003;13:344-346.

284. Fischer U, Vosshenrich R, Doler W, Hamadeh A, Oestmann JW, Grabbe E. MR imaging-guided breast intervention: experience with two systems. Radiology 1995;195:533-538.

285. Wald DS, Weinreb JC, Newstead G, Flyer M, Bose S. MR-guided fine needle aspiration of breast lesions: initial experience. J Comput Assist Tomogr 1996;20:1-8.

286. Fischer U, Kopka L, Grabbe E. Magnetic resonance guided localization and biopsy of suspicious breast lesions. Top Magn Reson Imaging 1998;9:44-59.

287. Giard RW, Hermans J. The value of aspiration cytologic examination of the breast: a statistical review of the medical literature. Cancer 1992;69:2104-2110.

288. Kuhl CK, Morakkabati N, Leutner CC, Schmiedel A, Wardelmann E, Schild HH. MR imaging-guided large-core (14-gauge) needle biopsy of small lesions visible at breast MR imaging alone. Radiology 2001;220:31-39.

289. Schneider JP, Schulz T, Horn LC, Leinung S, Schmidt F, Kahn T. MR-guided percutaneous core biopsy of small breast lesions: first experience with a vertically open 0.5T scanner. J Magn Reson Imaging 2002;15:374-385.

290. Viehweg P, Heinig A, Amaya B, Alberich T, Laniado M, Heywang-Kobrunner SH. MR-guided interventional breast procedures considering vacuum biopsy in particular. Eur J Radiol 2002;42:32-39.

291. Heywang-Kobrunner SH, Heinig A, Schaumloffel U, et al. MR-guided percutaneous excisional and incisional biopsy of breast lesions. Eur Radiol 1999;9:1656-1665.

292. Kuhl CK, Elevelt A, Leutner CC, Gieseke J, Pakos E, Schild HH. Interventional breast MR imaging: clinical use of a stereotactic localization and biopsy device. Radiology 1997;204:667-675.

293. Fischer U, Vosshenrich R, Bruhn H, Keating D, Raab BW, Oestmann JW. MR-guided localization of suspected breast lesions detected exclusively by postcontrast MRI. J Comput Assist Tomogr 1995;19:63-66.

294. Morris EA, Liberman L, Dershaw DD, et al. Preoperative MR imaging-guided needle localization of breast lesions. AJR Am J Roentgenol 2002;178:1211-1220.

295. Warren R, Kessar P. A method of coil localization for breast lesions seen only on MRI. Br J Radiol 2001;74:548-551.

296. Muralidharan V, Christophi C. Interstitial laser thermotherapy in the treatment of colorectal liver metastases. J Surg Oncol 2001;76:73-81.

297. Hill CR, ter Haar GR. Review article: high intensity focused ultrasound—potential for cancer treatment. Br J Radiol 1995;68: 1296-1303.

298. Janzen N, Zisman A, Pantuck AJ, Perry K, Schulam P, Belldegrun AS. Minimally invasive ablative approaches in the treatment of renal cell carcinoma. Curr Urol Rep 2002;3:13-20.

299. Hynynen K, Pomeroy O, Smith DN, et al. MR imaging-guided focused ultrasound surgery of fibroadenomas in the breast: a feasibility study. Radiology 2001;219:176-185.

300. Hall-Craggs MA. Interventional MRI of the breast: minimally invasive therapy. Eur Radiol 2000;10:59-62.

301. Huber PE, Jenne JW, Rastert R, et al. A new noninvasive approach in breast cancer therapy using magnetic resonance imaging-guided focused ultrasound surgery. Cancer Res 2001;61:8441-8447.

302. Gianfelice D, Khiat A, Amara M, Belblidia A, Boulanger Y. MR imaging-guided focused US ablation of breast cancer: histopathologic assessment of effectiveness—initial experience. Radiology 2003;227:849-855.

11

MR Imaging and MR Arteriography of the Aorta

David Roberts, MD, PhD
Evan S. Siegelman, MD

IMAGING THE AORTA

The aorta presents several imaging challenges. It is a large anatomic structure, and to provide a comprehensive assessment the arterial structures must be visualized from the level of the aortic valve to the femoral heads. The branch vessels of the aorta are relatively small and centrally located deep within the chest and abdomen. Artifacts from both respiratory and cardiac motion can limit image quality.

Several imaging modalities have been employed for evaluation of the aorta, including contrast-enhanced magnetic resonance angiography (CE MRA), catheter angiography, transesophageal echocardiography, and computed tomographic angiography (CTA). To provide all the information necessary for patient management, an imaging test should evaluate the extent of disease, aortic dimensions, status of the aortic wall, and presence of complications. CE MRA is an accurate imaging modality in the evaluation of aortic disease.[1-5] MR offers several advantages over other noninvasive imaging modalities including direct multiplanar imaging, intrinsically high soft-tissue contrast, sensitivity to flow, and capability of evaluating both the aortic lumen and its wall. The gadolinium chelates used as intravenous (IV) MR contrast media have less renal toxicity and better patient tolerance than iodinated contrast.[6,7] CE MRA examination may be performed safely in patients with underlying renal dysfunction,

making it the examination of choice in this patient population.

Coils and Patient Position

Patients are usually placed into the magnet supine and feet first, although the use of prone positioning may alleviate claustrophobia. Local coils should be used whenever possible because they provide an increased intrinsic signal-to-noise ratio, thereby allowing for improved resolution through the use of smaller fields of view.[6] Typically, a multielement anteroposterior phased-array coil is placed around the chest. In patients with suspected acute aortic syndromes, noninvasive monitoring of the heart rate, blood pressure, and oxygen saturation is recommended. In patients in whom electrocardiographic (ECG) gating is desired, lead placement that results in a well-defined QRS complex allows for accurate triggering. Secure IV access allows for bolus injection. Contrast should not be injected ipsilateral to a suspected abnormality of the aortic arch or great vessels, since artifact can occur from concentrated gadolinium in the adjacent subclavian vein (Fig. 11-1).[7,8]

MR Pulse Sequences

The basic elements of an MR protocol for aortic disease appear in Box 11-1. In hemodynamically stable patients, most of the protocol sequences can

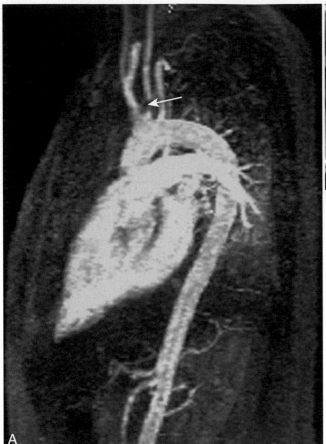

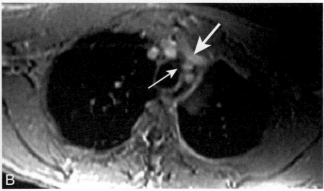

Figure 11-1 ■ MR depiction of artifactual left common carotid stenosis secondary to hyperconcentrated gadolinium in the adjacent left subclavian vein. A, Focal stenosis is present in the proximal left common carotid artery on this maximum intensity projection (MIP) image from a dynamic CE MRA *(arrow)*. The stenosis was not present on the later acquisitions. **B,** Delayed CE T1-WI shows the close relationship between the left subclavian vein *(large arrow)* and carotid artery *(small arrow)*. Contrast was injected through the patient's left antecubital vein. T2* effects from concentrated gadolinium caused the pseudostenosis of the adjacent carotid artery in **A.**

11-1 MRI Protocol Elements for Aortic Evaluation

Sequence (Generic Name)	Sequence (Common Trade Name)	Plane	Characteristics	Comments
Localizer T2-WI	HASTE (Siemens) SSFSE (GE)	Coronal Sagittal	Breath hold T2-weighted	Sensitive to pleural/ pericardial effusion
T1-GRE	FLASH (Siemens) SPGR (GE)	Axial	Breath hold May run in- or out-of-phase TE (or both)	Acute/subacute hemorrhage shows high SI
T2-WI	TSE (Siemens) FSE (GE)	Axial	Often acquired with fat suppression	Time-consuming May use single-shot methods in unstable patients
CINE (gated)	True-FISP (Siemens) FASTCARD, FIESTA (GE)	Variable	Bright-blood sequences Gradient echo	Aortic valve assessment
Black-blood (gated)	Multiple IR (Siemens) Double IR (GE)	Axial	Nulls signal from arterial lumen to provide structural assessment	Time consuming Not advisable in unstable patients
CE-MRA	FISP (Siemens) FGRE (GE)	Variable	Run dynamically during gadolinium injection Choose plane to match patient anatomy	Fat suppression should not be used in thorax Centric acquisition useful in poor breath holders
Delayed CE T1-W GRE	FLASH (Siemens) SPGR (GE)	Axial	Chemical fat suppression and out-of-phase TE	Excellent visualization of arterial wall structures

be acquired. However, physician judgment becomes important in the evaluation of unstable patients, and in all patients a careful risk-benefit assessment should be taken to determine the necessary level of imaging detail. It is important to minimize examination time in potentially unstable patients.

T1-WEIGHTED IMAGE (T1-WI)

T1-WIs should be acquired in all patients. There are two forms of T1-WI: spin-echo (SE) and gradient echo (GRE). GRE sequences can be modified such that they show bright-blood contrast and can be acquired in a breath hold. Before the introduction and implementation of CE MRA in the evaluation of vascular disease, "time-of-flight" imaging (a subtype of T1-W GRE sequences) was the most commonly used technique for MRA. T1-W SE sequences reveal flowing blood as low signal intensity (SI; "flow void") and offer excellent delineation of the aortic wall. SE acquisitions are usually acquired using ECG gating that requires longer acquisition times (see below).

T1-WIs are valuable for the detection of hemorrhagic complications of aortic disease (Fig. 11-2). The SI on T1-WI is a useful tool in determination of the chronicity of a hematoma—high SI within a hematoma is secondary to the T1 shortening effects of methemoglobin and is present in the setting of subacute blood.[9,10] T1-WIs also provide excellent visualization of mediastinal and retroperitoneal pathology (such as fibrosis and adenopathy) due to the contrast provided by surrounding fat.

Fat-suppressed T1-WI is are more sensitive than routine T1-WI in the detection of high SI methemoglobin within subacute hemorrhage and can demonstrate whether T1 hyperintensity is secondary to fat or blood. Similar pulse sequences are routinely obtained in the female pelvis to distinguish between hemorrhagic and fat-containing adnexal masses.[11]

T2-WEIGHTED IMAGE (T2-WI)

T2-W imaging of the aorta is challenging owing to the presence of motion and flow artifact. However, T2-WIs can accurately evaluate for the presence of free fluid and edema and so can reveal pleural

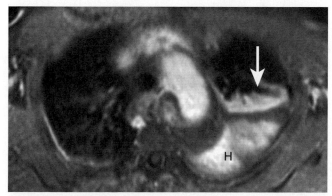

Figure 11-2 ■ MR depiction of hemorrhagic complications of aortic disease. Fat-saturated CE T1-WI shows a large hemorrhagic left pleural effusion (H) and adjacent enhancing atelectasis *(arrow)* in a patient with a ruptured aneurysm.

and pericardial effusions. T2-WIs are important in the assessment of patients with vasculitis, as T2 hyperintensity has been shown in the aortic wall and periaortic tissue in patients with active disease.[12-14] Conventional and fast spin-echo (FSE) T2-WIs require longer acquisition times and are obtained using cardiac gating or breathing-averaged techniques. Single-shot T2 methods (e.g., rapid acquisition with relaxation enhancement [RARE]) allow for the acquisition of images in less than 1 second thus minimize or eliminate motion artifact. Single-shot T2-WIs may be acquired in two orthogonal planes as "localizer" sequences that can delineate the vascular anatomy adequately for the placement of imaging volumes for subsequent angiographic pulse sequences. The use of cardiac gated RARE imaging has been described as a method of performing black-blood MRA.[15-17]

CARDIAC GATED MRI

In patients who are hemodynamically stable, cardiac gated MRI can provide structural and functional information about the aorta and its branches. Cardiac gated methods may be divided into "black-blood" and "bright-blood" techniques. Black-blood pulse sequences exploit flow phenomena to suppress intravascular signal and are usually based on spin echoes.[16] Both spin-echo and double inversion recovery black-blood techniques have been described.[18] In all these methods, suppression of the intravascular signal is achieved by motion of the blood during the application of the imaging pulses. Black-blood MRI provides excellent delineation of vascular morphology and is useful in the evaluation of suspected aortic dissection.[17]

Bright-blood MRI methods use GRE techniques that result in high SI within vessels secondary to flow-related enhancement.[19] Bright-blood MRI sequences are usually acquired in cine mode in which multiple temporally resolved images throughout the cardiac cycle are reconstructed at each slice location. Several different cine MRI methods have been described, including conventional spoiled GRE, segmented k-space, and true-FISP (fast imaging with steady-state precession) acquisition.[20-23] Cine pulse sequences can be acquired in selected planes to assess aortic valve function and to evaluate dissection flap extension. Cine pulse sequences may be used to distinguish between slow flow and thrombosis in the setting of acute dissection.[24-26] Bright-blood MRI may be used to provide a rapid assessment of the aorta without need for contrast injection.[22]

CONTRAST-ENHANCED MRA (CE MRA)

Three-dimensional (3D) CE MRA has become the predominant method of evaluating diseases of the aorta.[27-29] The CE MRA method is based on the use of a 3D GRE pulse sequence with a minimally short repetition time (TR), resulting in severe T1-weighting. The dynamic injection of gadolinium chelates selectively shortens the T1 of blood in the intravascular space. As a result of the short repetition time, such acquisitions may usually be performed within a 10- to 30-second breath hold. Although cardiac triggering

11-2 CE-MRA Parameter Choices for the Aorta

Parameter	Single Station	Multistation	
		Chest	*Abdomen*
Field-of-view (FOV)	44–48 cm	36–40 cm	32–38 cm
Slice thickness	4	2–3	3–4
Matrix	512 × (128–160)	512 × (128–160)	512 × (128–192)
Number of slices	28–48	28–36	28–36
Plane	Sagittal	Oblique sagittal	Coronal
Fat suppression	No	No	Yes
Coil	Phased-array	Phased-array	Body

reduces artifacts,[30] it results in longer scan times and thus cannot be recommended with current MR systems.

CE MRA is performed dynamically in sequential breath holds following dynamic intravenous contrast administration, providing arterial-, venous-, and delayed-phase images. A total dose of 0.1 to 0.2 mmol/kg of an extravascular gadolinium chelate is given as a bolus injection at a typical rate of 2 to 3 cc/sec. Power injectors are useful for standardization of examinations.[31] Suggested acquisition parameters for CE MRA are provided in Box 11-2. The use of chemical fat suppression should be avoided in the chest because it may create artifactual suppression of the vascular lumen, mimicking thrombotic or occlusive disease.[7] The CE MRA images are transferred via a high-speed network to a dedicated workstation where multiplanar reformatted (MPR) and maximum-intensity pixel (MIP) images are created using postprocessing techniques.[32] In the future, virtual aortic endoscopy (similar to CT and MR colonography[33]) may facilitate the evaluation of aortic plaque and occlusive disease.[34]

Accurate bolus timing is a necessary component of high-quality CE MRA of the aorta.[35] The goal is to acquire the low-frequency content of the Fourier transform (also called k-space) of the image during the peak phase of selective arterial enhancement. Acquisition of MRA data during either the wash-in or the washout of aortic enhancement can result in undesired "ringing" artifacts (Fig. 11-3).[36] Several strategies for bolus timing have been described, including the use of timing runs,[31] automated bolus detection,[37] and fluoroscopically triggered CE MRA.[38] Automated bolus detection methods are based on the repetitive sampling of a "tracker" volume that is usually defined in a large vessel such as the aorta.[39] The signal in the tracker volume is monitored dynamically as contrast is injected and, upon detection of the upstroke of initial enhancement, data acquisition is automatically initiated after a brief delay. CE MRA data may be acquired using either a "centric" or a "noncentric" acquisition strategy.[40]

In centric acquisition, the most important data, the low frequencies, are acquired near the beginning of the breath hold. In a noncentric acquisition, the low-frequency information is sampled toward the middle of the breath hold. Centric acquisition is useful for patients who may not be able to complete the breath-holding maneuver.[41] The actual timing of the resulting CE MRA image is a function of three parameters: (1) the location of the tracker volume, (2) the delay between bolus-detection and image acquisition, and (3) the data acquisition order. Choice of these variables must be coordinated such that the proper phase of enhancement is obtained. For patients with large aortic aneurysms, the tracker volume usually is placed in the descending thoracic aorta and a centric acquisition is performed after an acquisition delay of 10 to 20 seconds. This usually results in complete filling of the aneurysm in the arterial phase. It is important to adjust the acquisition parameters so that an early acquisition is avoided, especially in patients with aneurysm, since there is increased transit time. An alternative method of bolus timing is the use of "fluoroscopically triggered" MRA in which a time-resolved two-dimensional pulse sequence is used to

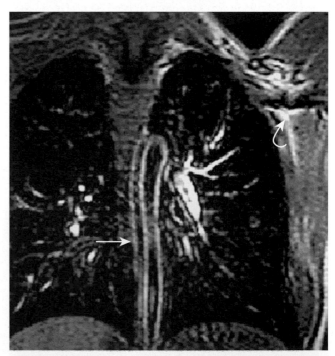

Figure 11-3 ■ MR illustration of "ringing artifact." The "edgy" appearance of the descending thoracic aorta *(arrow)* on this dynamic CE MRA acquisition results from an early acquisition and poor bolus timing. The low SI within the left axillary vein *(curved arrow)* is secondary to concentrated gadolinium. Blooming from T2* effects can result in artifactual stenosis of adjacent arterial segments (see Fig. 11-1).

track aortic enhancement.[38,42] When enhancement is observed in the desired arterial segment, data acquisition is initiated.

In many patients, it is desirable to obtain angiographic images of the entire aorta and iliac arteries, to the level of the femoral heads, most notably in patients who are candidates for potential stent-graft repair.[43] This coverage is extremely difficult to achieve in a single-station examination because of coil coverage limitations. Multistation CE MRA has been described for evaluation of the aorta.[44,45] In the multistation approach, the aorta is imaged in two or three separate acquisitions ("stations") with the table moving between stations after gadolinium injection.[46] The multistation technique has several distinct advantages over single-station examination: it allows for (1) imaging of the entire aorta and the iliac arteries with greater coverage than in a single-station examination, (2) the use of fat suppression selectively in the abdomen, thereby avoiding potential artifacts in the chest, (3) the use of a local coil to increase signal-to-noise ratio, and (4) higher resolution imaging through the use of smaller volumes tailored to each station. Suggested parameter choices for both single- and multistation CE MRA evaluation of the aorta appear in Box 11-2.

DELAYED-ENHANCED T1-WI

Delayed CE T1-WIs should be acquired in all patients who have dynamic CE-MRA of the aorta. The use of concomitant fat suppression results in an image contrast that is largely dependent on gadolinium distribution, and this acquisition often provides important information about the aortic wall and unsuspected nonvascular pathology.[47,48] Delayed CE images are an accurate and sensitive method for the evaluation of the aortic wall (Fig. 11-4) and for the diagnosis of venous disease.

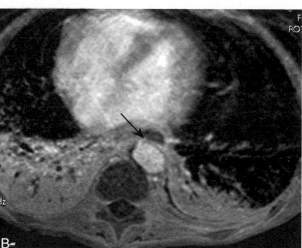

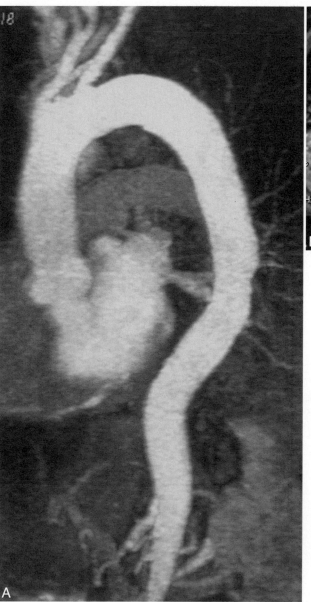

Figure 11-4 ▪ **Value of delayed imaging in suggesting site of leak in a patient with a proven aorto-esophageal fistula. A,** MIP image from CE MRA does not show contrast extravasation. **B,** Delayed fat-suppressed T1-WI shows a focal disruption of the anterior aortic wall *(arrow)* that was confirmed surgically as the location of the fistula. Bibasilar atelectasis/consolidation is present.

THE NORMAL AORTA

Anatomy

The aorta is the largest artery in the human body, extending from the aortic valve to the iliac bifurcation. The ascending aorta consists of the following components: aortic annulus, sinus portion, sinotubular junction, and tubular portion. The term aortic root refers to the annulus and sinus portion. The aortic arch classically gives rise to the innominate artery, the left common carotid artery, and the left subclavian artery. Variations in aortic arch anatomy are common and are described below. The ligamentum arteriosum inserts on the anteromedial aspect of the aorta, just distal to the origin of the left subclavian artery. The ligamentum arteriosum is the remnant of the ductus arteriosus and is an important site of potential injury in cases of trauma. The descending thoracic aorta passes through the aortic hiatus in the diaphragm at the level of T10. The celiac trunk is the first branch of the abdominal aorta, arising anteriorly at the L1–L2 disk space. The superior mesenteric artery is the next branch, arising anteriorly at the superior aspect of L2. The renal arteries usually arise less than 1 cm inferior to the origin of the superior mesenteric artery, approximately at the mid-body of L2. The inferior mesenteric artery is the final major branch of the abdominal aorta, arising from the left anterolateral aspect at L3.

Anatomic Variants

Anatomic variation in the aortic arch is common, with more than 25 known variants (Box 11-3).[49]

11-3 Congenital Variants of the Aortic Arch
(Adapted from reference 49)

Aortic Arch Variants (with Population Incidence in Parentheses)

Left arch with variant great-vessel branching
  "Bovine arch" (22%)
  Left vertebral artery (6%)
  Thyroid ima artery directly from arch (1%)
  Aberrant right subclavian artery (0.5%)
    Retroesophageal (80%)
    Between esophagus/trachea (15%)
    Pretracheal (5%)
Right-sided arch (<1%)
  Aberrant left subclavian/innominate artery
  Mirror-image branching
  Situs inversus totalis
Double arch (<1%)
  Patent hemi-arches
  Atretic hemi-arch (unilateral)
Coarctation (<1%)
  Preductal
  Postductal
  Patent ductus arteriosus
Interrupted arch (<1%)
Cervical arch (<1%)
  Ductus diverticulum

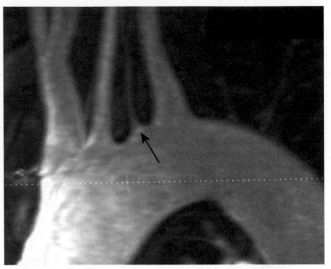

Figure 11-5 ■ CE MRA illustration of a separate origin of the left vertebral artery *(arrow)* from the aortic arch. This variant is present in 6% of the population.

CE MRA is an accurate method for the detection of abnormalities of the aortic arch.[50] A "bovine arch," in which the left common carotid artery arises from a common trunk shared with the innominate artery (see Fig. 11-12A) is the most common variant and is present in 20% to 25% of individuals. The left vertebral artery arises as a separate branch from the arch in 6% of the population (Fig. 11-5). An aberrant right subclavian artery, in which the right subclavian artery arises as the last branch of the arch and courses in the posterior mediastinum to the right upper extremity (Fig. 11-6), occurs in 0.5% of individuals. The aberrant vessel may pass either posterior to the esophagus (80%), between the trachea and esophagus (15%), or anterior to the trachea (5%). An aberrant right subclavian artery does not comprise a vascular ring and therefore usually is asymptomatic unless there is an associated aneurysm at the origin of the aberrant vessel.[51] Symptomatic patients may have with dysphagia, dyspnea, or upper extremity ischemia.[52] A right-sided aortic arch is an uncommon variant, occurring in less than 1% of the population.

Aortic Size

Aortic size is the outer, or "adventitial," diameter. This measurement therefore includes the aortic wall. Aortic size is of critical importance in surgical planning and should be reported accurately. The size of the aorta is a function of age, sex, and body surface area (BSA).[53] Normal ranges for aortic dimensions are provided in Box 11-4. The diameter of the aorta should taper uniformly and gradually with increasing distance from the aortic valve plane. Expansion of the outer diameter to less than 150% of the normal value is termed *ectasia*, while *aneurysm* is defined as dilation to greater than 150% of the normal value.[54] Aneurysm extension into the iliac arteries is important in surgical planning, and size measurements of the iliac arteries also should be provided in any evaluation of the aorta.

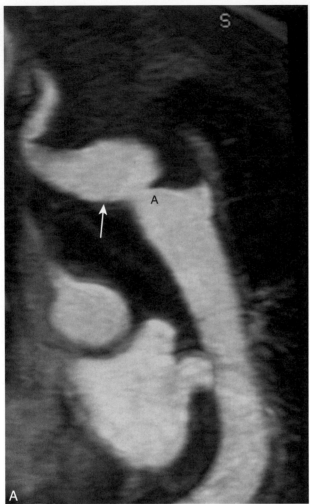

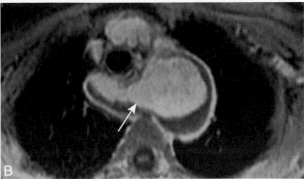

Figure 11-6 ■ **Aberrant right subclavian artery revealed on CE MRA and MRI. A,** CE MRA coronal MIP image shows a large aneurysmal right subclavian artery *(arrow)* arising as the last branch of the aortic arch (A) and coursing to the right shoulder. **B,** Delayed fat-suppressed CE T1-WI depicts the aneurysmal origin (diverticulum of Kommerell) of the vessel *(arrow)* that contains eccentric mural thrombus.

AORTIC ANEURYSM

Aortic aneurysm is a relatively common disorder, affecting 1% to 5% of the population of the U. S. each year, with an increasing incidence over the past 30 years.[55] Approximately 5% of men aged 65 years have aortic aneurysms.[56,57] Although the incidence of aortic aneurysm is increasing, there is also an improved prognosis, largely due to advances in diagnosis and surgical therapy.[58] Clinical factors such as age, sex, and body size should be assessed when evaluating for aneurysm. Elective surgery for aneurysms that are 4 to 5.5 cm in size does not improve long-term survival.[59-62] Interval change in aortic diameter is important, since patients with a rapid (>1 cm/yr) increase in aortic diameter are often treated surgically[54] as are patients with aneurysms larger than 6 cm.[57]

Patients should be encouraged to quit smoking, since cigarettes are the only documented risk factor associated with aneurysm growth.[63] The results of ongoing randomized studies comparing endovascular repair and open surgical repair of aortic aneurysms are not available yet.[64] Evidenced-based techniques suggest that endovascular repair has fewer short-term

11-4 Normal Aortic Dimensions
(Adapted from references 53, 169)

Location of Aorta	Body Surface Area (m²)	Diameter (cm)* Males	Females
Ascending (sinus)	1.3	N/A	N/A
	1.7 to 1.9	3.0	2.9
	2.5	N/A	N/A
Ascending (mid-tubular)	1.3	N/A	N/A
	1.7 to 1.9	3.2	2.9
	2.5	N/A	N/A
Descending (carina)	1.3	2.1 to 2.5	2.0 to 2.4
	1.9	2.7 to 3.1	2.6 to 3.1
	2.5	3.3 to 3.7	3.2 to 3.6
Celiac	1.3	1.9 to 2.3	1.7 to 2.1
	1.9	2.2 to 2.6	2.0 to 2.4
	2.5	2.6 to 2.9	2.4 to 2.7
Renals	1.3	1.7 to 1.9	1.5 to 1.7
	1.9	2.0 to 2.2	1.7 to 2.0
	2.5	2.3 to 2.5	2.0 to 2.3
Infrarenal	1.3	1.6 to 1.8	1.3 to 1.5
	1.9	1.8 to 2.0	1.6 to 1.8
	2.5	2.0 to 2.2	1.8 to 2.0

*Ranges, where given, represent values for patients aged 55 and 85 years old.

complications than open repair. However, endovascular treatments cost more and do not perform as well as surgical grafts at mid-term and long-term follow-up.[64,65] In addition, there is no documented decreased risk of aneurysm rupture after endovascular stent placement[66] compared with surveillance alone.[59,61]

Differential diagnostic considerations in aortic aneurysm appear in Box 11-5. Atherosclerosis accounts for approximately 80% of aortic aneurysms.[54] *Inflammatory abdominal aortic aneurysm* (IAAA) is an important variant that is characterized by marked wall thickening and inflammation in association with dense perianeurysmal fibrosis. The incidence of IAAA is from 5% to 23% of all aortic aneurysms.[67] Inflammatory aneurysm is more commonly symptomatic, and patients often have abdominal, flank, or back pain; weight loss; and elevated sedimentation rate. MRI findings of inflammatory aneurysm include a thickened, aneurismal wall with a layered appearance and homogeneous enhancement.[68,69] The relationship of IAAA to retroperitoneal fibrosis is further discussed in Chapter 6.

The classification of aortic aneurysm depends on extent of disease. *Thoracoabdominal aortic aneurysm* (TAAA) is classified according to the Crawford scheme (Fig. 11-7),[70] which provides a useful means for risk stratification and surgical planning. *Abdominal aortic aneurysm* (AAA) is classified as suprarenal, juxtarenal, or infrarenal depending on the proximal extent.[55] A suprarenal AAA involves the renal artery origins but not the superior

mesenteric artery. A juxtarenal AAA extends proximally to within 10 mm of the most inferior renal artery (excluding small accessory arteries and does not allow for safe clamping of the infrarenal aorta. An infrarenal aneurysm originates below the renal arteries and allows safe clamp placement.

11-5 Differential Diagnosis of Aortic Aneurysm

- Atherosclerosis (most common)
  Cystic medial necrosis
    Primary
    Marfan's syndrome
    Ehlers-Danlos syndrome
- Vasculitis
    Takayasu's arteritis
    Giant cell arteritis
    Ankylosing spondylitis
    Rheumatoid arthritis
    Reiter's syndrome
    Relapsing polychondritis
- Infection ("mycotic")
    Tuberculosis
    Bacterial
    Fungal
    Syphilis
- Congenital
    Aberrant subclavian artery
- Traumatic/iatrogenic

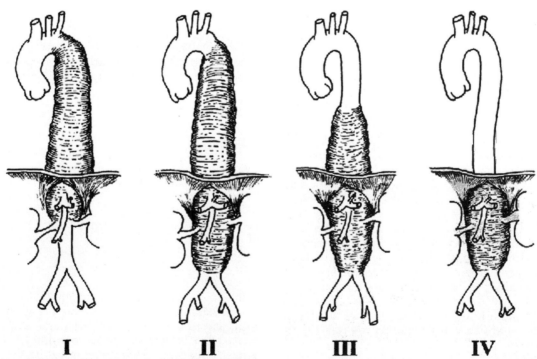

I   II   III   IV

Figure 11-7 ▪ The Crawford classification of thoracoabdominal aortic aneurysm. This classification is based solely on the anatomic extent of the aneurysm and has important implications for both surgical treatment and prognosis. Type I, proximal descending to suprarenal abdominal aorta; Type II, proximal descending to infrarenal abdominal aorta; Type III, distal thoracic to abdominal aorta; Type IV, primarily abdominal aorta.

MR has high accuracy in the assessment of aortic aneurysm, and CE MRA is an important component of the examination.[2,4] CE MRA provides excellent visualization of complex branch-vessel involvement (Fig. 11-8), which may be difficult to evaluate on conventional aortography. Complications of aortic aneurysm, including rupture, embolization, fistula, and branch vessel occlusion/stenosis, usually are well shown with MR and CE MRA. Aortocaval fistula is a major complication that occurs in 0.2% to 1.3% of patients with aortic aneurysm.[54] The most frequent site is fistula between the distal aorta and the inferior vena cava, just superior to the confluence of the iliac veins (Fig. 11-9). Findings associated with ruptured aneurysm include hemorrhagic pleural effusion (see Fig. 11-2), mediastinal/retroperitoneal hematoma (Fig. 11-10), prominent mural enhancement, intramural hematoma, abnormal aortic contour (Fig. 11-11), and active contrast extravasation.[71] The use of multistation examination allows for high-resolution MRA of the iliac arteries to the level of the femoral heads (Fig. 11-12). This is important in the era of stent-graft repair, since the luminal diameter of the iliac arteries is an important determinant of candidacy for minimally invasive therapy.[54]

Limitations of CE MRA in the evaluation of patients with aneurysm include insensitivity to calcium.[72] CE MRA may still overestimate some vascular stenoses secondary to phase-induced turbulence or inadequate contrast bolus.[73] Finally, CE MRA is not sensitive to the presence of aneurysm because it is a luminal imaging technique. Specifically, the adventitia is not visualized well at CE MRA and thus the outer aortic diameter may not be accurately measurable. For this reason, it is important to acquire delayed CE T1-WIs to define the extent and size of an aneurysm.

AORTIC DISSECTION

Aortic dissection is a life-threatening condition that must be diagnosed promptly and accurately.[74] The mortality rate in acute type A aortic dissection is 1% per hour during the initial 24 hours and 80% in 2 weeks.[75] The incidence of aortic dissection is estimated to be more than 2,000 cases per year in the U. S. Dissecting thoracoabdominal aortic aneurysm (TAAA) differs fundamentally from atherosclerotic TAAA with respect to natural history, epidemiology, risk factors, and treatment.[54] Risk factors for the development of aortic dissection include hypertension, connective tissue disorder (Marfan's syndrome, Ehlers-Danlos syndrome), bicuspid aortic valve, coarctation, Turner's syndrome,[76] vasculitis, pregnancy, cocaine use, and trauma. Complications due to dissection include stroke, renal failure, mesenteric ischemia, lower extremity ischemia, and paraplegia.

Pathologically, aortic dissection is identified as a disruption of the inner layer of the media, associated with an intimal tear. Fenestrations of the intimal flap are frequently present in chronic dissection and provide communication between the true and false lumens. Aneurysmal dilation of the aortic lumen can be present secondary to loss of structural integrity, creating a so-called dissecting aneurysm. The etiology of aortic dissection is unclear. Proposed mechanisms include atherosclerosis, cystic medial necrosis, spontaneous rupture of the vasa vasorum, and disorders of elastin. However, degenerative changes do not completely explain the development of dissection, and mechanical factors associated with increased focal stress on the wall of the aorta are thought to contribute as well. The most common sites of intimal laceration are the right lateral wall of the ascending aorta and the descending aorta in the region of the insertion of the ligamentum arteriosum. These are also the sites of greatest movement during the

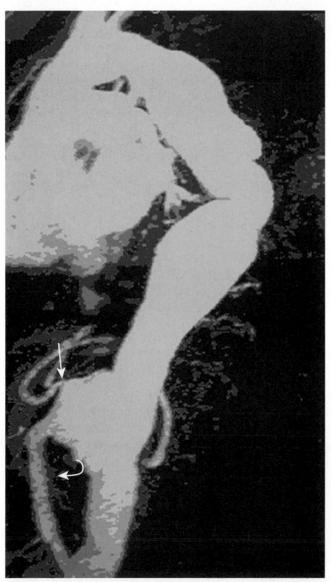

Figure 11-8 ▪ MR illustration of branch-vessel disease in a patient with a thoracoabdominal aortic aneurysm. MIP image from CE MRA shows that both the celiac trunk *(arrow)* and superior mesenteric artery *(curved arrow)* originate from the aneurysm.

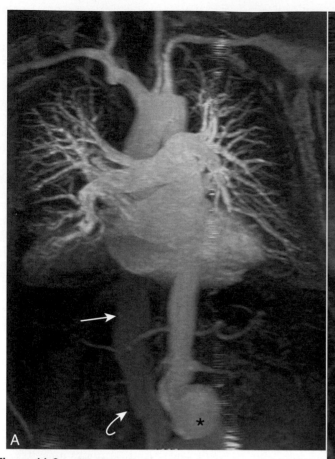

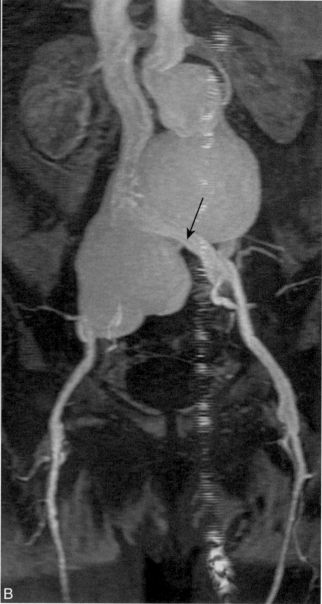

Figure 11-9 ▪ **CE MRA illustration of an aortocaval fistula as a complication of a mycotic abdominal aortic aneurysm.** **A,** Coronal MIP image from multistation CE MRA shows early enhancement of the inferior vena cava (IVC) during the arterial phase without contrast within the renal veins. There is greater enhancement within the peripheral IVC *(curved arrow)* compared with the proximal, central IVC *(arrow)*. In the setting of elevated right-sided heart pressures and/or tricuspid regurgitation one would expect higher SI within the central, superior IVC. A saccular aneurysm of the infrarenal abdominal aorta is present (∗). **B,** Abdominal station redemonstrates abnormal enhancement of the IVC and left common iliac vein *(arrow)*. Surgery confirmed an aortocaval fistula just above the confluence of the iliac veins.

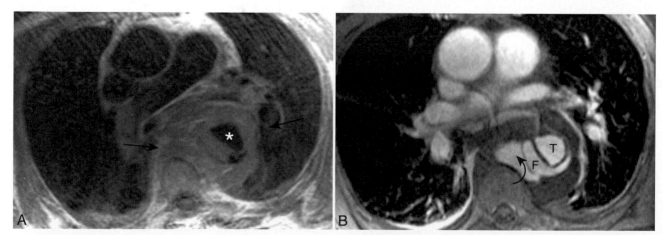

Figure 11-10 ▪ **MR depiction of a periaortic posterior mediastinal hematoma from a ruptured type B aortic dissection. A,** Axial T1-W spin-echo image shows circumferential soft tissue SI *(arrows)* around the descending aorta. Flow void is present in the anterior aspect of the aorta (∗), while both lower and higher SI regions are present posteriorly. **B,** Delayed fat-suppressed T1-W GRE image shows the presence of flow within both true (T) and false (F) lumens of an aortic dissection (determination of the true lumen was established on dynamic CE MRA). An active leak is present from the false lumen *(curved arrow)*, resulting in the posterior mediastinal hematoma.

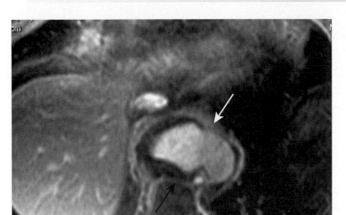

Figure 11-11 ■ **MR illustration of an abnormal aortic contour in a patient with a documented contained rupture.** Delayed CE T1-WI shows a markedly abnormal aortic contour with pronounced asymmetric sacculation *(arrows)* in this patient with a contained aortic rupture.

cardiac cycle and experience the greatest shear stress. Atherosclerosis is not considered a primary causative factor in the development of dissection. Aortic dissection often arises in the ascending aorta, an infrequent site of atherosclerosis, and dissection in the region of an atheroma is frequently limited by surrounding fibrosis and calcification.

Aortic dissection is classified according to the Stanford system as type A or type B.[77] Type A dissection involves the ascending aorta, and type B does not. Type A aortic dissection generally requires immediate surgical repair, while type B aortic dissections are managed medically, principally through control of hypertension or by the use of aortic stents.[43,78] In this system, dissection limited to the aortic arch would be classified as type B; however, such dissections may necessitate surgical intervention. Therefore, the radiologist should not rely on such classification schemes and should instead convey clearly and explicitly the extent of dissection.

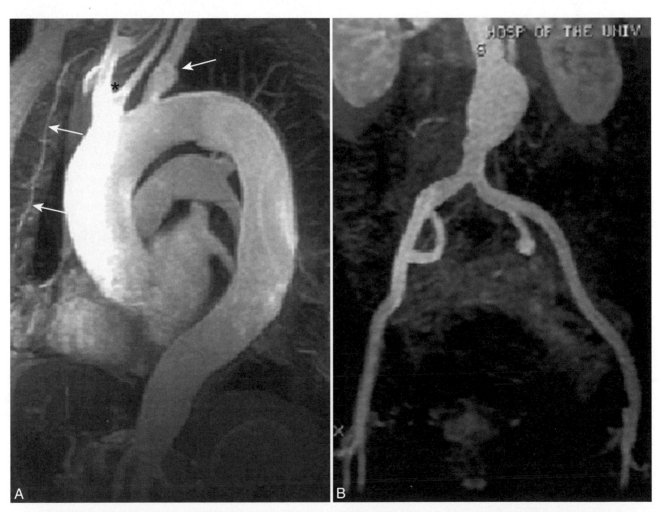

Figure 11-12 ■ **Multistation CE MRA of a thoracoabdominal aortic aneurysm (TAAA). A** and **B,** Oblique sagittal MIP image from a chest station (**A**) and coronal MIP image from an abdominal station (**B**) obtained in a patient with a Crawford type II TAAA shows a dilated aorta extending from the ascending aorta to above the aortic bifurcation. A fusiform aneurysm of the origin of the left subclavian artery *(top arrow)* and a bovine arch (∗) are present. A segment of a normal-caliber right internal thoracic artery is well illustrated *(arrows)*. The lower signal-to-noise ratio of the upper abdomen in **A** is secondary to limited coverage of the phased-array coil.

MRI is a highly accurate method for the evaluation of aortic dissection.[79] CE MRA has increased its accuracy by providing excellent delineation of the type and extent of disease, branch-vessel involvement, and vascular dimensions, all of which must be identified prior to planning surgical therapy.[80-82] MRI is a sensitive technique for detection of the complications of dissection, including pericardial hematoma mediastinal hematoma (see Fig. 11-11), branch-vessel occlusion, and rupture (Fig. 11-13; see Fig. 11-2).

Aortic dissection commonly involves both the thoracic and abdominal aorta, with extension commonly into one or both iliac arteries. MRI is a useful method for following patients with type B or surgically repaired type A dissection[83-85] because it provides comprehensive evaluation of the entire aorta, allowing assessment of progressive thrombosis and residual flow in the false lumen.[86] The SI characteristics of the false lumen may be used to estimate the chronicity of the lesion.[26] Change in the size of the aorta and progressive branch-vessel involvement can be shown with MRI.

Multistation CE MRA is particularly useful for the evaluation of the extension of aortic dissection into the iliac vessels. In addition to providing excellent resolution of the aortic arch branch vessels, celiac, superior mesenteric and renal arteries, a dedicated lower abdominal-pelvic station may be chosen to provide full coverage of the iliac arteries to detect flap involvement with high accuracy (Fig. 11-14).[45]

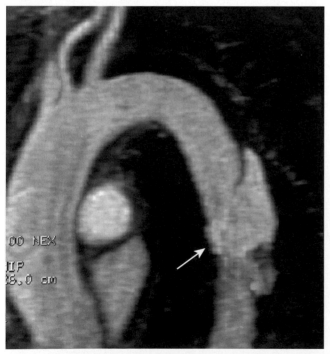

Figure 11-13 ■ MR depiction of a ruptured of type B dissection. CE MRA MIP image shows active contrast extravasation in the setting of a ruptured dissection *(arrow)*.

PENETRATING AORTIC ULCER (PAU)

In 1934 Shennan gave the first description of the clinical entity of penetrating aortic ulcer (PAU). PAU is characterized by ulceration of an atheroma with subsequent disruption of the internal elastic lamina and extension into the inner media. The ulcerated plaque may produce a localized intramedial dissection with variable amounts of associated intramural hematoma, ultimately placing the patient at risk for adventitial disruption, pseudoaneurysm formation, and free rupture.

PAU is most frequently present in a background of advanced atherosclerosis. The clinical presentation of PAU mimics that of aortic dissection. Patients usually have severe chest or back pain. However, symptoms and signs associated with branch vessel involvement and hypoperfusion are not typically present. Most cases (90%) of PAU involve the descending aorta. As for aortic dissection, anterior chest pain has been associated with anterior aortic involvement, and posterior (back) pain with PAU of the descending aorta.[87]

Approximately 10% of patients with acute aortic syndromes on presentation were found on imaging studies to have PAU.[87] A background of severe atherosclerosis was observed in all patients. Contrast-filled outpouchings of the aortic lumen were present in all patients, with varying degrees of associated focal intramural hematoma. PAU typically presented in older patients with larger aortic diameter than in dissection and often was associated with abdominal aortic aneurysm.[88] PAU had a higher incidence of rupture (42%) than either aortic dissection or intramural hematoma (see below). Persistent pain, hemodynamic instability, and any evidence of expansion should prompt treatment with an aortic graft[89] or stent placement.[90,91]

The MR appearance of PAU is principally defined by the identification of focal ulceration or outpouching of the aortic lumen, often associated with localized intramural hematoma and inflammatory change (Fig. 11-15).[92-94] Hemorrhagic processes are well depicted on fat-suppressed T1-WI, which should be acquired in all patients suspected of having PAU. Unlike simple ulcerated plaque, PAU extends beyond the elastic lamina of the aortic wall. However, this distinction is sometimes difficult, and ulcerated plaque can mimic PAU. Therefore, care should be taken in making the diagnosis of PAU in asymptomatic patients, particularly in the absence of findings of intramural hemorrhage.[94]

INTRAMURAL HEMATOMA (IMH)

Intramural hematoma (IMH) was first described by Krukenberg in 1920 as "dissection without intimal tear."[95] However, it is now believed that IMH is a distinct clinical entity with a different etiology from that of classic aortic dissection. The cause of IMH is thought to be rupture of the vasa vasorum in the

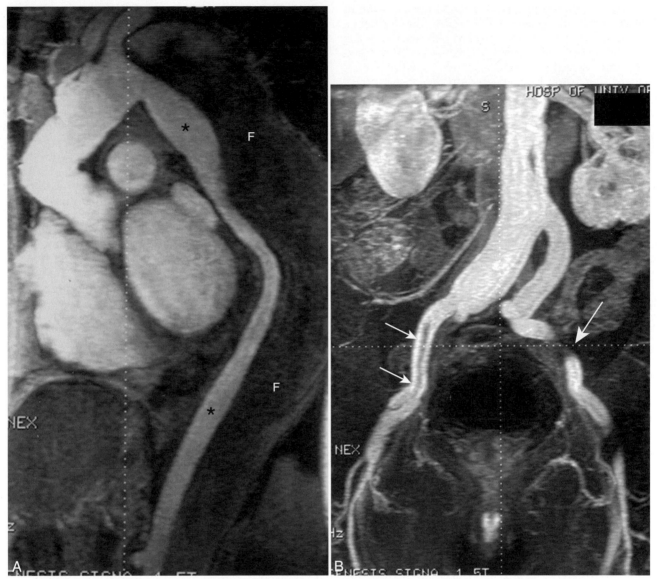

Figure 11-14 ■ **MR findings of aortic dissection on multistation CE MRA. A,** Chest station MIP image shows prompt enhancement of the true lumen (*) with a large, posterior false lumen (F). **B,** MIP coronal image from the abdominopelvic station reveals termination of the flap in the right external iliac artery *(small arrows).* There is also segmental occlusion of the left external iliac artery *(large arrow).*

outer two thirds of the aortic wall. The vasa vasorum are small arterioles that penetrate the outer half of the media and then arborize. IMH is not associated with either intimal disruption or focal ulceration of the aortic lumen.

IMH may occur spontaneously in hypertensive patients, after blunt chest trauma, or secondary to atherosclerosis. Similarly to PAU, approximately 10% of patients with acute aortic syndromes were found on imaging studies to have IMH.[87] In these patients, the majority of lesions involved the descending thoracic aorta (71%), and there was a higher incidence of aortic rupture (35%) than observed for aortic dissection. All patients with IMH involving the ascending aorta went on to have a rupture. Intramural hematoma of the descending aorta

may resolve with conservative therapy (Fig. 11-16). At surgery, patients with IMH were found to have medial hematoma in close physical proximity to the adventitia. This differs in patients with aortic dissection who have hematoma limited to the inner portion of the media. IMH associated with acute trauma has a better prognosis than does nontraumatic IMH.[96]

Focal aortic wall thickening is the hallmark finding of IMH. Normally, the wall of the aorta is 3 mm or less in width. MR findings include a crescentic or circular distribution of wall thickening secondary to hemorrhage that is completely contained within the wall of the aorta (see Fig. 11-16). By definition, there is no free flap or focal ulceration. The MR SI characteristics are important in distinguishing IMH from

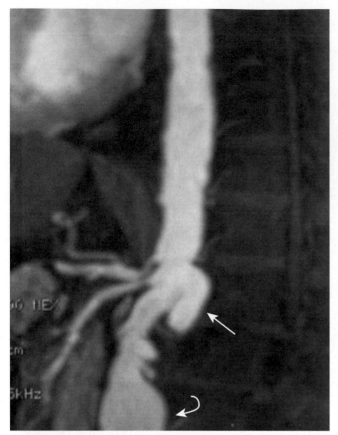

Figure 11-15 ▪ MR imaging findings of a penetrating aortic ulcer (PAU). MIP image from CE MRA shows a saccular ulcer extending from the posterior aspect of the aorta *(arrow)* in a background of diffuse atherosclerosis. The superior segment of an abdominal aortic aneurysm is also present *(curved arrow)*.

chronic mural thrombus and dissection. Intramural hematoma is revealed as a hyperintense thickened aortic wall on T1-WIs (see Fig. 11-16). Chronic mural thrombus shows low T1 SI and tends to have an irregular contour.

ACUTE AORTIC SYNDROMES: MANAGEMENT DECISIONS

Although the acute aortic syndromes of dissection, intramural hematoma, and penetrating aortic ulcer have distinguishing clinical features (Box 11-6), it is difficult to make management decisions without imaging evaluation.[97,98] Immediate surgical therapy is the accepted management of most lesions involving the ascending aorta, including IMH and PAU. However, the management of descending aortic lesions remains controversial. Surgery should be considered in patients with worsening symptoms, with a large associated aneurysm, and with progressive luminal enlargement or expanding hematoma on follow-up imaging.[87] In the absence of ominous imaging findings, a trial of medical management may be performed.[99] However, close interval follow-up imaging should be performed to document stability or resolution.

THE POSTOPERATIVE AORTA

It is important for the radiologist to recognize the common appearances of patients who have undergone aortic repair.[100] Detailed knowledge of the nature of the surgical procedure aids in the detection of complications after surgery. Surgical repair of the ascending aorta takes several forms, which may be broadly subdivided into those in which additional repair or replacement of the aortic valve is performed (composite repair) and those in which the aortic valve is preserved.[101] Bentall described the first successful composite repair of the ascending aorta in 1967.[102] The Bentall procedure is a composite graft repair consisting of a mechanical valve and a tube graft in the ascending aorta. The coronary ostia are sutured to the side to the graft. The Ross procedure is more complex, involving the use of the native pulmonic valve to replace the aortic valve. Homografts are human cadaveric tissue that in almost all cases are cryopreserved and sterilized. "Valve-sparing aortic root replacement" is a procedure in which there is prosthetic replacement of the sinus and tubular portions of the ascending aorta, with preservation of the aortic valve. In these valve-sparing procedures, the graft is sewn directly to the aortic valve annulus and coronary reimplantation is performed. Surgical repair of the descending thoracic or abdominal aorta typically consists of prosthetic replacement, often including wrapping of the adventitia around the graft. Detailed knowledge of the surgical anatomy is required to ensure that an adequate study is obtained.

MR plays an important role in the evaluation of patients who have had surgical aortic repair.[100,103,104] Postoperative complications that may be detected on MRI include anastomotic pseudoaneurysm, coronary occlusion, graft infection, perigraft fluid collections, and distal dissection. A common cause of death in patients who have had ascending aortic repair for dissection is distal extension of dissection with subsequent aneurysm formation and rupture. For this reason, it is imperative to image the entire thoracic aorta. Although enhancement within the adventitial wrap of a repaired aorta may be transiently present in the immediate postoperative period, follow-up imaging to confirm resolution of this finding should be performed.

Perigraft fluid is a relatively common finding in patients who have undergone graft repair within the prior 3 months and does not necessarily imply infection.[105,106] Simple fluid has low SI on T1-WI, whereas complex fluid (protein, hemorrhage) has higher T1 SI. Perigraft fluid of lymphatic origin likely occurs as the result of a delayed hypersensitivity reaction, while perigraft seromas are the result of direct plasma leakage from the graft. Perigraft seromas may be asymptomatic or symptomatic secondary to local mass effect and are deleted incidentally on postprocedural imaging.[106]

Most patients with graft infection have a fever and an elevated white blood cell count on presentation. After 3 months, the presence of perigraft fluid is considered abnormal and should raise suspicion of

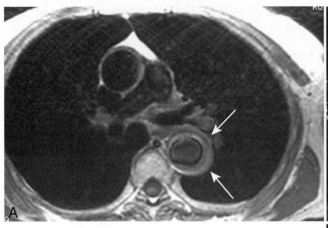

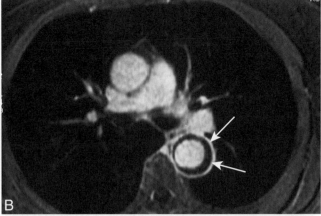

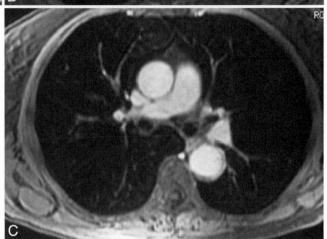

Figure 11-16 ■ **MR illustration of an intramural hematoma in a 66-year-old man. A,** Axial SE T1-WI shows circumferential intermediate SI tissue *(arrows)* surrounding the descending thoracic aorta. The ascending aortic wall has a normal appearance. **B,** Delayed enhanced T1-WI shows no enhancement of the intramural hematoma *(arrows)*. The apparent decrease in relative SI of the hematoma is secondary to differences in dynamic range with the presence of high SI contrast within the adjacent aortic lumen. **C,** Corresponding enhanced image obtained 5 months later shows complete resolution of the intramural hematoma. Atherosclerotic mural thrombus typically has lower T1 SI, has irregular contours, and does not resolve on follow-up imaging.

11-6 Acute Aortic Syndromes: Clinical and MRI Features *(Adapted from reference 87)*

Lesion	Demographic Features	Symptoms or Signs	MRI Features	Management/ Outcome
Type A, aortic dissection	Younger (mean age of 57 yr) AAA in 10%	Substernal chest pain Dyspnea Differential arm blood pressures	Intimal flap Ascending aortic involvement ± Pericardial effusion ± Aortic valve dysfunction	Surgical 1-year survival = 90%
Type B, aortic dissection	Older (mean age of 70 yr) Hypertension AAA in 30%	Back/chest pain Symptoms of branch-vessel occlusion and lower extremity ischemia	Intimal flap Variable flow/thrombosis in false lumen ± Branch vessel involvement	Medical (blood pressure control) 1-year survival = 90%
Intramural hematoma (IMH)	Older (mean age = 74) Hypertension AAA in 30%	Back/chest pain No hypoperfusion syndromes	Intramural hemorrhage No flap No branch vessel involvement Descending aorta > ascending	Ascending—surgery Descending—consider medical therapy Lowest 1-year survival (67%)
Penetrating aortic ulcer (PAU)	Older (mean age of 74 yr) Hypertension AAA in 40% to 45%	Back/chest pain No malperfusion syndromes	Focal luminal ulceration No flap Largest aortas (mean size = 6.2 cm) Severe atherosclerosis ± Intramural hemorrhage ± Pseudoaneurysm No branch vessel involvement Descending aorta > ascending	Ascending—surgery Descending—lower threshold for surgery 1-year survival = 75%

AAA, abdominal aortic aneurysm.

graft infection. Prosthetic graft infections are difficult to eradicate and can result in significant morbidity and mortality. The sensitivity of MR for graft infection is similar to that of CT.[103] Suggestive MRI findings of graft infection include thick perigraft enhancement, perigraft fluid, pseudoaneurysm formation, hydronephrosis, retroperitoneal/mediastinal fluid extension, perigraft air, and bowel thickening. The presence of perigraft air in association with bowel abnormalities should raise suspicion for aortoenteric fistula. Aortoenteric fistula most commonly occurs in the transverse duodenum.[107]

The use of covered stent-grafts is a minimally invasive therapy for aortic aneurysm and dissection.[43,78,108] MRI is useful in the preoperative evaluation of patients undergoing stent-graft repair[109,110] because it can delineate the morphology of the aortic lumen, allowing for measurement of key parameters such as length and diameter of the infrarenal neck (Fig. 11-17). For patients undergoing thoracic repair, the use of stepped-table technique allows for accurate depiction of the iliac arteries during a single injection (see Fig. 11-9). The luminal diameter of the iliac arteries is readily obtained.

The majority of patients who are treated with a stent-graft are followed by CT. However, MRI may be used to follow patients with renal dysfunction after stent-graft repair, since many devices are composed largely of nonferrous materials (e.g., tantalum and polyethylene) and do not cause significant artifact.[111-114]

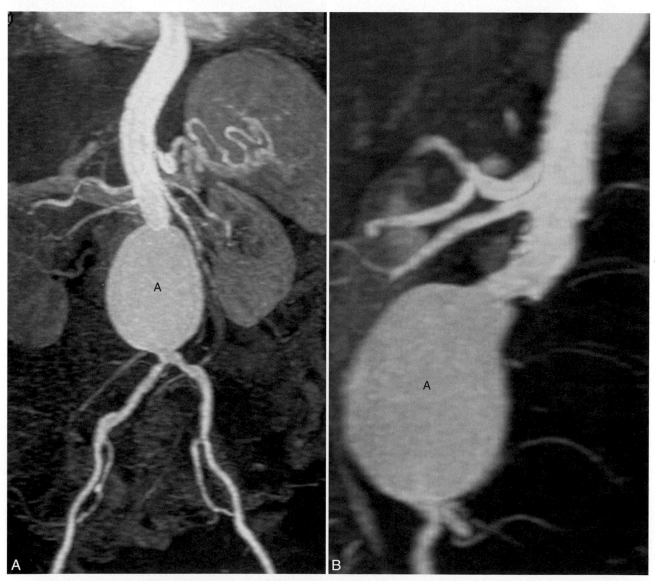

Figure 11-17 ■ CE MRA illustration of an infrarenal abdominal aortic aneurysm. Coronal (**A**) and sagittal (**B**) MIP images of a 3D CE MRA of the aorta shows the relationship of the abdominal aortic aneurysm (**A**) to the renal and iliac arteries to good advantage.

However, nitinol, steel, and cobalt-based stents may produce artifacts that preclude diagnostic MR evaluation after placement.[115-117] The primary role of imaging in this patient population is to define aortic size, confirm aneurysm shrinkage, and detect and characterize endoleaks.[113] An *endoleak* is defined as contrast enhancement within the aneurysm sac following stent-graft repair.[118,119] The classification scheme of endoleak is as follows: type I, related to graft attachment site; type II, collateral supply to sac; type III, leakage between graft components; and type IV, transgraft leakage seen acutely following placement. The most common is the type II endoleak, and the vessels most commonly implicated in type II endoleaks are the inferior mesenteric artery and lumbar arteries (Fig. 11-18). The presence of air within

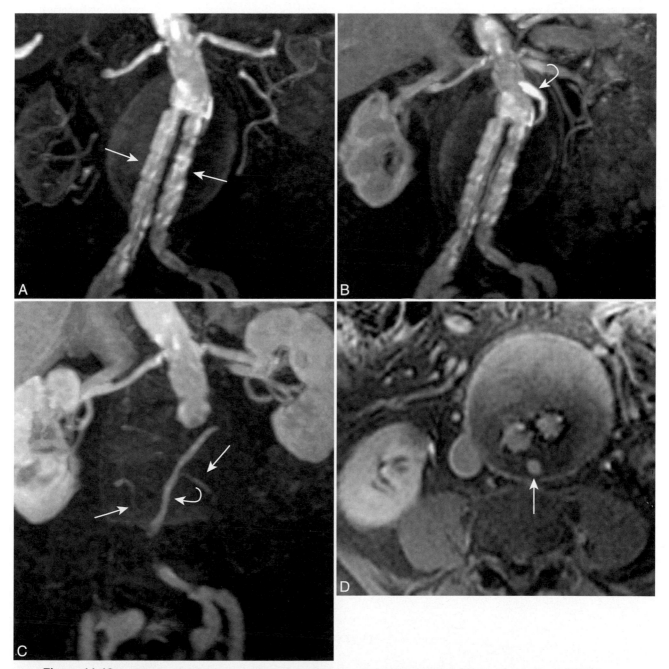

Figure 11-18 ■ MR depiction of a type II endoleak in a patient after stent graft repair. A, Coronal MIP image of a 3D CE MRA of the aorta shows a bifurcated aortic stent graft *(arrows)* without leak. **B** and **C**, Thick (**B**) and thin (**C**) section MIP images obtained 20 seconds later reveal contrast in the endoleak *(curved arrows)*, which is external to the stent. The thin section image reveals adjacent lumbar arteries *(arrows)* that were presumed to represent the source of this type II endoleak. **D**, Delayed axial fat-suppressed T1-WI shows contrast within the bifurcated graft and within the endoleak *(arrow)*, revealed in cross-section. The patient's endoleak was subsequently treated by embolization via a translumbar route.

the aneurysm sac after stent-graft repair is normal only in the immediate postoperative period.[120]

AORTOILIAC OCCLUSIVE DISEASE

MRI is a highly accurate method for the diagnosis of patients with occlusive disease of the aorta and iliac arteries.[121-124] The accuracy of CE MRA is equivalent to that of digital subtraction angiography (DSA) using pressure measurements as the gold standard for detection of hemodynamically significant iliac stenosis.[125] CE MRA provides an accurate depiction of the luminal morphology, including the length and degree of stenoses. In occlusive disease, CE MRA demonstrates collateral pathways (Fig. 11-19). CE MRA is a useful method for planning interventional therapy and also for following patients after stent placement, although luminal measurements within the treated vessel are not accurate.[117,122] A careful history

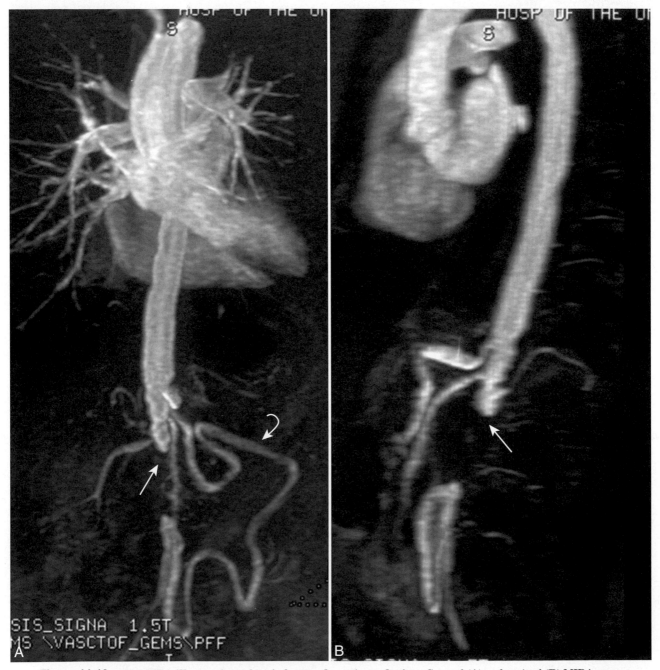

Figure 11-19 ■ CE MRA illustration of an infrarenal aortic occlusion. Coronal (**A**) and sagittal (**B**) MIP images show an infrarenal aortic occlusion *(arrow)* with a prominent arc of Riolan *(curved arrow)* that reconstitutes the inferior mesenteric artery. *(Continued)*

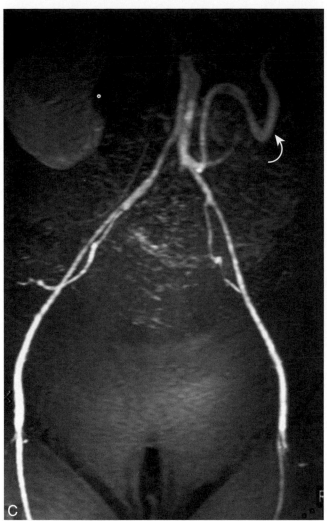

Figure 11-19 ▪ Cont'd The pelvic station MIP image (**C**) shows reconstitution of the distal aorta and iliac vessels.

should be obtained in all patients, since artifact from metallic stents can mimic occlusive disease (Fig. 11-20).

AORTIC TRAUMA

The most common site of traumatic aortic injury in patients who survive the immediate trauma is at the insertion of the ligamentum arteriosum, just distal to the left subclavian artery (Fig. 11-21). At this location, the aorta is relatively fixed, and deceleration/acceleration forces produce excessively high local shear stress on the aortic wall. Other common sites of aortic injury include the aortic root and the aortic hiatus. The aortic injury may extend either completely or partially through the aortic wall. Although CT is the most common cross-sectional imaging study performed in patients with acute trauma,[126,127] MR has also been shown to be a safe and accurate method for the evaluation of this patient population.[128] However, since CT is sensitive in detection of the direct findings of pseudoaneurysm, intimal flap, and periaortic hematoma,[129-131] MR should probably be

reserved for evaluation of equivocal findings revealed on an initial CT.

AORTIC INFECTION

The term mycotic aneurysm is misleading and does not imply a fungal etiology. The word mycotic refers to the mushroom-shaped configuration of many infected aneurysms. Mycotic aneurysms are frequently saccular rather than fusiform and most commonly affect the abdominal aorta. The differential diagnosis for a saccular aortic aneurysm is infection, pseudoaneurysm (Fig. 11-22), and atherosclerosis. The triad of fever, abdominal pain, and a pulsatile abdominal mass should suggest the diagnosis clinically.

Bacterial/Fungal Aortitis

Patients with bacterial or fungal injection of the aorta typically present with fever, pain, leukocytosis, and positive blood cultures. Most cases of bacterial or fungal infection of the aorta occur secondary to hematogenous spread of the organisms, such as from an infected valve (endocarditis) or from a complication of catheterization. Direct spread of an organism from an adjacent structure such as a disk space is possible.

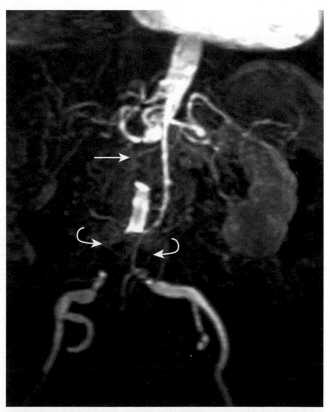

Figure 11-20 ▪ False-positive vascular occlusions secondary to susceptibility artifacts from vascular stents as revealed on CE MRA. The presence of wall stents in the aorta (*arrow*) and iliac bifurcation (*curved arrows*) mimic occlusive disease.

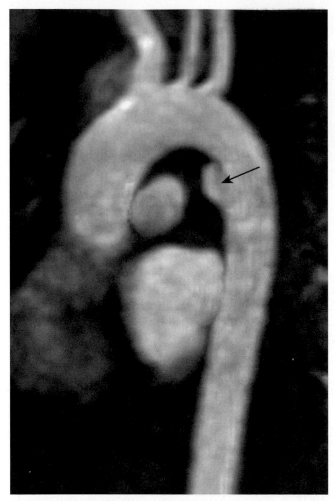

Figure 11-21 ▪ **MR illustration of an aortic transection in a 16-year-old after a motor vehicle accident.** Sagittal CE MRA shows a contained transection *(arrow)* of the aorta near the isthmus.

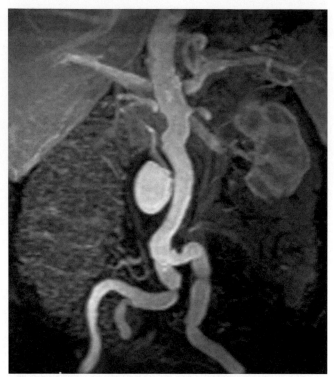

Figure 11-22 ▪ **MR depiction of a postprocedural pseudo-aneurysm at the origin of an occluded renal artery bypass graft.** Coronal MIP image from CE MRA shows a saccular pseudoaneurysm *(arrow)* that displaces the adjacent aorta to the left. There is an absent right nephrogram secondary to renal infarction due to occlusion of the bypass graft.

Common bacterial pathogens affecting the aorta are *Staphylococcus, Salmonella, Streptococcus,* and *Pseudomonas* species.[132-134] Gram-negative bacteria and fungal infections are also possible. The most common fungal pathogen affecting the aorta is *Aspergillus.*

Infectious (mycotic) aneurysms are often saccular; however, many patients with this entity do not have specific features to allow for definitive diagnosis. An infectious cause may be suggested when there is thick delayed periaortic enhancement,[135] sometimes associated with erosion into adjacent structures. Mycotic aneurysm can be complicated by aortocaval[136] (see Fig. 11-10) or aortoesophageal fistula.[137]

Tuberculous Aortitis

Tuberculous infection of the aorta may result in true aneurysm formation, pseudoaneurysm, or stenosis.[67] Most mycotic tuberculous aneurysms are saccular pseudoaneurysms.[138,139] Tuberculous aneurysm results from direct contiguous spread in 75% of patients, either from infected lymph nodes or a para-aortic abscess.[138] Hematogenous seeding of the adventitia

or of the vasa vasorum of the media occurs in the other 25%. The abdominal and thoracic aorta are involved with equal frequency. Other clinical evidence, including abnormal chest X-ray and sputum analysis, often suggests the diagnosis. Miliary tuberculosis when present is thought to be the result, and not the cause, of the mycotic aneurysm.[140]

VASCULITIS OF THE AORTA: TAKAYASU'S ARTERITIS (PULSELESS DISEASE)

Many different vasculitic conditions can affect the aorta, including Takayasu's arteritis, ankylosing spondylitis, rheumatoid aortitis, and giant cell arteritis (temporal arteritis). The most commonly encountered is Takayasu's arteritis. The incidence is relatively high in younger women (aged 15 to 40 years) and in Asia. In histologic studies, the arterial wall is infiltrated by a dense band of inflammatory cells. The local immune reaction leads to chronic wall thickening and subsequent luminal obliteration. Treatment usually consists of immunosuppression with oral corticosteroids.

The American College of Rheumatology has established criteria for the clinical diagnosis of Takayasu's arteritis. Specifically, a patient must meet three or more of the following criteria: onset by age 40, claudication of an extremity, diminished brachial pulses, greater than 10 mm Hg difference in arm blood pressure, and subclavian/aortic bruit. There are four subtypes of Takayasu's arteritis. Type I involves the aortic arch and great vessels. Type II involves the descending and the abdominal aorta with relative sparing of the arch. Type III has features of both types I and II. Type IV involves the pulmonary artery. This classification system, although commonly used, provides little prognostic information.

MRI is an accurate imaging modality in the anatomic assessment of patients with Takayasu's arteritis [12-14,141-143] Results have been mixed concerning the capability of MRI to predict disease activity.[12,144,145] In active phases of the disease, there is marked wall thickening (Fig. 11-23) that shows intermediate T1 SI, high T2 SI, and avid enhancement. In chronic, inactive disease, the wall is relatively thin with luminal narrowing. CE MRA is a useful technique for surgical planning in these patients.[142]

CONGENITAL ANOMALIES OF THE AORTA

Marfan's Syndrome

Marfan's syndrome is an autosomal dominant disorder of connective tissue in which cardiovascular, skeletal, ocular, and other abnormalities are present to a variable degree.[146-148] Prevalence has been estimated to

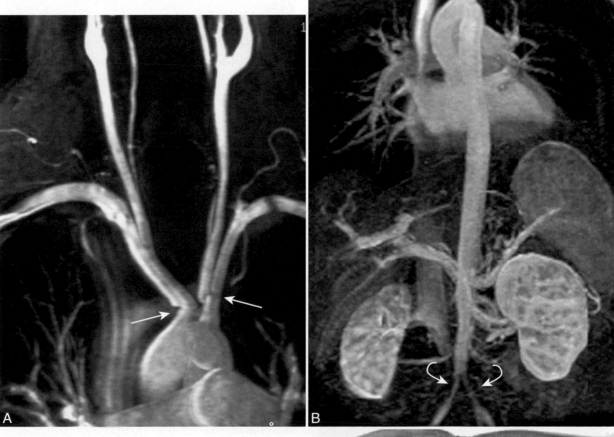

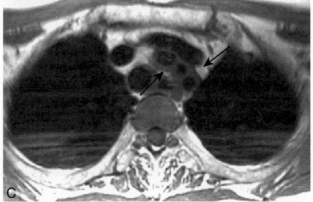

Figure 11-23 ▪ **MR illustration of Takayasu's arteritis in a 46-year-old man who had left recurrent nerve palsy on presentation. A** and **B**, Multistation CE MRA demonstrates involvement of the aortic arch, with web-like stenosis present *(arrows)*, as well as unsuspected involvement of the aortic bifurcation *(curved arrows)*. **C**, Cardiac gated black-blood MRI shows circumferential thickening of the walls of the branch vessels of the affected arch *(arrows)*.

be 1 in 3,000 to 5,000. Clinical diagnosis is based on the Ghent criteria.[149] Affected individuals are commonly tall and thin with long extremities and fingers (arachnodactyly). Scoliosis, pectus carinatum, pectus excavatum, and dural ectasia are associated orthopedic conditions. Ectopia of the lens is observed in 50% to 80% of affected individuals. By age 21, more than half of patients with Marfan's syndrome will have cardiovascular involvement. New mutations account for 25% to 30% of cases. The clinical features are the result of a weakening of connective tissues due to defects in the gene (FBN1) on chromosome 15 that codes for fibrillin-1, a glycoprotein and a principal component of the extracellular matrix microfibril.[148-150] More than 200 mutations in FBN1 have been described.

The mean survival of patients with Marfan's syndrome who are not treated is 40 years.[151] Both medical and surgical therapies have improved life expectancy significantly. The risk of type A dissection increases with increasing aortic root diameter. However, dissection may occur even in the absence of aneurysm. The use of beta blockade and the avoidance of high-stress sports activity are generally recommended. Indications for surgery in Marfan's syndrome include the following: (1) maximal aortic root diameter greater than 55 mm, (2) maximal aortic root dimension greater than 44 mm if pregnancy is desired, (3) aneurysm greater than 5 cm involving other parts of the aorta, and (4) severe mitral regurgitation associated with symptoms of progressive left ventricular dysfunction. Surgical intervention may also be employed in patients who have a prior history of dissection or who do not have involvement of the aortic valve. The surgical procedure of choice in patients with Marfan's syndrome is composite graft repair, and outcomes continue to improve.[152-154]

The most common site of vascular involvement in patients with Marfan's syndrome is the aortic root. There is disruption of the elastic media of the aortic wall, leading to the characteristic finding on pathology of cystic medial necrosis. This usually results in marked dilation of the aortic annulus and sinus portion, so-called annuloaortic ectasia. Myxomatous changes may be observed in the tricuspid valves, and associated valvular dysfunction (aortic insufficiency, aortic stenosis) also is common. These patients are at high risk for superimposed aortic dissection, which is commonly seen affecting the ascending aorta (type A).

The classic imaging finding in patients with Marfan's syndrome is the tulip-shaped aorta, in which there is aneurismal dilation of the aortic root. Cine images often show jet phenomena secondary to superimposed aortic insufficiency and aortic stenosis. Calcification of the aortic wall or valve annulus may be present. Meticulous inspection for the presence of superimposed dissection must be performed. MRI can provide a complete evaluation of the aorta and its branch vessels in patients with Marfan's syndrome both before and after surgery.[155]

Bicuspid Aortic Valve

Bicuspid aortic valve occurs when there are only two cusps in the aortic valve and the noncoronary cusp is absent. The incidence in the general population is 1% to 2%.[156] Individuals are usually asymptomatic until the valve orifice area is reduced to below 40% of normal. Clinical symptoms and signs include a palpable thrill and murmur, angina pectoris, exertional dyspnea, syncope, and reduction in systemic blood pressure. Sudden death occurs in 10% to 20% of cases at an average age of 60 years, presumably owing to arrhythmia. MRI findings in patients with bicuspid aortic valve may include jet phenomena on cine images secondary to aortic valvular dysfunction, valve calcification, and aneurysm of the ascending aorta.[157] Aneurysms are usually confined to the tubular portion of the ascending aorta, and involvement of the root is less common.

Coarctation

Coarctation is narrowing in the aorta that usually occurs in the region of the ligamentum arteriosum. Rarely, it can occur in the arch or distally in the descending thoracic/abdominal aorta. It is most commonly a discrete lesion; however, a variant may be seen in which there is more diffuse hypoplasia of the aorta (Fig. 11-24). Coarctation has an incidence of approximately 1/10,000 (0.01%). It is more common in males (M/F=1.5) and is usually sporadic. However, genetic influences can play a role (up to 35% of individuals with Turner's syndrome [45,X] have aortic coarctation).

Coarctation typically presents in adult life with symptoms and signs attributable to chronic aortic occlusive disease, including upper limb hypertension, differential arm-leg pulses, headache, and claudication. Murmurs secondary to aortic valve disease may be detected. Symptoms are often absent. The mean survival of patients with untreated coarctation is 35 years, with 75% mortality by 46 years of age. Most patients had systemic hypertension and subsequent cardiac failure. Associated complications include heart failure, aortic rupture/dissection, infection, aortic valve dysfunction, and cerebral hemorrhage. Surgery is the gold standard therapy for coarctation.[158]

The most common form of coarctation detected in adult life is "simple" coarctation, which arises in the absence of associated congenital heart disease. "Complex" coarctation occurs in the presence of other important congenital cardiac anomalies and usually is diagnosed in infancy. Cardiovascular abnormalities that have an association with coarctation include ventricular septal defect (VSD), bicuspid aortic valve (up to 85%),[157] intracranial berry aneurysm (3% to 5%), anomalous right subclavian artery (5%), and cystic medial necrosis of the ascending aorta. Nonvascular abnormalities involving the respiratory, gastrointestinal, or genitourinary tracts or the musculoskeletal system have been reported in up to 25% of patients.

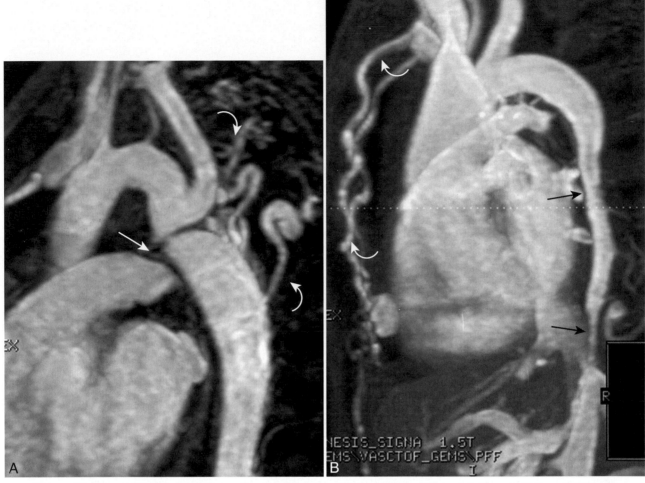

Figure 11-24 ▪ CE MRA depictions of two different patients with aortic coarctation. A, Oblique MIP image of a classic juxtaductal coarctation of the descending aorta at the insertion of the ligamentum arteriosum *(arrow).* Prominent posterior mediastinal collateral vessels are present *(curved arrows).* **B,** Oblique MIP image of another patient with a variant long-segment coarctation consisting of long-segment hypoplasia of the descending thoracic aorta *(arrows).* Aneurysmal dilation of the right internal mammary artery is present *(curved arrows).*

MR plays a useful role in the evaluation of patients with aortic coarctation.[159,160] CE MRA accurately provides morphologic data regarding the primary lesion; specifically, it allows for accurate computation of the percent reduction in cross-sectional area at the site of stenosis. In addition, CE MRA helps in surgical planning because it accurately depicts both extent of disease and presence of enlarged collateral vessels (see Fig. 11-24).[161] The presence of poststenotic aneurysm may lower the threshhold for performing surgical repair. MRI is also useful in the assessment of patients who have undergone surgical repair, in the detection of complications including pseudoaneurysm formation, restenosis, and dissection.

The term *pseudocoarctation* refers to a variant anatomy of the aortic arch in which there is an acute "kink" in the aorta just distal to the arch. This lesion is usually not of hemodynamic significance and does not typically create a pressure gradient. MR findings of pseudocoarctation have been reported.[162,163]

Right-sided Aortic Arch

Right-sided aortic arch is an uncommon condition with an estimated incidence of less than 1%. A modified version of the Stewart system is a currently used classification method, in which five major anatomic types of right-sided aortic arch are recognized based on the arrangement of the arch vessels.[164] Type I consists of a mirror-image arch branching configuration (left innominate, right common carotid, right subclavian). Type II is also a mirror-image branching pattern, with an additional left ductus arteriosus extending from the proximal descending aorta to the left pulmonary artery. Type III is distinctive for an aberrant left subclavian artery that is not derived from a left innominate, instead arising as a separate

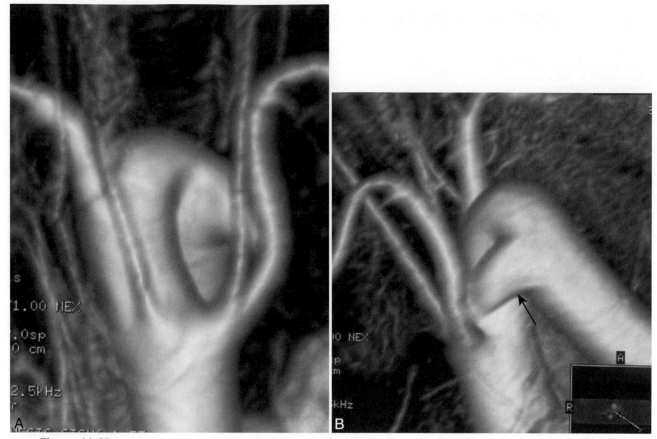

Figure 11-25 ▪ MR illustration of a type II right aortic arch. Coronal (**A**) and oblique (**B**) views on CE MRA reveal a right aortic arch with mirror-image branching of the great vessels. An asymptomatic ductal diverticulum *(arrow)* also is present. This study was reformatted using a shaded-surface display algorithm. Studies suggest that this method does not offer advantages over routine MIP techniques for CE MRA of the thoracic and abdominal aorta.[170]

branch of the descending aorta after the other arch vessels. Type IV consists of an aberrant left innominate artery that arises as the third arch vessel and courses behind the esophagus. Type V contains an isolated left subclavian artery that is a branch from the left pulmonary artery (via left ductus arteriosus) rather than the aorta. The most common type is one in which there is an aberrant left subclavian artery (type III).

The clinical presentation of patients with right-sided aortic arch is variable. While the aberrant arch anatomy itself does not cause symptoms per se, its associated abnormalities do. In types in which there is mirror-image branching of the great vessels (types I and II), there is a high frequency (96% to 98%) of cyanotic congenital heart disease; types III to V have an accompanying cardiac abnormality in 10% to 15%.[165,166] The most common associated cardiac abnormalities are tetralogy of Fallot, truncus arteriosus, tricuspid atresia, and situs inversus.[167] Another commonly observed constellation of symptoms occurs when the abnormal vascular configuration, referred to as a vascular ring or sling, results in encirclement of the trachea and esophagus.

MRI is an accurate method for the diagnosis of right aortic arch variants.[168] Black-blood MRI is useful for delineation of the arch anatomy and for vessel measurements (Fig. 11-25). CE MRA accurately depicts luminal morphologic features. Delayed postcontrast images aid in the detection of associated aneurysms.

REFERENCES

1. Quinn SF, Sheley RC, Semonsen KG, Leonardo VJ, Kojima K, Szumowski J. Aortic and lower-extremity arterial disease: evaluation with MR angiography versus conventional angiography. Radiology 1998;206:693-701.
2. Hartnell GG, Finn JP, Zenni M, et al. MR imaging of the thoracic aorta: comparison of spin-echo, angiographic, and breath-hold techniques. Radiology 1994;191:697-704.
3. Krinsky G, Reuss PM. MR angiography of the thoracic aorta. Magn Reson Imaging Clin North Am 1998;6:293-320.
4. Prince MR, Narasimham DL, Jacoby WT, et al. Three-dimensional gadolinium-enhanced MR angiography of the thoracic aorta. AJR Am J Roentgenol 1996;166:1387-1397.
5. Yucel EK, Anderson CM, Edelman RR, et al. AHA scientific statement. Magnetic resonance angiography: update on applications for extracranial arteries. Circulation 1999;100:2284-2301.
6. Huber A, Scheidler J, Wintersperger B, et al. Moving-table MR angiography of the peripheral runoff vessels: comparison of body coil and dedicated phased array coil systems. AJR Am J Roentgenol 2003;180:1365-1373.

7. Siegelman ES, Charafeddine R, Stolpen AH, Axel L. Suppression of intravascular signal on fat-saturated contrast-enhanced thoracic MR arteriograms. Radiology 2000;217:115-118.

8. Axel L, Kolman L, Charafeddine R, Hwang SN, Stolpen AH. Origin of a signal intensity loss artifact in fat-saturation MR imaging. Radiology 2000;217:911-915.

9. Bradley WG, Jr. MR appearance of hemorrhage in the brain. [Comments.] Radiology 1993;189:15-26.

10. Bluemke DA. Definitive diagnosis of intramural hematoma of the thoracic aorta with MR imaging. Radiology 1997;204:319-321.

11. Ha HK, Lim YT, Kim HS, Suh TS, Song HH, Kim SJ. Diagnosis of pelvic endometriosis: fat-suppressed T1-weighted vs conventional MR images. AJR Am J Roentgenol 1994;163:127-131.

12. Choe YH, Kim DK, Koh EM, Do YS, Lee WR. Takayasu arteritis: diagnosis with MR imaging and MR angiography in acute and chronic active stages. J Magn Reson Imaging 1999;10:751-757.

13. Hata A, Numano F. Magnetic resonance imaging of vascular changes in Takayasu arteritis. Int J Cardiol 1995;52:45-52.

14. Matsunaga N, Hayashi K, Sakamoto I, et al. Takayasu arteritis: MR manifestations and diagnosis of acute and chronic phase. J Magn Reson Imaging 1998;8:406-414.

15. Yu BC, Jara H, Melhem ER, Caruthers SD, Yucel EK. Black-blood MR angiography with GRASE: measurement of flow-induced signal attenuation. J Magn Reson Imaging 1998;8:1334-1337.

16. Jara H, Barish MA. Black-blood MR angiography: techniques, and clinical applications. Magn Reson Imaging Clin North Am 1999;7:303-317.

17. Stemerman DH, Krinsky GA, Lee VS, Johnson G, Yang BM, Rofsky NM. Thoracic aorta: rapid black-blood MR imaging with half-Fourier rapid acquisition with relaxation enhancement with or without electrocardiographic triggering. Radiology 1999;213:185-191.

18. Campos S, Martinez Sanjuan V, Garcia Nieto JJ, et al. New black blood pulse sequence for studies of the heart. Int J Cardiac Imaging. 1999;15:175-183.

19. Bradley WG, Jr., Waluch V, Lai KS, Fernandez EJ, Spalter C. The appearance of rapidly flowing blood on magnetic resonance images. AJR Am J Roentgenol 1984;143:1167-1174.

20. Boxerman JL, Mosher TJ, McVeigh ER, Atalar E, Lima JA, Bluemke DA. Advanced MR imaging techniques for evaluation of the heart and great vessels. Radiographics 1998;18:543-564.

21. Epstein FH, Wolff SD, Arai AE. Segmented k-space fast cardiac imaging using an echo-train readout. Magn Reson Med 1999;41:609-613.

22. Pereles FS, McCarthy RM, Baskaran V, et al. Thoracic aortic dissection and aneurysm: evaluation with nonenhanced true FISP MR angiography in less than 4 minutes. Radiology 2002;223:270-274.

23. Reeder SB, Atalar E, Faranesh AZ, McVeigh ER. Multi-echo segmented k-space imaging: an optimized hybrid sequence for ultrafast cardiac imaging. Magn Reson Med 1999;41:375-385.

24. Rumancik WM, Naidich DP, Chandra R, et al. Cardiovascular disease: evaluation with MR phase imaging. Radiology 1988;166:63-68.

25. Miller SW, Holmvang G. Differentiation of slow flow from thrombus in thoracic magnetic resonance imaging, emphasizing phase images. J Thorac Imaging 1993;8:98-107.

26. Kaminaga T, Yamada N, Takamiya M, Nishimura T. Sequential MR signal change of the thrombus in the false lumen of thrombosed aortic dissection. Magn Reson Imaging 1995;13:773-779.

27. Prince MR, Yucel EK, Kaufman JA, Harrison DC, Geller SC. Dynamic gadolinium-enhanced three-dimensional abdominal MR arteriography. J Magn Reson Imaging 1993;3:877-881.

28. Carr JC, Finn JP. MR imaging of the thoracic aorta. Magn Reson Imaging Clin N Am 2003;11:135-148.

29. Tatli S, Lipton MJ, Davison BD, Skorstad RB, Yucel EK. From the RSNA refresher courses: MR imaging of aortic and peripheral vascular disease. Radiographics 2003;23(Spec No.):S59-78.

30. Arpasi PJ, Bis KG, Shetty AN, White RD, Simonetti OP. MR angiography of the thoracic aorta with an electrocardiographically triggered breath-hold contrast-enhanced sequence. Radiographics 2000;20:107-120.

31. Earls JP, Rofsky NM, DeCorato DR, Krinsky GA, Weinreb JC. Breath-hold single-dose gadolinium-enhanced three-dimensional MR aortography: usefulness of a timing examination and MR power injector. Radiology 1996;201:705-710.

32. Davis CP, Hany TF, Wildermuth S, Schmidt M, Debatin JF. Postprocessing techniques for gadolinium-enhanced three-dimensional MR angiography. Radiographics 1997;17:1061-1077.

33. Geenen RW, Hussain SM, Cademartiri F, Poley JW, Siersema PD, Krestin GP. CT and MR colonography: scanning techniques, postprocessing, and emphasis on polyp detection. Radiographics 2004;24:e18.

34. Glockner JF. Navigating the aorta: MR virtual vascular endoscopy. Radiographics 2003;23:e11.

35. Ho VB, Corse WR. MR angiography of the abdominal aorta and peripheral vessels. Radiol Clin North Am 2003;41:115-144.

36. Svensson J, Petersson JS, Stahlberg F, Larsson EM, Leander P, Olsson LE. Image artifacts due to a time-varying contrast medium concentration in 3D contrast-enhanced MRA. J Magn Reson Imaging 1999;10:919-928.

37. Ho VB, Foo TK. Optimization of gadolinium-enhanced magnetic resonance angiography using an automated bolus-detection algorithm (MR SmartPrep): original investigation. Invest Radiol 1998;33:515-523.

38. Wilman AH, Riederer SJ, King BF, Debbins JP, Rossman PJ, Ehman RL. Fluoroscopically triggered contrast-enhanced three-dimensional MR angiography with elliptical centric view order: application to the renal arteries. Radiology 1997;205:137-146.

39. Hussain HK, Londy FJ, Francis IR, et al. Hepatic arterial phase MR imaging with automated bolus-detection three-dimensional fast gradient-recalled-echo sequence: comparison with test-bolus method. Radiology 2003;226:558-566.

40. Shetty AN, Bis KG, Vrachliotis TG, Kirsch M, Shirkhoda A, Ellwood R. Contrast-enhanced 3D MRA with centric ordering in k space: a preliminary clinical experience in imaging the abdominal aorta and renal and peripheral arterial vasculature. J Magn Reson Imaging 1998;8:603-615.

41. Maki JH, Chenevert TL, Prince MR. The effects of incomplete breath-holding on 3D MR image quality. J Magn Reson Imaging 1997;7:1132-1139.

42. Riederer SJ, Bernstein MA, Breen JF, et al. Three-dimensional contrast-enhanced MR angiography with real-time fluoroscopic triggering: design specifications and technical reliability in 330 patient studies. Radiology 2000;215:584-593.

43. Nienaber CA, Fattori R, Lund G, et al. Nonsurgical reconstruction of thoracic aortic dissection by stent-graft placement. N Engl J Med 1999;340:1539-1545.

44. Ho VB, Choyke PL, Foo TK, et al. Automated bolus chase peripheral MR angiography: initial practical experiences and future directions of this work-in-progress. J Magn Reson Imaging 1999;10:376-388.

45. Earls JP, DeSena S, Bluemke DA. Gadolinium-enhanced three-dimensional MR angiography of the entire aorta and iliac arteries with dynamic manual table translation. Radiology 1998;209:844-849.

46. Hentsch A, Aschauer MA, Balzer JO, et al. Gadobutrol-enhanced moving-table magnetic resonance angiography in patients with peripheral vascular disease: a prospective, multi-centre blinded comparison with digital subtraction angiography. Eur Radiol 2003;13:2103-2114.

47. Kelekis NL, Semelka RC, Molina PL, Warshauer DM, Sharp TJ, Detterbeck FC. Immediate postgadolinium spoiled gradient-echo MRI for evaluating the abdominal aorta in the setting of abdominal MR examination. J Magn Reson Imaging 1997;7:652-656.

48. Kelekis NL, Semelka RC, Worawattanakul S, Molina PL, Mauro MA. Magnetic resonance imaging of the abdominal aorta and iliac vessels using combined 3-D gadolinium-enhanced MRA and gadolinium-enhanced fat-suppressed spoiled gradient echo sequences. Magn Reson Imaging 1999;17:641-651.

49. Kadir S. Atlas of Normal and Variant Angiographic Anatomy. Philadelphia, WB Saunders, 1991.

50. Carpenter JP, Holland GA, Golden MA, et al. Magnetic resonance angiography of the aortic arch. J Vasc Surg 1997;25:145-151.

51. Kent PD, Poterucha TH. Images in clinical medicine. Aberrant right subclavian artery and dysphagia lusoria. N Engl J Med 2002;346:1637.

52. Myers JL, Gomes MN. Management of aberrant subclavian artery aneurysms. J Cardiovasc Surg (Torino) 2000;41:607-612.

53. Pearce WH, Slaughter MS, LeMaire S, et al. Aortic diameter as a function of age, gender, and body surface area. Surgery 1993;114:691-697.

54. Moore WS. Vascular Surgery: A Comprehensive Review. Philadelphia, WB Saunders, 1998.

55. Ernst CB, Stanley JC. Current Therapy in Vascular Surgery. St. Louis, Mosby-Year Book, 1995.

56. Singh K, Bonaa KH, Jacobsen BK, Bjork L, Solberg S. Prevalence of and risk factors for abdominal aortic aneurysms in a population-based study: the Tromso study. Am J Epidemiol 2001;154:236-244.

57. Powell JT, Greenhalgh RM. Clinical practice. Small abdominal aortic aneurysms. N Engl J Med 2003;348:1895-1901.

58. Clouse WD, Hallett J, Schaff HV, Gayari M, Ilstrup DM, Joseph ML. Improved prognosis of thoracic aortic aneurysms: a population-based study. JAMA 1998;280:1926-1929.

59. Lederle FA, Wilson SE, Johnson GR, et al. Immediate repair compared with surveillance of small abdominal aortic aneurysms. N Engl J Med 2002;346:1437-1444.

60. United Kingdom Small Aneurysm Trial Participants. Long-term outcomes of immediate repair compared with surveillance of small abdominal aortic aneurysms. N Engl J Med 2002;346:1445-1452.

61. United Kingdom Small Aneurysm Trial Participants. Mortality results for randomised controlled trial of early elective surgery or ultrasonographic surveillance for small abdominal aortic aneurysms. Lancet 1998;352:1649-1655.

62. Brady AR, Fowkes FG, Greenhalgh RM, Powell JT, Ruckley CV, Thompson SG. Risk factors for postoperative death following elective surgical repair of abdominal aortic aneurysm: results from the UK Small Aneurysm Trial—on behalf of the UK Small Aneurysm Trial participants. Br J Surg 2000;87:742-749.

63. Wilmink TB, Quick CR, Day NE. The association between cigarette smoking and abdominal aortic aneurysms. J Vasc Surg 1999;30:1099-1105.

64. Maher MM, McNamara AM, MacEneaney PM, Sheehan SJ, Malone DE. Abdominal aortic aneurysms: elective endovascular repair versus conventional surgery—evaluation with evidence-based medicine techniques. Radiology 2003;228:647-658.

65. Ohki T, Veith FJ, Shaw P, et al. Increasing incidence of midterm and long-term complications after endovascular graft repair of abdominal aortic aneurysms: a note of caution based on a 9-year experience. Ann Surg 2001;234:323-334; discussion 334-325.

66. Harris PL, Vallabhaneni SR, Desgranges P, Becquemin JP, van Marrewijk C, Laheij RJ. Incidence and risk factors of late rupture, conversion, and death after endovascular repair of infrarenal aortic aneurysms: the EUROSTAR experience—European Collaborators on stent/graft techniques for aortic aneurysm repair. J Vasc Surg 2000;32:739-749.

67. Loscalzo J, Creager MA, Dzau VJ, Chobanian A. Vascular Medicine: A Textbook of Vascular Biology and Diseases, 2nd ed. Philadelphia, Lippincott Williams & Wilkins, 1996.

68. Hayashi H, Kumazaki T. Case report: inflammatory abdominal aortic aneurysm—dynamic Gd-DTPA enhanced magnetic resonance imaging features. Br J Radiol 1995;68:321-323.

69. Anbarasu A, Harris PL, McWilliams RG. The role of gadolinium-enhanced MR imaging in the preoperative evaluation of inflammatory abdominal aortic aneurysm. Eur Radiol 2002;12(Suppl 4):S192-195.

70. Crawford ES, Crawford JL, Safi HJ, et al. Thoracoabdominal aortic aneurysms: preoperative and intraoperative factors determining immediate and long-term results of operations in 605 patients. J Vasc Surg 1986;3:389-404.

71. Reddy GP, Higgins CB. MR imaging of the thoracic aorta. Magn Reson Imaging Clin North Am 2000;8:1-15.

72. Carriero A, Palumbo L, Tonni AG, D'Angelo C, Magarelli N, Bonomo L. [Diagnostic pitfalls in magnetic resonance angiography.] Radiol Med 1995;90:719-725.

73. Chiowanich P, Mitchell DG, Ortega HV, Mohamed F. Arterial pseudostenosis on first-pass gadolinium-enhanced three-dimensional MR angiography: new observation of a potential pitfall. AJR Am J Roentgenol 2000;175:523-527.

74. Nienaber CA, Eagle KA. Aortic dissection: new frontiers in diagnosis and management. 1. From etiology to diagnostic strategies. Circulation 2003;108:628-635.

75. Hagan PG, Nienaber CA, Isselbacher EM, et al. The International Registry of Acute Aortic Dissection (IRAD): new insights into an old disease. JAMA 2000;283:897-903.

76. Bordeleau L, Cwinn A, Turek M, Barron-Klauninger K, Victor G. Aortic dissection and Turner's syndrome: case report and review of the literature. J Emerg Med 1998;16:593-596.

77. Daily PO, Trueblood HW, Stinson EB, Wuerflein RD, Shumway NE. Management of acute aortic dissections. Ann Thorac Surg 1970;10:237-247.

78. Dake MD, Kato N, Mitchell RS, et al. Endovascular stent-graft placement for the treatment of acute aortic dissection. N Engl J Med 1999;340:1546-1552.

79. Nienaber CA, von Kodolitsch Y, Nicolas V, et al. The diagnosis of thoracic aortic dissection by noninvasive imaging procedures. N Engl J Med 1993;328:1-9.

80. Krinsky GA, Rofsky NM, DeCorato DR, et al. Thoracic aorta: comparison of gadolinium-enhanced three-dimensional MR angiography with conventional MR imaging. Radiology 1997;202:183-193.

81. Hartnell GG. Imaging of aortic aneurysms and dissection: CT and MRI. J Thorac Imaging 2001;16:35-46.

82. Roberts DA. Magnetic resonance imaging of thoracic aortic aneurysm and dissection. Semin Roentgenol 2001;36:295-308.

83. Bogaert J, Meyns B, Rademakers FE, et al. Follow-up of aortic dissection: contribution of MR angiography for evaluation of the abdominal aorta and its branches. Eur Radiol 1997;7:695-702.

84. Cesare ED, Giordano AV, Cerone G, De Remigis F, Deusanio G, Masciocchi C. Comparative evaluation of TEE, conventional MRI and contrast-enhanced 3D breath-hold MRA in the post-operative follow-up of dissecting aneurysms. Int J Cardiac Imaging 2000;16:135-147.

85. Gaubert JY, Caus T, Dahan M, et al. MRI for follow-up after surgery for thoracic aorta dissection. Magma 2000;11:78-79.

86. Inoue T, Watanabe S, Sakurada H, et al. Evaluation of flow volume and flow patterns in the patent false lumen of chronic aortic dissections using velocity-encoded cine magnetic resonance imaging. Jpn Circ J 2000;64:760-764.

87. Coady MA, Rizzo JA, Elefteriades JA. Pathologic variants of thoracic aortic dissections. Penetrating atherosclerotic ulcers and intramural hematomas. Cardiol Clin 1999;17:637-657.

88. Macura KJ, Corl FM, Fishman EK, Bluemke DA. Pathogenesis in acute aortic syndromes: aortic aneurysm leak and rupture and traumatic aortic transection. AJR Am J Roentgenol 2003;181:303-307.

89. Tittle SL, Lynch RJ, Cole PE, et al. Midterm follow-up of penetrating ulcer and intramural hematoma of the aorta. J Thorac Cardiovasc Surg 2002;123:1051-1059.

90. Schoder M, Grabenwoger M, Holzenbein T, et al. Endovascular stent-graft repair of complicated penetrating atherosclerotic ulcers of the descending thoracic aorta. J Vasc Surg 2002;36:720-726.

91. Kos X, Bouchard L, Otal P, et al. Stent-graft treatment of penetrating thoracic aortic ulcers. J Endovasc Ther 2002;9(Suppl 2):II25-31.

92. Krinsky GA. Diagnostic imaging of aortic atherosclerosis and its complications. Neuroimaging Clin N Am 2002;12:437-443.

93. Mohiaddin RH, McCrohon J, Francis JM, Barbir M, Pennell DJ. Contrast-enhanced magnetic resonance angiogram of penetrating aortic ulcer. Circulation 2001;103:E18-19.

94. Hayashi H, Matsuoka Y, Sakamoto I, et al. Penetrating atherosclerotic ulcer of the aorta: imaging features and disease concept. Radiographics 2000;20:995-1005.

95. Krukemberg E. Beitrage zur Frage des Aneurysma dissecans. Beitr Pathol Anat Allg Pathol 1920;67.

96. Vilacosta I, San Roman JA, Ferreiros J, et al. Natural history and serial morphology of aortic intramural hematoma: a novel variant of aortic dissection. Am Heart J 1997;134:495-507.

97. Macura KJ, Corl FM, Fishman EK, Bluemke DA. Pathogenesis in acute aortic syndromes: aortic dissection, intramural hematoma, and penetrating atherosclerotic aortic ulcer. AJR Am J Roentgenol 2003;181:309-316.

98. Macura KJ, Szarf G, Fishman EK, Bluemke DA. Role of computed tomography and magnetic resonance imaging in assessment of acute aortic syndromes. Semin Ultrasound CT MR 2003;24:232-254.

99. Song JK, Kim HS, Song JM, et al. Outcomes of medically treated patients with aortic intramural hematoma. Am J Med 2002;113:181-187.

100. Riley P, Rooney S, Bonser R, Guest P. Imaging the post-operative thoracic aorta: normal anatomy and pitfalls. Br J Radiol 2001;74:1150-1158.

101. Cameron DE. Surgical techniques: ascending aorta. Cardiol Clin 1999;17:739-750.

102. Bentall H, De Bono A. A technique for complete replacement of the ascending aorta. Thorax 1968;23:338-339.

103. Orton DF, LeVeen RF, Saigh JA, et al. Aortic prosthetic graft infections: radiologic manifestations and implications for management. Radiographics 2000;20:977-993.

104. Loubeyre P, Delignette A, Bonefoy L, Douek P, Amiel M, Revel D. Magnetic resonance imaging evaluation of the ascending aorta after graft-inclusion surgery: comparison between an ultrafast contrast-enhanced MR sequence and conventional cine-MRI. J Magn Reson Imaging 1996;6:478-483.

105. Spartera C, Morettini G, Petrassi C, Di Cesare E, La Barbera G, Ventura M. Healing of aortic prosthetic grafts: a study by magnetic resonance imaging. Ann Vasc Surg 1994;8:536-542.

106. Kat E, Jones DN, Burnett J, Foreman R, Chok R, Sage MR. Perigraft seroma of open aortic reconstruction. AJR Am J Roentgenol 2002;178:1462-1464.

107. Amin S, Luketich J, Wald A. Aortoesophageal fistula: case report and review of the literature. Dig Dis Sci 1998;43:1665-1671.

108. Blum U, Voshage G, Lammer J, et al. Endoluminal stent-grafts for infrarenal abdominal aortic aneurysms. N Engl J Med 1997;336:13-20.

109. Neschis DG, Velazquez OC, Baum RA, et al. The role of magnetic resonance angiography for endoprosthetic design. J Vasc Surg 2001;33:488-494.

110. Thurnher SA, Dorffner R, Thurnher MM, et al. Evaluation of abdominal aortic aneurysm for stent-graft placement: comparison of gadolinium-enhanced MR angiography versus helical CT angiography and digital subtraction angiography. Radiology 1997;205:341-352.

111. Kramer SC, Gorich J, Pamler R, Aschoff AJ, Wisianowski C, Brambs HJ. [The contribution of MRI to the detection of endovascular aneurysm repair.] Rofo Fortschr Geb Rontgenstr Neuen Bildgeb Verfahr 2002;174:1285-1288.

112. Merkle EM, Klein S, Kramer SC, Wisianowsky C. MR angiographic findings in patients with aortic endoprostheses. AJR Am J Roentgenol 2002;178:641-648.

113. Insko EK, Kulzer LM, Fairman RM, Carpenter JP, Stavropoulos SW. MR imaging for the detection of endoleaks in recipients of abdominal aortic stent-grafts with low magnetic susceptibility. Acad Radiol 2003;10:509-513.

114. Lookstein RA, Goldman J, Pukin L, Marin ML. Time-resolved magnetic resonance angiography as a noninvasive method to characterize endoleaks: initial results compared with conventional angiography. J Vasc Surg 2004;39:27-33.

115. Maintz D, Tombach B, Juergens KU, Weigel S, Heindel W, Fischbach R. Revealing in-stent stenoses of the iliac arteries: comparison of multidetector CT with MR angiography and digital

radiographic angiography in a Phantom model. AJR Am J Roentgenol 2002;179:1319-1322.

116. Maintz D, Kugel H, Schellhammer F, Landwehr P. In vitro evaluation of intravascular stent artifacts in three-dimensional MR angiography. Invest Radiol 2001;36:218-224.

117. Meyer JM, Buecker A, Schuermann K, Ruebben A, Guenther RW. MR evaluation of stent patency: in vitro test of 22 metallic stents and the possibility of determining their patency by MR angiography. Invest Radiol 2000;35:739-746.

118. Wain RA, Marin ML, Ohki T, et al. Endoleaks after endovascular graft treatment of aortic aneurysms: classification, risk factors, and outcome. J Vasc Surg 1998;27:69-78; discussion 78-80.

119. Veith FJ, Baum RA, Ohki T, et al. Nature and significance of endoleaks and endotension: summary of opinions expressed at an international conference. J Vasc Surg 2002;35:1029-1035.

120. Velazquez OC, Carpenter JP, Baum RA, et al. Perigraft air, fever, and leukocytosis after endovascular repair of abdominal aortic aneurysms. Am J Surg 1999;178:185-189.

121. Winterer JT, Laubenberger J, Scheffler K, et al. Contrast-enhanced subtraction MR angiography in occlusive disease of the pelvic and lower limb arteries: results of a prospective intraindividual comparative study with digital subtraction angiography in 76 patients. J Comput Assist Tomogr 1999;23:583-589.

122. Link J, Steffens JC, Brossmann J, Graessner J, Hackethal S, Heller M. Iliofemoral arterial occlusive disease: contrast-enhanced MR angiography for preinterventional evaluation and follow-up after stent placement. Radiology 1999;212:371-377.

123. Fenchel S, Wisianowsky C, Schams S, et al. Contrast-enhanced 3D MRA of the aortoiliac and infrainguinal arteries when conventional transfemoral arteriography is not feasible. J Endovasc Ther 2002;9:511-519.

124. Torreggiani WC, Varghese J, Haslam P, McGrath F, Munk PL, Lee MJ. Prospective comparison of MRA with catheter angiography in the assessment of patients with aortoiliac occlusion before surgery or endovascular therapy. Clin Radiol 2002;57:625-631.

125. Wikstrom J, Holmberg A, Johansson L, et al. Gadolinium-enhanced magnetic resonance angiography, digital subtraction angiography and duplex of the iliac arteries compared with intra-arterial pressure gradient measurements. Eur J Vasc Endovasc Surg 2000;19:516-523.

126. Fishman JE. Imaging of blunt aortic and great vessel trauma. J Thorac Imaging 2000;15:97-103.

127. Gavelli G, Canini R, Bertaccini P, Battista G, Bna C, Fattori R. Traumatic injuries: imaging of thoracic injuries. Eur Radiol 2002;12:1273-1294.

128. Mirvis SE, Shanmuganathan K. MR imaging of thoracic trauma. Magn Reson Imaging Clin North Am 2000;8:91-104.

129. Cleverley JR, Barrie JR, Raymond GS, Primack SL, Mayo JR. Direct findings of aortic injury on contrast-enhanced CT in surgically proven traumatic aortic injury: a multi-centre review. Clin Radiol 2002;57:281-286.

130. Downing SW, Sperling JS, Mirvis SE, et al. Experience with spiral computed tomography as the sole diagnostic method for traumatic aortic rupture. Ann Thorac Surg 2001;72:495-501; discussion 501-492.

131. Parker MS, Matheson TL, Rao AV, et al. Making the transition: the role of helical CT in the evaluation of potentially acute thoracic aortic injuries. AJR Am J Roentgenol 2001;176:1267-1272.

132. Feigl D, Feigl A, Edwards JE. Mycotic aneurysms of the aortic root: a pathologic study of 20 cases. Chest 1986;90:553-557.

133. Rubery PT, Smith MD, Cammisa FP, Silane M. Mycotic aortic aneurysm in patients who have lumbar vertebral osteomyelitis: a report of two cases. J Bone Joint Surg Am 1995;77:1729-1732.

134. Hsu RB, Tsay YG, Wang SS, Chu SH. Surgical treatment for primary infected aneurysm of the descending thoracic aorta, abdominal aorta, and iliac arteries. J Vasc Surg 2002;36:746-750.

135. Walsh DW, Ho VB, Haggerty MF. Mycotic aneurysm of the aorta: MRI and MRA features. J Magn Reson Imaging 1997;7:312-315.

136. Torigian DA, Carpenter JP, Roberts DA. Mycotic aortocaval fistula: efficient evaluation by bolus-chase MR angiography. J Magn Reson Imaging 2002;15:195-198.

137. Molina PL, Strobl PW, Burstain JM. Aortoesophageal fistula secondary to mycotic aneurysm of the descending thoracic aorta: CT demonstration. J Comput Assist Tomogr 1995;19:309-311.

138. Long R, Guzman R, Greenberg H, Safneck J, Hershfield E. Tuberculous mycotic aneurysm of the aorta: review of published medical and surgical experience. Chest 1999;115:522-531.

139. Choudhary SK, Bhan A, Talwar S, Goyal M, Sharma S, Venugopal P. Tubercular pseudoaneurysms of aorta. Ann Thorac Surg 2001;72:1239-1244.

140. Felson B, Akers PV, Hall GS, Schreiber JT, Greene RE, Pedrosa CS. Mycotic tuberculous aneurysm of the thoracic aorta. JAMA 1977;237:1104-1108.

141. Choe YH, Lee WR. Magnetic resonance imaging diagnosis of Takayasu arteritis. Int J Cardiol 1998;66:S175-S179; discussion S181.

142. Atalay MK, Bluemke DA. Magnetic resonance imaging of large vessel vasculitis. Curr Opin Rheumatol 2001;13:41-47.

143. Yamada I, Nakagawa T, Himeno Y, Kobayashi Y, Numano F, Shibuya H. Takayasu arteritis: diagnosis with breath-hold contrast-enhanced three-dimensional MR angiography. J Magn Reson Imaging 2000;11:481-487.

144. Tso E, Flamm SD, White RD, Schvartzman PR, Mascha E, Hoffman GS. Takayasu arteritis: utility and limitations of magnetic resonance imaging in diagnosis and treatment. Arthritis Rheum 2002;46:1634-1642.

145. Aluquin VP, Albano SA, Chan F, Sandborg C, Pitlick PT. Magnetic resonance imaging in the diagnosis and follow up of Takayasu's arteritis in children. Ann Rheum Dis 2002;61:526-529.

146. Pyeritz RE. The Marfan syndrome. Annu Rev Med 2000;51:481-510.

147. Aburawi EH, O'Sullivan J, Hasan A. Marfan's syndrome: a review. Hosp Med 2001;62:153-157.

148. Collod-Beroud G, Boileau C. Marfan syndrome in the third millennium. Eur J Hum Genet 2002;10:673-681.

149. Maron BJ, Moller JH, Seidman CE, et al. Impact of laboratory molecular diagnosis on contemporary diagnostic criteria for genetically transmitted cardiovascular diseases: hypertrophic cardiomyopathy, long QT syndrome and Marfan syndrome. Circulation 1998;98:1460-1471.

150. Robinson PN, Godfrey M. The molecular genetics of Marfan syndrome and related fibrillinopathies. J Med Genet 2000;37:9-25.

151. Murdoch JL, Walker B, Halpern BL, et al. Life expectancy and causes of death in the Marfan syndrome. N Engl J Med 1992;286:804-808.

152. LeMaire SA, Coselli JS. Aortic root surgery in Marfan syndrome: current practice and evolving techniques. J Cardiac Surg 1997;12:137-141.

153. Safi HJ, Vinnerkvist A, Bhama JK, Miller CC III, Koussayer S, Haverich A. Aortic valve disease in Marfan syndrome. Curr Opin Cardiol 1998;13:91-95.

154. Gott VL, Greene PS, Alejo DE, et al. Replacement of the aortic root in patients with Marfan's syndrome. N Engl J Med 1999;340:1307-1313.

155. Kawamoto S, Bluemke DA, Traill TA, Zerhouni EA. Thoracoabdominal aorta in Marfan syndrome: MR imaging findings of progression of vasculopathy after surgical repair. Radiology 1997;203:727-732.

156. Fedak PW, Verma S, David TE, Leask RL, Weisel RD, Butany J. Clinical and pathophysiological implications of a bicuspid aortic valve. Circulation 2002;106:900-904.

157. Bruce CJ, Breen JF. Images in clinical medicine: aortic coarctation and bicuspid aortic valve. N Engl J Med 2000;342:249.

158. Corno AF, Botta U, Hurni M, et al. Surgery for aortic coarctation: a 30 years experience. Eur J Cardiothorac Surg 2001;20:1202-1206.

159. Godart F, Labrot G, Devos P, McFadden E, Rey C, Beregi JP. Coarctation of the aorta: comparison of aortic dimensions between conventional MR imaging, 3D MR angiography, and conventional angiography. Eur Radiol 2002;12:2034-2039.

160. Vogt FM, Goyen M, Debatin JF. MR angiography of the chest. Radiol Clin North Am 2003;41:29-41.

161. Julsrud PR, Breen JF, Felmlee JP, Warnes CA, Connolly HM, Schaff HV. Coarctation of the aorta: collateral flow assessment with phase-contrast MR angiography. AJR Am J Roentgenol 1997;169:1735-1742.

162. Soler R, Pombo F, Bargiela A, Gayol A, Rodriguez E. MRI of pseudocoarctation of the aorta: morphological and cine-MRI findings. Comput Med Imaging Graph 1995;19:431-434.

163. Munjal AK, Rose WS, Williams G. Magnetic resonance imaging of pseudocoarctation of the aorta: a case report. J Thorac Imaging 1994;9:88-91.

164. Juhl JH, Crummy AB, Kuhlman JE. Paul and Juhl's Essentials of Radiologic Imaging. Philadelphia, Lippincott-Raven, 1998.

165. Felson B, Palayew MJ. The two types of right aortic arch. Radiology 1963;81:745-759.

166. Stewart JR, Kincaid OW, Titus JL. Right aortic arch: plain film diagnosis and significance. Am J Roentgenol Radium Ther Nucl Med 1966;97:377-389.

167. Keith JD, Rowe RD, Vlad P. Heart Disease in Infancy and Childhood. New York, Macmillan, 1978.

168. Kleinman PK, Spevak MR, Nimkin K. Left-sided esophageal indentation in right aortic arch with aberrant left subclavian artery. Radiology 1994;191:565-567.

169. Hager A, Kaemmerer H, Rapp-Bernhardt U, et al. Diameters of the thoracic aorta throughout life as measured with helical computed tomography. J Thorac Cardiovasc Surg 2002;123:1060-1066.

170. Fink C, Hallscheidt PJ, Hosch WP, et al. Preoperative evaluation of living renal donors: value of contrast-enhanced 3D magnetic resonance angiography and comparison of three rendering algorithms. Eur Radiol 2003;13:794-801.

Index

Note: Numbers followed by f indicate figures; those followed by b indicate boxed material.

A

Abdomen, of fetus, 362–366
Abdominal aortic aneurysm (AAA), 488
  classification of, 488
  complications of, 489, 490f, 491f
  inflammatory, 250–252, 252b, 488
  infrarenal, 496f
"Abdominal cocoon," in sclerosing encapsulating peritonitis, 261
Abdominal cysts, nonparenchymal, 239–244, 240b
Abdominal hemangioma, 244, 244b
Abdominal lipoma, 235–236, 236b
Abdominal neurofibroma, 230–231, 230b, 231f
Abdominal paraganglioma, 224–225, 225b, 226f
Abdominal schwannoma, 227–230, 227b, 229f
Abdominal tuberculosis, 246, 246b
Abdominal wall fibromatosis, 232–235, 234b, 235f
Abdominopelvic fat-containing lesions, benign nonparenchymal, 235–236, 236b
Abdominopelvic lymphadenopathy, 244–248, 245b
Abscess(es)
  hepatic, 16–19
    amebic, 19
    fungal, 17–19, 17b, 19f
    pyogenic, 16–17, 17b, 18f
  pelvic, 328, 329f
  psoas muscle, 258
  retroperitoneal and intraperitoneal, 253b, 256–258, 259f
  scrotal, 380
  splenic, 190b, 196–197, 196b
    fungal, 197
    pyogenic, 196
  tubo-ovarian, 328, 329f
Acinar cell carcinoma, pancreatic, 98
Acquired cystic kidney disease (ACKD), and renal cell carcinoma, 159–160, 160b
Acquired immunodeficiency syndrome (AIDS), cholangiopathy due to, 74
Acute tubular necrosis (ATN), after renal transplantation, 177
Adenocarcinoma, of prostate. *See* Prostate cancer.
Adenoma(s)
  adrenocortical, 130–133, 130f–132f
    hypersecreting, 133
    nonhypersecreting, 133–134
    vs. adrenal metastasis, 132–133, 132b, 134
  hepatocellular, 4–5, 4b, 6f, 7f
  microcystic, of pancreas, 100–101, 101b, 102f, 103f
Adenoma malignum, of cervix, 290
Adenomatoid tumor, paratesticular, 382b, 383, 384f
Adenomatosis, liver, 5, 6f
Adenomatous polyposis, familial, desmoid tumors in, 232, 234, 234b
Adenomucinosis, disseminated peritoneal, 220
Adenomyomatosis, of gallbladder, 83–84, 83b, 83f
Adenomyosis, uterine, 273f, 275–277, 278f
  vs. leiomyoma, 271, 276, 277b
  with tamoxifen use, 284f
Adnexal masses, nonovarian causes of, 326–328, 326b, 327f, 329f
ADPCKD. *See* Autosomal dominant polycystic kidney disease (ADPCKD).

Adrenal adenomas, 130–133, 130f–132f
  hypersecreting, 133
  nonhypersecreting, 133–134
  vs. adrenal metastasis, 132–133, 132b, 134
Adrenal cortex
  neoplasms of, 130–134
  normal anatomy of, 129
Adrenal cysts, 139–141, 145f
  in fetal neuroblastoma, 363
Adrenal gland, 129–145
  chemical shift imaging of, 129–130, 130f
  fetal, 363
  metastasis to, 134–135, 138f–140f
    adrenal adenoma vs., 132–133, 132b, 134
    of renal cell carcinoma, 140f, 156
  normal anatomy of, 129
Adrenal gland hemorrhage, after liver transplantation, 42–43
Adrenal hematoma, 139, 145f
Adrenal medulla, normal anatomy of, 129
Adrenal metastases, 134–135, 138f–140f
  adrenal adenoma vs., 132–133, 132b, 134
  of renal cell carcinoma, 140f, 156
Adrenal myelolipoma, 137–139, 143f, 144f
Adrenal pheochromocytoma, 135–137, 139b, 140f–142f
Adrenal pseudocyst, 145f
Adrenal rests, testicular, 376–377, 379f
Adrenalectomy, for pheochromocytoma, 136–137
Adrenocortical adenomas, 130–133, 130f–132f
  hypersecreting, 133
  nonhypersecreting, 133–134
  vs. adrenal metastasis, 132–133, 132b, 134
Adrenocortical carcinoma, 134, 134b, 135f–137f
AIDS (acquired immunodeficiency syndrome), cholangiopathy due to, 74
AIS (androgen insensitivity syndrome), 299
Alprostadil, for penile imaging, 372
Amebic hepatic abscess, 19
AMLs. *See* Angiomyolipomas (AMLs).
Ampullary carcinoma, 76–77, 77f
Ampullary lesions, of bile ducts, 76–77, 77f
Ampullary neoplasms, 76–77, 77f
Ampullary stenosis, 76
Amyloidosis, of seminal vesicles, 400–401
Androgen insensitivity syndrome (AIS), 299
Aneurysm(s)
  aortic. *See* Aortic aneurysm.
  defined, 486
  pseudoaneurysm. *See* Pseudoaneurysm.
  splenic artery, 197–198
Angiofollicular lymph node hyperplasia, 247–248, 248b
Angiomyolipomas (AMLs)
  hepatic, 26–27
  renal, 153f, 154f, 160b, 169–170
    vs. renal cell carcinoma, 156
    vs. retroperitoneal liposarcoma, 210
Angiosarcoma, of spleen, 202
Ann Arbor Staging System, for lymphoma, 245, 246b
Annular pancreas, 90
Annuloaortic ectasia, 502